Evidence-Based Cardiology Consult

Kathleen Stergiopoulos • David L. Brown
Editors

Evidence-Based Cardiology Consult

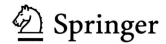 Springer

Editors
Kathleen Stergiopoulos, MD, PhD, FASE, FACC,
FAHA
Division of Cardiology
Department of Medicine
Stony Brook University
School of Medicine
Stony Brook, NY
USA

David L. Brown, MD, FACC
Division of Cardiology
Department of Medicine
Stony Brook University
School of Medicine
Stony Brook, NY
USA

ISBN 978-1-4471-4440-3   ISBN 978-1-4471-4441-0   (eBook)
DOI 10.1007/978-1-4471-4441-0
Springer London Heidelberg New York Dordrecht

To my parents, Mom and Dad
My husband, George and our children, Anna and John

–Kathleen Stergiopoulos

Preface

Cardiology consultation occupies an expanding role in clinical medicine. Cardiologists are increasingly being asked to be involved in the care of complex general medical patients with concurrent cardiac problems, pregnancy, cancers and their treatment, noncardiac surgery, and systemic diseases, among others. Although cardiology consultation is the most commonly performed task by the cardiology clinician in practice, few books address the issues specific and relevant to a cardiology consultation in one place. We have, therefore, created a new textbook, *Evidence-Based Cardiology Consult*, that addresses these new and increasing demands for clinicians to adequately take care of their patients. It provides an up-to-date, detailed, evidence-based approach to key issues facing the consultant including practical clinical advice on the prevention, diagnosis, and treatment of heart disease.

Part I focuses on cardiac issues in the general medical patient such as the evaluation of chest pain, acute coronary syndromes, acute decompensated heart failure, infective endocarditis, sudden cardiac death, primary prevention of cardiovascular disease, and the role of imaging in cardiology in cardiology consultation. Video clips and high-quality images accompany the chapters on imaging.

Part II addresses cardiac problems in specific populations and includes topics such as cardiac problems in women, the elderly, and the athlete; thoracic aortic disease; cardiovascular disease in patients with chronic kidney disease; and right heart failure.

Cardio-oncology has recently emerged as a new discipline at the intersection of cardiology and oncology. Therefore, we have devoted a section to this rapidly evolving subject. Part III addresses cardiac disease resulting from chemotherapy and radiation in oncology patients.

Part IV addresses cardiac diseases in patients with concurrent pregnancy including hypertensive disorders, cardiomyopathies, valvular heart disease, and congenital heart disease. This part addresses specific issues as they relate to both mother and fetus. Assistance with perioperative management of patients with concurrent cardiovascular disease may be the most common reason for cardiology consultation. Part V addresses these topics as well as cardiovascular risk assessment prior to noncardiac surgery and the management of patients of antiplatelet or anticoagulant therapy who require surgery.

Part VI includes topics on the evaluation and management of patients with cardiac disease as a source of neurologic sequelae, such as cardiovascular source of embolism and syncope.

The editors gratefully acknowledge the work of each of the contributors to this textbook for their superb chapters.

Stony Brook, NY, USA   Kathleen Stergiopoulos, MD, PhD, FASE, FACC, FAHA
Stony Brook, NY, USA   David L. Brown, MD, FACC

Contents

Contributors

J. Dawn Abbott, MD Department of Medicine, Division of Cardiology, Brown Medical School, Rhode Island Hospital, Providence, RI, USA

Alexander J. Abramowicz, BS Department of Radiology, Stony Brook University Medical Center, Stony Brook, NY, USA

Ali O. Abualsaud, MBBS Department of Cardiology, McGill University Health Center/McGill Univesrity, Montreal, QC, Canada

Letitia Acquah, MD, MSc, FACP Divisions of General and Obstetric Medicine, Department of Medicine, Mayo Clinic, Rochester, MN, USA

Ahsanuddin Ahmad, MD Division of Cardiology, Tufts Medical Center, Boston, MA, USA

Ibrahim O. Almasry, MD, FACC, FHRS Section of Cardiac Electrophysiology, Division of Cardiology, SUNY/Stony Brook University Medical Center, Stony Brook, NY, USA

Stavros Z. Apostolakis, MD, PhD Department of Cardiology, Democritus University of Thrace, Alexandroupolis, Greece

Usman Baber, MD, MS Department of Cardiology, Mount Sinai School of Medicine, New York, NY, USA

Nitish Badhwar, MBBS, FACC, FHRS Cardiac Electrophysiology Training Program, Department of Medicine/Cardiology, University of California, San Francisco, CA, USA

Aaron L. Baggish, MD Department of Cardiology, Massachusetts General Hospital, Boston, MA, USA

George L. Bakris, MD Department of Medicine, ASH Hypertension Center, The University of Chicago Medicine, Chicago, IL, USA

David L. Brown, MD, FACC Division of Cardiology, Department of Medicine, Stony Brook University School of Medicine, Stony Brook, NY, USA

Kimberly D. Brunisholz, MST, CRCC Department of Cardiovascular Research, Intermountain Medical Center, Intermountain Heart Institute, Salt Lake City, UT, USA

Ammar Chaudhry Department of Diagnostic Radiology, Stony Brook University Medical Center, Stony Brook, NY, USA

Jack M. Colman, MD, FRCPC Department of Cardiology, University of Toronto, Toronto, ON, Canada

Jérôme Cornette, MD Department of Obstetrics and Gynaecology, Erasmus MC, Rotterdam, The Netherlands

Anthony R. Cucci, MD Pulmonary Fellow, Indiana University, Pulmonary/Critical Care, Indianapolis, IN, USA

Gabriel A. Delgado, MD Interventional Cardiology Fellow, Department of Medicine, Cardiology, Brown Medical School, Providence, RI, USA

Mark J. Eisenberg, MD, MPH, FACC, FAHA Divisions of Cardiology and Clinical Epidemiology, Jewish General Hospital/McGill University, Montreal, QC, Canada

Lea El Hage, MD Department of Medicine/Cardiology, University of California, San Francisco, Dublin, CA, USA

John A. Elefteriades, MD Department of Cardiac Surgery, Aortic Institute of Yale-New Haven, Yale University School of Medicine, New Haven, CT, USA

N.A. Mark Estes III, MD Division of Cardiology, Tufts University School of Medicine, Boston, MA, USA

Suzanne B. Evans, MD, MPH Department of Therapeutic Radiology, Yale School of Medicine, Yale University School of Medicine, New Haven, CT, USA

Roger Fan, MD Cardiac Arrhythmia Consult Service, Department of Medicine, Stony Brook University School of Medicine, Stony Brook, NY, USA

Lee A. Fleisher, MD Department of Anesthesiology and Critical Care, Perelman School of Medicine at the University of Pennsylvania, Philadelphia, PA, USA

JoAnne M. Foody, MD, FACC, FAHA Cardiovascular Wellness Program, Department of Medicine, Brigham and Women's Hospital, Boston, MA, USA

Valentin Fuster, MD, PhD Zena and Michael A. Wiener Cardiovascular Institute and the Marie-Josée and Henry R. Kravis Center for Cardiovascular Health, New York, NY, USA

Centro Nacional de Investigaciones Cardiovasculares Carlos III (CNIC), Madrid, Spain

Department of Cardiology, Mount Sinai Medical Center, New York, NY, USA

Adriana Quiñones, MD Leon H. Charney Division of Cardiology, New York University Langone Medical Center, New York, NY, USA

Santiago Garcia, MD, FACC, FSCAI Department of Cardiology, University of Minnesota/ Minneapolis VA Healthcare System, Minneapolis, MN, USA

Ania Garlitski, MD Division of Cardiology, Tufts University School of Medicine, Boston, MA, USA

Vesna D. Garovic, MD Division of Nephrology and Hypertension, Mayo Clinic, Rochester, MN, USA

Nora Goldschlager, MD Cardiology Division, Department of Medicine, University of California, San Francisco, San Francisco General Hospital, San Francisco, CA, USA

Nilush Gukathasan, MD Department of Cardiology, Mount Sinai School of Medicine, New York, NY, USA

M. Azam Hadi, MD Department of Cardiology, Indiana University, Indianapolis, IN, USA

Philip G. Haines, BM, Bch, MPH, MRCP (UK) Department of Cardiology, Hospital of the University of Pennsylvania, Philadelphia, PA, USA

Adam A. Harris, MD Department of Internal Medicine, NYU Langone Medical Center, New York, NY, USA

Usman Hashmi, MD Department of Cardiology, St. John Providence Health System, Detroit, MI, USA

Rachel Hatton, BMed, FRACP Department of Adult Cardiology, University of Toronto/University Health Network, Toronto, ON, Canada

Munther K. Homoud, MD Division of Cardiology, Tufts University School of Medicine, Boston, MA, USA

Benjamin D. Horne, PhD, MPH Division of Genetic Epidemiology, Intermountain Medical Center and University of Utah, Intermountain Heart Institute, Salt Lake City, UT, USA

Massimo Imazio, MD, FESC Department of Cardiology, Maria Vittoria Hospital, Torino, Italy

Sei Iwai, MD, FACC, FHRS Cardiac Electrophysiology, Division of Cardiology, Westchester Medical Center, New York Medical College, Valhalla, NY, USA

Stuart D. Katz, MD, MS Leon H. Charney Division of Cardiology, New York University Langone Medical Center, New York, NY, USA

Abdallah Georges Kfoury, MD, FACC Department of Cardiology, Intermountain Medical Center, Salt Lake City, UT, USA

Todd L. Kiefer, MD Department of Cardiology, Duke University Medical Center, Durham, NC, USA

James N. Kirkpatrick, MD Department of Cardiology, Hospital of the University of Pennsylvania, Philadelphia, PA, USA

George J. Klein, MD Division of Cardiology/Arrhythmia Service, University of Western Ontario/University Hospital, London, ON, Canada

Stavros V. Konstantinides, MD, PhD, FESC Department of Cardiology, Democritus University of Thrace, Alexandroupolis, Greece

Andrew D. Krahn, MD Division of Cardiology/Electrophysiology Service, University of Western Ontario/University Hospital, London, ON, Canada

Eric V. Krieger, MD Division of Cardiology, Department of Medicine and Pediatrics, University of Washington/University of Washington Medical Center and Seattle Children's Hospital, Seattle, WA, USA

Tim Lahm, MD Division of Pulmonary, Allergy, Critical Care, Occupational, and Sleep Medicine, Department of Medicine, Indiana University School of Medicine and Richard L. Roudebush VA Medical Center, Indianapolis, IN, USA

Cheng Ting Lin, MD Department of Radiology, Stony Brook University Medical Center, Stony Brook, NY, USA

Mark Link, MD Division of Cardiology, Tufts University School of Medicine, Boston, MA, USA

Peter A. McCullough, MD, MPH, FACC, FACP, FAHA Department of Providence Park Clinical Research, St. John Providence Health System, Novi, MI, USA

Edward O. McFalls, MD, PhD Department of Cardiology, University of Minnesota/Minneapolis VA Healthcare System, Minneapolis, MN, USA

Judith L. Meadows, MD, MPH Department of Internal Medicine/Cardiology, Yale School of Medicine, Yale University/VACT Healthcare System, West Haven, CT, USA

Nidhi Mehta, MD Department of Cardiovascular Diseases, University of Pennsylvania, Philadelphia, PA, USA

Edward J. Miller, MD, PhD Section of Cardiovascular Medicine, Boston University School of Medicine, Boston, MA, USA

Muzammil H. Musani, MD Department of Radiology, Stony Brook University, Stony Brook, NY, USA

Karthiek Narala, MD Department of Internal Medicine, St. John Providence Health System, Detroit, MI, USA

Catherine M. Otto, MD Echocardiographic Laboratory, Division of Cardiology, Department of Medicine, University of Washington School of Medicine, Seattle, WA, USA

Michael Poon, MD Advanced Cardiovascular Imaging, Department of Radiology, Stony Brook University Medical Center, Stony Brook, NY, USA

T. Flint Porter, MD, MPH Division of Maternal-Fetal Medicine, Department of Obstetrics and Gynecology, Intermountain Medical Center, University of Utah, Salt Lake City, UT, USA

Eric J. Rashba, MD Cardiac Electrophysiology, Department of Medicine, Stony Brook University School of Medicine, Stony Brook, NY, USA

Kismet D. Rasmusson, MSN, FNP-BC Heart Failure Program Development Lead, Intermountain Medical Center, University of Utah- College of Nursing, The Heart Institute, Heart Failure and Transplant Program, Salt Lake City, UT, USA

Alex Reyentovich, MD Leon H. Charney Division of Cardiology, New York University Langone Medical Center, New York, NY, USA

Michael W. Rich, MD Department of Internal Medicine/Cardiology, Washington University, St. Louis, MO, USA

Kenneth B. Roberts, MD Department of Therapeutic Radiology, Yale School of Medicine, Yale University, New Haven, CT, USA

Fatima Rodriguez, MD, MPH Department of Medicine, Resident of Internal Medicine, Brigham and Woman's Hospital, Boston, MA, USA

Jolien W. Roos-Hesselink, MD, PhD Department of Cardiology, Thoraxcenter, Erasmus MC, Rotterdam, The Netherlands

Lisa Rosenbaum, MD Division of Cardiology, University of Pennsylvania, Philadelphia, PA, USA

Kerry Strong Russell, MD, PhD, FACC, FAHA Internal Medicine, Department of Cardiovascular Medicine, Yale University School of Medicine, New Haven, CT, USA

Raymond R. Russell III, MD, PhD Division of Cardiovascular Medicine, Department of Internal Medicine, Yale School of Medicine, New Haven, CT, USA

Pradyot Saklani, MBBS Division of Cardiology/Electrophysiology Service, University of Western Ontario/University Hospital, London, ON, Canada

Matthew Sermer, MD, FRCSC Departments of Obstetrics, Gynecology and Medicine, University of Toronto, Toronto, ON, Canada

Shimoli V. Shah, MD Department of Cardiology, Washington University School of Medicine – St. Louis/Barnes Jewish Hospital, St. Louis, MO, USA

Candice K. Silversides, MD, MS, FRCPC Department of Cardiology, University of Toronto, Mount Sinai Hospital, Toronto, ON, Canada

Samuel C. Siu, MD, SM Department of Medicine, Schulich School of Medicine and Dentistry, London, ON, Canada

Matthew Sorrentino, MD, FACC, FASH Department of Medicine/Cardiology, University of Chicago, Chicago, IL, USA

Robert Soufer, MD Department of Internal Medicine/Cardiology, Yale School of Medicine, Yale University/VACT Healthcare System, West Haven, CT, USA

Kathleen Stergiopoulos, MD, PhD, FASE, FACC, FAHA Division of Cardiology, Department of Medicine, Stony Brook University School of Medicine, Stony Brook, NY, USA

Karen K. Stout, MD Division of Cardiology, Department of Medicine and Pediatrics, University of Washington/University of Washington Medical Center and Seattle Children's Hospital, Seattle, WA, USA

B. Frazier Taylor, MD, PhD Department of Therapeutic Radiology, Yale New Haven Hospital, Yale School of Medicine, New Haven, CT, USA

Szilard Voros, MD Department of Radiology, Stony Brook Medicine, Stony Brook, NY, USA

Andrew Wang, MD Department of Medicine, Duke University Hospital, Durham, NC, USA

James A. White, MD Cardiovascular MRI Clinical Research Program, Division of Cardiology/Cardiovascular Imaging, Robart's Research Institute, University of Western Ontario/University Hospital, London, ON, Canada

Malissa J. Wood, MD, FACC, FASE, FAHA Department of Medicine/Cardiology, Harvard/Massachusetts General Hospital, Boston, MA, USA

Justina C. Wu, MD, PhD, FACC Department of Medicine, Harvard Medical School, Brigham and Women's Hospital, Boston, MA, USA

Henry Yaun, MD Department of Nephrology, Johns Hopkins Hospital, Detroit, MI, USA

Firas Yazigi, MD Department of Cardiology, St. John Providence Health System, Detroit, MI, USA

Elisa Zaragoza-Macias, MD Division of Cardiology, Department of Medicine, University of Washington School of Medicine, Seattle, WA, USA

Bulat A. Ziganshin, MD Section of Cardiac Surgery, Department of Surgery, Yale University School of Medicine, New Haven, CT, USA

Department of Surgical Diseases, Kazan State Medical University, Kazan, Russia

Jodi L. Zilinski, MD Department of Cardiology, Massachusetts General Hospital, Boston, MA, USA

List of Videos

Part I

Cardiac Issues in the General Medical Patient

Edward J. Miller

Abstract

The evaluation of patients with chest pain is a common task for medical practitioners. This commonly occurs in the context of an emergency department or inpatient hospital encounter and requires a comprehensive yet focused approach to provide a rapid diagnosis and assessment of risk. This chapter outlines the key elements of this evaluation: history and symptoms, physical exam, and ancillary testing, with a particular focus on imaging strategies that can be employed for the evaluation of chest pain and their use in settings such as chest pain evaluation units.

Keywords

Chest pain • Angina • Stress testing • Stress echocardiography • CT angiography • Myocardial perfusion imaging

Introduction

The evaluation of chest pain is a critical skill in current medical practice as chest pain remains one of most common chief complaints for patients presenting to the emergency department, as well as one of the top medicine admission diagnoses. A correct diagnosis of the cause of chest pain, particularly to ensure the absence of an acute coronary syndrome (ACS), is especially important as the missed diagnosis of this condition is a significant source of malpractice litigation for the emergency department/acute care physician. Not only must the evaluation of chest pain establish an accurate diagnosis, but the testing strategy must be timely, efficient, and cost-effective. A concept key to this evaluation is the necessity of not only making the correct diagnosis but also understanding the implication of this diagnosis for the patient's risk of having a major adverse cardiac event. While it is important to provide diagnostic certainty, it is equally important to understand how this evaluation allows for risk stratification of a future cardiac problem.

This chapter provides a framework for the understanding of the biology of various causes of chest pain, focusing on angina. Specifically, this chapter emphasizes the role of ancillary testing and chest pain units, either in the emergency department or inpatient hospital settings, in an expedient, efficient, and evidence-based approach to the evaluation and risk stratification of patients with chest pain.

Pathophysiology of Cardiac Chest Pain

Chest pain can occur from many cardiac and noncardiac conditions. Chest pain of cardiac origin is most commonly a nociceptive response originating from stimulation of afferent innervation of the heart, with the prototypical example being chest pain occurring as a consequence of myocardial ischemia in the presence of coronary artery disease (CAD). During myocardial ischemia, myocardial oxygen demand outpaces oxygen delivery, either during acute stress in the setting of a fixed coronary stenosis, due to acute plaque rupture leading to coronary occlusion in the setting of an acute

E.J. Miller, MD, PhD
Section of Cardiovascular Medicine,
Boston University School of Medicine,
88 E. Newton Street,
Boston, MA 02118, USA
e-mail: ejmiller@bu.edu

Fig. 1.1 Ischemic cascade. The first event in the ischemic cascade is decreased coronary perfusion, leading to contractile dysfunction, ECG changes, and angina

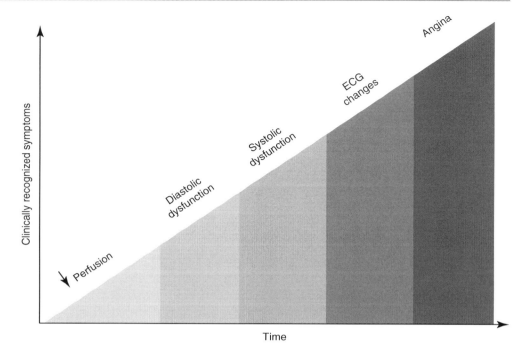

myocardial infarction, coronary vasospasm, or coronary dissection. This leads to the release and accumulation of local metabolites such as adenosine, lactate, histamine, and bradykinin. These metabolites lead to stimulation of lower cervical and thoracic sympathetic afferent dorsal root ganglia. The diffuse location of these sensory afferents is likely the cause of the variable localization of chest pain among patients.

Ischemic Cascade

The clinical presentation of myocardial ischemia depends on both the severity and duration of the ischemic stimulus. Classically, this continuum of events begins with the mismatch of perfusion in relation to myocardial work, progressing to electrical repolarization abnormalities visualized on the surface electrocardiogram, then to mechanical cardiomyocyte contractile dysfunction, and finally to onset of chest pain symptoms. This process is termed the "ischemic cascade," shown graphically in Fig. 1.1. While this provides a general framework for understanding the pathophysiology of the ischemic process, it is not uncommon for variation in the time or severity of various aspects of the ischemic cascade to occur. For example, some patients may not recognize their symptoms or have atypical symptoms that precede other evidence of myocardial ischemia, such as electrocardiographic, perfusion, or contractile abnormalities. In others, myocardial ischemia can be clinically silent, without manifest angina. Therefore, it is imperative that the evaluating physician be familiar with both classic and atypical presentations of cardiac chest pain, realizing a patient's anginal symptoms can be quite individualized.

Diagnosis

A comprehensive evaluation of chest pain requires attention to all phases of the medical encounter: history and symptoms, physical exam, and ancillary testing. This includes an evaluation and attention of potential noncardiac causes of chest pain. Each of these aspects will be described below, focusing particularly on testing and imaging strategies that allow for rapid risk stratification of patients presenting with presumed cardiac chest pain.

Causes of Noncardiac Chest Pain

In addition to cardiac causes, symptoms of chest discomfort can arise from a plethora of noncardiac causes. It is imperative that the evaluating physician be familiar with this differential diagnosis and pay attention to whether the patient has a history of conditions in Table 1.1 that may cause noncardiac chest pain. A list of commonly encountered causes of noncardiac chest pain is listed in Table 1.1.

History and Symptoms

When interviewing a patient regarding their chest pain symptoms, it is important to pay attention to a patient's history of medical conditions putting them at risk for the development of coronary artery disease. Chief among these are a history of smoking, diabetes mellitus, hyperlipidemia, hypertension, and family history of premature CAD. In addition to

Table 1.1 Differential diagnosis of chest pain

Cardiac	Noncardiac
Angina	Pulmonary embolism
Acute coronary syndrome (ACS)	Costochondritis
Pericarditis	Pulmonary contusion or infarction
Aortic dissection	Pneumonia
	Pneumothorax
	Pleurisy
	Rib fracture
	Gastroesophageal reflux disease or peptic ulcer disease
	Herpes zoster

List includes common causes of chest pain and is not exhaustive. ACS includes unstable angina, NSTEMI (non-ST elevation myocardial infarction), and STEMI (ST elevation myocardial infarction)

Table 1.2 Characteristics of various types of chest pain

Definite (typical) angina	Probable (atypical) angina	Nonspecific (noncardiac) chest pain
Substernal discomfort of characteristic quality	Meets two features of definite angina, plus	Meets one or no characteristics of definite or probable angina
Precipitated by exertion or emotional stress	Radiation to neck, jaw, or arm	Can be positional, fleeting, non-exertional, or reproduced on palpation
Relieved by rest or nitroglycerin in < 10 min.	Unpredictable relief with nitroglycerin	
	Variable duration	

Modified from Chaitman et al. [3, 4]

prior coronary revascularizations or surgery, conditions that serve as "coronary artery disease equivalents" based on the ACC/AHA 2007 Guidelines for the Management of Patients With Unstable Angina/Non–ST-Elevation Myocardial Infarction (ACC/AHA UA/NSTEMI) include peripheral vascular disease, a history of diabetes mellitus in patients over the age of 40, and a multiplicity of risk factors that predict a 20 % likelihood of developing CAD estimated by the Framingham Risk Score [1].

A complete history of chest pain symptoms should include details regarding the quality, duration (minutes to hours), time of onset and/or resolution, associated symptoms such as dyspnea or diaphoresis, and aggravating or alleviating factors. The time of onset and/or resolution can be particularly important when deciding whether additional acute imaging (particularly echocardiography and/or nuclear perfusion imaging) can assist with the diagnostic evaluation. Also, aggravating factors such as chest pain that occurs with exertion or exercise and is alleviated with rest may point towards a cardiac cause. Unfortunately, resolution of chest pain with nitroglycerin is a relatively nonspecific discriminator of cardiac versus noncardiac chest pain, in that nitroglycerin has been shown to relieve chest pain in approximately 40 % of patients who do not have CAD as the cause of their discomfort [2].

The character of chest pain symptoms can either be described as "definite angina," "probable angina," or "nonspecific chest pain," based on classic definitions proposed by the Coronary Artery Surgery Study (CASS) study investigators in 1981 [3]. Angina is defined as a clinical syndrome characterized by discomfort in the chest, jaw, shoulder, back, or arm; is typically aggravated by exertions or emotional stress, with adjectives such as squeezing, grip-like, pressure-like, suffocating, and heavy; and is rarely sharp or stabbing [4]. This definition is important not only because it assists with establishing a differential diagnosis but also because many risk stratification schemes that use symptoms in their schemes depend on an accurate characterization of anginal symptoms. For example, in the CASS

study, patients with definite angina had a CAD prevalence of 72–93 %, while those with probable angina had a CAD prevalence of 36–66 %, and nonspecific chest pain had a 6–14 % risk of CAD [3]. Definite angina is defined as substernal chest discomfort precipitated by exertion and relieved by rest or nitroglycerin in <10 min. Probable angina is similar to definite angina but has some atypical features, while nonspecific chest pain has features that are distinct from either definite or probable angina. Common characteristics associated with definite angina, probable angina, and nonspecific chest pain are listed in Table 1.2. It is important to realize that certain patient groups (women and elderly) may present less frequently with definite anginal symptoms.

The history and symptom characterization described above can provide an initial assessment of the patient's risk of having either coronary disease or an acute ischemic event. This can be used to further develop a diagnostic strategy based on a patient's pretest risk [5]. Pretest risk can be estimated using the age, gender, and quality of symptoms for define risk. This approach was combined with CASS study data in the ACC/AHA/ACP-ASIM Guidelines for the Management of Patients with Chronic Stable Angina (ACC/AHA Chronic Stable Angina guidelines) in 1999 (updated in 2002) to provide a pretest likelihood of CAD in symptomatic patients (Table 1.3) [4, 6]. In general, older patients with more classic symptoms have a higher pretest likelihood of CAD, and men are more likely to have CAD at any age than women with similar symptoms.

Physical Exam

After obtaining a focused history and a thorough understanding of the patient's chest pain symptoms, the physical exam should focus on establishing whether features are present that suggest a cardiac or noncardiac cause of the chest pain. A general inspection of the patient can provide clues such as cool, pale extremities (acute CHF), diaphoresis (nonspecific

Table 1.3 Pretest likelihood of CAD in symptomatic patients according to age and sex, combined Diamond/Forrester, and CASS data

Age (years)	Nonanginal chest pain		Atypical angina		Typical angina	
	Men	Women	Men	Women	Men	Women
30–39	4	2	34	12	76	26
40–49	13	3	51	22	87	55
50–59	20	7	65	31	93	73
60–69	27	14	72	51	94	86

(Reproduced with permission from Gibbons et al. [6])
Values are percent with significant CAD on angiography

finding in acute myocardial infarction), and/or respiratory distress. Basic vital signs should be evaluated for features such as an unstable pulse rate, hypotension or hypertension, and hypoxemia.

A focused cardiovascular exam should include precordial auscultation to examine for features of cardiac pump failure (i.e., S3), stiff ventricle (S4), ischemia-mediated murmurs (i.e., the holosystolic murmur of acute mitral regurgitation from ischemic papillary muscle dysfunction), acute aortic regurgitation (acute aortic dissection), distant heart sounds/pericardial friction rub (suggestive of a pericardial effusion), pulmonary rales (acute CHF), egophony (pneumonic consolidation), or dullness (pleural effusion). Further, a focused vascular exam can provide insight into processes such as acute aortic dissection (differential blood pressures in the upper extremities), acute aortic regurgitation ("water hammer" carotid pulsations), or obstructive peripheral vascular disease (bruits and/or diminished carotid, femoral, popliteal, dorsalis pedis, posterior tibial arterial pulses). A focused chest and upper abdominal palpation can provide clues about reproducible chest/rib/cartilage pain with palpation (costochondritis) or upper abdominal pathology such as cholecystitis or pancreatitis.

Lastly, while not directly part of the physical examination, a chest radiograph (preferably with posterior-anterior and lateral views) should be obtained in all patients with chest pain. This is recommended by the ACC/AHA Chronic Stable Angina guidelines (Class IB) [4] and can provide information such as an enlarged cardiac silhouette (left ventricular hypertrophy and/or pericardial effusion), enlarged mediastinal silhouette (aortic aneurysm and/or dissection), pulmonary vascular congestion, pleural effusion, pneumonia, lung masses, or rib fractures.

Management: Ancillary Testing in the Evaluation of Acute Chest Pain

While a patient's history, symptoms, and physical exam are useful, the crucial task in the evaluation of chest pain of presumed cardiac origin is the appropriate use of ancillary testing.

The additional information gained by the use of ancillary testing assists the clinician to determine both the diagnosis and the level of aggressiveness needed for further therapeutic interventions. It is crucial that a patient presenting with chest pain not only receive a timely diagnosis but also not be subjected to over-testing strategies that may impart some additional risk (e.g., contrast dye, radiation, invasive procedures). Therefore, the appropriate testing strategy will not be the same in all patients. Instead, the best testing strategies will be tailored to take into account a patient's pretest risk of CAD, institutional capabilities and expertise, cost, safety, and patient satisfaction in order to provide the best information to the clinician in a timely manner. This section reviews many commonly employed testing modalities endorsed by ACC/AHA guidelines.

Electrocardiogram (ECG)

The standard 12-lead ECG can be rapidly and serially performed, is noninvasive, poses no risk to the patient, and is nearly universally available. Electrocardiography plays a central and critical role in the initial evaluation of chest pain because it can rapidly and with reasonable sensitivity help to differentiate patients who are experiencing active myocardial ischemia. A resting ECG, preferably during symptoms, receives a Class 1B recommendation from both the ACC/AHA Chronic Stable Angina [4] and UA/NSTEMI guidelines [1]. In addition, in the setting of ST-segment elevation myocardial infarction (STEMI), the ECG is the singular triage modality for determining which patients require acute reperfusion therapy. The standard definition of ST-segment elevation on ECG is the presence of greater than 1 mm of ST-segment elevation in two or more contiguous ECG leads [1]. It has been well validated that patients presenting with STEMI should receive either prompt pharmacological thrombolysis or percutaneous coronary intervention (PCI) in order to restore target vessel patency and salvage at-risk ischemic myocardium (see ACC/AHA UA/NSTEMI guidelines [1]).

However, only a small minority of patients presenting with acute chest pain have ST-segment elevation present on their 12-lead ECG. Therefore, the task of the interpreting physician is to evaluate the ECG for evidence of current myocardial ischemia and/or previous myocardial infarction. Dynamic ST-segment changes of ≥ 0.5 mm are strongly associated with the presence of underlying CAD [1]. However, other ECG findings are suggestive of a cardiac cause of chest pain. These include the presence of pathological Q waves (≥ 0.04 s) suggestive of prior myocardial infarction, T-wave inversions ≥ 2 mm, QT interval prolongation due to altered myocardial repolarization during myocardial ischemia, and the development of a new left bundle branch block (LBBB) suggestive of diffuse myocardial ischemia.

It is especially important to obtain a 12-lead ECG while the patient is symptomatic, if possible, as 50 % of patients with normal resting ECGs have abnormal ECGs during angina [4]. If dynamic ECG changes are present during symptoms, this strongly suggests myocardial ischemia. However, a normal ECG during symptoms can place the patient into a lower-risk category. Indeed, in patients presenting with angina, the probability of acute MI can be as low as approximately 3 % but is highly dependent on the patient's age and symptoms (classic angina vs. nonspecific chest pain) [7]. Another exception is patients presenting with left circumflex coronary artery distribution ischemia which can be missed on the standard 12-lead ECG.

Stress Electrocardiography

Because many patients present for evaluation after cessation of symptoms and without ongoing ECG abnormalities, further provocative testing may be needed in order to evaluate for underlying obstructive coronary artery disease. Guidelines for the use of exercise testing are available from the ACC/AHA [8]. Stress electrocardiography (ECG) is a central component of many initial diagnostic and risk stratification strategies because it is simple and easy to perform, has reasonable diagnostic yield, exposes the patient to minimal risk (rate of death or MI ~ 1:2500), and provides validated prognostic information about future CAD outcomes. Contraindications to stress ECG testing include acute MI within 2 days, unstable cardiac arrhythmias, symptomatic and severe aortic stenosis, symptomatic heart failure, acute pulmonary embolus, pericarditis, aortic dissection, Wolff-Parkinson-White (WPW) syndrome, paced rhythm, >1 mm resting ST depression, or LBBB on ECG [4, 8, 9].

Stress ECG is most commonly performed using treadmill exercise, although bicycle ergometers can also be employed. In brief, a patient is attached to a 12-lead ECG, and graded exercise is performed until an appropriate workload target is obtained. Stress ECG testing should be symptom limited, with the goal to reach an appropriate level of metabolic stress (typically >85 % of age-predicted maximal heart rate, 6–12 min of exercise, and/or ≥7 METs) to improve test sensitivity. Indications for cessation of a stress ECG test include ≥2 mm ST-segment depression, ≥1 mm ST elevation, moderate/severe angina, patient's inability to continue exercise due to severe fatigue or dyspnea, development of LBBB, fall in systolic blood pressure >10 mmHg, severe hypertension (>250/>115 mmHg), or sustained cardiac arrhythmia [8, 9].

A positive stress ECG test is reflected by either the development of anginal symptoms or ischemic changes on ECG. The most common definition of ischemic ECG changes is 1 mm of horizontal or downsloping ST depression ≥60–80 ms after the end of the QRS [4], realizing the interpretation of a stress ECG test includes not only symptoms and ECG changes but also exercise duration and hemodynamic response. One common method of integrating exercise duration, symptoms, and ECG changes seen on exercise ECG testing to give a quantitative estimate of CAD prognostic risk is the Duke Treadmill Score (DTS) [10]. The DTS is calculated by:

$$\text{Exercise time} - 5 \times (\text{ST-segment deviation(mm)} - 4 \times \text{angina score}^*$$

*angina score = 0 for no angina, 1 for any angina, 2 if angina was reason for cessation of exercise

The DTS is able to reasonably risk stratify patients undergoing stress ECG, showing those with a DTS score of ≥+5 have an average annual CV mortality of 0.5 % while those in the highest risk group (DTS ≤ −11) have an annual CV mortality of >5 %. Stress ECG has a reasonable overall sensitivity (68 %) and specificity (77 %) for the detection of CAD [4]. However, other analyses suggest the sensitivity of stress ECG is below 50 % [11], and there are particular patient groups in whom the test performs less optimally for risk stratification. For example, patients with significant baseline ECG abnormalities (LVH, digoxin effect, LBBB, resting ST-segment depression) should not undergo stress ECG testing for the diagnosis of CAD due to the lack of specificity of the test in these groups [11]. Test sensitivity is also reduced in patients receiving beta-blockers for treatment of hypertension. In addition, stress ECG testing is less sensitive in women for complex, multifactorial reasons including the lower prevalence of CAD and the tendency to develop nonspecific ECG changes. Nonetheless, stress ECG testing has a Class IB recommendation for the diagnosis of CAD in patients with an intermediated pretest risk, including patients with RBBB and <1 mm of resting ST depression [4].

Biomarkers of Myocardial Injury

While a normal ECG during symptoms can help distinguish patients having active myocardial ischemia and/or infarction, many patients present for evaluation after their symptoms have abated. Determination of the presence of myocardial necrosis is critical to risk stratification and acute therapeutic interventions. Therefore, patients require testing with a method that can help to determine whether or not an acute coronary syndrome has occurred in the past several hours to days. This can be accomplished using circulating biomarkers, such as myoglobin, creatine kinase isoforms (CK-MB), and troponin. Each of these biomarkers has different specificities, kinetics of appearance in the blood stream, and clearance (Fig. 1.2), so an understanding of the use of biomarkers relative to time of symptom onset is critical. Myoglobin is present in both heart and skeletal muscle and is rapidly released from damaged tissue (<2 h). Therefore, early myoglobin release into the blood is suggestive of myocardial

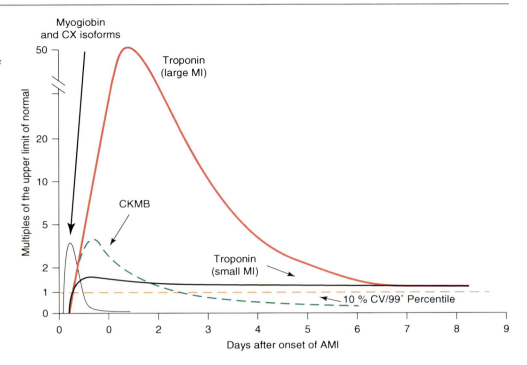

Fig. 1.2 Blood stream kinetics of commonly used cardiac biomarkers. Myoglobin rises rapidly in acute MI (AMI), while troponin rises slightly later but remains detectable for days following AMI (Reproduced with permission from Anderson et al. [1] ©2007 American Heart Association, Inc.)

damage, but this should be confirmed using a more cardiac-specific marker such as troponin. CK-MB is present in both heart and skeletal muscle and is normally present in small quantities in normal blood, making it less specific for myocardial injury. However, because CK-MB rises quickly in the blood, it can be used as a rapid assay for reinfarction and/or periprocedural MI [1].

Troponin has many attributes that make it the preferred biomarker for determination of de novo myocardial necrosis. Of the three subunits of troponin (TnC, TnT, and TnI), the expression of troponin I and T subunits is restricted to the cardiomyocyte, and these are not measureable in blood from normal persons. This makes them both sensitive and specific markers of myocardial injury when released into the bloodstream. This has led to a recent update on the definition of myocardial necrosis by the European Society of Cardiology, American College of Cardiology, American Heart Association, and World Heart Federation [12] as "an elevation of troponin above the 99th percentile of normal." Myocardial infarction is defined as myocardial necrosis that occurs within a clinical context of myocardial ischemia [12].

Troponin detection in the bloodstream usually occurs within 2–4 h of the ischemic event and persists for up to 2 weeks. An elevation of troponin is not just a diagnostic aid, but it also serves as a marker of increased clinical risk. In general, a positive troponin level in the context of a presentation consistent with myocardial ischemia increases the relative risk of death three to five-fold. In addition, patients with a positive troponin level benefit from an invasive angiographic coronary evaluation, based on data from the FRISC

[13] and TIMI-18 [14] studies and others. Therefore, the ACC/AHA UA/NSTEMI guidelines give measurement of troponin a Class IC recommendation for initial assessment, risk stratification, and repeat assessment [1].

Echocardiography

Assessment of left ventricular systolic function and regional wall motion abnormalities provide very useful data when evaluating a patient with chest pain. While not specific for coronary artery disease, abnormal LV function and regional contractile dysfunction place the patient into an elevated risk category and can increase the likelihood of requiring an invasive assessment to rule out obstructive CAD. In patients with acute chest pain, echocardiography performed during symptoms or with adjunctive stress following cessation of symptoms can be used for the diagnosis of obstructive CAD.

Resting Echocardiography

Regional left ventricular systolic dysfunction is one of the markers of recent or ongoing myocardial ischemia and is visualized on the echocardiogram as hypokinesis, akinesis, or dyskinesis. These regional wall motion abnormalities (RWMAs) are quite transient, usually subsiding within minutes of resolution of the ischemic event. Nonetheless, if a patient is having ongoing chest pain symptoms, the presence of regional LV dysfunction has a 50 % positive predictive value for obstructive CAD. However, the best use of resting echocardiography during symptoms is to rule out obstructive

CAD in the setting of normal regional LV function. If no RWMAs are present during symptoms, the negative predictive value of echocardiography is 95 % [4, 15, 16]. The use of resting echocardiography for the detection of regional ischemia receives a Class IC recommendation from the ACC/AHA Chronic Stable Angina guidelines if it can be performed during chest pain or within 30 min of cessation of symptoms [4].

Stress Echocardiography

The addition of imaging techniques, such as echocardiography or nuclear imaging, is particularly important and useful in patients who cannot exercise and/or have ECGs that are uninterpretable for ischemia (LBBB, pacemakers, WPW, etc.). In addition, imaging also improves the diagnostic characteristics of stress testing, improving both sensitivity and specificity when compared to stress ECG alone. Multisociety appropriate use criteria for stress echocardiography are published and provide detailed guidance for the use of this technique [17].

Stress echocardiography is performed following either exercise or dobutamine stress (5, 10, 20, 40 mcg/kg/min ± atropine). Images are obtained from standard views: short axis, parasternal long axis, apical four-chamber, and apical two-chamber. The rest and stress views are visually compared side by side using computer-assisted displays to evaluate for induction of abnormal regional wall motion at peak stress.

The strengths of stress echocardiography are that it is easily available at most centers and provides additional useful information to the referring physician. Namely, it can give information on global left ventricular function, cardiac valve structure and function, and the presence of a pericardial effusion. In addition, stress echocardiography does not expose the patient to ionizing radiation and has lower up-front costs. The weakness of stress echocardiography includes difficulty in acquiring images in patients with poor acoustic windows (obese, large breasts, obstructive lung disease), the qualitative nature of its interpretation, and difficulty in differentiating infarct from ischemia in patients with previous myocardial infarction.

Overall, the sensitivity and specificity of stress echocardiography are reported to be 75 and 88 %, respectively [18], with exercise echo performing better (sensitivity 83 %, specificity 91 %) than dobutamine echo (sensitivity 75 %, specificity 85 %) [4].

Computed Tomography Coronary Angiography

Computed tomography coronary angiography (CTA) is a noninvasive, ECG-gated, contrast-utilizing method for visualizing coronary anatomy and the presence of major epicardial coronary artery disease. CTA is most commonly employed using 64-slice (or greater) CT cameras, enabling faster acquisitions. To compensate for cardiac motion, a regular heart rate (preferably <70 beats per minute) is required, usually necessitating premedication with beta-blockers. Commonly employed CTA techniques use between 60 and 100 ml of iodinated contrast to opacify the coronary arteries, which limits the use of this technique in patients with impaired renal reserve.

CTA offers an accurate, noninvasive method to effectively and accurately rule out the presence of major epicardial coronary artery disease. The overall sensitivity and specificity of 64-slice CTA for >70 % diameter stenosis are 94 and 83 %, respectively, with corresponding negative predictive value of 99 % [19]. The positive predictive value of CTA in unselected patients is only 48 % and is significantly worse in patients with coronary calcium scores >400 [19]. These data support the use of CTA for effectively "ruling out" significant CAD in patients presenting with chest pain. Other recent data validate the concept that an increase in CAD disease burden on CTA increases the likelihood of CAD-related events [20], providing emerging data that CTA may assist in prognostication.

With further advances in CTA techniques, including reductions in radiation exposure through tube current modulation and prospective gating, increasing multi-detector technologies, recently updated appropriate use criteria (AUC) [21], and improving outcomes data, it is likely CTA will become more frequently utilized in the future. Recent appropriateness criteria give an appropriate indication for the use of CTA in patients who have either an interpretable or uninterpretable ECG, including those who are able to exercise in the setting of chest pain syndromes, as long as biomarkers are not elevated [21]. This recommendation builds on the most recent ACC/AHA UA/NSTEMI guidelines to give a Class IIa recommendation for CTA in patients with a low/intermediate probability of CAD and normal ECG/biomarkers as an alternative to stress testing [1]. It is likely the appropriate indications for CTA will expand as further data become available. This increased use of CTA will likely be tempered by the continued need for iodinated contrast, as well as a necessity to show improved outcomes and decreased resource utilization when using CTA-based testing strategies.

Nuclear Myocardial Perfusion Imaging

Myocardial perfusion imaging (MPI) assesses myocardial blood flow using either planar, single-photon computed tomography (SPECT), or positron emission tomography (PET) techniques and radiopharmaceuticals such as thallium-201, Tc-99m sestamibi, Tc-99m tetrofosmin, rubidium-82,

Fig. 1.3 Principle of perfusion imaging: induction of flow heterogeneity. In this schematic model, two arteries perfuse the heart. One artery has a stenosis that is flow limiting at stress (*left side*), while the other artery is normal. At rest, blood flow through both arteries is normal, but at peak stress blood flow through the diseased artery cannot increase to the degree present in the normal (*right side*) artery

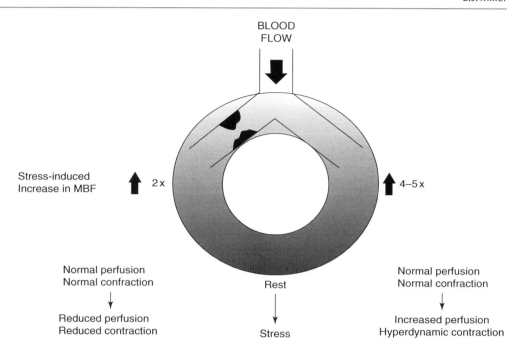

and N-13 ammonia. Since the acquisition of emitted photons is inherently quantitative, this enables comparison of perfusion data to standard normal databases as well as ECG-gated functional assessment, which enhance the sensitivity and specificity of the technique.

Resting Perfusion During Symptoms

Since abnormal myocardial perfusion is the sine qua non of myocardial ischemia, the ability to evaluate perfusion during symptoms consistent with an acute coronary syndrome can assist in diagnosis. Multiple studies have evaluated the utility of injection of Tc-99m-based perfusion tracers to patients during (or within 30 min of) an episode of acute chest pain and found the absence of perfusion places these patients into a low-risk category (0–1 % 30-day event rate) [22–25]. These studies are particularly helpful in patients who have nondiagnostic or non-interpretable ECGs. While the injection of radiotracer occurs during symptoms, the actual imaging can occur 1–2 h later, after the patient has been clinically stabilized. While this technique is quite helpful, decreases resource utilization, and provides a wealth of information, it requires close coordination with nuclear cardiology imaging staff to ensure timely delivery and injection of the tracer, followed by rapid imaging and reporting.

Stress Myocardial Perfusion Imaging

Stress MPI is an extremely well-validated method for evaluating patients with chest pain, with over 10,000 published articles describing its use. As with stress echocardiography and CTA, appropriate use criteria provide recommendations for use of this technique [17]. The majority of the data on stress MPI describes the use of SPECT imaging tracers such

as Tc-99m and thallium-201, although outcomes and prognostic data are also published for the PET tracers, rubidium-82 and N-12 ammonia [26]. Stress modalities that can be used for stress MPI include exercise or pharmacologic stress with either vasodilators (dipyridamole, adenosine, and regadenoson) or inotropes (dobutamine). However, due to decreased diagnostic sensitivity with MPI and inotropic stress, dobutamine should be reserved for patients in whom vasodilator stress is contraindicated (active severe asthma, severe obstructive lung disease, and/or advanced AV nodal conduction system disease).

MPI relies on the principle of imaging myocardial blood flow heterogeneity in response to stress, where blood flow increases disparately in territories perfused by arteries with functionally significant stenoses compared to normal arteries (Fig. 1.3). In general, exercise is the preferred stress modality, except for rubidium-82 PET which requires pharmacologic stress due to the short half-life of the isotope. For pharmacologic stress, vasodilator stress is preferred due to an increased maximal myocardial blood flow with these agents and fewer side effects (particularly arrhythmias) compared with dobutamine [9].

The strengths of MPI are that it can accurately and reproducibly define the ischemic burden, largely due to its inherently quantitative methodology that allows for comparison to normal patients. Quantitative analysis provides greater confidence in interpretation, decreases intra-/interobserver variability, and provides a reproducible measure of the ischemic burden that can be tracked over time. However, MPI has a number of weaknesses. Paramount among them is a concern about radiation exposure, as MPI has been cited as primary driver for an increase in exposure of patients to medical ionizing radiation.

In addition, reimbursement for MPI is currently higher than for stress echocardiography in the United States, which increases overall medical costs to society. Lastly, MPI can be adversely affected by differential photon attenuation from larger breasts, subdiaphragmatic activity, and obesity.

While traditional MPI has evolved dramatically from its initial development in the 1970s, recent advances in new methods, tracers, and technology continue to improve the technique. Chief among the methodological improvements has been growth in the use of cardiac PET. This has been driven by an increase in the number of PET scanners in US hospitals for use in oncologic imaging and by the availability of the PET perfusion tracer, rubidium-82 (Rb-82), which does not require an on-site cyclotron. Rb-82 PET has advantages over traditional SPECT imaging in that its higher energy (511 KeV) photons lead to improved spatial and contrast resolution. Its use of robust attenuation correction, rapid imaging protocols (approximately 45 min for complete rest/stress Rb-82 study), lower radiation exposure (~3–4 mSv for a 40 mCI×2 rest/stress Rb-82 study), and the ability to measure a peak-stress ejection fraction (as opposed to a post-stress ejection fraction traditionally measured with SPECT) are other potential advantages over SPECT imaging.

The overall diagnostic accuracy of PET is superior to SPECT, with reported sensitivity and specificity of 92 and 85 % [27]. In addition, Rb-82 PET has superior diagnostic accuracy in women, obese subjects (BMI >30), and those with multivessel CAD [28]. Furthermore, the ability to measure peak-stress ejection fraction adds significant prognostic accuracy [26]. Lastly, recently validated and FDA-approved software for dynamic PET-acquired estimates of myocardial blood flow will likely add further utility to noninvasively identifying CAD severity, improving diagnostic certainty in multivessel CAD and allowing routine measures of vascular response to medical interventions [29].

Comparison of Stress Modalities and Imaging Techniques

Given the multiple options for stress and imaging modalities, the evaluating physician should tailor their testing strategy to best evaluate the individual patient and answer the clinical question. This approach recognizes that factors such as cost, safety, availability, diagnostic characteristics, and institutional expertise all play a role in test selection. The American Society of Nuclear Cardiology has recently attempted to address how to best use various nuclear stress testing imaging methods and protocols, focusing on "patient-centered imaging" [30].

This concept is also addressed in the ACC/AHA UA/NSTEMI guidelines which provide a Class IC recommendation that the:

"Choice of stress test is based on the resting ECG, ability to perform exercise, local expertise, and technologies available. Treadmill exercise is useful in patients able to exercise in whom the ECG is free of baseline ST-segment abnormalities, bundle-branch block, LV hypertrophy, intraventricular conduction delay, paced rhythm, pre-excitation, and digoxin effect" [1].

In addition, the ACC/AHA Chronic Stable Angina guidelines provide specific recommendations regarding which patients should also receive imaging as part of their exercise stress ECG. These include a Class IB recommendation for imaging in patients with pre-excitation, >1mm resting ST-segment depression, and prior revascularization (PCI or CABG) [4]. In these patients, imaging improves sensitivity in the setting of resting ECG abnormalities and assists in the localization of ischemia in patients with prior revascularization.

In patients who are unable to exercise, pharmacologic stress imaging (adenosine, regadenoson, or dipyridamole nuclear imaging; or dobutamine stress echocardiography) receives a Class IB recommendation in intermediate risk patients, a Class IC recommendation in patients with a paced ventricular rhythm, and a Class IB recommendation in patients with LBBB [4].

In the evaluation of acute chest pain, particularly in a CPU setting, the trade-off between sensitivity and specificity should be weighted towards improved sensitivity so as to not miss. This is especially true when considering the choice between MPI and exercise echo for localization of disease (esp. left circumflex territory ischemia). For example, the lower sensitivity of stress echocardiography versus MPI for the diagnosis of CAD has been suggested to decrease the level of confidence that a normal stress echocardiogram imparts the same low-risk event rate as a normal MPI. Some have reported event rates as high as 5 % per year for patients following a normal stress echo compared to <1 % per year for a normal MPI [31]. This low event rate following a normal MPI has been reproduced in multiple studies [32], including in patients with known CAD [33]. Further, it is likely that the use of PET-based MPI imaging strategies will further advance the evaluation of acute chest pain due to its greater sensitivity for overall CAD, multivessel CAD, and the ability of PET/CT-based cameras to provide quantitative assessments of coronary calcium which can further define low-risk patients when coronary calcium is absent.

The Role of Chest Pain Observation Units

Chest Pain Units (CPUs) are specialized units and/or patient care clinical pathways that serve to rapidly assess whether a patient presenting with chest pain is undergoing an acute coronary syndrome. A majority of the over 600 accredited CPUs in the US are located in the hospital Emergency Department, but CPUs can also be located in a telemetry ward of a inpatient hospital. CPUs offer the advantage of systematic, protocol-driven patient evaluations, and randomized controlled trial data support their utility in reducing costs, use of resources, and lengths of stay [34]. To accomplish these advantages, CPUs generally attempt to evaluate patients within 6–24 hours of presentation using serial observations of ECGs and biomarkers (troponin). If the initial evaluation period is completed without recurrence of classical anginal symptoms and the ECG and biomarkers remain negative for findings consistent with ACS, patients are then risk stratified by either stress ECG, stress imaging (nuclear or echo), or CTA. The choice of the stress and/or imaging modality should be based on the strengths and weaknesses of that particular test for a given a patient and clinical scenario, realizing institutional expertise and test availability play a significant role in choosing a particular testing strategy.

Patients with recurrent chest pain consistent with ACS, positive biomarkers, ECG changes, or stress test should be admitted and undergo further evaluation [1]. Alternatively, patients who symptoms do not recur, have negative biomarkers and ECGs, and low-risk findings on stress testing can be discharged with recommended close follow-up with their primary care physician. The current ACC/AHA UA/NSTEMI Guidelines detail a Class IB recommendation for patients with probable or possible ACS to undergo observation and repeat ECG and biomarker monitoring in a CPU telemetry ward, and a Class IC recommendation for stress testing in a CPU (or outpatient within 72 hours) in patients with suspected ACS as an alternative to admission [1].

Cardiac Catheterization

While cardiac catheterization remains the gold standard for the diagnosis of epicardial coronary artery disease, only a small minority of patients who present with chest pain undergo this test. Current recommendations for the appropriate use of coronary angiography in patients with suspected angina include patients with high-risk criteria on noninvasive testing for risk stratification (Class I, B), patients with an uncertain diagnosis after noninvasive testing for risk stratification (I, B) or with increasing symptoms (IIa, C), patients with LV dysfunction (EF < 45 %) (IIa, C), patients who cannot undergo noninvasive testing (IIA, C) or who have inadequate prognostic information after noninvasive testing (IIa, C), patients with an occupational requirement for definitive diagnosis (IIa, C), and patients with a high pretest probability of left main or 3-vessel CAD (IIa, C) [4]. More specifically, an early invasive angiographic assessment for CAD is recommended in patients with recurrent angina at rest/low-level exercise while on medical therapy, elevated biomarkers, worsening CHF and/or reduced LV function, hemodynamic instability, prior PCI within 6 months, prior CABG, and an elevated TIMI risk score.

Key Points
- The evaluation of chest pain should include a complete history, physical exam, and target ancillary testing.
- In addition to providing a diagnosis, a complete evaluation of chest pain should provide an assessment of cardiovascular risk.
- Ancillary testing strategies include ECG, echocardiography, myocardial perfusion imaging, and/or CT angiography.
- Protocol-driven chest pain evaluation units can provide a rapid, evidence-based method of screening patients for acute coronary syndromes.

References

1. Anderson JL, Adams CD, Antman EM, et al. ACC/AHA 2007 guidelines for the management of patients with unstable angina/non ST-elevation myocardial infarction: a report of the American College of Cardiology/American Heart Association Task Force on Practice Guidelines (Writing Committee to Revise the 2002 Guidelines for the Management of Patients With Unstable Angina/Non ST-Elevation Myocardial Infarction): developed in collaboration with the American College of Emergency Physicians, the Society for Cardiovascular Angiography and Interventions, and the Society of Thoracic Surgeons: endorsed by the American Association of Cardiovascular and Pulmonary Rehabilitation and the Society for Academic Emergency Medicine. Circulation. 2007;116(7):e148–304.
2. Henrikson CA, Howell EE, Bush DE, et al. Chest pain relief by nitroglycerin does not predict active coronary artery disease. Ann Intern Med. 2003;139(12):979–86.
3. Chaitman BR, Bourassa MG, Davis K, et al. Angiographic prevalence of high-risk coronary artery disease in patient subsets (CASS). Circulation. Aug 1981;64(2):360–7.
4. Gibbons RJ, Abrams J, Chatterjee K, et al. ACC/AHA 2002 guideline update for the management of patients with chronic stable angina–summary article: a report of the American College of Cardiology/American Heart Association Task Force on Practice Guidelines (Committee on the Management of Patients With Chronic Stable Angina). Circulation. 2003;107(1):149–58.
5. Diamond GA, Forrester JS. Analysis of probability as an aid in the clinical diagnosis of coronary-artery disease. N Engl J Med. 1979; 300(24):1350–8.
6. Gibbons RJ, Chatterjee K, Daley J, et al. ACC/AHA/ACP-ASIM guidelines for the management of patients with chronic stable angina: a report of the American College of Cardiology/American Heart Association Task Force on Practice Guidelines (Committee on Management of Patients With Chronic Stable Angina). J Am Coll Cardiol. Jun 1999;33(7):2092–197.
7. Rouan GW, Lee TH, Cook EF, Brand DA, Weisberg MC, Goldman L. Clinical characteristics and outcome of acute myocardial infarction in patients with initially normal or nonspecific electrocardiograms (a report from the Multicenter Chest Pain Study). Am J Cardiol. 1989;64(18):1087–92.
8. Gibbons RJ, Balady GJ, Beasley JW, et al. ACC/AHA Guidelines for Exercise Testing. A report of the American College of Cardiology/American Heart Association Task Force on Practice Guidelines (Committee on Exercise Testing). J Am Coll Cardiol. Jul 1997;30(1):260–311.

9. Henzlova MJ, Cerqueira MD, Mahmarian JJ, Yao SS. Stress protocols and tracers. J Nucl Cardiol. Nov 2006;13(6):e80–90.

10. Mark DB, Hlatky MA, Harrell Jr FE, Lee KL, Califf RM, Pryor DB. Exercise treadmill score for predicting prognosis in coronary artery disease. Ann Intern Med. Jun 1987;106(6):793–800.

11. Fearon WF, Lee DP, Froelicher VF. The effect of resting ST segment depression on the diagnostic characteristics of the exercise treadmill test. J Am Coll Cardiol. Apr 2000;35(5):1206–11.

12. Thygesen K, Alpert JS, Jaffe AS, et al. Third universal definition of myocardial infarction. J Am Coll Cardiol. 2012;60(16):1581–98.

13. Invasive compared with non-invasive treatment in unstable coronary-artery disease: FRISC II prospective randomised multicentre study. FRagmin and Fast Revascularisation during InStability in Coronary artery disease Investigators. Lancet. 1999;354(9180):708–15.

14. Kleiman NS, Lakkis N, Cannon CP, et al. Prospective analysis of creatine kinase muscle-brain fraction and comparison with troponin T to predict cardiac risk and benefit of an invasive strategy in patients with non-ST-elevation acute coronary syndromes. J Am Coll Cardiol. 2002;40(6):1044–50.

15. Horowitz RS, Morganroth J, Parrotto C, Chen CC, Soffer J, Pauletto FJ. Immediate diagnosis of acute myocardial infarction by two-dimensional echocardiography. Circulation. Feb 1982;65(2):323–9.

16. Peels CH, Visser CA, Kupper AJ, Visser FC, Roos JP. Usefulness of two-dimensional echocardiography for immediate detection of myocardial ischemia in the emergency room. Am J Cardiol. 1990;65(11):687–91.

17. Douglas PS, Khandheria B, Stainback RF, et al. ACCF/ASE/ACEP/AHA/ASNC/SCAI/SCCT/SCMR 2008 appropriateness criteria for stress echocardiography: a report of the American College of Cardiology Foundation Appropriateness Criteria Task Force, American Society of Echocardiography, American College of Emergency Physicians, American Heart Association, American Society of Nuclear Cardiology, Society for Cardiovascular Angiography and Interventions, Society of Cardiovascular Computed Tomography, and Society for Cardiovascular Magnetic Resonance: endorsed by the Heart Rhythm Society and the Society of Critical Care Medicine. Circulation. 2008;117(11):1478–97.

18. Geleijnse ML, Elhendy A. Can stress echocardiography compete with perfusion scintigraphy in the detection of coronary artery disease and cardiac risk assessment? Eur J Echocardiogr. Mar 2000;1(1):12–21.

19. Budoff MJ, Dowe D, Jollis JG, et al. Diagnostic performance of 64-multidetector row coronary computed tomographic angiography for evaluation of coronary artery stenosis in individuals without known coronary artery disease: results from the prospective multicenter ACCURACY (Assessment by Coronary Computed Tomographic Angiography of Individuals Undergoing Invasive Coronary Angiography) trial. J Am Coll Cardiol. 2008;52(21):1724–32.

20. Min JK, Dunning A, Lin FY, et al. Age- and sex-related differences in all-cause mortality risk based on coronary computed tomography angiography findings results from the International Multicenter CONFIRM (Coronary CT Angiography Evaluation for Clinical Outcomes: An International Multicenter Registry) of 23,854 patients without known coronary artery disease. J Am Coll Cardiol. 2011;58(8):849–60.

21. Taylor AJ, Cerqueira M, Hodgson JM, et al. ACCF/SCCT/ACR/AHA/ASE/ASNC/NASCI/SCAI/SCMR 2010 appropriate use criteria for cardiac computed tomography. A report of the American College of Cardiology Foundation Appropriate Use Criteria Task Force, the Society of Cardiovascular Computed Tomography, the American College of Radiology, the American Heart Association, the American Society of Echocardiography, the American Society of Nuclear Cardiology, the North American Society for Cardiovascular Imaging, the Society for Cardiovascular Angiography and Interventions, and the Society for Cardiovascular Magnetic Resonance. J Am Coll Cardiol. 2010;56(22):1864–94.

22. Hilton TC, Thompson RC, Williams HJ, Saylors R, Fulmer H, Stowers SA. Technetium-99m sestamibi myocardial perfusion imaging in the emergency room evaluation of chest pain. J Am Coll Cardiol. Apr 1994;23(5):1016–22.

23. Hilton TC, Fulmer H, Abuan T, Thompson RC, Stowers SA. Ninety-day follow-up of patients in the emergency department with chest pain who undergo initial single-photon emission computed tomographic perfusion scintigraphy with technetium 99m-labeled sestamibi. J Nucl Cardiol. 1996;3(4):308–11.

24. Varetto T, Cantalupi D, Altieri A, Orlandi C. Emergency room technetium-99m sestamibi imaging to rule out acute myocardial ischemic events in patients with nondiagnostic electrocardiograms. J Am Coll Cardiol. Dec 1993;22(7):1804–8.

25. Heller GV, Stowers SA, Hendel RC, et al. Clinical value of acute rest technetium-99m tetrofosmin tomographic myocardial perfusion imaging in patients with acute chest pain and nondiagnostic electrocardiograms. J Am Coll Cardiol. Apr 1998;31(5):1011–7.

26. Dorbala S, Hachamovitch R, Curillova Z, et al. Incremental prognostic value of gated Rb-82 positron emission tomography myocardial perfusion imaging over clinical variables and rest LVEF. JACC Cardiovasc Imaging. Jul 2009;2(7):846–54.

27. Nandalur KR, Dwamena BA, Choudhri AF, Nandalur SR, Reddy P, Carlos RC. Diagnostic performance of positron emission tomography in the detection of coronary artery disease: a meta-analysis. Acad Radiol. Apr 2008;15(4):444–51.

28. Bateman TM, Heller GV, McGhie AI, et al. Diagnostic accuracy of rest/stress ECG-gated Rb-82 myocardial perfusion PET: comparison with ECG-gated Tc-99m sestamibi SPECT. J Nucl Cardiol. 2006;13(1):24–33.

29. El Fakhri G, Kardan A, Sitek A, et al. Reproducibility and accuracy of quantitative myocardial blood flow assessment with (82)Rb PET: comparison with (13)N-ammonia PET. J Nucl Med. Jul 2009;50(7):1062–71.

30. Depuey EG, Mahmarian JJ, Miller TD, et al. Patient-centered imaging. J Nucl Cardiol. Apr 2012;19(2):185–215.

31. Brown KA. Do stress echocardiography and myocardial perfusion imaging have the same ability to identify the low-risk patient with known or suspected coronary artery disease? Am J Cardiol. 1998;81(8):1050–3.

32. Brown KA. Prognostic value of thallium-201 myocardial perfusion imaging. A diagnostic tool comes of age. Circulation. 1991;83(2):363–81.

33. Iskandrian AE, Verani MS. Nuclear cardiac imaging: principles and applications. 3rd ed. New York: Oxford University Press; 2003.

34. American College of Emergency Physicians. State of the Art: Observation Units in the Emergency Department. Policy Resource and Education Paper. 2011; http://www.acep.org/Search.aspx?searchtext=chest+pain&folderId=2144&isRecursive=True. Accessed 6 Apr 2012.

Acute Coronary Syndromes

2

Gabriel A. Delgado and J. Dawn Abbott

Abstract

Acute coronary syndromes (ACS) are responsible for over 1.4 million hospital admissions in the USA each year and are associated with considerable mortality. ACS encompasses a group of three related clinical entities: unstable angina (UA), non-ST-elevation myocardial infarction (NSTEMI), and ST-elevation myocardial infarction (STEMI). A comprehensive description of the definitions and clinical classification of the diseases will be followed by a review of disease pathophysiology. The role of inflammation, endothelial dysfunction, and plaque vulnerability and rupture are presented. The ability to rapidly and accurately diagnose ACS is paramount to patient care as early initiation of therapy improves outcomes. The diagnostic criteria will be covered including methods of clinical risk stratification. The treatment of ACS has evolved rapidly over the last 10 years, with a focus on achieving timely reperfusion in STEMI and the approval of several new antiplatelet and antithrombin therapies. This chapter will provide a categorized review of medical treatment options and interventional strategies for ACS and guide clinicians in determining appropriate patients for invasive therapies. Additionally, a review of recently published ACS guidelines will be provided.

Keywords

Acute coronary syndrome • Unstable angina • Myocardial infarction • Plaque rupture • Percutaneous coronary intervention • Thrombus

Introduction

Definition and Classification

ACS encompasses a group of three related clinical entities: unstable angina (UA), non-ST-elevation myocardial infarction (NSTEMI), and ST-elevation myocardial infarction (STEMI).

They represent different manifestations of a common underlying disorder, acute myocardial ischemia. The UA/NSTEMI and STEMI classifications of ACS have replaced the older terms "Q wave" and "non-Q wave" myocardial infarction (MI).

The clinical presentation of UA/NSTEMI is characterized by new onset or a worsening pattern of prior angina, originating from a mismatch between myocardial oxygen requirements and a limited supply due to an acute impediment to coronary blood flow, usually from nonocclusive intracoronary thrombosis. The two syndromes are differentiated based on the presence or absence of myocardial necrosis. In UA there is no evidence of myocardial necrosis, whereas in NSTEMI the degree of ischemia is sufficiently severe to cause circulatory release of cardiac biomarkers. Patients with UA/NSTEMI can be further classified according to Braunwald's classification as having primary angina, secondary angina occurring in the setting of an extracardiac condition that intensifies ischemia,

G.A. Delgado, MD
Interventional Cardiology Fellow,
Department of Medicine, Cardiology, Brown Medical School,
593 Eddy Street, Providence, RI 02903, USA
e-mail: gdelgado@lifespan.org

J.D. Abbott, MD (✉)
Department of Medicine, Division of Cardiology,
Brown Medical School, Rhode Island Hospital,
593 Eddy Street, Providence, RI 02903, USA
e-mail: jabbott@lifespan.org

or angina within 2 weeks of a myocardial infarction known as post-infarct angina [1]. All UA/NSTEMI patients require aggressive therapy, but the classification provides prognostic information with secondary angina associated with a higher risk of 1-year death or MI than primary angina [2]. STEMI arises from a complete occlusion of the infarct-related artery and it is differentiated form NSTEMI on the basis of the electrocardiogram (ECG) finding of ST-segment elevation.

Prevalence and Mortality

Approximately every 25 s an American will have a coronary event, and every minute, someone will die of one. There are 1.4 million ACS-related hospitalizations every year in the USA. Approximately 40 % of which are for UA and the remainder are for MI. Of the latter, nearly two-thirds are NSTEMI and one third STEMI [3, 4].

Pathophysiology

Role of Inflammation and Endothelial Dysfunction

An ACS is the final manifestation of a process of progressive atherosclerotic plaque formation within the intima of medium and large-sized arteries that develops over decades. Risk factors such as hyperlipidemia, smoking, hypertension, diabetes, and genetic susceptibilities facilitate endothelial damage with subendothelial migration of inflammatory cells, predominantly monocytes, which differentiate into macrophages. This inflammatory process results in increased production of adhesion molecules, endothelin-1, and decreased production of nitric oxide further disrupting endothelial homeostasis. Low-density lipoprotein (LDL) penetrates the arterial wall and is digested by macrophages which then become highly atherogenic foam cells that release cytokines (TNF-alpha, interleukins, among others) that recruit more macrophages and smooth muscle cells [5, 6].

Vulnerable Plaque and Plaque Rupture

Smooth muscle cells synthesize the extracellular matrix which provides stability to the atherosclerotic plaque and fibrous cap. Macrophages do the opposite, by elaborating matrix metalloproteinases such as collagenase and gelatinase that digest the collagen foundation of the interstitial matrix. A preponderance of macrophages over smooth muscle cells, along with a thin fibrous cap and a rich lipid core, make the plaque vulnerable to rupture. These plaque characteristics along with physiologic parameters such as coronary vasomotor tone and the hemodynamic, hemostatic, and hormonal milieu contribute to the risk of plaque disruption. If the plaque ruptures or fissures, exposure of the highly thrombogenic

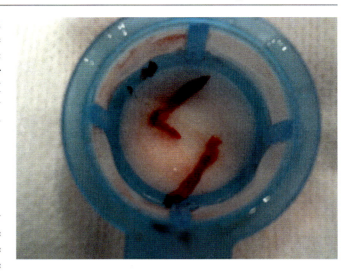

Fig. 2.1 Gross appearance of intracoronary "*red*" thrombus extracted from a patient with an acute STEMI by manual thrombectomy

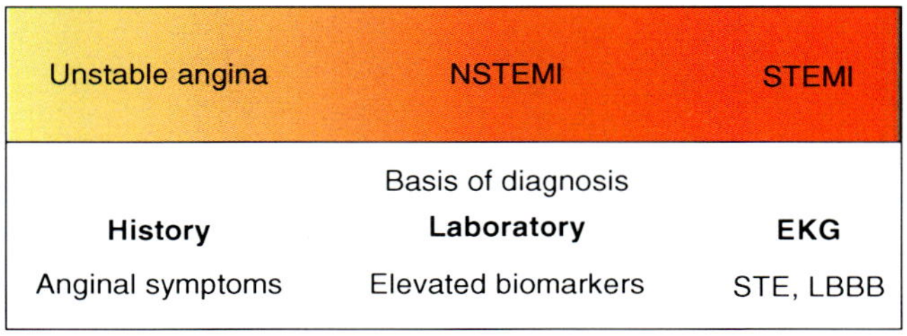

Unstable angina	NSTEMI	STEMI
	Basis of diagnosis	
History	**Laboratory**	**EKG**
Anginal symptoms	Elevated biomarkers	STE, LBBB

Fig. 2.2 The acute coronary syndrome continuum of unstable angina, non-ST-elevation myocardial infarction (*NSTEMI*), and ST-elevation myocardial infarction (*STEMI*)

subendothelium to circulating leukocytes and platelets activates the coagulation cascade and promotes platelet adhesion and aggregation resulting in thrombus formation. A thrombus that only partially occludes the artery (usually a platelet-rich or "white clot") causes UA or NSTEMI, while a completely occlusive clot (usually a fibrin-rich or "red clot") causes STEMI [7, 8] (Fig. 2.1). The preexisting degree of coronary stenosis by the atherosclerotic plaque is not a predictor of its vulnerability, in fact, most ACS cases are caused by atherosclerotic lesions with only mild-moderate stenosis [9, 10]. Furthermore, patients with ACS may have multiple areas of plaque rupture distinct from the culprit lesion [11].

Diagnosis

In general, UA is diagnosed by history on the basis of symptoms of an unstable pattern of angina as detailed below, and NSTEMI is a laboratory diagnosis provided by detectable levels of cardiac biomarkers (troponin, CK-MB, myosin). Only about 50 % of patients with UA/NSTEMI have ECG changes. Conversely, the diagnosis of STEMI requires the presence of ST elevations or new left bundle branch block (LBBB) on an ECG in association with symptoms (Fig. 2.2).

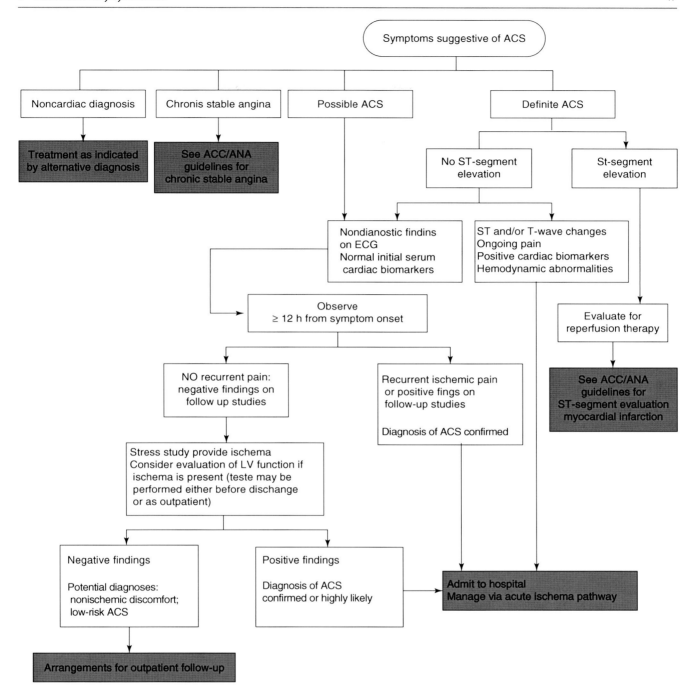

Fig. 2.3 Algorithm for evaluation and management of patients with suspected acute coronary syndrome (From Little et al. [10] with permission from Elsevier)

Prompt diagnosis is essential for the initiation of adequate therapy, to limit or save the myocardium at risk, and to prevent the complications of ACS.

The information gathered from the following three main diagnostic elements: history and physical examination, ECG, and laboratory evaluation should be used to assign patients to one of four diagnostic categories suggested by the ACC/AHA: 1. noncardiac diagnosis, 2. chronic stable angina, 3. possible ACS, or 4. definite ACS [12] (Fig. 2.3).

History and Physical Examination

The most common manifestation of myocardial ischemia is chest discomfort or angina. Typically it is substernal in location with radiation to the jaw, neck, left arm, or shoulder. However, atypical presentations and even silent ischemia are not infrequent, particularly in women, diabetics, and the elderly [13]. Some patients present with epigastric discomfort or with "anginal equivalents" such as fatigue, back pain, or shortness of breath. Associated symptoms are often

Table 2.1 Differential diagnosis of chest pain

Cardiac nonischemic
Aortic dissection
Pericarditis, myocarditis
Cardiomyopathies, e.g., hypertrophic, Takotsubo
Pulmonary
Pneumothorax
Pulmonary embolism
Pneumonia, pleuritis
Musculoskeletal
Disc disease
Costochondritis
Trauma, rib fracture
Gastrointestinal
Pancreatitis
Cholecystitis
Peptic ulcer disease
Gastroesophageal reflux
Esophageal spasm, perforation
Others
Zoster and other neuropathic disorders
Psychiatric (anxiety, panic attack, somatization disorders)

reported, the most common being dyspnea, but anxiety, diaphoresis, nausea, and vomiting are also common, with gastrointestinal type complaints more prominent in patients with MI involving the inferior wall [14]. The history and physical examination should also aim to elucidate the diagnosis of ACS from nonischemic causes of chest pain, particularly those that also pose a life-threatening risk such as aortic dissection or pulmonary embolism (Table 2.1).

Stable angina is defined by a level of angina (or its equivalent) that is triggered by a relatively reproducible degree of physical activity or emotional stress and is relieved by rest or sublingual nitroglycerin. In contrast, UA is characterized by the presence of one or more of the following features: rest angina (generally lasting more than 20 min), new onset (within the preceding 2 months), or crescendo (increasing frequency, duration, intensity, or triggered by a lower activity level) [1]. NSTEMI and STEMI patients can present with variable symptoms but when angina is present, pain at rest lasting more than 20 min is characteristic. It may be intermittent or "stuttering" in NSTEMI but it is commonly unrelenting in STEMI.

Syncope by itself, pleuritic pain, or pain that can be localized with the tip of one finger, reproducible with movement or by palpation, is seldom ischemic [15]. Relief of chest pain by sublingual nitroglycerin in the emergency department is an unreliable predictor of ACS [16]. Although traditional cardiovascular risk factors increase the likelihood that underlying atherosclerotic disease exists, they have been found to be weak predictors of acute ischemia. However, their presence in a patient with an established diagnosis of ACS is related to poor outcomes [17, 18].

The physical exam in a patient with ACS can be normal and should be aimed at risk stratification and recognizing the potential complications of myocardial ischemia, especially in patients with STEMI, and those presenting late after the onset of the ischemic event. High-risk findings suggestive of a large area of myocardial ischemia include sinus tachycardia, signs of hypoperfusion (oliguria, clammy skin, confusion), jugular venous distention, third or fourth heart sounds, pulmonary congestion, and hypotension. A loud systolic murmur, often associated with a palpable thrill, signals ventricular septal rupture. Although it may be audible as a soft systolic murmur radiating to the back or left axilla, acute ischemic mitral regurgitation is often silent.

Electrocardiogram

An ECG should be done and read by an experienced emergency physician within 10 min of presentation with symptoms suggestive of ACS [19]. ECG changes are present in approximately 40 % of ACS patients including T-wave inversions (21 %), ST-segment deviation ≥1 mm (14 %), and new LBBB (7 %) [20]. These changes may occur in combination, be transient, or dynamic. ST-segment deviations are particularly specific for acute ischemia and their presence is related to adverse outcomes [21, 22]. T-wave inversions, unless pronounced (≥3 mm), are less specific [23]. Complete occlusion of a coronary artery creates a current of epicardial injury that manifests as ST-segment elevations (Fig. 2.4). ST elevations of ≥1 mm in two or more anatomically contiguous leads or new LBBB establish the diagnosis of STEMI. The anatomic grouping of leads includes inferior (II, III, aVF), lateral (I, aVL), and anterior (V1-V6). The diagnosis of UA or NSTEMI does not require ECG changes but their presence support the diagnosis. If the initial ECG is unremarkable or nondiagnostic and there is a high clinical suspicion for ACS, an ECG should be repeated every 5–10 min [19]. Patients with confirmed absence of ECG changes have a better prognosis and are at significantly lower risk of major adverse cardiac events (MACE) during their index hospitalization and follow-up [24–26].

Laboratory Evaluation

Cardiac biomarkers are released into the circulation following cardiomyocyte death, and their presence defines NSTEMI, distinguishing the diagnosis from UA [27]. Elevation of cardiac biomarkers is not a requirement for the diagnosis of STEMI as these patients often present before their levels become detectable. The two most commonly used biomarkers are the cardiac isoform of creatine kinase (CK-MB) and troponins T and I. Troponins are highly sensitive and cardiac-specific, providing an accurate measure of the degree of myocardial necrosis. However, they typically do not become detectable until approximately 6 h after the onset of the ischemic event. Because of this, they need to be rechecked at 4–8 h intervals, typically three times, to detect deviations from normal. If the biomarker level continues to increase, daily measurements can be made to determine the peak level. Measuring more than one biomarker is probably not necessary or cost-effective and therefore measurement of troponin only is a reasonable approach. Troponins peak at 12–48 h after symptom onset and remain elevated for 7–14 days. CK-MB is less specific than troponins with elevated levels following skeletal muscle injury. However, their short half-life (24–48 h) allows laboratory assessment of recurrent, extending, or periprocedural MI. Reinfarction can also be determined with troponin and is defined by a 20 % increase in troponin level within 3–6 h from the onset of clinical signs or symptoms of recurrent ischemia [28]. The degree of elevation of cardiac biomarkers, and of troponin in particular, is independently related to short- and long-term outcomes including the risk of death within the first 42 days

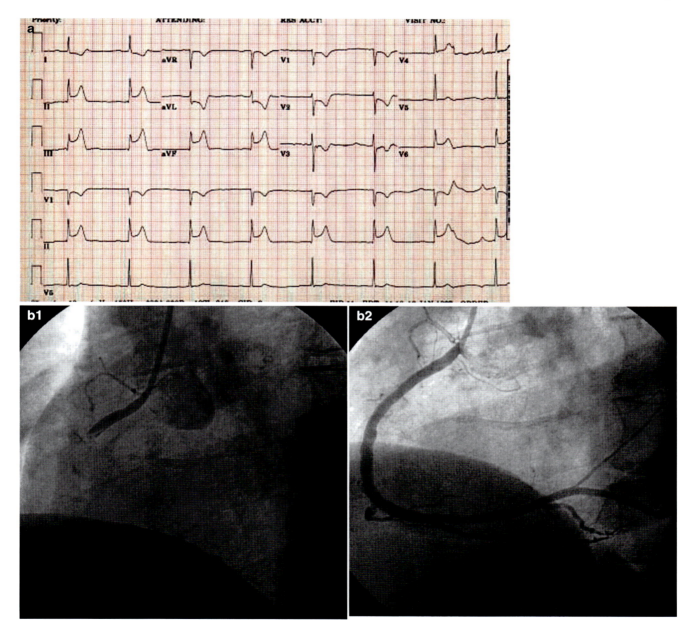

Fig. 2.4 STE or STD EKG with matching angiogram. (**a**) 12 lead EKG demonstrates ST segment elevation in leads II, III, aVF, and V6 indicating an acute inferior wall ST elevation myocardial infarction (**b1**) right coronary artery angiography confirms coronary occlusion with thrombolysis in myocardial infarction (TIMI) grade 0 flow (**b2**) after percutaneous coronary intervention with a stent TIMI grade 3 flow is restored (**c**) 12 lead EKG demonstrates ST segment depressions in multiple limb and precordial leads suggestive of diffuse subendocardial ischemia (**d**) left coronary angiography identified a ciritical stenosis in the distal left main coronary artery with TIMI grade III flow

Fig. 2.4 (continued)

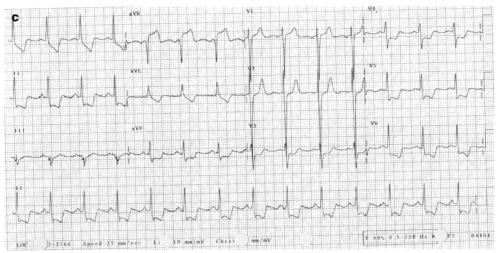

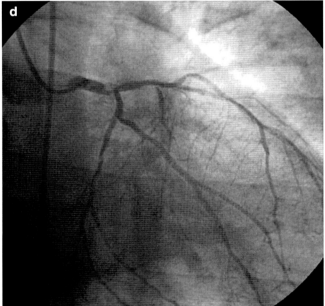

after an MI [29, 30] (Fig. 2.5). Myoglobin is a highly sensitive cardiac biomarker with a very early rise and short half-life following myocardial necrosis. This makes it useful as a screening test with the limitation of its very low specificity in the setting of skeletal muscle damage (Fig. 2.6).

Treatment

Risk Stratification

Early risk stratification is essential to identify UA/NSTEMI patients at a high acute and long-term risk of recurrent MI and death in which prompt initiation of more aggressive therapies has been shown to improve outcomes. Conversely, identification of low-risk patients allows not only adequate prioritization of therapy but also prevents these patients from

receiving more costly and potentially harmful interventions from which no or limited benefit may be obtained.

Several risk stratification tools have been developed. The Thrombolysis in Myocardial Infarction (TIMI) [32] and the Global Registry of Acute Coronary Events (GRACE) risk scores have been extensively validated [33]. The TIMI risk score for UA/NSTEMI uses seven variables to assess the risk of death, MI, or recurrent ischemia within 14 days after hospitalization. Those with ≥3 variables present are considered to be at high risk. The GRACE score uses eight independent variables to assess the likelihood of death and MI in-hospital or on the following 6 months. A GRACE score of >140 is considered high risk. The GRACE score has the advantages of assigning an individualized value to each variable and the inclusion of a variable for renal dysfunction. However, it requires a nomogram or a computer to calculate it as opposed to the simpler TIMI risk score (Table 2.2). Both scores have been shown

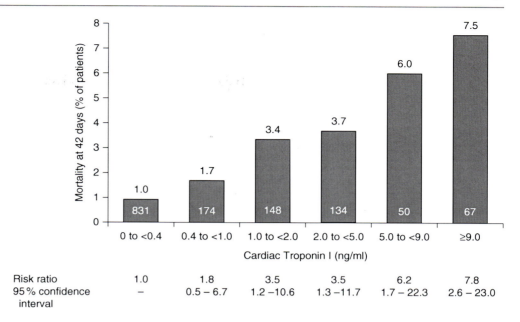

Fig. 2.5 Mortality rates according to cardiac troponin level. Mortality rates at 42 days are shown for ranges of cardiac troponin I levels. The numbers at the bottom of each bar are the numbers of patients with cardiac troponin I levels in each range, and the numbers above the bars are percentages. $P = 0.001$ for the increase in the mortality rate with increasing levels of cardiac troponin I (From Antman et al. [30])

	0 to <0.4	0.4 to <1.0	1.0 to <2.0	2.0 to <5.0	5.0 to <9.0	≥9.0
Risk ratio	1.0	1.8	3.5	3.5	6.2	7.8
95 % confidence interval	–	0.5 – 6.7	1.2 –10.6	1.3 –11.7	1.7 – 22.3	2.6 – 23.0

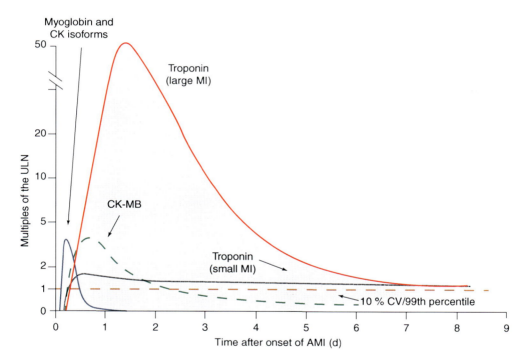

Fig. 2.6 Timing of biomarkers release following an acute myocardial infarction (AMI). The biomarkers are plotted with the multiples of the cutoff for AMI over time. The dashed horizontal line shows the upper limit of normal (ULN, defined as the 99th percentile from a normal reference population; the coefficient of variation [CV] of the assay should be 10 % or less). The earliest rising biomarkers are myoglobin and creatine kinase (CK) isoforms. The muscle/brain fraction of CK (CK-MB, dashed curve) rises to a peak of 2–5 times the ULN and returns to the normal range within 2–3 days. Troponin exhibit small elevations in small infarctions but may rise to 20–50 times the ULN in the setting of larger infarctions and remain elevated above the ULN for 7 days or more (Adapted from Mayo Clinic Cardiology: Concise Textbook, 3rd ed. [31])

to be helpful management guides with patients classified as high-risk deriving the most benefit from more aggressive treatment strategies including percutaneous coronary intervention (PCI) [34, 35]. Online calculators are available at www.TIMI. org and at www.outcomes-umassmed.org/grace.

Therapy in UA/NSTEMI is primarily pharmacological aimed at angina relief, decreasing myocardial oxygen demand, stabilization of the thrombus, and facilitation of the endogenous fibrinolytic mechanisms which prevents further growth of the nonocclusive coronary thrombus. This initial

Table 2.2 Scoring models to identify level of risk in acute coronary syndrome

TIMI variables	GRACE variables
Age >65 years	Age
Three or more cardiac risk factors	Killip class
Known coronary artery disease	Systolic arterial blood pressure
ST-segment deviation ≥0.5 mm	Cardiac arrest during presentation
Elevated cardiac biomarkers	Serum creatinine level
Two or more anginal episodes in the preceding 24 h	Elevated cardiac biomarkers

period of pharmacological stabilization is followed by two distinct management pathways: early invasive or initial conservative therapy (described below). In STEMI, the infarct-related artery is already completely occluded and therefore emergent revascularization with thrombolytic therapy (fibrinolysis) or PCI is mandatory. Unless stated otherwise, the recommendations given below follow the latest available set of guidelines by the American College of Cardiology/ American Heart Association (ACC/AHA) for patients in whom the diagnosis of ACS (UA/NSTEMI and STEMI) is likely or definite [12, 36, 37].

Anticoagulants

Also referred to in the literature as "antithrombins," these agents often inhibit other proteins proximal to thrombin in the coagulation cascade. Anticoagulants constitute one of the two pillars of antithrombotic therapy in ACS (the other being antiplatelets) and should be given to all patients without contraindications as soon as possible after presentation (Class I recommendation) [12]. There are three main types of anticoagulants approved for ACS: heparin based (unfractionated and low molecular weight), fondaparinux (a factor Xa inhibitor), and bivalirudin (a direct thrombin inhibitor). Despite the similarities between these agents, they are pharmacologically different and appropriate selection varies depending on the clinical risk and the management pathway chosen, i.e., early invasive versus initial conservative (for UA/NSTEMI).

Unfractionated Heparin

The two heparin-based anticoagulants: unfractionated heparin (UFH) and low-molecular-weight heparins (LMWH) exert their effect by coupling with antithrombin (AT, formerly ATIII) and accelerating the inhibitory effect of AT on thrombin (factor IIa). UFH also has inhibitory effects on factor Xa and to a lesser extent on factors XIIa, XIa, and IXa.

The effect achieved is largely prevention of thrombus propagation, rather than degradation. When tested in earlier ACS trials, UFH decreased the rates of refractory angina, death, and MI compared to ASA alone [38–40]. Its benefits include a long record of effective anticoagulation in ACS and its reversibility with protamine (1–1.5 mg protamine per 100 units heparin). The intrinsic limitations to UFH include the inability to inactivate clot-bound thrombin and its variable pharmacodynamics requiring frequent monitoring and titration. In addition, UFH activates platelets and carries an overall risk of heparin-induced thrombocytopenia (HIT) of approximately 2.6 % [41]. The incidence of HIT decreases to only 0.2 % for those treated for less than 4 days but is higher in individuals with previous exposure to heparin [42]. For UA/NSTEMI the ACC/AHA guidelines recommend a weight-adjusted intravenous (IV) bolus of 60 U/kg (max 4,000 U) followed by an infusion of 12 U/kg/h (max 1,000 U/h) adjusted to a goal for the activated partial thrombin time (aPTT) of 1.5–2 times control or approximately 50–70 s, and continued for 48 h or until the end of PCI for uncomplicated cases [12].

Low-Molecular-Weight Heparin

The LMWH are smaller, depolymerized fragments of UFH that retain anticoagulant properties. LMWH have enhanced anti-factor Xa activity and a more predictable pharmacodynamic profile negating the need for routine monitoring. In addition, LMWH carries a lower risk of HIT and even full therapeutic doses can be administered subcutaneously [43]. Although other LMWH (e.g., dalteparin) [44] have been studied, the existing body of literature supports the ACC/AHA guidelines recommendation for enoxaparin as the only LMWH to be used in ACS. In a meta-analysis of six randomized trials comparing enoxaparin to UFH in UA/NSTEMI, enoxaparin lowered the risk of death or MI without a significant difference in major bleed using an initial conservative strategy [45]. The evidence for its use if an early invasive strategy is employed is not as compelling. Despite initial promising results from trials such as ESSENCE (Efficacy and Safety of Subcutaneous Enoxaparin in Unstable Angina and Non-Q-wave MI) [46] and TIMI 11B (Enoxaparin vs. Unfractionated Heparin for Unstable Angina or Non-Q-wave Myocardial Infarction) [47], more recent studies such as SYNERGY (Superior Yield of the New Strategy of Enoxaparin, Revascularization and Glycoprotein IIb/IIIa Inhibitors) [48] and A to Z (Aggrastat to Zocor) [49] revealed a lack of significant benefit and an increase in bleeding rates on patients treated with enoxaparin and an early invasive approach. A caveat with the latter two trials, however, was their unblinded design, the coadministration of other antithrombotics before allocation to the enoxaparin arm, and the high rates of crossover [50]. The benefits of enoxaparin seem to be greater for higher-risk patients such as those with elevated troponin levels [51], ST-segment deviation [47], and high TIMI risk scores [35]. The incidence of HIT with enoxaparin is significantly lower than with UFH (0.2 %) but it increases with prior exposure to any form of heparin [43].

The ACC/AHA guidelines give enoxaparin a Class I recommendation for the treatment of UA/NSTEMI employing either an early invasive or an initial conservative approach [36]. For STEMI, the optimal anticoagulant depends on whether reperfusion is achieved by fibrinolysis or primary PCI. With fibrinolysis, the ExTRACT-TIMI 25 (Enoxaparin and Thrombolysis Reperfusion for Acute Myocardial Infarction Treatment—Thrombolysis in Myocardial Infarction 25) trial [52] and a large meta-analysis of trials comparing UFH to enoxaparin [53] showed a benefit of enoxaparin with a 16 % lower risk than UFH for the primary end point of death, MI, or major bleed at 30 days, despite more major bleeding with enoxaparin (2.6 % vs. 1.8 %). In the setting of primary PCI the data is less clear. The largest randomized trial, ATOLL (STEMI Treated with Primary Angioplasty and Intravenous Lovenox or UFH) [54], was open labeled and included 910 patients. Enoxaparin was administered IV at a dose of 0.5 mg/kg and UFH bolus IV with a variable dose range of 50–00 IU, depending on planned use of a glycoprotein IIb/IIIa inhibitor (GPI). Particulars of this trial included a high use of radial access and GPIs. At 30 days there was a lower risk of the combined end point of death, recurrent MI or ACS, or urgent revascularization with enoxaparin (relative risk [RR] 0.59, 95 % CI 0.38–0.91) without a difference in bleeding. A subsequent meta-analysis that included ATOLL similarly found enoxaparin had better outcomes compared to UFH in primary PCI [55]. Enoxaparin has not been adopted over UFH for primary PCI in the USA, and this is probably the result of concerns about the limited data available, limitations of published studies, use of bivalirudin, and common use of femoral access.

The dosing schedule of anticoagulants varies according to the clinical situation (Table 2.4). For UA/NSTEMI enoxaparin is given as 1 mg/kg subcutaneous every 12 h for the duration of hospitalization (max 8 days) or until the end of an uncomplicated PCI. If the creatinine clearance (CrCl) is <30 ml/min, dosing should be decreased to once a day. With fibrinolysis, a 30 mg IV bolus should be given with the subcutaneous dose in patients less than 75 years of age. Enoxaparin is used less often in the setting of primary PCI due to concerns about inadequate anticoagulation and bleeding risk. Enoxaparin can be reversed with 1 mg protamine for each mg of enoxaparin (1 mg of enoxaparin is equal to 100 IU of anti-Xa activity); however, the reliability of its reversal with protamine is less than for UFH.

Fondaparinux

Fondaparinux is a synthetic pentasaccharide with specific, direct factor Xa inhibitor effects. It has high specificity and bioavailability that allows for once-daily administration without the need for monitoring or titration. In the OASIS-5 trial (the Fifth Organization to Assess Strategies in Acute Ischemic Syndromes) [56], over 20,000 patients with high-risk UA/NSTEMI were randomized to fondaparinux or standard dose enoxaparin. Although fondaparinux was found to be similar to enoxaparin with regard to the primary composite end point of death, MI, refractory ischemia, or major bleed at 9 days, the rate of major bleeding was nearly 50 % lower in the fondaparinux arm (2.2 % vs. 4.1 %, p<0.001). Revascularization was common in the trial, with 40 % undergoing PCI and 15 % coronary artery bypass grafting (CABG). In the subset of patients who underwent PCI, the incidence of catheter-related thrombosis was more than three times higher in the fondaparinux arm (0.9 % vs. 0.3 %, OR=3.59), requiring an in-study amendment to supplement fondaparinux with UFH during PCI cases [57]. Based predominantly on the OASIS-5 trial, fondaparinux was given a Class I recommendation by the ACC/AHA for the management of UA/NSTEMI with either an early invasive or an initial conservative approach. In a cautionary note the guidelines mention that patients treated with fondaparinux should receive an additional anticoagulant if undergoing PCI, that UFH is the only anticoagulant evaluated for that purpose to date, and that this recommendation is not fully evidence-based, originating from the inconsistent and uncontrolled use of UFH in OASIS-5 [36]. The dose of UFH in the setting of fondaparinux is 50–60 U per kg IV bolus. The efficacy of fondaparinux in STEMI patients was evaluated in the OASIS-6 (The Sixth Organization to Assess Strategies in Acute Ischemic Syndromes) trial, which included over 12,000 patients. This complex trial included patients treated with fibrinolysis, primary PCI, or without reperfusion. There was a trend towards harm with fondaparinux in primary PCI patients, while the other patients had a lower risk of ischemic events with a non-significantly lower rate of bleeding [58]. Fondaparinux is given as a once-daily dose of 2.5 mg subcutaneously. It has a long half-life and is not reversible with protamine. It may be used with caution in mild-moderate renal dysfunction (CrCl 30–50 ml/min) without dose adjustment but it is contraindicated in severe renal disease (CrCl <30 ml/min). Since it is not a heparin-based anticoagulant, fondaparinux is not associated with HIT.

Direct Thrombin Inhibitors

The direct thrombin inhibitors (DTI) offer several advantages over heparin-based anticoagulants including more predictable pharmacodynamics, lack of interaction with other plasma proteins, no need for a cofactor for their effect (i.e., antithrombin), activity on clot-bound thrombin, and no incidence of HIT. In fact, DTIs are used for the treatment of HIT. The initial studies of DTI in ACS were done with hirudin (lepirudin) with mixed results [59–61]. Subsequent studies done with bivalirudin demonstrated significant reductions in bleeding rates without an increase in ischemic end points leading to its approval for the treatment of both UA/NSTEMI and STEMI ACS [62]. The landmark study for bivalirudin in UA/NSTEMI was the ACUITY (the Acute Catheterization and Urgent Intervention Triage Strategy) trial. ACUITY was a randomized but open-label study assigning ACS patients managed with an early invasive strategy to one of three antithrombotic regimens: UFH or enoxaparin plus a glycoprotein IIb/IIIa inhibitor (GPI), bivalirudin plus a GPI, or bivalirudin alone. At 30 days, bivalirudin alone compared to UFH (or enoxaparin) plus GPI resulted in markedly reduced rates of major bleeding (3 % vs. 5.7 %, $p < 0.001$) with non-inferior rates of a composite ischemic end point. The net clinical outcome inclusive of death, MI, unplanned revascularization for ischemia, and major bleeding at 30 days favored bivalirudin (10.1 % vs. 11.7 %, $p = 0.015$) driven primarily by a reduction in bleeding rates. Of note, these benefits disappeared (but without harm) in the bivalirudin plus GPI arm compared to UFH [63]. As with heparin-based anticoagulants, patients who undergo PCI treated with bivalirudin should receive an antiplatelet agent as early as possible, preferably prior to arrival to the cath lab. This was underscored by results from the ACUITY PCI substudy that showed that patients who did not receive a thienopyridine pre-PCI had higher rates of the composite ischemic end point compared to the UFH plus GPI group [64]. Based on these findings, the ACC/AHA guidelines give bivalirudin a Class I recommendation for the treatment of UA/NSTEMI patients assigned to an early invasive management strategy and state that it is reasonable (Class IIa recommendation) to omit the administration of a GPI if a thienopyridine is given prior to catheterization [36].

Data supporting the use of bivalirudin in STEMI patients treated with primary PCI comes from the HORIZONS (the Harmonizing Outcomes with Revascularization and Stents in Acute Myocardial Infarction) [65] and ISAR-REACT 4 (Randomized Comparison of Abciximab Plus Heparin with Bivalirudin in Acute Coronary Syndrome) [66] trials. Patients in the HORIZONS trial were randomized, with open-labeled methodology, to bivalirudin plus provisional GPI or UFH plus planned GPI. Approximately 65 % of patients received UFH prior to randomization and the majority of patients were treated with dual antiplatelet therapy prior to catheterization. Bailout GPI use was uncommon in the bivalirudin group (7.5 %). At 30 days, the composite end point of MACE (death, reinfarction, target vessel revascular-

ization, or stroke) was similar in the two groups, but major bleeding was significantly lower with bivalirudin [65]. In addition, mortality was significantly lower at 30 days and this persisted out to 3 years (5.9 % vs. 7.7 %, hazard ratio (HR) 0.75 [0.58–0.97]; $p = 0.03$) [67]. While these results provide strong evidence for the selection of bivalirudin over UFH plus GPI, an increase in stent thrombosis within 24 h was noted in the bivalirudin group leading some to recommend a more prolonged infusion of bivalirudin, but this has not been tested. In ISAR-REACT 4, a double-blind study of bivalirudin versus UFH/GPI, similar findings were observed with a reduction in bleeding with bivalirudin without a difference in ischemic events [66]. Bivalirudin has a class I recommendation in STEMI patients treated with primary PCI.

Hirudin and other DTI such as argatroban remain options for deep venous thrombosis prophylaxis and for the management of HIT, but compared to UFH they are ineffective antithrombotics for the treatment of ACS and their use is not recommended [68].

Bivalirudin is given as a 0.75 mg/kg IV bolus followed by an infusion at 1.75 mg/kg/h up to 4 h, then 0.2 mg/kg/h up to 24 h total. However, as with other antithrombotics discussed above, it should be stopped at the completion of an uncomplicated PCI. Bivalirudin is metabolized in plasma through the CYP450 pathway but its excretion is renal and the infusion rate should be reduced if the CrCl is <30 to 1 mg/kg/h up to 4 h. The initial bolus dose does not have to be adjusted. There is no reversal agent for bivalirudin.

Antiplatelet Agents

Antiplatelet agents, together with anticoagulants, form the basis of pharmacologic therapy in ACS. The antiplatelet agents used in ACS can be divided into two broad groups: aspirin and the adenosine diphosphate (ADP) P2Y12 receptor blockers. The thienopyridines (clopidogrel and prasugrel) and the non-thienopyridine ticagrelor belong to this latter category. Unless contraindicated, both aspirin and a P2Y12 receptor blocker are used concomitantly in the management of ACS due to their synergistic effects. This combination is referred to as dual antiplatelet therapy.

Aspirin

Aspirin irreversibly acetylates cyclooxygenase I, irreversibly blocking the synthesis of thromboxane A2 resulting in decreased platelet aggregation. Its critical role on inhibition of acute thrombosis across the spectrum of ACS is reflected in studies demonstrating a reduction in the rates of death or MI of 30 % to greater than 50 % [38, 39, 69–71]. In fact, the occurrence of an ACS on a patient already taking aspirin is a marker of adverse outcomes (as included in the TIMI score). This "breakthrough" thrombosis may be due to a degree of resistance to the antithrombotic effects of aspirin, a large thrombotic stimulus that overcomes the effects of aspirin, or a combination of both [72–74]. With regard to dosing, studies have demonstrated no difference in efficacy with a wide range of doses, from 75 mg to more than 1,500 mg daily [75]. A wide geographic variation in the pattern of aspirin dosing has been noted with the common use of higher daily doses of aspirin after PCI in the USA (162–325 mg) compared to outside the USA (<100 mg). In patients with ACS treated with an early invasive strategy standard versus lower-dose aspirin was compared in the CURRENT-OASIS-7 (Clopidogrel and Aspirin Optimal Dose Usage to Reduce Recurrent Events—Seventh Organization to Assess Strategies in Ischemic Syndromes) [76] trial. In over 25, 000 patients, with concomitant standard or double-dose clopidogrel, no significant difference between higher-dose and lower-dose aspirin was observed for the primary outcome of cardiovascular death, myocardial infarction, or stroke at 30 days (4.2 % vs. 4.4 %; HR, 0.97; 95 % CI, 0.86–1.09; $p = 0.61$) with a major bleeding rate of 2.3 % that did not differ according to dose. An analysis from the CURE (Clopidogrel in Unstable Angina to Prevent Recurrent Events) trial found no difference in the rate of thrombotic events according to aspirin dose, but in patients on aspirin monotherapy there was a dose-dependent increase in major bleeding [77]. The ACC/AHA guidelines recommend an initial dose of 325 mg to be given as early as possible in ACS. After the index hospitalization, patients treated medically (without PCI) should continue aspirin 75–162 mg daily indefinitely. Among those treated with PCI, the initial dose is 162–325 mg daily for 1 month if a bare-metal stent (BMS) was used, and 3 months if a drug-eluting stent (DES) was used. Thereafter, it can be lowered to 75–162 mg. Of note, the European Society of Cardiology guidelines recommend low doses of aspirin (≤100 mg daily) after PCI and this is reasonable for patients at high risk of bleeding on dual antiplatelet therapy or with the use of more potent ADP receptor blockers than clopidogrel [78].

Ticlopidine

Ticlopidine is a first generation thienopyridine seldom used currently due to its multiple side effects including rash, nausea, vomiting, diarrhea, thrombocytopenia, and neutropenia (in 2.4 % of patients, severe in 0.8 %) as well as fatal cases of thrombotic thrombocytopenic purpura [79]. In combination with aspirin, it reduced rates of MI and vascular death by 46 % in NSTEMI patients and was proven of benefit in the secondary prevention of stent thrombosis and graft occlusion when compared to warfarin [80, 81]. Its current use may be

limited to patients allergic or with contraindications to the other more contemporary antiplatelet agents described below.

Clopidogrel

Clopidogrel is the most studied thienopyridine to date. Initial evidence of its benefits was obtained from the CURE trial [82]. CURE studied patients with UA/NSTEMI and randomized within 24 h of presentation to placebo or clopidogrel (loading dose of 300 mg followed by 75 mg/day) in addition to aspirin. The primary end point, a composite of cardiovascular death, MI, or stroke at 3–12 months, was decreased by 20 % (9.3 % vs. 11.5 %, $p < 0.001$) with clopidogrel. With dual antiplatelet therapy, there was an increase in the rates of minor and major bleeding (2.7 % in the placebo group vs 3.7 % in the clopidogrel group, $p = 0.003$) but without an increment in life-threatening bleeding. There were also higher bleeding rates if CABG was performed less than 5 days after stopping clopidogrel. Most patients in CURE were managed conservatively (77 %), providing strong evidence for the addition of clopidogrel to aspirin in this group. In the PCI-CURE substudy, patients that underwent revascularization with PCI had an even greater benefit, with a 31 % reduction in the rate of cardiovascular death, MI, or target vessel revascularization within 30 days. This study also demonstrated the benefits of clopidogrel pretreatment and post-PCI dual antiplatelet therapy for up to 1 year [83]. When treatment with thienopyridines is used in ACS, a loading dose is required to shorten the delay in attainment of the maximal antiplatelet effect. Most studies have examined a 300 mg loading dose, but in patients undergoing PCI, more favorable outcomes were observed with a 600 mg loading dose [84]. The clopidogrel maintenance dose is 75 mg/day.

Clopidogrel is also beneficial in patients with STEMI. The CLARITY-TIMI 28 (Clopidogrel as Adjunctive Reperfusion Therapy—Thrombolysis in Myocardial Infarction 28) trial randomized patients 18–75 years of age, who presented within 12 h after the onset of a STEMI to clopidogrel (300-mg loading dose, followed by 75 mg once daily) or placebo [85]. The addition of clopidogrel improved the patency rate of the infarct-related artery and reduced ischemic complications. In the PCI substudy of the trial, there was a 46 % reduction in the composite end point of cardiovascular death, MI, or stroke after PCI at 30 days in the clopidogrel pretreatment arm [86].

Clopidogrel Resistance

Clopidogrel is a prodrug that requires metabolism into its active metabolite through a 2-step process involving the cytochrome P450 system. Only 15 % of the original amount administered is metabolized into its active compound while the rest undergoes ester hydrolization in plasma into an inactive subproduct. Genetic polymorphisms of the involved liver enzymes, particularly the CYP2C19 subclass, and differences in gastric absorption produce significant variability in the antiplatelet response to clopidogrel [87]. Studies on the prevalence of clopidogrel resistance vary depending on the laboratory test and threshold employed, loading and maintenance doses received, and ethnicity of the population studied, ranging between 5 and 31 % [88–90]. Observational studies have demonstrated that the inadequate clopidogrel response associated with the presence of one or more of the loss-of-function alleles coding for the CYP2C19 isoenzyme is associated with an increased risk of adverse cardiac events [91–93]. However, these studies have been limited by the heterogeneity of the assessment method, nonuniform clopidogrel dosing, wide interindividual variation in platelet response, and lack of an identified optimal level of clopidogrel-induced platelet inhibition [94–96]. In 2010, the FDA announced a "boxed warning" regarding the decreased effect of clopidogrel in patients with metabolic deficiencies for conversion into its active form, generating a great deal of interest regarding testing for the involved mutations or laboratory confirmation of platelet inhibition by clopidogrel. In the latest 2011 ACC/AHA guideline update however, routine testing for CYP2C19 mutations or clopidogrel-induced antiplatelet effect was not recommend, stating that it may be considered on a case-by-case basis, particularly for patients with recurrent thrombotic events despite adequate clopidogrel therapy [36]. There is also uncertainty about what is the best therapeutic option if clopidogrel resistance is identified. The GRAVITAS (Gauging Responsiveness with a VerifyNow Assay—Impact on Thrombosis and Safety) study randomized patients with a poor response to clopidogrel (as measured by the VerifyNow P2Y12 test) to low (no loading and 75 mg/day maintenance) versus high (600 mg load and 150 mg/day) clopidogrel dose after PCI with a DES. The primary end point of death from cardiovascular causes, nonfatal myocardial infarction, or stent thrombosis at 6 months was the same (2.3 %) regardless of treatment arm [96]. Using one of the newer, more potent thienopyridines listed below with a more reliable bioavailability profile, although attractive in concept, has not been tested as part of a tailored approach in patients with antiplatelet resistance in any clinical trial to date.

Clopidogrel and Proton Pump Inhibitors

Proton pump inhibitors (PPI) interfere with the metabolism of clopidogrel with retrospective studies reporting adverse cardiac outcomes if used simultaneously. However, subsequent studies such as PRINCIPLE [97] and the randomized COGENT [98] trial demonstrated that even though there is pharmacodynamic attenuation of the effects of clopidogrel

(and prasugrel but to a lesser extent) when used with a PPI, it does not translate into adverse clinical outcomes. These results held true regardless of PPI studied, including omeprazole and pantoprazole. The ACC/AHA released a statement clarifying that the use of a PPI in combination with clopidogrel is not prohibitive and mentions the benefits of such combination in appropriate clinical settings to reduce gastrointestinal bleeding [99].

Prasugrel

Prasugrel is a newer oral thienopyridine with a more rapid, potent, and consistent antiplatelet effect than clopidogrel. The TRITON-TIMI 38 (Trial to Assess Improvement in Therapeutic Outcomes by Optimizing Platelet Inhibition with Prasugrel—Thrombolysis in Myocardial Infarction) studied moderate- to high-risk ACS patients (UA/NSTEMI and STEMI) with planned PCI randomized to prasugrel or clopidogrel. At a median follow-up of 15 months, prasugrel treatment resulted in a 19 % reduction in the composite end point of cardiac death, nonfatal MI, or nonfatal ($p < 0.001$). Prasugrel also decreased the individual risks of MI by 24 %, need for urgent target vessel revascularization by 34 %, and stent thrombosis by 52 %. The trade-off is an increase in the absolute risk of non-CABG related TIMI major bleeding of 0.5 and a 0.3 % increase in the absolute risk of fatal bleeding [100]. Importantly, a post-hoc analysis of this study demonstrated that patients with a history of transient ischemic attacks (TIA) or stroke of any kind had an even higher risk of bleeding, and a net harm from prasugrel compared to clopidogrel. In addition, patients older than 74 years of age and those weighting less than 60 kg failed to obtain a favorable net clinical benefit due to higher bleeding rates [101, 102]. This led the FDA to cite a contraindication to prasugrel for patients with a history of TIA or stroke and a general warning against its use in patients older than 74 years of age. For patients weighing less than 60 kg or over age 74, a reduced dose of 5 mg daily (following a standard loading dose of 60 mg) has been recommended; however, this dose has not been tested in clinical trials. In the 2011 ACC/AHA guidelines update, prasugrel was given a Class I recommendation for UA/NSTEMI patients treated with an invasive approach or for whom PCI is planned (Class I) [36].

Even though prasugrel is also a prodrug that requires conversion into its active metabolite, it is a single CYP-mediated step independent of the CYP2C19 isoenzyme and the genetic polymorphisms responsible for clopidogrel resistance. Observational studies have demonstrated no significant decrease on the platelet-inhibiting effects of prasugrel in carriers of the loss-of-function allele that affects clopidogrel [103, 104]. As a consequence, prasugrel has been proposed as a therapeutic alternative for clopidogrel nonresponders or those experiencing a thrombotic event while on clopidogrel therapy. Prasugrel has not been tested on ACS patients treated with an initial conservative approach and in the setting of elective PCI for stable angina. Currently, prasugrel is only approved for ACS patients intended to be managed with PCI. Prasugrel is given as a 60-mg loading dose followed by 10-mg daily maintenance. It does not require adjustment in mild-moderate renal insufficiency. Doses for severe renal failure or hemodialysis are not defined.

Ticagrelor

Ticagrelor is a non-thienopyridine P2Y12 receptor blocker and the latest antiplatelet agent approved for the treatment of ACS. As opposed to clopidogrel and prasugrel, it does not require enzymatic activation and its binding to the P2Y12 receptor is reversible. Similar to prasugrel, the degree of platelet inhibition is greater and the onset of action more rapid than clopidogrel. The use of ticagrelor in ACS was evaluated in the PLATO (PLATelet inhibition and patient Outcomes) trial, which randomized patients with UA/NSTEMI and STEMI to ticagrelor or clopidogrel, in addition to aspirin. All patients with STEMI were intended to be managed by PCI, but a conservative approach was permitted for UA/NSTEMI. At 12 months the primary end point of cardiovascular death, MI, or stroke occurred in 9.8 % of ticagrelor patients versus 11.7 % of patients on clopidogrel (HR 0.84, $p<0.001$). Mortality from any cause was also decreased with ticagrelor (4.5 % vs. 5.9 %, $p<0.001$). Compared to clopidogrel there was no increase in the rates of TIMI major or fatal bleeding (11.6 % vs. 11.2 %) [105]. Interestingly, a pre-specified subgroup analysis showed a greater incidence of the primary end point in patients taking aspirin at doses greater than 100 mg (12.6 % vs. 10.1 %, HR: 1.27, 95 % CI: 0.93–1.75). This led to the FDA recommendation that after the initial loading dose of 325 mg, aspirin should be decreased to 81 mg daily [106]. Ticagrelor is given as a single 180 mg loading dose, followed by a 90 mg twice a day as maintenance. Ticagrelor has no specific restrictions in patients with low body weight, or age over 74. Use in patients with prior stroke or TIA is cautioned due to the results of the randomized MATCH (Management of Atherothrombosis with Clopidogrel in High-Risk Patients with TIA or Stroke) trial which showed no benefit of dual antiplatelet therapy over clopidogrel alone, but a 1.3 % absolute increase in life-threatening bleeding in this patient population [107]. Ticagrelor can also be administered to patients with renal dysfunction but, given its metabolism, it should be used with caution in patients with moderate hepatic impairment. The most common side effect is dyspnea which occurs in 14 % of patients, compared to 8 % of clopidogrel-treated patients.

Although ticagrelor's inhibition of the platelet receptor is reversible, the antiplatelet effect persists for several days;

therefore, the reversibility does not translate into safer outcomes if CABG is required. All non-aspirin antiplatelet agents should ideally be discontinued prior to CABG to avoid excessive bleeding. However, an effort should be made to continue aspirin, particularly in the first month after a BMS, and for the first year after a DES. Clopidogrel and ticagrelor can be stopped 5 days prior to CABG, prasugrel needs to be stopped at least 7 days in advance. Ticagrelor received its FDA approval after the release of the latest 2011 UA/NSTEMI ACC/AHA guidelines update, thus it is not included as a therapeutic option.

Because of the importance of dual antiplatelet therapy with aspirin and an ADP receptor antagonist in ACS patients who undergo PCI, particularly with a drug-eluting stent, the ability to comply with dual antiplatelet therapy for at least 1 year is an important consideration. Patient with ACS should therefore be questioned about medication compliance, history and risk factors for major bleeding, and upcoming surgical procedures within 1 year. Patients should also be instructed not to discontinue their antiplatelet therapy without contacting their treating cardiologist, because premature discontinuation of antiplatelet therapy significantly increases the risk of stent thrombosis, which often results in MI or death. Health care providers should be aware that elective surgical procedures should be delayed 12 months after drug-eluting stent implantation or if performed sooner, the patient should be maintained on at least one but preferably both antiplatelet agents. When temporarily discontinued, the duration of antiplatelet agents should be minimized.

Glycoprotein IIb/IIIa Inhibitors

The GPI exert their antiplatelet effect at the end of the common pathway of platelet activation by blocking the glycoprotein (GP) IIb/IIIa heterodimer complex which is abundant and localized on the surface of the platelet. The GP IIb/IIIa molecule is the platelet fibrinogen receptor and plays a key role in clot formation through fibrinogen-mediated platelet cross-linking. Inhibition of this final step leads to potent inhibition of platelet aggregation. There are three GPI: abciximab, a monoclonal antibody, and eptifabitide and tirofiban which are synthetic small molecule antagonists. Abciximab is only indicated for ACS patients intended for PCI and should not be used in UA/NSTEMI patients treated with conservative therapy. Multiple trials and a meta-analysis have demonstrated the effectiveness of GPI in the management of ACS [108–111]; however, these studies were conducted before the current era of routine use of dual antiplatelet and early invasive therapy. A more contemporary trial, ISAR-REACT 2 (Intracoronary Stenting and Antithrombotic Regimen: Rapid Early Action for Coronary Treatment 2), evaluated UA/NSTEMI patients undergoing PCI and pretreated with clopidogrel (600 mg load at least 2 h prior to PCI) and randomized to abciximab or placebo. Even though abciximab was associated with a significant reduction in the primary end point of death, MI, or urgent target vessel revascularization, a subgroup analysis demonstrated that this benefit was limited to patients with an elevated troponin level [112]. Patients in the highest risk categories, i.e., those with elevated cardiac biomarkers [113, 114], diabetes [115], ST-segment changes [23], recurrent angina [116], and elevated TIMI risk score (four or greater) [117], undergoing PCI seem to derive the most benefit from antiplatelet therapy with GPI. No randomized study has directly compared the use of an oral antiplatelet agent (clopidogrel, prasugrel, or ticagrelor) versus a GPI, in addition to aspirin, for the management of UA/NSTEMI.

The ACC/AHA guidelines recommend that for patients with UA/NSTEMI treated with an invasive approach, clopidogrel or a GPI (eptifabitide or tirofiban preferred), in addition to aspirin and anticoagulant therapy, should be given prior to PCI (Class I). However, two trials, EARLY ACS [118] and ACUITY [119], addressed the issue of when to administer GPI to patients with UA/NSTEMI. "Upstream" refers to the administration of GPI at presentation and before angiography, and "deferred" or "downstream", when it is given in the cath lab, at the time of angiography or PCI. Overall, these studies suggest that there is no benefit to a routine strategy of upstream use. A strategy of deferred, selective use of GPI in the cath lab, at the discretion of the interventional cardiologist, and dictated by factors such as intracoronary clot burden, complicated PCI, and bleeding risk is a reasonable approach that does not increase the risk of adverse ischemic outcomes. UA/NSTEMI patients treated with an initial conservative approach should receive clopidogrel, in addition to aspirin and anticoagulant therapy. If clopidogrel is withheld due to suspected need for urgent CABG, or if clopidogrel-treated patients have recurrent ischemia, heart failure, or serious arrhythmia then a GPI should be initiated (Class I). The use of both a thienopyridine and a GPI, in addition to aspirin and an anticoagulant, receives a "may be reasonable" Class IIb recommendation and is reserved for patients with high-risk features such as elevated troponin levels, diabetes, and ST-segment depression who do not have a high bleeding risk [36].

Early Invasive Versus Initial Conservative Management of NSTEMI

Unlike the well-established benefits of urgent reperfusion therapy in STEMI, the optimal timing of revascularization in NSTEMI ACS is less clear. Keeping in mind that therapy with anticoagulants, antithrombotic, and other antianginal measures is otherwise largely unchanged, two distinct and often overlapping treatment strategies can be employed in regard to timing of angiography. "Early invasive" therapy refers to initial diagnos-

tic angiography with the intention to perform PCI within 24–48 h of presentation. An "initial conservative" approach, on the other hand, refers to a period of optimal medical management with angiographic evaluation dictated by recurrence of ischemia on optimal medical therapy, the presence of significant arrhythmias, or demonstration of residual ischemia or LV dysfunction on noninvasive testing. In general, a growing body of evidence seems to demonstrate reduced rates of death or nonfatal MI in NSTEMI ACS patients with high-risk features, or a high score in a predictive model (TIMI, GRACE), treated with an early invasive approach. High-risk criteria, as defined by the ACC/AHA and the European Society of Cardiology, include diabetes, elevated cardiac biomarkers, ST-segment depression or transient ST-segment elevation, recurrent ischemic symptoms, history of CABG, or PCI within the preceding 6 months [12]. Three large meta-analyses, conducted in the current era of stents and newer pharmacologic agents (thienopyridines, LMWH, GPI), compared early invasive and initial conservative strategies: Mehta at al. [120] found that early invasive therapy reduced the end point of death or MI by 2.2 % (12.2 % vs. 14.4 %, $p=0.001$); Bavry et al. [121] showed a 25 % relative risk reduction in all-cause mortality (6.5 % vs. 4.9 %, $p=0.001$) at 2 years follow-up; and Hoenig et al. [122] reported a 33 % relative risk reduction in the incidence of refractory angina and rehospitalization. Data supporting very early invasive therapy is less conclusive. TIMACS randomized patients to angiography ≤24 h (median 14 h) or ≥36 h (median 50 h) after randomization. At 6 months there was no significant difference in the primary composite end point of death, MI, or stroke (9.6 % vs. 11.3 %) in the early versus delayed groups. However, post-hoc analysis suggested benefit for intervention among patients at the highest risk. Due to the high incidence of adverse cardiac events among them, NSTEMI ACS patients with very high-risk features including cardiogenic shock, hemodynamic instability, severe LV dysfunction (Killip Class $\geq$III), sustained ventricular arrhythmias, and mechanical complications of MI such as worsening mitral regurgitation should probably be treated with urgent revascularization akin to that employed in STEMI patients. On the other end of the spectrum, patients with significant comorbidities (malignancy, advanced dementia, etc.), with a life expectancy of less than 1 year, or with a low quality of life that is not expected to be improved by PCI, should be treated in a conservative manner (Table 2.3).

Reperfusion Therapy for STEMI

While for UA/NSTEMI treatment focuses on "stabilizing" a partially occlusive thrombus, in STEMI the thrombus is fully occlusive and the management is aimed at urgent reperfusion. This can be accomplished by pharmacological (fibrinolysis) or invasive ("primary" PCI) means. Urgent CABG as a method of primary revascularization in the setting of STEMI is rarely used due to the significant risk and delays inherent

Table 2.3 Factors influencing the decision between early invasive and initial conservative therapy in UA/NSTEMI

Invasive	Conservative
Recurrent angina	Patient or physician preference in the absence of high-risk features
Elevated cardiac biomarkers	Low-risk TIMI or GRACE scores
High-risk TIMI or GRACE scores	Significant comorbidities
New or worse ST-segment depression	Life expectancy <1 year
Signs or symptoms of heart failure	Low quality of life unlikely to be improved by PCI
New or worsening mitral regurgitation	
High-risk findings on noninvasive testing	
Hemodynamic instability	
Sustained ventricular arrhythmias	
Prior CABG or PCI within 6 months	
Reduced left ventricular function	

Table 2.4 Absolute and relative contraindications to fibrinolysis

Absolute	Relative
Prior intracranial hemorrhage	Pregnancy
Intracranial neoplasm	Active peptic ulcer disease
Suspected aortic dissection	Recent (within 2–4 weeks) internal bleeding
Known cerebral vascular lesion	Noncompressible vascular puncture
Active bleeding or bleeding diathesis	Systolic blood pressure >180 mmHg
Ischemic stroke during the prior 3 months	Ischemic stroke >3 months prior
Significant head trauma during the prior 3 months	Dementia or other intracranial pathology
	Current anticoagulant use
	For streptokinase or anistreplase: prior use (>5 days) or prior allergic reaction to these agents

to this complex surgical procedure. An exception is in the presence of a mechanical complication of STEMI such as a ventricular septal defect or acute papillary muscle rupture with severe mitral regurgitation for which surgical correction, while high risk, is emergently indicated.

Fibrinolysis

Fibrinolysis is generally indicated, in the absence of contra-indications, for patients presenting within 12 h of symptom onset and either left bundle branch block (LBBB) or ST elevations of 1 mm or more in at least two anatomically contiguous leads. The absolute and relative contraindications for fibrinolysis are outlined below (Table 2.4). Although fibrinolysis has been largely replaced by primary PCI as the main method of reperfusion therapy for STEMI, it retains an ACC/AHA Class I recommendation for patients presenting to a facility without the capability to provide primary PCI or, in a PCI-capable facility, when the difference between "door-to-needle" and "door-to-balloon" time exceeds 1 h [37]. A collective review of 9 fibrinolysis trials by the Fibrinolytic Therapy Trialists' Collaborative Group demonstrated an absolute mortality reduction of 2 % for patients presenting between 7 and 12 h after symptom onset and of 3 % for those presenting within the first 6 h of symptom onset. The greatest benefit was derived by patients presenting with a ST elevations in the anterior leads or with LBBB and occurred regardless of gender, age, prior history of MI, or diabetes. Patients presenting with ST depressions obtained no benefit (and a trend toward harm) from fibrinolysis [123]. Several fibrinolytic agents have been introduced since the original advent of streptokinase.

The TIMI I (Thrombolysis in Myocardial Infarction) and GUSTO I (Global Utilization of Streptokinase and Tissue-Type Plasminogen Activator for Occluded Coronary Arteries) trials compared streptokinase to alteplase revealing significantly improved rates of reperfusion at 90 min and lower 30-day mortality (6.3 % vs. 7.3 %, $p=0.001$), respectively, with alteplase [124, 125]. The newer fibrin-specific agents, reteplase and tenecteplase, have the advantage of abbreviated, bolus administration but have demonstrated no incremental survival advantage [126].

Primary PCI

Primary PCI has become the mainstay of reperfusion therapy for STEMI. A meta-analysis of 23 randomized trials comparing fibrinolytic therapy to primary PCI revealed the superiority of the latter in decreasing short-term, long-term outcomes, and mortality [127]. Primary PCI, however, is a critically time-dependent intervention with multivariate analysis showing that "door-to-balloon" times >90 min, and greater than 2 h in particular, are associated with higher mortality rates [128]. In settings where PCI is not immediately available, the decision to perform thrombolysis versus transfer for PCI depends on the timeliness of fibrinolytic administration, the delay introduced by transfer to another institution, and clinical variables. In general, transfer for PCI remains a preferred option if "door-to-balloon" time is ≤90 min and the difference compared to fibrinolytic administration is ≤1 h. In addition, patients in whom the diagnosis of STEMI is in doubt, those with contraindication to or high bleeding risk from thrombolytics, presenting late (>3 h) after symptom onset, or with a STEMI complicated by pulmonary edema or cardiogenic shock are probably best treated with PCI (Table 2.5).

Table 2.5 Factors influencing the choice of reperfusion therapy in ST-elevation myocardial infarction (STEMI)

Primary PCI preferred	Fibrinolysis preferred
Late-presenting STEMI (>3 h since symptom onset)	Early-presentation STEMI (≤3 h since symptom onset)
High-risk STEMI (shock, hemodynamic instability, Killip class ≥3)	Lack of access to or unavailable PCI laboratory
Contraindications to fibrinolytics	Anticipated difficulty with vascular access
Increased risk of intracranial bleeding	Delay to primary PCI (door-to-balloon time >90 min or difference with door-to-needle time >1 h)
Diagnosis of STEMI is in doubt	
PCI-capable facility available with door-to-balloon time ≤90 min and difference with door-to-needle time ≤1 h	

PCI percutaneous coronary intervention

Facilitated PCI, Rescue PCI, and Pharmacoinvasive Management

Even though the terms "facilitated" and "rescue" PCI have fallen out of favor, and have been replaced with the term "pharmacoinvasive" strategy, a brief review of their meaning is in order. Facilitated PCI refers to the use of partial or full-dose fibrinolytic therapy, with or without a GPI, followed immediately by PCI. The purpose was to increase the chance of an open artery by the time of PCI thereby limiting myonecrosis. Two studies, ASSENT-4 (Assessment of the Safety and Efficacy of a New Treatment Strategy with Percutaneous Coronary Intervention) and FINESSE (Facilitated Intervention with Enhanced Reperfusion Speed to Stop Events) addressed this issue. ASSENT-4 was designed to determine if fibrinolysis prior to delayed PCI would compensate for the negative impact associated with that delay. It randomized patients to full-dose tenecteplase plus PCI (the facilitated arm) or routine primary PCI. The trial was stopped prematurely due to an increase in the primary end point (death, cardiogenic shock, or congestive heart failure at 90 days) in the facilitated arm (13.7 % vs. 18.8 %, p <0.005) [129]. Similarly, FINESSE, randomized patients to reduced-dose tenecteplase plus abciximab followed by PCI (combination-facilitated PCI), abciximab only followed by PCI (facilitated PCI), or placebo (primary PCI). Despite improved rates of early ST-segment resolution in the combined arm, the composite ischemic end point including all-cause mortality was no different among the groups at 90 days. Furthermore, the incidence of transfusion, minor, and major bleeding was greater in the combined group [130].

Rescue PCI refers to PCI performed after fibrinolytic therapy fails to achieve reperfusion defined as at least 50 % reduction in ST-segment elevation at 90 min in the lead with the greatest elevation, or by evidence of persistent or recurrent ischemia. A meta-analysis of rescue PCI trials demonstrated a significant benefit with rescue PCI compared to repeat doses of fibrinolytics, in moderate to high-risk STEMI patients who fail reperfusion with fibrinolytics [131].

A reasonable alternative is to reserve a "pharmacoinvasive" management strategy for high-risk STEMI patients presenting to non-PCI-capable hospitals. The benefits of such approach in this group were demonstrated in the CARESS-in-AMI (Combined Abciximab Reteplase Stent Study in Acute Myocardial Infarction) [132] and TRANSFER-AMI (Trial of Routine Angioplasty and Stenting and After Fibrinolysis to Enhance Reperfusion in Acute Myocardial Infarction) [133] trials. CARESS-in-AMI studied patients ≤75 years old with at least one high-risk feature (extensive ST-segment elevation, new-onset LBBB, prior MI, Killip class >2, or EF ≤35 %) all of whom were given half-dose reteplase plus abciximab followed by randomization to either immediate transfer for PCI or expectant treatment with transfer for rescue PCI if needed. Despite a median transfer time of 110 min, the primary outcome of all-cause mortality, refractory ischemia, and reinfarction was significantly reduced in the immediate PCI arm. TRANSFER-AMI studied patients with at least one high-risk feature (≥2 mm ST-segment elevation or depression in anterior leads, systolic blood pressure less than 100 mmHg, heart rate >100 bpm, Killip class ≥2, evidence of right ventricular infarction) treated with full-dose tenecteplase and randomized to immediate transfer for PCI (within 6 h of lytic therapy) or standard management with rescue PCI as needed. Based on this data, the AHA/ACC guidelines grant a Class IIa recommendation to high-risk patients who receive fibrinolysis at a non-PCI-capable hospital to be transferred as soon as possible to a PCI-capable facility for PCI to be performed as part of a pharmacoinvasive strategy [37].

Ancillary Therapy

Oxygen

The administration of supplemental oxygen in the absence of objective evidence of hypoxia is of unclear value. A Cochrane review of MI trials in which patients were randomly assigned to oxygen or room air showed no mortality difference with a trend toward harm, particularly in normoxic patients [134] Inadvertent hyperoxia has been observed to have direct coronary vasoconstrictor effects and there is some evidence of potentially deleterious effects in cardiac patients [135].

Nitrates

Nitroglycerin can be administered to patients with persistent chest pain despite other anti-ischemic and routine ACS therapy. It also has a role in the acute management of significant hypertension and to decrease preload in acutely decompensated heart failure (ADCHF) or pulmonary edema associated with ACS. It should be used with caution in patients with right ventricular infarction as reductions in preload may cause hemodynamic decompensation in this setting. In the acute setting nitroglycerin is best administered as an IV infusion, with a typical range between 20 and 100 (max 400) mcg/min. Nitrates are contraindicated in patients who have taken a phosphodiesterase inhibitor for erectile dysfunction during the preceding 24 h due to the risk of severe hypotension. In addition to its analgesic and anxiolytic properties, morphine has a mild preload reducing effect and may be given as an adjunctive antianginal measure and with nitroglycerin for ADCHF.

Beta Blockers

Several studies and pooled data analyses conducted in the fibrinolytic, pre-PCI era revealed reductions in morbidity and acute mortality (13 % relative risk reduction) with early beta blocker use in acute MI patients. The benefits of beta blockers in non-STEMI patients are less clear. However, given the substantial potential benefit, the absence of demonstrable harm in non-STEMI patients and the common underlying effects through which beta blockers exert their benefits have led to the acute use of beta blockers in ACS patients in general. The ACC/AHA guidelines recommend beta blockers to all ACS patients, regardless of type, in the absence of contraindications [36]. The routine, indiscriminate use of IV beta blockers, however, can be harmful. The large, placebo-controlled COMMIT/CCS2 trial randomized acute STEMI patients to placebo or 3 IV doses of 5 mg of metoprolol tartrate (on presentation), followed by extended-release metoprolol succinate PO 200 mg/day for 30 days [136]. Even though 50 % of patients were treated with fibrinolytics (the therapeutic method used in the original beta blocker studies showing benefit), COMMIT/CCS2 failed to demonstrate a mortality difference for beta blockade compared to placebo (7.8 % for both arms). Furthermore, in patients with hemodynamic compromise there was a 30 % increase in the relative risk of cardiogenic shock and a trend toward higher mortality rates. It has been postulated that the indiscriminate beta blocker use and the relatively rapid dose up-titration may account for the untoward results observed. In the absence of hemodynamic compromise (HR >100 bpm, SBP <100 mmHg, rales, jugular venous distention, or other evidence of LV failure) a cardioselective beta blocker such as metoprolol or atenolol may be given. Patients requiring more rapid beta blockade onset such as those with significant hypertension, atrial fibrillation with rapid heart rates, or ongoing ischemia despite routine ACS therapy may be treated initially with IV beta blockers. In the absence of

contraindications as discussed above, the ACC/AHA guidelines give a Class I recommendation to the initiation of oral beta blockers within 24 h for all ACS patients, and a Class IIb to the initial administration of IV beta blockers for hypertensive ACS patients.

Statins

Cholesterol-lowering therapy, particularly with HMG-CoA reductase inhibitors (also known as statins), are an essential component in the comprehensive management of CAD. In addition, there is data suggesting improved outcomes with early initiation of high-dose statin therapy in ACS patients. The MIRACL [137] and PROVE IT-TIMI 22 [138] trials revealed a reduction in ischemic end points with a regimen of atorvastatin 80 mg/day versus placebo or pravastatin 40 mg/day, respectively. Subgroup analysis of PROVE IT-TIMI 22 showed improved outcomes as early as 30 days after initiation of "intensive" statin therapy but, in general, limited to patients with a LDL cholesterol level of ≥125 mg/ dl.

Key Points

- Unstable angina, NSTEMI, and STEMI are part of the continuum that encompasses ACS and are differentiated by the presence of myonecrosis and ECG findings of acute coronary occlusion (ST elevation/LBBB).
- ACS results primarily from atherosclerotic plaque rupture and coronary thrombosis.
- Patients with ACS should be rapidly evaluated and risk stratified based on clinical, ECG, and laboratory parameters.
- Early initiation of antiplatelet therapy is of paramount importance in ACS:
  - In addition to aspirin, patients should receive a loading and maintenance dose of clopidogrel, prasugrel, or ticagrelor.
  - A GPI should be considered in patients who are not treated with an ADP receptor antagonist or as an adjunctive therapy during PCI.
- Early initiation of antithrombin therapy is of paramount importance in ACS:
  - For patients with STEMI treated with primary PCI or with UA/NSTEMI treated with an early invasive strategy, either bivalirudin or UFH with GPI is recommended over treatment with LMWH or fondaparinux.
  - For patients with STEMI treated with fibrinolysis or UA/NSTEMI treated with a conservative strategy LMWH or fondaparinux is preferred over UFH and bivalirudin.

- In UA/NSTEMI treatment is aimed at relieving ischemic symptoms and plaque stabilization through anticoagulant, antiplatelet, and ancillary interventions. Patients with high-risk features should be approached with an early invasive strategy with intent for PCI whereas low-risk patients can be managed with a conservative ischemia guided approach.
- STEMI patients require immediate reperfusion therapy with primary PCI when an adequate PCI laboratory is available in a timely manner or fibrinolysis when PCI is not available.
- The optimal duration of antiplatelet therapy in ACS patients managed either conservatively or with PCI has not been clearly determined, but the favorable results of thienopyridine therapy for 1 year or more suggest that at least 1 year of dual antiplatelet therapy is a reasonable goal.
- ACS patients should be initiated on a statin and beta blockade unless a contraindication exists.

References

1. Braunwald E. Unstable angina. A classification. Circulation. 1989;80(2):410–4.
2. Scirica BM, Cannon CP, McCabe CH, et al. Prognosis in the thrombolysis in myocardial ischemia III registry according to the Braunwald unstable angina pectoris classification. Am J Cardiol. 2002;90:821–6.
3. Roger VL, Go AS, Lloyd-Jones DM, et al. Executive summary: heart disease and stroke statistics—2012 update: a report from the American Heart Association. Circulation. 2012;125(1):188–97.
4. Lloyd-Jones D, Adams R, Carnethon M, et al. American Heart Association Statistics Committee and Stroke Statistics Subcommittee. Heart disease and stroke statistics—2009 update. A report from the American Heart Association Statistics Committee and Stroke Statistics Subcommittee. Circulation. 2009;119(3):480–6.
5. Fuster V, Badimon L, Badimon JJ, et al. The pathogenesis of coronary artery disease and the acute coronary syndromes. N Engl J Med. 1992;326(5):310–8.
6. Libby P. Current concepts of the pathogenesis of the acute coronary syndromes. Circulation. 2001;104(3):365–72.
7. Sullivan E, Kearney M, Isner JM, et al. Pathology of unstable angina: analysis of biopsies obtained by directional coronary atherectomy. J Thromb Thrombolysis. 1994;1(1):63–71.
8. Mizuno K, Satumo K, Miyamoto A, et al. Angioscopic evaluation of coronary artery thrombi in acute coronary syndromes. N Engl J Med. 1992;326(5):287–91.
9. Chen L, Chester MR, Crook R, Kaski JC. Differential progression of complex culprit stenoses in patients with stable and unstable angina pectoris. J Am Coll Cardiol. 1996;28(3):597–603.
10. Little WC, Constantinescu M, Applegate RJ, et al. Can coronary angiography predict the site of a subsequent myocardial infarction in patients with mild-to-moderate coronary artery disease? Circulation. 1988;78:1157–66.
11. Rioufol G, Finet G, Ginon I, et al. Multiple atherosclerotic plaque rupture in acute coronary syndrome: a three-vessel intravascular ultrasound study. Circulation. 2002;106(7):804–8.
12. Anderson JL, Adams CD, Antman EM, et al. ACC/AHA 2007 guidelines for the management of patients with unstable angina/non-ST-elevation myocardial infarction. J Am Coll Cardiol. 2007;50(7):e1–157.
13. Summers RL, Cooper GJ, Carlton FB, et al. Prevalence of atypical chest pain descriptions in a population from the southern United States. Am J Med Sci. 1999;318(3):142–5.
14. Pope JH, Ruthazer R, Beshansky JR, et al. Clinical features of emergency department patients presenting with symptoms suggestive of acute cardiac ischemia: a multicenter study. J Thromb Thrombolysis. 1998;6(1):63–74.
15. Braunwald E, Mark DB, Jones RH, et al. Unstable angina: diagnosis and management, AHCPR Publication No. 94-0602. Rockville: Agency for Health Care Policy and Research and the National Heart, Lung, and Blood Institute, US Public Health Service, US Department of Health and Human Services; 1994.
16. Henrikson CA, Howell EE, Bush DE, et al. Chest pain relief by nitroglycerin does not predict active coronary artery disease. Ann Intern Med. 2003;139:979–86.
17. Jayes Jr RL, Beshansky JR, D'Agostino RB, Selker HP. Do patients' coronary risk factor reports predict acute cardiac ischemia in the emergency department? A multicenter study. J Clin Epidemiol. 1992;45(6):621–6.
18. Pryor DB, Shaw L, McCants CB, et al. Value of the history and physical in identifying patients at increased risk for coronary artery disease. Ann Intern Med. 1993;118(2):81–90.
19. Antman EM, Anbe DT, Armstrong PW, et al. ACC/AHA guidelines for the management of patients with ST-elevation myocardial infarction-executive summary: a report of the American College of Cardiology/American Heart Association Task Force on Practice Guidelines. Circulation. 2004;110(5):588–636.
20. Cannon CP, McCabe CH, Stone PH, et al. The electrocardiogram predicts one-year outcome of patients with unstable angina and non-Q wave myocardial infarction: results of the TIMI III Registry ECG Ancillary Study. Thrombolysis in Myocardial Ischemia. J Am Coll Cardiol. 1997;30(1):133–40.
21. Manari A, Albiero R, De Servi S. High-risk non-ST-segment elevation myocardial infarction versus ST-segment elevation myocardial infarction: same behaviour and outcome? J Cardiovasc Med. 2009;10 Suppl 1:S13–6.
22. Savonitto S, Ardissino D, Granger CB, et al. Prognostic value of the admission electrocardiogram in acute coronary syndromes. JAMA. 1999;281(8):707–13.
23. Platelet Receptor Inhibition for Ischemic Syndrome Management in Patients Limited by Unstable Signs and Symptoms (PRISM-PLUS) Trial Investigators. Inhibition of the platelet glycoprotein IIb/IIIa receptor with tirofiban in unstable angina and non-Q-wave myocardial infarction. N Engl J Med. 1998;338(21):1488–97.
24. Brush YE, Brand DA, Acamporci D, et al. Use of the initial electrocardiogram to predict in-hospital complications of acute myocardial infarction. N Engl J Med. 1985;312:1137–41.
25. Slater DK, Hlatky MA, Mark DB, et al. Outcome in suspected acute myocardial infarction with normal or minimally abnormal admission electrocardiographic findings. Am J Cardiol. 1987;60:766–70.
26. Boden WE, Kleiger RE, Gibson RS, et al. Favourable long term prognosis in patients with non-Q wave acute myocardial infarction not associated with specific electrocardiographic changes. Br Heart J. 1989;61:396–402.
27. Alpert JS, Thygesen K, Antman E, Bassand JP. Myocardial infarction redefined–a consensus document Of The Joint European Society of Cardiology/American College of Cardiology Committee for the redefinition of myocardial infarction. J Am Coll Cardiol. 2000;36(3):959–69.
28. Thygesen K, Alpert JS, White HD, et al. Universal definition of myocardial infarction. Circulation. 2007;116:2634–53.

29. Ottani F, Galvani M, Nicolini FA, et al. Elevated cardiac troponin levels predict the risk of adverse outcome in patients with acute coronary syndromes. Am Heart J. 2000;140(6):917–27.
30. Antman EM, Tanasijevic MJ, Thompson B, et al. Cardiac-specific troponin I levels to predict the risk of mortality in patients with acute coronary syndromes. N Engl J Med. 1996;335(18):1342–9.
31. Shapiro BP, Babuin L, Jaffe AS. Cardiac biomarkers. In: Murphy JG, Lloyd MA, editors. Mayo clinic cardiology: concise textbook. 3rd ed. Rochester/Boca Raton: Mayo Clinic Scientific Press and New York/Informa Healthcare; 2007. p. 773–80.
32. Sabatine MS, Antman EM. The thrombolysis in myocardial infarction risk score in unstable angina/non-ST-segment elevation myocardial infarction. J Am Coll Cardiol. 2003;41(S):89S–95.
33. Eagle KA, Lim MJ, Dabbous OH, et al. A validated prediction model for all forms of acute coronary syndrome: estimating the risk of 6-month post discharge death in an international registry. JAMA. 2004;291:2727–33.
34. de Araujo GP, Ferreira J, Aguiar C, et al. TIMI, PURSUIT, and GRACE risk scores: sustained prognostic value and interaction with revascularization in NSTE-ACS. Eur Heart J. 2005;26: 865–72.
35. Antman EM, Cohen M, Bernink PJ, et al. The TIMI risk score for unstable angina/non-ST elevation MI: a method for prognostication and therapeutic decision making. JAMA. 2000;284: 835–42.
36. Wright RS, Anderson JL, Adams CD, et al. 2011 ACCF/AHA focused update incorporated into the ACC/AHA 2007 guidelines for the management of patients with unstable angina/ Non-ST-elevation myocardial infarction: a report of the American College of Cardiology Foundation/American Heart Association Task Force on Practice Guidelines developed in collaboration with the American Academy of Family Physicians, Society for Cardiovascular Angiography and Interventions, and the Society of Thoracic Surgeons. J Am Coll Cardiol. 2011;57(19):e215–367.
37. Kushner FG, Hand M, Smith Jr SC, et al. 2009 focused updates: ACC/AHA guidelines for the management of patients with ST-elevation myocardial infarction and ACC/AHA/SCAI guidelines on percutaneous coronary intervention a report of the American College of Cardiology Foundation/American Heart Association Task Force on Practice Guidelines. J Am Coll Cardiol. 2009;54(23):2205–41.
38. Théroux P, Ouimet H, McCans J, et al. Aspirin, heparin or both to treat unstable angina. N Engl J Med. 1988;319(17):1105–11.
39. Group RISC. Risk of myocardial infarction and death during treatment with low dose aspirin and intravenous heparin in men with unstable coronary artery disease. Lancet. 1990;336(8719): 827–30.
40. Oler A, Whooley MA, Oler J, Grady D. Adding heparin to aspirin reduces the incidence of myocardial infarction and death in patients with unstable angina. A meta-analysis. JAMA. 1996;276(10):811–5.
41. Martel N, Lee J, Wells PS. Risk for heparin-induced thrombocytopenia with unfractionated and low-molecular-weight heparin thromboprophylaxis: a meta-analysis. Blood. 2005;106(8): 2710–5.
42. Smythe MA, Koerber JM, Mattson JC. The incidence of recognized heparin-induced thrombocytopenia in a large, tertiary care teaching hospital. Chest. 2007;131(6):1644–7.
43. Warkentin TE, Levine MN, Hirsh J, et al. Heparin-induced thrombocytopenia in patients treated with low-molecular-weight heparin or unfractionated heparin. N Engl J Med. 1995;332(20): 1330–5.
44. Swahn E, Wallentin L. Low-molecular-weight heparin (Fragmin) during instability in coronary artery disease (FRISC). FRISC study group. Am J Cardiol. 1997;80(5A):25E–9.
45. Petersen JL, Mahaffey KW, Hasselblad V, et al. Efficacy and bleeding complications among patients randomized to enoxaparin or unfractionated heparin for antithrombin therapy in non-ST- segment elevation acute coronary syndromes: a systematic overview. JAMA. 2004;292(1):89–96.
46. Cohen M, Demers C, Gurfinkel EP, et al. A comparison of low-molecular-weight heparin with unfractionated heparin for unstable coronary artery disease. Efficacy and Safety of Subcutaneous Enoxaparin in Non-Q-Wave Coronary Events Study Group. N Engl J Med. 1997;337(7):447–52.
47. Antman EM, McCabe CH, Gurfinkel EP, et al. Enoxaparin prevents death and cardiac ischemic events in unstable angina/non-Q-wave myocardial infarction. Results of the thrombolysis in myocardial infarction (TIMI) 11B trial. Circulation. 1999;100(15):1593–601.
48. Ferguson JJ, Califf RM, Antman EM, et al. Enoxaparin vs unfractionated heparin in high-risk patients with non-ST-segment elevation acute coronary syndromes managed with an intended early invasive strategy: primary results of the SYNERGY randomized trial. JAMA. 2004;292(1):45–54.
49. de Lemos JA, Blazing MA, Wiviott SD, A to Z Investigators, et al. Enoxaparin versus unfractionated heparin in patients treated with tirofiban, aspirin and an early conservative initial management strategy: results from the a phase of the A-to-Z trial. Eur Heart J. 2004;25(19):1688–94.
50. Califf RM, Petersen JL, Hasselblad V, et al. A perspective on trials comparing enoxaparin and unfractionated heparin in the treatment of non-ST-elevation acute coronary syndromes. Am Heart J. 2005;149(4 Suppl):S91–9.
51. de Lemos JA, Rifai N, Morrow DA, et al. Elevated baseline myoglobin is associated with increased mortality in acute coronary syndromes, even among patients with normal baseline troponin I: a TIMI 11B substudy. Circulation. 1999;100(suppl I): I372–3.
52. Antman EM, Morrow DA, McCabe CH, et al. Enoxaparin versus unfractionated heparin with fibrinolysis for ST-elevation myocardial infarction. N Engl J Med. 2006;354:1477–88.
53. Murphy SA, Gibson CM, Morrow DA, et al. Efficacy and safety of the low-molecular weight heparin enoxaparin compared with unfractionated heparin across the acute coronary syndrome spectrum: a meta-analysis. Eur Heart J. 2007;28:2077–86.
54. Montalescot G, Zeymer U, Silvain J, et al. Intravenous enoxaparin or unfractionated heparin in primary percutaneous coronary intervention for ST-elevation myocardial infarction: the international randomised open-label ATOLL trial. Lancet. 2011;378(9792): 693–703.
55. Navarese EP, De Luca G, Castriota F, et al. Low-molecular-weight heparins vs. unfractionated heparin in the setting of percutaneous coronary intervention for ST-elevation myocardial infarction: a meta-analysis. J Thromb Haemost. 2011;9:1902–15.
56. Fifth Organization to Assess Strategies in Acute Ischemic Syndromes Investigators, Yusuf S, Mehta SR, Chrolavicius S, Afzal R, Pogue J, et al. Comparison of fondaparinux and enoxaparin in acute coronary syndromes. N Engl J Med. 2006;354(14): 1464–76.
57. MICHELANGELO OASIS-5 Steering Committee, Mehta SR, Yusuf S, Granger CB, et al. Design and rationale of the MICHELANGELO Organization to Assess Strategies in Acute Ischemic Syndromes (OASIS)-5 trial program evaluating fondaparinux, a synthetic factor Xa inhibitor, in patients with non-ST-segment elevation acute coronary syndromes. Am Heart J. 2005;150(6):1107.
58. Yusuf S, Mehta SR, Chrolavicius S, et al. Effects of fondaparinux on mortality and reinfarction in patients with acute ST-segment elevation myocardial infarction: the OASIS-6 randomized trial. JAMA. 2006;295:1519–30.

59. The Global Use of Strategies to Open Occluded Coronary Arteries (GUSTO) IIa Investigators. Randomized trial of intravenous heparin versus recombinant hirudin for acute coronary syndromes. Circulation. 1994;90:1631–7.

60. Antman EM. Hirudin in acute myocardial infarction: Thrombolysis and Thrombin Inhibition in Myocardial Infarction (TIMI) 9B trial. Circulation. 1996;94:911–21.

61. Organisation to Assess Strategies for Ischemic Syndromes (OASIS-2) Investigators. Effects of recombinant hirudin (lepirudin) compared with heparin on death, myocardial infarction, refractory angina, and revascularisation procedures in patients with acute myocardial ischaemia without ST elevation: a randomised trial. Lancet. 1999;353:429–38.

62. Lincoff AM, Bittl JA, Harrington RA, et al. Bivalirudin and provisional glycoprotein IIb/IIIa blockade compared with heparin and planned glycoprotein IIb/IIIa blockade during percutaneous coronary intervention: REPLACE-2 randomized trial. JAMA. 2003;289:853–63.

63. Stone GW, McLaurin BT, Cox DA, et al. Bivalirudin for patients with acute coronary syndromes. N Engl J Med. 2006;355:2203–16.

64. Stone GW, White HD, Ohman EM, et al. Bivalirudin in patients with acute coronary syndromes undergoing percutaneous coronary intervention: a subgroup analysis from the Acute Catheterization and Urgent Intervention Triage strategy (ACUITY) trial. Lancet. 2007;369:907–19.

65. Stone GW, Witzenbichler B, Guagliumi G, et al. Bivalirudin during primary PCI in acute myocardial infarction. N Engl J Med. 2008;358:2218–30.

66. Kastrati A, Neumann F, Schulz S, et al. Abciximab and heparin versus bivalirudin for non–ST-elevation myocardial infarction. N Engl J Med. 2011;365:1980–9.

67. Stone GW, Witzenbichler B, Guagliumi G, et al. Heparin plus a glycoprotein IIb/IIIa inhibitor versus bivalirudin monotherapy and paclitaxel-eluting stents versus bare-metal stents in acute myocardial infarction (HORIZONS-AMI): final 3-year results from a multicentre, randomised controlled trial. Lancet. 2011;377:2193–204.

68. The Direct Thrombin Inhibitor Trialists' Collaborative Group. Direct thrombin inhibitors in acute coronary syndromes: principal results of a meta-analysis based on individual patients' data. Lancet. 2002;359:294–302.

69. Lewis HD, Davis JW, Archibald DG, et al. Protective effects of aspirin against acute myocardial infarction and death in men with unstable angina. N Engl J Med. 1983;309(7):396–403.

70. Cairns JA, Gent M, Singer J, et al. Aspirin, sulfinpyrazone, or both in unstable angina; results of a Canadian multicenter trial. N Engl J Med. 1985;313(22):1369–75.

71. Collaborative overview of randomised trials of antiplatelet therapy-I: Prevention of death, myocardial infarction, and stroke by prolonged antiplatelet therapy in various categories of patients. Antiplatelet Trialists' Collaboration. BMJ. 1994; 308(6921):81–106.

72. Alexander JH, Harrington RA, Tuttle RH, et al. Prior aspirin use predicts worse outcomes in patients with non-ST-elevation acute coronary syndromes. PURSUIT Investigators. Platelet IIb/IIIa in Unstable angina: Receptor Suppression Using Integrilin Therapy. Am J Cardiol. 1999;83(8):1147–51.

73. Michelson AD, Cattaneo M, Eikelboom JW, Gurbel P, Kottke-Marchant K, Kunicki TJ, et al. Aspirin resistance: position paper of the working group on aspirin resistance. J Thromb Haemost. 2005;3(6):1309–11.

74. Hankey GJ, Eikelboom JW. Aspirin resistance. Lancet. 2006; 367(9510):606–17.

75. Antithrombotic Trialists' Collaboration. Collaborative meta-analysis of randomised trials of antiplatelet therapy for prevention of death, myocardial infarction, and stroke in high risk patients. BMJ. 2002;324(7329):71–86.

76. The CURRENT-OASIS Investigators. Dose comparisons of clopidogrel and aspirin in acute coronary syndromes. N Engl J Med. 2010;363:930–42.

77. Peters RJ, Mehta SR, Fox KA, et al. Effects of aspirin dose when used alone or in combination with clopidogrel in patients with acute coronary syndromes: observations from the clopidogrel in unstable angina to prevent recurrent events (CURE) study. Circulation. 2003;108(14):1682–7.

78. Silber S, Albertsson P, Avilés FF, et al. Guidelines for percutaneous coronary interventions. The Task Force for Percutaneous Coronary Interventions of the European Society of Cardiology. Eur Heart J. 2005;26(8):804–47.

79. Love BB, Biller J, Gent M. Adverse haematological effects of ticlopidine. Prevention, recognition and management. Drug Saf. 1998;19:89–98.

80. Balsano F, Rizzon P, Violi F, et al. Antiplatelet treatment with ticlopidine in un- stable angina. A controlled multicenter clinical trial. The Studio della Ticlopidina nell'Angina Instabile Group. Circulation. 1990;82(1):17–26.

81. Urban P, Macaya C, Rupprecht HJ, et al. Randomized evaluation of anticoagulation versus antiplatelet therapy after coronary stent implantation in high-risk patients: the multicenter aspirin and ticlopidine trial after intracoronary stenting (MATTIS). Circulation. 1998;98(20):2126–32.

82. Yusuf S, Zhao F, Mehta SR, et al. Effects of clopidogrel in addition to aspirin in patients with acute coronary syndromes without ST-segment elevation. N Engl J Med. 2001;345(7):494–502.

83. Mehta SR, Yusuf S, Peters RJ, et al. Effects of pretreatment with clopidogrel and aspirin followed by long-term therapy in patients undergoing percutaneous coronary intervention: the PCI-CURE study. Lancet. 2001;358(9281):527–33.

84. Patti G, Colonna G, Pasceri V, et al. Randomized trial of high loading dose of clopidogrel for reduction of periprocedural myocardial infarction in patients undergoing coronary intervention. Results from the ARMYDA-2 (Antiplatelet therapy for Reduction of MYocardial Damage during Angioplasty) study. Circulation. 2005;111:2099–106.

85. Sabatine MS, Cannon CP, Gibson CM, et al. Addition of clopidogrel to aspirin and fibrinolytic therapy for myocardial infarction with ST-segment elevation. N Engl J Med. 2005;352(12):1179–89.

86. Sabatine MS, Cannon CP, Gibson CM, et al. Effect of clopidogrel pretreatment before percutaneous coronary intervention in patients with ST-elevation myocardial infarction treated with fibrinolytics. The PCI-CLARITY study. JAMA. 2005;294:1224–32.

87. Oqueli E, Hiscock M, Dick R. Clopidogrel resistance. Heart Lung Circ. 2007;16 Suppl 3:S17–28.

88. Lev EI, Patel RT, Maresh KJ, et al. Aspirin and clopidogrel drug response in patients undergoing percutaneous coronary intervention: the role of dual drug resistance. J Am Coll Cardiol. 2006;47(1):27–33.

89. Gurbel PA, Bliden KP, Hiatt BL, O'Connor CM. Clopidogrel for coronary stenting: response variability, drug resistance, and the effect of pretreatment platelet reactivity. Circulation. 2003;107(23):2908–13.

90. Müller I, Besta F, Schulz C, et al. Prevalence of clopidogrel non-responders among patients with stable angina pectoris scheduled for elective coronary stent placement. Thromb Haemost. 2003;89(5):783–7.

91. Shuldiner AR, O'Connell JR, Bliden KP, et al. Association of cytochrome P450 2C19 genotype with the antiplatelet effect and clinical efficacy of clopidogrel therapy. JAMA. 2009;302:849–57.

92. Simon T, Verstuyft C, Mary-Krause M, et al. Genetic determinants of response to clopidogrel and cardiovascular events. N Engl J Med. 2009;360:363–75.

93. Trenk D, Hochholzer W, Fromm MF, et al. Cytochrome P450 2C19 681G>a polymorphism and high on-clopidogrel platelet reactivity associated with adverse 1-year clinical outcome of elective percutaneous coronary intervention with drug-eluting or bare-metal stents. J Am Coll Cardiol. 2008;51:1925–34.

94. Nguyen TA, Diodati JG, Pharand C. Resistance to clopidogrel: a review of the evidence. J Am Coll Cardiol. 2005;45(8):1157–64.

95. Sweeny JM, Gorog DA, Fuster V. Antiplatelet drug 'resistance'. Part 1: mechanisms and clinical measurements. Nat Rev Cardiol. 2009;6(4):273–82.

96. Price MJ, Berger PB, Teirstein PS, et al. Standard- vs high-dose clopidogrel based on platelet function testing after percutaneous coronary intervention: the GRAVITAS randomized trial. JAMA. 2011;305(11):1097–105.

97. O'Donoghue ML, Braunwald E, Antman EM, et al. Pharmacodynamic effect and clinical efficacy of clopidogrel and prasugrel with or without a proton-pump inhibitor: an analysis of two randomised trials. Lancet. 2009;374:989–97.

98. Bhatt DL, Cryer BL, Contant CF, et al. Clopidogrel with or without omeprazole in coronary artery disease. N Engl J Med. 2010; 363:1909–17.

99. Abraham NS, Hlatky MA, Antman EM, et al. ACCF/ACG/AHA 2010 expert consensus document on the concomitant use of proton pump inhibitors and thienopyridines: a focused update of the ACCF/ACG/AHA 2008 expert consensus document on reducing the gastrointestinal risks of antiplatelet therapy and NSAID use. J Am Coll Cardiol. 2010;56:2051–66.

100. Wiviott SD, Braunwald E, McCabe CH, et al. Prasugrel versus clopidogrel in patients with acute coronary syndromes. N Engl J Med. 2007;357(20):2001–15.

101. Wiviott SD, Braunwald E, McCabe CH, et al. Intensive oral anti-platelet therapy for reduction of ischaemic events including stent thrombosis in patients with acute coronary syndromes treated with percutaneous coronary intervention and stenting in the TRITON-TIMI 38 trial: a subanalysis of a randomised trial. Lancet. 2008;371(9621):1353–63.

102. Murphy SA, Antman EM, Wiviott SD, et al. Reduction in recurrent cardiovascular events with prasugrel compared with clopidogrel in patients with acute coronary syndromes from the TRITON- TIMI 38 trial. Eur Heart J. 2008;29(20):2473–9.

103. Mega JL, Close SL, Wiviott SD, et al. Cytochrome P450 genetic polymorphisms and the response to prasugrel: relationship to pharmacokinetic, pharmacodynamic, and clinical outcomes. Circulation. 2009;119:2553–60.

104. Varenhorst C, James S, Erlinge D, et al. Genetic variation of CYP2C19 affects both pharmacokinetic and pharmacodynamic responses to clopidogrel but not prasugrel in aspirin-treated patients with coronary artery disease. Eur Heart J. 2009;30: 1744–52.

105. Wallentin L, Becker RC, Budaj A, et al. Ticagrelor versus clopidogrel in patients with acute coronary syndromes. N Engl J Med. 2009;361(11):1045–57.

106. Ticagrelor [package insert]. London, UK: AstraZeneca. Available at: www.brillinta.com. Accessed 31 Jan2012.

107. Diener HC, Bogousslavsky J, Brass LM, et al. Aspirin and clopidogrel compared with clopidogrel alone after recent ischaemic stroke or transient ischaemic attack in high-risk patients (MATCH): randomised, double-blind, placebo-controlled trial. Lancet. 2004;364(9431):331–7.

108. Effects of platelet glycoprotein IIb/IIIa blockade with tirofiban on adverse cardiac events in patients with unstable angina or acute myocardial infarction undergoing coronary angioplasty. The RESTORE Investigators. Randomized Efficacy Study of Tirofiban for Outcomes and Restenosis. Circulation. 1997;96(5):1445–53.

109. Platelet Receptor Inhibition in Ischemic Syndrome Management (PRISM) Study Investigators. A comparison of aspirin plus tirofiban with aspirin plus heparin for unstable angina. N Engl J Med. 1998;338(21):1498–505.

110. Lincoff AM, Califf RM, Anderson KM, et al. Evidence for prevention of death and myocardial infarction with platelet membrane glycoprotein IIb/IIIa receptor blockade by abciximab (c7E3 Fab) among patients with unstable angina undergoing percutaneous coronary revascularization. EPIC Investigators. Evaluation of 7E3 in preventing ischemic complications. J Am Coll Cardiol. 1997;30(1):149–56.

111. Boersma E, Harrington RA, Moliterno DJ, et al. Platelet glycoprotein IIb/IIIa inhibitors in acute coronary syndromes: a meta-analysis of all major randomised clinical trials. Lancet. 2002;359(9302):189–98.

112. Kastrati A, Mehilli J, Neumann FJ, et al. Abciximab in patients with acute coronary syndromes undergoing percutaneous coronary intervention after clopidogrel pretreatment: the ISAR-REACT 2 randomized trial. JAMA. 2006;295(13):1531–8.

113. Hamm CW, Heeschen C, Goldmann B, et al. c7E3 Fab Antiplatelet Therapy in Unstable Refractory Angina (CAPTURE) Study Investigators. Benefit of abciximab in patients with refractory unstable angina in relation to serum troponin T levels. N Engl J Med. 1999;340(21):1623–9.

114. Heeschen C, Hamm CW, Goldmann B, PRISM Study Investigators. Troponin concentrations for stratification of patients with acute coronary syndromes in relation to therapeutic efficacy of tirofiban. Lancet. 1999;354(9192):1757–62.

115. Théroux P, Alexander Jr J, Pharand C, et al. Glycoprotein IIb/IIIa receptor blockade improves outcomes in diabetic patients presenting with unstable angina/non-ST-elevation myocardial infarction: results from the platelet receptor inhibition in ischemic syndrome management in patients limited by unstable signs and symptoms (PRISM-PLUS) study. Circulation. 2000;102(20): 2466–72.

116. Klootwijk P, Meij S, Melkert R, et al. Reduction of recurrent ischemia with abciximab during continuous ECG-ischemia monitoring in patients with unstable angina refractory to standard treatment (CAPTURE). Circulation. 1998;98(14):1358–64.

117. Morrow DA, Antman EM, Snapinn SM, et al. An integrated clinical approach to predicting the benefit of tirofiban in non-ST elevation acute coronary syndromes: application of the TIMI risk score for UA/NSTEMI in PRISM-PLUS. Eur Heart J. 2002;23(3): 223–9.

118. Giugliano RP, White JA, Bode C, et al. Early versus delayed, provisional eptifibatide in acute coronary syndromes. N Engl J Med. 2009;360:2176–90.

119. Stone GW, Bertrand ME, Moses JW, et al. Routine upstream initiation vs deferred selective use of glycoprotein IIb/IIIa inhibitors in acute coronary syndromes: the ACUITY timing trial. JAMA. 2007;297:591–602.

120. Mehta SR, Cannon CP, Fox KA, et al. Routine vs selective invasive strategies in patients with acute coronary syndromes: a collaborative meta-analysis of randomized trials. JAMA. 2005; 293(23):2908–17.

121. Bavry AA, Kumbhani DJ, Rassi AN, et al. Benefit of early invasive therapy in acute coronary syndromes: a meta-analysis of contemporary randomized clinical trials. J Am Coll Cardiol. 2006; 48(7):1319–25.

122. Hoenig MR, Doust JA, Aroney CN, Scott IA. Early invasive versus conservative strategies for unstable angina & non-ST- elevation myocardial infarction in the stent era. Cochrane Database Syst Rev. 2006;3, CD004815.

123. Fibrinolytic Therapy Trialists' (FTT) Collaborative Group. Indications for fibrinolytic therapy in suspected acute myocardial infarction: collaborative overview of early mortality and major morbidity results from all randomised trials of more than 1000 patients. Lancet. 1994;343(8893):311–22.
124. Chesebro JH, Knatterud G, Roberts R, et al. Thrombolysis in myocardial infarction (TIMI) trial, phase I: a comparison between intravenous tissue plasminogen activator and intravenous streptokinase: clinical findings through hospital discharge. Circulation. 1987;76(1):142–54.
125. Investigators GUSTO. An international randomized trial comparing four thrombolytic strategies for acute myocardial infarction. N Engl J Med. 1993;329(10):673–82.
126. Assessment of the Safety and Efficacy of a New Thrombolytic (ASSENT-2) Investigators. Single-bolus tenecteplase compared with front-loaded alteplase in acute myocardial infarction: the ASSENT-2 double-blind randomised trial. Lancet. 1999; 354(9180):716–22.
127. Keeley EC, Boura JA, Grines CL. Primary angioplasty versus intra- venous thrombolytic therapy for acute myocardial infarction: a quantitative review of 23 randomised trials. Lancet. 2003; 361(9351):13–20.
128. Cannon CP, Gibson CM, Lambrew CT, et al. Relationship of symptom-onset-to-balloon time and door-to-balloon time with mortality in patients undergoing angioplasty for acute myocardial infarction. JAMA. 2000;283(22):2941–7.
129. ASSENT-4 PCI investigators. Primary versus tenecteplase-facilitated percutaneous coronary intervention in patients with ST-segment elevation acute myocardial infarction (ASSENT-4 PCI): randomised trial. Lancet. 2006;367(9510):569–758.
130. Ellis SG, Armstrong P, Betriu A, et al. Facilitated percutaneous coronary intervention versus primary percutaneous coronary intervention: design and rationale of the facilitated intervention with enhanced reperfusion speed to stop events (FINESSE) trial. Am Heart J. 2004;147(4):E16.
131. Wijeysundera HC, Vijayaraghavan R, Nallamothu BK, et al. Rescue angioplasty or repeat fibrinolysis after failed fibrinolytic therapy for ST-segment myocardial infarction: a meta-analysis of randomized trials. J Am Coll Cardiol. 2007;49:422–30.
132. Di Mario C, Dudek D, Piscione F, et al. Immediate angioplasty versus standard therapy with rescue angioplasty after thrombolysis in the combined abciximab reteplase stent study in acute myocardial infarction (CARESS-in-AMI): an open, prospective, randomised, multicentre trial. Lancet. 2008;371:559–68.
133. Cantor WJ, Fitchett D, Borgundvaag B, et al. Routine early angioplasty after fibrinolysis for acute myocardial infarction. N Engl J Med. 2009;360:2705–18.
134. Cabello JB, Burls A, Emparanza JI, et al. Oxygen therapy for acute myocardial infarction. Cochrane Database Syst Rev. 2010; (6):CD007160.
135. Moradkhan R, Sinoway LI. Revisiting the role of oxygen therapy in cardiac patients. J Am Coll Cardiol. 2010;56(13):1013–6.
136. Chen ZM, Pan HC, Chen YP, et al. Early intravenous then oral metoprolol in 45,852 patients with acute myocardial infarction: randomised placebo-controlled trial. Lancet. 2005;366(9497): 1622–32.
137. Schwartz GG, Olsson AG, Ezekowitz MD, et al. Effects of atorvastatin on early recurrent ischemic events in acute coronary syndromes: the MIRACL study: a randomized controlled trial. JAMA. 2001;285(13):1711–8.
138. Cannon CP, Braunwald E, McCabe CH, et al. Pravastatin or atorvastatin evaluation and infection therapy-thrombolysis in myocardial infarction 22 investigators. N Engl J Med. 2004;350(15): 1495–504.

Acute Decompensated Heart Failure: Systolic and Diastolic

Adriana Quiñones, Alex Reyentovich, and Stuart D. Katz

Abstract

Heart failure is a chronic disease characterized in part by intermittent exacerbations of worsening symptoms that increase in frequency with disease progression. Despite a trend towards reduced heart failure hospitalization over the last decade, heart failure remains the most common cause of hospitalization in the Medicare population. Hospitalization for worsening symptoms is a sentinel event that identifies heart failure patients at high risk for subsequent morbidity and mortality. Initial assessment should include confirmation of the diagnosis (recognizing that patient may present with atypical signs and symptoms), measurement of left ventricular function with appropriate imaging procedures, identification of precipitating factors, clinical assessment of the hemodynamic status based on physical findings of congestion and tissue perfusion, and formulation of an individualized treatment plan. Decongestion therapy with intravenous loop diuretics is the most common therapeutic intervention with similar treatment approaches in patients with preserved or reduced ejection fraction. The cardiology consultant should also assess prognosis based on clinical findings and biomarkers and make recommendations for palliative care options in patients with poor prognosis who are not eligible for advanced therapies such as left ventricular assist device or cardiac transplantation. The cardiology consultant should also arrange appropriate transition of care at discharge with plans for post-discharge optimization of medical and device therapy and for high-risk patients, referral to a heart failure disease management program.

Keywords

Heart failure • Ventricular function • Diuretics • Positive inotropic agents • Vasodilator agents • Disease management

A. Quiñones, MD
Leon H. Charney Division of Cardiology,
New York University Langone Medical Center,
530 First Avenue HCC 4F,
New York 10016, NY, USA
e-mail: adriana.quinones@nyumc.org

A. Reyentovich, MD • S.D. Katz, MD, MS (✉)
Leon H. Charney Division of Cardiology,
New York University Langone Medical Center,
530 First Avenue Skirball 9R,
New York 10016, NY, USA
e-mail: alex.reyentovich@nyumc.org;
stuart.katz@nyumc.org

Epidemiology

Heart failure is a chronic and progressive disease with an estimated prevalence in the United States (US) of 5,700,000 [1]. It is estimated that by 2030, an additional three million people will suffer from heart failure [2]. The incidence of heart failure increases with age and is approximately 10 per 1,000 people over the age of 65. At age 40, the lifetime risk of developing heart failure is 1 in 5 [3]. Heart failure was the underlying cause of death in 56,830 deaths in 2008. Heart failure also accounts for a significant number of hospital admissions. Based on National Institutes of Health (NIH) data, in 2009, there were approximately one million hospital discharges for heart failure [1]. Despite the population-based data indicating increasing prevalence of heart failure in the United States, Medicare data from 1998 to 2008 has shown a 29.5 % decline in risk-adjusted heart failure hospitalizations. There has also been a decline in risk-adjusted 1-year mortality during this decade [4]. It is thought that greater use of guideline-recommended therapies may be contributing to these trends, but changes in administrative coding over time and other unmeasured factors may be confounding interpretation of these data.

Hospitalization for heart failure is a sentinel event that identifies patients at high risk for subsequent morbidity and mortality. However, it is important to recognize that heart failure is a chronic condition characterized by progression of disease and discrete episodes of decompensation. Accordingly, there is increasing focus on understanding the impact of acute care during a hospitalization on the subsequent clinical course of disease.

Pathophysiology

Heart failure occurs when the heart is unable to pump sufficient oxygenated blood to meet the metabolic needs of the body tissues. Most heart failure encountered in clinical practice is attributable to diminished pump reserve due to myocardial injury or overload. Myocardial injury or overload reduces effective arterial volume and triggers a complex process of systemic neurohormonal and local autocrine and paracrine signals that mediate pathological changes in cardiac structure and function, known as left ventricular remodeling. Left ventricular remodeling is characterized by progressive myocyte hypertrophy associated with changes in contractile protein gene expression, intracellular calcium regulation, and interstitial fibrosis. The progression of left ventricular remodeling is associated with increased symptoms and increased risk of mortality and, thus, has been identified as an important therapeutic target.

Renal hypoperfusion due to cardiac pump dysfunction contributes to activation of the renin-angiotensin-aldosterone system with consequent sodium and water retention. Increased intravascular volume in excess of the capacitance of the systemic venous system results in elevation of cardiac filling pressures with associated symptoms of pulmonary congestion. Accordingly, enhancement of renal perfusion and reduction in sodium and water overload are useful therapeutic strategies in patients with symptomatic congestion.

Acute heart failure usually occurs in the setting of chronic heart failure and, in many cases, can be identified as a subacute event. In most cases, excess sodium and water retention either due to excess sodium intake, inadequate sodium excretion, or both, is an important contributing factor to heart failure exacerbation. Other common contributing factors include cardiovascular stressors (hypertension, ischemia, and/or arrhythmia), metabolic stressors (infection, anemia, thyroid disease), comorbid conditions such as chronic kidney disease and lung disease, and drugs with negative inotropic (calcium channel blockers) or sodium-retaining effects (nonsteroidal anti-inflammatory agents). Less common entities associated with ventricular dysfunction and heart failure such as myocarditis and Takotsubo cardiomyopathy should also be considered in the differential diagnosis.

Diagnosis

Severity of symptoms in the acute setting is related to the degree of volume overload and concomitant increase in ventricular filling pressures. Most of the symptoms of congestion are nonspecific, so other causes of sodium and water retention including kidney disease and hypoxic lung disease must also be considered. Symptoms of orthopnea and paroxysmal nocturnal dyspnea (PND) are more specific for heart failure. Many patients with decompensated heart failure also present with atypical symptoms of abdominal pain and anorexia, likely related to underlying splanchnic congestion. The recorded medical history should also include a summary of the etiology of ventricular dysfunction, severity of preadmission chronic heart failure symptoms, and concomitant conditions contributing to the acute or subacute worsening of symptoms.

Physical examination documentation should include direct measurement of blood pressure and pulse for accurate detection of signs of low cardiac output (low pulse pressure and pulsus alternans). Respirations should be observed long enough to determine if a cyclical pattern consistent with Cheyne-Stokes respirations is present. Signs of cardiac cachexia are associated with poor prognosis and should be recorded if present. Volume status should be carefully assessed with evaluation of filling pressures by assessment of jugular venous pressure (JVP), abdominojugular reflux, presence of an S3 or S4 gallop, pulmonary rales, and peripheral edema. The location and nature of the point of maximal impulse and intensity of the first and second heart sounds should be routinely recorded.

Electrocardiogram (ECG) should be performed, as it may be helpful in identifying coronary artery disease or arrhythmia as the precipitant for the exacerbation. Chest x-ray can confirm the presence of pulmonary vascular congestion and/or pulmonary edema. It is important to note that the typical signs of congestion on physical examination and chest radiography are absent approximately 50 % of the time in patients with chronic heart failure with documented severe elevation of pulmonary capillary wedge pressure [5, 6]. Increased JVP is the most sensitive and specific predictor of increased pulmonary capillary wedge pressure. Accordingly it is important to accurately assess JVP at the bedside and maintain a high level of suspicion for a cardiac cause of dyspnea, even in patients with a paucity of typical signs of lung congestion.

Basic laboratory evaluation should routinely include assessment of serum electrolytes, renal and hepatic function, hemoglobin and white blood cell count, and thyroid function tests. Measurement of brain natriuretic peptide (BNP or NT-pro-BNP assay) can be a useful diagnostic aid when evaluating a patient with dyspnea, as low levels have strong negative predictive value for excluding a cardiac cause of dyspnea (except in patients with severe obesity) [7].

Heart failure with preserved vs. reduced ejection fraction cannot be reliably discerned based on history, physical examination, laboratory, and radiographic tests. An assessment of left ventricular function should be obtained in all patients with worsening heart failure to quantitate left ventricular function. If a patient has a recent study (within 6 months) and there is no suspicion for an interim myocardial injury since the prior study, it is reasonable to proceed with clinical decision making based on the most recent assessment. Echocardiography is most often used for assessment of left ventricular function based on its ability to provide real-time noninvasive assessment of ventricular and valve function without ionizing radiation. Other modalities of left ventricular function measurement, such as ventriculogram, radionuclide imaging, and magnetic resonance imaging, may also be useful in selected patients.

Risk Assessment

Patients at high risk for adverse outcomes can be readily identified from information routinely obtained from the physical examination and admission laboratory data. Based on observational data obtained from the Acute Decompensated Heart Failure National Registry (ADHERE) of patients hospitalized with heart failure, a blood urea nitrogen (BUN) value ≥43 mg/dl was the single best discriminator of in-hospital survival. Systolic blood pressure <115 mmHg was the next best predictor of in-hospital mortality, regardless of BUN levels. In those with elevated BUN and systolic blood pressure <115 mmHg, a serum creatinine level ≥2.75 mg/dl provided additional prognostic value. The overall in-hospital mortality in the cohort with none of these risk factors was 2.1 % but increased to 21.9 % when all three prognostic markers were present [8].

Serum BNP levels are associated with in-hospital mortality in both patients with normal and impaired systolic function. BNP remained a significant predictor of in-hospital mortality even after adjustment for other risk factors such as age, systolic blood pressure, BUN, creatinine, sodium, pulse, and dyspnea at rest [9].

A meta-analysis of 22 studies evaluating the relationship of hyponatremia and mortality in heart failure indicates that hyponatremia is a powerful predictor of mortality in patients with heart failure with systolic dysfunction as well as preserved ejection fraction. It is uncertain if correction of hyponatremia translates into improved outcomes [10]. However, a retrospective study of patients hospitalized with heart failure and hyponatremia, with mean follow-up of 20 months, reported a significant improvement in survival in patients whose serum sodium increased after discharge, suggesting that hyponatremia is a modifiable risk factor. Overall mortality in this report was 69.6 %, highlighting the fact that hyponatremic patients hospitalized for heart failure comprise a very high-risk group [11].

Elevated levels of cardiac troponin T have also been found to be associated with an increased risk of in-hospital mortality in heart failure patients. The mechanism of troponin elevation in the setting of heart failure is not fully characterized. Several mechanisms have been proposed, including subendocardial ischemia, myocyte damage from inflammatory cytokines or oxidative stress, hibernating myocardium, myocardial stretch, and/or other mechanisms leading to apoptosis [12].

Several other biomarkers, including galectin-3, ST2, adrenomedullin, and copeptin, are elevated in patients with heart failure and have been shown to have prognostic implications, although the clinical utility of these new markers has not yet been determined [13–16].

Management

Volume Management

Symptoms associated with volume overload are the most common cause for heart failure hospitalization. Adequate decongestion is essential for improvement in heart failure symptoms and may be associated with a reduced risk of recurrent hospitalization.

Diuretics

Intravenous administration of loop diuretics is the mainstay treatment for decongestion in patients hospitalized with decompensated heart failure. Several small studies have evaluated the efficacy of continuous infusion of loop diuretics vs. multiple bolus doses. Meta-analysis of these data does not demonstrate compelling evidence for superiority of either treatment strategy [17]. In the Diuretic Optimization Strategies Evaluation (DOSE) trial, the largest prospective randomized trial comparing strategies of multiple bolus doses of loop diuretics vs. continuous infusion, there was no difference in patient-reported symptoms, net fluid loss, renal function, or post-discharge outcomes in patients treated with bolus vs. continuous

Table 3.1 Recommended dose range for diuretic agents for patients hospitalized with heart failure

Drug	Initial dose	Dose range	Half life	Class
Furosemide PO	20–80 mg	20–480 mg/day divided daily to BID	2 h	Loop diuretic
Furosemide IV bolus	20–40 mg	20–480 mg/day daily or BID	2 h	Loop diuretic
Furosemide IV drip	0.1 mg/kg bolus, followed by 0.1 mg/kg/h	0.1–0.4 mg/kg/h	2 h	Loop diuretic
Bumetanide PO	0.5–2 mg	0.5–10 mg/day divided daily to BID	1–1.5 h	Loop diuretic
Bumetanide IV	05–1 mg	0.5–10 mg/day divided daily to BID	1–1.5 h	Loop diuretic
Torsemide IV or PO	10–20 mg	10–200 mg/day	3.5 h	Loop diuretic
Metolazone	5 mg	5–20 mg/day	14 h	Thiazide diuretic
Chlorothiazide IV or PO	500–1,000 mg	500–1,000 mg daily to BID	45–120 min	Thiazide diuretic
Spironolactone	25 mg	25–50 mg/day	1.4[a]	Aldosterone antagonist
Eplerenone	25 mg	25–50 mg/day	4–6 h	Aldosterone antagonist

mg milligram, *kg* kilogram, *IV* intravenous, *PO* oral, *BID* twice a day
[a]Spironolactone has active metabolites with longer half-life 14–17 h

infusion treatment strategies [18]. Since continuous infusions require a volumetric pump attached to a support pole, this approach should be used with caution in elderly patients at greater risk for falls. Moreover, higher-dose diuretics were associated with greater weight loss, greater risk of worsening renal function, but no difference in post-discharge outcomes. These findings support the safety of higher-dose loop diuretics as a tool to achieve rapid decongestion therapy. Therapeutic dose ranges of available loop diuretics are provided in Table 3.1.

The therapeutic response to loop diuretics in heart failure is limited by the high rates of sodium resorption in proximal and distal portions of the nephron [19]. Thiazide diuretics (and related compounds such as metolazone) can be used in combination with loop diuretics to overcome this mechanism of diuretic resistance. Combination therapy should be prescribed with caution and close monitoring of hemodynamics and electrolytes, as the synergistic effects of the two classes of diuretics can result in a very large increase in urine volume with associated risk for hypokalemia, hypomagnesemia, hyponatremia, and hypotension.

Worsening renal function occurs commonly in patients hospitalized with heart failure undergoing decongestion therapy. The pathophysiology of this phenomenon likely involves a complex interplay of the hemodynamic effects of decongestion therapy on renal blood flow and glomerular filtration rate, intrarenal pharmacologic effects of loop diuretics, inflammatory mediators that may impact both cardiac and renal function, and other intrinsic renal factors associated with comorbid kidney disease. These complex factors may impact glomerular and/or renal tubular function. While many studies have demonstrated that worsening renal function during hospitalization for heart failure, defined as an increase in creatinine >0.3 mg/dl, is associated with increased risk of in-hospital and post-discharge adverse outcomes [20], other studies have demonstrated that effective decongestion therapy, assessed by evidence of hemoconcentration during

hospitalization, is associated with improved post-discharge outcomes regardless of the presence of worsening renal function [21, 22]. Accordingly, the current evidence suggests that diuretic therapy in hospitalized heart failure patients with volume overload should be individualized to optimize decongestion as the primary treatment endpoint. While monitoring for worsening renal function as marker of worse prognosis, but not as a primary guide to diuretic dosing.

Ultrafiltration

Ultrafiltration is the mechanical removal of isotonic filtrate from the intravascular space by application of hydrostatic pressure to blood across a semipermeable membrane in an extracorporeal circuit. Ultrafiltration can be performed with standard continuous venovenous hemofiltration (CVVH) devices or related devices developed specifically for the heart failure population. The heart failure device has lower flow rates and lower extracorporeal blood volume when compared with standard equipment so that it may be better tolerated in patients with low cardiac output. Potential benefits of ultrafiltration when compared with diuretic therapy include greater sodium removal per liter of fluid with ultrafiltration (as the ultrafiltrate is isotonic with greater sodium concentration than urine) and less potassium loss per liter of fluid removal. Potential risks include the need for placement of an indwelling catheter for the duration of treatment and risk of bleeding with full-dose heparinization required for treatment. In a small prospective randomized trial comparing ultrafiltration to standard diuretic therapy in patients hospitalized with heart failure, ultrafiltration was associated with greater weight reduction when compared with standard care but similar improvement in dyspnea score and similar risk of worsening renal function [23]. In contrast, another small, randomized study demonstrated equal amounts of weight loss between groups assigned to diuretic therapy vs. ultrafiltration, with a greater increase in serum creatinine present in the ultrafiltration group [24]. These studies had substantial

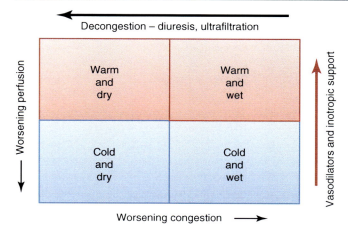

Fig. 3.1 Hemodynamic subsets of patients hospitalized with worsening heart failure based on clinical assessment of volume status and tissue perfusion can be used to guide initial therapeutic approach (Adapted from Thomas and Nohria [26])

differences in the protocols used for both treatment modalities, so the optimal target population and treatment regimen for ultrafiltration remains uncertain. Ultrafiltration can be considered in patients resistant to high-dose diuretic therapy or as primary decongestion treatment in patients with massive volume overload. Ultrafiltration can also be considered in collaboration with a nephrologist in patients with comorbid kidney disease.

Vasopressin Antagonists

Tolvaptan, a selective V_2-vasopressin receptor antagonist, has been studied in patients admitted with worsening heart failure and evidence of volume overload. It has been useful in accelerating fluid removal and providing short-term improvement in symptoms without significant harm; however, long-term outcomes were not different than placebo [25]. This agent is not routinely recommended in clinical practice for decongestion therapy but can be safely used in the subset of hypervolemic heart failure patients with severe hyponatremia (serum sodium <125 meq/l).

Hemodynamic Management

Assessing Hemodynamics

Bedside evaluation can provide important information about the degree and cause of decompensation. Based on the assessment of volume status and peripheral perfusion, four hemodynamic profiles have been previously described (Fig. 3.1). The overwhelming majority of patients admitted with worsening heart failure are categorized as warm and wet [26]. Therapy is primarily directed at decongestion therapy in this subset as described above. Patients with evidence of tissue hypoperfusion represent a group at higher risk of

in-hospital and post-discharge mortality and require a more complex therapeutic strategy with multiple drugs and/or devices.

The Evaluation Study of Congestive Heart Failure and Pulmonary Artery Catheterization Effectiveness (ESCAPE) trial prospectively investigated the impact of hemodynamic monitoring with pulmonary artery catheters in patients with impaired LV systolic function who had been hospitalized for heart failure within the preceding year, had an urgent visit to the emergency room, or had been treated with high doses of loop diuretics after hospital admission for heart failure with evidence of volume overload. Although pulmonary artery catheter placement in experienced centers was overall considered safe, the addition of pulmonary artery catheter for hemodynamic monitoring had no effect on survival. Based on these data, routine pulmonary artery catheter placement is not routinely recommended during heart failure hospitalization. Hemodynamic monitoring with pulmonary artery catheter may be considered in patients with evidence of severe tissue hypoperfusion (impending shock) and patients who fail to respond to initial therapy determined by clinical assessment as described below [27].

Positive Inotropic Agents

Dobutamine was approved for treatment of acute heart failure characterized by low cardiac output and elevated filling pressures in 1978. Dobutamine acts directly on beta-1 adrenergic receptors in the myocardium, producing positive inotropic and chronotropic effects [28]. Dobutamine has a balanced direct action in peripheral blood vessels, as it is both a beta-2 and alpha-1 agonist. Early clinical trials with dobutamine clearly demonstrate improvement in resting hemodynamics, but the effects of short-term dobutamine on outcomes have never been assessed in a prospective trial.

Milrinone is a specific type 3 phosphodiesterase inhibitor (PDE) with potent positive inotropic and vasodilating effects. There are several important pharmacological differences between milrinone and dobutamine. Since milrinone acts intracellularly on the type 3 PDE isozyme, this agent maintains its myocardial effects in patients treated with beta-adrenergic blockers. Due to its direct vasodilating effects in vascular smooth muscle, milrinone does not increase myocardial oxygen consumption to the same extent as dobutamine. The direct vasodilating action of milrinone may also enhance its therapeutic profile in patients with severe mitral regurgitation and/or marked secondary pulmonary hypertension. The serum half-life of milrinone (2 h) is substantially longer than dobutamine (6 min) and thus requires a loading dose if rapid onset of hemodynamic support is required. The half-life of milrinone, but not dobutamine, is increased in patients with severe renal insufficiency (estimated GFR <30 ml/min), hence the chronic infusion dose must be adjusted in this population.

The Outcomes of Prospective Trial of Intravenous Milrinone for Exacerbations of Chronic Heart Failure (Optime-CHF) was the first large randomized trial addressing the use of intravenous milrinone in patients hospitalized with acute decompensated heart failure (ADHF) without evidence of low cardiac output or tissue hypoperfusion. There was no difference in length of hospitalization for cardiac causes; however, there were a significantly higher number of patients experiencing hypotension as well as atrial arrhythmias in the treatment arm. There was also a trend towards increased rates of mortality or rehospitalization in those with ischemic cardiomyopathy. Routine use of milrinone is not recommended in patients hospitalized with heart failure without signs of low cardiac output or tissue hypoperfusion [29].

Levosimendan is a calcium-sensitizing agent with complex pharmacological action including positive inotropy, positive chronotropy, and vasodilation. The Survival of Patients With Acute Heart Failure in Need of Intravenous Inotropic Support (SURVIVE) trial compared levosimendan, which increases inotropy by augmenting the affinity of troponin C to calcium, to dobutamine in patients with ADHF with EF $\leq$30 % who required inotropic support based on lack of response to intravenous diuretics with or without the use of vasodilators. There was no difference in all-cause mortality [30]. Levosimendan is currently marketed in Europe but not the United States.

Vasodilators

Nitroglycerin is an organic nitrate that reduces preload and afterload by activation of the soluble form of cyclic guanosine monophosphate (cGMP) in vascular smooth muscle. Its main effects at low doses are in the venous circulation, so higher doses are usually required for arterial afterload reduction in heart failure patients. In a subset of the Vasodilator in the Management of Acute Heart Failure(VMAC) study, nitroglycerin was noted to produce a significant decrease in pulmonary capillary wedge pressure (PCWP) when administered at doses >160 mcg/min [31]. Other studies indicate that doses as high as 600 mcg/min may be required in some patients. Nitroglycerin is generally well tolerated and, due to its very short half-life, can be quickly reversed if hypotension occurs. The clinical utility of nitroglycerin is limited by the development of tachyphylaxis to its hemodynamic effects within 24 h in many patients. Nitroprusside is another nitrosovasodilator that has proven short-term hemodynamic benefit in heart failure patients with high systemic vascular resistance. In contrast to nitroglycerin, tachyphylaxis has not been described with this agent, but risk of thiocyanate toxicity during longer-term infusion limits its clinical utility.

Nesiritide, a recombinant form of human BNP, is chemically indistinguishable from the native cardiac-derived peptide hormone and has venous and arterial vasodilatory properties mediated by membrane-bound receptors coupled to cGMP signaling pathways in vascular smooth muscle. It can reduce preload and afterload and causes an increase in cardiac output without direct inotropic effects in the heart. Nesiritide is cleared from the circulation by a combination of specific receptors and circulating enzymes resulting in a half-life of approximately 20 min. When compared to nitroglycerine and placebo in the VMAC study, nesiritide resulted in a reduction in PCWP, pulmonary vascular resistance (PVR), and right atrial pressure (RAP). It also induced a more significant improvement in cardiac index (CI) and reduction in systemic vascular resistance (SVR) when compared to placebo. Nesiritide was also associated with improvement in dyspnea [31]. In a large-scale clinical trial, Acute Study of Clinical Effectiveness of Nesiritide in Decompensated Heart Failure (ASCEND-HF), nesiritide was comparable to placebo with respect to clinical outcomes and was associated with an increased rate of hypotension. These findings suggest that nesiritide should not be routinely used in patients hospitalized with heart failure but can be considered in patients with an appropriate hemodynamic profile in closely monitored settings [32].

There are no prospective data comparing the initial strategy of a positive inotropic agent to a vasodilator agent in patients hospitalized with heart failure. To some extent, such a trial is not feasible, as the hemodynamic subset of ideal candidates for these approaches differs. Observational data from the Acute Decompensated Heart Failure National Registry (ADHERE) indicated that patients treated with vasodilating agents such as nitroglycerin or nesiritide had reduced hospital and intensive care unit lengths of stay, as well as lower in-hospital mortality than those who were treated with inotropic agents such as milrinone or dobutamine [33]. These differences persisted even after adjustment with a propensity score to account for the clinical characteristics that led to the decision to prescribe different classes of drugs. Although interpretation of these findings could be confounded by unmeasured variables, these data support a strategy of preferential use of vasodilator agents before positive inotropic agents in patients with a suitable hemodynamic profile. Dosing recommendations for commonly used positive inotropic and vasodilating agents are listed in Table 3.2.

Mechanical Circulatory Support

In the presence of tissue hypoperfusion and low cardiac output refractory to medical therapy, mechanical support with intra-aortic balloon pump or left ventricular assist device (LVAD) can be considered. The cardiology consultant should engage subspecialists in advanced heart failure and cardiac transplantation for discussion of available treatment options in patients with refractory disease.

Table 3.2 Recommended dose range for positive inotropic and vasodilation agents for patients hospitalized with heart failure

Drug	Initial dose	Dose range	Half life	Class
Dobutamine	2.5 mcg/kg/min	2.5–20 mcg/kg/min	2 min	Beta-agonist
Milrinone	50 mcg/kg IV bolus over 10 min 0.5 mcg/kg/min	0.375–0.75 mcg/kg/min[a]	2.3 h	cAMP PDE type III inhibitor
Nitroglycerin	10–20 mcg/min	10–600 mcg/min	1–3 min	Organic nitrate
Nitroprusside	0.1 mcg/kg/min	0.1–10 mcg/kg/min	2 min	Inorganic nitrosovasodilator
Nesiritide	2 mcg/kg IV bolus 0.01 mcg/kg/min	0.01–0.03 mcg/kg/min	18 min	NP receptor agonist

cAMP cyclic AMP, *NP* neuropeptide
[a]Lower dose range for patients with >stage 3 chronic kidney disease

Noninvasive Ventilation

Noninvasive ventilation, with continuous or bi-level positive airway pressure (CPAP or BiPAP), induces more rapid improvement in dyspnea and acid/base disturbances when compared to standard oxygen delivery in patients with acute cardiogenic pulmonary edema without effect on short-term mortality [34].

Adjustment of Chronic Medical Therapy During Hospitalization

Beta-blockers should be continued during admission for acutely decompensated heart failure unless clinical indications for dobutamine therapy or catecholamine pressors are present. The B-Convinced study was a randomized trial where patients with ejection fraction <40 % admitted with acutely decompensated heart failure who were chronically on beta-blockers were randomized to continuation or cessation of beta-blocker therapy. There was no difference in symptom resolution, BNP levels, length of hospital stay, rehospitalization, or death. Continuation of beta-blocker therapy at 3-month follow-up was higher in the group who continued beta-blocker therapy through the hospitalization [35].

For patients with a new diagnosis of systolic heart failure not previously treated with beta-blockers, therapy should be initiated after the patient is stabilized before hospital discharge. Patients who are started on beta-blockers prior to discharge are more likely to be treated with beta-blockers at 60 days post discharge. There is no significant increase in length of hospitalization or risk of side effects in those started on beta-blockers prior to discharge [36]. Discharge plans should include appropriate follow-up visits for dose up-titration as tolerated.

There are no prospective studies of strategies comparing continuation vs. discontinuation of angiotensin converting enzyme (ACE) inhibitors in patients hospitalized with heart failure. Randomized withdrawal trials in ambulatory outpatients indicate that the worsening heart failure symptoms do not occur until many weeks after withdrawal [37]. Observational data suggests that the risk of worsening renal function is independent of the use of ACE inhibitors [20]. Accordingly, it is reasonable to routinely continue ACE inhibitors during hospitalization for heart failure except in setting of symptomatic hypotension and/or oliguric renal failure.

Heart Failure with Preserved Ejection Fraction

Clinical features of ADHF in patients with normal ejection fraction are comparable to those with systolic dysfunction. The ADHERE database analyzed the subgroup of patients in this registry with preserved ejection fraction. In this cohort, patients with preserved EF were more commonly older women and had history of hypertension, coronary artery disease, or diabetes mellitus.

When compared to those with systolic dysfunction, several differences in clinical presentation were identified. On admission, patients with preserved ejection fraction are more likely to be hypertensive and to have atrial fibrillation and peripheral edema. There was no difference in dyspnea at rest and renal function.

Management during hospitalization frequently includes intravenous diuretics. The use of ACEi, angiotensin receptor blockers (ARB), beta-blockers, digoxin, and spironolactone at the time of discharge was lower than in those with systolic dysfunction.

In-hospital mortality is significantly lower for patients with preserved ejection fraction, when compared to those with systolic dysfunction [38].

A prospective registry of hospitalized with ADHF patients with preserved ejection fraction characterized this population as mostly elderly women with chronic NYHA class II or III symptoms prior to admission with a high prevalence of comorbid conditions including hypertension, diabetes, and obesity. In-hospital mortality was 4.2 % with older patients being at higher risk of death. Echocardiogram findings were notable for increased LV mass. Most patients were on chronic diuretics prior to admission. A low percentage of these patients were treated with beta-blockers, ACE inhibitors, or spironolactone. Therapeutic adjustments during the hospitalization included an increase in patients receiving diuretics, ACE inhibitors, aldosterone receptor antagonists, and beta-blockers [39].

Perioperative Management of Heart Failure

Noncardiac Surgery

A history of heart failure is known to be associated with increased risk of perioperative complications after noncardiac surgery [40]. Patients with heart failure who undergo noncardiac surgery have an increased risk of morbidity and mortality when compared to patients with coronary artery disease or the general population [41]. Among 174 patients with a history of heart failure undergoing intermediate and high-risk noncardiac surgery, 31 % had at least one adverse postoperative event including death (8.1 %), myocardial infarction (14.9 %), and heart failure exacerbation (25.3 %). Patients with preserved ejection fraction and mild to moderately reduced ejection fractions had comparable rates of adverse events. The presence of an ejection fraction <30 %, age >80 years, and diabetes mellitus were identified as independent predictors of adverse perioperative events in this population [42]. Rates of adverse events did not differ by type of anesthesia or type of surgery.

Volume status, ventricular function, and functional capacity should be carefully assessed in heart failure patients in the preoperative evaluation. In patients with evidence of volume overload, diuretic therapy should be optimized to eliminate signs and symptoms of congestion before surgery. In patients with systolic dysfunction, doses of neurohormonal antagonists should also be optimized before surgery. Routine exercise stress testing or invasive hemodynamic monitoring does not add prognostic information prior to surgical intervention [43].

Controversy remains in how to manage chronic heart failure therapies in the perioperative period. Patients treated with ACE inhibitors may be at greater risk for hypotension during induction and maintenance of general, spinal, or epidural anesthesia. Temporary withdrawal of ACE inhibitor therapy may reduce the risk of hypotension in the perioperative period [44]. However, perioperative administration of ACE inhibitors has been shown to have specific organ-protective benefits. Patients given enalapril prior to aortic-abdominal surgery had a smaller reduction in cardiac output and more favorable renal function on the first postoperative day [45]. Although there is conflicting evidence on the benefits of continuation of this therapy in the perioperative period, the general recommendation is to continue ACE inhibitor therapy perioperatively as the benefit of ACE inhibition in the setting of heart failure is well established and brief episodes of hypotension can be treated with vasoactive agents [44].

Doses of aldosterone receptor blockade used for heart failure are not felt to contribute to intraoperative hypotension; however, the risk of hyperkalemia is increased, especially when used in combination with ACE inhibitors or ARBs and in the setting of preexisting renal insufficiency, diabetes, or anemia. Intraoperative monitoring of serum potassium is suggested, especially when red blood cell transfusion is necessary [44].

Preoperative administration of beta-blocker therapy has been extensively studied in surgical patients who are at high risk for cardiovascular complications. There is conflicting evidence on the role of initiation of therapy prior to surgical intervention; however, it is generally suggested to continue such therapy on patients chronically maintained on beta-blockers. Beta-blockers are also indicated for the treatment of perioperative hypertension, ischemia, or tachyarrhythmias [46].

For patients with advanced heart failure symptoms or those with persistent signs of congestion, perioperative invasive hemodynamic monitoring to assist in volume and blood pressure management may be considered [43]. A retrospective observational study of patients undergoing major elective noncardiac surgery who had perioperative right heart catheterization found an increase in the rate of adverse events and a longer length of hospitalization in those undergoing right heart catheterization even after multivariate adjustment. Patients who underwent preoperative right heart catheterization were found to have an increased rate of postoperative cardiogenic pulmonary edema [47]. These findings may be attributable to the confounding effects of the patient characteristics that led to the clinical decision for hemodynamic monitoring. However, a prospective randomized trial of the use of pulmonary artery catheterization in high-risk patients undergoing urgent or elective major surgery found no benefit over standard of care when the primary outcome was all-cause mortality. A higher rate of pulmonary artery embolism was seen in the intervention group [48]. Accordingly, right heart catheters should be used only in selected patients in whom the hemodynamic information is thought to be important for patient management.

Noncardiac Surgery in Patients with Mechanical Circulatory Support

An increasing number of patients with chronic LVAD support are being referred for noncardiac surgery. LVAD therapy poses several risks for those undergoing noncardiac surgery. Risk of bleeding should be considered as continuous flow LVAD support requires systemic anticoagulation. Patients with destination therapy LVAD also tend to be older and have a higher prevalence of comorbidities. A retrospective study examining outcomes in patients with continuous flow LVAD undergoing noncardiac surgery has concluded that noncardiac surgery can safely be performed in this population. There were no deaths or LVAD-related morbidity events in this series. The LVAD speed may need to be adjusted in response to reduced preload during anesthesia induction, so the presence of support personnel familiar with the LVAD operations and the hemodynamic effects of the LVAD is essential. Transient reduction in perioperative anticoagulation goals may be considered to reduce the risk of perioperative bleeding [49].

Cardiac Surgery

Impaired systolic function is a significant risk factor for mortality during cardiac surgery. In the European System for Cardiac Operative Risk Evaluation (EUROSCORE), an LVEF <30 % is scored 3 points, placing the patient in a medium-risk category associated with 3 % mortality [50]. Controversy exists regarding management of chronic heart failure therapy in the perioperative period in the setting of cardiac surgery. Administration of ACE inhibitors prior to cardiopulmonary bypass resulted in lower levels of cardiac enzyme release when compared to clonidine, enoximone, or placebo [51]. Coronary bypass patients treated with ACE inhibitors in the perioperative period have also been found to have better-preserved renal function during cardiopulmonary bypass [52].

The role of surgical therapy for management of patients with impaired systolic function and coronary artery disease remains controversial. The Surgical Treatment for Ischemic Heart Failure (STICH) trial studied surgical outcomes in patients with coronary artery disease amenable to coronary artery bypass surgery (CABG) and left ventricular dysfunction amenable to surgical reconstruction by randomizing them to coronary artery bypass surgery alone or coronary artery bypass surgery with surgical ventricular reconstruction. Surgical ventricular reconstruction reduced end-systolic volume index by 19 %, while CABG alone reduced end-systolic volume index by 6 %. There was similar improvement in heart failure symptoms in both groups. There was no significant difference among the groups in the composite endpoint of death from any cause or hospitalization for cardiac causes [53]. A subset of this trial, assessing the role for viability assessment prior to CABG in patients with left ventricular dysfunction, randomized patients after assessment of viability using SPECT or dobutamine stress echo to CABG and medical therapy or medical therapy alone. There was no significant mortality difference identified between viability status as established by SPECT or dobutamine stress echo and treatment assignment. Presence of viability was associated with greater likelihood of survival; however, after multivariate adjustment, this difference was no longer present [54].

End of Life Care

Heart failure is a progressive disease with high mortality in patients hospitalized with worsening symptoms. Advance directive counseling should be offered to all heart failure patients. In the acute care setting, the cardiology consultant is often in the best position to assess prognosis and recommend consideration of palliative care approaches in patients with less than 6 months expected survival. The cardiology consultant also has a more extensive knowledge base and thus can provide the best information on treatment options and risks of adverse outcomes to the patient and patient's family. Many of the chronic neurohormonal antagonists recommended for patients with less severe disease are poorly tolerated in patients with advanced disease and may be discontinued. Deactivation of the implantable cardiovert or defibrillator should also be considered in this population [55].

Transition of Care

Heart failure is a chronic condition that requires coordinated care after hospital discharge. The cardiology consultant should arrange for appropriate post-discharge cardiology care in accordance with the patient's needs. For high-risk patients, referral to a specialized heart failure disease management program should be considered [56].

Key Points
- Heart failure is a progressive chronic disease characterized by long periods of relative stability punctuated by episodes of decompensation.
- Heart failure is the most common cause for hospitalization in the Medicare population.
- Symptoms of volume overload are the most common presenting complaints in acute care settings.
- Effective decongestion therapy is essential for improvement of symptoms.
- Invasive hemodynamic monitoring and inotropic support are not recommended in patients who are responding to noninvasive strategies.
- Initiation of beta-blockers prior to discharge is associated with increased rates of adherence and improved post-discharge outcomes.
- Heart failure with preserved ejection fraction accounts for approximately half of all heart failure presentations. Evidence-based treatment strategies are lacking; optimization of volume status and control of hypertension and other comorbid conditions are recommended.
- Presentation and management during episodes of acute decompensation in patients with preserved ejection fraction are similar to those with systolic dysfunction and should focus on effective decongestion therapy.

- Heart failure patients are considered high-risk candidates for noncardiac surgery. Careful assessment of volume and hemodynamic status in the perioperative period is recommended. Routine invasive hemodynamic monitoring is not recommended. Continuation of chronic heart failure therapies during the perioperative period is recommended.
- Viability assessment prior to surgical revascularization has not been shown to translate into mortality benefit.
- Surgical ventricular reconstructive surgery has not been shown to result in improved mortality.

Summary of the Key Guidelines from Professional Societies

Diagnosis

Primarily based on signs and symptoms derived from a thorough history and physical examination. Clinicians should determine adequacy of systemic perfusion, volume status, contribution of precipitating factors and/or comorbidities, if heart failure is new onset or exacerbation of existing disease, and whether it is associated with preserved ejection fraction. Chest radiographs, electrocardiogram, and echocardiogram are key tests in this assessment. Class 1, level of evidence (LOE) C

Concentrations of B-type natriuretic peptide (BNP) or N-terminal pro-B-type natriuretic peptide (NT-pro-BNP) should be measured in patients with dyspnea in whom the contribution from heart failure is not known. These results should be evaluated in the context of all available clinical data. Class 1 LOE A

Identification of Etiology for Deterioration of Clinical Status

Acute coronary syndrome precipitating heart failure hospitalization should be promptly identified by ECG and troponin testing, and treated, as appropriate to the overall condition and prognosis of the patient. Class 1 LOE C

When patients present with ADHF and known or suspected acute myocardial ischemia due to occlusive coronary disease, especially when there are signs and symptoms of inadequate systemic perfusion, urgent cardiac catheterization and revascularization is reasonable where it is likely to prolong meaningful survival. Class IIa LOE C

Common potential precipitating factors for ADHF, such as coronary ischemia, severe hypertension, atrial and ventricular arrhythmias, infections, pulmonary emboli, renal

failure and medical or dietary non compliance should be identified as their recognition is critical to guide therapy. Class 1 LOE C

Management

Hemodynamics

Patients who present with rapid decompensation and hypoperfusion associated with decreasing urine output and other manifestations of shock are critically ill, and rapid intervention should be used to improve systemic perfusion. Class 1 LOE C

In patients with clinical evidence of hypotension associated with hypoperfusion and obvious evidence of elevated cardiac filling pressures (e.g., elevated jugular venous pressure, elevated pulmonary artery wedge pressure), intravenous inotropic or vasopressor drugs should be administered to maintain systemic perfusion and preserve end-organ performance while more definitive therapy is considered. Class 1 LOE C

Invasive hemodynamic monitoring should be performed to guide therapy in patients who are in respiratory distress or with clinical evidence of impaired perfusion in whom the adequacy or excess of intracardiac filling pressures cannot be determined from clinical assessment. Class 1 LOE C

In patients with reduced ejection fraction experiencing a symptomatic exacerbation of heart failure requiring hospitalization during chronic maintenance treatment with oral therapies known to improve outcomes, particularly ACE inhibitors or ARBs and beta-blocker therapy, it is recommended that these therapies be continued in most patients in the absence of hemodynamic instability or contraindications. Class 1 LOE C

In patients hospitalized with ADHF with reduced ejection fraction not treated with oral therapies known to improve outcomes, particularly ACE inhibitors or ARBs and beta-blocker therapy, initiation of these therapies is recommended in stable patients prior to hospital discharge. Class 1 LOE B

Initiation of beta-blocker therapy is recommended after optimization of volume status and successful discontinuation of intravenous diuretics, vasodilators, and inotropic agents. Beta-blocker therapy should be initiated at a low dose and only in stable patients. Particular caution should be used when initiating beta-blockers in patients who have required inotropes during their hospital course. Class 1 LOE B

In patients with evidence of severely symptomatic fluid overload in the absence of systemic hypotension, vasodilators such as intravenous nitroglycerin, nitroprusside, or nesiritide can be beneficial when added to diuretics and/or in those who do not respond to diuretics alone. Class IIa LOE C

Invasive hemodynamic monitoring can be useful for carefully selected patients with ADHF who have persistent symptoms despite empiric adjustment of standard therapies; whose fluid status, perfusion, or systemic or pulmonary vascular resistances are uncertain; whose systolic pressure remains low, or is associated with symptoms, despite initial therapy; whose renal function is worsening with therapy; who require parenteral vasoactive agents; or who may need consideration for advanced device therapy or transplantation. Class II a LOE C

Intravenous inotropic drugs such as dopamine, dobutamine, or milrinone might be reasonable for patients presenting with documented severe systolic dysfunction, low blood pressure, and evidence of low cardiac output, with or without congestion, to maintain systemic perfusion and preserve end-organ performance. Class IIb LOE C

Use of parenteral inotropes in normotensive patients with ADHF without evidence of decreased organ perfusion is not recommended. Class III LOE B

Routine use of invasive hemodynamic monitoring in normotensive patients with ADHF and congestion with symptomatic response to diuretics and vasodilators is not recommended. Class III LOE B

Volume Overload

Patients admitted with ADHF and with evidence of significant fluid overload should be treated with intravenous loop diuretics. Therapy should begin in the emergency department or outpatient clinic without delay, as early intervention may be associated with better outcomes for patients hospitalized with ADHF. Class 1, LOE B

If patients are already receiving loop diuretic therapy, the initial intravenous dose should equal or exceed their chronic oral daily dose. Urine output and signs and symptoms of congestion should be serially assessed, and diuretic dose should be titrated to relieve symptoms and to reduce extracellular fluid volume excess. Class 1 LOE C

Effect of ADHF treatment should be monitored with careful measurement of fluid intake and output; vital signs; body weight, determined at the same time each day; clinical signs (supine and standing); and symptoms of systemic perfusion and congestion. Daily serum electrolytes, urea nitrogen, and creatinine concentrations should be measured during the use of intravenous diuretics or active titration of HF medications. Class 1 LOE C

When diuresis is inadequate to relieve congestion, as evidenced by clinical evaluation, the diuretic regimen should be intensified using either higher doses of loop diuretics, addition of a second diuretic (such as metolazone, spironolactone, or intravenous chlorothiazide), or continuous infusion of a loop diuretic. Class 1 LOE C

In all patients hospitalized with ADHF, both with preserved and low EF, transition should be made from intravenous to oral diuretic therapy with careful attention to oral diuretic dosing and monitoring of electrolytes. With all medication changes, the patient should be monitored for supine and upright hypotension, worsening renal function and HF signs/symptoms. Class 1 LOE C

Ultrafiltration is reasonable for patients with refractory congestion not responding to medical therapy. Class IIa LOE B

Discharge and Transition of Care

Medications should be reconciled in every patient and adjusted as appropriate on admission to and discharge from the hospital. Class 1 LOE C

Comprehensive written discharge instructions for all patients with a hospitalization for ADHF and their caregivers are strongly recommended, with special emphasis on the following six aspects of care: diet; discharge medications, with a special focus on adherence, persistence, and up-titration to recommended doses of ACE inhibitor/ARB and beta-blocker medication; activity level; follow-up appointments; daily weight monitoring; and what to do if symptoms worsen. Class 1 LOE C

Post-discharge systems of care, if available, should be used to facilitate the transition to effective outpatient care for patients hospitalized with ADHF. Class 1 LOE B

References

1. Roger VL, Go AS, Lloyd-Jones DM, et al. Heart disease and stroke statistics – 2012 update: a report from the American Heart Association. Circulation. 2012;125(1):e2–220.
2. Heidenreich PA, Trogdon JG, Khavjou OA, et al. Forecasting the future of cardiovascular disease in the United States: a policy statement from the American Heart Association. Circulation. 2011;123(8):933–44.
3. Lloyd-Jones DM, Larson MG, Leip EP, et al. Lifetime risk for developing congestive heart failure: the Framingham Heart Study. Circulation. 2002;106(24):3068–72.
4. Chen J, Normand SL, Wang Y, Krumholz HM. National and regional trends in heart failure hospitalization and mortality rates for Medicare beneficiaries, 1998-2008. JAMA. 2011;306(15):1669–78.
5. Butman SM, Ewy GA, Standen JR, Kern KB, Hahn E. Bedside cardiovascular examination in patients with severe chronic heart failure: importance of rest or inducible jugular venous distension. J Am Coll Cardiol. 1993;22(4):968–74.
6. Androne AS, Hryniewicz K, Hudaihed A, Mancini D, Lamanca J, Katz SD. Relation of unrecognized hypervolemia in chronic heart failure to clinical status, hemodynamics, and patient outcomes. Am J Cardiol. 2004;93(10):1254–9.
7. Onwuanyi A, Taylor M. Acute decompensated heart failure: pathophysiology and treatment. Am J Cardiol. 2007;99(6B):25D–30.
8. Fonarow GC, Adams Jr KF, Abraham WT, Yancy CW, Boscardin WJ. Risk stratification for in-hospital mortality in acutely decompensated heart failure: classification and regression tree analysis. JAMA. 2005;293(5):572–80.
9. Fonarow GC, Peacock WF, Phillips CO, Givertz MM, Lopatin M. Admission B-type natriuretic peptide levels and in-hospital mortality in acute decompensated heart failure. J Am Coll Cardiol. 2007;49(19):1943–50.
10. Rusinaru D, Tribouilloy C, Berry C, et al. Relationship of serum sodium concentration to mortality in a wide spectrum of heart failure patients with preserved and with reduced ejection fraction:

an individual patient data meta-analysis: Meta-Analysis Global Group in Chronic heart failure (MAGGIC). Eur J Heart Fail. 2012;14:1139–46.

11. Madan VD, Novak E, Rich MW. Impact of change in serum sodium concentration on mortality in patients hospitalized with heart failure and hyponatremia. Circ Heart Fail. 2011;4(5):637–43.

12. Kociol RD, Pang PS, Gheorghiade M, Fonarow GC, O'Connor CM, Felker GM. Troponin elevation in heart failure prevalence, mechanisms, and clinical implications. J Am Coll Cardiol. 2010; 56(14):1071–8.

13. Ueland T, Aukrust P, Broch K, et al. Galectin-3 in heart failure: high levels are associated with all-cause mortality. Int J Cardiol. 2011;150(3):361–4.

14. Manzano-Fernandez S, Januzzi JL, Pastor-Perez FJ, et al. Serial monitoring of soluble interleukin family member ST2 in patients with acutely decompensated heart failure. Cardiology. 2012;122(3): 158–66.

15. Maisel A, Xue Y, Shah K, et al. Increased 90-day mortality in patients with acute heart failure with elevated copeptin: secondary results from the Biomarkers in Acute Heart Failure (BACH) study. Circ Heart Fail. 2011;4(5):613–20.

16. Braunwald E. Biomarkers in heart failure. N Engl J Med. 2008; 358(20):2148–59.

17. Salvador DR, Rey NR, Ramos GC, Punzalan FE. Continuous infusion versus bolus injection of loop diuretics in congestive heart failure. Cochrane Database Syst Rev. 2005;(3):CD003178.

18. Felker GM, Lee KL, Bull DA, et al. Diuretic strategies in patients with acute decompensated heart failure. N Engl J Med. 2011; 364(9):797–805.

19. Brater DC. Diuretic therapy. N Engl J Med. 1998;339(6):387–95.

20. Damman K, Navis G, Voors AA, et al. Worsening renal function and prognosis in heart failure: systematic review and meta-analysis. J Card Fail. 2007;13(8):599–608.

21. Davila C, Reyentovich A, Katz SD. Clinical correlates of hemoconcentration during hospitalization for acute decompensated heart failure. J Card Fail. 2011;17(12):1018–22.

22. Testani JM, Chen J, McCauley BD, Kimmel SE, Shannon RP. Potential effects of aggressive decongestion during the treatment of decompensated heart failure on renal function and survival. Circulation. 2010;122(3):265–72.

23. Costanzo MR, Guglin ME, Saltzberg MT, et al. Ultrafiltration versus intravenous diuretics for patients hospitalized for acute decompensated heart failure. J Am Coll Cardiol. 2007;49(6):675–83.

24. Bart BA, Goldsmith SR, Lee KL, et al. Ultrafiltration in decompensated heart failure with cardiorenal syndrome. N Engl J Med. 2012; 367:2296–304.

25. Konstam MA, Gheorghiade M, Burnett Jr JC, et al. Effects of oral tolvaptan in patients hospitalized for worsening heart failure: the EVEREST Outcome Trial. JAMA. 2007;297(12):1319–31.

26. Thomas SS, Nohria A. Hemodynamic classifications of acute heart failure and their clinical application – an update. Circ J. 2012;76(2): 278–86.

27. Binanay C, Califf RM, Hasselblad V, et al. Evaluation study of congestive heart failure and pulmonary artery catheterization effectiveness: the ESCAPE trial. JAMA. 2005;294(13):1625–33.

28. Sonnenblick EH, Frishman WH, LeJemtel TH. Dobutamine: a new synthetic cardioactive sympathetic amine. N Engl J Med. 1979; 300(1):17–22.

29. Cuffe MS, Califf RM, Adams Jr KF, et al. Short-term intravenous milrinone for acute exacerbation of chronic heart failure: a randomized controlled trial. JAMA. 2002;287(12):1541–7.

30. Mebazaa A, Nieminen MS, Packer M, et al. Levosimendan vs dobutamine for patients with acute decompensated heart failure: the SURVIVE Randomized Trial. JAMA. 2007;297(17):1883–91.

31. Publication Committee for the VMAC Investigators (Vasodilatation in the Management of Acute CHF). Intravenous nesiritide vs nitroglycerin for treatment of decompensated congestive heart failure: a randomized controlled trial. JAMA. 2002;287(12): 1531–40.

32. O'Connor CM, Starling RC, Hernandez AF, et al. Effect of nesiritide in patients with acute decompensated heart failure. N Engl J Med. 2011;365(1):32–43.

33. Abraham WT, Adams KF, Fonarow GC, et al. In-hospital mortality in patients with acute decompensated heart failure requiring intravenous vasoactive medications: an analysis from the Acute Decompensated Heart Failure National Registry (ADHERE). J Am Coll Cardiol. 2005;46(1):57–64.

34. Gray A, Goodacre S, Newby DE, Masson M, Sampson F, Nicholl J. Noninvasive ventilation in acute cardiogenic pulmonary edema. N Engl J Med. 2008;359(2):142–51.

35. Jondeau G, Neuder Y, Eicher JC, et al. B-CONVINCED: Betablocker CONtinuation vs. INterruption in patients with congestive heart failure hospitalizED for a decompensation episode. Eur Heart J. 2009;30(18):2186–92.

36. Gattis WA, O'Connor CM, Gallup DS, Hasselblad V, Gheorghiade M. Predischarge initiation of carvedilol in patients hospitalized for decompensated heart failure: results of the initiation management predischarge: Process for Assessment of Carvedilol Therapy in Heart Failure (IMPACT-HF) trial. J Am Coll Cardiol. 2004;43(9): 1534–41.

37. Pflugfelder PW, Baird MG, Tonkon MJ, DiBianco R, Pitt B. Clinical consequences of angiotensin-converting enzyme inhibitor withdrawal in chronic heart failure: a double-blind, placebo-controlled study of quinapril. The Quinapril Heart Failure Trial Investigators. J Am Coll Cardiol. 1993;22(6):1557–63.

38. Yancy CW, Lopatin M, Stevenson LW, De Marco T, Fonarow GC. Clinical presentation, management, and in-hospital outcomes of patients admitted with acute decompensated heart failure with preserved systolic function: a report from the Acute Decompensated Heart Failure National Registry (ADHERE) Database. J Am Coll Cardiol. 2006;47(1):76–84.

39. Klapholz M, Maurer M, Lowe AM, et al. Hospitalization for heart failure in the presence of a normal left ventricular ejection fraction: results of the New York Heart Failure Registry. J Am Coll Cardiol. 2004;43(8):1432–8.

40. Goldman L, Caldera DL, Nussbaum SR, et al. Multifactorial index of cardiac risk in noncardiac surgical procedures. N Engl J Med. 1977;297(16):845–50.

41. Hernandez AF, Whellan DJ, Stroud S, Sun JL, O'Connor CM, Jollis JG. Outcomes in heart failure patients after major noncardiac surgery. J Am Coll Cardiol. 2004;44(7):1446–53.

42. Healy KO, Waksmonski CA, Altman RK, Stetson PD, Reyentovich A, Maurer MS. Perioperative outcome and long-term mortality for heart failure patients undergoing intermediate- and high-risk noncardiac surgery: impact of left ventricular ejection fraction. Congest Heart Fail. 2010;16(2):45–9.

43. Hernandez AF, Newby LK, O'Connor CM. Preoperative evaluation for major noncardiac surgery: focusing on heart failure. Arch Intern Med. 2004;164(16):1729–36.

44. Groban L, Butterworth J. Perioperative management of chronic heart failure. Anesth Analg. 2006;103(3):557–75.

45. Licker M, Bednarkiewicz M, Neidhart P, et al. Preoperative inhibition of angiotensin-converting enzyme improves systemic and renal haemodynamic changes during aortic abdominal surgery. Br J Anaesth. 1996;76(5):632–9.

46. Eagle KA, Berger PB, Calkins H, et al. ACC/AHA guideline update for perioperative cardiovascular evaluation for noncardiac surgery – executive summary: a report of the American College of Cardiology/ American Heart Association Task Force on Practice Guidelines (Committee to Update the 1996 Guidelines on Perioperative Cardiovascular Evaluation for Noncardiac Surgery). J Am Coll Cardiol. 2002;39(3):542–53.

47. Polanczyk CA, Rohde LE, Goldman L, et al. Right heart catheterization and cardiac complications in patients undergoing noncardiac surgery: an observational study. JAMA. 2001;286(3):309–14.
48. Sandham JD, Hull RD, Brant RF, et al. A randomized, controlled trial of the use of pulmonary-artery catheters in high-risk surgical patients. N Engl J Med. 2003;348(1):5–14.
49. Morgan JA, Paone G, Nemeh HW, et al. Non-cardiac surgery in patients on long-term left ventricular assist device support. J Heart Lung Transplant. 2012;31(7):757–63.
50. Nashef SA, Roques F, Michel P, Gauducheau E, Lemeshow S, Salamon R. European system for cardiac operative risk evaluation (EuroSCORE). Eur J Cardiothorac Surg. 1999;16(1):9–13.
51. Boldt J, Rothe G, Schindler E, Doll C, Gorlach G, Hempelmann G. Can clonidine, enoximone, and enalaprilat help to protect the myocardium against ischaemia in cardiac surgery? Heart. 1996;76(3):207–13.

52. Colson P, Ribstein J, Mimran A, Grolleau D, Chaptal PA, Roquefeuil B. Effect of angiotensin converting enzyme inhibition on blood pressure and renal function during open heart surgery. Anesthesiology. 1990;72(1):23–7.
53. Jones RH, Velazquez EJ, Michler RE, et al. Coronary bypass surgery with or without surgical ventricular reconstruction. N Engl J Med. 2009;360(17):1705–17.
54. Bonow RO, Maurer G, Lee KL, et al. Myocardial viability and survival in ischemic left ventricular dysfunction. N Engl J Med. 2011;364(17):1617–25.
55. Allen LA, Stevenson LW, Grady KL, et al. Decision making in advanced heart failure: a scientific statement from the American Heart Association. Circulation. 2012;125(15):1928–52.
56. McAlister FA, Lawson FM, Teo KK, Armstrong PW. A systematic review of randomized trials of disease management programs in heart failure. Am J Med. 2001;110(5):378–84.

Diagnosis, Prevention, and Treatment of Hypertensive Heart Disease

4

Matthew Sorrentino and George L. Bakris

Abstract

Hypertension is an independent risk factor for cardiovascular disease events. There is a continuous relationship between both systolic and diastolic blood pressure levels and the chance of a heart attack or heart failure beginning at a blood pressure of 115/75 mmHg (Lewington et al., Lancet 360:1903–1913, 2002). The heart, central nervous system, kidneys, and peripheral arterial system are the major target organs that are susceptible to hypertensive disease. The most important treatment goal, however, is blood pressure control, and the choice of agent used to reach treatment goals may be less important. Although clinical trial data is lacking, a treatment target of 130/80 mmHg as recommended by the AHA is a reasonable target until further studies better define the optimal blood pressure in patients with established heart disease. Care may be needed in the elderly and patients with advanced diabetes and severe CAD to avoid treating too low blood pressure with the possibility of increasing adverse effects.

Keywords

Hypertension • Antihypertensive therapy • Resistant hypertension

Introduction

Blood pressure is an independent risk factor for cardiovascular disease events. There is a continuous relationship between both systolic and diastolic blood pressure levels and the chance of a heart attack or heart failure beginning at a blood pressure of 115/75 mmHg [1]. The heart, central nervous system, kidneys, and peripheral arterial system are the major target organs that are susceptible to hypertensive

M. Sorrentino, MD, FACC, FASH (✉)
Department of Medicine/Cardiology,
University of Chicago, 5841 S. Maryland Ave, MC 6080,
Chicago, IL 60305, USA
e-mail: msorrent@medicine.bsd.uchcago.edu

G.L. Bakris, MD
Department of Medicine, ASH Hypertension Center,
The University of Chicago Medicine,
5841 S. Maryland Ave, MC 1027, Chicago, IL 46321, USA
e-mail: gbakris@gmail.com

disease. Overt target organ involvement of the heart includes the development of left ventricular hypertrophy (LVH), coronary artery disease (CAD) including the risk for myocardial infarction (MI) and the need for revascularization, and heart failure (Table 4.1).

Hypertension has traditionally been classified by defining discrete blood pressure categories. In 2005, the Hypertension Writing Group of the American Society of Hypertension proposed incorporating cardiovascular risk factors, early disease markers, and target organ damage into a classification scheme of hypertension [2]. This expanded definition of hypertension recognizes that early target organ damage can be detected before overt clinical disease is manifested. The presence of these early markers of target organ involvement may suggest the need for earlier blood pressure treatment or more aggressive blood pressure treatment goals to prevent further progression of target organ damage. Early markers of hypertensive cardiovascular disease are listed in Table 4.2.

Table 4.1 Hypertensive cardiac target organ damage and overt disease

Left ventricular hypertrophy (moderate to severe)
Systolic or diastolic cardiac dysfunction
Symptomatic heart failure (Heart failure with preserved ejection fraction and heart failure with reduced ejection fraction)
Myocardial infarction
Angina pectoris
Ischemic heart disease/coronary revascularization

Adapted from Giles et al. [2]

Table 4.2 Early markers of hypertensive cardiovascular disease

Blood pressure	Loss of nocturnal blood pressure dipping
	Exaggerated blood pressure response to exercise
	Salt sensitivity
	Wide pulse pressure
Cardiac	Left ventricular hypertrophy (mild)
	Increased atrial filling pressure
	Decreased diastolic relaxation
Vascular	Increased central arterial stiffness or pulse wave velocity
	Small artery stiffness
	Increased systemic vascular resistance
	Increased wave reflection and systolic pressure augmentation
	Increased carotid intima-media thickness
	Coronary calcification
	Endothelial dysfunction
Renal	Microalbuminuria
	Elevated serum creatinine
	Reduced glomerular filtration rate
Eye	Hypertensive retinal changes

Adapted from Giles et al. [2]

Hypertension and Coronary Artery Disease

Hypertension is an independent risk factor for the development of coronary artery disease (CAD). The Multiple Risk Factor Intervention Trial of over 316,000 men showed a strong graded relationship for both systolic and diastolic blood pressure and coronary death with systolic blood pressure, the stronger predictor for CAD than diastolic blood pressure [3]. The National Cholesterol Education Program has recognized hypertension as one of the major modifiable risk factors used to estimate future cardiovascular risk [4]. The Framingham Heart Study examined blood pressure as a continuous variable and after adjustment for other risk factors showed that about 28 % of CAD events in men and women can be attributed to blood pressure levels of 130/85 mmHg or greater [5]. The Pathobiological Determinants of Atherosclerosis in Youth (PDAY) study showed that hypertension is a potent risk factor for the development of advanced atherosclerotic lesions in the coronary arteries and the abdominal aorta in 15–34-year-olds [6]. Finally, it appears that the prevalence of

silent MI may be increased in individuals with hypertension [7]. Once CAD is established, the presence of hypertension may adversely affect prognosis. An elevated blood pressure before or after an MI significantly increases the death rate [8].

Risk factor reduction to prevent the development of CAD has been a major focus of multiple clinical trials. Once CAD has developed, the management of hypertension should focus on the reduction of myocardial ischemia to prevent coronary events and relief of symptoms.

Blood Pressure Treatment Goals in Patients with Coronary Artery Disease

The seventh report of the Joint National Committee on Prevention, Detection, Evaluation, and Treatment of High Blood Pressure (JNC 7) recommended a blood pressure treatment goal of less than 140/90 mmHg except in individuals with diabetes or renal disease where the recommended goal is less than 130/80 mmHg [9]. Recent evidence based on newer clinical trials suggests that reassessment of this data is needed and supports a higher blood pressure goal in those with diabetes and kidney disease [10, 11]. In addition, an American Heart Association (AHA) Scientific Statement published in 2007 suggested a blood pressure target of less than 130/80 for patients with documented CAD [12].

There is very little evidence to support a blood pressure goal lower than 130/80 mmHg in patients with hypertension and CAD. The International Verapamil-Trandolapril Study (INVEST) compared morbidity and mortality outcomes in patients with hypertension and CAD treated with either a calcium channel blocker or a beta blocker [13]. The calcium channel blocker strategy was as effective as therapy using a beta blocker in preventing the primary outcome of death, MI, and stroke. Subgroup analysis was performed in the diabetic cohort evaluating individuals with tight blood pressure control defined as an achieved systolic blood pressure of <130 mmHg, a usual control group with achieved systolic blood pressure of 130–139 mmHg, and an uncontrolled blood pressure group defined as a systolic blood pressure 140 mmHg or greater [14]. Tight systolic blood pressure control was not associated with better cardiovascular outcomes than usual control.

In contrast, the CAMELOT (Comparison of Amlodipine versus Enalapril to Limit Occurrences of Thrombosis) study suggested that blood pressure goals lower than recommended by JNC 7 treatment guidelines may further reduce risk in CAD patients [15]. The CAMELOT trial was a double-blind, randomized study comparing amlodipine or enalapril with placebo in patients with angiographically documented CAD and normal blood pressure. Blood pressure averaged 129/78 mmHg for all patients and decreased approximately 5/2.5 mmHg in the treatment groups. There was a significant reduction in cardiovascular events in the amlodipine group with similar but not statistically significant effects observed in the enalapril group. This study suggests that patients with CAD may benefit from blood pressure treatment even when resting blood pressures are at what have been traditionally accepted as normal levels.

Excessive lowering of diastolic blood pressure may paradoxically increase coronary events by reducing coronary artery perfusion and cause ischemia. Studies attempting to demonstrate the presence of a J-shaped relationship between a reduction in diastolic blood pressure and an increase in coronary events are inconclusive. A meta-analysis of seven randomized clinical trials observed a J-shaped relationship between diastolic blood pressure and mortality in *both* treated and untreated subjects suggesting that the increased risk was not a blood pressure treatment effect [16]. Patients with a low pretreatment diastolic blood pressures or wide pulse pressures may represent a less healthy cohort accounting for the observation of the J-curve. Since coronary artery blood flow occurs predominantly during diastole, it is prudent to lower blood pressure slowly in patients with advanced CAD and to use caution in older hypertensive individuals or patients with diabetes when lowering the diastolic pressure below 60 mmHg.

Prevention and Treatment Recommendations

In addition to a therapeutic lifestyle program, the JNC 7 recommends pharmacological therapy for certain antihypertensive medications for high-risk conditions based on favorable outcome data from clinical trials [9]. Thiazide-type diuretics are considered first-line agents for the treatment of hypertension and are especially useful in patients with signs of volume overload. In the primary prevention Antihypertensive and Lipid-Lowering Treatment to Prevent Heart Attack Trial (ALLHAT), chlorthalidone was found to be equivalent to the angiotensin converting enzyme (ACE) inhibitor lisinopril and the calcium channel blocker (CCB) amlodipine for cardiovascular event reduction [17]. In addition, chlorthalidone reduced the risk of nonfatal MI and coronary death by 27 % in the Systolic Hypertension in the Elderly Program (SHEP) [18]. In patients without cardiometabolic risk factors or compelling reasons for specific pharmacological therapy, diuretics are an effective first-choice medication for controlling blood pressure. Diuretics, however, may worsen dyslipidemia and glucose tolerance suggesting that metabolically neutral agents may be preferred in individuals with cardiometabolic risk factors.

High cardiometabolic risk patients or patients with CAD may achieve greater benefit from a strategy using different classes of medications than diuretics. The Avoiding Cardiovascular Events through Combination Therapy in Patients Living with Systolic Hypertension (ACCOMPLISH) trial was a large randomized multicenter double-blind trial of 11,506 high-risk hypertensive individuals that compared the ACE inhibitor benazepril plus the CCB amlodipine versus benazepril plus hydrochlorothiazide. The ACE inhibitor-CCB combination was superior in reducing cardiovascular events compared with the ACE inhibitor-diuretic cohort despite a nearly identical reduction in blood pressure [19]. This study suggested either that the beneficial pleiotropic effects of the ACE inhibitor-CCB combination provided better cardiovascular disease outcomes than the ACE inhibitor-diuretic combination or that the diuretic partially negated some of the blood pressure lowering benefit of the ACE inhibitor.

Beta blockers are first-line therapy to control hypertension in patients with the compelling indications of congestive heart failure (CHF), a previous MI, established CAD, or high risk for CAD. Beta blockers reduce ischemia and relieve angina by negative inotropic effects and by reducing the heart rate. Cardioselective beta blockers are most frequently used in part to avoid side effects although nonselective beta blockers have also been shown to be effective. A number of investigators have recently questioned the value of first generation beta blockers and of atenolol in particular in the primary prevention of cardiovascular events in hypertensive patients [20]. These concerns, however, likely do not apply to secondary prevention patients since randomized studies in patients with CAD have clearly demonstrated clinical benefits with most of the available beta blockers.

Beta blockers are indicated in patients after an MI and for heart failure with a low left ventricular ejection fraction. Beta blockers should continue indefinitely in patients following an MI. For patients with heart failure and hypertension, the beta blockers carvedilol, metoprolol succinate, and bisoprolol have been shown to improve outcomes and are the preferred agents for these patients.

Calcium channel blockers (CCBs) may also be useful in patient with CAD since they reduce myocardial oxygen demand and dilate coronary arteries. In the Anglo-Scandinavian Cardiac Outcomes Trial (ASCOT), a strategy using the CCB amlodipine compared with standard blood pressure treatment using the beta blocker atenolol in high-risk hypertensive patients showed that the amlodipine-based regimen prevented more cardiovascular events than the beta blocker-based treatment [21]. The nondihydropyridine CCBs diltiazem and verapamil slow the sinus heart rate and decrease conduction through the AV node making them useful in patients with atrial arrhythmias such as atrial fibrillation. CCBs in combination with beta blockers further reduce blood pressure and can alleviate angina. CCBs may be substituted for beta blockers in patients who have a contraindication to beta blockers. CCBs also relieve angina in patients with vasospastic angina. Short-acting agents, such as short-acting nifedipine, should be avoided since they may increase the risk of MI. Verapamil and diltiazem should not be used in patients with left ventricular systolic dysfunction since they have negative inotropic effects and may worsen heart failure.

ACE inhibitors and angiotensin receptor blockers (ARBs) are first-line treatment for hypertensive patients with heart failure, a previous MI, high cardiovascular risk, diabetes, and chronic kidney disease and for recurrent stroke prevention. Several studies such as the Heart Outcomes Prevention Evaluation (HOPE) study [22] and the European Trial on Reduction of Cardiac Events with Perindopril in Stable Coronary Artery Disease (EUROPA) study [23] have shown reductions in cardiovascular events in individuals with established CAD or at high risk for the development of cardiovascular disease with the use of ACE inhibitors compared with placebo. This benefit was observed in patients with and without hypertension at baseline. ARBs are generally used in patients who are intolerant of ACE inhibitors.

Hypertension and Left Ventricular Hypertrophy

LVH develops in response to the elevated systemic vascular resistance found in patients with hypertension. Initially, hypertrophy may be an adaptive response to the increase in afterload but over time can be maladaptive leading to noncompliance of the ventricle, subendocardial ischemia, ventricular arrhythmias, and reduced cardiac function. The presence of LVH is associated with an increased risk of heart failure, atrial and ventricular arrhythmias, MI, sudden death, and cerebrovascular events [24–27]. The increased cardiovascular risk associated with LVH is likely due to myocardial ischemia. A reduced density of myocardial capillaries, compression of capillaries by hypertrophied muscle, and a limited ability of epicardial blood vessels to dilate under stress have all been implicated as causes of ischemia [28]. LVH is generally global and concentric, but at times eccentric remodeling with left ventricular enlargement and the development of heart failure may occur. In the Framingham Heart Study, hypertension was the most common preexisting risk factor for the development of heart failure [29].

LVH can be diagnosed with either an electrocardiogram (ECG) or echocardiogram. Echocardiography is a more sensitive test for the diagnosis of LVH. In the Framingham Heart Study, ECG criteria for LVH was seen in about 2–3 % of the population studied, whereas echocardiography diagnosed LVH in 14–18 % [30]. In populations of patients with hypertension, the prevalence of LVH can approach 30 [31].

Lowering blood pressure with antihypertensive therapy can induce regression of LVH. In general, most antihypertensive agents will bring about LVH regression with the exception of

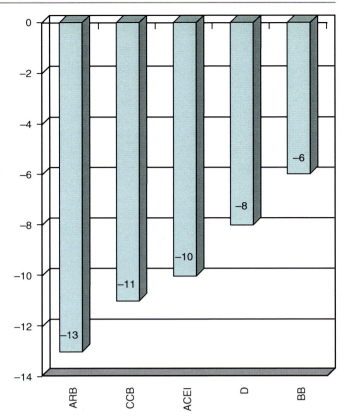

Fig. 4.1 Percent change in left ventricular mass index with different antihypertensive classes. *ARB* angiotensin receptor blocker, *CCB* calcium channel blocker, *ACEI* angiotensin converting enzyme inhibitor, *D* diuretic, *BB* beta blocker (Data from Klingbeil et al. [32])

peripheral vasodilators possibly because of the development of a sympathetic tachycardia as a result of the peripheral vasodilatation. ARBs, CCBs, and ACE inhibitors appear to cause more regression of LVH than diuretics and beta blockers for the same degree of blood pressure lowering (Fig. 4.1) [32]. Regression of LVH occurs slowly usually over many months to years. Regression of LVH may also be accompanied by a reduction in left atrial size and improvement in diastolic dysfunction [33]. Worsening diastolic dysfunction is an independent predictor of mortality. Preliminary evidence suggests that improvement in diastolic dysfunction may be associated with a lower mortality [34].

The Losartan Intervention for Endpoint reduction in hypertension study (LIFE) randomized over 9,000 essential hypertension patients with ECG-diagnosed LVH into beta blocker versus ARB treatment arms [35]. Cardiovascular morbidity and mortality was significantly reduced in the losartan arm compared with the beta blocker arm for a similar reduction in blood pressure. Those individuals that achieved greater reductions in left ventricular mass had fewer cardiovascular events [36]. This large prospective study verified findings from earlier studies and meta-analyses that indicted that regression of LVH is associated with a marked reduction in risk for subsequent cardiovascular events [37].

Blood pressure reduction may be the most important determinant of LVH regression. A study comparing 2 beta blocker/ACE inhibitor combination therapies and an ACE inhibitor alone showed similar reductions in LV mass assessed by MRI in individuals achieving blood pressure goals suggesting that achieving the targeted blood pressure goal is more important than the particular treatment regimen [38].

Prevention and Treatment Recommendations

LVH is an independent risk factor for cardiovascular morbidity and mortality. It is reasonable to screen for LVH in hypertensive individuals especially if hypertension has been long standing and resistant to treatment or there are physical signs suggesting target organ involvement. An ECG can be used as a screening test but has poor sensitivity for detecting LVH. A limited echocardiogaphic exam has been advocated to measure LVH and may be considered in individuals when there is concern about target organ damage.

ACE inhibitors, ARBs, and CCBs are preferred initial agents to use in patients with LVH since these agents are associated with greater LVH regression than beta blockers and diuretics. Many patients will require combination therapy to achieve blood pressure goals. Reaching recommended blood pressure goals is more important than the drug regimen chosen to reach the goal. Further research is needed to determine the optimal blood pressure goal to achieve the greatest degree of LVH regression.

Hypertension and Heart Failure with Preserved Ejection Fraction

Hypertension is a common risk factor for the development of heart failure. An increasing number of patients are presenting with clinical heart failure symptoms and preserved cardiac contractility. This entity, previously called diastolic heart failure, has been termed heart failure with preserved ejection fraction (HFpEF). Patients with HFpEF typically have a history of hypertension. A survey of nearly 6,000 patients with hospital admission for heart failure determined that 31 % had a preserved ejection fraction [39]. Patients with HFpEF were more likely to be older and female and have a history of hypertension and atrial fibrillation. Mortality rates were similar for patients with HFpEF and patients with an ejection fraction of less than 40 %. A Mayo clinic survey showed that the proportion of patients with HFpEF is increasing over time and accounts for 55 % of community patients admitted to the hospital with clinical heart failure [40].

Diastolic dysfunction is implicated as a cause of HFpEF. Diastolic dysfunction refers to an abnormality of diastolic distensibility affecting filling and relaxation of the left ventricle [41]. In order to preserve left ventricular stroke volume, left atrial filling pressures need to increase for adequate filling of the noncompliant ventricle. Elevated left ventricular diastolic pressures lead to elevated pulmonary venous pressures, reduced lung compliance, and symptoms of dyspnea. Many patients will develop an inadequate stroke volume during exertion causing fatigue and breathlessness. Increased muscle mass (hypertrophy) increases chamber stiffness requiring a further increase in left atrial pressure to adequately fill the ventricle. Since hypertension is the leading cause of left ventricular hypertrophy, it is a common underlying factor associated with HFpEF. Atrial fibrillation, by preventing left atrial contraction and reducing left ventricular filling, can also precipitate HFpEF. Hypertension is a common risk factor for the occurrence of atrial fibrillation [42].

Medications that target the renin-angiotensin-aldosterone system (RAAS) reduce morbidity and mortality in patients with heart failure and reduced ejection fraction and are useful in regression of left ventricular hypertrophy. These agents have been recommended for patients with HFpEF. Clinical trial results using these agents, however, have been disappointing. Three large trials using ACE inhibitors and ARBs (PEP-CHF [43], CHARM-preserved [44], and I-PRESERVE [45] using perindopril, candesartan, and irbesartan, respectively) failed to show an improvement in outcomes using these agents in contrast to the positive outcomes observed in patients with low ejection fraction.

Despite these findings, hypertension treatment studies have shown a reduction in the incidence of heart failure. For example, the SHEP trial using the diuretic chlorthalidone observed a greater than 50 % decrease in heart failure in the treatment group [18]. A large meta-analysis reported a significant reduction in heart failure in 64 blood pressure difference trials and 31 drug combination trials except for beta blockers without cardioselective or alpha blocking properties [46]. The incidence of heart failure was reduced by 24 % on average although the reduction was slightly lower with calcium channel blockers at 19 %. The effect of the drugs was similar in primary and secondary prevention trials including a reduction in hospitalization or death in individuals already diagnosed with heart failure. This suggests that blood pressure lowering and not necessarily the type of blood pressure agent used is important in the treatment of hypertensive patients with HFpEF.

Prevention and Treatment Recommendations

Treatment of hypertension has been shown in many clinical trials to reduce the incidence of heart failure. In patients with HFpEF, targeting the blood pressure can improve symptoms. At this point, there are no studies that suggest that one treatment strategy is better than another in preventing adverse outcomes. Diuretics are commonly needed to help relieve symptoms of volume overload and have been shown to prevent heart failure admissions in primary prevention trials. Agents that target the renin-angiotensin system are reasonable choices to use because of their proven efficacy in patients with heart failure and reduced ejection fraction even though they have not been shown to be superior to standard hypertensive therapies. These agents have also been noted to improve diastolic parameters. Most important, however, is achieving adequate blood pressure control and not necessarily the blood pressure agent chosen to achieve the goal.

Resistant Hypertension with High Coronary Disease Risk

Resistant hypertension is defined as blood pressure >140/90 mmHg despite adherence to therapy with maximum doses of at least *three* antihypertensive agents with complementary modes of action, one of which being a diuretic appropriate for kidney function [47]. This would then exclude combinations such as ACE inhibitors and ARBs or clonidine and beta blockers but would include RAAS blockers with either diuretics or calcium antagonists or calcium antagonists with beta blockers [48].

The exact prevalence of resistant hypertension is not well defined in the literature but ranges between 8.5 and 10 % of all hypertensive patients [49]. Resistant hypertension is more common in older patients, those with chronic kidney disease, i.e., eGFR <60 ml/min/1.73 m^2, and is associated with high sympathetic tone; increased long-term risk of cardiovascular events such as myocardial infarction, congestive heart failure, and stroke; and progressive nephropathy.

Resistant hypertension is a diagnosis of exclusion thus, there are a number of issues to consider before labeling a person as resistant. These factors include the following: (a) *pseudoresistance:* a white-coat phenomenon defined as persistently elevated blood pressure in the physician's clinic office but normal blood pressure at home must be excluded with repeated home blood pressure measurements or 24-h ambulatory blood pressure monitoring. These patients typically have no evidence of target organ damage, but if they have primary hypertension with a white-coat component, they very well would have target organ injury. Also in older patients pseudohypertension due to severely calcified and sclerotic arteries may simulate resistant hypertension. This diagnosis should be suspected by the presence of palpable radial pulse while the brachial artery is occluded by the cuff (the Osler maneuver). An intra-arterial blood pressure measurement confirms this condition. (b) *Patient adherence*: Adherence to lifestyle modifications, especially

low-sodium diet, and antihypertensive therapy must be carefully evaluated and confirmed with pharmacy records. Although difficult to recognize, suggestive symptoms include missed clinic appointments, lack of use of medication refills, and in patients on beta blockers presence of normal heart rate. (c) *Physician inaction* (inertia): Some patients receive inadequate or insufficient antihypertensive drug dose titration despite multiple clinic visits. In other patients, non-initiation or use of inappropriate diuretics, e.g., thiazide in a patient with an estimated GFR <30 ml/min, may be an important reason for the poorly controlled blood pressure. (d) *Drug-drug interaction or exogenous substances:* A detailed drug history including over-the-counter pain medicines, herbal preparations, and nutritional supplements must be obtained routinely in these patients. Nonsteroidal anti-inflammatory agents will antagonize the effects of some antihypertensive agents secondary to local prostaglandin inhibition and impairment of sodium excretion which induces volume expansion. (e) *Secondary hypertension:* True secondary hypertension is uncommon but must be evaluated if the conditions discussed above have been excluded. Of note, chronic kidney disease, renovascular disease, hyperaldosteronism, pheochromocytoma, and sleep apnea are conditions that must be screened for and if detected managed appropriately before labeling the patient as resistant.

Treatment Recommendations

These patients all require a minimum of 4 drugs at maximally tolerated doses so most common combinations recommended include a blocker of the renin-angiotensin system combined with a diuretic and calcium antagonist and in obese people addition of spironolactone at 25–50 mg a day. If that still fails to control BP, additional therapies including vasodilating beta blockers like carvedilol or bisoprolol may be given and consideration to a nondihydropyridine calcium antagonist or agents like hydralazine with a nitrate or minoxidil.

Newer experimental therapies such as renal denervation and Barostim therapy are in the research stages but renal denervation is approved in Europe [50]. These are interventional therapies one involving radiofrequency to denervate the renal nerves and the Barostim places an electrode on the carotid body and uses electrical stimulation to inhibit central sympathetic output. The Symplicity HTN-3 trial is ongoing in the United States, and the design of the study includes 24-h ambulatory monitoring, and it is the largest study to investigate this procedure for the resolution of resistant hypertension, recruiting 542 participants [51].

Key Points

- The most important treatment goal, however, is blood pressure control and the choice of agent used to reach treatment goals may be less important.
- Although clinical trial data is lacking, a treatment target of 130/80 mmHg as recommended by the AHA is a reasonable target until further studies better define the optimal blood pressure in patients with established heart disease.
- Care may be needed in the elderly and patients with advanced diabetes and severe CAD to avoid treating too low blood pressure with the possibility of increasing adverse effects.
- Resistant hypertension is defined as blood pressure >140/90 mmHg despite adherence to therapy with maximum doses of at least *three* antihypertensive agents with complementary modes of action, one of which being a diuretic appropriate for kidney function.

References

1. Lewington S, Clarke R, Qizilbash N, Peto R, Collins R. Age-specific relevance of usual blood pressure to vascular mortality: a meta-analysis of individual data for one million adults in 61 prospective studies. Lancet. 2002;360(9349):1903–13.
2. Giles TD, Berk BC, Black HR, et al. Expanding the definition and classification of hypertension. J Clin Hypertens (Greenwich). 2005;7(9):505–12.
3. Neaton JD, Blackburn H, Jacobs D, et al. Serum cholesterol level and mortality findings for men screened in the Multiple Risk Factor Intervention Trial. Multiple Risk Factor Intervention Trial Research Group. Arch Intern Med. 1992;152(7):1490–500.
4. Executive Summary of The Third Report of The National Cholesterol Education Program (NCEP) Expert Panel on Detection, Evaluation, And Treatment of High Blood Cholesterol In Adults (Adult Treatment Panel III). JAMA. 2001;285(19):2486–97.
5. Wilson PW, D'Agostino RB, Levy D, Belanger AM, Silbershatz H, Kannel WB. Prediction of coronary heart disease using risk factor categories. Circulation. 1998;97(18):1837–47.
6. McMahan CA, Gidding SS, Fayad ZA, et al. Risk scores predict atherosclerotic lesions in young people. Arch Intern Med. 2005;165(8):883–90.
7. Boon D, Piek JJ, van Montfrans GA. Silent ischaemia and hypertension. J Hypertens. 2000;18(10):1355–64.
8. Njolstad I, Arnesen E. Preinfarction blood pressure and smoking are determinants for a fatal outcome of myocardial infarction: a prospective analysis from the Finnmark Study. Arch Intern Med. 1998;158(12):1326–32.
9. Chobanian AV, Bakris GL, Black HR, et al. The Seventh Report of the Joint National Committee on Prevention, Detection, Evaluation, and Treatment of High Blood Pressure: the JNC 7 report. JAMA. 2003;289(19):2560–72.
10. Kalaitzidis RG, Bakris GL. Pros and cons of aggressive blood pressure lowering in patient with type 2 diabetes. Curr Vasc Pharmacol. 2012;10:156–61.
11. Upadhyay A, Early A, Haynes SM, Uhlig K. Systematic review: blood pressure target in chronic kidney disease and proteinuria as an effect modifier. Ann Intern Med. 2011;154:541–8.
12. Rosendorff C, Black HR, Cannon CP, et al. Treatment of hypertension in the prevention and management of ischemic heart disease: a scientific statement from the American Heart Association Council for High Blood Pressure Research and the Councils on Clinical Cardiology and Epidemiology and Prevention. Circulation. 2007;115(21):2761–88.
13. Pepine CJ, Handberg EM, Cooper-DeHoff RM, et al. A calcium antagonist vs a non-calcium antagonist hypertension treatment strategy for patients with coronary artery disease. JAMA. 2003;290:2805–16.
14. Cooper-DeHof RM, Gong Y, Handberg EM, et al. Tight blood pressure control and cardiovascular outcomes among hypertensive patients with diabetes and coronary artery disease. JAMA. 2010;304:61–8.
15. Nissen SE, Tuzcu EM, Libby P, et al. Effect of antihypertensive agents on cardiovascular events in patients with coronary disease and normal blood pressure: the CAMELOT study: a randomized controlled trial. JAMA. 2004;292(18):2217–25.
16. Boutitie F, Gueyffier F, Pocock S, Fagard R, Boissel JP. J-shaped relationship between blood pressure and mortality in hypertensive patients: new insights from a meta-analysis of individual-patient data. Ann Intern Med. 2002;136(6):438–48.
17. Major outcomes in high-risk hypertensive patients randomized to angiotensin-converting enzyme inhibitor or calcium channel blocker vs diuretic: The Antihypertensive and Lipid-Lowering Treatment to Prevent Heart Attack Trial (ALLHAT). JAMA. 2002;288(23):2981–97.
18. Prevention of stroke by antihypertensive drug treatment in older persons with isolated systolic hypertension. Final results of the Systolic Hypertension in the Elderly Program (SHEP). SHEP Cooperative Research Group. JAMA. 1991;265(24):3255–64.
19. Jamerson K, Weber MA, Bakris GL, et al. Benazepril plus amlodipine or hydrochlorothiazide for hypertension in high-risk patients. N Engl J Med. 2008;359(23):2417–28.
20. Ong HT. Beta blockers in hypertension and cardiovascular disease. BMJ. 2007;334(7600):946–9.
21. Dahlof B, Sever PS, Poulter NR, et al. Prevention of cardiovascular events with an antihypertensive regimen of amlodipine adding perindopril as required versus atenolol adding bendroflumethiazide as required, in the Anglo-Scandinavian Cardiac Outomes Trial-Blood Pressure Lowering Arm (ASCOT-BPLA): a mulitcentre randomised controlled trial. Lancet. 2005;366:895–906.
22. Yusuf S, Sleight P, Pogue J, Bosch J, Davies R, Dagenais G. Effects of an angiotensin-converting-enzyme inhibitor, ramipril, on cardiovascular events in high-risk patients. The Heart Outcomes Prevention Evaluation Study Investigators. N Engl J Med. 2000;342(3):145–53.
23. Fox KM. Efficacy of perindopril in reduction of cardiovascular events among patients with stable coronary artery disease: randomised, double-blind, placebo-controlled, multicentre trial (the EUROPA study). Lancet. 2003;362(9386):782–8.
24. Kannel WB, Dannenberg AL, Levy D. Population implications of electrocardiographic left ventricular hypertrophy. Am J Cardiol. 1987;60(17):85I–93.
25. Levy D, Anderson KM, Savage DD, Balkus SA, Kannel WB, Castelli WP. Risk of ventricular arrhythmias in left ventricular hypertrophy: the Framingham Heart Study. Am J Cardiol. 1987;60(7):560–5.
26. Levy D, Garrison RJ, Savage DD, Kannel WB, Castelli WP. Prognostic implications of echocardiographically determined left ventricular mass in the Framingham Heart Study. N Engl J Med. 1990;322(22):1561–6.

27. Verdecchia P, Porcellati C, Reboldi G, et al. Left ventricular hypertrophy as an independent predictor of acute cerebrovascular events in essential hypertension. Circulation. 2001;104(17): 2039–44.

28. Beache GM, Herzka DA, Boxerman JL, et al. Attenuated myocardial vasodilator response in patients with hypertensive hypertrophy revealed by oxygenation-dependent magnetic resonance imaging. Circulation. 2001;104(11):1214–7.

29. Levy D, Larson MG, Vasan RS, Kannel WB, Ho KK. The progression from hypertension to congestive heart failure. JAMA. 1996;275(20):1557–62.

30. Levy D, Labib SB, Anderson KM, Christiansen JC, Kannel WB, Castelli WP. Determinants of sensitivity and specificity of electrocardiographic criteria for left ventricular hypertrophy. Circulation. 1990;81(3):815–20.

31. Verdecchia P, Carini G, Circo A, et al. Left ventricular mass and cardiovascular morbidity in essential hypertension: the MAVI study. J Am Coll Cardiol. 2001;38(7):1829–35.

32. Klingbeil AU, Schneider M, Martus P, Messerli FH, Schmieder RE. A meta-analysis of the effects of treatment on left ventricular mass in essential hypertension. Am J Med. 2003;115(1):41–6.

33. Franz IW, Tonnesmann U, Muller JF. Time course of complete normalization of left ventricular hypertrophy during long-term antihypertensive therapy with angiotensin converting enzyme inhibitors. Am J Hypertens. 1998;11(6 Pt 1):631–9.

34. Aljaroudi W, Alraies MC, Halley C, et al. Impact of progression of diastolic dysfunction on mortality in patients with normal ejection fraction. Circulation. 2012;125(6):782–8.

35. Dahlof B, Devereux RB, Kjeldsen SE, et al. Cardiovascular morbidity and mortality in the Losartan Intervention For Endpoint reduction in hypertension study (LIFE): a randomised trial against atenolol. Lancet. 2002;359(9311):995–1003.

36. Devereux RB, Wachtell K, Gerdts E, et al. Prognostic significance of left ventricular mass change during treatment of hypertension. JAMA. 2004;292(19):2350–6.

37. Verdecchia P, Angeli F, Borgioni C, et al. Changes in cardiovascular risk by reduction of left ventricular mass in hypertension: a meta-analysis. Am J Hypertens. 2003;16(11 Pt 1):895–9.

38. Miller AB, Reichek N, St John SM, et al. Importance of blood pressure control in left ventricular mass regression. J Am Soc Hypertens. 2010;4(6):302–10.

39. Bhatia RS, Tu JV, Lee DS, et al. Outcome of heart failure with preserved ejection fraction in a population-based study. N Engl J Med. 2006;355(3):260–9.

40. Owan TE, Hodge DO, Herges RM, Jacobsen SJ, Roger VL, Redfield MM. Trends in prevalence and outcome of heart failure with preserved ejection fraction. N Engl J Med. 2006;355(3):251–9.

41. Aurigemma GP, Gaasch WH. Clinical practice. Diastolic heart failure. N Engl J Med. 2004;351(11):1097–105.

42. Benjamin EJ, Levy D, Vaziri SM, D'Agostino RB, Belanger AJ, Wolf PA. Independent risk factors for atrial fibrillation in a population-based cohort. The Framingham Heart Study. JAMA. 1994;271(11):840–4.

43. Cleland JG, Tendera M, Adamus J, Freemantle N, Polonski L, Taylor J. The Perindopril in Elderly People with Chronic Heart Failure (PEP-CHF) study. Eur Heart J. 2006;27:2338–45.

44. Yusuf S, Pfeffer MA, Swedberg K, et al. Effects of candesartan in patients with chronic heart failure and preserved left-ventricular ejection fraction: the CHARM-Preserved Trial. Lancet. 2003;362:777–81.

45. Massie BM, Carson PE, McMurray JJ, et al. Irbesartan in patients with heart failure and preserved ejection fraction. N Engl J Med. 2008;359:2456–67.

46. Law MR, Morris JK, Wald NJ. Use of blood pressure lowering drugs in the prevention of cardiovascular disease: meta-analysis of 147 randomised trials in the context of expectations from prospective epidemiological studies. BMJ. 2009;338:b1665.

47. Gonzaga CC, Calhoun DA. 2008 American Heart Association Statement on diagnosis, evaluation, and treatment of resistant hypertension: what should we remember in everyday practice? Pol Arch Med Wewn. 2008;118:196–7.

48. Gradman AH, Basile JN, Carter BL, Bakris GL. Combination therapy in hypertension. J Clin Hypertens. 2011;13:146–54.

49. Egan BM, Zhao Y, Axon RN, Brzezinski WA, Ferdinand KC. Uncontrolled and apparent treatment resistant hypertension in the United States, 1998 to 2008. Circulation. 2011;124:1046–58.

50. Bakris GL, et al. Baroreflex activation therapy provides durable benefit in patients with resistant hypertension: results of long-term follow-up in the Rheos Pivotal Trial. J Am Soc Hypertens. 2012;6:152–8.

51. Kandzari DE, et al. Catheter-based renal denervation for resistant hypertension: rationale and design of the SYMPLICITY HTN-3 trial. Clin Cardiol. 2012;35:528–35.

Valvular Heart Disease

5

Elisa Zaragoza-Macias and Catherine M. Otto

Abstract

Significant valvular heart disease is present in about 2 % of the population. The most common serious valve condition is calcific aortic stenosis (AS), with severe disease presenting in older adults with symptoms of decreased exercise tolerance or dyspnea and a systolic murmur. Valve replacement is lifesaving and is recommended regardless of patient age. Mitral stenosis is a late consequence of rheumatic heart disease and now is treated with percutaneous balloon commissurotomy in most patients. Mitral valve regurgitation often is secondary to other cardiac conditions, such as dilated cardiomyopathy and coronary disease, with treatment directed toward the underlying disease process. In patients with primary mitral regurgitation, for example, due to mitral valve prolapse, surgical repair often provides durable relief of valve dysfunction without the need for a prosthetic valve. Aortic regurgitation may be due to disease of the valve leaflets, such as a bicuspid valve, or to dilation of the aorta; treatment depends on the cause of valve dysfunction. Acute aortic or mitral regurgitation is a medical and surgical emergency with a range of causes including aortic dissection, endocarditis, and spontaneous mitral chordal rupture. Acute valve regurgitation often is misdiagnosed because a typical murmur may not be present; echocardiography should be considered in all patients with acute pulmonary decompensation. Patients with prosthetic heart valves require careful management to prevent endocarditis and to provide optimal antithrombotic therapy, as well as to monitor valve function. Endocarditis has mortality rate as high as 40 % at 1 year; management requires collaborative care by cardiologists, cardiac surgeons, and infectious disease specialists.

Keywords

Aortic stenosis • Aortic regurgitation • Mitral stenosis • Mitral regurgitation • Endocarditis • Prosthetic heart valve

E. Zaragoza-Macias, MD
Division of Cardiology, Department of Medicine,
University of Washington School of Medicine,
1959 NE Pacific St., HSB Rm AA522, Seattle 98195, WA, USA
e-mail: ezargoza-macias@cardiology.washington.edu

C.M. Otto, MD (✉)
Echocardiographic Laboratory,
Division of Cardiology, Department of Medicine,
University of Washington School of Medicine,
1959 NE Pacific St., HSB Rm AA522, Seattle 98195, WA, USA
e-mail: cmotto@u.washington.edu

Introduction

The prevalence of significant valvular heart disease in the general population is between 1.8 and 2.5 % [1]. In developing countries, rheumatic valve disease remains common in contrast to developed countries where the major causes of valve disease are calcific aortic stenosis (AS) and mitral valve prolapse (MVP). Some patients with valve disease are initially diagnosed due to symptom onset with decreased exercise tolerance, palpitations, syncope, new onset atrial fibrillation (AF), endocarditis, or frank heart failure. Cardiac auscultation is helpful for detection of valve dysfunction, and the location, timing, quality, and change in intensity with certain maneuvers can help guide diagnosis.

Valve disease often is secondary to a systemic or inherited condition so it is important to inquire about diseases such as rheumatic fever, connective tissue disorders, rheumatologic diseases, or a family history of valve disease. Echocardiography is the primary modality for diagnosis, follow-up, and management of patients with valvular heart disease. In addition to defining the location and severity of valve dysfunction, echocardiography provides information of left ventricular (LV) size and function, pulmonary pressures, and associated cardiac conditions. Rarely, other diagnostic approaches are needed, such as cardiac magnetic resonance imaging when more precise measurements of ventricular size and function are needed or cardiac catheterization at the time of an interventional valve procedure.

Valve Stenosis

Aortic Stenosis

The most common cause of valvular AS is calcification of a normal trileaflet or congenially bicuspid valve, typically presenting after 60 years of age. In young adults, AS more often is due to a congenital stenotic valve [2]. Calcific AS is characterized by deposition of calcium on the aortic side of leaflets without commissural fusion, and it is estimated that 2–4 % of adults over 65 years of age have some degree of calcific AS [3, 4]. Men tend to have higher rates of calcific AS than women. Inflammation, lipid accumulation, and activation of pro-osteogenic signaling cascades are thought to be important mechanisms in initiation of calcific AS [5]. Risk factors for development and progression of calcific AS include age, hypertension, hyperlipidemia, metabolic syndrome, and smoking [3, 6].

Pathophysiology

The three main effects of AS on the LV are pressure overload, diastolic dysfunction, and supply–demand ischemia. Pressure overload results from the obstruction of blood flow through the LV outflow tract to the aorta with a compensatory increase in LV wall thickness and a normal chamber size (e.g., concentric hypertrophy). Hypertrophy is associated with decreased myocardial compliance and diastolic dysfunction. Ischemia results from increased myocardial O_2 consumption due to LV hypertrophy in conjunction with decreased myocardial O_2 supply due to a rise in LV diastolic pressure. Aortic valve obstruction occurs gradually over several years, and patients remain asymptomatic until progressive narrowing results in severe stenosis. However, disease progression is inevitable once even mild AS is present (aortic velocity over 2.5 m/s) with an average increase in aortic velocity of 0.3 m/s/year, an increase in gradient of 7 mmHg/year, and a decrease in valve area of 0.12 cm^2/year. Symptom onset in adults with severe AS leads to heart failure with a very high (about 80 %) mortality at 2 years unless valve replacement is performed [7, 8].

Diagnosis

In adults with mild to moderate AS, management focuses on careful follow-up and standard medical therapy for comorbid conditions. Even with severe AS, annual mortality remains low at <2 % in asymptomatic patients so that close clinical follow-up and education about reporting any symptoms promptly is imperative [9, 10].

Historically, the triad of symptoms associated with severe AS included angina, syncope, and heart failure. However, the majority of patients present earlier in the disease course with decreased exercise tolerance, exertional dyspnea, dizziness, or chest tightness (Table 5.1).

Physical exam demonstrates a crescendo-decrescendo systolic ejection murmur, best heard at the base of the heart, usually radiating to the carotids but rarely to the LV apex (Gallavardin phenomenon). A late peaking murmur, longer murmur duration, and a single S2 (absence of A2 component) indicate severe AS, whereas the intensity of the murmur does not correlate with severity. Carotid pulses that are delayed, slow rising, and with low amplitude "parvus et tardus" also indicate severe AS.

Echocardiography is the main diagnostic modality to determine the severity of AS and to follow patients. Morphology of the aortic valve, number of cusps, degree of calcification, peak velocity, transvalvular gradient, and valve area all can be assessed by echocardiography. Additionally, echocardiography provides evaluation of LV hypertrophy, systolic and diastolic LV function, aortic root dimensions, and other intracardiac structures (Table 5.2).

Magnetic resonance imaging or computed tomography may helpful when further measurements of the ascending aorta are needed. Hemodynamic measurements at cardiac catheterization are rarely needed, although coronary angiography is recommended prior to valve replacement.

Management

The treatment for severe symptomatic AS is aortic valve replacement. Despite initial hopes for medical therapy to prevent disease progression, randomized controlled trials showed no effect of statins in halting the hemodynamic progression or time to valve replacement for calcific AS or patients with congenital AS [11–14] (Table 5.3).

Table 5.1 Diagnosis of valvular heart disease

	Physical exam	Symptoms	Key echo findings
Aortic stenosis	Crescendo-decrescendo systolic ejection murmur best heard base of the heart radiating to carotids Delayed, slow rising, and low amplitude carotid pulse	Exercise intolerance Dizziness Dyspnea Angina Syncope Heart failure	Cause of stenosis Degree of leaflet calcification Severity of stenosis LV hypertrophy LV systolic function LV diastolic function Aortic sinus dilation
Mitral stenosis	Opening snap followed by diastolic murmur best heard in the apex RV heave and loud P2 if PA pressures elevated	Exertional dyspnea Orthopnea Paroxysmal nocturnal dyspnea Fatigue Palpitations	Mitral valve morphology Candidacy for percutaneous valvotomy Severity of stenosis Associated mitral regurgitation Left atrial size Left atrial thrombus (TEE) Pulmonary pressures
Aortic regurgitation	Wide pulse pressure Hyperdynamic pulse Blowing decrescendo murmur best heard at left sternal border Hyperdynamic pulse	Exercise intolerance Exertional dyspnea Orthopnea Paroxysmal nocturnal dyspnea	Cause of regurgitation Associated valve stenosis Severity of regurgitation LV dimensions, volumes, and ejection fraction Dimension of aortic sinuses and ascending aorta
Mitral regurgitation	Holosystolic murmur best heard at the apex radiating to the axilla	Dyspnea Paroxysmal nocturnal dyspnea Exercise intolerance	Cause of regurgitation Regurgitant severity Likelihood of valve repair LV dimensions, volumes, and ejection fraction Pulmonary pressures

LV left ventricular, *PA* pulmonary artery, *TEE* transesophageal echocardiography

Table 5.2 Severity of left-sided valve disease

	Mild	Moderate	Severe
Aortic stenosis	Mild leaflet calcification and reduced leaflet motion Doppler $V_{max} < 3$ m/s Mean $\Delta P < 25$ mmHg Valve area >1.5 cm^2	Moderate leaflet calcification and reduced leaflet motion Doppler V_{max} 3–4 m/s Mean ΔP 25–40 mmHg Valve area 1–1.5 cm^2	Severe leaflet calcification with nearly immobile leaflets Doppler $V_{max} > 4$ m/s Mean $\Delta P > 40$ mmHg Valve area <1 cm^2
Mitral stenosis	Mild commissural fusion with leaflet doming in diastole Valve area >1.5 cm^2 Mean $\Delta P < 5$ mmHg Normal PASP (<30 mmHg)	Commissural fusion, chordal shortening and fusion Valve area 1–1.5 cm^2 Mean ΔP 5–10 mmHg PASP 30–50 mmHg	Severe commissural fusion, leaflet doming in diastole, and chordal shortening Valve area <1 cm^2 Mean $\Delta P > 10$ mmHg PASP >50 mmHg
Aortic regurgitation	VC <0.3 cm RV <30 ml RF <30 % ROA 0.1–0.29 cm^2 Normal distal aortic flow patterns CWD AR signal density weak, often incomplete	VC 0.3–0.6 cm RV 30–59 ml RF 30–49 % ROA 0.1–0.29 cm^2 Holodiastolic flow reversal in the descending thoracic (but not proximal abdominal) aorta CWD AR signal density $<$ systolic flow	VC >0.6 cm RV ≥ 60 ml RF ≥ 50 % ROA ≥ 0.3 cm^2 Holodiastolic flow reversal in the abdominal aorta CWD AR signal density $=$ systolic flow *Left ventricular dilation is present*
Mitral regurgitation[a]	VC <0.3 cm RV <30 ml RF <30 % ROA <0.2 cm^2 CWD AR signal density weak, often incomplete	VC 0.3–0.69 cm RV 30–59 ml RF 30–49 % ROA 0.2–0.39 cm^2 CWD AR signal density $<$ systolic flow	VC ≥ 0.7 cm RV ≥ 60 ml RF ≥ 50 % ROA ≥ 0.4 cm^2 CWD AR signal density $=$ systolic flow *Increased left atrial and ventricular size*

AR aortic regurgitation, *CWD* continuous wave Doppler, *Mean ΔP* mean transvalvular pressure gradient, *MR* mitral regurgitation, *PASP* pulmonary artery systolic pressure, *RF* regurgitant fraction, *RV* regurgitant volume, *ROA* regurgitant orifice area, *VC* vena contracta (width of the jet on color Doppler), *V_{max}* maximum velocity

[a]These hemodynamic criteria are for primary mitral regurgitation. Lower thresholds may be used for functional regurgitation

Table 5.3 Long-term management of valvular heart disease

Valve	Prevention	Considerations when following patients	Patient follow-up*
Aortic stenosis	*General principles*: Evaluate and treat CAD risk factors Encourage routine dental care and optimal dental hygiene Educate patient about likely disease course and symptoms	*Medical management*: Avoid hypovolemia and lowering systemic vascular resistance due to fixed cardiac output Evaluate disease severity prior to noncardiac surgery *Physical activity*: in severe AS avoid vigorous athletic activity	*Clinical f/u*: every 6–12 months in severe AS, every 12 months in mod AS *Echocardiogram*: every 3–5 years for mild, 1–2 years for moderate, and every year for severe AS or when there is a change in symptoms
Mitral stenosis	*General principles*: Evaluate and treat CAD risk factors Encourage routine dental care and optimal dental hygiene Educate patient about likely disease course and symptoms *Rheumatic fever prophylaxis*: if MS present daily oral penicillin V or monthly benzathine penicillin with duration of 10 years since last RF attack or until age 40. Lifelong if high risk of reinfection	*Medical management*: Rate control with beta blockers, calcium channel blockers, or digoxin can reduce symptoms in decompensated patients especially if atrial arrhythmias encountered Coumadin anticoagulation in atrial fibrillation *Physical activity*: avoid vigorous athletic activity in moderate to severe MS, symptom limited exercise is the main recommendation	*Clinical f/u*: once a year if moderate to severe MS *Echocardiogram* every year for severe MS (to assess PAP), every 1–2 years for moderate MS, and every 3–5 years for mild MS or when there are changes in symptoms or intervention is planned
Aortic regurgitation	*General principles*: Evaluate and treat CAD risk factors Encourage routine dental care and optimal dental hygiene Educate patient about likely disease course and symptoms *Screening family members*: evaluate aorta and recommend family screening if dilated or if positive family history for bicuspid valve disease	*Medical management*: no therapy delays progression. Treat hypertension if present *Physical activity*: avoid vigorous activity and isometric exercises with severe AR	*Clinical f/u*: Every 6 months in severe AR. If moderate AR every 2–3 years *Echocardiogram*: every 6–12 months for severe AR and 2–3 years for moderate and mild AR or if there is change in symptoms
Mitral regurgitation	*General principles*: Evaluate and treat CAD risk factors Encourage routine dental care and optimal dental hygiene Educate patient about likely disease course and symptoms	*Medical management*: no treatment will delay progression of MR. Treat hypertension if present Warfarin when atrial fibrillation and more than mild MR is present *Physical activity*: avoid vigorous activity and isometric exercises if severe MR	*Clinical f/u*: every 6–12 months for severe MR No follow-up with mild MR and normal LV function *Echocardiogram*: every 6–12 months for severe MR or if change in symptoms
Prosthetic valve	*General principles*: Evaluate and treat CAD risk factors Encourage routine dental care and optimal dental hygiene *Endocarditis prophylaxis for dental procedures* (*see text*)	*Medical management*: monitor anticoagulation with mechanical valves. Aspirin for bioprosthetic valves *Physical activity*: no limitations except as related to long term warfarin anticoagulation	*Clinical f/u*: annual evaluation with cardiology *Echocardiogram*: baseline after surgery, then only for changes in signs or symptoms with mechanical valves. After 5 years, annual studies may be considered for bioprosthetic valves

AR aortic regurgitation, *AS* aortic stenosis, *F/u* follow-up, *LV* left ventricle, *MPV* mitral valve prolapse, *MR* mitral regurgitation, *MS* mitral stenosis, *PAP* pulmonary arterial pressure, *RF* rheumatic fever
*General recommendations for all valve disease patients include optimal dental hygiene, evaluation and treatment of coronary disease risk factors, and patient education about the disease course to ensure early symptom reporting. Endocarditis prophylaxis is no longer recommended in patients with native valve disease. Currently there are no medical therapies to prevent progression of valve disease

Usually clinical history is adequate for detection of symptom onset, but a treadmill stress test can be used when symptoms are uncertain to identify an abnormal blood pressure response to exercise or exercise-related symptoms. Other indications for valve replacement can be found in Table 5.4.

Balloon valvotomy has no impact on mortality or morbidity in adults with AS and, therefore, is rarely indicated. Its use is reserved for children, young adults, and adults who are hemodynamically unstable or have serious morbid conditions either as a bridge to surgery or as palliative therapy. For patients with very high surgical mortality, the United States Food and Drug

Table 5.4 Surgical management of valvular heart disease

Valve	Indications for intervention[a]	Choice of intervention
Aortic stenosis	*Class I* Severe symptomatic AS Severe asymptomatic AS at time of CABG, aortic surgery, or other valve surgery Severe asymptomatic AS and an EF <50 % *Class II* Severe AS with hypotensive response to exercise Severe asymptomatic AS if surgery might be delayed or there is rapid progression "Extremely" severe asymptomatic AS (velocity >5 m/s or valve area <0.6 cm^2) Moderate AS at the time of CABG, aortic surgery, or other valve surgery	Aortic valve replacement Bioprosthetic valve in older adults or when anticoagulation in contraindicated Mechanical valve when longer durability is preferred Transcatheter valve implantation only in very high-risk patients
Mitral stenosis	*Class I* Symptomatic moderate or severe MS Asymptomatic moderate to severe MS if PASP >50 mmHg at rest or >60 mmHg with exercise *Class II* Asymptomatic moderate to severe MS with atrial fibrillation Asymptomatic moderate to severe MS with recurrent embolic stroke	Percutaneous mitral balloon valvotomy is preferred Mitral valve replacement only if valvotomy cannot be performed Mechanical usually preferred for durability because anticoagulation needed for concurrent AF
Aortic regurgitation	*Class I* Severe symptomatic AR Severe asymptomatic AR with EF <50 % Severe asymptomatic AR if undergoing CABG, surgery of the aorta, or other valves *Class II* Severe asymptomatic AR with ESD >55 mm or EDD >75 Severe asymptomatic AR with progressive dilation and ESD >50 mm and EDD >70 mm Moderate AR at the time of CABG or surgery of the aorta	Surgical aortic valve replacement Aortic valve repair only in selected cases at experienced valve centers
Mitral regurgitation	*Class I* Asymptomatic severe MR Asymptomatic severe MR with ESD >40 mm or EF <60 % *Class II* Asymptomatic severe MR when likelihood of repair is >90 % Asymptomatic severe MR with new onset atrial fibrillation Asymptomatic severe MR and PASP >50 mmHg at rest or >60 mmHg with exercise	Mitral valve repair is preferred Mitral valve replacement if repair is not possible

Class I indicates the procedure *should* be performed because the benefit clearly outweighs the risk based on current evidence. Class II indicated that the procedure *is reasonable* to perform; current data supports a favorable benefit to risk ratio but additional studies with focused objectives are needed

AS aortic stenosis, *CABG* coronary artery bypass graft surgery, *EF* ejection fraction, *EDD* end-diastolic dimension, *ESD* end-systolic dimension, *PASP* pulmonary arterial systolic pressure

[a]These recommendations are summarized from BONOW 2006 [35]

Administration has approved the transcatheter aortic valve implanted via the femoral artery or the LV apical approach. A randomized study showed that in patients who were not candidates for surgery, transcatheter valve was associated with higher survival at 1 year and decreased hospitalization compared with balloon valvuloplasty. In addition, in high-risk patients randomized to surgical versus transcatheter valve replacement, survival was similar at 1-year follow-up. Surgery was associated with a higher risk of bleeding complications, but transcatheter valve replacement was associated with a higher risk of stroke and vascular complications [15, 16].

Individuals with concurrent AS and LV systolic dysfunction represent a challenge. Some of these patients have only moderate AS, with a small calculated valve area due to low transvalvular flow secondary to primary LV dysfunction. Others have true severe AS with LV dysfunction due to high afterload. In order to differentiate these two entities, a low-dose dobutamine stress echocardiogram can be performed. If the AS aortic velocity increases to over 4 m/s and valve area remains less than 1.0 cm^2, true severe AS is present and valve replacement is appropriate [17]. This test will also provide information regarding contractile reserve, which is the ability to increase stroke volume by 20 %, which identifies patients with better outcomes after surgery.

Mitral Stenosis

Rheumatic carditis from beta-hemolytic streptococci accounts for nearly all mitral stenosis (MS) cases and is more prevalent in developing countries. Approximately 60 % of patients who have rheumatic fever will go on to develop valvular involvement with fusion of the commissures, leaflet thickening, and chordal fusion [18].

Prevalence of rheumatic MS is more common in females with a ratio of 2:1. Other less frequent causes of MS include mitral annular calcification, rheumatoid arthritis, systemic lupus erythematosus, congenital MS, and mucopolysaccharidoses.

Pathophysiology

The hallmark of MS is a decrease in mitral valve area; in order to move blood flow through the narrower orifice, a greater pressure gradient is needed. A higher diastolic transvalvular gradient increases left atrial filling pressure and is reflected to the pulmonary circulation leading to pulmonary hypertension and pulmonary edema due to the low pulmonary venous compliance. Patients with MS rely on atrial contraction to generate the increased transvalvular gradient and as such do not tolerate atrial fibrillation or atrioventricular dyssynchrony. Transvalvular gradient is dependent on transvalvular flow rate which is determined by the diastolic filling period. An increase in heart rate from exercise, pregnancy, or infection reduces the diastolic filling period and worsens the symptoms of MS.

With rheumatic MS, there is a long latency period without symptoms. The interval between acute rheumatic fever and symptomatic MS shows marked geographical variability, likely related to recurrent infection, ranging from only a few years in Africa to as long as 20–40 years in North America [19, 20]. Mortality is high once severe symptoms develop in MS patients with less than 15 % survival at 5 years unless the valve obstruction is relieved [19, 21].

Diagnosis

Typical symptoms of MS include dyspnea during exertion, orthopnea, paroxysmal nocturnal dyspnea, and fatigue. Rarely hemoptysis and hoarseness from severe left atrial dilatation may occur. Atrial arrhythmias, especially AF, due to severe left atrial dilatation may cause palpitations as the presenting symptom. On physical exam, MS is characterized by a diastolic murmur preceded by an opening snap that will be best heard at the apex. Duration but not intensity of the murmur correlates with MS severity.

Echocardiographic characteristics of rheumatic MS include reduced excursion of the valve leaflets, fusion of the commissures, and variable degrees of valve and chordal calcification. The left atrium is usually enlarged, sometimes massively, and there is a high risk of atrial thrombus, even in patients in sinus rhythm. Measurements of valve area, mean gradients, and pulmonary arterial systolic pressure will determine the severity of MS (see Table 5.2).

Management

Percutaneous balloon valvotomy is the main therapeutic option for symptomatic moderate or severe MS. Success with balloon valvotomy increases when the valve has favorable morphology by echocardiographic criteria, which include mobile leaflets with fusion only at the leaflet tips, mild valve thickening, mild chordal fusion and shortening, and minimal calcification.

Balloon valvotomy is recommended for moderate as well as severe MS because of its efficacy and relatively low risk as a nonsurgical intervention (see Table 5.3). Indications for mitral valve surgery include symptomatic moderate or severe MS when balloon valvotomy is not available or contraindicated due to left atrial clot, significant mitral regurgitation, or unfavorable valve morphology.

While awaiting surgical or percutaneous intervention, symptom relief can be achieved with diuresis if the patient has evidence of pulmonary edema, heart rate control with a beta blocker or calcium channel blocker, and avoiding physical stress that would result in tachycardia which is poorly tolerated.

In patients with previous rheumatic fever, antibiotic prophylaxis to avoid recurrent rheumatic fever is recommended. This secondary prophylaxis can be with penicillin G 1,200,000 U IM every 4 weeks, penicillin V 1 g oral daily, sulfadiazine 1 g oral daily, or, in those allergic to penicillin, a macrolide taken daily. The duration of secondary prophylaxis for rheumatic fever for those with carditis and residual valvular heart disease is 10 years or until 40 years of age; sometimes, lifelong prophylaxis is recommended if risk of reinfection is high [22].

Follow-up of patients that do not meet criteria for balloon valvotomy or valve replacement is outlined in Table 5.3.

Valve Regurgitation

Aortic Regurgitation

Aortic regurgitation (AR) is due either to intrinsic disease of the valve or to aortic root disease. Etiologies of valve-related AR include congenitally malformed valves (i.e., bicuspid valves), infective endocarditis, and rheumatic disease. AR from aortic root disease can occur with aortic dilatation due to a connective tissue disorder (i.e., Marfan syndrome), aortic dissection, or aortitis. The true prevalence of AR is unknown, but from echocardiographic studies the estimated prevalence of moderate AR is 0.8 % [23, 24].

Pathophysiology

Regurgitation of blood back into the LV in diastole results in increased LV preload, whereas ejection of an increased total stroke volume into the high resistance aorta results in increased LV wall tension or afterload. With chronic AR, the LV compensates by dilating while maintaining normal wall thickness and contractile function (e.g., eccentric hypertrophy). Compensatory LV dilation both increases total stroke volume, conserving effective forward stroke volume, and minimizes left ventricular end-diastolic pressure. With time, a subset of patients develops asymptomatic LV contractile dysfunction, emphasizing the importance of close clinical and echocardiographic follow-up to avoid irreversible LV dysfunction.

Diagnosis

Many patients present with an asymptomatic murmur and are followed for many years prior to symptom onset. Exercise intolerance may be the presenting symptom in some patients. In severe, symptomatic AR, the main symptoms are exertional dyspnea, orthopnea, and paroxysmal nocturnal dyspnea.

On exam, patients have a wide pulse pressure, hyperdynamic pulse, and a high-frequency blowing decrescendo diastolic murmur best heard at the left sternal border. There might be an associated mid systolic ejection murmur and a late diastolic rumble, known as an Austin Flint murmur. The intensity of S2 is often decreased. Peripheral findings due to the hyperdynamic pulse include pulsation in the retinal arteries and pupils (Becker's sign), capillary pulsations in the nail beds (Quincke's sign), systolic murmur over the femoral artery (Duroziez's sign), pulsation of the uvula (Muller's sign), and head bob with each heartbeat (De Musset's sign), among others.

Echocardiography provides information on the severity and mechanism of AR, degree of LV dilation, LV ejection fraction, and aortic dimensions. AR severity is assessed by color Doppler, in conjunction with evidence for diastolic flow reversal in the descending and abdominal aorta and the degree of LV dilation.

MRI can provide accurate quantification of regurgitant flow, regurgitant volumes, LV volumes, and ejection fraction, but this is usually reserved for patients with poor echocardiographic images or when aortic diameters need to be accurately determined.

Management

Medical management of chronic AR patients focuses on careful periodic clinical and echocardiographic evaluation to detect symptom onset and to evaluate for asymptomatic LV contractile dysfunction.

The main indication for surgery is severe symptomatic AR. In those who are asymptomatic, avoiding irreversible changes in the LV is critical. Thus, the criteria for surgery include LV end-systolic diameter of more than 55 mm and ejection fraction of less than 50 %. End-systolic LV dimension is thought to be a more reliable measurement since it is load independent. The only available treatment for AR is surgical valve replacement; repair is rarely possible and percutaneous approaches are not available. Thus, the threshold for intervention is higher than for valve lesions with effective percutaneous approaches (such as MS) or repair procedures (such as mitral regurgitation).

Medical management does not improve survival or morbidity and is used only for symptom relief in those who are not candidates for surgery. This includes diuresis to reduce pulmonary edema and vasodilators such as ACE inhibitors, angiotensin receptor blockers, or calcium channel blockers to reduce LV afterload.

Mitral Regurgitation

Mitral valve regurgitation (MR) either is due to primary valve pathology or is considered functional due to LV dilation and dysfunction with distortion of the normal relationship between the valve apparatus and the LV. The most common causes of primary MR are myxomatous mitral valve or mitral valve prolapse (MVP), endocarditis, and rheumatic heart disease. In the Framingham study, the prevalence of moderate MR was 1.6 %. The prevalence of MVP is estimated at 1–2.5 % in the general population [25, 26].

Pathophysiology

The hallmark of MR is regurgitant volume flowing into the low-pressure left atrium during systole. Compensatory mechanisms include a decrease in afterload or wall tension of the LV which will allow for more complete emptying of the LV lower end-systolic dimensions and an increase in preload with the dilated LV accommodating a larger total stroke volume. In addition, the left atrium enlarges to accommodate the regurgitant volume at a normal filling pressure. Initially, LV contractile function is preserved, but long term, LV contractile dysfunction occurs in some patients and may be obscured by the altered loading conditions with MR. Despite the limitations in clinical measures of LV systolic function, demonstration of contractile dysfunction is based on assessment of LV end-systolic dimensions and ejection fraction.

Diagnosis

Most patients with MR are diagnosed following detection of an asymptomatic murmur; symptomatic patients may present with pulmonary edema, dyspnea on exertion, and PND. On exam, a holosystolic murmur is heard at the apex that radiates to the axilla. Depending on the mechanism of regurgitation, the murmur may radiate to the back if the regurgitant jet is more posteriorly directed as in patients with anterior leaflet prolapse. When the jet is anteriorly directed (with posterior leaflet prolapse), the murmur may radiate to the left parasternal border or even the top of the head (Merendino's sign).

Echocardiography allows determination of the mechanism of regurgitation including prolapse, chordal rupture, vegetations, or LV dysfunction. Echocardiography also allows measurement of parameter keys to clinical decision-making, including LV size and systolic function, left atrial size, and pulmonary pressures. If severe MR is present but the LV and left atrium are not dilated, acute MR should be considered.

Management

The goal when monitoring patients with MR is to improve survival and preserve LV function. Periodic clinical and echocardiographic monitoring is recommended. In patients who develop AF, warfarin anticoagulation is recommended.

Criteria for valve surgery include severe symptomatic MR. In asymptomatic severe mitral regurgitation, the goal is to avoid irreversible LV dysfunction; LV end-systolic dimension should be followed since it is less influenced by loading conditions and thus is a more reliable measurement than end-diastolic LV dimension. Long-term outcomes after mitral valve surgery are known to be better when LV ejection fraction is >60 % and LV end-systolic diameter is <40 mm [27, 28].

There is no role for medical treatment in delaying progression or improving mortality in patients with primary MR. In adults with secondary or functional MR and LV dysfunction, afterload reduction may decrease regurgitation due to a reduction in LV size and improvement in systolic function. Biventricular pacing also may decrease the severity of functional MR. For ischemic MR, the primary focus is on treating the underlying coronary disease.

Acute Valvular Regurgitation

Acute valvular regurgitation is a surgical emergency and is associated with a high mortality if not identified and treated in a timely fashion. Hemodynamically, significant acute valvular regurgitation involves the aortic and mitral valves, whereas acute tricuspid and pulmonic valvular regurgitation are better tolerated. The etiology for acute valvular regurgitation includes infective endocarditis (IE), ischemic heart disease, blunt trauma, chordal rupture, prosthetic valve dysfunction, ascending aortic dissection, and iatrogenic from procedural complications. Acute MR may be primarily due to a structural disruption of the valve, such as spontaneous chordal rupture or endocarditis, and secondarily from an abnormality of the LV or associated structures with resultant valve dysfunction. Primary or valvular causes represent a surgical emergency while secondary etiologies treatment will be directed to the underlying disease process such as heart failure management or revascularization.

Pathophysiology

The pathophysiology of acute valvular regurgitation involves a sudden increase of volume into a LV that has not had time to adapt. This abrupt volume load into a small stiff chamber leads to a significant increase in end-diastolic pressure that is reflected into the pulmonary circulation causing acute increase in pulmonary pressures and pulmonary edema. Moreover, forward stroke volume is also decreased resulting in symptoms of low cardiac output, including heart failure and cardiogenic shock.

Diagnosis

Acute valvular regurgitation should be included in the differential diagnosis of all patients presenting with acute pulmonary edema, even when a cardiac cause is not initially suspected. Patients may present with shortness of breath and new onset of heart failure or cardiogenic shock or may be thought to have an acute pulmonary process. Chest pain may be the initial symptom with aortic dissection or an acute coronary syndrome. On physical exam, the murmur may not reflect the true severity of valvular dysfunction or might be absent because the low velocity flow across the valve does not generate a typical murmur. Other signs include tachycardia, diaphoresis, altered mental status, cool extremities, and pulmonary congestion.

Diagnosis depends on echocardiography where severe mitral or aortic regurgitation will be detected by color and Doppler flow imaging. Characteristics suggestive of acute regurgitation include valve vegetations, flail leaflets, aortic dissection, or simply the finding of significant regurgitation with a small LV. An exception to the finding of a non-dilated LV occurs in patients with acute or chronic regurgitation, such as mitral valve prolapse with chronic moderate regurgitation with new chordal rupture or endocarditis. Whenever acute regurgitation is seen without a clear mechanism, blood cultures should be obtained to evaluate for endocarditis.

Management

The only treatment for primary acute valvular regurgitation is prompt surgical intervention. Medical management is mainly used for hemodynamic stabilization of the patient while awaiting surgery. To decrease the regurgitant volume and improve forward stroke volume, afterload reduction with vasodilators such as nitroprusside is helpful in some cases. An intra-aortic balloon pump is helpful for stabilization with acute MR but is contraindicated with acute AR because regurgitation worsens with diastolic balloon inflation.

Right-Sided Valve Disease

Tricuspid Regurgitation

Tricuspid regurgitation (TR) of some degree is present in more than 80 % of echocardiograms but typically is mild and of no clinical significance [25]. More severe TR is associated with worse survival independent of biventricular systolic function [29]. The majority of pathological TR is from secondary causes such as LV dysfunction, right ventricular (RV) dilatation or dysfunction, pulmonary hypertension, severe mitral regurgitation, and pulmonary stenosis. Primary or intrinsic valvular causes of TR include Ebstein's anomaly, ventricular septal defects that damage the tricuspid valve, rheumatic valve disease, endocarditis, and iatrogenic from pacemaker or defibrillator implantation damaging or deforming the tricuspid valve.

Pathophysiology

Significant TR causes an increase in right atrial pressure that is translated into the systemic venous circulation leading to significant edema and liver congestion. To compensate for the increased volume, the RV enlarges with subsequent tricuspid annular dilatation and worsening TR generating a vicious cycle of more TR. RV volume overload and dilatation with time leads to RV dysfunction.

Diagnosis

Patients with isolated TR present with exercise intolerance, fatigue due to decreased cardiac output, and signs of right-sided heart failure such as edema, ascites, and congestive hepatopathy from high right atrial pressure.

The murmur of tricuspid regurgitation is a systolic murmur best heard at the left parasternal border with inspiratory accentuation. If TR is severe, marked V waves are seen in the jugular pulsation and a pulsatile liver may be identified.

On echocardiography, valve morphology, severity, and the mechanism of tricuspid regurgitation can be determined. By color and pulsed Doppler, the degree of TR is estimated taking into consideration that in functional TR, severity can be affected by loading conditions and afterload. Evidence of right ventricular and atrial dilatation suggests chronicity of TR. Finally, in patients in sinus rhythm, Doppler in the hepatic veins shows systolic flow reversal with severe TR.

Management

Outcomes with surgery for TR are suboptimal so that intervention is deferred unless severe symptomatic TR is refractory to medical therapy or when valve repair is likely. In addition, tricuspid annuloplasty or repair is recommended in patients with severe TR who are undergoing mitral valve surgery.

Tricuspid Stenosis

Tricuspid stenosis (TS) is rare and it is usually secondary to rheumatic disease, occurring in about 9 % of patients with rheumatic mitral valve disease. Carcinoid syndrome also can cause tricuspid stenosis, although regurgitation is more common.

Pathophysiology

In TS there is a diastolic pressure gradient between the right atrium and RV that raises right atrial pressure causing systemic venous congestion with resultant hepatic congestion, ascites, and edema. Due to the fixed valve area and fixed cardiac output, patients present with fatigue.

Diagnosis

Symptoms of TS include edema, ascites, fatigue, and decreased exercise capacity. On physical exam there is a tricuspid opening snap with a diastolic crescendo-decrescendo murmur best heard in the lower left parasternal border augmented with inspiration. Jugular venous distention is present reflecting the elevated right atrial pressure.

Management

Diuresis decreases congestive symptoms, but the ultimate therapy will be surgical open valvotomy or valve replacement if open valvotomy does not yield good results.

Pulmonic Stenosis

Pulmonic stenosis is rare and usually congenital. The management consist of balloon valvotomy unless it is associated with subvalvular or supravalvular stenosis where surgery might be needed.

Pulmonic Regurgitation

The majority of isolated pulmonary regurgitation (PR) cases are from congenital heart disease. Most PR will be secondary to tetralogy of Fallot repair, especially when a transannular patch is placed at the time of repair or after balloon valvotomy for pulmonic stenosis. Rarely there will be isolated PR related to endocarditis.

Pathophysiology

Although previously thought to be benign, PR is now recognized as deleterious due to volume overload of the RV, RV dilatation that leads to RV failure, and increased risk for ventricular arrhythmias [30].

Diagnosis

Symptoms of PR include fatigue and peripheral edema. On exam there is wide splitting of S2 and a midsystolic ejection murmur best heard in the 2nd left intercostal space. The main diagnostic modality for evaluating PR is echocardiography, with magnetic resonance imaging used when accurate assessment of right ventricular volumes and function is needed.

Treatment

Indications for surgery include severe symptomatic PR or severe asymptomatic PR with significant RV enlargement and systolic dysfunction. Valve replacement with a bioprosthetic valve is the preferred treatment, which may be via a surgical or transcatheter approach.

Prosthetic Valves

The type of valve implanted at the time of surgery will depend on age of the patient, valve affected, lifestyle, comorbidities, and patient preference.

Mechanical valves are characterized by their longevity with a durability of 20–30 years compared to bioprostheses that have 10- to 15-year durability [31, 32]. The durability of a bioprosthesis is dependent on a patient's age such that patients more than 65 years old tend to have lower rates of primary bioprosthetic valve failure compared to those less than 65 [31]. Mechanical valves, although durable, are more thrombogenic with an annual risk of thrombosis of 1.4 % compared to 0.87 % with a bioprosthesis and, thus, require lifelong anticoagulation with warfarin [33].

Current guidelines recommend anticoagulation with warfarin for mechanical valves with a goal INR of 2–3 for bileaflet or tilting disc aortic valves and 2.5–3.5 for cage and ball aortic valves or any type of valve in the mitral position. If there is high risk of thromboembolic complications, the target INR may be raised and aspirin can be added. For bioprosthetic valves, anticoagulation is recommended with warfarin for the first 3 months although many centers use only aspirin anticoagulation for this type of valve.

For "bridging" anticoagulation at the time of surgical interventions, in procedures with low bleeding risk, it may be appropriate to continue anticoagulation. When interruption of warfarin therapy is needed, heparin is recommended during the time period of a subtherapeutic INR. If there is history of prior thromboembolism, AF, hypercoagulable condition, older-generation mechanical valves, or a mechanical valve in the mitral or tricuspid position, heparin is started when the INR falls below 2, then is stopped for 4–6 h before surgery and resumed postoperatively as soon as bleeding risk allows. For mechanical valves in the aortic position with no other risk factors, bridging is not required. In these lower risk patients, warfarin is stopped 48–72 h before the procedure and then restarted 24 h later. Most guidelines recommend intravenous heparin for bridging therapy, but some centers use subcutaneous low molecular weight heparin with close monitoring of levels. Although currently the only anticoagulant that has been studied and approved for anticoagulation of patients with mechanical prostheses is warfarin, ongoing trials of new anticoagulants might change practice in the future.

Clinical follow-up of patients with prosthetic valves is recommended yearly with echocardiography once after surgery and a subsequent echocardiogram only if there is a change in symptoms or physical exam. Patient education is important during clinical visits emphasizing anticoagulation compliance, good dental hygiene, antibiotic prophylaxis prior to dental procedures, and the need to obtain blood cultures if there is ever a concern for bloodstream infections.

Endocarditis Prophylaxis

In patients with prosthetic valves, antibiotic prophylaxis against endocarditis is recommended prior to dental procedures that involve manipulation of the gingival tissue, periapical region, or perforation of the oral mucosa [34]. The guidelines recommend against antibiotic prophylaxis for gastrointestinal or genitourinary procedures unless there is associated infections of these organs. The recommended antimicrobial regimen for those without penicillin allergy is amoxicillin 2 g oral or ampicillin 2 g IM or IV 30 min–1 h prior to the procedure. For those allergic to penicillin, cephalexin 2 g oral, clindamycin 600 mg oral, azithromycin 500 mg oral, clarithromycin 500 mg oral, ceftriaxone 1 g IV or IM, cefazolin 1 g IV or IM, or clindamycin 600 mg IV or IM can be used.

Key Points

- Calcific aortic stenosis is the main etiology of valvular AS. Common symptoms of severe AS are exercise intolerance and dyspnea on exertion. Treatment for severe symptomatic AS is aortic valve replacement.
- Most MS is secondary to rheumatic heart disease. Patients with rheumatic MS should receive secondary prophylaxis to avoid another episode of rheumatic fever. Balloon valvotomy is indicated for moderate to severe symptomatic MS.
- Common etiologies of acute valvular regurgitation include endocarditis, spontaneous chordal rupture, ischemia, and prosthetic valve dysfunction. Acute severe valve regurgitation is a surgical emergency.
- Congenitally abnormal valves and aortic root disease are the main causes of AR. Aortic valve replacement is indicated in severe symptomatic AR.
- In asymptomatic AR, close monitoring with intervention when EF <50 % or LV end-systolic dimension of >55 mm is important to avoid irreversible LV changes.
- The main etiologies of chronic primary mitral regurgitation are mitral valve prolapse and rheumatic heart disease. Mitral valve repair or surgical valve replacement is indicated in severe symptomatic MR.
- In asymptomatic severe MR with EF <60 % or LV end-systolic dimension of >40 mm, repair or replacement is indicated in order to preserve LV function.
- Mechanical valves are very durable but require lifelong anticoagulation with warfarin. Bioprosthetic valves have limited durability with valve longevity inversely related to patient age.

References

1. Nkomo VT, Gardin JM, Skelton TN, Gottdiener JS, Scott CG, Enriquez-Sarano M. Burden of valvular heart diseases: a population-based study. Lancet. 2006;368:1005–11.
2. Roberts WC, Ko JM. Frequency by decades of unicuspid, bicuspid, and tricuspid aortic valves in adults having isolated aortic valve replacement for aortic stenosis, with or without associated aortic regurgitation. Circulation. 2005;111:920–5.
3. Stewart BF, Siscovick D, Lind BK, Gardin JM, Gottdiener JS, Smith VE, Kitzman DW, Otto CM. Clinical factors associated with calcific aortic valve disease. Cardiovascular Health Study. J Am Coll Cardiol. 1997;29:630–4.
4. Otto CM, Lind BK, Kitzman DW, Gersh BJ, Siscovick DS. Association of aortic-valve sclerosis with cardiovascular mortality and morbidity in the elderly. N Engl J Med. 1999;341:142–7.
5. Miller JD, Weiss RM, Heistad DD. Calcific aortic valve stenosis: methods, models, and mechanisms. Circ Res. 2011;108:1392–412.
6. Katz R, Wong ND, Kronmal R, Takasu J, Shavelle DM, Probstfield JL, Bertoni AG, Budoff MJ, O'Brien KD. Features of the metabolic syndrome and diabetes mellitus as predictors of aortic valve calcification in the Multi-Ethnic Study of Atherosclerosis. Circulation. 2006;113:2113–9.
7. Otto CM. Valvular aortic stenosis: disease severity and timing of intervention. J Am Coll Cardiol. 2006;47:2141–51.
8. Rosenhek R, Klaar U, Schemper M, Scholten C, Heger M, Gabriel H, Binder T, Maurer G, Baumgartner H. Mild and moderate aortic stenosis. Natural history and risk stratification by echocardiography. Eur Heart J. 2004;25:199–205.
9. Otto CM, Burwash IG, Legget ME, Munt BI, Fujioka M, Healy NL, Kraft CD, Miyake-Hull CY, Schwaegler RG. Prospective study of asymptomatic valvular aortic stenosis. Clinical, echocardiographic, and exercise predictors of outcome. Circulation. 1997;95:2262–70.
10. Rosenhek R, Binder T, Porenta G, Lang I, Christ G, Schemper M, Maurer G, Baumgartner H. Predictors of outcome in severe, asymptomatic aortic stenosis. N Engl J Med. 2000;343:611–7.
11. Cowell SJ, Newby DE, Prescott RJ, Bloomfield P, Reid J, Northridge DB, Boon NA. Scottish Aortic Stenosis and Lipid Lowering Trial IpoRSI. A randomized trial of intensive lipid-lowering therapy in calcific aortic stenosis. N Engl J Med. 2005;352:2389–97.
12. Dichtl W, Alber HF, Feuchtner GM, Hintringer F, Reinthaler M, Bartel T, Süssenbacher A, Grander W, Ulmer H, Pachinger O, Müller S. Prognosis and risk factors in patients with asymptomatic aortic stenosis and their modulation by atorvastatin (20 mg). Am J Cardiol. 2008;102:743–8.
13. van der Linde D, Yap SC, van Dijk AP, Budts W, Pieper PG, van der Burgh PH, Mulder BJ, Witsenburg M, Cuypers JA, Lindemans J, Takkenberg JJ, Roos-Hesselink JW. Effects of rosuvastatin on progression of stenosis in adult patients with congenital aortic stenosis (PROCAS Trial). Am J Cardiol. 2011;108:265–71.
14. Chan KL, Teo K, Dumesnil JG, Ni A, Tam J, Investigators A. Effect of lipid lowering with rosuvastatin on progression of aortic stenosis: results of the aortic stenosis progression observation: measuring effects of rosuvastatin (ASTRONOMER) trial. Circulation. 2010;121:306–14.
15. Leon MB, Smith CR, Mack M, Miller DC, Moses JW, Svensson LG, Tuzcu EM, Webb JG, Fontana GP, Makkar RR, Brown DL, Block PC, Guyton RA, Pichard AD, Bavaria JE, Herrmann HC, Douglas PS, Petersen JL, Akin JJ, Anderson WN, Wang D, Pocock S, Investigators PT. Transcatheter aortic-valve implantation for aortic stenosis in patients who cannot undergo surgery. N Engl J Med. 2010;363:1597–607.
16. Smith CR, Leon MB, Mack MJ, Miller DC, Moses JW, Svensson LG, Tuzcu EM, Webb JG, Fontana GP, Makkar RR, Williams M, Dewey T, Kapadia S, Babaliaros V, Thourani VH, Corso P, Pichard AD, Bavaria JE, Herrmann HC, Akin JJ, Anderson WN, Wang D, Pocock SJ, Investigators PT. Transcatheter versus surgical aortic-valve replacement in high-risk patients. N Engl J Med. 2011;364:2187–98.
17. Baumgartner H, Hung J, Bermejo J, Chambers JB, Evangelista A, Griffin BP, Iung B, Otto CM, Pellikka PA, Quiñones M. Echocardiography ASo, Echocardiography EAo. Echocardiographic assessment of valve stenosis: EAE/ASE recommendations for clinical practice. J Am Soc Echocardiogr. 2009;22:1–23; quiz 101–2.
18. Carapetis JR, Steer AC, Mulholland EK, Weber M. The global burden of group A streptococcal diseases. Lancet Infect Dis. 2005;5:685–94.
19. Horstkotte D, Niehues R, Strauer BE. Pathomorphological aspects, aetiology and natural history of acquired mitral valve stenosis. Eur Heart J. 1991;12 Suppl B:55–60.
20. Series WTR. Rheumatic fever and rheumatic heart disease: report of a WHO expert panel. Geneva: WHO; 2004.
21. Rowe JC, Bland EF, Sprague HB, White PD. The course of mitral stenosis without surgery: ten- and twenty-year perspectives. Ann Intern Med. 1960;52:741–9.
22. Gerber MA, Baltimore RS, Eaton CB, Gewitz M, Rowley AH, Shulman ST, Taubert KA. Prevention of rheumatic fever and diagnosis and treatment of acute Streptococcal pharyngitis: a scientific statement from the American Heart Association Rheumatic Fever, Endocarditis, and Kawasaki Disease Committee of the Council on Cardiovascular Disease in the Young, the Interdisciplinary Council on Functional Genomics and Translational Biology, and the Interdisciplinary Council on Quality of Care and Outcomes Research: endorsed by the American Academy of Pediatrics. Circulation. 2009;119:1541–51.
23. Roberts WC, Ko JM, Moore TR, Jones WH. Causes of pure aortic regurgitation in patients having isolated aortic valve replacement at a single US tertiary hospital (1993 to 2005). Circulation. 2006;114:422–9.
24. Reid CL, Anton-Culver H, Yunis C, Gardin JM. Prevalence and clinical correlates of isolated mitral, isolated aortic regurgitation, and both in adults aged 21 to 35 years (from the CARDIA study). Am J Cardiol. 2007;99:830–4.
25. Singh JP, Evans JC, Levy D, Larson MG, Freed LA, Fuller DL, Lehman B, Benjamin EJ. Prevalence and clinical determinants of mitral, tricuspid, and aortic regurgitation (the Framingham Heart Study). Am J Cardiol. 1999;83:897–902.
26. Freed LA, Levy D, Levine RA, Larson MG, Evans JC, Fuller DL, Lehman B, Benjamin EJ. Prevalence and clinical outcome of mitral-valve prolapse. N Engl J Med. 1999;341:1–7.
27. Enriquez-Sarano M, Tajik AJ, Schaff HV, Orszulak TA, Bailey KR, Frye RL. Echocardiographic prediction of survival after surgical correction of organic mitral regurgitation. Circulation. 1994;90:830–7.
28. Wisenbaugh T, Skudicky D, Sareli P. Prediction of outcome after valve replacement for rheumatic mitral regurgitation in the era of chordal preservation. Circulation. 1994;89:191–7.
29. Nath J, Foster E, Heidenreich PA. Impact of tricuspid regurgitation on long-term survival. J Am Coll Cardiol. 2004;43:405–9.
30. Huehnergarth KV, Gurvitz M, Stout KK, Otto CM. Repaired tetralogy of Fallot in the adult: monitoring and management. Heart. 2008;94:1663–9.
31. Hammermeister K, Sethi GK, Henderson WG, Grover FL, Oprian C, Rahimtoola SH. Outcomes 15 years after valve replacement with a mechanical versus a bioprosthetic valve: final report of the Veterans Affairs randomized trial. J Am Coll Cardiol. 2000;36:1152–8.

32. O'Brien MF, Stafford EG, Gardner MA, Pohlner PG, Tesar PJ, Kear L, Smith SE. The Medtronic Intact xenograft: an analysis of 342 patients over a seven-year follow-up period. Ann Thorac Surg. 1995;60:S253–7.

33. van Geldorp MW, Eric Jamieson WR, Kappetein AP, Ye J, Fradet GJ, Eijkemans MJ, Grunkemeier GL, Bogers AJ, Takkenberg JJ. Patient outcome after aortic valve replacement with a mechanical or biological prosthesis: weighing lifetime anticoagulant-related event risk against reoperation risk. J Thorac Cardiovasc Surg. 2009;137:881–6, 886e1–5.

34. Nishimura RA, Carabello BA, Faxon DP, Freed MD, Lytle BW, O'Gara PT, O'Rourke RA, Shah PM. ACC/AHA 2008 guideline update on valvular heart disease: focused update on infective endocarditis: a report of the American College of Cardiology/ American Heart Association Task Force on Practice Guidelines endorsed by the Society of Cardiovascular Anesthesiologists, Society for Cardiovascular Angiography and Interventions, and Society of Thoracic Surgeons. J Am Coll Cardiol. 2008;52: 676–85.

35. Bonow RO, Carabello BA, Chatterjee K et al. ACC/AHA 2006 guidelines for the management of patients with valvular heart disease: a report of the American College of Cardiology/American Heart Association Task Force on Practice Guidelines (writing Committee to Revise the 1998 guidelines for the management of patients with valvular heart disease) developed in collaboration with the Society of Cardiovascular Anesthesiologist endorsed by the Society for Cardiovascular Angiography and Interventions and the Society of Thoracic Surgeons. J Am Coll Cardiol. 2006;48:e1–148.

Infective Endocarditis

Todd L. Kiefer and Andrew Wang

Abstract

Infective endocarditis is defined as infection of a heart valve or other cardiac tissue. This diagnosis has broadened beyond infections involving native cardiac tissue or prosthetic heart valves to include infections of implanted intracardiac devices. Despite progress in the ability to accurately diagnose infective endocarditis in the modern era, the outcomes are still quite poor with respect to its associated morbidity and mortality. The focus of this chapter will be to review the pathophysiology, diagnosis, and guideline-focused management of infective endocarditis and intracardiac device infections. In addition, the current recommendations for antibiotic prophylaxis of infective endocarditis will be reviewed.

Keywords

Infective endocarditis • Intracardiac device infection • Surgery • Valve disease • Antimicrobial therapy • Prophylaxis

Introduction

Infective endocarditis was first described in the seventeenth century by Lazarus Riverius [1]. The history of medicine is replete with descriptions of the many complications associated with infective endocarditis. The technological advances of modern medicine have improved our ability to diagnose infective endocarditis. But its associated morbidity and mortality remain high, including the need for cardiac surgery in approximately 50 % of cases, in-hospital mortality of 15–20 %, and 1-year mortality of 30–40 % in modern observational series [2].

T.L. Kiefer, MD (✉)
Department of Cardiology,
Duke University Medical Center,
2301 Erwin Road, 7412A Duke North,
DUMC Box 3126, Durham, NC 27712, USA
e-mail: todd.kiefer@duke.edu

A. Wang, MD
Department of Medicine,
Duke University Hospital, DUMC 3428,
Durham, NC 27710, USA
e-mail: a.wang@duke.edu

From an epidemiologic perspective, endocarditis is uncommon with an incidence of 3–9 episodes/100,000 person-years [3, 4]. Although the incidence of endocarditis has remained stable over recent decades, the epidemiology has shifted toward more virulent causative organisms (*Staphylococcus aureus*) and older hosts with increased comorbid medical problems. A number of patient characteristics have been associated with the development of infective endocarditis. Infective endocarditis is more common in men than women with a gender ratio of 3–9:1 [5–7]. Intravenous drug abuse (IVDA) is associated with tricuspid valve and, also, left-sided valvular infective endocarditis, even in the absence of underlying valve disease [8]. There has also been an increase in the incidence of endocarditis in the elderly population with one study showing 20 episodes/100,000 person-years in the Medicare population [9]. Although a high percentage of patients has some form of valvular or congenital structural heart disease predisposing them to development of infective endocarditis [10, 11], infection of apparently normal native valves may develop from virulent organisms. A variety of conditions are associated with acquisition of infective endocarditis such as poor dentition, immunosuppression, liver cirrhosis, malignancies, or solid

K. Stergiopoulos, D.L. Brown (eds.), *Evidence-Based Cardiology Consult*,
DOI 10.1007/978-1-4471-4441-0_6, © Springer-Verlag London 2014

organ transplant [12]. Increasingly, exposure to medical care such as hemodialysis, indwelling central venous catheters, and outpatient medical care, termed health-care-associated infection, is recognized as contributing to endocarditis in approximately one-third of cases.

The aortic valve is the most commonly infected valve (38 % of cases) [13]. This is followed closely by the mitral valve which is involved in 34 % of cases [13]. Isolated tricuspid valve endocarditis is less common but is linked to IVDA, chronic hemodialysis, and the presence of pacemaker or ICD leads that cross the valve [13].

Pathophysiology

The basis for the development of infective endocarditis is endothelial damage. This initial lesion promotes the deposition of fibrin and platelets to which bacteria or fungal microorganisms may adhere. Common locations of endothelial injury are valve coaptation sites, with the atrial side of the mitral and tricuspid valves and the ventricular side of the aortic and pulmonary valves most commonly affected [14]. In addition, endothelial damage and subsequent infective endocarditis may occur at sites of turbulent jet lesions such as the left atrial wall with mitral regurgitation, the mitral chordal apparatus with aortic regurgitation, or the septal leaflet of the tricuspid valve with a ventricular septal defect [14]. The hallmark lesion of infective endocarditis, an infected vegetation, results from this process of microorganism attachment to platelet-fibrin complexes in areas of endothelial damage.

Any underlying cardiac abnormality serves as a host factor associated with the microbiology of endocarditis. Native valve infective endocarditis is most commonly caused by *Staphylococcus, Streptococcus, or Enterococcus* species [15]. Much less frequent are cases of infective endocarditis caused by HACEK (Haemophilus, Actinobacillus, Cardiobacterium, Eikenella, Kingella species) organisms or gram-negative bacilli. As mentioned previously, IVDA is a strong risk factor for developing endocarditis, and the vast majority (>80 %) of IVDA-associated tricuspid valve infections are caused by *S. aureus* [15]. *S. aureus* is also associated with infection of normal heart valves in the absence of predisposing lesion.

The microbiology of prosthetic valve endocarditis is a function of the time interval since valve surgery. The three categories are early (<2 months), mid (2–12 months), and late (>12 months) after valve replacement [16]. Nosocomial organisms, such as *S. aureus*, coagulase-negative species, and gram-negative bacilli, account for the majority of cases of early prosthetic valve infective endocarditis [16]. Midterm prosthetic valve endocarditis infections are a mixture of nosocomial organisms and microorganisms that are commonly associated with native valve infective endocarditis [16]. The microbiology of late prosthetic valve infective endocarditis is quite similar to that

seen with native valve infections with *Staphylococcus* species, Viridans Streptococci, and *Enterococcus* species responsible for the vast majority of cases [16].

Finally, intracardiac device-related infective endocarditis with implanted defibrillators and pacemakers is increasing in incidence [17, 18]. The majority of these cases are caused by *Staphylococcus* species (coagulase-negative *Staphylococci* or *S. aureus*) [19].

Diagnosis

The diagnosis of infective endocarditis can be challenging as many other infections and systemic processes have similar clinical manifestations. Fever is the most common symptom reported on presentation in 60–90 % of patients [20]. The detection of a heart murmur with auscultation is reported in 80–85 % of patients with confirmed infective endocarditis [16]. On physical examination, classic cutaneous sequelae of infective endocarditis such as Janeway lesions, splinter hemorrhages, conjunctival/mucosal hemorrhage, and the tender Osler's nodes related to an underlying immunologic reaction may be found but are not sensitive diagnostic findings. Sustained bacteremia with an organism typical for infective endocarditis is present in approximately 90 % of cases, so multiple sets of blood cultures should be drawn before administering antibiotics to a patient with suspected endocarditis.

Given the protean manifestations of this condition, several case definitions have been developed to aid in correctly diagnosing patients with infective endocarditis. The most validated criteria are the Duke Criteria originally proposed in 1994 [21] and later modified to improve sensitivity. Since that time the diagnostic algorithm has been revised and validated in multiple populations [22–27]. The Duke Criteria consists of major and minor criteria (Table 6.1). The major criteria include positive blood cultures with a characteristic microorganism and evidence for endocardial infection. The minor criteria provide supporting clinical evidence of infective endocarditis based on predisposing conditions, immunologic, and/or vascular manifestations. A diagnosis of *definite endocarditis* is made if 2 major criteria, 1 major and 3 minor criteria, 5 minor criteria or pathologic evidence are present [25]. A diagnosis of *possible endocarditis* is made if 1 major and 1 minor or 3 minor criteria are present [25]. Finally, a diagnosis of *rejected endocarditis* is made when there is a complete resolution of the clinical features suggesting endocarditis with ≤4 days of antibiotic therapy and absence of pathologic evidence for endocarditis on a surgical or autopsy specimen with ≤4 days of antibiotic therapy or an alternative diagnosis has been made [25].

Echocardiography is critical to the diagnosis and evaluation of patients with suspected or definite infective endocarditis. This is reflected by the echocardiographic

Table 6.1 Modified Duke Criteria for the diagnosis of infective endocarditis

Major	Growth of typical bacterium from two separate blood cultures
	Viridans Streptococci
	Streptococcus bovis
	HACEK organism
	Staphylococcus aureus
	Community-acquired enterococci
	Persistent blood culture growth with a bacterium consistent with IE:
	Two positive blood cultures >12 h apart
	3 of 3 or a majority of ≥4 blood cultures
	Coxiella burnetii IgG titer >1:800 or growth from blood culture
	Echocardiographic evidence:
	Oscillating mass
	Intracardiac abscess
	New prosthetic valve dehiscence
	New murmur of valve regurgitation
	Endocardial involvement
Minor	Fever greater than 38 °C
	Predisposing condition:
	I.V. drug abuse
	Prior valve disease
	Immunologic manifestation:
	Roth's spots
	Osler's nodes
	Positive rheumatoid factor serology
	Glomerulonephritis
	Vascular manifestation:
	Janeway lesion
	Embolic event
	Intracranial hemorrhage
	Mycotic aneurysm
	Microbiologic data not satisfying the major criteria

features listed as a major criterion of the Duke Criteria. The diagnostic utility of transthoracic (TTE) and transesophageal echocardiography (TEE) has been evaluated in multiple studies. The sensitivity of TTE for the detection of vegetations is approximately 40 % [28]. The sensitivity of TTE for the detection of tricuspid valve vegetations is the highest given the proximity of the tricuspid valve to the chest wall. As expected, the diagnostic utility of TTE is greatest in patients with the greater pretest probability (intermediate to high likelihood) of having infective endocarditis [21]. It should be noted that a TTE examination that fails to document vegetations does not conclusively exclude the diagnosis of endocarditis.

TEE provides greater spatial imaging resolution and, thus, higher sensitivity and specificity to detect smaller vegetations and other anatomic findings of endocarditis. A TEE should be pursued in patients with high pretest probability of endocarditis, such as patients with a prosthetic heart valve, persistent *Staphylococcus* bacteremia without a clear source of infection, and suspected cardiac implantable electronic device (CIED) endocarditis or patients with a high pretest probability but a negative TTE study [29–32]. An algorithm to guide the use of TTE and/or TEE in the evaluation of suspected infective endocarditis is illustrated in Fig. 6.1. TEE may also offer better assessment of valvular regurgitation severity and mechanism, particularly for mitral valve endocarditis, and help guide the decision for surgical treatment.

Based upon the available evidence and expert opinion, guideline statements for the use of echocardiography in the evaluation of suspected infective endocarditis have been published. The Class I American College of Cardiology/American Heart Association (ACC/AHA) indications for transthoracic echocardiography related to endocarditis are for the detection of vegetations, to assess valve and ventricular function in patients with definite endocarditis, to diagnose mechanical cardiac complications of endocarditis, and for the repeat imaging of patients with definite infective endocarditis [15]. The Class I ACC/AHA indications for transesophageal echocardiography (TEE) are in the evaluation of patients with inconclusive TTE findings with symptomatic infective endocarditis, for diagnostic evidence in patients with suspected endocarditis and equivocal TTE findings, for the evaluation of mechanical cardiac complications, to evaluate suspected prosthetic valve endocarditis, and in the preoperative and intraoperative evaluation of definite infective endocarditis [15].

Management

Given the significant morbidity and mortality associated with infective endocarditis, it is imperative to initiate appropriate empiric antimicrobial therapy as soon as the diagnosis is considered. However, in order to accurately diagnose endocarditis, it is necessary to obtain the requisite blood culture samples prior to starting antibiotic therapy. Initial empiric antibiotic selections can be narrowed based upon blood culture and sensitivity data and also input from infectious diseases consultation.

Detailed empiric and culture-specific antimicrobial treatment regimens have been defined based on a synthesis of the available clinical data and expert opinion in several society guidelines [15, 33]. The various antimicrobial regimens for a broad range of different infections are delineated in these documents [15, 33]. Native valve infective endocarditis is usually treated for 4 weeks with intravenous antimicrobial therapy, whereas prosthetic valve infective endocarditis is managed with 6 weeks of intravenous antibiotic therapy. After initial inpatient therapy, selected patients can be successfully treated with outpatient intravenous antibiotic infusion. This approach utilizing outpatient antibiotic management has

Fig. 6.1 Algorithm for the use of echocardiography in the diagnosis and management of infective endocarditis

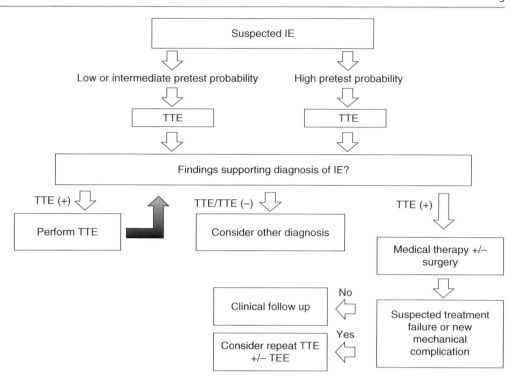

demonstrated success in the management of patients with Staphylococcal, Streptococcal, and Enterococcal infective endocarditis [34–37].

The issue of anticoagulation often arises in the care of a patient with infective endocarditis. There is controversy with respect to this issue since no randomized clinical trial data exists to guide management. Older observational data suggests that there is a higher mortality due to neurologic complications in patients receiving anticoagulation [38]. However, more recent prospective cohort data analysis reported no increase in cerebrovascular complications in patients on anticoagulant therapy [39]. In many centers, the standard of care is to discontinue chronic warfarin therapy at the time of endocarditis diagnosis and then initiate unfractionated heparin when the international normalized ratio (INR) is less than 2.0. Furthermore, warfarin can usually be restarted after 7 days of antibiotic therapy if valve surgery is not anticipated. If intracranial hemorrhage occurs and valve surgery is indicated, the Society of Thoracic Surgeons (STS) Clinical practice guidelines advise waiting at least 4 weeks to pursue valve surgery [40].

Infective endocarditis is associated with a variety of clinical complications affecting multiple organ systems. Congestive heart failure related to valve dysfunction is the most common, occurring in one-third to one-half of cases [2, 41]. Systemic embolization with central nervous system embolic stroke, along with embolism to the liver, kidneys, spleen, extremities, vertebral arteries, and the coronary arteries, also complicates many cases of endocarditis. Subclinical embolic events are also common in

patients with definite infective endocarditis with brain magnetic resonance imaging (MRI) showing evidence of cerebral infarction 30–48 % of patients [42, 43]. Embolic events are more common with mitral valve than aortic valve endocarditis [44, 45]. Septic pulmonary embolism may occur in cases of tricuspid valve endocarditis. Other well-characterized cardiac complications of endocarditis include paravalvular abscess formation, valve leaflet perforation, fistula formation, and prosthetic valve dehiscence. Inflammatory and immune-mediated complications such as glomerulonephritis, arthritis, and tenosynovitis are seen in many patients.

Valve surgery is integral to the treatment of patients with endocarditis who develop these complications or have a poor response to antibiotic therapy. This is also another area where large randomized clinical trial data is lacking. There are, however, several observational analyses that examine the utility of valve surgery in patients with infective endocarditis. A statistically significant mortality benefit for valve surgery in patients with infective endocarditis at 6-month follow-up has been demonstrated for patients with moderate to severe heart failure [46], the most common indication for surgery in endocarditis. A recent publication reported on the variables associated with in-hospital and 1-year mortality using a prospective, multicenter cohort of patients with infective endocarditis [5]. This work analyzed data from 4,075 patients with definite infective endocarditis with 1,359 patients designated as having New York Heart Association (NYHA) Class I–IV heart failure using multivariate analysis with and without propensity score adjustment [5].

Table 6.2 Class I ACC/AHA recommendations for valve surgery in patients with native or prosthetic valve infective endocarditis

Symptomatic heart failure from valve dysfunction (stenosis or regurgitation)

Fungal IE or infection with other antimicrobial resistant organism

Mechanical or anatomic complications of endocarditis:

　Acute mitral or aortic regurgitation with evidence of increased left atrial or left ventricular end-diastolic pressures

　Abscess, including new high-grade atrioventricular (AV) node block

　Valve leaflet perforation

　Fistula

　Prosthetic valve dehiscence

Table 6.3 Class I ACC/AHA recommendations for the management of cardiac implantable electronic device (CIED) infections and CIED-related infective endocarditis

Diagnosis of CIED infection:

　Obtain two sets of blood cultures prior to initiation of antimicrobial therapy

　Gram's stain and culture of generator pocket tissue and lead tip at explant

　TEE with positive blood cultures or negative cultures and recent antibiotic administration

　TEE for careful evaluation of left-sided heart valves for evidence of concomitant valvular infective endocarditis

Management:

　Isolated pocket infection: 10–14 days of antibiotic therapy after removal of device

　Bacteremia and a device-related infection: minimum of 14 days after removal of device

　Device-related endocarditis: 4–6 weeks of antibiotic therapy

　Device and lead extraction:

　　Definite CIED infection with a complicated pocket infection and abscess/erosion/or sinus tract even without evidence of lead infection

　　Valvular infective endocarditis even in the absence of obvious lead or device infection

　　Unexplained *Staphylococcus* bacteremia

　New device implantation:

　　Assess need for intracardiac device

　　Place new device at a site distant from prior device

Once again, valve surgery during the index hospitalization was statistically associated with decreased in-hospital and 1-year mortality [5].

Other studies have used propensity score methodology to adjust for differences between patients treated with antibiotics only versus antibiotics and surgery and have found that surgery was associated with lower mortality [47]. Another prospective, multicenter, international registry data analysis of 1,552 patients with native valve infective endocarditis using propensity matching, survivor bias adjustment, and instrumental variable adjustment also showed a statistically significant mortality benefit for valve surgery during the initial hospitalization compared with antibiotic therapy alone [48].

Based on these observational data and expert clinical opinion, guidelines have been published by professional societies to identify patients who may benefit from valve surgery for infective endocarditis. The ACC/AHA Valvular Heart Disease Management Guidelines are summarized in Table 6.2 [15]. Surgical valve replacement should be considered for patients with a mobile vegetation greater than 10 mm, recurrent embolic events, or for organisms resistant to standard antimicrobial therapy. The STS guidelines recommend mitral and tricuspid valve repair (Class I), if feasible, over valve replacement for patients who undergo valve surgery for infective endocarditis [40].

Finally, there is data to support the use of a multidisciplinary management strategy employing professional society guidelines and infectious diseases, cardiology, and cardiac surgery consultation. Using this algorithm, a statistically significant decrease in renal failure, multisystem organ failure, death from embolic events, and overall mortality was observed when compared with outcomes from the same institution prior to using the systematic approach [49].

Over the last two decades, there has been a tremendous increase in the number of implanted cardiac devices. Correspondingly, the incidence of CIED infections has increased at an even faster pace [18, 50]. Clinical management of patients with CIED endocarditis is guided by ACC/AHA guideline recommendations published in 2010 [32].

The Class I recommendations for diagnosis and management of device-related endocarditis are detailed in Table 6.3. In addition, the issue of timing of device reimplantation is addressed in this guideline document [32]. The Class I recommendations suggest evaluation of clinical indication for reimplantation and, if necessary, to implant at an anatomic location distant from the prior site. Reimplantation, when clinically indicated, is advised after 72 h of negative blood cultures for device infections [32].

Given the lack of clinical evidence, the question of endocarditis prophylaxis prior to invasive procedures is an often-debated issue. Statistical modeling has shown that bacteremia and subsequent endocarditis from dental procedures is exceedingly rare with an estimated risk of 1 in 95,000 in the highest risk individuals [51]. Furthermore, there is no evidence that antibiotic prophylaxis prevents infective endocarditis.

Several professional society guidelines, based primarily on expert opinion, have been published over the last few years addressing the specific patients and procedures for which antibiotic prophylaxis may be indicated. The ACC/AHA antibiotic prophylaxis guidelines are listed in Table 6.4. This document narrowed the cardiac conditions for which antibiotic prophylaxis is recommended and restricted this only to invasive dental procedures [51]. For patients in whom antibiotic prophylaxis is indicated, a regimen of 2 g of amoxicillin, or 600 mg of clindamycin for penicillin-allergic

Table 6.4 Class I ACC/AHA recommendations for cardiac conditions warranting antibiotic prophylaxis before invasive dental procedures

Conditions:

History of prior episode of infective endocarditis

Prosthetic heart valve or valve repair

Cardiac transplant valvulopathy

Congenital heart disease with residual shunt adjacent to prosthetic material used in prior surgical repair, within the first 6 months following surgical or percutaneous repair, or unrepaired cyanotic disease states

patients, 30–60 min prior to dental work is recommended [51]. Meanwhile, the ACC/AHA guidelines on the management of adult congenital heart disease published in 2008 expand the recommendation for antibiotic prophylaxis prior to vaginal delivery for patients with prosthetic heart valves and prosthetic material as a component of cardiac repair or in surgically repaired (surgical shunt or conduit) or unrepaired cyanotic cardiac disease [52].

In a similar manner to the ACC/AHA guidelines, the European Society of Cardiology (ESC) advises prophylaxis only for invasive dental procedures in the highest risk populations defined in the ACC/AHA statement with the exception of the transplant valvulopathy group which is not included in the ESC document [53]. An even more conservative policy is now advocated in the United Kingdom by the British National Institute for Health and Clinical Excellence (NICE) with antibiotic prophylaxis to prevent infective endocarditis no longer recommended for any population undergoing any type of invasive dental procedure [54].

Key Points

• Early consultation and discussion of management with cardiology, cardiac surgery, and infectious diseases experts.

• Obtain blood cultures prior to initiating empiric antimicrobial therapy.

• Understand the modified Duke Criteria in the diagnostic evaluation of patients with suspected infective endocarditis.

• Utilize TEE for patients with suspected prosthetic valve endocarditis, if the TTE is nondiagnostic with a high index of clinical suspicion or for evaluation of cardiac complications of endocarditis.

• Consider valve surgery in patients with heart failure from valve dysfunction, infection with multidrug-resistant microorganisms, or mechanical complications from infective endocarditis.

• Recognize the increasing incidence of CIED-related infections.

Summary of Guidelines

Class I ACC/AHA indications for valve surgery with infective endocarditis: symptomatic heart failure, infection with a fungal organism or other multidrug-resistant organism, and cardiac complications (abscess, heart block, fistula).

Class I ACC/AHA indications for TTE in the evaluation of infective endocarditis: detection of vegetations, assess valve and ventricular function in patients with definite endocarditis, diagnose mechanical cardiac complications of endocarditis and for the repeat imaging of patients with definite infective endocarditis.

Class I ACC/AHA indications for TEE in the evaluation of infective endocarditis: inconclusive TTE findings with symptomatic infective endocarditis, diagnostic evidence in patients with suspected endocarditis and equivocal TTE findings, evaluation of mechanical cardiac complications, to evaluate suspected prosthetic valve endocarditis and in the preoperative and intraoperative evaluation of definite infective endocarditis.

Class I STS guideline recommendation for mitral or tricuspid valve repair over replacement, if technically feasible, in patients having valve surgery for infective endocarditis of the mitral or tricuspid valve.

Class I STS guideline recommendation to postpone valve surgery for at least 4 weeks following intracranial hemorrhage related to active infective endocarditis.

Class I ACC/AHA recommendations for CIED infections:

Four to six weeks of antibiotic therapy with device-related endocarditis.

Device and lead extraction with a CIED infection and a complicated pocket infection, in the presence of valvular infective endocarditis, or with unexplained *Staphylococcus* bacteremia.

New device implant, if clinically indicated, at a site distant from prior device.

Class I ACC/AHA indications for antibiotic prophylaxis prior to invasive dental work: prior infective endocarditis, prosthetic heart valve or repair, cardiac transplant valvulopathy or congenital heart disease with residual shunt adjacent to prosthetic material used in surgical repair, within the first 6 months after surgical or percutaneous repair or unrepaired cyanotic conditions.

References

1. Levy DM. Centenary of William Osler's 1885 Gulstonian lectures and their place in the history of bacterial endocarditis. J R Soc Med. 1985;78:1039–46.
2. Bashore TM, Cabell C, Fowler Jr V. Update on infective endocarditis. Curr Probl Cardiol. 2006;31:274–352.
3. Berlin JA, Abrutyn E, Strom BL, et al. Incidence of infective endocarditis in the Delaware Valley, 1988–1990. Am J Cardiol. 1995;76:933–6.

4. Hoen B, Selton-Suty C, Danchin N, et al. Evaluation of the Duke criteria versus the Beth Israel criteria for the diagnosis of infective endocarditis. Clin Infect Dis. 1995;21:905–9.
5. Hill EE, Herijgers P, Claus P, Vanderschueren S, Herregods MC, Peetermans WE. Infective endocarditis: changing epidemiology and predictors of 6-month mortality: a prospective cohort study. Eur Heart J. 2007;28:196–203.
6. Lerner PI, Weinstein L. Infective endocarditis in the antibiotic era. N Engl J Med. 1966;274:388–93.
7. Watanakunakorn C. Changing epidemiology and newer aspects of infective endocarditis. Adv Intern Med. 1977;22:21–47.
8. Graves MK, Soto L. Left-sided endocarditis in parenteral drug abusers: recent experience at a large community hospital. South Med J. 1992;85:378–80.
9. Cabell CH, Fowler VG, Engemann JJ, McClellan M, Heidenreich P. Endocarditis in the elderly: incidence, surgery, and survival in 16,921 patients over 12 years. Circulation. 2002;106:547.
10. Griffin MR, Wilson WR, Edwards WD, O'Fallon WM, Kurland LT. Infective endocarditis. Olmsted county, Minnesota, 1950 through 1981. JAMA. 1985;254:1199–202.
11. McKinsey DS, Ratts TE, Bisno AL. Underlying cardiac lesions in adults with infective endocarditis. The changing spectrum. Am J Med. 1987;82:681–8.
12. Baddour LM, Wilson WR, Bayer AS, et al. Infective endocarditis: diagnosis, antimicrobial therapy, and management of complications: a statement for healthcare professionals from the Committee on Rheumatic Fever, Endocarditis, and Kawasaki Disease, Council on Cardiovascular Disease in the Young, and the Councils on Clinical Cardiology, Stroke, and Cardiovascular Surgery and Anesthesia, American Heart Association: endorsed by the Infectious Diseases Society of America. Circulation. 2005;111: e394–434.
13. Stuesse DC, Vlessis AA. Epidemiology of native valve endocarditis. In: Vlessis AA, Bolling SF, editors. Endocarditis: a multidisciplinary approach to modern treatment. Armonk: Futura Publishing Company; 1999. p. 77–84.
14. Rodbard S. Blood velocity and endocarditis. Circulation. 1963; 27:18–28.
15. Bonow RO, Carabello BA, Chatterjee K, et al. 2008 focused update incorporated into the ACC/AHA 2006 guidelines for the management of patients with valvular heart disease: a report of the American College of Cardiology/American Heart Association Task Force on Practice Guidelines (Writing Committee to revise the 1998 guidelines for the management of patients with valvular heart disease). Endorsed by the Society of Cardiovascular Anesthesiologists, Society for Cardiovascular Angiography and Interventions, and Society of Thoracic Surgeons. J Am Coll Cardiol. 2008;52:e1–142.
16. Karchmer AW. Infective endocarditis. In: Zipes DP, Libby P, Bonow RO, Braunwald E, editors. Heart disease. Philadelphia: Elsevier Saunders; 2005. p. 1633–56.
17. Voigt A, Shalaby A, Saba S. Rising rates of cardiac rhythm management device infections in the United States: 1996 through 2003. J Am Coll Cardiol. 2006;48:590–1.
18. Voigt A, Shalaby A, Saba S. Continued rise in rates of cardiovascular implantable electronic device infections in the United States: temporal trends and causative insights. Pacing Clin Electrophysiol. 2010;33:414–9.
19. Sohail MR, Uslan DZ, Khan AH, et al. Management and outcome of permanent pacemaker and implantable cardioverter-defibrillator infections. J Am Coll Cardiol. 2007;49:1851–9.
20. Armstrong W, Shea M. Clinical diagnosis of infective endocarditis. In: Vlessis AA, Bolling SF, editors. Endocarditis: A Multidisciplinary Approach to Modern Treatmen. Armonk, NY: Futura Publishing; 1999:107–34.
21. Lindner JR, Case RA, Dent JM, Abbott RD, Scheld WM, Kaul S. Diagnostic value of echocardiography in suspected endocarditis. An evaluation based on the pretest probability of disease. Circulation. 1996;93:730–6.
22. Durack DT, Lukes AS, Bright DK. New criteria for diagnosis of infective endocarditis: utilization of specific echocardiographic findings. Duke Endocarditis Service. Am J Med. 1994;96:200–9.
23. Olaison L, Hogevik H. Comparison of the von Reyn and Duke criteria for the diagnosis of infective endocarditis: a critical analysis of 161 episodes. Scand J Infect Dis. 1996;28:399–406.
24. Cecchi E, Parrini I, Chinaglia A, et al. New diagnostic criteria for infective endocarditis. A study of sensitivity and specificity. Eur Heart J. 1997;18:1149–56.
25. Li JS, Sexton DJ, Mick N, et al. Proposed modifications to the Duke criteria for the diagnosis of infective endocarditis. Clin Infect Dis. 2000;30:633–8.
26. Palepu A, Cheung SS, Montessori V, Woods R, Thompson CR. Factors other than the Duke criteria associated with infective endocarditis among injection drug users. Clin Invest Med. 2002;25: 118–25.
27. Tissieres P, Gervaix A, Beghetti M, Jaeggi ET. Value and limitations of the von Reyn, Duke, and modified Duke criteria for the diagnosis of infective endocarditis in children. Pediatrics. 2003;112:e467.
28. Khandheria BK. Suspected bacterial endocarditis: to TEE or not to TEE. J Am Coll Cardiol. 1993;21:222–4.
29. Birmingham GD, Rahko PS, Ballantyne 3rd F. Improved detection of infective endocarditis with transesophageal echocardiography. Am Heart J. 1992;123:774–81.
30. Mugge A, Daniel WG, Frank G, Lichtlen PR. Echocardiography in infective endocarditis: reassessment of prognostic implications of vegetation size determined by the transthoracic and the transesophageal approach. J Am Coll Cardiol. 1989;14:631–8.
31. Chu VH, Bayer AS. Use of echocardiography in the diagnosis and management of infective endocarditis. Curr Infect Dis Rep. 2007; 9:283–90.
32. Baddour LM, Epstein AE, Erickson CC, et al. Update on cardiovascular implantable electronic device infections and their management: a scientific statement from the American Heart Association. Circulation. 2010;121:458–77.
33. Gould FK, Denning DW, Elliott TS, et al. Guidelines for the diagnosis and antibiotic treatment of endocarditis in adults: a report of the Working Party of the British Society for Antimicrobial Chemotherapy. J Antimicrob Chemother. 2012;67:269–89.
34. Rehm S, Campion M, Katz DE, Russo R, Boucher HW. Community-based outpatient parenteral antimicrobial therapy (CoPAT) for Staphylococcus aureus bacteraemia with or without infective endocarditis: analysis of the randomized trial comparing daptomycin with standard therapy. J Antimicrob Chemother. 2009;63: 1034–42.
35. Amodeo MR, Clulow T, Lainchbury J, et al. Outpatient intravenous treatment for infective endocarditis: safety, effectiveness and one-year outcomes. J Infect. 2009;59:387–93.
36. Hirai Y, Ainoda Y, Shoji T, Totsuka K. Ceftriaxone plus gentamicin or ceftriaxone alone for streptococcal endocarditis in Japanese patients as alternative first-line therapies. J Infect Chemother. 2010;16:186–92.
37. Larioza J, Heung L, Girard A, Brown RB. Management of infective endocarditis in outpatients: clinical experience with outpatient parenteral antibiotic therapy. South Med J. 2009;102:575–9.
38. Tornos P, Almirante B, Mirabet S, Permanyer G, Pahissa A, Soler-Soler J. Infective endocarditis due to Staphylococcus aureus: deleterious effect of anticoagulant therapy. Arch Intern Med. 1999;159: 473–5.
39. Snygg-Martin U, Rasmussen RV, Hassager C, Bruun NE, Andersson R, Olaison L. Warfarin therapy and incidence of cerebrovascular complications in left-sided native valve endocarditis. Euro J Clin Microbiol Infect Dis. 2011;30:151–7.

40. Byrne JG, Rezai K, Sanchez JA, et al. Surgical management of endocarditis: the society of thoracic surgeons clinical practice guideline. Ann Thorac Surg. 2011;91:2012–9.

41. Kiefer T, Park L, Tribouilloy C, et al. Association between valvular surgery and mortality among patients with infective endocarditis complicated by heart failure. JAMA. 2011;306:2239–47.

42. Snygg-Martin U, Gustafsson L, Rosengren L, et al. Cerebrovascular complications in patients with left-sided infective endocarditis are common: a prospective study using magnetic resonance imaging and neurochemical brain damage markers. Clin Infect Dis. 2008;47:23–30.

43. Cooper HA, Thompson EC, Laureno R, et al. Subclinical brain embolization in left-sided infective endocarditis: results from the evaluation by MRI of the brains of patients with left-sided intracardiac solid masses (EMBOLISM) pilot study. Circulation. 2009;120:585–91.

44. Cabell CH, Pond KK, Peterson GE, et al. The risk of stroke and death in patients with aortic and mitral valve endocarditis. Am Heart J. 2001;142:75–80.

45. Anderson DJ, Goldstein LB, Wilkinson WE, et al. Stroke location, characterization, severity, and outcome in mitral vs aortic valve endocarditis. Neurology. 2003;61:1341–6.

46. Vikram HR, Buenconsejo J, Hasbun R, Quagliarello VJ. Impact of valve surgery on 6-month mortality in adults with complicated, left-sided native valve endocarditis: a propensity analysis. JAMA. 2003;290:3207–14.

47. Aksoy O, Sexton DJ, Wang A, et al. Early surgery in patients with infective endocarditis: a propensity score analysis. Clin Infect Dis. 2007;44:364–72.

48. Lalani T, Cabell CH, Benjamin DK, et al. Analysis of the impact of early surgery on in-hospital mortality of native valve endocarditis: use of propensity score and instrumental variable methods to adjust for treatment-selection bias. Circulation. 2010;121:1005–13.

49. Botelho-Nevers E, Thuny F, Casalta JP, et al. Dramatic reduction in infective endocarditis-related mortality with a management-based approach. Arch Intern Med. 2009;169:1290–8.

50. Cabell CH, Heidenreich PA, Chu VH, et al. Increasing rates of cardiac device infections among Medicare beneficiaries: 1990–1999. Am Heart J. 2004;147:582–6.

51. Wilson W, Taubert KA, Gewitz M, et al. Prevention of infective endocarditis: guidelines from the American Heart Association: a guideline from the American Heart Association Rheumatic Fever, Endocarditis, and Kawasaki Disease Committee, Council on Cardiovascular Disease in the Young, and the Council on Clinical Cardiology, Council on Cardiovascular Surgery and Anesthesia, and the Quality of Care and Outcomes Research Interdisciplinary Working Group. Circulation. 2007;116:1736–54.

52. Warnes CA, Williams RG, Bashore TM, et al. ACC/AHA 2008 guidelines for the management of adults with congenital heart disease: a report of the American College of Cardiology/American Heart Association Task Force on Practice Guidelines (Writing Committee to Develop Guidelines on the Management of Adults With Congenital Heart Disease). Developed in Collaboration With the American Society of Echocardiography, Heart Rhythm Society, International Society for Adult Congenital Heart Disease, Society for Cardiovascular Angiography and Interventions, and Society of Thoracic Surgeons. J Am Coll Cardiol. 2008;52:e1–121.

53. Habib G, Hoen B, Tornos P, et al. Guidelines on the prevention, diagnosis, and treatment of infective endocarditis (new version 2009): the Task Force on the Prevention, Diagnosis, and Treatment of Infective Endocarditis of the European Society of Cardiology (ESC). Endorsed by the European Society of Clinical Microbiology and Infectious Diseases (ESCMID) and the International Society of Chemotherapy (ISC) for Infection and Cancer. Eur Heart J. 2009;30:2369–413.

54. Stokes T, Richey R, Wray D. Prophylaxis against infective endocarditis: summary of NICE guidance. Heart. 2008;94:930–1.

Pericardial Diseases

7

Massimo Imazio

Abstract

Pericardial diseases are relatively common in clinical practice and may occur either as isolated disease or as a manifestation of a systemic disorder. A targeted etiological search should be directed to the most likely cause on the basis of the clinical background, epidemiological issues, or specific presentations. Clinicians should consider neoplastic, tuberculous, and purulent causes, as well as forms related to a systemic disease. Most cases remain idiopathic, and empiric anti-inflammatory therapy should be considered as first-line therapy in most cases with the possible addition of colchicine in the setting of inflammatory pericardial diseases especially those that relapse or do not respond to first-line drugs. The prognosis is determined by the underlying cause, with bacterial and neoplastic forms having the worst prognosis. Contemporary optimal management of the patient with suspected pericardial disease often requires the selection and integration of different imaging modalities.

Keywords

Pericardial diseases • Cardiac tamponade • Pericardial constriction

Introduction

The pericardium consists of two sacs: the outer, fibrous pericardium and the inner, serous or visceral pericardium. The proximal portions of the aorta and pulmonary artery are enclosed within the pericardial sac. The normal pericardium prevents friction between the heart and surrounding structures, acts as a mechanical and immunological barrier, and limits distension of the heart which maintains a relatively fixed maximal heart volume. In normal hearts, these functions are achieved by the presence of a small amount of pericardial fluid (25–50 ml) produced by the visceral pericardium.

Pericardial diseases are relatively common in clinical practice and may present either as isolated disease or as a manifestation of a systemic disorder. Although the potential etiologies are varied and complex (Table 7.1), the pericardium has a relatively nonspecific response to these different causes with inflammation of the pericardial layers and possible increased production of pericardial fluid. Chronic inflammation with fibrosis and calcification can lead to a rigid, usually thickened, and calcified pericardium, with possible progression to pericardial constriction. On this basis, pericardial disease may present as acute and recurrent pericarditis, pericardial effusion, cardiac tamponade, and constrictive pericarditis [1–6]. At present there are no updated international guidelines on the management of pericardial diseases beyond the 2004 guidelines issued by the European Society of Cardiology [7].

Pathophysiology

Pericarditis

Pericarditis is the most common disease of the pericardium encountered in clinical practice. It is diagnosed in 0.1 % of all admissions and 5 % of emergency room admissions for chest pain [8].

M. Imazio, MD, FESC
Department of Cardiology, Maria Vittoria Hospital,
Via Cibrario 72, Torino 10141, Italy
e-mail: massimo_imazio@yahoo.it

K. Stergiopoulos, D.L. Brown (eds.), *Evidence-Based Cardiology Consult*,
DOI 10.1007/978-1-4471-4441-0_7, © Springer-Verlag London 2014

Table 7.1 Etiology of pericardial diseases. The pericardium may be affected by all categories of diseases including infectious, autoimmune, neoplastic, iatrogenic, traumatic, and metabolic

Infectious causes

Viral (coxsackievirus, echovirus, EBV, CMV, adenovirus, parvovirus B19, and human herpes virus 6-possible overlap with etiological viral agents of myocarditis)

Bacterial (tuberculosis, Coxiella burnetii, other bacterial rare may include Pneumo-, Meningo-, Gonococcus, Haemophilus, Streptococci, Staphylococci, Chlamydia, Mycoplasma, Legionella, Leptospira, Listeria)

Fungal (rare: Histoplasma more likely in immunocompetent patients, aspergillosis, blastomycosis, Candida more likely in immunosuppressed host)

Parasitic (very rare: Echinococcus, Toxoplasma)

Noninfectious causes

Autoimmune

    Pericardial injury syndromes (postmyocardial infarction syndrome, post-pericardiotomy syndrome, post-traumatic including forms after iatrogenic trauma)

    Systemic autoimmune and autoinflammatory diseases (systemic lupus erythematosus, Sjögren syndrome, rheumatoid arthritis, systemic sclerosis, systemic vasculitides, Behçet syndrome, sarcoidosis, familial Mediterranean fever)

Neoplastic

    Primary tumors (rare, above all pericardial mesothelioma)

    Secondary metastatic tumors (common, above all lung and breast cancer, lymphoma)

Metabolic (uremia, myxedema, other rare)

Traumatic and iatrogenic

    Direct injury (penetrating thoracic injury, esophageal perforation, iatrogenic)

    Indirect injury (non-penetrating thoracic injury, radiation injury)

    Drug-related (*procainamide, hydralazine, isoniazid, and phenytoin* as lupus-like syndrome, *penicillins* as hypersensitivity pericarditis with eosinophilia, *doxorubicin, and daunorubicin* often associated with a cardiomyopathy, may cause pericardiopathy)

    Post-interventions: e.g., coronary percutaneous intervention, pacemaker lead insertion, and radiofrequency ablation

Modified from Imazio et al. [1]

Table 7.2 Final etiological diagnosis in major published unselected series of acute pericarditis

	Permanyer-Miralda et al. [62]	Zayas et al. [63]	Imazio et al. [64]	Reuter et al.[a]
Patients	($n=231$)	($n=100$)	($n=453$)	($n=233$)
Years	1977–1983	1991–1993	1996–2004	1995–2001
Geographic area	Western Europe	Western Europe	Western Europe	Africa
Idiopathic	199 (86.0 %)	78 (78.0 %)	377 (83.2 %)	32 (13.7 %)
Specific etiology:	32 (14.0 %)	22 (22.0 %)	76 (16.8 %)	201 (86.3 %)
Neoplastic	13 (5.6 %)	7 (7.0 %)	23 (5.1 %)	22 (9.4 %)
Tuberculosis	9 (3.9 %)	4 (4.0 %)	17 (3.8 %)	161 (69.5 %)
Autoimmune	4 (1.7 %)	3 (3.0 %)	33 (7.3 %)	12 (5.2 %)
Purulent	2 (0.9 %)	1 (1.0 %)	3 (0.7 %)	5 (2.1 %)

Modified from Imazio et al. [1]
[a]Based on pericardial effusions

Globally, tuberculosis is the most important cause of pericardial diseases and pericarditis [9]. In this setting tuberculosis is often associated with HIV infection, especially in Sub-Saharan Africa [10]. On the contrary, idiopathic and viral forms are more common in developed countries (Table 7.2).

Recurrent pericarditis is the most common and troublesome complication of acute pericarditis affecting 20–30 % of patients after a first attack of acute pericarditis. The pathogenesis of recurrent pericarditis is not known. A new viral infection, a reinfection, or a chronic viral infection has been proposed as possible causes. In many cases, inadequate therapy of the first attack (low doses, short courses without complete resolution of symptoms, and markers of inflammation) may be causative [1, 3]. However, the pathogenesis of acute pericarditis is often presumed to be immune-mediated; genetic predisposition and autoimmune responses may be important in many cases. In a recently published study on idiopathic recurrent pericarditis, anti-heart (AHA) and anti-intercalated-disk (AIDA) antibodies were identified in two-thirds of patients supporting the autoimmune hypothesis of recurrent pericarditis [11].

Pericardial Effusion

Pericardial effusion, without evidence of inflammation and pericarditis, often presents a clinical dilemma. An idiopathic etiology is less common in patients who present with an isolated pericardial effusion than in those who have acute pericarditis. Specific diagnoses (nonidiopathic etiologies) have been reported in up to 90 % of patients with moderate to large pericardial effusions [12]. Although reported frequencies vary according to geographic location, selection criteria (how effusion severity is defined), and medical setting (general vs. tertiary referral centers), the etiology of pericardial effusion can often be suspected on the basis of the clinical presentation. Pericardial effusion is associated with a known systemic disease in up to 60 % of cases [13]. The presence of inflammatory signs, including elevated C-reactive protein (CRP) and erythrocyte sedimentation rates (which favor a diagnosis of pericarditis), and the size and hemodynamic importance of the effusion should also be considered. Large effusions and cardiac tamponade without inflammatory signs are often associated with a neoplastic etiology [12, 13].

Pericardial effusions can occur as a component of almost any pericardial disorder, but the majority results from one of the following causes conditions: pericarditis, systemic inflammatory diseases, post-injury pericardial syndromes (myocardial infarction, cardiac surgery, iatrogenic or accidental trauma), malignancies (especially lung cancer, breast cancer, and lymphomas), mediastinal radiation, metabolic diseases (especially renal failure and hypothyroidism), aortic dissection, and, rarely, with selected drugs (Table 7.1).

Patients with hemorrhagic pericardial effusions have more commonly a neoplastic, tuberculous, or iatrogenic cause. In this setting, the presentation with large pericardial effusions or cardiac tamponade is more frequent [12].

Cardiac Tamponade

Cardiac tamponade is a clinical pericardial syndrome characterized by compression of the heart due to accumulation of pericardial fluid, pus, blood, clots, gas within pericardial space, and subsequent impaired diastolic filling and reduced cardiac output [14, 15]. According to 2004 European Society of Cardiology guidelines, cardiac tamponade is defined as the decompensated phase of cardiac compression caused by effusion accumulation and the resultant increased intrapericardial pressure [7]. Cardiac tamponade presents with equal elevation of atrial and pericardial pressure, an exaggerated inspiratory decrease in arterial systolic pressure (pulsus paradoxus), distended jugular veins, and arterial hypotension [16].

The etiology of cardiac tamponade is varied reflecting the epidemiological background and different possible causes of pericardial disease. Pericardial diseases of any etiology may cause cardiac tamponade (Table 7.1); however, specific etiologies have a higher risk of evolution toward tamponade [13, 17, 18]. Bacterial pericarditis (especially tuberculous) and neoplastic pericardial disease are the most common causes of cardiac tamponade [19–21]. In developed countries an additional relevant cause is represented by iatrogenic pericardial effusion that occurs most frequently in percutaneous cardiac interventions (coronary interventions, mitral valvuloplasty, endomyocardial biopsy), pacemaker implantation, and radiofrequency ablation [22].

The pericardium has a limited distensibility essentially determined by the histological composition of the parietal pericardium with a limited amount of elastic fibers and more collagen fibers. However, if pericardial fluid accumulates slowly, a remodeling of pericardial connective tissue may allow pericardial distension with accumulation of up to 2,000 ml of fluid. On the contrary, acute tamponade occurs with accumulation of as little as 250 ml [14, 23].

The pressure-volume relation of normal pericardium is a J-shaped curve. After an initial short shallow portion that allows the pericardium to prevent cardiac chamber dilatation in response to physiological events such as posture changes, there is a minimal increase in pericardial pressure. Thereafter the pressure increase is extremely steep for sudden, acute changes of volume. Thus an acute increase of 100–200 ml may greatly elevate pericardial pressure to 20–30 mmHg and be responsible for cardiac tamponade. On the contrary, a slowly increasing pericardial volume is accompanied by only modest increases of pericardial pressure, even up to 1,000–2,000 ml before the development of cardiac tamponade.

Constrictive Pericarditis

Constrictive pericarditis occurs when the fibrotic pericardium impedes normal diastolic filling because of loss of elasticity. Usually the pericardium is considerably thickened, but it can be of normal thickness in up to 20 % of cases. Pericardiectomy is equally successful in patients with and without increased pericardial thickness. Histopathologic abnormalities, including mild and focal fibrosis, inflammation, calcification, fibrin deposition, and focal noncaseating granulomas, may be present. Pericardial constriction is typically chronic, but variants include subacute, transient, and occult constriction. The most common etiologies are idiopathic or viral (42–49 %), cardiac surgery (11–37 %), radiation therapy, mostly for Hodgkin's disease or breast cancer (9–31 %), connective tissue disorders (3–7 %), and infection (tuberculous or purulent pericarditis, 3–6 %) [1, 4]. Tuberculosis is a major cause of constrictive pericarditis in developing countries, and this etiology is particularly prevalent in Africa [20]. In developed countries, tuberculous pericarditis is rare but is being reported with increasing frequency among immigrants from developing nations and in patients with HIV infection [1].

Diagnosis

Pericarditis

The clinical diagnosis of acute pericarditis is relatively easy (Table 7.3), while the identification of the etiology may be more complex [24, 25]. Markers of inflammation are elevated in most cases at presentation and may confirm the clinical suspicion of pericarditis. In a recently published Italian study, high-sensitivity CRP (hs-CRP) was elevated in about 80 % of cases at presentation. Recognized causes of a negative hs-CRP at presentation were early assessment in 15 of 44 cases (34 %) and previous anti-inflammatory therapies in 22 of 44 cases (50 %). Hs-CRP normalization was achieved with the following time course: 120 of 200 (60 %) at week 1, 170 of 200 (85 %) at week 2, 190 of 200 (95 %) at week 3, and all cases (100 %) at week 4. Persistent elevation of hs-CRP was a risk factor for recurrences in multivariable analysis [26].

Pericardial Effusion

The diagnosis of pericardial effusion can be easily achieved by the use of transthoracic echocardiography. Echocardiography is the first-level diagnostic modality for the assessment of the presence, size, and hemodynamic importance of pericardial effusion. Echocardiography is able to detect pericardial effusions exceeding 15–35 ml. According to a common semi-quantitative assessment, pericardial effusions are graded according to the echo-free space in diastole [12] as:

- Small (<10 mm)
- Moderate (10–20 mm)
- Large (>20 mm)

Echocardiography is recommended for the evaluation of all patients with suspected pericardial disease [27].

Table 7.3 Diagnostic criteria for pericarditis (at least 2 of 4 should be present)

1. Typical chest pain
2. Pericardial friction rub
3. Suggestive ECG changes (typically widespread ST segment elevation, PR depression)
4. New or worsening pericardial effusion

Cardiac Tamponade

In a systematic review of the literature, five features have been reported in the majority of patients with cardiac tamponade: dyspnea (85–90 %), cardiomegaly on chest radiograph (89 %), pulsus paradoxus (82 %), tachycardia (77 %), and elevated jugular venous pressure (76 %). In the setting of a large pericardial effusion, the presence of pulsus paradoxus with an inspiratory decrease of systolic blood pressure >10 mmHg increases the likelihood of cardiac tamponade threefold [28]. Hypotension and diminished heart sounds were insensitive. Cardiac tamponade includes a hemodynamic spectrum ranging from mild to severe cases and with different onset (acute vs. subacute). Clinical examination is essential to suspect tamponade in a single patient. Cardiac tamponade is a clinical diagnosis that should be based on the combination of symptoms and signs and that can be confirmed noninvasively by echocardiography [28]. Most cases of cardiac tamponade have a moderate to large pericardial effusion, and swinging of the heart within the pericardial fluid is a common echocardiographic finding [12].

Echocardiographic findings in cardiac tamponade are essentially characterized by transient chamber collapse and increased ventricular interdependence [29]. Major echocardiographic signs include:

- *Diastolic collapse of the right atrium (RA)*: This is an early sign that can be detected with moderate to large pericardial effusions without cardiac tamponade; sensitivity range is 50–100 % and specificity range is 33–100 %.
- *Diastolic collapse of the right ventricle*: Right ventricular (RV) collapse is less sensitive for the presence of cardiac tamponade than RA collapse but it is more specific; sensitivity range is 48–100 % and specificity range is 72–100 %.
- *Left-sided chamber collapse*: Left atrial (LA) collapse is recorded in about 25 % of cases with cardiac tamponade and is a very specific sign. Left ventricular (LV) collapse is rare because LV pressures are higher and its wall is thicker than RV. This sign can be seen in case of regional or focal compression.
- *Respiratory variation in volumes and flows of cardiac chambers*: Increased ventricular interdependence observed in cardiac tamponade is responsible for reciprocal changes of LV and RV volumes and mitral and tricuspid flows during respiratory phases. Variations in E velocities during respiration across the mitral valve, tricuspid valve, and pulmonary outflow that are greater than 25, 50, and 30 %, respectively, indicate cardiac tamponade.
- *Inferior vena cava (IVC) plethora*: An inspiratory collapse of less than 50 % of the diameter of the dilated IVC reflects a marked elevation in central venous pressure and is frequently reported in patients with cardiac tamponade.

It is a very sensitive sign (97 %) but not very specific (40 %), being common in other pathologic conditions (i.e., heart failure, tricuspid regurgitation).

In most patients, cardiac tamponade should be diagnosed by a clinical examination that shows elevated systemic venous pressure, tachycardia, dyspnea, and paradoxical arterial pulse. Systemic blood pressure may be normal, decreased, or even elevated. The diagnosis is confirmed by echocardiographic demonstration of a moderately large or large circumferential pericardial effusion and, in most instances, of RA compression, abnormal respiratory variation in right and left ventricular dimensions and in tricuspid and mitral valve flow velocities [30].

Constrictive Pericarditis

Patients with suspected constrictive pericarditis, based on history and physical examination, should undergo initial evaluation with electrocardiography (ECG), chest radiography, and echocardiography. While the diagnosis of constrictive pericarditis is often made by echocardiography, patients commonly undergo cardiac catheterization prior to surgical intervention. Invasive hemodynamic evaluation during cardiac catheterization can confirm the diagnosis, and concurrent coronary angiography defines the patient's coronary anatomy prior to possible surgical intervention. In patients being evaluated for pericardiectomy, particularly those with prior radiation exposure, computed tomography or cardiac magnetic resonance imaging can provide additional detailed anatomic information about adjacent vascular structures and the extent of pericardial thickening, calcification, and scarring [16].

Pericardial inflammation may be a marker for reversibility. In a pilot study from the Mayo Clinic, pericardial late gadolinium enhancement (LGE) by cardiac magnetic resonance (CMR) and inflammatory biomarkers predicted the reversibility of constriction after anti-inflammatory therapy. In this study, about 50 % of patients receiving empiric anti-inflammatory therapies had resolution of constriction after 13 months of follow-up. The patients with reversible constriction had higher baseline CRP levels and erythrocyte sedimentation rates than the persistent constriction group [31]. A recent study also investigated the prevalence and histopathologic correlates of LGE seen with CMR among patients with constrictive pericarditis undergoing pericardiectomy. In this study 12 of 25 patients (48 %) with LGE had greater fibroblastic proliferation and neovascularization, as well as more prominent chronic inflammation and granulation tissue, while patients with constriction without pericardial LGE had more pericardial fibrosis and calcification, as well as lesser degrees of pericardial thickening [32].

Further studies in a larger number of patients are needed but growing evidence suggests the importance of assessing inflammation and reversibility of constriction in the setting of newly diagnosed constrictive pericarditis.

Although cardiac catheterization has historically been the principal diagnostic modality for the diagnosis of constrictive pericarditis, this diagnosis can now be made by noninvasive methods (echocardiography, CMR) in most cases. Cardiac catheterization may be useful to resolve discrepancies between clinical and other diagnostic data [33–36].

Management

Pericarditis

Idiopathic and viral pericarditis has a relatively benign outcome. It is often self-limiting or responds well to conventional anti-inflammatory therapy. On this basis, patients with pericarditis can be safely managed on an outpatient basis without a thorough diagnostic evaluation unless a specific cause is suspected or the patient has high-risk features (fever >38 °C, subacute course, severe pericardial effusion >20 mm, cardiac tamponade, and lack of response to empiric anti-inflammatory therapy). A targeted etiological search should be directed to the most common causes on the basis of the clinical background, epidemiological issues, or specific presentations. In developed countries the clinicians should rule out neoplastic, tuberculous, and purulent pericarditis, as well as pericarditis related to a systemic disease [1, 23, 24]. An algorithm has been proposed to select high-risk cases of acute pericarditis for admission and low-risk cases for outpatient management (Fig. 7.1) [1].

Treatment of pericarditis should be targeted at the specific cause as much as possible [1]. However, most cases remain idiopathic, and empiric anti-inflammatory therapy should be considered as first-line therapy in most cases. Aspirin and nonsteroidal anti-inflammatory (NSAID) are the mainstays of empiric anti-inflammatory therapy (Table 7.4) [1, 37]. Aspirin is a reasonable first choice for patients with ischemic heart disease or with any indication for aspirin use as antiplatelet therapy. Full anti-inflammatory doses should be used with administration every 8 h in order to control symptoms over the first 24 h. The ideal length of therapy is not well known. A proposed practical approach is to develop a tailored management providing the full anti-inflammatory dose until symptoms resolve and CRP levels return to normal [26]. Tapering may be considered after symptoms resolve and markers of inflammation normalize [26, 38]. Systemic corticosteroids are a second-choice therapy especially for patients with contraindications to aspirin or NSAIDs, incomplete response to or failure of first-line anti-inflammatory

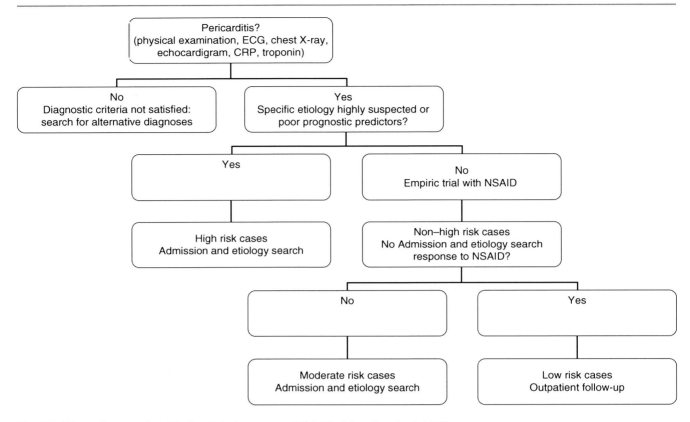

Fig. 7.1 Triage of acute pericarditis for clinical management (Modified from Imazio et al. [1])

therapy, and for specific indications such as systemic inflammatory diseases or pregnancy [39–41]. Use of low to moderate doses (i.e., prednisone 0.2–0.5 mg/kg/day) is associated with better outcomes than higher doses (i.e., prednisone 1.0–1.5 mg/kg/day). The initial dose should be continued until symptoms resolve and CRP normalizes after which these agents should be slowly tapered [1].

In a recently published systematic review of controlled clinical trials on pharmacologic treatments for acute and recurrent pericarditis, colchicine use was associated with a reduced risk of treatment failure (odds ratio (OR) = 0.23) and recurrent pericarditis (OR = 0.39) but with a trend toward more adverse effects (OR = 5.27). Corticosteroids were associated with a trend toward increased risk of recurrent pericarditis (OR = 7.50), possibly because steroids promote a chronic form of the disease, especially in the setting of idiopathic/viral forms. Moreover low-dose steroids may reduce the risk of treatment failure or further recurrences (OR = 0.29), readmissions (OR = 0.19), and adverse effects (OR = 0.07) compared to high-dose corticosteroids [37].

The prognosis of pericarditis is essentially determined by the etiology of the underlying disease. Idiopathic/viral pericarditis has an overall good prognosis, usually with a good response to empiric anti-inflammatory therapy and often self-limiting. Recurrences are possible and may affect the quality of life especially for patients on corticosteroid therapy. The mean recurrence rate is 30 % [1]. The most feared complication is the evolution toward constrictive pericarditis. In a recently prospective study on 500 consecutive cases with acute pericarditis of different etiologies, constriction developed in 9 of 500 patients (1.8 %): 2 of 416 patients with idiopathic/viral pericarditis (0.48 %) versus 7 of 84 patients with a nonviral/nonidiopathic etiology (8.3 %) during a median follow-up of 72 months. Although this complication was relatively rare for viral or idiopathic acute pericarditis (<0.5 %), the risk was quite high for bacterial pericarditis (20–30 %) and intermediate for autoimmune (systemic inflammatory diseases and post-injury pericardial syndromes) and neoplastic etiologies [42].

Some cases of pericarditis may show concomitant myocardial involvement, usually detected as troponin elevation. Generally these cases have a preserved or mildly reduced left ventricular function at presentation [43]. Cases with predominant pericarditis (myopericarditis) usually have a good prognosis without development of heart failure, constrictive pericarditis, or recurrence. In these cases normalization of the electrocardiogram (ECG), left ventricular function, and exercise capacity is reported within 12 months [44, 45].

Treatment of recurrences follows the same principles as treatment of the initial episode of acute pericarditis (Table 7.4).

Table 7.4 Empiric anti-inflammatory therapy for pericarditis

Drug	Attack dose	Treatment length[a]	Tapering[a]
Acetylsalicylic acid	750–1,000 mg TID	Until symptoms and CRP normalize	Each week when CRP is normalized (i.e., 1,000 mg TID for 1 week, 750 mg TID for 1 week, then 500 mg TID for 1 week)
Ibuprofen	600 mg TID	Same	Each week when CRP is normalized (i.e., 600 mg, 400 mg, 600 mg/day for 1 week, 600 mg, 400 mg, 400 mg/day for 1 week, then 400 mg TID for 1 week)
Indomethacin	50 mg TID	Same	Each week when CRP is normalized (i.e., 50 mg, 25 mg, 50 mg/day for 1 week, 50 mg, 25 mg, 25 mg/day for 1 week, then 25 mg TID for 1 week)
Prednisone	0.2–0.5 mg/kg/day	Same	Slow tapering when CRP is normalized[a]
Colchicine	Not necessary 0.5 mg BID (0.5 mg/day if <70 kg)	First attack: 3 months Recurrence: 6–12 months	May be required in recurrent form

[a]Treatment length is empirical. Generally 1–2 weeks but an individualized approach until symptoms resolve and CRP normalizes may be useful to reduce the subsequent recurrence rate. Very slow tapering is recommended only after stable remission with symptom resolution and normalization of CRP: 5–10 mg/day every 1–2 weeks (prednisone daily dose >25 mg), 2.5 mg/day every 2–4 weeks (prednisone daily dose 15–25 mg), and 1.0–2.5 mg/day every 2–6 weeks (prednisone daily dose <15 mg). NSAID and colchicine may be necessary during tapering of corticosteroids

However, in this setting colchicine has been proven to be a useful adjunct to conventional anti-inflammatory therapy (aspirin or NSAIDs). In the recently published multicenter, double-blind, randomized Colchicine for Recurrent Pericarditis (CORP trial), 120 patients with a first recurrence of pericarditis were randomly assigned to receive either placebo or colchicine, 1.0–2.0 mg on the first day followed by a maintenance dose of 0.5–1.0 mg/day for 6 months. At 18 months, the recurrence rate was 24 % in the colchicine group and 55 % in the placebo group (absolute risk reduction, 0.31 [95 % CI, 0.13–0.46]; relative risk reduction (RRR), 0.56 [CI, 0.27–0.73]; number needed to treat (NNT), 3 [CI, 2–7]). Colchicine also reduced the persistence of symptoms at 72 h (absolute risk reduction, 0.30 [CI, 0.13–0.45]; RRR 0.56 [CI, 0.27–0.74]) and the mean number of recurrences, increased the remission rate at 1 week, and prolonged the time to subsequent recurrence with similar rates of side effects and drug withdrawal between the study groups [46].

Colchicine has been used for centuries for the treatment of gouty attacks and rheumatic complaints. The exact mechanism of action as an anti-inflammatory agent is only partially known. Colchicine accumulates preferentially in neutrophils interfering with several cell functions through tubulin polymerization blockade and interference with microtubule function. In clinical practice, the use of colchicine for pericarditis is "off label," and interactions with drugs interfering with CYP3A4-dependent enzymes and P-glycoprotein may occur and are clinically important (especially statins and macrolide antibiotics). Renal impairment is a major risk factor for side effects. On this basis, the dosage should be reduced in patients with relevant hepatic and/or renal dysfunction as well as in the geriatric and pediatric settings. Concurrent use of colchicine and P-glycoprotein or strong CYP3A4 inhibitors is contraindicated in case of hepatic or renal impairment. Fatal toxicity has been reported in this setting. When appropriately used and contraindications have been excluded, oral colchicine is a safe and efficacious treatment for pericarditis and its prevention [47–49].

Recurrences may seriously affect the quality of life of patients especially those on corticosteroids. Severe side effects are reported in about 25 % of patients treated with high-dose oral corticosteroids. To avoid systemic side effects of corticosteroids, the intrapericardial route has been proposed. One case series and three open-label trials evaluating intrapericardial triamcinolone for the management of autoreactive pericarditis have been reviewed [50]. Available studies were limited by small sample sizes, lack of control groups, short durations of follow-up (<12 months), use of adjuvant agents, subjective reporting of symptoms, and variable doses of intrapericardial triamcinolone. However, although the available data suggest symptom resolution and reduced pericarditis recurrence with administration of intrapericardial triamcinolone to patients with autoreactive pericarditis, the appropriate regimen (dose and duration of treatment), adverse effect profile, and specific therapeutic role require further investigation [50]. Most cases respond to combined therapies including aspirin or NSAIDs, colchicine, and corticosteroids. For refractory cases, immunosuppressive drugs such as azathioprine may be required. Use of additional immunosuppressive therapies requires specific knowledge of the drugs and cooperation with a rheumatologist [51].

Pericardial Effusion

Isolated pericardial effusion may be detected as an incidental finding during echocardiography or a diagnostic imaging study. When a pericardial effusion is detected, the first step is to assess its size, hemodynamic importance, and possible associated diseases including infections (viral, bacterial,

Fig. 7.2 Triage of pericardial effusion (Modified from Imazio et al. [1])

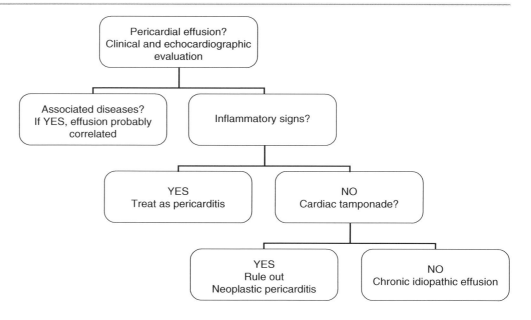

especially tuberculosis), cancer, connective tissue diseases, pericardial injury syndromes, metabolic causes (i.e., hypothyroidism), and myocardial, pericardial, and aortic diseases. The relative frequency of different causes depends on the local epidemiology, the hospital setting, and the diagnostic protocol that has been adopted [52]. Specific testing should be performed according to clinical suspicion. The presence of elevated inflammatory markers and other criteria (chest pain, pericardial rubs, ECG changes) suggest pericarditis, and management should be directed accordingly [12, 13].

Treatment should be targeted at the etiology as much as possible. Nevertheless, when diagnosis is still unclear, or idiopathic and inflammatory markers are elevated, empiric anti-inflammatory therapy may be worthwhile [4]. Patients with chronic massive idiopathic pericardial effusions represent a special management issue. A true isolated effusion may not require a specific treatment if the patient is asymptomatic, but large ones have a theoretical risk of progression to cardiac tamponade (up to one-third) because of concurrent events (i.e., pericarditis, trauma), especially if the effusion is associated with signs of right-sided collapse or chronic (>3 months) [1, 12, 13]. However, such practice is controversial and not accepted by all authors and experts in the field. Pericardiocentesis alone may be curative for large effusions, but recurrences are also common, and pericardiectomy or less invasive options (i.e., pericardial window) should be considered whenever fluid re-accumulates (especially with tamponade), becomes loculated, or biopsy material is required.

A practical approach and triage of pericardial effusion has been also proposed as for pericarditis (Fig. 7.2) [1, 12].

Postoperative and neoplastic pericardial effusions represent discrete entities with challenging management issues. Colchicine significantly reduces the incidence of postoperative pericardial (12.8 % vs. 22.8 %, P=0.019, RRR 43.9 %, NNT 10) and pleural effusions (12.2 % vs. 25.6 %, P=0.002, RRR 52.3 %, NNT 8) without significant side effects [53], while an NSAID failed [54].

Management of patients with neoplastic pericardial effusions constitutes another special challenge for clinicians. Pericardial effusions may develop from direct extension of a tumor, metastasis to the heart, opportunistic infections, or complications of oncologic therapies (i.e., radiation therapy or chemotherapeutic toxicity) [21, 55–57]. The clinical presentation is also variable ranging from asymptomatic effusions to cardiac tamponade. Management depends on cancer type and stage, available therapies, as well as patient prognosis. Re-accumulation of pericardial fluid is an important issue in this setting. Therapeutic possibilities include extended indwelling pericardial catheters, percutaneous pericardiostomy, and intrapericardial instillation of antineoplastic and sclerosing agents [56]. Lung cancer is one the most common cause of neoplastic pericardial effusion because of early lymphatic invasion. In this setting local chemotherapy, alone or with systemic chemotherapy, is effective in treating pericardial metastases from lung carcinoma, leading to a good control of pericardial effusion in >90 % of cases and to complete disappearance of effusion and masses in >60 %. Pericardiocentesis and intrapericardial chemotherapy should be used whenever possible in pericardial disease due to lung cancer, not only in cases of tamponade [56, 57].

Cardiac Tamponade

Cardiac tamponade is an absolute indication for pericardiocentesis that has a therapeutic and diagnostic role in this setting [1, 7].

Constrictive Pericarditis

Although the mainstay of treatment of chronic cases is surgery, medical therapy may have a role in at least three conditions [3, 4]. First, medical therapy of infectious pericarditis may prevent the progression to constriction. For example, antituberculosis antibiotics may reduce the risk of constriction from >80 to 10–20 %. Second, medical therapy (generally based on anti-inflammatory drugs, especially corticosteroids) may resolve the transient constriction that occurs in 10–20 % of cases during the resolution of pericarditis. Although constriction is transient or reversible only in a minority of patients with constrictive pericarditis, this finding is important to prevent unnecessary surgery [58, 59]. Third, medical therapy is supportive and aimed at controlling symptoms of congestion in advanced cases and when surgery is contraindicated associated with high risk. In these cases medical therapy should never delay surgery, if this option is feasible, because advanced cases have a higher mortality and a worse prognosis if surgery is delayed [4].

> **Key Points**
> - Pericardial diseases are relatively common in clinical practice and may present either as isolated disease or manifestations of a systemic disorder.
> - A targeted etiological search should be directed to the most common cause on the basis of the clinical background, epidemiological issues, or specific presentations. Clinicians should rule out neoplastic, tuberculous, and purulent causes, as well as forms related to other systemic diseases.
> - Most cases remain idiopathic and empiric anti-inflammatory therapy should be considered as first-line therapy in most cases with the possible addition of colchicine in the setting of inflammatory pericardial diseases particularly for relapse or patients who do not respond to first-line drugs.
> - The prognosis is essentially determined by the etiology of the underlying disease. Bacterial and neoplastic forms have a worse prognosis. The most feared complication is pericardial constriction, whose risk is higher in bacterial forms, intermediate for post-pericardiotomy syndromes and systemic inflammatory diseases, and low for viral and idiopathic cases.
> - Contemporary optimal management of the patient with suspected pericardial disease often requires the integration of different imaging modalities and the ability to choose the appropriate imaging test for each patient [59–61].

Summary of the Key Guidelines

At present there are no updated international guidelines on the management of pericardial diseases beyond the 2004 guidelines issued by the European Society of Cardiology [7]. A summary of the most important recommendations is (Level of Evidence – LOE: A multiple randomized trials or meta-analysis, B: a single randomized study or nonrandomized studies, C: experts opinion):

Acute and Recurrent Pericarditis

Diagnosis
Obligatory (class I, LOE C): auscultation, ECG, echocardiography, blood analyses, chest x-ray.

Pericardiocentesis and Drainage
Obligatory (cardiac tamponade: class I, LOE B), optional in large/recurrent effusions or if previous tests were inconclusive (class IIa, LOE B) in small effusions (class IIb, LOE C).

CT, MRI, pericardioscopy, pericardial biopsy: optional or if previous tests inconclusive (class IIa, LOE C).

Therapy
Aspirin or NSAIDs (class I, LOE A).

Corticosteroids (class IIa, LOE B).

Colchicine: class IIa, LOE B (acute pericarditis), I, LOE A (recurrent pericarditis).

Pericardial Effusion and Cardiac Tamponade

Indications for Pericardiocentesis
Class I, LOE B: cardiac tamponade, large effusions (>20 mm), suspected purulent, or tuberculous pericardial effusion.

Class IIa, LOE C: effusions 10–20 mm for diagnostic purposes other than purulent or tuberculous etiology, suspected neoplastic pericardial effusions.

Class IIb, LOE C: effusions <10 mm for diagnostic purposes other than purulent, tuberculous, or neoplastic etiology.

Class III, LOE C: aortic dissection, relative contraindications for uncorrected coagulopathy, anticoagulant therapy, thrombocytopenia (platelet count <50,000/mm³), small, posterior, loculated effusions, if the effusion is small and resolve with anti-inflammatory therapy.

Pericardial Fluid Analyses
Class I, LOE C: cytology (suspected neoplastic effusion), acid-fast bacilli staining, mycobacterium culture, adenosine deaminase, IFN-gamma, pericardial lysozyme, polymerase chain reaction (PCR) analyses (suspected tuberculous effusion), at least three cultures of pericardial fluid for aerobes,

and anaerobes as well as three blood cultures with sensitivity tests for antibiotics in case of positive cultures (suspected bacterial infection).

Class IIa, LOE C: PCR analyses for cardiotropic viruses (viral vs. autoreactive pericarditis), tumor markers (suspected neoplastic cause).

Class IIb, LOE C: pericardial fluid specific gravity >1.015, protein level >3.0 g/dl, fluid/serum ratio >0.5, LDH >200 mg/dl, fluid/serum ratio >0.6, and glucose (exudate vs. transudate).

Constrictive Pericarditis

Differential Diagnosis with Restrictive Cardiomyopathy (Essential Diagnostic Evaluation)

Clinical presentation, ECG, chest x-ray, echocardiography, CT/MRI, cardiac catheterization.

References

1. Imazio M, Spodick DH, Brucato A, et al. Controversial issues in the management of pericardial diseases. Circulation. 2010;121:916–28.
2. Khandaker MH, Espinosa RE, Nishimura RA, et al. Pericardial disease: diagnosis and management. Mayo Clin Proc. 2010;85:572–93.
3. Imazio M, Brucato A, Mayosi BM, et al. Medical therapy of pericardial diseases: part I: idiopathic and infectious pericarditis. J Cardiovasc Med (Hagerstown). 2010;11:712–22.
4. Imazio M, Brucato A, Mayosi BM, et al. Medical therapy of pericardial diseases: part II: noninfectious pericarditis, pericardial effusion and constrictive pericarditis. J Cardiovasc Med (Hagerstown). 2010;11:785–94.
5. Azam S, Hoit BD. Treatment of pericardial diseases. Cardiovasc Ther. 2011;29:308–14.
6. Imazio M, Brucato A, Trinchero R, Adler Y. Diagnosis and management of pericardial diseases. Nat Rev Cardiol. 2009;6:743–51. Epub 2009 Oct 27.
7. Maisch B, Seferović PM, Ristić AD, et al. Task Force on the Diagnosis and Management of Pericardial Diseases of the European Society of Cardiology. Guidelines on the diagnosis and management of pericardial diseases executive summary; The Task force on the diagnosis and management of pericardial diseases of the European Society of Cardiology. Eur Heart J. 2004;25:587–610.
8. Sheith S, Wang DD, Kasapis C. Current and emerging strategies for the treatment of acute pericarditis: a systematic review. J Inflamm Res. 2010;3:135–42.
9. Sia IG, Wieland ML. Current concepts in the management of tuberculosis. Mayo Clin Proc. 2011;86:348–61.
10. Sliwa K, Mocumbi AO. Forgotten cardiovascular diseases in Africa. Clin Res Cardiol. 2010;99:65–74. Epub 2009 Dec 11.
11. Caforio AL, Brucato A, Doria A, et al. Anti-heart and anti-intercalated disk autoantibodies: evidence for autoimmunity in idiopathic recurrent acute pericarditis. Heart. 2010;96:779–84.
12. Imazio M, Mayosi BM, Brucato A, et al. Triage and management of pericardial effusion. J Cardiovasc Med (Hagerstown). 2010;11:928–35.
13. Sagristà-Sauleda J, Mercé AS, Soler-Soler J. Diagnosis and management of pericardial effusion. World J Cardiol. 2011;3:135–43.
14. Spodick DH. Acute cardiac tamponade. N Engl J Med. 2003;349:684–90.
15. Seferović PM, Ristić AD, Imazio M, et al. Management strategies in pericardial emergencies. Herz. 2006;31:891–900.
16. Hoit BD. Pericardial disease and pericardial tamponade. Crit Care Med. 2007;35:S355–64.
17. Imazio M, Cecchi E, Demichelis B, Ierna S, Demarie D, Ghisio A, Pomari F, Coda L, Belli R, Trinchero R. Indicators of poor prognosis of acute pericarditis. Circulation. 2007;29(115):2739–44. Epub 2007 May 14.
18. Permanyer-Miralda G. Acute pericardial disease: approach to the aetiologic diagnosis. Heart. 2004;90:252–4.
19. Pankuweit S, Ristić AD, Seferović PM, Maisch B. Bacterial pericarditis: diagnosis and management. Am J Cardiovasc Drugs. 2005; 5:103–12.
20. Mayosi BM, Burgess LJ, Doubell AF. Tuberculous pericarditis. Circulation. 2005;112:3608–16.
21. Refaat MM, Katz WE. Neoplastic pericardial effusion. Clin Cardiol. 2011;34:593–8. doi:10.1002/clc.20936. Epub 2011 Sep 16.
22. Holmes Jr DR, Nishimura R, Fountain R, Turi ZG. Iatrogenic pericardial effusion and tamponade in the percutaneous intracardiac intervention era. JACC Cardiovasc Interv. 2009;2:705–17.
23. Shabetai R. Pericardial effusion: haemodynamic spectrum. Heart. 2004;90(3):255–6.
24. Imazio M, Spodick DH, Brucato A, et al. Diagnostic issues in the clinical management of pericarditis. Int J Clin Pract. 2010;64:1384–92. Epub 2010 May 10.
25. Imazio M. Evaluation and management of pericarditis. Expert Rev Cardiovasc Ther. 2011;9:1221–33.
26. Imazio M, Brucato A, Maestroni S, et al. Prevalence of C-reactive protein elevation and time course of normalization in acute pericarditis: implications for the diagnosis, therapy, and prognosis of Pericarditis. Circulation. 2011;123:1092–7. Epub 2011 Feb 28.
27. Cheitlin MD, Armstrong WF, Aurigemma GP, Beller GA, Bierman FZ, Davis JL, Douglas PS, Faxon DP, Gillam LD, Kimball TR, Kussmaul WG, Pearlman AS, Philbrick JT, Rakowski H, Thys DM, Antman EM, Smith Jr SC, Alpert JS, Gregoratos G, Anderson JL, Hiratzka LF, Hunt SA, Fuster V, Jacobs AK, Gibbons RJ, Russell RO, American College of Cardiology, American Heart Association, American Society of Echocardiography. ACC/AHA/ASE 2003 guideline update for the clinical application of echocardiography: summary article: a report of the American College of Cardiology/ American Heart Association Task Force on Practice Guidelines (ACC/AHA/ASE committee to update the 1997 guidelines for the clinical application of echocardiography). Circulation. 2003;108: 1146–62.
28. Roy CL, Minor MA, Brookhart MA, Choudhry NK. Does this patient with a pericardial effusion have cardiac tamponade? JAMA. 2007;297:1810–8.
29. Guntheroth WG. Sensitivity and specificity of echocardiographic evidence of tamponade: implications for ventricular interdependence and pulsus paradoxus. Pediatr Cardiol. 2007;28:358–62.
30. Fowler NO. Cardiac tamponade. A clinical or an echocardiographic diagnosis? Circulation. 1993;87:1738–41.
31. Feng D, Glockner J, Kim K, et al. Cardiac magnetic resonance imaging pericardial late gadolinium enhancement and elevated inflammatory markers can predict the reversibility of constrictive pericarditis after antiinflammatory medical therapy: a pilot study. Circulation. 2011;124:1830–7. Epub 2011 Oct 3. *First evidence of criteria to identify reversibility in pericardial constriction.
32. Zurick AO, Bolen MA, Kwon DH, et al. Pericardial delayed hyperenhancement with CMR imaging in patients with constrictive pericarditis undergoing surgical pericardiectomy: a case series with histopathological correlation. JACC Cardiovasc Imaging. 2011;4:1180–91.
33. Young PM, Glockner JF, Williamson EE, et al. MR imaging findings in 76 consecutive surgically proven cases of pericardial disease

with CT and pathologic correlation. Int J Cardiovasc Imaging. 2012;28:1099–109.

34. Ntsekhe M, Shey Wiysonge C, et al. The prevalence and outcome of effusive constrictive pericarditis: a systematic review of the literature. Cardiovasc J Afr. 2012;22:1–5. doi:10.5830/CVJA-2011-072.

35. Almeida AR, Lopes LR, Cotrim C, et al. Effusive-constrictive pericarditis: the role of noninvasive imaging. Rev Port Cardiol. 2011;30:433–43.

36. Sorajja P. Invasive hemodynamics of constrictive pericarditis, restrictive cardiomyopathy, and cardiac tamponade. Cardiol Clin. 2011;29:191–9.

37. Lotrionte M, Biondi-Zoccai G, Imazio M, et al. International collaborative systematic review of controlled clinical trials on pharmacologic treatments for acute pericarditis and its recurrences. Am Heart J. 2010;160:662–70.

38. Imazio M. Pericarditis: pathophysiology, diagnosis, and management. Curr Infect Dis Rep. 2011;13:308–16.

39. Sparano DM, Ward RP. Pericarditis and pericardial effusion: management update. Curr Treat Options Cardiovasc Med. 2011;13:543–55.

40. Imazio M. Pericardial involvement in systemic inflammatory diseases. Heart. 2011;97:1882–92.

41. Imazio M, Brucato A, Rampello S, et al. Management of pericardial diseases during pregnancy. J Cardiovasc Med (Hagerstown). 2010;11:557–62.

42. Imazio M, Brucato A, Maestroni S, et al. Risk of constrictive pericarditis after acute pericarditis. Circulation. 2011;124:1270–5. Epub 2011 Aug 15.

43. Imazio M, Trinchero R. The spectrum of inflammatory myopericardial diseases. Int J Cardiol. 2010;144:134. Epub 2009 Jan 28.

44. Imazio M, Cecchi E, Demichelis B, et al. Myopericarditis versus viral or idiopathic acute pericarditis. Heart. 2008;94:498–501. Epub 2007 Jun 17.

45. Imazio M, Brucato A, Barbieri A, Ferroni F, Maestroni S, Ligabue G, Chinaglia A, Cumetti D, Casa GD, Bonomi F, Mantovani F, Di Corato P, Lugli R, Faletti R, Leuzzi S, Bonamini R, Modena MG, Belli R. Good prognosis for pericarditis with and without myocardial involvement: results from a multicenter, prospective cohort study. Circulation. 2013 Jul 2;128(1):42–9. doi:10.1161/CIRCULATIONAHA.113.001531. Epub 2013 May 24. PubMed PMID: 23709669.

46. Imazio M, Brucato A, Cemin R, et al. CORP (COlchicine for Recurrent Pericarditis) Investigators. Colchicine for recurrent pericarditis (CORP): a randomized trial. Ann Intern Med. 2011;155:409–14. Epub 2011 Aug 28.

47. Cocco G, Chu DC, Pandolfi S. Colchicine in clinical medicine. A guide for internists. Eur J Intern Med. 2010;21:503–8. Epub 2010 Nov 5.

48. Farand P, Bonenfant F, Belley-Côté EP, Tzouannis N. Acute and recurring pericarditis: more colchicine, less corticosteroids. World J Cardiol. 2010;2:403–7.

49. Finkelstein Y, Aks SE, Hutson JR, et al. Colchicine poisoning: the dark side of an ancient drug. Clin Toxicol (Phila). 2010;48:407–14.

50. Frasiolas JA, Cahoon WD. Intrapericardial triamcinolone administration for autoreactive pericarditis. Ann Pharmacother. 2010;44:1641–6.

51. Vianello F, Cinetto F, Cavraro M, et al. Azathioprine in isolated recurrent pericarditis: a single centre experience. Int J Cardiol. 2011;147:477–85. Epub 2011 Feb 5.

52. Schairer JR, Biswas S, Keteyian SJ, Ananthasubramaniam K. A systematic approach to evaluation of pericardial effusion and cardiac tamponade. Cardiol Rev. 2011;19:233–8.

53. Imazio M, Brucato A, Rovere ME, et al. Colchicine prevents early postoperative pericardial and pleural effusions. Am Heart J. 2011;162:527–32.e1.

54. Meurin P, Tabet JY, Thabut G, French Society of Cardiology, et al. Nonsteroidal anti-inflammatory drug treatment for postoperative pericardial effusion: a multicenter randomized, double-blind trial. Ann Intern Med. 2010;152:137–43.

55. Lee GY, Ahn KT, Jung CW, Chang SA. Recurrent pericarditis after chemotherapy for acute myeloid leukemia: a case report and a modern approach to chemotherapy-induced pericarditis. Cardiology. 2011;120:130–4.

56. Lestuzzi C. Neoplastic pericardial disease: old and current strategies for diagnosis and management. World J Cardiol. 2010;2:270–9.

57. Lestuzzi C, Bearz A, Lafaras C, et al. Neoplastic pericardial disease in lung cancer: impact on outcomes of different treatment strategies. A multicenter study. Lung Cancer. 2011;72:340–7. Epub 2010 Nov 30.

58. Akyuz S, Yaylak B, Ergelen M, Uyarel H. Transient constrictive pericarditis: an elusive diagnosis. Future Cardiol. 2010;6:785–90.

59. Kim JB, Park NH, Choi SY, Kim H. Transient constrictive pericarditis after coronary bypass surgery. Korean J Thorac Cardiovasc Surg. 2011;44:64–7.

60. Verhaert D, Gabriel RS, Johnston D, et al. The role of multimodality imaging in the management of pericardial disease. Circ Cardiovasc Imaging. 2010;3:333–43.

61. Yared K, Baggish AL, Picard MH, et al. Multimodality imaging of pericardial diseases. JACC Cardiovasc Imaging. 2010;3:650–60.

62. Permanyer-Miralda G, Sagristá-Sauleda J, Soler-Soler J. Primary acute pericardial disease: a prospective series of 231 consecutive patients. Am J Cardiol. 1985;56(10):623–30.

63. Zayas R, Anguita M, Torres F, Giménez D, Bergillos F, Ruiz M, Ciudad M, Gallardo A, Vallés F. Incidence of specific etiology and role of methods for specific etiologic diagnosis of primary acute pericarditis. Am J Cardiol. 1995;75(5):378–82.

64. Imazio M, Cecchi E, Demichelis B, Ierna S, Demarie D, Ghisio A, Pomari F, Coda L, Belli R, Trinchero R. Indicators of poor prognosis of acute pericarditis. Circulation. 2007;115(21):2739–44.

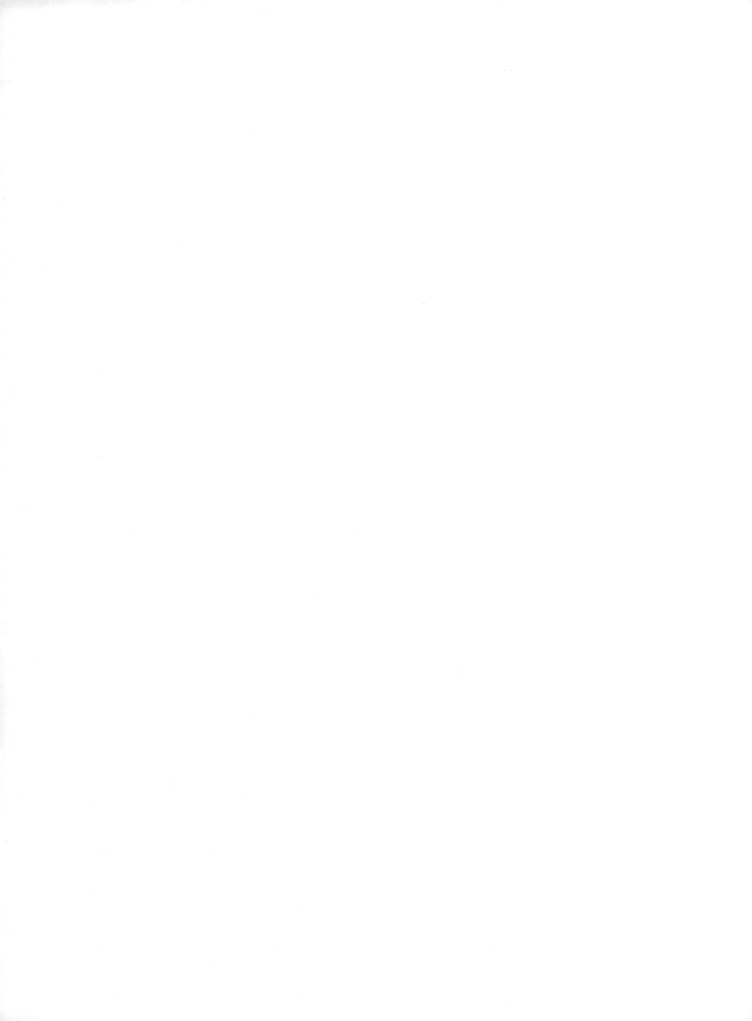

Atrial Fibrillation and Supraventricular Tachycardias

Roger Fan and Eric J. Rashba

Abstract

Atrial fibrillation (AF) can cause significant symptoms and diminished quality of life, but, more importantly, is associated with increased risks of stroke, congestive heart failure, and mortality. It is the most common arrhythmia, and its prevalence continues to increase. Its prevalence in 2005 was 3.03 million and is projected to rise to 7.56 million by 2050. Already AF accounts for 350,000 annual hospitalizations and $6.65 billion dollars in annual healthcare costs in the United States. The medical management of atrial fibrillation can be challenging and needs to encompass evaluation and treatment of underlying causes, thromboembolic prophylaxis, and decision-making regarding rate or rhythm control.

Supraventricular tachycardia (SVT) is a term that encompasses atrioventricular nodal reentrant tachycardia (AVNRT), atrioventricular reentrant tachycardia (AVRT), atrial tachycardia (AT), and inappropriate sinus tachycardia (IST). Although these disorders are generally considered benign, they can cause significant morbidity. In certain instances (Wolff-Parkinson-White syndrome), they can be life-threatening, and almost all tachyarrhythmias, if left untreated for extended periods of time, can lead to tachycardia-mediated cardiomyopathies. The prognostic implications for the patient, subsequent evaluation, and treatment may vary considerably depending on the etiology of the arrhythmia. The aim of this chapter is to provide a framework to successfully diagnose and manage these arrhythmias.

Keywords

Atrial fibrillation • SVT • AVNRT • AVRT • Catheter ablation • Inappropriate sinus tachycardia

Introduction

Atrial fibrillation (AF) can cause significant symptoms and diminished quality of life, but, more importantly, is associated with increased risks of stroke, congestive heart failure, and mortality [1–3]. It is the most common arrhythmia, and its prevalence continues to increase. In 2005, its prevalence was 3.03 million and is projected to rise to 7.56 million by 2050 [4]. Already AF accounts for 350,000 annual hospitalizations and $6.65 billion dollars in annual healthcare costs in the United States [5]. The medical management of atrial fibrillation can be challenging and needs to encompass evaluation and treatment of underlying causes, thromboembolic prophylaxis, and decision-making regarding a rate or rhythm control strategy.

R. Fan, MD (✉)
Cardiac Arrhythmia Consult Service, Department of Medicine, Stony Brook University School of Medicine, HSC 16-080, Stony Brook, NY 11794, USA
e-mail: roger.fan@stonybrookmedicine.edu

E.J. Rashba, MD
Cardiac Electrophysiology, Department of Medicine, Stony Brook University School of Medicine, HSC 16-080, Stony Brook, NY 11794, USA
e-mail: eric.rashba@stonybrookmedicine.edu

K. Stergiopoulos, D.L. Brown (eds.), *Evidence-Based Cardiology Consult*, DOI 10.1007/978-1-4471-4441-0_8, © Springer-Verlag London 2014

Supraventricular tachycardia (SVT) is a term that encompasses atrioventricular nodal reentrant tachycardia (AVNRT), atrioventricular reentrant tachycardia (AVRT), atrial tachycardia (AT), and inappropriate sinus tachycardia (IST). Although these disorders are generally considered benign, they can cause significant morbidity. In certain instances (Wolff-Parkinson-White syndrome), they can be life-threatening, and almost all tachyarrhythmias, if left untreated for extended periods of time, can lead to tachycardia-mediated cardiomyopathies [6]. The prognostic implications for the patient, subsequent evaluation, and treatment may vary considerably depending on the etiology of the arrhythmia. The aim of this chapter is to provide a framework to successfully approach and manage these arrhythmias.

The etiologies of AF and SVTs are disorders of impulse formation or conduction. Abnormal impulse formation is due to either abnormal automaticity or triggered activity. Abnormal automaticity occurs when cardiac tissue assumes pacemaker activity due to abnormal acceleration of phase 4 activity. This can occur in cells that normally have automatic activity (sinus node or AV junction), as well as other ectopic cells within the atrium. Triggered activity is provoked by prior beats or series of beats, which cause abnormal leak of current into the cell, leading to afterdepolarizations. Disorders of impulse conduction can cause reentry, which is the most common mechanism for tachyarrhythmias including atrial fibrillation, atrial flutter, AVNRT, AVRT, and some ATs. Reentry occurs in tissue with heterogeneous conduction properties, where a propagated impulse fails to extinguish, leading to a repetitive circuit of impulse conduction in adjacent tissue that has regained excitability. Although most arrhythmias have a single mechanism, some arrhythmias may be caused by multiple mechanisms, independently or in concert, such as AT or AF, respectively.

Atrial Fibrillation

AF is characterized by disorganized atrial activity with an irregular ventricular response. Symptoms and adverse consequences from AF are due to the irregular ventricular rate, tachycardia, bradycardia, diminished cardiac output, and thromboembolism. The etiology of AF is complex and incompletely understood but is thought to be due to a combination of triggers, substrate, and autonomic influences on the atria. The field of AF was revolutionized when Haissaguerre et al. documented that the majority of AF was triggered by ectopic firing from within the pulmonary veins [7]. In addition to triggers for AF, an atrial substrate has to be present which allows AF to perpetuate. It is believed that atrial stretch results in both anatomic and electrical remodeling that creates a substrate rich for reentry, where multiple wave fronts coexist and collide in a chaotic manner [8]. Atrial

stretch can be due to a vast number of causes, including hypertension, congestive heart failure, cardiomyopathies, valvular disease, pericarditis, pulmonary disease, hyperthyroidism, infections, and drugs including caffeine and alcohol. Lastly, the autonomic nervous system is thought to play a role in both the genesis and maintenance of AF, likely mediated by ganglionic plexuses that insert into the left atrium [9].

AF is diagnosed by electrocardiogram (ECG) when there is a lack of organized P wave activity and irregular RR intervals. In certain patients there may be an appearance of P wave organization in V1, which may be confused with atrial flutter or atrial tachycardia, but this organization will not be seen in other leads. Additionally, the appearance of organization will be irregular, and the atrial cycle length will typically be less than 200 ms (or greater than 300 bpm). AF is characterized as being paroxysmal, persistent, long-standing persistent, or permanent. Paroxysmal AF is defined as recurrent AF that terminates within 7 days. Persistent AF is defined as recurrent AF that is sustained for ≥7 days. Long-standing persistent AF is defined as continuous AF of greater than 12 months' duration. The term permanent AF refers to patients for whom a decision has been made not to restore or maintain sinus rhythm by any means, including catheter or surgical ablation [10].

All patients with newly diagnosed AF should be evaluated and treated for precipitating or reversible causes. A transthoracic echocardiogram to identify left atrial (LA) and right atrial (RA) size and to evaluate for structural heart disease should be performed. In addition, blood tests for thyroid, renal, and hepatic functions should be sent. The primary goals for management of AF are prevention of thromboembolism and symptom control, which may be achieved by either a rate control or rhythm control strategy.

Anticoagulation

The etiology of stroke in atrial fibrillation is primarily due to blood stasis in the left atrial appendage and systemic hypercoagulability, with resultant thrombus formation. The yearly risk for stroke in patients with AF varies from 1.9 to 18.2 % depending on risk factors and is independent of whether the AF is paroxysmal, persistent, or permanent [11, 12]. Treatment with warfarin and antiplatelet agents reduces stroke risk by 64 and 22 %, respectively, but warfarin is associated with an increased major bleeding risk compared to aspirin (2.2 % vs. 1.3 %) [13, 14]. The decision to anticoagulate patients with nonvalvular AF depends on the risk factors for stroke that are present. The risk model for stroke that is most commonly used and validated is the CHADS$_2$ risk score (Table 8.1) [11]. 1 point is given for each risk factor of congestive heart failure, hypertension, age ≥75, and diabetes

Table 8.1 Stroke risk in patients with nonvalvular atrial fibrillation not treated with anticoagulation according to the $CHADS_2$ risk score

$CHADS_2$ risk factors		Score
Cardiac failure		1
Hypertension		1
Age >75 years		1
Diabetes mellitus		1
Prior Stroke or TIA		2
$CHADS_2$ score	Patients (n = 1,733)	Adjusted stroke rate (%/year) (95 % CI)
0	120	1.9 (1.2–3.0)
1	463	2.8 (2.0–3.8)
2	523	4.0 (3.1–5.1)
3	337	5.9 (4.6–7.3)
4	220	8.5 (6.3–11.1)
5	65	12.5 (8.2–17.5)
6	5	18.2 (10.5–27.4)

Adapted from Gage et al. [11]

mellitus; 2 points are given for a history of transient ischemic attack, stroke, or systemic thromboembolism. For $CHADS_2$ score of 0, aspirin 81–325 mg daily is recommended. For $CHADS_2$ score ≥2, oral anticoagulation is recommended. For $CHADS_2$ score of 1, patients can be treated with either aspirin or an oral anticoagulant, depending on physician assessment of stroke risk, risk of bleeding, and patient preference [15]. A modified CHA_2DS_2VASc risk score has been proposed to improve the accuracy of risk stratification for stroke in patients with a $CHADS_2$ score of 0–1 and has been adopted by the European Society of Cardiology (ESC) [16]. In addition to the risk factors for the $CHADS_2$ score, CHA_2DS_2VASc places emphasis on female sex (1 point), age (1 point for ages 65–74; 2 points for age ≥75), and presence of atherosclerotic cardiovascular disease (1 point). For a CHA_2DS_2VASc score of 0, no anticoagulation is recommended; for a score of 1, aspirin or oral anticoagulant is recommended; and for a score ≥2, oral anticoagulation is recommended. There are certain other patients with AF who are at high risk for stroke who are indicated for anticoagulation with warfarin, which includes patients with valvular heart disease and prosthetic heart valves.

In the past several years, several new alternatives to warfarin have emerged for nonvalvular AF. Dabigatran is an oral direct thrombin inhibitor which has been shown in the Randomized Evaluation of Long-Term Anticoagulation Therapy (RE-LY) trial to significantly decrease the risk of stroke and systemic embolism compared to warfarin with a similar risk for major hemorrhage (150 mg dosing), but with a trend towards increased risk of bleeding in patients >74 years [17]. Rivaroxaban and apixaban are oral factor Xa inhibitors. In the Rivaroxaban Once Daily Oral Direct Factor Xa Inhibition Compared with Vitamin K Antagonism for Prevention of Stroke and Embolism Trial in Atrial Fibrillation

(ROCKET AF), rivaroxaban was shown to be noninferior to warfarin but with a decreased risk for intracerebral hemorrhage and fatal bleeds [18]. In the Apixaban for Reduction in Stroke and Other Thromboembolic Events in Atrial Fibrillation (ARISTOTLE) trial, apixaban was superior to warfarin in preventing stroke and systemic embolism in addition to having a lower risk for major bleeding and all-cause mortality [19]. Although these novel drugs are more convenient than warfarin since they do not require international normalized ratio (INR) monitoring, there are some significant disadvantages, notably higher cost, need for dose adjustment for dabigatran and rivaroxaban in patients with impaired renal function, and lack of an antidote or reversal agent.

Initial Management

For patients who present with AF with rapid ventricular rates and hemodynamic instability or coronary ischemia, immediate electrical cardioversion is indicated. For other patients who are stable, but are unable to be successfully rate controlled with AV node-blocking agents or who remain symptomatic in AF despite adequate rate control, an attempt at restoring sinus rhythm with pharmacologic or electrical cardioversion should be considered. It is believed that most left atrial thrombi form in patients who are in AF for more than 48 h, and most thromboembolic events occur within 10 days of cardioversion due to atrial stunning [15].

Patients who have been in AF less than 48 h may be cardioverted without need for transesophageal echocardiography (TEE) to rule out left atrial thrombus. Few studies have evaluated the need for short- or long-term anticoagulation in these patients. Our practice is to administer intravenous heparin, enoxaparin, or dabigatran prior to cardioversion only in patients with high-risk factors for stroke and to continue oral anticoagulation according to risk-based guidelines.

In patients who have been in AF for longer than 48 h, or if there is uncertainty regarding the time of onset, therapeutic oral anticoagulation is recommended for 3 weeks prior to cardioversion and for a minimum of 4 weeks after anticoagulation (ACC/AHA/ESC Class I recommendation, Level of Evidence B). Alternatively, TEE can be performed to rule out left atrial thrombus prior to cardioversion (ACC/AHA ESC Class IIa recommendation, Level of Evidence B) [15]. Cardioversion should be performed when the INR is therapeutic in patients treated with warfarin or after administration of therapeutic doses of heparin (PTT 60–90 s), Lovenox 1 mg/kg SC BID, or dabigatran [15, 20]. If a thrombus is seen, therapeutic oral anticoagulation should be documented for a minimum of 4 weeks before a repeat TEE is performed. After cardioversion, anticoagulation should be continued for a minimum of 4 weeks and potentially longer according to risk-based guidelines.

Rate Versus Rhythm Control

There are two main pharmacologic strategies for the long-term management of AF. Rate control refers to using medications to slow conduction in the AV node to control the heart rate during AF. Rhythm control involves using antiarrhythmic drugs to prevent recurrences of AF. No study has shown one strategy to be superior to the other; patients may often fail one strategy, requiring attempts at the other. The decision for anticoagulation is independent of the decision for a rate or rhythm control strategy.

The mainstays of rate control therapy include beta-blockers, non-dihydropyridine calcium channel blockers, and digoxin. To control the rapid heart rates, occasionally these medications can cause symptomatic bradycardia that may warrant pacemaker implantation. The Rate Control Efficacy in Permanent Atrial Fibrillation: a Comparison between Lenient versus Strict Rate Control II (RACE II) trial compared patients with permanent AF randomized either to a lenient rate control strategy (resting heart rate (HR) <110 bpm) or to a strict rate control strategy (resting HR <80 bpm and HR with moderate exercise <110 bpm) and found the lenient strategy to be noninferior (composite outcome of death, heart failure, stroke, systemic embolism, bleeding, and life-threatening arrhythmias) with a higher success rate in reaching target heart rates [21]. Whether or not this lenient strategy can apply to patient with congestive heart failure or cardiomyopathies is unknown. In patients who cannot be rate-controlled pharmacologically and who are not candidates for rhythm control, AV nodal ablation with implantation of a pacemaker can be considered. If the patient has a reduced left ventricular ejection fraction (LVEF) or congestive heart failure (CHF) symptoms, implantation of a biventricular pacemaker may prevent deterioration in LVEF or CHF [22].

Antiarrhythmics typically used for rhythm control are the class IC agents, propafenone and flecainide, and the class III agents sotalol, dofetilide, dronedarone, and amiodarone. The class IC agents are the usual first-line antiarrhythmics in younger patients with structurally normal heart and are convenient because they can be started in an outpatient setting. However, they are contraindicated in patients with CAD or structural heart disease due to the risk of fatal proarrhythmia [23]. Because of the potential for IC agents to organize AF into atrial flutter that can conduct 1:1 to the ventricle, they must be used in conjunction with beta-blockers or calcium channel blockers. The IC agents are also associated with use dependence (the faster the HR, the greater the antiarrhythmic effect due to drug binding), and consequently, routine treadmill stress testing should be performed to evaluate for exercise-induced QRS widening >150 % of baseline, or proarrhythmia [15]. The class III agents sotalol and dofetilide are associated with QTc prolongation and torsades de pointes

and therefore must be initiated in the hospital setting. Telemetry monitoring for arrhythmias is required for 5 doses; ECGs should be obtained 2 h after each dose to monitor for QTc prolongation. Sotalol should be avoided in patients with CHF or renal insufficiency and, because of its beta-blocker effects, may exacerbate bronchospasm, bradycardia, or hypotension. Dofetilide is a useful agent because it has no negative hemodynamic effects and only mild negative chronotropic effects. However, it must also be used with caution in patients with renal insufficiency with appropriate dose adjustment. Dronedarone should be avoided in patients with NYHA class III–IV CHF, recent hospitalization for CHF, or LVEF ≤ 35 % [24]. It is associated with increased rates of heart failure, stroke, and death from cardiovascular causes in patients with risk factors for vascular events and permanent AF [25]. Amiodarone is the most effective antiarrhythmic in treating AF, but is associated with many long-term side effects such as pulmonary toxicity (1–17 %), hepatotoxicity (15–30 % with elevated AST/ALT, <3 % with hepatitis and cirrhosis), hypothyroidism (6 %), hyperthyroidism (0.9–2 %), photosensitivity (25–75 %), skin discoloration (4–9 %), optic neuritis (≤1–2 %), and tremors and ataxia (3–35 %) [26].

The Atrial Fibrillation Follow-up Investigation of Rhythm Management (AFFIRM) trial randomized patients with AF to a rate control or rhythm control strategy and found no survival advantage with a rhythm control strategy [27]. A major limitation of the AFFIRM trial is that younger, healthier patients were excluded from the study as well as patients with highly symptomatic AF. It is possible that a more aggressive strategy for rhythm control in this population of patients may be beneficial. The Atrial Fibrillation and Congestive Heart Failure (AF-CHF) trial randomized patients with AF, CHF, and LVEF ≤ 35 % to a rate control or rhythm control strategy and also found no difference in death from cardiovascular causes or worsening CHF [28]. Although these trials showed similar outcomes between rate control and rhythm control strategies, substudies of the AFFIRM trial and Danish Investigations of Arrhythmia and Mortality ON Dofetilide (DIAMOND) trial (comparison of dofetilide to placebo in patients with LV dysfunction) showed that the presence of sinus rhythm was associated with significant reductions in mortality [29, 30]. These results suggest that maintaining sinus rhythm may improve outcomes if there were a safer and more effective way of maintaining sinus rhythm than using medications, such as catheter ablation of AF.

Catheter Ablation of AF

Catheter ablation of AF has developed into a relatively safe and effective alternative for treating AF in select patients. The basic principle behind catheter ablation of AF is to electrically isolate the pulmonary veins from the left atrium, preventing pulmonary vein ectopic firings from triggering AF. There are additional techniques used to target the substrate underlying AF, such as creating linear lesions within the LA and targeting sites of complex fractionated electrograms. A meta-analysis of 8 randomized controlled trials comparing AF ablation to antiarrhythmic medications demonstrated a 76.8 % success rate in preventing atrial tachyarrhythmia recurrence in the ablation group compared to a 23.4 % success rate in the antiarrhythmic group [31]. In general, success rates from AF ablation are higher in patients with paroxysmal AF compared to patients with persistent AF. Predictors of poorer outcome include sleep apnea, obesity, increased LA size, increased age, and HTN. AF ablation is associated with a major complication rate of 4.5 %, which is mainly comprised of cardiac tamponade (1.3 %) and femoral vascular pseudoaneurysm/AV fistula (0.9 %/0.5 %). Other risks include pulmonary vein stenosis requiring intervention (0.3 %), stroke/TIA (0.2 %/0.7 %), atrioesophageal fistula (0.02 %), and death (0.15 %) [32].

Catheter ablation of AF has been clearly demonstrated to be superior to antiarrhythmic medications in preventing recurrences of AF and improving quality of life. In addition, catheter ablation results in reverse remodeling of the LA and, in patients with AF and CHF, improves exercise capacity, symptoms, quality of life, and ejection fraction [33]. Because of these outcomes, catheter ablation of AF performed in experienced centers is recommended to maintain sinus rhythm in selected patients with significantly symptomatic, paroxysmal AF who have failed treatment with an antiarrhythmic drug and have normal or mildly dilated left atria, normal or mildly reduced LVEF, and no severe pulmonary disease (American College of Cardiology (ACC)/American Heart Association (AHA)/European Society of Cardiology (ESC) Class I recommendation, Level of Evidence A). Catheter ablation is also reasonable to treat symptomatic persistent AF (ACC/AHA ESC Class IIa recommendation, Level of Evidence A) [15]. One major question that remains is whether catheter ablation of AF is associated with improved survival, which is expected to be answered with ongoing multicenter, prospective, randomized clinical trials comparing catheter ablation with medical management of AF.

Postoperative AF

Atrial fibrillation and flutter is very common in the early postoperative period following open heart surgery with an incidence between 10 and 65 %. The incidence is lower in patients undergoing coronary artery bypass graft surgery (CABG) alone and higher in patients undergoing valve surgery or combined CABG and valve operations [34]. The likely pathophysiology includes the underlying predisposition for AF, such as age-related degenerative changes in the myocardium and perioperative conditions that alter the electrophysiological properties of the atria, such as adrenergic tone, vasoactive medications and inotropes, volume overload, inflammation, pericarditis, atrial ischemia, and electrolyte imbalance. The majority of AF episodes occur within postoperative days 2–3 and usually self-terminate within 24 h. Ninety percent of patients are in sinus rhythm 6–8 weeks following surgery [35]. However, postoperative AF after CABG is associated with increased in-hospital mortality (7.4 % vs. 3.4 %) and long-term mortality at 4 years (26 vs. 13 %) [36].

Prophylactic therapy with beta-blockers and amiodarone has been shown to decrease the incidence of post-CABG AF by 77 and 45 %, respectively [34]. Because no study has directly compared amiodarone to beta-blockers for prophylaxis of postoperative AF and due to the cost and incidence of side effects with amiodarone, beta-blockers are recommended as first-line prophylactic therapy (ACC/AHA/ESC Class I recommendation, Level of Evidence A). Angiotensin converting enzyme (ACE) inhibitors, statins, and colchicine have also been shown to prevent postoperative AF [37–39]. Postoperative continuous atrial overdrive pacing using temporary epicardial wires can also decrease the incidence of postoperative AF after CABG [40]. For rate control of AF, beta-blockers are recommended as first-line therapy (ACC/AHA/ESC Class I recommendation, Level of Evidence A), particularly because they counter the heightened sympathetic postoperative state [15]. Calcium channel blockers and digoxin may also be used.

If the ventricular rate cannot be controlled, the patient remains symptomatic despite rate control, or if anticoagulation needs to be avoided, pharmacologic or electrical cardioversion can be performed if the duration of AF is less than 48 h. If the duration of AF is ≥48 h, a TEE is recommended to rule out LA thrombus, and cardioversion should be performed on therapeutic anticoagulation. In patients requiring cardioversion, short-term amiodarone can be a useful agent for both cardioversion and maintenance of sinus rhythm in the postoperative setting. We generally stop amiodarone by postoperative week 4.

Patients who develop AF after cardiac surgery have a small but significant increase in the risk for stroke [41]. Because of this, patients who develop AF after cardiac surgery lasting for >48 h should be treated with antithrombotic medications, as recommended for nonsurgical patients (ACC/AHA/ESC Class IIa recommendation, Level of Evidence B) [15]. The decision for bridging with heparin should be made on a case-by-case basis according to bleeding risk. Patients who had preexisting AF or have evidence of AF after the postoperative period should be treated with oral anticoagulation according to their risk factors for thromboembolism.

Key Points
- All patients with AF should be evaluated for oral anticoagulation according to risk factors for thromboembolism.
- Patients not on therapeutic anticoagulation who are in AF for >48 h require either 3 weeks of therapeutic anticoagulation or TEE prior to cardioversion.
- Patients with AF can be managed with either rate control or rhythm control strategies.
- Catheter ablation of AF is an effective alternative to antiarrhythmic medications and the side effects associated with them.

Atrial Flutter

Atrial flutter is the second most common atrial tachyarrhythmia. It is a macroreentrant arrhythmia originating in the right atrium. The arrhythmic wave front typically travels in a circular loop behind the tricuspid annulus, involving the cavotricuspid isthmus. The underlying disorders that typically precipitate AF can also be associated with atrial flutter. In addition, patients with atrial flutter often have coexisting AF.

Atrial flutter is classified as being typical or atypical. Typical atrial flutters originate in the right atrium, involve the cavotricuspid isthmus, and rotate behind the tricuspid valve in either a counterclockwise (more common) or clockwise direction. Atypical atrial flutters do not involve the cavotricuspid isthmus, can originate in both the right and left atria, and usually are due to reentry around surgical scars or as a consequence of extensive catheter ablation, such as seen after ablation for atrial fibrillation.

The atrial rate of typical atrial flutter is typically 300 bpm, and conduction to the ventricle usually occurs in a 2:1 or 4:1 ratio. Because of this, any supraventricular tachycardia at ~150 bpm should trigger the suspicion for atrial flutter, especially since every other flutter wave may be hidden within the QRS complex or ST segment. Vagal maneuvers or adenosine may transiently increase the degree of AV block, making the flutter waves more apparent. The ECG characteristics of typical counterclockwise atrial flutter include a negative sawtooth pattern in the inferior leads and a positive flutter wave in V1 with transition to negative by V3. Typical clockwise atrial flutter has the opposite pattern, with positive flutter waves in the inferior leads, with negative flutter wave in V1 and transition to positive by V3. Additionally, clockwise flutter exhibits a sine wave pattern in the inferior leads rather than a sawtooth pattern (Fig. 8.1).

The management strategies of typical atrial flutter generally mirror that of AF, but there are several important differences. Atrial flutter is associated with increased thromboembolic risk, but comparisons to AF are limited as patients often have both atrial flutter and AF. Consequently, recommendations for anticoagulation for atrial flutter are the same as those for AF [15]. Rate control of atrial flutter is often more difficult and requires higher doses of AV node-blocking medications than AF. This is because the slower atrial flutter rate results in less concealed conduction and refractoriness in the AV node than in AF. Rhythm control of typical atrial flutter with antiarrhythmic medications has fallen out of favor because of the efficacy of catheter ablation. A meta-analysis of 158 studies comprising 10,719 patients reported a 93 % long-term ablation success rate [42]. In patients who present with symptomatic recurrent atrial flutter without a reversible cause or have a history of CHF or cardiomyopathy, catheter ablation of atrial flutter is the first-line therapy (ACC/AHA/ESC Class I, Level of Evidence B) [43]. Similar to the recommendations for AF, if the patient has been in atrial flutter for >48 h without therapeutic anticoagulation, a TEE is recommended to rule out LA clot prior to catheter ablation and should be continued for a minimum of 4 weeks. After successful ablation of atrial flutter, 34 % of patients are found to have occurrences of AF [42]. Because of this, in patients with risk factors for thromboembolism, our practice is to monitor for asymptomatic occurrences of AF prior to discontinuation of anticoagulation.

Key Points
- Catheter ablation is first-line therapy for symptomatic recurrent atrial flutter.
- After successful ablation of atrial flutter, patients have a relatively high incidence of AF.

Atrioventricular Nodal Reentrant Tachycardia

AVNRT is the most common SVT and accounts for 60 % of all SVTs. It originates in the AV node due to the presence of two anatomically and functionally distinct pathways of conduction, called the fast and slow pathways. Typical AVNRT is initiated by atrial premature beats that block in the fast pathway and conduct with enough delay in the slow pathway that the fast pathway recovers from refractoriness and is then able to conduct retrograde, initiating intranodal reentry. The arrhythmic circuit involves only the AV node; the atria and ventricle are passively activated. Atypical AVNRT, which is less common, conducts antegrade down the fast pathway and retrograde up the slow pathway.

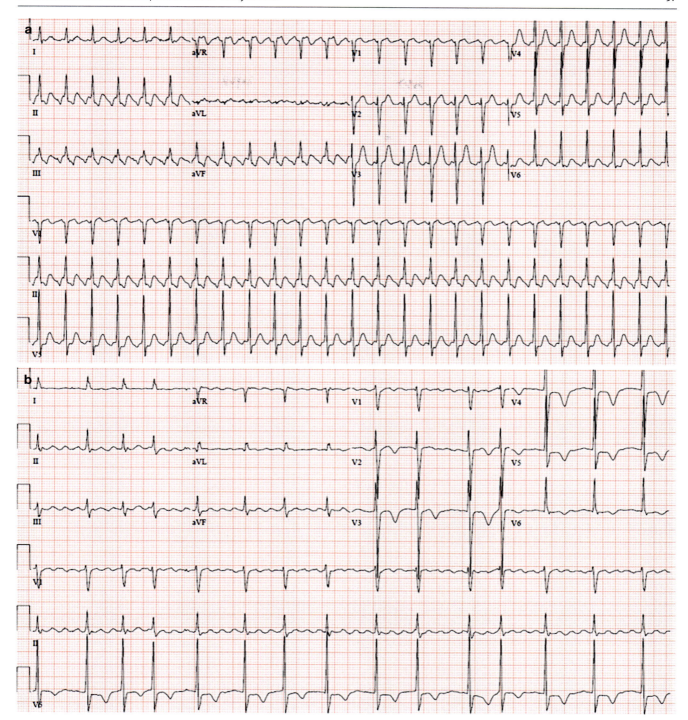

Fig. 8.1 Twelve-lead electrocardiograms of typical atrial flutters. (**a**) Counterclockwise atrial flutter with 2:1 ventricular response, with characteristic negative sawtooth f waves in leads *II, III,* and F and positive f wave in *V1.* (**b**) Clockwise atrial flutter with variable ventricular response, with positive sine waves in leads *II, III,* and F and negative f wave in *V1*

ECG characteristics of typical AVNRT are a narrow complex tachycardia, usually 140–250 bpm, with a short RP interval (in the first half of the RR interval). However, often the P wave is not readily seen because it is hidden within the QRS complex as the RP interval is usually ≤70 ms. If the P wave is able to be identified, it usually appears at the end of the QRS complex or early in the ST segment, causing a pseudo-R′ at the end of the QRS in V1 or pseudo-S′ in the inferior leads (Fig. 8.2). Atypical AVNRT is associated with a long RP interval (the second half of the RR interval) with

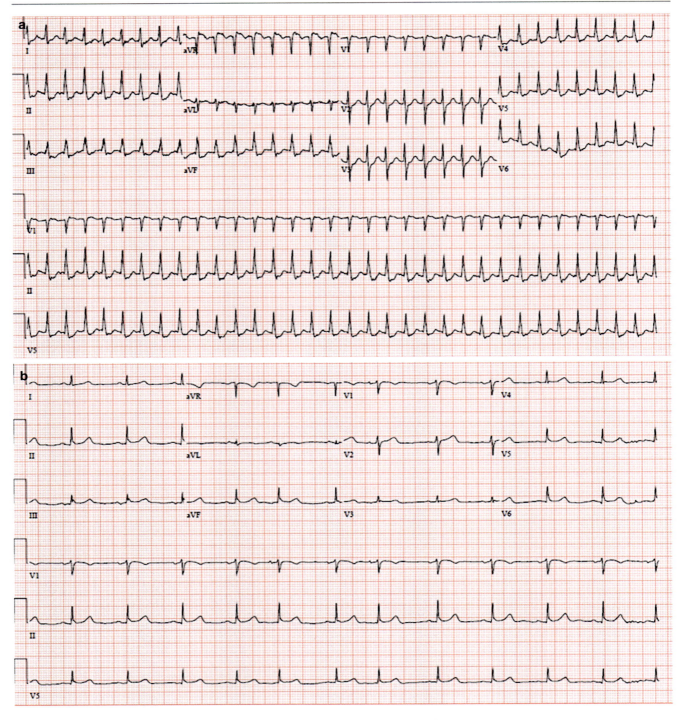

Fig. 8.2 Twelve-lead electrocardiogram of atrioventricular nodal reentry tachycardia (*AVNRT*). (**a**) Typical AVNRT with short RP interval, represented by pseudo-R′ in lead *V1* and pseudo-S′ in leads *II*, *III*, and F. (**b**) Same patient in sinus rhythm with resolution of pseudo-R′ in *V1* and pseudo-S′ in the inferior leads

the retrograde P wave occurring after inscription of the T wave. The P wave is typically inverted in leads II, III, and F. The response to vagal maneuvers or adenosine can be informative. If the tachycardia terminates abruptly with a P wave, it favors AVNRT or AVRT and excludes AT, as it is unlikely

that the AT will terminate coincidentally with AV node block. If it terminates abruptly with a QRS, AT is favored.

If AVNRT is not acutely terminated with vagal maneuvers or adenosine, intravenous beta-blockers and calcium channel blockers can be used. Cardioversion is rarely required, but may be necessary if AVNRT is not hemodynamically tolerated. For long-term therapy, treatment is determined by the frequency and severity of symptoms. Some patients with infrequent and well-tolerated symptoms may not need chronic medications if vagal maneuvers are successful in terminating the arrhythmia. If required, beta-blockers, calcium channel blockers, or digoxin can be used. Class IC and III antiarrhythmics are an option in treating AVNRT but are rarely used due to the efficacy and safety profile of catheter ablation. Since overall drug efficacy is in the range of 30–50 %, catheter ablation is considered the preferred therapy for patients with AVNRT (ACC/AHA/ESC Class I, Level of Evidence B) [43]. Catheter ablation targets the slow pathway of the AV node and is associated with a 96 % success rate. The only significant complication rate is a 1 % risk of second- or third-degree heart block [43].

> **Key Points**
> • Catheter ablation is first-line therapy for patients with AVNRT.

Preexcitation Syndromes and Atrioventricular Reentrant Tachycardia

Preexcitation is present in up to 0.25 % of the general population and is due to the presence of an accessory pathway (AP) connecting the atrium and ventricle across the AV groove [44]. APs can have variable patterns of conduction, either antegrade, retrograde, or both. When APs conduct antegrade, they result in manifest preexcitation in the form of a delta wave on ECG, due to fusion of conduction through the AV node and the AP. The degree and pattern of preexcitation depends on the location of the AP, conduction properties of the AP, and conduction properties of the AV node. If the AP is on the left side of the heart and is slowly conducting or if the AV node is rapidly conducting, there may only be a small degree of preexcitation. Wolff-Parkinson-White (WPW) syndrome is diagnosed when preexcitation is associated with tachyarrhythmias, typically atrioventricular reentrant tachycardia (AVRT). AVRT is characterized as being orthodromic or antidromic. Orthodromic AVRT, which is more common, conducts antegrade over the AV node and retrogradely up the AP, resulting in a normal QRS pattern. Antidromic AVRT conducts antegrade down the AP and retrograde up the AP, resulting in a fully preexcited QRS complex. Atrial fibrillation, which may be initiated by rapid AVRT, is a potentially lethal arrhythmia in patients with WPW if rapid conduction to the ventricles over the AP degenerates into ventricular fibrillation. If the

AP conducts retrograde only, which is called a concealed bypass tract, the surface ECG will have a normal QRS pattern. The only clinical evidence of a concealed bypass tract may be SVT.

Orthodromic AVRT is recognized on ECG as an SVT with a short RP interval. As opposed to AVNRT, the RP interval is usually longer than 70 ms, and the retrograde P wave is usually identified in the ST segment (Fig. 8.3). Antidromic AVRT can be confused with ventricular tachycardia (VT) because the AP inserts directly into ventricular myocardium and the resulting ECG pattern is similar to that of a VT that originates in the same myocardial location. ECG criteria for distinguishing between the two are imperfect, but if the precordial QRS in V4–6 is predominantly negative or there is evidence of AV dissociation, the diagnosis is likely VT. Preexcited AF can also be confused with VT, but it is recognized as having irregular RR intervals with varying degrees of preexcitation (Fig. 8.4).

Patients with preexcited AF who are hemodynamically unstable require immediate electrical cardioversion. If the patient is stable, intravenous ibutilide or procainamide is recommended to restore sinus rhythm and/or to slow conduction of the AP. Beta-blockers, calcium channel blockers, and digoxin are contraindicated in preexcited AF as inhibition of AV node conduction can accelerate AP conduction by decreasing retrograde concealed conduction into the AP. The medical management of orthodromic AVRT is similar to AVNRT. Intravenous adenosine, beta-blockers, or calcium channel blockers can be used to acutely terminate the tachycardia in the AV node. Antidromic AVRT can also be acutely terminated with AV nodal blockade. However, it is often difficult to distinguish between antidromic tachycardia and VT; inadvertent treatment of VT with adenosine, beta-blockers, or calcium channel blockers may lead to hemodynamic collapse. Thus, intravenous procainamide or amiodarone are recommended.

Patients who present with preexcitation and have a history of palpitations, syncope, atrial fibrillation, or SVT are candidates for catheter ablation of the AP because of the increased risk for sudden death (ACC/AHA/ESC Class I, Level of Evidence B) [43]. In patients without preexcitation and suspected AVRT due to a concealed bypass tract, an individual decision can be made between using beta-blockers, calcium channel blockers, class IC and III antiarrhythmics, and catheter ablation, depending on the frequency and severity of the patient's symptoms. Similar to the management of AVNRT, because of its safety and efficacy profile, catheter ablation is favored in order to avoid long-term medications (ACC/AHA/ESC Class IIa, Level of Evidence B) [43]. Overall success rate of the procedure is 93 %, with higher success associated with AP location on the left free wall compared to the right free wall or posteroseptum. Major complications include complete heart block (1 %), stroke (0.2 %), and death (0.2 %) [45].

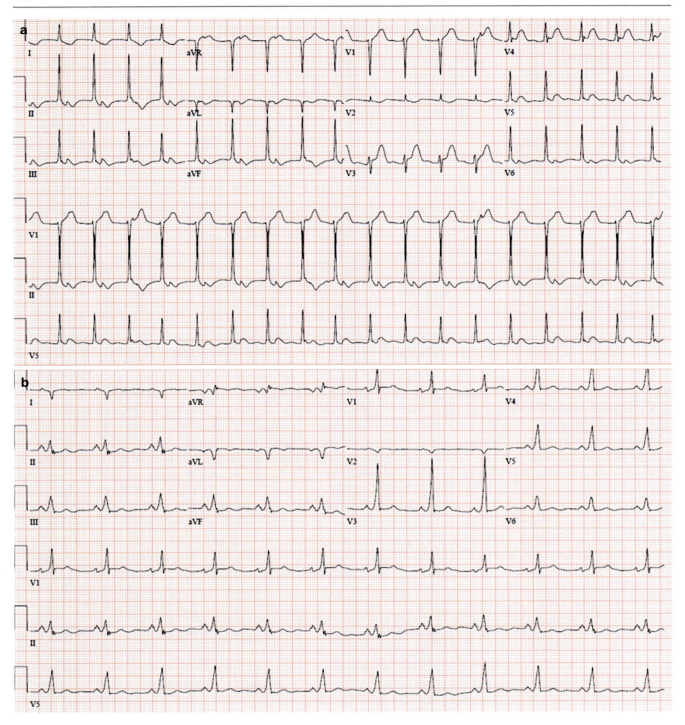

Fig. 8.3 Twelve-lead electrocardiogram of atrioventricular reentry tachycardia (AVRT). (**a**) AVRT with short RP interval which is >70 ms, as opposed to AVNRT, which is typically ≤70 ms. Preexcitation is not seen because of orthodromic conduction down the AV node and retrograde conduction up the accessory pathways. (**b**) Same patient in sinus rhythm with return of preexcitation

The management of patients with asymptomatic preexcitation is problematic as there is no consensus of expert opinion. Overall, the risk of sudden death with asymptomatic preexcitation is very low (estimated 0.1 % annual risk), which is "front loaded" in the first part of life, with the majority of patients between 10 and 40 years [46]. The risk in older individuals may be attenuated by the tendency for APs to weaken over time. Clinical features indicating low risk are intermittent preexcitation at rest and sudden loss of preexcitation on treadmill stress testing, which indicates a

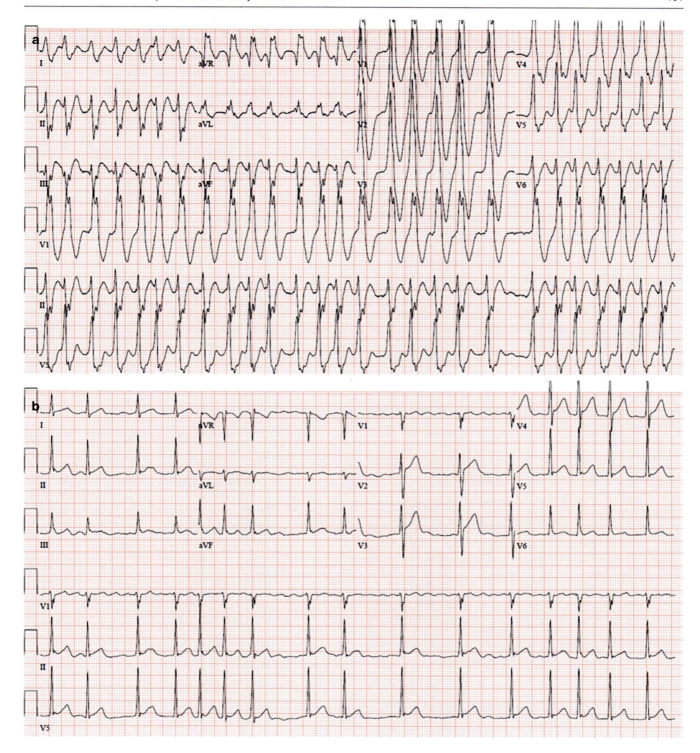

Fig. 8.4 Twelve-lead electrocardiogram of preexcited atrial fibrillation (*AF*). (**a**) Preexcited AF is recognized as a wide complex tachycardia with irregular RR intervals and variable preexcitation. (**b**) After admin- istration of procainamide, the patient remains in AF, but the accessory pathway is blocked with loss of preexcitation

weakly conducting pathway that will not conduct rapidly in AF. In patients who do not exhibit these low-risk features, an electrophysiologic (EP) study for further risk stratification can be considered. High-risk features on EP study that are associated with development of VF are SVT, multiple APs, AP antegrade refractory period ≤250 ms, and the shortest preexcited RR interval in AF <200 ms [47]. In patients with high-risk features, catheter ablation should be performed. Patients in high-risk occupations, which includes school bus drivers, pilots, and scuba divers, should be evaluated for catheter ablation [43].

> **Key Points**
> - In patients with preexcited AF, AV nodal blocking medications are contraindicated.
> - Asymptomatic patients with preexcitation can be risk stratified for risk of sudden death using noninvasive testing or EP study.

Atrial Tachycardia

Atrial tachycardias (ATs) account for 10–15 % of SVT and can be caused by increased automaticity, triggered activity, or micro-reentry. Focal ATs arise from a single ectopic site within the atria and while associated with the same underlying causes as AF and atrial flutter, can also be found in patients without any other underlying cardiac or extracardiac abnormalities. The most common sites of origin of focal ATs are the crista terminalis, pulmonary veins, atrial septum, and mitral annulus. Multifocal ATs (MAT) are characterized by multiple foci of atrial ectopic depolarizations and are usually the result of an underlying etiology, most commonly, pulmonary disease.

Focal ATs usually occur at a rate of 100–250 bpm and are recognized as a long RP tachycardia on ECG. At higher heart rates, the P wave can be obscured by the T wave. The differential diagnosis of a long RP tachycardia includes atrial flutter, sinus tachycardia, atypical AVNRT, and permanent junctional reciprocating tachycardia (PJRT), which is a type of AVRT which utilizes a retrograde conducting AP with decremental conduction properties. The response to vagal maneuvers or adenosine can be used to help differentiate AT from the other arrhythmias. AT is differentiated from atrial flutter if an isoelectric interval between P waves is present. Evidence of AV block with continuation of the tachycardia in the atrium favors AT, excludes PJRT (because the ventricle is a critical part of the arrhythmic circuit), and usually argues against AVNRT (although occasionally AVNRT can have a 2:1 AV or VA relationship as the atrium and ventricle are passively activated). Acute termination of the SVT with a P wave rules out AT. If the tachycardia transiently slows then reaccelerates (cool down, warm up), atrial tachycardia or sinus tachycardia is favored. AT can be differentiated from sinus tachycardia if the P wave morphology is distinct from the P wave morphology in normal sinus rhythm. MAT is diagnosed by a heart rate >100 bpm and the presence of at least three different P wave morphologies.

Occasionally focal ATs can be terminated with vagal maneuvers or adenosine. Most commonly, focal ATs are treated with beta-blockers and calcium channel blockers. If unsuccessful, class IC or class III antiarrhythmics can be used. Cardioversion can be attempted, but AT often recurs, especially if the arrhythmia mechanism is increased automaticity. For patients with drug refractory AT or in patients who have incessant tachycardia or tachycardia-induced cardiomyopathy, catheter ablation is recommended (ACC/AHA/ESC Class I, Level of Evidence B) [43]. Regardless of whether the mechanism of focal AT is increased automaticity, triggered activity, and micro-reentry, catheter ablation can be successful in treating the AT. The success rate of the ablation largely depends on whether or not the arrhythmia is present or inducible at the time of the procedure, especially since sedation and analgesics administered during the procedure can suppress the arrhythmia due to their effects on reducing autonomic tone. Ablation of focal AT has an 86 % success rate with a 1–2 % risk of complications [43]. MAT is usually treated by correcting the underlying pulmonary, metabolic, or electrolyte abnormality. Calcium channel blockers are an option because beta-blockers often cannot be used due to underlying pulmonary disease. There is usually no role for antiarrhythmics, DC cardioversion, or catheter ablation.

> **Key Points**
> - The mechanism of focal atrial tachycardia can be due to abnormal automaticity, triggered activity, or micro-reentry.

Sinus Tachycardia

Sinus tachycardia is defined as sinus rhythm with a rate >100 bpm and is almost always an appropriate physiologic response to an underlying cause, such as pain, anxiety, fever, infection, hypovolemia, anemia, thyrotoxicosis, pheochromocytoma, CHF, acute myocardial ischemia or infarction, pulmonary embolism and other pulmonary diseases, medications (caffeine, nicotine), or alcohol withdrawal. Inappropriate sinus tachycardia (IST) occurs in patients without cardiac abnormalities or other underlying reasons for sinus tachycardia and can be manifested as an elevated resting heart rate or an exaggerated heart rate response to physical activity or emotional stress. The mechanism of IST is unknown but is presumed to be the result of defects in autonomic tone or abnormalities within the sinus node.

ECG characteristics of sinus tachycardia include a P wave that matches the morphology in normal sinus rhythm, which typically is positive in leads I and II. However, the P wave morphology may be difficult to determine due to overlap with the prior T wave in tachycardic patients. To distinguish sinus tachycardia from other SVTs or 2:1 atrial flutter, vagal maneuvers or adenosine can be used. By slowing the sinus rate and/or causing transient AV block, they can allow proper identification of the P wave morphology as well as unmasking 2:1 atrial flutter if it is present. Additionally, the response of the arrhythmia to the maneuver may be informative as sinus tachycardia will characteristically slow then reaccelerate.

When confronted with a persistent sinus tachycardia, the initial step is to evaluate for and treat the underlying cause. If no other explanation for sinus tachycardia is found, the diagnosis of IST is made. Beta-blockers are the first-line therapy for IST (ACC/AHA/ESC Class I, Level of Evidence C), followed by verapamil and diltiazem (ACC/AHA/ESC Class IIa, Level of Evidence C) [43]. However, these measures are often unsuccessful in controlling symptoms and elevated heart rates. Ivabradine appears to be a promising drug for treatment of IST. It decreases the I_f current in cells in the SA node, decreasing the heart rate and was shown in 1 study to significantly lower the resting and exercise heart rate in 18 patients [48]. Catheter ablation to perform sinus node modification can be considered if medical therapies fail (ACC/AHA/ESC Class IIb, Level of Evidence C). The long-term success rate is 66 %; potential complications include pericarditis, phrenic nerve injury, SVC syndrome, and bradycardia requiring permanent pacing [43].

> **Key Points**
> - In patients with persistent sinus tachycardia, the initial step is to evaluate and treat potential underlying causes.

References

1. Wolf PA, Abbott RD, Kannel WB. Atrial fibrillation as an independent risk factor for stroke: the Framingham study. Stroke. 1991;22(8):983–8.
2. Maisel WH, Stevenson LW. Atrial fibrillation in heart failure: epidemiology, pathophysiology, and the rationale for therapy. Am J Cardiol. 2003;91(6A):2D–88.
3. Benjamin EJ, Wolf PA, D'Agostino RB, Silbershatz H, Kannel WB, Levy D. Impact of atrial fibrillation on the risk of death: the Framingham study. Circulation. 1998;98:946–52.
4. Naccarelli GV, Varker H, Lin J, Schulman KL. Increasing prevalence of atrial fibrillation and flutter in the United States. Am J Cardiol. 2009;104(11):1534–9.
5. Coyne KS, Paramore C, Grandy S, Mercader M, Reynolds M, Zimetbaum P. Assessing the direct costs of treating nonvalvular atrial fibrillation in the United States. Value Health. 2006;9(5):348–56.
6. Shinbane JS, Wood MA, Jensen DN, Ellenbogen KA, Fitzpatrick AP, Scheinman MM. Tachycardia-induced cardiomyopathy: a review of animal models and clinical studies. J Am Coll Cardiol. 1997;29(4):709–15.
7. Haissaguerre M, Jais P, Shah DC, et al. Spontaneous initiation of atrial fibrillation by ectopic beats originating in the pulmonary veins. N Engl J Med. 1998;339(10):659–66.
8. Thijssen VL, Ausma J, Liu GS, Allessie MA, Van Eys GH, Borgers M. Structural changes of atrial myocardium during chronic atrial fibrillation. Cardiovasc Pathol. 2000;9(1):17–28.
9. Shen MJ, Choi EK, Tan AY, Lin SF, Fishbein MC, Chen LS, Chen PS. Neural mechanisms of atrial arrhythmias. Nat Rev Cardiol. 2011;9(1):30–9.
10. Calkins H, Kuck KH, Cappato R, et al. 2012 HRS/EHRA/ECAS expert consensus statement on catheter and surgical ablation of atrial fibrillation: recommendations for patient selection, procedural techniques, patient management and follow-up, definition, endpoints, and research trial design: a report of the Heart Rhythm Society (HRS) Task Force on Catheter and Surgical Ablation of Atrial Fibrillation. Heart Rhythm. 2012;9(4):632–96.
11. Gage BF, Waterman AD, Shannon W, Boechler M, Rich MW, Radford MJ. Validation of clinical classification schemes for predicting stroke: results from the National Registry of Atrial Fibrillation. JAMA. 2001;285(22):2864–70.
12. Hart RG, Pearce LA, Rothbart RM, McAnulty JH, Asinger RW, Halperin JL. Stroke with intermittent atrial fibrillation: incidence and predictors during aspirin therapy. J Am Coll Cardiol. 2000;35(1):183–7.
13. Hart RG, Pearce LA, Aguilar MI. Meta analysis: antithrombotic therapy to prevent stroke in patients who have nonvalvular atrial fibrillation. Ann Intern Med. 2007;146(12):857–67.
14. Van Walraven C, Hart RG, Singer DE, et al. Oral anticoagulants vs aspirin in nonvalvular atrial fibrillation: an individual patient meta-analysis. JAMA. 2002;288(19):2441–8.
15. Fuster V, Ryden LE, Cannom DS, et al. ACC/AHA/ESC 2006 guidelines for the management of patients with atrial fibrillation: a report of the American College of Cardiology/American Heart Association Task Force on Practice Guidelines and the European Society of Cardiology Committee for Practice Guidelines. J Am Coll Cardiol. 2006;48:e149–246.
16. European Heart Rhythm Association, European Association for Cardio-Thoracic Surgery, Camm AJ, et al. Guidelines for the management of atrial fibrillation: the Task Force for the Management of Atrial Fibrillation of the European Society of Cardiology (ESC). Europace. 2010;12(10):1360–420.
17. Connolly SJ, Ezekowitz MD, Yusuf S, et al. Dabigatran versus warfarin in patients with atrial fibrillation. N Engl J Med. 2009;361:1139–51.
18. Patel MR, Mahaffey KW, Garg J, et al. Rivaroxaban versus warfarin in nonvalvular atrial fibrillation. N Engl J Med. 2011;365(10):883–91.
19. Granger CB, Alexander JH, McMurray JJ, et al. Apixaban versus warfarin in patients with atrial fibrillation. N Engl J Med. 2011;365(11):981–92.
20. Nagarakanti R, Ezekowitz MD, Oldgren J, et al. Dabigatran versus warfarin in patients with atrial fibrillation: an analysis of patients undergoing cardioversion. Circulation. 2011;123(2):131–6.
21. Van Gelder IC, Groenveld HF, Crijns HJ, et al. Lenient versus strict rate control in patients with atrial fibrillation. N Engl J Med. 2010;362(15):1363–73.
22. Doshi RN, Daoud EG, Fellows C, et al. Left ventricular-based cardiac stimulation post AV nodal ablation evaluation (the PAVE study). J Cardiovasc Electrophysiol. 2005;16(11):1160–5.
23. Echt DS, Liebson PR, Mitchell LB, et al. Mortality and morbidity in patients receiving encainide, flecainide, or placebo: the Cardiac Arrhythmia Suppression Trial. N Engl J Med. 1991;324(12):781–8.
24. Kober L, Torp-Pedersen C, McMurray JJ, et al. Increased mortality after dronedarone therapy for severe heart failure. N Engl J Med. 2008;358(25):2678–87.

25. Connolly SJ, Camm AJ, Halperin JL, et al. Dronedarone in high-risk permanent atrial fibrillation. N Engl J Med. 2011;365(24):2268–76.

26. Vassallo P, Trohman RG. Prescribing amiodarone: an evidence-based review of clinical indications. JAMA. 2007;298(11):1312–22.

27. Wyse DG, Waldo A, DiMarco JP, et al. A comparison of rate control and rhythm control in patients with atrial fibrillation. N Engl J Med. 2002;347(23):1825–33.

28. Roy D, Talajic M, Nattel S, et al. Rhythm control versus rate control for atrial fibrillation and heart failure. N Engl J Med. 2008;358(25):2667–77.

29. Corley SD, Epstein AE, DiMarco JP. Relationships between sinus rhythm, treatment and survival in the Atrial Fibrillation Follow-Up Investigation of Rhythm Management (AFFIRM) Study. Circulation. 2004;109(12):1509–13.

30. Pederson OD, Bagger H, Keller N, Marchant B, Kober L, Torp-Pedersen C. Efficacy of dofetilide in the treatment of atrial fibrillation-flutter in patients with reduced left ventricular function: a Danish investigations of arrhythmia and mortality on dofetilide (diamond) substudy. Circulation. 2001;104(3):292–6.

31. Bonanno C, Paccanaro M, La Vecchia L, Ometto R, Fontanelli A. Efficacy and safety of catheter ablation versus antiarrhythmic drugs for atrial fibrillation: a meta-analysis of randomized trials. J Cardiovasc Med. 2010;11(6):408–18.

32. Cappato R, Calkins H, Chen SA, et al. Updated worldwide survey on the methods, efficacy, and safety of catheter ablation for human atrial fibrillation. Circ Arrhythm Electrophysiol. 2010;3(1):32–8.

33. Hsu LF, Jais P, Sanders P, et al. Catheter ablation for atrial fibrillation in congestive heart failure. N Engl J Med. 2004;351(23):2373–83.

34. Maisel WH, Rawn JD, Stevenson WG. Atrial fibrillation after cardiac surgery. Ann Intern Med. 2001;135:1061–73.

35. Kowey PR, Stebbins D, Igidbashian L, et al. Clinical outcome of patients who develop PAF after CABG surgery. Pacing Clin Electrophysiol. 2001;24:191–3.

36. Villareal RP, Hariharan R, Liu BC, et al. Postoperative atrial fibrillation and mortality after coronary artery bypass surgery. J Am Coll Cardiol. 2004;43(5):742–8.

37. Mathew JP, Fontes ML, Tudor IC, et al. A multicenter risk index for atrial fibrillation after cardiac surgery. JAMA. 2004;291(14):1720–9.

38. Patti G, Chello M, Candura D, Pasceri V, D'Ambrosio A, Covino E, Di Sciascio G. Randomized trial of atorvastatin for reduction of postoperative atrial fibrillation in patients undergoing cardiac surgery: results of the ARMYDA-3 (Atorvastatin for Reduction of MYocardial Dysrhythmia after cardiac surgery) study. Circulation. 2006;114(14):1455–61.

39. Imazio M, Brucato A, Ferrazzi P, et al. Colchicine reduces postoperative atrial fibrillation: results of the Colchicine for the Prevention of the Postpericardiotomy Syndrome (COPPS) atrial fibrillation substudy. Circulation. 2011;124(21):2290–5.

40. Crystal E, Garfinkle MS, Connolly SS, Ginger TT, Sleik K, Yusuf SS. Interventions for preventing post-operative atrial fibrillation in patients undergoing heart surgery. Cochrane Database Syst Rev. 2004;4, CD003611.

41. Creswell LL, Schuessler RB, Rosenbloom M, Cox JL. Hazards of post-operative atrial arrhythmias. Ann Thorac Surg. 1993;56(3):539–49.

42. Perez FJ, Schubert CM, Parvez B, Pathak V, Ellenbogen KA, Wood MA. Long-term outcomes after catheter ablation of cavo-tricuspid isthmus dependent atrial flutter: a meta-analysis. Circ Arrhythm Electrophysiol. 2009;2(4):393–401.

43. Blomstrom-Lundqvist C, Scheinman MM, Aliot EM, et al. ACC/AHA/ESC guidelines for the management of patients with supraventricular arrhythmias – executive summary: a report of the American College of Cardiology/American Heart Association Task Force on practice guidelines and the European Society of Cardiology Committee for practice guidelines (writing committee to develop guidelines for the management of patients with supraventricular arrhythmias developed in collaboration with NASPE-Heart Rhythm Society). J Am Coll Cardiol. 2003;42(8):1493–531.

44. Krahn AD, Manfreda J, Tate RB, Mathewson FA, Cuddy TE. The natural history of electrocardiographic preexcitation in men. The Manitoba follow-up study. Ann Intern Med. 1992; 116(6):456–60.

45. Calkins H, Yong P, Miller JM, et al. Catheter ablation of accessory pathways, atrioventricular nodal reentrant tachycardia, and the atrioventricular junction: final results of a prospective, multicenter clinical trial. Circulation. 1999;99(2):262–70.

46. Klein GJ, Gula LJ, Krahn AD, Skanes AC, Yee R. WPW pattern in the asymptomatic individual: has anything changed? Circulation. 2009;2:97–9.

47. Wellens HJ. Should catheter ablation be performed in asymptomatic patients with Wolff-Parkinson-White syndrome? When to perform catheter ablation in asymptomatic patients with a Wolff-Parkinson-White electrocardiogram. Circulation. 2005;112(14):210–7.

48. Calo L, Rebecchi M, Sette A, et al. Efficacy of ivabradine administration in patients affected by inappropriate sinus tachycardia. Heart Rhythm. 2010;7(9):1318–23.

Evidenced-Based Approach to Bradyarrhythmias

9

Ibrahim O. Almasry

Abstract

Bradycardia can be caused by a wide variety of factors that affect the sinoatrial or the atrioventricular nodes. The sinus node is the main pacemaker of the heart and is extremely sensitive to autonomic influences as it is richly innervated by sympathetic and parasympathetic nerve inputs. Sinus node dysfunction is a result of various intrinsic or extrinsic causes, most commonly aging and medications. The clinical presentation can vary widely with electrocardiographic (ECG) manifestations including sinus bradycardia, sinus arrest, sinoatrial exit block, hypersensitive carotid sinus syndrome, chronotropic incompetence, and tachycardia-bradycardia syndrome. The key to the diagnosis is correlating symptoms to ECG findings. The only effective management is by pacing. The atrioventricular (AV) conduction axis has complex anatomical and physiological characteristics and the AV node is also strongly influenced by autonomic inputs. There are multiple causes of AV block divided into three ECG classifications – first-, second-, and third-degree AV block – based on the P wave to QRS complex relationship. Additional forms include 2:1, high-grade, and paroxysmal AV block which do not fit within those ECG classifications. Definitive therapy is pacemaker implantation which is indicated for treatment of symptoms with any form of AV block or an infranodal site of conduction block regardless of symptoms.

Keywords

Bradycardia • Sinus node dysfunction • Sinus bradycardia • Sinus arrest • Sinoatrial exit block • Chronotropic incompetence • Carotid sinus hypersensitivity • Tachycardia-bradycardia syndrome • Sick sinus syndrome • Type 1 second-degree block • Type 2 second-degree block • Mobitz I • Mobitz II • Wenckebach • 2:1 AV block • High-grade AV block • Complete AV block • Infranodal AV block • Pacemaker implantation

Introduction

Bradycardia is arbitrarily defined as a heart rate less than 60 beats per minute (bpm), although a rate below 50 bpm has been suggested by some authors [1]. Bradyarrhythmias are a commonly encountered problem and their spectrum may range from the benign and physiologically normal to pathological life-threatening conditions. This can make their management a challenge for the consulting physician. A careful evaluation of the patient's presenting rhythm and associated symptoms is the key to accurate diagnosis and appropriate intervention.

Many causes of bradycardia are the result of extrinsic and intrinsic factors that can influence the cardiac conduction system either by directly affecting its structures or by affecting the balance of sympathetic and parasympathetic influences upon those structures. The summation of these effects

I.O. Almasry, MD, FACC, FHRS
Section of Cardiac Electrophysiology,
Division of Cardiology, SUNY/Stony Brook
University Medical Center, HSC Level 16 Rm 080,
Stony Brook, NY 11794, USA
e-mail: ibrahim.almasry@stonybrookmedicine.edu

K. Stergiopoulos, D.L. Brown (eds.), *Evidence-Based Cardiology Consult*,
DOI 10.1007/978-1-4471-4441-0_9, © Springer-Verlag London 2014

can be categorized into conditions that affect the sinoatrial node (SA node) or the atrioventricular node (AV node). From an electrophysiological standpoint, they may be viewed as either abnormalities of impulse formation or abnormalities of impulse propagation.

While not all bradyarrhythmias require intervention, definitive therapy of pathological bradycardia due to either sinus node dysfunction or AV node conduction abnormalities is achieved by pacemaker implantation. Pacemakers have become increasingly sophisticated with complex pacing algorithms aimed at maintaining atrioventricular and interventricular synchrony. These algorithms have been derived from outcomes-based findings of a number of important clinical trials. The aim of this chapter is to discuss the various forms of bradycardia commonly encountered in practice, outline their key diagnostic features, and present an evidenced-based approach to their management.

Bradycardia Due to the SA Node

Anatomy and Physiology of the SA Node

The sinus node is the main pacemaker of the heart. It is a spindle-shaped structure composed of groups of cells called P cells (named due to their pale appearance on electron microscopy) which possess automaticity, allowing for spontaneous depolarization. These groups or nests of P cells are interspersed within connective tissue composed of collagen and fibroblasts. The SA node measures 10–20 mm long and starts epicardially in the lateral part of the right atrium in the sulcus terminalis at the junction with the superior vena cava and extends endocardially [2].

The arterial blood supply to the SA node is variable accounting for vulnerability to damage during surgical procedures. The SA nodal artery provides the principal blood supply and originates from the right coronary artery in 55–60 % of patients and from the left circumflex artery in the remainder. A more recent publication suggests that the SA nodal artery may take several different routes and that two or more branches to the SA node may be present in about 54 % of hearts [3]. This collateralization may explain the rarity of SA node infarction.

Pacemaker activity is not confined to a single set of cells within the sinus node. It occurs as a result of integrated activity of the cells throughout the region where cells affect each other through cell-to-cell coupling, called mutual entrainment, to depolarize simultaneously [4]. The more rapidly depolarizing cells are the predominant pacemakers, while other, more slowly depolarizing cells are backup or subsidiary pacemakers. These subsidiary pacemakers only take over under certain conditions such as changes in autonomic tone or electrolyte imbalances.

The SA node is richly innervated by both sympathetic and parasympathetic nervous inputs in the form of postganglionic adrenergic and cholinergic nerve terminals [5]. These inputs have a profound effect on the rate of depolarization within pacemaker cells, causing a shift in the origin of the predominant pacemaker cell group that can vary by as much as 3 cm along the SA node region. These shifts then cause a change in the exit site of the sinus impulse to the surrounding atrial tissue and may be associated with subtle changes in P wave morphology [6]. Activation mapping has demonstrated that sympathetic influences, resulting in faster rates, cause a shift of impulse origin to the superior portion of the SA node, whereas vagal influences produce slower rates and cause a shift to the lower portion [7, 8].

Pathophysiology of Sinus Node Dysfunction

Ferrer was the first to describe sinus node dysfunction (SND) as a distinct clinical entity in 1968 [9], although Wenckebach had reported on its electrocardiographic (ECG) manifestations in 1923. SND refers to a wide range of abnormalities affecting sinus node impulse formation or propagation. These various abnormalities are detailed below. The causes of sinus node dysfunction can be categorized as either extrinsic or intrinsic and are detailed in Table 9.1.

Table 9.1 Intrinsic and extrinsic causes of sinus node dysfunction

Intrinsic causes	Extrinsic causes
Idiopathic degenerative (sick sinus syndrome)	Hypervagotonia (cardioinhibitory influence with neurocardiogenic syncope, athletic training)
Ischemic (acute and chronic coronary artery disease)	Medications (calcium channel blockers, beta-blockers, digitalis, class I and III antiarrhythmics)
Inflammatory (collagen vascular disease, SLE, myocarditis)	Hypoxia (obstructive sleep apnea, mucus plugging)
Infiltrative (amyloidosis, sarcoid, hemochromatosis)	Metabolic disorders (hypothyroidism, hypothermia)
Iatrogenic (surgical trauma, Mustard and Fontan repairs, radiation therapy)	Electrolyte abnormalities (hypo- and hyperkalemia)
Inherited (myotonic dystrophy, Friedreich's ataxia, Kearns-Sayre)	Neurological disorders (increased intracranial pressure and CNS tumors)

Intrinsic Causes

Idiopathic degenerative disease is by far the most common cause of intrinsic SND [10]. Primarily seen in the elderly, it is predominantly due to aging and degeneration of the sinus node. Data from multiple studies suggests that associated AV block is uncommon, implying that the degenerative process does not affect the remainder of the conduction system to the same degree [11]. SND is also commonly seen in ischemic heart disease which is more common in the elderly. It is associated with acute inferior wall myocardial infarction from occlusion of the right coronary artery proximal to the origin of the SA node artery. Nevertheless, SND may be diagnosed at any age due to any of the listed causes.

Extrinsic Causes

While numerous causes for extrinsic SND exist, the most common are drug effects and autonomic nervous system influences. Drugs that typically depress sinus node function include beta-blockers, calcium channel blockers, digoxin, several classes of antiarrhythmic agents, and sympatholytic antihypertensive agents.

Autonomic influences are typically due to increased vagal tone as seen in well-trained athletes with sinus bradycardia or normal individuals with bradycardia during sleep. These influences also play a large role in hypervagotonic conditions such as hypersensitive carotid sinus syndrome or various forms of neurocardiogenic syncope.

Diagnosis

Presentation

The clinical presentation of SND can vary widely. The most significant symptom is syncope, which typically occurs as a result of continued suppression of sinus node impulse formation after sudden termination of a tachycardia such as atrial fibrillation. The range of clinical findings can include asymptomatic electrocardiographic findings or a wide array of nonspecific symptoms including dizziness, lightheadedness, pre-syncope, shortness of breath, or fatigue.

The natural history can be variable with the majority of patients exhibiting slow progression over many years. Prognosis frequently depends on other comorbidities and the presence or absence of concomitant structural heart disease. Syncope is associated with recurrent events and a worse prognosis [12]. Atrial fibrillation occurs in about 40–45 % [13–15] of SND patients with thromboembolic events occurring in 15 % in untreated patients. Acute arterial thromboembolism may be the first manifestation of SND. The incidence of thromboembolic events is 13 % in ventricularly paced patients and 1.6 % in atrially paced patients [16]. This underscores the relative protective effect of atrial pacing in patients

with SND. The incidence of sudden cardiac death is extremely low [12] and SND does not appear to affect mortality whether treated or untreated with pacemaker therapy [17, 18].

Diagnostic Evaluation

The gold standard for the diagnosis of SND is the correlation between symptoms and ECG evidence of SND on 12-lead ECGs, inpatient telemetry, or ambulatory monitoring such as 24–48-h Holter recordings. These are typically low-yield tools unless the patient has very frequent or, at least, daily symptoms. More commonly, the diagnosis can be made utilizing cardiac event monitors worn for 30-day intervals in association with interactive patient recording of symptoms. Exercise stress testing can be useful in documenting evidence of chronotropic incompetence. In patients with very infrequent symptoms, electrophysiology (EP) testing with a careful evaluation of SA node function may be required; however, these tests have limited specificity and do not correlate with the patient's symptoms. Therefore, the role of EP testing in the management of sinus node dysfunction is limited. Implantable loop recorders are becoming an increasingly important tool in the diagnostic evaluation of sinus node dysfunction. They can now be implanted for periods of up to 3 years, allowing a diagnosis even in patients with very infrequent symptoms.

Electrocardiographic Manifestations of SND

Sinus Bradycardia

Sinus bradycardia is generally defined as a heart rate of less than 60 bpm with P wave morphology consistent with sinus node origin (Fig. 9.1). It is often associated with sinus arrhythmia. In most circumstances, this is a benign condition and should not be considered a true arrhythmia in certain patients. For example, asymptomatic sinus bradycardia can frequently be seen in young healthy adults and trained athletes as a result of increased vagal tone. It is not uncommon for heart rates to drop to 30–40 bpm during sleep in younger patients. It may also be seen in conditions associated with increased parasympathetic stimulation such as neurocardiogenic syncope, carotid sinus stimulation, and vomiting. In older patients, however, it is mostly seen as a result of medications. Beta-blockers and calcium channel blockers are the most common, but sinus bradycardia can be caused by a wide variety of medications including antiarrhythmics, antihypertensives, and a variety of psychotropic medications.

Pathological sinus bradycardia occurs in a setting where the heart rate is inappropriate for the physiological condition at the time, such as bradycardia in the setting of sepsis or heart failure. Heart rates less than 40 bpm are generally

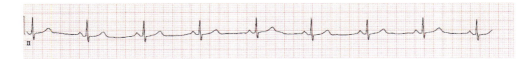

Fig. 9.1 Sinus bradycardia. No other abnormalities noted here except for sinus bradycardia at 50 bpm which may be physiological or pathological

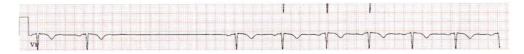

Fig. 9.2 Sinus arrest. Note sudden cessation of sinus impulse for 3 s prior to resumption of normal sinus rhythm once more

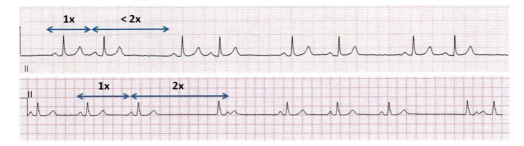

Fig. 9.3 *Top panel*: Type I second-degree sinoatrial exit block. Note the pause that is less than two times the PP interval. Also note the group beating consistent with Wenckebach periodicity. *Bottom panel*: Type II second-degree sinoatrial exit block. The pause here is two times the PP interval, with the occurrence of a junctional beat prior to the return of a sinus P wave which is followed by unperturbed sinus mechanism before there is another recurrence

considered to be abnormal. Sinus bradycardia has also been noted in patients presenting with an acute myocardial infarction (MI), particularly inferior wall MI. Unless associated with hemodynamic compromise, treatment is generally not required. Persistent sinus bradycardia that does not resolve with discontinuation of potentially causative medications may be seen in elderly patients who complain of fatigue. In these circumstances, treatment is warranted.

Sinus Arrest

As the name implies, sinus arrest occurs as a result of complete cessation of automaticity and, therefore, impulse formation in the sinus node. The term is often used interchangeably with sinus pause. Differentiation between sinus arrest and sinoatrial exit block (see below) on the basis of the surface ECG, and without direct recordings, can be difficult. The duration of sinus arrest is typically random and, as a rule, is not a multiple of the underlying sinus rate. There is no consensus on the exact duration required to meet the definition of sinus arrest. For practical purposes, pauses of 2–3 s during sinus rhythm can be termed sinus arrest (Fig. 9.2). While these can rarely be seen in normal individuals with a high degree of vagal tone, pauses greater than 3 s are typically a marker of sinus node dysfunction. In the absence of subsidiary pacemakers that can provide escape

beats, prolonged sinus pauses can result in periods of ventricular asystole. While a thorough evaluation of the patient is necessary in these situations, treatment is only warranted if symptoms can be correlated to these pauses.

Sinoatrial Exit Block

Sinoatrial exit block refers to either impulse conduction delay or block between the sinus node and the surrounding perinodal or atrial tissue. Similar to AV conduction block, it may be categorized into first-, second-, and third-degree block. In first-degree sinoatrial exit block, there is a fixed delay between the sinus node and the atrial tissue. In third-degree sinoatrial exit block, sinus impulses are not conducted to the atrial tissue and therefore no P waves appear on the surface ECG, with a subsidiary pacemaker typically taking over. Neither of these can be distinguished on the basis of the surface ECG alone and require direct recordings from the sinus node to make the diagnosis.

Second-degree sinoatrial exit block can either be type I or type II (Fig. 9.3). In type I, typical Wenckebach behavior is seen with shortening of the PP intervals before the dropped P wave is noted. The resultant pause is less than twice the shortest preceding PP interval. Type II sinoatrial exit block is similar to Mobitz type II AV block with no change in the preceding PP intervals before the dropped P

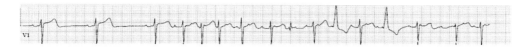

Fig. 9.4 Tachy-brady syndrome. Note the patient has sinus bradycardia at the beginning of the strip and quickly transforms into atrial fibrillation with a rapid ventricular response with PVCs occasionally noted

wave. The resultant pause is typically twice the preceding PP interval. If more than one P wave is blocked, then the resultant pause is a multiple of the baseline PP interval.

Hypersensitive Carotid Sinus Syndrome
Hypersensitive carotid sinus syndrome is characterized by an exaggerated vagal response to carotid stimulation and is associated with sinus arrest or exit block. In the cardioinhibitory form, a sinus pause of greater than 3 s typically occurs without the appearance of subsidiary pacemakers resulting in asystole. AV node conduction is typically affected as well, although this is not easily elucidated due to lack of atrial impulse formation. In the cardiodepressor form, a 30–50 mmHg drop of systolic blood pressure with reproduction of the patient's symptoms may be elicited. The classic clinical presentation is syncope or pre-syncope associated with head turning or tight shirt collars and is more commonly observed in males.

Chronotropic Incompetence
Chronotropic incompetence refers to a form of sinus node dysfunction in which there is an inability to increase the heart rate in response to sympathetic stimulation to meet increased physiological demands such as exercise. Treadmill exercise testing can be very useful in unmasking this form of sinus node dysfunction which is defined as an inability to achieve a heart rate greater than 100 bpm at maximal exercise or a failure to reach 70 % of the maximal predicted heart rate (220-age).

Tachycardia-Bradycardia Syndrome
Tachycardia-bradycardia syndrome is the most common form of SND and is sometimes termed sick sinus syndrome or tachy-brady syndrome. It refers to patients with sinus bradycardia alternating with various tachyarrhythmias, typically atrial fibrillation (Fig. 9.4). Tachycardia-bradycardia syndrome is often manifested by prolonged pauses after sudden cessation of the tachyarrhythmia and is likely the most common cause of syncope in patients with SND. Functional bradycardia may be an element in this syndrome since rapid atrial rates can result in sinus node suppression and remodeling [19]. This syndrome is further exacerbated by the management of the tachyarrhythmia component which frequently necessitates utilizing medications that further suppress the sinus node and exacerbate the bradycardia. Pacemaker implantation is often the only solution to facilitate safe and effective rate control.

Table 9.2 Indications for pacing in sinus node dysfunction

Recommendations for permanent pacing in sinus node dysfunction
Class I indication
Documented symptomatic sinus bradycardia
Documented symptomatic chronotropic incompetence
Symptomatic sinus bradycardia resulting from necessary drug therapy
Class IIa indications
SND with heart rate less than 40 beats/min, when a clear association between bradycardic symptoms and actual bradycardia has not been established
Unexplained syncope with clinical evidence of significant SND
Class IIb indications
Minimally symptomatic patients with heart rate less than 40 beats/min while awake
Class III indications
Asymptomatic patients with SND
Symptomatic patients with documented symptoms occurring in the absence of bradycardia
Symptomatic bradycardia due to nonessential drug therapy

Adapted from Epstein et al. [20]

Management

Since SND is not associated with increased mortality, the goal of therapy should be to alleviate symptoms. Therefore, it is imperative to correlate symptoms with the electrocardiographic findings of SND. Patients may have symptoms that are unrelated to the electrocardiographic evidence of this disease and some patients may have evidence of the disease and be completely asymptomatic. In either of these cases, pacemaker implantation is not indicated.

The indications for pacemaker implantation are listed in Table 9.2. The general rule is that only symptomatic patients with SND should undergo pacemaker implantation. Prior to committing to pacemaker implantation, every effort should be made to remove any extrinsic factor or offending medication. Patients with SND and concomitant atrial fibrillation are at high risk of thromboembolic complications and long-term anticoagulation should be considered [16].

In patients who require pacing, pacemaker selection is the next critical step. Patients with long-standing persistent or permanent atrial fibrillation require only a single right ventricular lead programmed to the VVI pacing mode. In patients with sinus mechanism and intact AV conduction, atrial-based pacing systems appear to be more effective at reducing stroke, systemic embolization [21], atrial fibrillation, stroke, heart failure, and cardiovascular mortality [22]. Due to the 1–3 % annual incidence of AV block, however, most patients in the United States receive dual-chamber pacing systems.

While it would seem logical that, for patients in sinus rhythm, maintaining AV synchrony with dual-chamber pacing would be superior to ventricular-based pacing alone, there has been a paucity of evidence of any survival benefit in that regard. DDDR pacing was associated with less atrial fibrillation than VVIR pacing in the Canadian Trial of Physiological Pacing (CTOPP) [23]. In the Mode Selection Trial (MOST), there was a reduction in the incidence of heart failure and atrial fibrillation but no difference in mortality [24]. There is increasing evidence of the association between chronic right ventricular pacing and the development of heart failure. In the MOST study, ventricular pacing more than 40 % of the time in DDDR mode was associated with a 2.6-fold increase in heart failure compared to similar patients with less pacing. This has led to novel patented pacing modes such as the Managed Ventricular Pacing Mode (MVP) which provides AAIR pacing with DDDR backup allowing atrial pacing, while maintaining native conduction and providing AV synchrony only when required.

Bradycardia Due to the Atrioventricular (AV) Node

Anatomy and Physiology of the AV Node

The AV node is a subendocardial structure originating in the transitional zone in the inferior portion of the right atrium. This zone receives atrial input from 3 preferential pathways of conduction (superior, medial, and posterior) that connect to the compact AV node located at the apex of the triangle of Koch. This triangle is formed by the tendon of Todaro superiorly, the septal leaflet of the tricuspid valve medially, and the os of the coronary sinus posteriorly and inferiorly. The AV node continues as the penetrating AV bundle through the central fibrous body, penetrating the annulus fibrosis and emerging along the left ventricular septum as the bundle of His. It immediately divides into the right and left bundle branches, both of which connect to an extensive endocardial His-Purkinje network, constituting the AV conduction axis.

From an electrophysiological standpoint, the AV node and perinodal area can be divided into 3 distinct regions. The atrionodal (AN) region is made up of transitional zone cells possessing electrophysiological and histological characteristics distinct from those of atrial myocytes. The AN region connects to the nodal (N) region made up of N cells. These represent the typical AV node cells with their characteristic decremental conduction properties. The last region is the nodal-His (NH) region with cell characteristics that combine those of the nodal region and the His-Purkinje system.

Under normal circumstances, the AV node is the only conduction pathway from the atria to the ventricles. Its primary function is to regulate and limit atrial impulses being conducted to the ventricles. This buffering action is protective as it prevents potentially harmful rapid impulses, such as those occurring in atrial fibrillation, from being conducted to the ventricles possibly resulting in ventricular fibrillation. In addition, utilizing the properties of automaticity in the cells of its distal portion, the AV node may function as a subsidiary pacemaker under certain circumstances such as sinus node dysfunction or proximal AV node conduction block.

The blood supply of the AV node is primarily supplied by the AV nodal artery, originating from the right coronary artery in 85–90 % of patients and from the left circumflex artery in the remainder. The penetrating AV bundle receives a dual blood supply from the AV nodal artery and the first septal perforator of the left anterior descending coronary artery. This dual blood supply can be protective in situations of myocardial ischemia. Like the SA node, the AV node is richly innervated by both sympathetic and parasympathetic nervous inputs in the form of postganglionic adrenergic and cholinergic nerve fibers. Sympathetic stimulation causes shorter AV node conduction time and refractoriness, whereas parasympathetic stimulation results in the opposite. Neither the bundle of His nor the His-Purkinje system is influenced by the autonomic nervous system [25].

Pathophysiology of Atrioventricular (AV) Block

Delay or block of a cardiac impulse may occur anywhere along the AV conduction axis. AV block may be either congenital or acquired. Congenital AV block is a result of embryonic developmental abnormalities. Acquired AV block may be classified based on its severity as either first-, second-, or third-degree AV block and may result from a variety of physiological or pathophysiological causes. Physiological causes of AV block include increased vagal tone such as in young athletic patients, during sleep, or in painful situations. This form of physiological response typically results in first-degree or type I second-degree (Wenckebach) AV block. Pathophysiological causes may be either intrinsic or extrinsic (Table 9.3) and can produce any form of AV block. The following are some of the most important causes.

Degenerative Disease
Degenerative disease is the most common cause of acquired AV block accounting for about 50 % of cases. Idiopathic progressive sclerosis seen with aging is referred to as Lev's

Table 9.3 Causes of acquired AV block

Idiopathic degenerative: Lev's disease, Lenegre's disease
Ischemic disease: Acute MI, chronic CAD
Iatrogenic: Post cardiac surgery, TAVI, radiofrequency ablation
Medications: Calcium channel and beta-blockers, digoxin, antiarrhythmics, adenosine
Infectious: Lyme disease, endocarditis, Chagas, syphilis, TB, toxoplasmosis, diphtheria
Autonomic: Neurocardiogenic, carotid hypersensitivity
Infiltrative: Amyloidosis, hemochromatosis, sarcoidosis, lymphoma, melanoma
Rheumatic: Scleroderma, ankylosing spondylitis, rheumatoid arthritis, SLE
Heritable: Kearns-Sayre, myotonic dystrophy, facioscapulohumeral, Emery-Dreifuss

disease and is commonly due to the degenerative effects of long-standing hypertension, diabetes, and atherosclerosis. The resulting impairment in blood supply causes fibrosis and calcification at the ventricular septum, central fibrous body, and the aortic and mitral valve annuli, which subsequently extends to the adjacent conduction tissues of the AV node [26, 27]. Lenegre's disease is a progressive fibrotic degenerative process usually affecting younger individuals. It is typically associated with a slow progression to complete AV block and may have a hereditary component.

Ischemic Heart Disease

Ischemic heart disease may account for 40 % of acquired AV block [28]. In acute myocardial infarction (MI), the rate of AV block is almost 20 %, including 8 % with first-degree, 5 % with second-degree, and 6 % with third-degree AV block [29–31].

First-degree AV block and type I second-degree AV block are more commonly seen with inferior myocardial infarction. They are typically associated with increased vagal tone, respond to atropine (as the level of block is usually at the AV node), and are transient, typically resolving within 72 h. They rarely progress to more advanced AV block. Type II second-degree AV block (seen more commonly with anterior MI) and complete AV block may occur with either inferior or anterior MI. In inferior MI, the level of block is typically the AV node and is associated with stable narrow junctional escape complexes and has a better prognosis. In anterior MI, the level of block is at the level of the His-Purkinje system and is typically not transient. The ECG demonstrates an unstable wide QRS escape rhythm and is associated with a more hemodynamically unstable presentation related to a larger infarct size. Patients may present with severe hypotension, pulmonary edema, and ventricular tachyarrhythmias. These patients are critically ill requiring urgent intervention including revascularization and temporary pacemaker support during the initial presentation and have a worse prognosis [32–34].

Iatrogenic

A variety of medications can impair AV conduction and give rise to AV block. Among the most common are cardiac medications specifically used for management of tachyarrhythmias such as digoxin, calcium channel blockers, and beta-blockers. Type I and type III antiarrhythmic agents (with the exception of dofetilide) can cause delayed infranodal conduction with resultant AV block. Patients that progress to AV block typically have underlying conduction system disease to begin with that is further exacerbated by these medications. Discontinuation of medications can resolve the AV block transiently but recurrence may occur at a later date requiring pacing [35].

Cardiac surgery can be complicated by the development of various degrees of AV block. This is seen more commonly with aortic valve replacement, with up to 3–4 % of patients requiring permanent pacing compared with coronary artery bypass surgery in which permanent pacing may be required in less than 1 % [36, 37]. The AV block appears to be due to trauma or ischemia affecting the AV node conduction system which is in close proximity to the aortic valve. More recently, transcatheter aortic valve implantation (TAVI) has been offered to patients with aortic stenosis who are poor surgical candidates. This procedure has been associated with a high rate of AV block, with up to one-third of patients receiving the CoreValve device requiring permanent pacing; the incidence may be lower with the Edwards SAPIEN™ valve [38, 39]. Alcohol septal ablation for the treatment of hypertrophic cardiomyopathy has also been associated with a high rate of AV block. The incidence of pacemaker requirement ranges from 14 to 22 % [40, 41]. Complete AV block may also complicate radiofrequency ablation of atrioventricular nodal reentrant tachycardia (AVNRT) or septal accessory pathways with an incidence of about 1 % (range 0–3 %) [42].

Infectious Disease

Infectious endocarditis may result from viral, bacterial, and parasitic infections. The most common cause in the northeastern region of the United States is Lyme disease due to tick bites transmitting *Borrelia burgdorferi*. Lyme disease is one of the most important causes of reversible AV block. AV block may progress and fluctuate rapidly from first-degree to complete AV block. The level of block is typically at the AV node but may occur throughout the conduction system and is usually associated with symptoms. Complete AV block typically improves within 1 week after initiation of appropriate intravenous antibiotics [43]. Other causes include rheumatic fever, tuberculosis, Chagas disease, measles, syphilis, and bacterial endocarditis. The development of AV block is associated with a worse prognosis in these patients.

Diagnosis

Presentation

The clinical presentation of AV block can vary from being asymptomatic to dramatic presentations with syncope. First-degree AV block is typically asymptomatic, although in cases of extreme PR interval prolongation, some patients may present with symptoms of AV dyssynchrony similar to those seen with pacemaker syndrome. Patients with type I second-degree AV block may be asymptomatic for prolonged periods of time. Sedentary patients may only be noted to be in complete AV block incidentally upon presentation for an unrelated medical evaluation. Depending on the etiology of the AV block, patients may present with the symptoms associated with the triggering cause such as acute MI or symptoms of endocarditis. In general, the symptoms tend to be those associated with decreased cardiac output and may initially be noted in association with exertion only or may occur at rest from the very beginning. These may include decreased exercise capacity, chest pain, dyspnea, dizziness, light headedness, pre-syncope, or syncope. Patients presenting with syncope require urgent intervention as opposed to a more elective management approach in relatively asymptomatic patients. Patients with heart failure may be more affected, with worsening of heart failure being the primary symptom. AV block and its associated symptoms may occur intermittently, making the diagnosis elusive.

Diagnostic Evaluation

The primary goal of a diagnostic evaluation in AV block is to determine the site of conduction block as this may sometimes determine if pacemaker implantation is warranted. When patients are symptomatic, this is less important from a clinical standpoint since symptomatic patients require pacemaker implantation. The primary tool in this evaluation is electrocardiography, including inpatient and ambulatory telemetry, to diagnose intermittent conduction block and to determine how it correlates with symptoms. Bedside evaluation maneuvers in conjunction with electrocardiography can also be helpful, since increasing adrenergic stimulation may help improve the conduction ratio of AV block where the site of block is at the level of the AV node, but worsen the ratio of block if it is at the infranodal level. Exercise testing may also be helpful in demonstrating the differential response to adrenergic stimulation. Increased vagal stimulation, such as with Valsalva maneuvers or carotid sinus massage, may improve the ratio of conduction block with infranodal disease and worsen AV block at the level of the AV node. These maneuvers may be especially useful in assessing 2:1 AV block (Table 9.4). Electrophysiology testing may be of additional benefit in patients with intermittent symptoms suspicious for AV block but without documented bradyarrhythmias.

Table 9.4 Differentiating AV node from His-Purkinje site of block

Observation/maneuver	AV node block	His-Purkinje system block
PR interval	>300 ms	<160 ms
QRS width	Narrow QRS	Wide QRS or BBB
Atropine or exercise	Improves conduction	Worsens conduction
Carotid sinus massage	Worsens conduction	Improves conduction

Electrocardiographic Manifestations of AV Block

First-Degree AV Block

First-degree AV block is defined as a PR interval greater than 200 milliseconds (ms) following a normally timed atrial impulse. This is a misnomer considering that there is no true "block" of any atrial impulses. Instead, there is a fixed conduction delay that may occur anywhere along the AV conduction axis. The site of delay may be at the level of the atrium especially in cases of atriopathies associated with structural heart disease such as Ebstein's anomaly or endocardial cushion defects. PR prolongation with a narrow QRS is typically noted in these cases. The AV node is the most common site of conduction delay in first-degree AV block, accounting for 90 % of cases with PR intervals greater than 300 ms [44]. The infranodal His-Purkinje system may be the site of first-degree AV block and should be suspected in cases with first-degree AV block and concomitant bundle branch block (Fig. 9.5). The bundle branches are involved in the majority of these cases [45], and in about two-thirds of cases, there is a combination of delay in both the AV node and the infranodal tissue. Both exercise and atropine can shorten the PR interval when the site of delay is at the level of the AV node and prolong it at the level of the infranodal tissue. Vagal stimulation will have the opposite effect. An EP study can be helpful in accurately identifying the site of conduction delay by evaluating both the AH and HV intervals. In patients with an HV interval exceeding 100 ms, pacemaker implantation has been advocated as 25 % of these patients progress to complete AV block over the next 22 months [46].

Second-Degree AV Block

Second-degree AV block indicates intermittent conduction of atrial impulses to the ventricles along the AV conduction axis. This intermittent conduction may be associated with a fixed or variable pattern. Type I and type II (Mobitz I and II) patterns describe the presence or absence of PR interval changes when at least two conducted P waves occur prior to interruption of AV conduction. Other forms of intermittent conduction include the

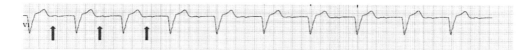

Fig. 9.5 First-degree AV block. Note the P waves were indicated by the arrows demonstrating sinus rhythm with first-degree AV block with a PR interval of 480 ms and a left bundle branch block with a QRS width of 190 ms. While first-degree AV block typically occurs at the level of the AV node, the presence of such a wide QRS in accompaniment should alert the consultant to the high likelihood of infranodal conduction disease as well

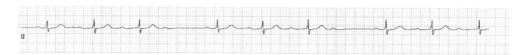

Fig. 9.6 Mobitz type I (Wenckebach) AV block. Notice the classic form of AV Wenckebach in a 4:3 pattern. The PP intervals are fixed, with lengthening of each successive PR interval with progressively decreasing increments and shorter RR intervals prior to the dropped beat. The pause is less than a multiple of the shortest RR interval, the return-cycle PR interval is shorter than the PR interval prior to the dropped beat, and there is obvious group beating periodicity

2:1 AV conduction pattern which cannot be definitively categorized as type I or II second-degree AV block, as well as high-grade AV block where more than one consecutive P wave is intermittently blocked.

Mobitz Type I (Wenckebach) Second-Degree AV Block

Wenckebach first described this phenomenon of progressive delay between atrial and ventricular beats prior to failure of conduction of one beat to the ventricles [47]. On the surface ECG, it is manifested by progressive prolongation of the PR interval with each normally timed P wave, prior to a nonconducted P wave. The longest PR interval is the one that occurs just prior to the nonconducted P wave and the shortest is the one that occurs immediately thereafter. This phenomenon is due to increased AV node refractoriness with each successive beat increasing the relative refractory period of the AV node until a beat arrives at the absolute effective refractory period of the AV node and fails to conduct. This allows a return to the baseline refractoriness of the AV node allowing it to conduct the subsequent beat with maximal conduction velocity, which corresponds to the shortest PR interval, before it starts to become progressively refractory again. Wenckebach periodicity may occur in a classic or nonclassic fashion. In the classic form, in addition to the above features, lengthening of the PR interval occurs with progressively decreasing increments with resultant shorter RR intervals, the pause is less than the sum of two RR intervals, and group beating patterns are observed (Fig. 9.6). In the nonclassic form, these additional features may not be noted.

Wenckebach AV block may occur due to physiological or pathological reasons. Under physiological conditions and in the absence of structural heart disease, it may be seen with increased vagal tone, such as that seen in well-trained athletes or during sleep. This is associated with an excellent prognosis and almost never advances to complete AV block [48, 49]. In patients with underlying heart disease, Wenckebach AV block may be associated with a worse prognosis such as when it occurs in conjunction with inferior myocardial infarction.

The site of block is at the level of the AV node in about 75 % of cases [45] and occurs below the AV node at the level of the His-Purkinje system in the remainder. Clues indicating the site of block to be the AV node include a classic form of Wenckebach periodicity, a narrow QRS, and a long PR interval at baseline. The presence of bundle branch block may point to disease at the level of the His-Purkinje system, but AV node disease is still more common.

Wenckebach AV block occurring at the level of the AV node will respond to sympathetic influences such as increased adrenergic tone with exercise or the administration of atropine, dopamine, or isoproterenol in emergent situations. If the site of block is below the AV node, these influences will worsen the ratio of AV block.

Mobitz Type II AV Block

Twenty-five years after Wenckebach published his findings on AV block, Mobitz further subdivided second-degree AV block on the basis of the ECG [50]. Mobitz type II AV block is defined as the sudden failure to conduct a normally timed P wave without prior PR prolongation. The PR interval immediately following the nonconducted P wave is identical to the PR interval of the last conducted beat prior to the AV block. The PP interval must remain constant and the resultant pause is two times the PP interval (Fig. 9.7). These features exclude atypical Wenckebach periodicity and must be present to make the diagnosis since it has serious implications.

Mobitz type II AV block is due to conduction disease in the infranodal tissue and has never been proven to be due to conduction block at the level of the AV node. It is therefore typically associated with a wide QRS or bundle branch block.

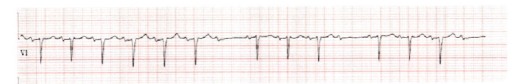

Fig. 9.7 Mobitz type II second-degree AV block. Note that there is ongoing sinus rhythm with a fixed PP interval before there is a sudden failure of conduction to the ventricles demonstrated by a dropped QRS. Note that there is no change in the PR interval preceding and following the dropped QRS, and this recurs later in the strip. The resultant pause is exactly twice the PP interval. Note the narrow QRS in this example that may suggest an intra-Hisian site of conduction block

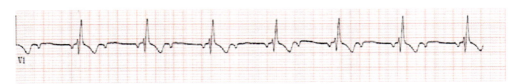

Fig. 9.8 2:1 AV block. 2:1 conduction with a short PR interval of 150 ms and the presence of RBBB. While not diagnostic currently, the ECG is suggestive for an infranodal site of conduction block. Further differentiation with maneuvers may be required to identify the level of block (see Table 9.4)

It is rarely associated with a narrow QRS and, in such cases, is indicative of intra-Hisian conduction block which accounts for only 20 % of all Mobitz type II AV block cases [45].

Since the level of block is below the AV node, increased adrenergic tone as with exercise or administration of atropine, dopamine, or isoproterenol only serves to worsen the ratio of AV block as the sinus rate speeds up while the infranodal conduction tissue remains refractory. Alternatively, vagal influences that slow the sinus rate down may allow for an improved conduction ratio of AV block, including a return of 1:1 conduction transiently.

Patients with Mobitz type II AV block are typically older and the etiology is often related to advanced degenerative cardiac disease or myocardial infarction. Unlike Wenckebach block, this type of AV block is permanent and frequently progresses to complete AV block requiring pacemaker implantation [51].

2:1 AV Block

This type of block describes a condition where only every second P wave is conducted to the ventricles. It is associated with a constant PP interval as well as a fixed PR interval in the conducted beats. It cannot be referred to as either type I or type II AV block since those designations require a minimum of 2 consecutive conducted P waves to observe the PR interval behavior. This type of block may occur at the level of the AV node or below the node and, as such, may represent a diagnostic challenge. Occasionally, running a rhythm strip for an extended period of time will allow the level of block to be revealed when the ratio of block spontaneously improves thereby allowing 2 consecutive P waves to be conducted. In the absence of such spontaneous observations, there are certain clues that may aid in identifying the level of

block (see Table 9.4). In the absence of symptoms, 2:1 AV block at the level of the AV node may be managed the same as Wenckebach AV block while that below the AV node should be managed in the same was as type II AV block (Fig. 9.8). Presence of symptoms mandates pacemaker insertion in the absence of a reversible cause.

High-Grade AV Block

Sometimes referred to as advanced AV block, high-grade AV block refers to the failure to conduct two or more consecutive P waves that arrive at the normal time. This cannot be confused with vagal episodes that sometimes occur during sleep or with neurocardiogenic syncope where there is associated sinus rate slowing prior to the occurrence of AV block. It must also be differentiated from block that occurs due to retrograde concealment of conduction into the AV node as a result of ventricular or junctional escape beats. Identifying the site of block may be difficult, but it may occur at either the level of the AV node or the His-Purkinje system. The same maneuvers in Table 9.3 may be required to elucidate the site of block.

Paroxysmal AV Block

Paroxysmal AV block is defined as a sudden failure of P wave conduction despite otherwise normal conduction [52]. Episodes are associated with prolonged periods of ventricular asystole. Thought to be due to phase 4 block, it must be assumed that the location of block is distal to the His-Purkinje system and that escape subsidiary pacemakers are unreliable, necessitating pacing [32].

Third-Degree (Complete) AV Block

Third-degree AV block is a complete lack of conduction of any P waves to the ventricles despite having plenty of

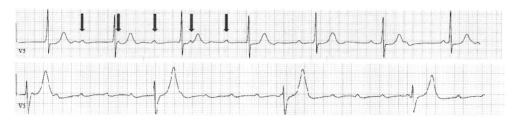

Fig. 9.9 Complete heart block. *Top panel*: Ongoing sinus rhythm at a rate of 75 bpm with complete heart block and a narrow junctional escape at just over 40 bpm. *Bottom panel*: Sinus tachycardia at a rate of 125 bpm with a wide ventricular escape focus at 24 bpm. The sinus tachycardia indicates that this patient may be in distress and is far more likely to be symptomatic upon presentation

opportunity for conduction, resulting in AV dissociation and a regular atrial rate that is faster than the regular ventricular rate. This cannot be confused with conditions that simply result in AV dissociation such as when fast junctional rhythms compete with a slower atrial rate. The site of block may be either at the level of the AV node or the His-Purkinje system. The QRS morphology of the subsidiary pacemaker provides important clues to the site of the conduction block. In the absence of preexisting bundle branch block, a narrow QRS indicates that the level of block is at the level of the AV node with an escape focus firing from either the lower portion of the AV node or the bundle of His. These subsidiary pacemakers are typically faster (40–60 bpm) and more reliable than those that occur at the more distal level of the conduction system. In patients with a preexisting bundle branch block, if the QRS morphology resembles that of the preexisting bundle branch, then the site of block is at the level of the AV node as well. In the absence of a preexisting bundle branch or in those patients with a preexisting bundle branch, a new wide QRS of different morphology indicates a site of block at the level of the His-Purkinje system. These subsidiary pacemakers are typically slower (20–40 bpm), far less reliable, and associated with more severe symptoms on presentation (Fig. 9.9). This presentation should prompt a more urgent management approach, with temporary pacemaker insertion. Notably, block at the His-Purkinje level will not improve with administration of atropine or dopamine as this will only worsen the ratio of AV block. A search for a reversible cause should be undertaken with discontinuation of any offending drugs, correction of metabolic derangements, and ruling out myocardial infarction. In the absence of a reversible cause, the only safe and definitive therapy is pacemaker implantation.

Management

In the acute or emergent setting, drugs such as atropine, dopamine, or isoproterenol may provide transient improvement in conduction only if the site of block is at the level of the AV node. This may provide the time needed for proceeding with pacing. If there is hemodynamic instability, this can be quickly achieved either by percutaneous or transvenous temporary pacing. A search for reversible causes such as Lyme disease or ischemia, as well as the removal of offending medications, should be undertaken prior to permanent pacing.

In the non-emergent situation, decisions regarding pacemaker implantation in patients with AV block depend on the presence of symptoms as well as the degree of AV block. Asymptomatic patients with first-degree or type I second-degree AV block should not receive pacemakers as these patients do not commonly progress to advanced AV block and pacing is not associated with any survival benefit [51, 53, 54]. However, it is now recognized that there is a subset of patients with PR intervals greater than 300 ms who have significant symptoms, similar to those of pacemaker syndrome, and have functional improvement with pacing and shorter PR intervals [55]. The same is true for patients with symptomatic type I second-degree AV block, and while controversial, pacemaker implantation should be considered in these patients [20, 56–58].

Patients with type II second-degree AV block should undergo pacemaker implantation regardless of symptoms since sudden progression to complete AV block is common and associated with an unfavorable prognosis [54, 59]. In patients with complete AV block, especially when associated with syncope, nonrandomized studies have shown improved survival following pacemaker implantation [59]. These patients should undergo pacemaker implantation regardless of symptoms. AV block provoked by exercise is indicative of diffuse conduction system disease, is associated with a poor prognosis, and thus necessitates pacing [60]. Pacing is also indicated in patients with infranodal 2:1 AV block as well as advanced and paroxysmal AV block in the absence of a clear and reversible cause. A summary of recommendations for pacemaker implantation for AV block is provided in Table 9.5.

In patients presenting with acute myocardial infarction, the decision to place a temporary pacemaker can be difficult. Patients with inferior MI often present with first-degree or type I second-degree AV block. They typically do not require

Table 9.5 Indications for pacing in acquired AV block

Recommendations for pacing in acquired AV block
Class I indication
Third-degree and advanced second-degree AV block at any level associated with:
Symptomatic bradycardia including heart failure
Ventricular arrhythmias due to AV block
Arrhythmias requiring drug therapy resulting in symptomatic bradycardia
Asymptomatic patients with greater than 3-s pauses, escape rate <40 bpm, and/or escape rhythm below the AV node
In atrial fibrillation patients with pauses >5 s
After catheter ablation of the AV node
Postoperative block that is not expected to resolve
Neuromuscular disorders such as muscular dystrophy, Kearns-Sayre, or Erb's dystrophy
During exercise in the absence of reversible ischemia
Symptomatic second-degree AV block regardless of site of block
Asymptomatic third-degree AV block regardless of site of block with average awake heart rates of 40 bpm if associated with LV dysfunction or in infranodal without LV dysfunction
Class IIa indication
Asymptomatic third-degree AV block, with heart rate >40 bpm without LV dysfunction
Asymptomatic second-degree AV block at the infranodal level found on electrophysiology study
First- or second-degree AV block and symptoms similar to pacemaker syndrome
Asymptomatic type II second-degree AV block with narrow QRS (wide QRS is class I)
Class IIb indication
Asymptomatic neuromuscular dystrophy with any AV block including first-degree
AV block associated with drug use that is expected to recur even after drug withdrawal
Class III indication
Asymptomatic first-degree AV block
Asymptomatic type I second-degree AV block at the level of AV node
AV block expected to resolve due to a reversible cause such as Lyme disease or increased vagal tone

Adapted from Epstein et al. [20]

Table 9.6 Indications for pacing in AV block accompanying MI

Recommendations for permanent pacing in atrioventricular (AV) block associated with acute myocardial infarction
Class I indications
Persistent second- or third-degree infranodal AV block after ST segment elevation MI
Transient advanced second-degree or third-degree AV block associated with bundle branch block
Persistent symptomatic second- or third-degree AV block
Class IIb indications
Asymptomatic persistent second- or third-degree AV block at the level of the AV node
Class III indications
Transient AV block without bundle branch block
Transient AV block with left anterior fascicular block only
New bundle branch or fascicular block without AV block
First-degree AV block with bundle branch or fascicular block

Adapted from Epstein et al. [20]

pacing as the site of block is at the level of the AV node and is usually transient, without hemodynamic instability and associated with a good prognosis. Type II second-degree AV block associated with inferior MI is rare and the site of block is at the level of the His-Purkinje system. These patients may have hemodynamic instability, sudden progression to complete AV block, and frequently require pacing. Patients with anterior MI may present with type II second-degree AV block or complete AV block. The site of block is at the level of the His-Purkinje system with a resultant wide unstable escape rhythm that is frequently associated with hemodynamic instability and requires pacing. This usually portends a worse

prognosis since the infarct size is usually large [32]. In these patients, permanent pacing will be required if the AV block persists beyond the peri-infarct period or if there is persistent intraventricular conduction delay, regardless of symptoms, as they have an increased risk of sudden death [61–64]. In patients that require permanent pacing following myocardial infarction and an ejection fraction (EF) less than or equal to 35 %, consideration should be given to implantation of a defibrillator device with biventricular pacing ability to provide cardiac resynchronization (CRT-D). Alternatively, a biventricular pacing device could also be considered (CRT-P) if a defibrillator device is not indicated. A summary of recommendations for pacemaker implantation for AV block associated with acute MI is provided in Table 9.6.

Key Points

- The sinus node is the main pacemaker of the heart and is richly innervated by sympathetic and parasympathetic nerve inputs.
- Sinus node dysfunction can be a result of a variety of intrinsic and extrinsic causes, most commonly aging and medications.
- The key to the diagnosis is correlating symptoms to electrocardiographic findings.
- The only effective management is by pacing and the main indication is for symptoms associated with sinus node dysfunction.
- The AV conduction axis has complex anatomical and physiological characteristics, some of which are not yet completely understood.

- There are a wide variety of causes of AV block, the most common of which are idiopathic, ischemic, iatrogenic, and infectious.
- AV block is divided into 3 ECG classifications called first-, second-, and third-degree AV block based on the P to QRS relationship.
- The electrocardiogram is the cornerstone of the diagnostic workup with electrophysiological testing having a limited role in regard to clinical management.
- Definitive management for acquired AV block is pacemaker implantation but is dependent on the presence of symptoms with any AV block or an infranodal site of conduction block regardless of symptoms.

References

1. Spodick DH. Normal sinus heart rate: sinus tachycardia and sinus bradycardia redefined. Am Heart J. 1992;124:1119–21.
2. Rubart M, Zipes DP. Genesis of cardiac arrhythmias: electrophysiological considerations. In: Zipes DP, Libby P, Bonow R, Braunwald E, editors. Braunwald's heart disease: a textbook of cardiovascular medicine. 7th ed. Philadelphia: WB Saunders; 2004. p. 653–88.
3. Kawashima T. The morphological significance of the human sinuatrial nodal branch (artery). Heart Vessels. 2003;18(4):213.
4. Jalife J. Mutual entrainment and electrical coupling as mechanisms for synchronous firing of rabbit sino-atrial pace-maker cells. J Physiol. 1984;356:221–43.
5. Schwartz PJ, Zipes DP. Autonomic modulation of cardiac arrhythmias. In: Zipes DP, Jalife J, editors. Cardiac electrophysiology: from cell to bedside. 3rd ed. Philadelphia: WB Saunders; 1999. p. 300–14.
6. Lee RJ, Kalmasn JM, Fitzpatrick AP, et al. Radiofrequency catheter modification of the sinus node for "inappropriate" sinus tachycardia. Circulation. 1995;92:2919–28.
7. Boyett MR, Honjo H, Kodama I. The sinoatrial node, a heterogeneous pacemaker structure. Cardiovasc Res. 2000;47:658.
8. Lee RJ, Shinbane JS. Advances in supraventricular tachycardia. Cardiol Clin. 1997;15:599–605.
9. Ferrer I. The sick sinus syndrome in atrial disease. JAMA. 1968;206:645–52.
10. Dobrzynski H, Boyett MR, Anderson RH. New insights into pacemaker activity: promoting understanding of sick sinus syndrome. Circulation. 2007;115:1921.
11. Rosenqvist M, Obel IW. Atrial pacing and the risk of AV block: is there a time for change in attitude? Pacing Clin Electrophysiol. 1989;12:97–101.
12. Mennozi C, Brignole M, Alboni P, et al. The natural course of untreated sick sinus syndrome and identification of variables predictive of unfavorable outcome. Am J Cardiol. 1998;82:1205–9.
13. Anderson HR, Thuesen L, Bagger JP, et al. Prospective randomized trial of atrial versus ventricular pacing in sick sinus syndrome. Lancet. 1994;344:1523–8.
14. Santini M, Alexidou G, Ansalone G, et al. Relation of prognosis in sick sinus syndrome to age, conduction defects and modes of permanent cardiac pacing. Am J Cardiol. 1990;65:729–35.
15. Simonsen E, Nielsen JS, Nielsen BL. Sinus node dysfunction in 128 patients. A retrospective study with followup. Acta Med Scand. 1980;208:343–8.
16. Sweeney MO. Sinus node dysfunction. In: Zipes D, Jalife J, editors. Cardiac electrophysiology: from cell to bedside. Philadelphia: WB Saunders; 2004. p. 879–83.
17. Alt E, Volker R, Witzfeld A, Ulm K. Survival and follow up after pacemaker implantation: a comparison of patients with sick sinus syndrome, complete heart block and atrial fibrillation. Pacing Clin Electrophysiol. 1985;8:849–55.
18. Simon AB, Janz N. Symptomatic bradyarrhythmias in the adult: natural history following ventricular pacemaker implantation. Pacing Clin Electrophysiol. 1982;5:372–83.
19. Elvan A, Wylie K, Zipes DP. Pacing-induced chronic atrial fibrillation impairs sinus node function in dogs: electrophysiological remodeling. Circulation. 1996;94:2953–60.
20. Epstein AE, DiMarco JP, Ellenbogen KA, et al. ACC/AHA/HRS 2008 guidelines for device-based therapy of cardiac rhythm abnormalities: a report of the American College of Cardiology/American Heart Association Task Force on Practice Guidelines (Writing Committee to Revise the ACC/AHA/NASPE 2002 Guideline Update for Implantation of Cardiac Pacemakers and Antiarrhythmia Devices): developed in collaboration with the American Association for Thoracic Surgery and Society of Thoracic Surgeons. Circulation. 2008;117:e350–408 [Erratum, Circulation 2009;120(5):e34–5].
21. Andersen HR, Thuesen L, Bagger JP, et al. Prospective randomized trial of atrial versus ventricular pacing in sick sinus syndrome. Lancet. 1994;344:1523–8.
22. Andersen HR, Nielsen JC, Rhomsen PEB, et al. Long term follow-up of patients from a randomized trial of atrial versus ventricular pacing for sick sinus syndrome. Lancet. 1997;350:1210–6.
23. Ac S, Krahn AD, Yee R, et al. Progression to chronic atrial fibrillation after pacing: the Canadian Trial of Physiological Pacing. CTOPP Investigators. J Am Coll Cardiol. 2001;38:167–72.
24. Lamas GA, Lee KL, Sweeney MO, et al. Ventricular pacing or dual chamber pacing for sinus node dysfunction. N Engl J Med. 2002;346:1854–62.
25. Rubart M, Zipes DP. Genesis of cardiac arrhythmias: electrophysiological considerations. In: Zipes DP, Libby P, Bonow R, Braunwald E, editors. Braunwalds heart disease: a textbook of cardiovascular medicine. 7th ed. Philadelphia: WB Saunders; 2004. p. 653–88.
26. Lev M. Anatomic basis for atrioventricular block. Am J Med. 1964;37:742.
27. Lev M. The pathology of complete atrioventricular block. Prog Cardiovasc Dis. 1964;6:317.
28. Zoob M, Smith KS. The aetiology of complete heart-block. Br Med J. 1963;2(5366):1149.
29. Levine SA, Miller H, Penton GB. Some clinical features of complete heart block. Circulation. 1956;13(6):801.
30. Hejtmancik MR, Herrmann GR, Shields AH, Wright JC. A clinical study of complete heart block. Am Heart J. 1956;52(3):369.
31. Rowe JC, White PD. Complete heart block: a follow-up study. Ann Intern Med. 1958;49(2):260.
32. Schwartzman D. Atrioventricular block and atrioventricular dissociation. In: Zipes DP, Jalife J, editors. Cardiac electrophysiology: from cell to bedside. 4th ed. Philadelphia: WB Saunders; 2004. p. 485–9.
33. Wellens HJJ. Atrioventricular nodal and subnodal ventricular disturbances. In: Willerson J, Cohn J, Wellens Jr H, Holmes D, editors. Cardiovascular medicine. New York: Springer; 2007. p. 1991–8.

34. Olgin JE, Zipes DP. Specific arrhythmias: diagnosis and treatment. In: Zipes DP, Libby P, Bonow R, Braunwald E, editors. Braunwald's heart disease: a textbook of cardiovascular medicine. 7th ed. Philadelphia: WB Saunders; 2004. p. 803–64.

35. Zeltser D, Justo D, Halkin A, Rosso R, Ish-Shalom M, Hochenberg M, Viskin S. Drug-induced atrioventricular block: prognosis after discontinuation of the culprit drug. J Am Coll Cardiol. 2004; 44(1):105.

36. Erdogan HB, Kayalar N, Ardal H, Omeroglu SN, Kirali K, Guler M, Akinci E, Yakut C. Risk factors for requirement of permanent pacemaker implantation after aortic valve replacement. J Card Surg. 2006;21:211–5.

37. Limongelli G, Ducceschi V, D'Andrea A, Renzulli A, Sarubbi B, De Feo M, Cerasuolo F, Calabro R, Cotrufo M. Risk factors for pacemaker implantation following aortic valve replacement: a single centre experience. Heart. 2003;89:901–4.

38. Khawaja MZ, Rajani R, Cook A, Khavandi A, Moynagh A, Chowdhary S, Spence MS, Brown S, Khan SQ, Walker N, Trivedi U, Hutchinson N, De Belder AJ, Moat N, Blackman DJ, Levy RD, Manoharan G, Roberts D, Khogali SS, Crean P, Brecker SJ, Baumbach A, Mullen M, Laborde JC, Hildick-Smith D. Permanent pacemaker insertion after CoreValve transcatheter aortic valve implantation: incidence and contributing factors (the UK CoreValve collaborative). Circulation. 2011;123(9):951.

39. Roten L, Wenaweser P, Delacrétaz E, Hellige G, Stortecky S, Tanner H, Pilgrim T, Kadner A, Eberle B, Zwahlen M, Carrel T, Meier B, Windecker S. Incidence and predictors of atrioventricular conduction impairment after transcatheter aortic valve implantation. Am J Cardiol. 2010;106(10):1473.

40. Chang SM, Nagueh SF, Spencer 3rd WH, Lakkis NM. Complete heart block: determinants and clinical impact in patients with hypertrophic obstructive cardiomyopathy undergoing nonsurgical septal reduction therapy. J Am Coll Cardiol. 2003;42(2):296.

41. Nagueh SF, Ommen SR, Lakkis NM, Killip D, Zoghbi WA, Schaff HV, Danielson GK, Quiñones MA, Tajik AJ, Spencer WH. Comparison of ethanol septal reduction therapy with surgical myectomy for the treatment of hypertrophic obstructive cardiomyopathy. J Am Coll Cardiol. 2001;38(6):1701.

42. Scheinman MM, Huang S. The 1998 NASPE prospective catheter ablation registry. Pacing Clin Electrophysiol. 2000;23(6):1020.

43. Fish AE, Pride YB, Pinto DS. Lyme carditis. Infect Dis Clin North Am. 2008;22(2):275.

44. Josephson ME. Atrioventricular conduction. In: Clinical cardiac electrophysiology: techniques and interpretations. 4th ed. Philadelphia: Lea & Febiger; 1993.

45. Peuch P, Groileau R, Guimond C. Incidence of different types of A-V block and their localization by His bundle recordings. In: Wellens HJJ, Lie KI, Janse MJ, editors. The conduction system of the heart. Leiden: Stenfert; 1976. p. 467.

46. Scheinman MM, Peters RW, Suavé MJ, Desai J, Abbott JA, Cogan J, Wohl B, Williams K. Value of the H-Q interval in patients with bundle branch block and the role of prophylactic permanent pacing. Am J Cardiol. 1982;50(6):1316–22.

47. Wenckebach KF. Zur analyse der unregelmässigen pulses. Ztschr klin Med. 1899;36:181.

48. Meytes I, Kaplinsky E, Yahini JH, Hanne-Paparo N, Neufeld HN. Wenckebach A-V block: a frequent feature following heavy physical training. Am Heart J. 1975;90(4):426.

49. Zeppilli P, Fenici R, Sassara M, Pirrami MM, Caselli G. Wenckebach second-degree A-V block in top-ranking athletes: an old problem revisited. Am Heart J. 1980;100(3):281.

50. Mobitz W. Über die unvollständige Störung der Erregungsüberleitung zwischen Vorhof und Kammer des menschlichen Herzens. Z Gesamte Exp Med. 1924;41:180.

51. Strasberg B, Amat-Y-Leon F, Dhingra RC, Palileo E, Swiryn S, Bauernfeind R, Wyndham C, Rosen KM. Natural history of chronic second-degree atrioventricular nodal block. Circulation. 1981; 63(5):1043.

52. Barold SS. Atrioventricular block revisited. Compr Ther. 2002;28:74–8.

53. Mymin D, Mathewson FA, Tate RB, Manfreda J. The natural history of primary first-degree atrioventricular heart block. N Engl J Med. 1986;315:1183–7.

54. Dhingra RC, Denes P, Wu D, Chuquimia R, Rosen KM. The significance of second degree atrioventricular block and bundle branch block. Observations regarding site and type of block. Circulation. 1974;49:638–46.

55. Barold SS. Indications for permanent cardiac pacing in first-degree AV block: class I, II, or III? Pacing Clin Electrophysiol. 1996; 19:747–51.

56. Recommendations for pacemaker prescription for symptomatic bradycardia. Report of a working party of the British Pacing and Electrophysiology Group. Br Heart J. 1991;66:185–91.

57. Connelly DT, Steinhaus DM. Mobitz type I atrioventricular block: an indication for permanent pacing? Pacing Clin Electrophysiol. 1996;19:261–4.

58. Shaw DB, Kekwick CA, Veale D, Gowers J, Whistance T. Survival in second degree atrioventricular block. Br Heart J. 1985;53: 587–93.

59. Donoso E, Adler LN, Friedberg CK. Unusual forms of second-degree atrioventricular block, including mobitz type-II block, associated with the Morgagni-Adams-Stokes Syndrome. Am Heart J. 1964;67:150–7.

60. Chokshi SK, Sarmiento J, Nazari J, Mattioni T, Zheutlin T, Kehoe R. Exercise-provoked distal atrioventricular block. Am J Cardiol. 1990;66:114–6.

61. Hindman MC, Wagner GS, JaRo M, et al. The clinical significance of bundle branch block complicating acute myocardial infarction. 2. Indications for temporary and permanent pacemaker insertion. Circulation. 1978;58:689–99.

62. Col JJ, Weinberg SL. The incidence and mortality of intraventricular conduction defects in acute myocardial infarction. Am J Cardiol. 1972;29:344–50.

63. Ginks WR, Sutton R, Oh W, Leatham A. Long-term prognosis after acute anterior infarction with atrioventricular block. Br Heart J. 1977;39:186–9.

64. Petrina M, Goodman SG, Eagle KA. The 12–lead electrocardiogram as a predictive tool of mortality after acute myocardial infarction: current status in an era of revascularization and reperfusion. Am Heart J. 2006;152:11–8.

Cardiac Arrest and Sudden Cardiac Death

10

Pradyot Saklani, James A. White, George J. Klein, and Andrew D. Krahn

Abstract

Sudden cardiac death (SCD) is a major public health issue and ranks among the leading causes of mortality in the developed world. The mechanism of death is mostly malignant ventricular arrhythmia. The underlying etiology is primarily ischemic heart disease, although susceptibility to SCD is a complex process with multiple interactions between genes that regulate cardiac and vascular function and other physiological factors. A minority of cases of cardiac arrest or SCD occur in the context of hereditary channelopathies, without overt structural heart disease, such as Brugada syndrome, long QT syndrome, or catecholaminergic polymorphic VT. Prevention of SCD is hampered by our inability to predict who is at risk at an individual level, since the majority of cases occur as the index event without associated high-risk features. In patients with high-risk features for SCD, antiarrhythmic drugs do not reduce mortality and, in fact, can contribute to arrhythmic death, particularly in those with impaired left ventricular systolic function. The ICD is the only proven treatment for prevention of SCD. The advent of the ICD has been perceived as a panacea for SCD, although in reality the degree of residual risk is significant. Ongoing research into genetic susceptibilities and the development of complex computer modeling may provide us with a better understanding of this complex disease process in the future. Until such time, SCD is destined to remain a significant public health threat that requires further study.

Keywords

Cardiac arrest • Sudden cardiac death • Ischemic heart disease • Brugada • Long QT syndrome • Implantable cardioverter/defibrillator • Antiarrhythmic drugs

P. Saklani, MBBS • A.D. Krahn, MD (✉)
Division of Cardiology/Electrophysiology Service, University of Western Ontario/University Hospital, 339 Windermere Road, London, ON N6A 5A5, Canada
e-mail: pradyotsaklani@gmail.com; akrahn9@gmail.com

J.A. White, MD
Cardiovascular MRI Clinical Research Program, Division of Cardiology/Cardiovascular Imaging, Robart's Research Institute, University of Western Ontario/University Hospital, 339 Windermere Road, London, ON N6A 5A5, Canada
e-mail: jwhite@robarts.ca

G.J. Klein, MD
Division of Cardiology/Arrhythmia Service, University of Western Ontario/University Hospital, 339 Windermere Road, London, ON N6A 5A5, Canada
e-mail: gklein@uwo.ca

Introduction

Sudden cardiac death (SCD) is defined as death from an unexpected circulatory arrest, usually presumed due to a cardiac arrhythmia occurring within an hour of the onset of symptoms [1]. SCD ranks among the leading causes of mortality in the developed world. Conservative estimates categorize up to 13 % of deaths as SCD [1]. SCD is responsible for more than 450,000 deaths annually in the United States alone [2] and accounts for more deaths than stroke, lung cancer, breast cancer, and AIDS combined [3].

Up to 80 % of cardiac arrests and SCDs are due to ischemic heart disease (IHD) [4]. Cardiomyopathies, principally

K. Stergiopoulos, D.L. Brown (eds.), *Evidence-Based Cardiology Consult*,
DOI 10.1007/978-1-4471-4441-0_10, © Springer-Verlag London 2014

although not limited to dilated cardiomyopathy, comprise another 10–15 %. Less than 5 % of cases of SCD involve hereditary channelopathies or primary electrical diseases [1, 4].

The average annual risk of SCD in the general population is 0.1–0.2 %. This risk increases as a function of advancing age. The greatest increase in risk of SCD is among those aged 40–65 years [4]. In those with established advanced cardiac disease, who have an average annual risk of SCD between 10 and 25 %, the age-related increase in risk is attenuated [4], stemming from the principles of absolute and relative risk. Whereas absolute risk refers to the probability of an adverse outcome occurring in a population, relative risk is a comparison of risk expressed as a percentage or ratio between two separate populations. Importantly, relative risk does not give any indication as to the actual risk of an event. It follows then that a large increase in relative risk may be associated with a small increase in absolute risk, and, conversely, a large increase in absolute risk may be associated with a small increase in relative risk. The two values need to be interpreted in context for useful information to be gleaned. The inverse of the absolute risk reduction with any given intervention is equal to the number needed to treat (NNT) to prevent one outcome. This value is of particular relevance in the case of SCD, where the intervention is potentially an invasive and costly ICD, which may be lifesaving.

The relative risk of SCD in adolescents and young adults (10–30 years of age) is 1/100th that of the general adult population. There is a modest but significant inverse relationship in risk of SCD between the ages of 10 and 30 years [4]. This resonates with the genetic/hereditary nature of the so-called inherited "channelopathies" and certain cardiomyopathies. These genetic disorders are more likely to manifest earlier in life than acquired heart disease. Consequently, primary electrical diseases and certain hereditary cardiomyopathies account for a disproportionate number of cases in this age group. Other conditions such as anomalous coronary arteries and myocarditis are also more common causes of SCD in younger individuals than in those older than 35 years of age.

The mechanism of death is predominantly malignant ventricular arrhythmia such as ventricular fibrillation (VF), polymorphic ventricular tachycardia (VT), or monomorphic VT. In up to 16.5 % of cases, advanced atrioventricular block or asystole has been observed [5]. These data need to be interpreted cautiously, as the initiating arrhythmia may degenerate into another. Pulseless electrical activity (PEA) can also lead to SCD. Survival data indicate even poorer outcomes from these forms of cardiac arrests that cannot be defibrillated or cardioverted, compared to tachyarrhythmia [6].

Risk Stratification in SCD

In spite of improvements in public health education, management of chronic heart disease and the availability of emergency medical services, survival rates for out-of-hospital cardiac arrests remain poor. Less than 5 % of patients survive an out-of-hospital cardiac arrest [2, 4]. Furthermore, while the overall rates of cardiac mortality in the United Sates have decreased, the proportion of sudden deaths has increased, accounting for 48 % of all cardiac mortality [2].

The use of implantable cardioverter/defibrillators (ICDs) has revolutionized the management of survivors of cardiac arrest. Because surviving cardiac arrest is clearly the exception and not the rule, the challenge is to be able to identify those at risk of SCD before their fatal index event. The majority (>80 %) of SCD occurs as the first presentation in an asymptomatic individual or patients with known cardiac disease but with an otherwise low-risk profile (LVEF >40 %, no prior history of arrhythmia or congestive cardiac failure) [1, 4, 6]. Traditional risk factors for SCD (LVEF <35 % and clinical congestive cardiac failure) are valid for a population-based risk prediction but not at an individual risk assessment level due to the low overall incidence of SCD. Consequently the positive predictive value of a traditional risk factor such as LVEF <35 % is poor. In spite of this, it is marginally better at predicting SCD than other traditional risk factors and is easily assessable and reproducible making it the accepted standard of risk stratification upon which management decisions are based. Individual risk stratification may be improved by the assessment for left ventricular hypertrophy (LVH) on electrocardiogram(ECG) or echocardiography, left bundle branch block (LBBB), ischemic burden, abnormal signal-averaged ECG, microvolt T wave alternans, abnormal heart rate variability and baroreceptor response, and invasive electrophysiology study for inducible VT [3]. The vast majority of cases of SCD will inevitably still occur among the low-risk population, even as the greatest rates of SCD are observed in the high-risk population as defined by current risk stratification (Fig. 10.1a, b). Thus, general prevention strategies that prevent progression of atherosclerosis and recognition of left ventricular dysfunction may be more likely to affect the population burden of sudden death than successfully targeting the highest risk minute fraction of the population. Consequently the use of ICDs in their current breadth will not significantly alter the rates of SCD at a population level. ICDs do however play an important primary and secondary prevention role, albeit in a select high-risk population.

The pathophysiology, management, and prognosis of resuscitated cardiac arrest patients are largely determined by the underlying etiology. These shall be discussed separately in greater detail.

Fig. 10.1 (**a**, **b**) Demonstrates the relative and absolute risks of sudden cardiac death (*SCD*) among the various subgroups. It is apparent that the greatest proportion of SCD occurs in those patients with the lowest relative risk of SCD (Adapted from Myerburg et al. [51])

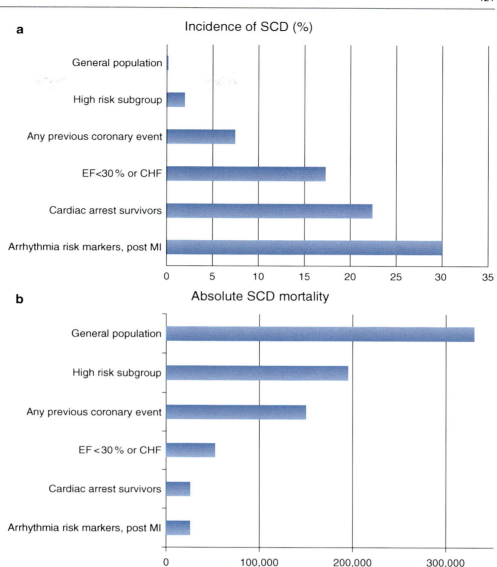

Ischemic Heart Disease

IHD is responsible for the majority of cases of SCD. Most patients with IHD have multivessel disease combined with evidence of acute plaque rupture or intra-intimal thrombosis [1]. Ischemia and infarction alter myocardial tissue refractoriness and conduction properties in a heterogeneous pattern. These changes promote various mechanisms of tachycardia, principally reentry, but including triggered activity and increased automaticity [7]. All forms of IHD including acute coronary syndrome (ACS), hibernating myocardium, and ischemic scar have been shown to be proarrhythmic [6–8]. There is also evidence of an interaction between the acute or chronic ischemic substrate and the selective genetic predisposition to arrhythmogenesis. The Paris Prospective Study demonstrated a nearly twofold increase in relative risk of

SCD as the expression of an acute coronary syndrome in those with a parental history of SCD [9]. The genetic basis is strongly suggested by the observation that if both parents had a history of SCD, the relative risk to the individual was 9.4, consistent with a dose-dependent relationship. A similar familial predisposition to SCD as the initial presentation of ACS, but not nonfatal myocardial infarction, has been borne out in other studies [10, 11]. This genetic predisposition likely represents arrhythmogenic mutations or polymorphisms in the genes that regulate cardiac ion channel function, which in the baseline state do not produce a pathologic phenotype. An arrhythmogenic phenotype is unmasked however during acute ischemia due to changes in autonomic tone, metabolic milieu, and other environmental factors [6]. In reality every element in the pathophysiology of ACS has a genetic component that is modified not only by environmental triggers but also by other genes. The process is thus complex and only partially understood in a conceptual framework.

A trigger and substrate concept for SCD therefore, while seemingly simplistic, is conceptually accurate. Effective prevention of SCD needs to focus on targeting both these factors. This includes risk factor modification and potential reduction in triggers such as infrequent vigorous exercise (shoveling snow). While complex, it is important to try and identify candidate genes, mutations, and polymorphisms that predispose to SCD to allow better risk stratification and treatment.

Traditional vascular risk factors such as hypertension, dyslipidemia, diabetes mellitus, obesity, and cigarette smoking are also independent risk factors for SCD that can be "inherited" environmentally from parental lifestyle or by conventional genetic means [9]. Aggressive treatment of these risk factors therefore not only reduces rates of ACS but also SCD [12].

Treatment

Primary and secondary prevention of SCD in both ischemic and nonischemic cardiomyopathy has been studied using medications and ICDs. It is worth noting that the relevant primary endpoint in the majority of studies is all-cause mortality. SCD data was often reported as a secondary outcome. Antiarrhythmic drugs do not reduce the risk of SCD and in many cases increase mortality when used in a primary prevention role. The following is a brief summary of the landmark trials.

The Cardiac Arrhythmia Suppression Trial (CAST) study was a randomized placebo-controlled trial that assessed the effect of class Ic agents (encainide, flecainide, and moricizine) on the suppression of asymptomatic or mildly symptomatic ventricular ectopy after myocardial infarction. The study was discontinued prematurely due to an increased mortality in the treatment arm [13]. Not surprisingly, the treatment of the marker of SCD risk such as PVCs is not the same as reducing SCD itself. This is intrinsically linked with the concept of cause and effect. While markers are associated with the primary outcome, the challenge is identifying those that are a cause of SCD rather than an effect of the process that leads to SCD. Only treatment of the former would be expected to result in a favorable outcome.

The Survival With Oral D-Sotalol (SWORD) trial was a randomized, placebo-controlled trial that assessed the effect of D-Sotalol on mortality in patients with ischemic cardiomyopathy. This trial was discontinued prematurely due to increased mortality (presumed arrhythmic) in the treatment arm [14].

The Sudden Cardiac Death in Heart Failure Trial (SCD-HeFT) demonstrated that amiodarone offered no benefit over placebo in reducing all-cause mortality in patients with class

II or III heart failure and an EF < 35 % from either ischemic or nonischemic cardiomyopathy [15].

Despite the failure of antiarrhythmic drugs to reduce SCD, a number of medications that are routinely used in the treatment of heart failure have shown a reduction in SCD when used in high-risk patients [16]. Beta-blockers have consistently been shown to reduce mortality and rates of SCD [7]. Aldosterone antagonists spironolactone and eplerenone reduce rates of SCD by up to 30 % [7]. Angiotensin-converting enzyme (ACE) inhibitors reduce rates of SCD in both ischemic and nonischemic cardiomyopathies. A meta-analysis of ACE inhibitor use following myocardial infarction verified a reduction in SCD of 20 % [16]. Similarly, statins have repeatedly been shown to reduce rates of cardiovascular mortality including SCD. The benefit within each family of drug appears to be a class effect.

The *antiarrhythmic* mechanism of the various classes of medications is complex and incompletely understood. Potential mechanisms include favorable remodeling of LV dimensions, reduction of myocardial fibrosis, antiadrenergic properties, improved autonomic tone by improving baroreceptor sensitivity, as well as protection against hypokalemia with concomitant diuretic use (ACE inhibitors and aldosterone antagonists) [16]. Perhaps the most important antiarrhythmic mechanism is the effect on reducing ischemic burden via reductions in blood pressure, modifications of endothelial function, as well as anti-inflammatory properties leading to plaque stability and reduced platelet aggregation [16].

Secondary Prevention ICD Trials

The utility of ICDs in the secondary prevention of SCD has been prospectively evaluated in three randomized controlled trials, Antiarrhythmics Versus Implantable Defibrillator (AVID) study, the Cardiac Arrest Study Hamburg (CASH), and the Canadian Implantable Defibrillator Study (CIDS, Table 10.1) [17]. All three studies compared ICD to antiarrhythmic medications, primarily amiodarone. The largest of these trials, AVID was terminated early due to the interim analysis showing clear superiority of ICD therapy. The other two smaller trials had a trend towards benefit but did not show a statistically significant benefit for ICD over antiarrhythmic medication in the secondary prevention of SCD. The follow-up in these studies was longer with more combined deaths than the AVID trial. Early termination in the AVID trial could have potentially biased the result in favor of a positive result for ICD. A meta-analysis of the three studies has allowed a more accurate and balanced determination of benefit for ICD in the secondary prevention of SCD [17]. Fixed effects analysis demonstrated a statistically significant benefit of ICD in reducing all-cause mortality

Table 10.1 Secondary prevention ICD trials

Study	AVID	CASH	CIDS
n	1,016	288	659
Inclusion criteria	Resuscitated cardiac arrest or symptomatic VT + syncope or + EF ≤40 %	Resuscitated cardiac arrest	Resuscitated cardiac arrest, symptomatic VT + EF ≤35 %, unmonitored syncope with documented or induced VT
Intervention	ICD vs. class III drugs (mainly amiodarone)	1:1:1ICD:amiodarone:beta-blocker	ICD vs. amiodarone
Mean follow-up	1.51 years	4.75 years	2.96 years
HR all-cause mortality	0.62 ($P < 0.05$)	0.77 ($P = 0.081$)	0.82 ($P = 0.142$)
HR arrhythmic mortality	0.43 ($P < 0.05$)	0.42 ($P = 0.005$)	0.68 ($P = 0.094$)

AVID Antiarrhythmics Versus Implantable Defibrillator trial, *CASH* Cardiac Arrest Study Hamburg, *CIDA* Canadian Implantable Defibrillator Study, *HR* hazard ratio, *n* number of patients enrolled, *ICD* implantable cardioverter/defibrillator, *VT* ventricular tachycardia, *EF* ejection fraction

(HR 0.72) and arrhythmic mortality (HR 0.5). It should be highlighted that this result, while encouraging, still suggests that at least half the cases of SCD are not preventable by ICDs. The residual risk of SCD is not insignificant and should not be underestimated, even after ICD implantation. The mortality benefit associated with ICD implantation starts to diminish after approximately 4 years when the survival curves between the two arms start to converge. The reduction in arrhythmic mortality however continues past 6 years. This is an expected outcome since survival from arrhythmic death increases the potential for mortality from other competing causes including heart failure and malignancy. ICDs reduce annual mortality from 12.3 to 8.8 % for an absolute risk reduction of 3.5 % [17]. This translates to an annual number needed to treat (NNT) of 29 to save one life. The average prolongation of life is 4.4 months at 6 years, a modest but not trivial effect [17].

Predefined subgroup analysis shows that patients with greater left ventricular systolic dysfunction (EF ≤35 %) derived greater mortality benefit from ICD implantation. Post-randomization beta-blocker use in CIDS and AVID patients was much greater in the ICD group than in the anti-arrhythmic group. However, ICD benefit was maintained even allowing for this discrepancy.

Primary Prevention ICD Trials

The initial primary prevention studies, Multicenter Automatic Defibrillator Implantation Trial (MADIT) and Multicenter Unsustained Tachycardia Trial (MUSTT), demonstrated a survival advantage of primary prevention ICD in the prevention of SCD in high-risk patients with ischemic cardiomyopathy. Eligibility required inducibility of VT during an electrophysiology (EP) study with programmed ventricular stimulation. The external validity of these studies in contemporary practice is debatable since an EP study with programmed ventricular stimulation is not the current standard

of care in patients with cardiomyopathy. Furthermore, the results of these studies have been confirmed by large randomized controlled studies that do not require risk stratification with an EP study (Table 10.2).

The Multicenter Automatic Defibrillator Implantation Trial II (MADIT II) study was a randomized controlled trial (RCT) comparing ICD to conventional medical management in patients with an ischemic cardiomyopathy (EF < 30 %). The trial was discontinued prematurely when a 30 % relative risk reduction in all-cause mortality was observed in the ICD group [18]. The SCD-HeFT trial was an RCT comparing ICD to amiodarone to placebo in patients with NYHA class II or III, ischemic or nonischemic cardiomyopathy, and EF < 35 %. There was a 23 % relative risk reduction in overall mortality in the ICD arm relative to placebo [15].

While the majority of primary prevention ICD studies in patients with ischemic cardiomyopathy have confirmed a mortality benefit, there are two notable detractors that highlight certain issues relating in particular to timing of ICD implantation. The Coronary Artery Bypass Graft (CABG) Patch study randomized 900 patients with ischemic cardiomyopathy (EF < 36 %) and an abnormal signal-averaged ECG (SAECG) scheduled for CABG to routine medical care or adjunctive ICD with an epicardial coil/lead. More than 80 % of patients had experienced a recent MI. No significant difference in mortality was observed. The Defibrillator in Acute Myocardial Infarction Trial (DINAMIT) study randomized 675 patients 4–40 days post-MI with EF < 35 % and abnormal heart rate variability to standard medical therapy or adjunctive ICD implantation. Once again, no mortality benefit was observed in the ICD group. One reason proposed to explain the neutral result in the CABG Patch trial was that revascularization at the time of randomization lead to a dramatic reduction in rates of SCD, dramatically reducing the power of the study to detect a difference in mortality [8]. In the DINAMIT trial the lack of mortality benefit may be understood by appreciating the observed mechanism of

Table 10.2 Primary prevention ICD trials

Study	N	Inclusion criteria	Mean follow-up (months)	Intervention	1° outcome	Results (ICD arm)
SCD-HeFT	2,521	NYHA II or III	45.5	Randomized 1:1:1	All-cause mortality	ICD vs. placebo HR 0.77 ($P = 0.007$)
RCT		LVEF < 35 %		Placebo, amiodarone, and ICD		Amiodarone vs. placebo HR 1.06 ($P = 0.53$)
		Ischemic or nonischemic cardiomyopathy				
MADIT II	1,232	MI > 1/12 ago	20	Randomized 3:2	All-cause mortality	HR 0.69 ($P = 0.016$)
RCT		EF < 30 %		ICD vs. medical Rx		Study stopped early
DINAMIT	674	Recent MI (6–40 days)	30 ± 13	ICD vs. medical Rx	All-cause mortality	HR 1.08 ($P = 0.66$)
RCT		EF < 35 %				
		Impaired autonomic function				
CABG patch	900	EF < 36 %, planned CABG (positive SAECG)	32 ± 16	CABG with or without ICD	All-cause mortality	HR 1.07 ($P = 0.64$)
RCT						

SCD-HeFT Sudden Cardiac Death in Heart Failure Trial, *MADIT II* Multicenter Automatic Defibrillator Implantation Trial II, *DINAMIT* Defibrillator In Acute Myocardial Infarction Trial, *CABG patch* Coronary Artery Bypass Graft patch trial, *RCT* randomized controlled trial, *N* number of patients enrolled, *NYHA* New York Heart Association heart failure score, *MI* myocardial infarction, *EF* ejection fraction, *SAECG* signal-averaged ECG, *ICD* implantable cardioverter/defibrillator, *Rx* treatment, *HR* hazard ratio

death early after an MI. Multiple studies have shown that the dominant cause of death in this period is reinfarction or progressive heart failure rather than primary arrhythmia [8]. Therefore, ventricular arrhythmia in the early post-infarct period is most likely a marker or surrogate for recurrent acute coronary syndromes. An ICD would be expected to be significantly less effective in this context. Revascularization and appropriate heart failure treatment would be expected to improve LV function, once again diminishing the risk of SCD and the potential benefit of an ICD. In principal therefore, primary prevention ICDs should not be implanted for at least 3 months after revascularization or commencement of heart failure medications.

Investigation of Aborted SCD

Investigation into the cause of aborted SCD needs to be comprehensive and systematic. A detailed history is essential (Table 10.3). Patients often are not able to provide this due to amnesia or more profound neurological deficits as a consequence of hypoxic cerebral injury. Collateral history from family members, witnesses, or attending emergency medical service (EMS) personnel is often very informative. An attempt should always be made to analyze the EMS rhythm strip at the scene. Physical examination is rarely revealing as to the cause of cardiac arrest [1].

The sequence in which testing is performed is guided by the clinical scenario (Fig. 10.2).

The ECG often provides the initial clues as to the etiology of cardiac arrest. Changes consistent with myocardial ischemia or infarction need to be diagnosed promptly to allow timely revascularization. The ECG should also be scrutinized

Table 10.3 Salient features of history in the investigation of sudden cardiac death or cardiac arrest

Relevant history
History of ischemic or structural heart disease
Preceding chest pain
Circumstances of the arrest: exercise/emotional distress/rest/sleep
History of syncope/epilepsy/sleep disordered breathing
Medications/recreational drug use
Family history of sudden cardiac death, unexplained drowning, accidents, or sudden infant death syndrome

for other abnormal patterns of depolarization and repolarization. Serial ECGs should be performed since both depolarization and repolarization are often transiently and nonspecifically abnormal in the post-resuscitation setting. The QT interval in particular is affected by the infusion of adrenergic drugs and induced hypothermia in the intensive care unit setting [19]. Marked QT prolongation is often observed with anoxic brain injury, subarachnoid hemorrhage, and traumatic brain injury. Osborn J waves are observed in hypothermic patients. Pathological depolarization patterns include preexcitation, bundle branch block, and frequent monomorphic or polymorphic ventricular ectopy. Abnormal repolarization patterns include long and short QT intervals, Brugada pattern, and early repolarization, especially in the inferolateral leads.

Cardiomyopathies are characterized by the presence of myocardial fibrosis with or without impairment in systolic function and overt structural change. Depolarization of viable myocardial tissue within scar is delayed and produces low amplitude, high frequency diastolic potentials referred to as late potentials. These late potentials are not usually distinguishable from background noise on a standard 12-lead

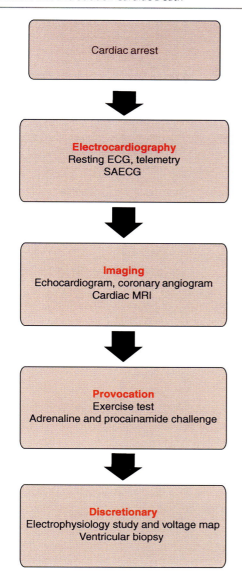

Fig.10.2 Flow diagram for systematic investigation of cardiac arrest victims. *SAECG* signal-averaged ECG, *MRI* magnetic resonance imaging

ECG. The signal-to-noise ratio is amplified when several hundred QRS complexes are averaged. Background noise by definition is random and cancels out when averaged, whereas late potentials are constant and remain [7]. The SAECG measures these late potentials and is a sensitive marker of occult cardiomyopathy and even Brugada syndrome [19].

The commonest cause of cardiac arrest is an acute coronary syndrome (ACS). As such, coronary angiography needs to be performed as a priority if the ECG does not manifest primary electrical disease. Moreover, an ACS can mimic both long QT and Brugada on the ECG. In select low-risk groups, computed tomography (CT) coronary angiography is an alternative to invasive coronary angiography, as this modality has a high negative predictive value for coronary

artery disease. In low-risk young populations, CT angiography can also rule out congenital coronary anomalies.

Cardiomyopathies in aggregate are the second most common cause of cardiac arrest. Consequently assessment of myocardial structure and function is paramount. The transthoracic echo (TTE) is widely available, inexpensive, and simple to perform and interpret [1]. TTE provides accurate information on valvular and myocardial dimensions and function. The quality of TTE imaging however can be strongly influenced by patient comorbidities such as morbid obesity and chronic obstructive lung disease. Cardiac MRI is increasingly becoming the imaging modality of choice for the identification and characterization of underlying cardiomyopathy [20]. This increasingly available modality is useful for the assessment of suspected arrhythmogenic right ventricular cardiomyopathy (ARVC) where regional or global functional abnormalities may be optimally identified. Cardiac MRI's capacity to incrementally assess for abnormal tissue characteristics, such as irreversible fibrosis or "scar," fat infiltration, or myocardial edema (consistent with recent myocardial injury), provides a robust diagnostic yield in this patient population [21]. Up to one-third of patients with resuscitated SCD demonstrate evidence for an acute myopathic process when studied early following their event, typically either acute viral injury or clinically unrecognized ischemic injury [21]. Mature, irreversible fibrosis can also characterize unsuspected chronic cardiomyopathies, such as cardiac sarcoid or variant forms of hypertrophic cardiomyopathy. The presence and burden of fibrosis in these diseases has been associated with arrhythmic events [20, 21]. This characterization of an underlying myopathic process may have important implications for future disease management and family counseling. For example, the identification of cardiac sarcoid may provide alternate therapeutic strategies, while the identification of ARVC or hypertrophic cardiomyopathy may be relevant for risk assessment in first-degree relatives. Cardiac MRI is also valuable for the identification of coronary anomalies and other rarer causes of arrhythmia, such as cardiac masses. Therefore, this versatile imaging test is rapidly being considered a standard of care in the assessment of cardiac arrest survivors, particularly when it occurs in the absence of clinically overt ischemia.

In the absence of ischemic heart disease, structural heart disease, or profound metabolic derangements, occult primary electrical cardiac disease should be suspected. These are predominantly hereditary channelopathies. Testing is initially directed at unmasking an inherited disease phenotype using provocation testing. The treadmill exercise stress test (EST) is the initial modality chosen in cases of suspected long QT syndrome (LQTS) and catecholaminergic polymorphic VT (CPVT) [22–25]. Inadequate QT shortening as a result of change in posture or exercise is suggestive of LQTS 1 or 2 [24]. Increasing frequency of ventricular ectopy or development of polymorphic or bidirectional VT with increasing workload during EST is suggestive of CPVT. Provocation testing with intravenous adrenaline is usually performed if the EST is negative. Provocation with a sodium channel blocker such as procainamide may be warranted if the clinical history and baseline ECG are suspicious for Brugada syndrome [26, 27].

Genetic testing is performed only when an inherited disease phenotype is observed. Blanket genetic testing is not currently advised outside of a research setting [19]. Direct-to-consumer marketing of genetic testing has led to the perception that broad panels of testing of genes related to sudden death are both feasible and simple. Unfortunately, the complexity of interpretation of multiple variants that are not necessarily pathogenic makes this strategy fraught with danger until we have a better mechanism to connect the genetic findings with phenotype. The diagnosis of a hereditary channelopathy has important implications beyond the care of the index patient, extending to their biologic relatives. A detailed family history or pedigree should be completed. A history of SCD can often be masked by seemingly unrelated deaths particularly at a young age. Specifically a history of infant cot/crib death, miscarriages or suspicious drownings, and single-vehicle accidents should be sought.

It should be recognized that in those patients without overt cardiac disease, extensive investigation fails to find a cause for cardiac arrest in nearly half of such cases [19].

Aborted SCD in a Structurally Normal Heart

The majority of cases of aborted SCD in a structurally normal heart involve hereditary channelopathies. A minority of cases involve occult structural heart disease from ARVD, sarcoidosis, amyloidosis, or myocarditis or miscellaneous conditions such as anomalous coronary arteries and coronary vasospasm (Table 10.4). These uncommon conditions will not be discussed in this chapter; suffice to mention that cardiac MRI should be performed to rule out these conditions if a clear diagnosis is not apparent (Fig. 10.3).

Long QT Syndrome

Long QT syndrome (LQTS) is a hereditary channelopathy that primarily affects the delayed rectifier potassium channels or the inward sodium channels. The estimated prevalence of LQTS is 1:2,000 [19]. The two main phenotypes described are the autosomal dominant Romano–Ward syndrome and the rare autosomal recessive Jervell and Lange–Nielsen syndrome, which is associated with sensorineural deafness. Mutations in the KCNQ1, KCNH2, and SCN5A genes are responsible for LQT1, LQT2, and LQT3,

Table 10.4 Causes of sudden cardiac death or cardiac arrest

Coronary artery disease	Acute plaque rupture
	Anomalous coronary artery
	Coronary artery vasospasm
	Type A aortic dissection
Overt cardiomyopathies	Hypertrophic cardiomyopathy
	Dilated cardiomyopathy
	Restrictive cardiomyopathy
	Left ventricular non-compaction cardiomyopathy
Occult cardiomyopathies	Sarcoidosis
	Arrhythmogenic right ventricular dysplasia
	Amyloidosis
	Myocarditis
Channelopathies	Long and short QT syndromes
	Brugada syndrome
	Catecholaminergic polymorphic ventricular tachycardia
	Idiopathic ventricular fibrillation
Miscellaneous	Commotio cordis
	Wolf–Parkinson–White syndrome
Metabolic	Electrolyte abnormalities/acidosis
	Drug overdose/proarrhythmia
	Hypoxia
Noncardiac	Massive pulmonary embolus
	Acute intracranial hemorrhage
	Epilepsy

respectively. Collectively these account for the vast majority of cases of LQTS. On average up to 13 % of patients with LQTS have a cardiac arrest before the age of 40, although 30–50 % of patients are symptomatic at some point, typically presenting with syncope [19, 28]. It is not uncommon for LQTS patients, especially those with LQT2, to be mistakenly diagnosed with epilepsy [29]. The hallmark arrhythmia is torsades de pointes (twisting of the points), a form of polymorphic VT, that is pause dependent and often non-sustained. Self-terminating arrhythmic episodes present with syncope, whereas more sustained events present with cardiac arrest or SCD. Triggers for symptoms are genotype specific, such as swimming and physical exertion in LQT1, sudden noises or emotional situations in LQT2, and sleep in LQT3. The postpartum state has also been recognized as being associated with a higher risk of SCD especially in LQT2. Drug-induced QT prolongation can potentially unmask latent LQTS [30]. Therefore, suspicion should be raised in patients with QT prolongation and cardiac arrest who have recently been prescribed medication.

The ECG is the initial diagnostic modality. The QT interval is typically measured in lead II or V5, from the start of the QRS to the end of the T wave. The end of the T wave is defined by the intersection of the steepest portion of the T wave with the baseline (Fig. 10.4). Defining the end of the T wave can be challenging, especially when a U wave is present. Ordinarily the U wave

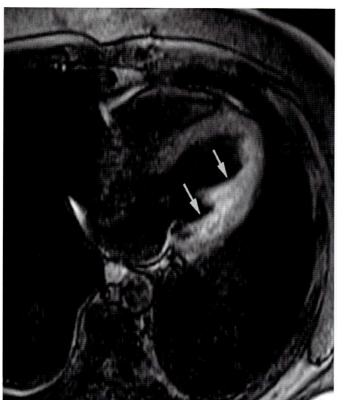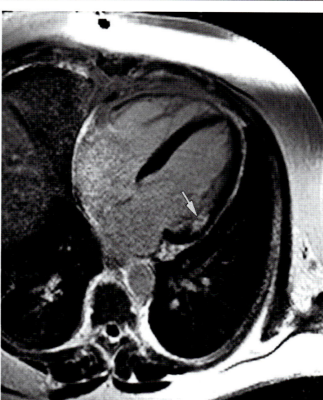

Fig. 10.3 Cardiac magnetic resonance imaging (MRI) in a 46-year-old man who presented with chest pain and subsequent ventricular fibrillation (VF) arrest. Despite a mild elevation in troponin, he was found to have a structurally normal heart by echocardiography and angiographically normal coronary arteries. Cardiac MRI however demonstrated marked edema throughout the lateral wall (*arrows*), as evidenced by T2-weighted imaging (*left image*). A small, subendocardial infarction was identified within the core of this region, evidenced by late gadolinium enhancement (*right image*). These images, in conjunction with his clinical presentation, lead to a diagnosis of coronary vasospasm, highlighting the incremental utility of cardiac MRI in the investigation of aborted sudden cardiac death

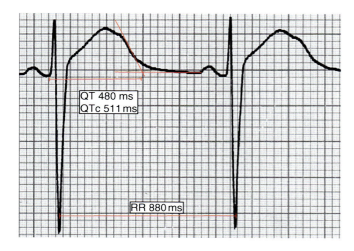

Fig. 10.4 Measurement of the *QT* interval from the onset of the QRS complex to the intersection of the steepest segment of the T wave with the isoelectric line. The measurement has been corrected using Bazett's formula: $QTc = QT \div \sqrt{R-R}\,(s)$

is not included in the measurement if it is distinct from the T wave. The end of a secondary deflection should be included if it abuts the T wave or if the T wave is bifid [31]. The QT interval should be measured as an average over 3–5 beats. Heart rate influences the QT interval and needs to be taken into consideration. The Bazett's formula corrects for this although it is less reliable at the extremes of heart rate. The corrected QT (QTc) interval can be within normal limits in 40 % of carriers of LQTS gene mutations [32]. In these cases provocation testing is helpful. Paradoxical lengthening of the uncorrected QT interval during brisk tachycardia induced by standing is observed in LQTS patients, especially LQT2 [33]. A similar paradoxical lengthening of the uncorrected QT interval is seen with low-dose epinephrine infusion and during an exercise stress test in patients with LQT1 [34] (Fig. 10.5). Genotyping confirms the phenotype in approximately 75 % of cases of LQTS. Risk stratification for SCD is based primarily on genotype and length of corrected long QT, with LQT3 and QTc > 500 ms carrying the worst prognosis [28]. Female sex carries a worse prognosis in LQT2, whereas the opposite is true for LQT3 [28].

Fig. 10.5 QT interval measured in a patient with long QT 1 syndrome in the supine position, immediately upon standing, and after treadmill exercise. Note the corrected QT interval begins within the normal range, but is markedly prolonged with provocation. This example highlights the dynamic nature of the QT interval in the long QT syndrome

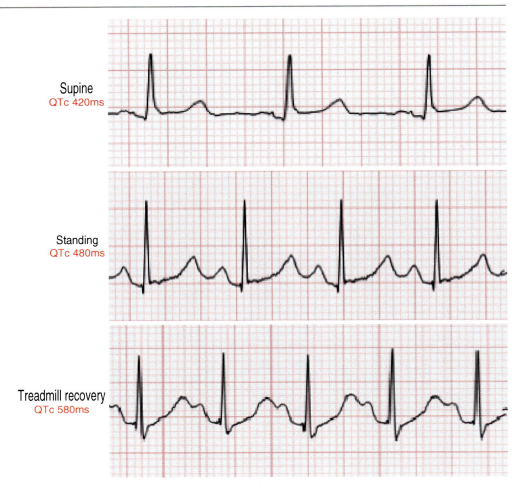

Treatment of LQTS centers on educating patients to be compliant with beta-blockers and to avoid gene-specific triggers as well as medications that have the potential to prolong the QT interval. A comprehensive list of such medications can be found at www.qtdrugs.org. Treatment with beta-blockers reduces the risk of SCD especially in patients with LQT1 and LQT2 [35]. Among symptomatic patients, there is a 32 % residual risk of SCD or recurrent symptoms within 5 years despite beta-blocker therapy [35]. Flecainide and mexiletine are beneficial in patients with LQT3 [19]. Patients with resuscitated SCD, recurrent symptoms despite beta-blocker therapy, or a constellation of high-risk features should have an ICD implanted. Programming a faster anti-bradycardia rate; avoiding the use of pacing avoidance algorithms that permit dropped beats and, thus, pauses; and increasing detection times using a rate-smoothing algorithm and algorithms that avoid T wave oversensing may reduce the number of inappropriate shocks [36]. Adjuvant therapy in the form of left cervicothoracic sympathectomy has been shown to reduce the rates of syncope and SCD in high-risk patients with LQTS [37]. Participation in competitive sports should be discouraged, especially in patients with LQT1. As is the

case with other hereditary conditions, screening and counseling of family members is an important component of management.

Brugada Syndrome

First described in 1989, this syndrome, caused by a loss of function mutation in the alpha subunit of the cardiac sodium channel encoded by the SCN5A gene, is associated with sudden cardiac death, particularly among young males. A prevalence of up to 12/10,000 has been reported. In certain parts of Southeast Asia where the condition is endemic, it is second only to motor vehicle accidents as a cause of mortality in those <40 years of age [38]. Presentation with cardiac arrest, syncope, or nocturnal agonal respiration typically occurs in adulthood with a mean age of SCD of 41 ± 15 years [38]. SVT, primarily atrial fibrillation, occurs in 10–20 % of patients. The pathognomonic feature of the syndrome is syncope or cardiac arrest associated with coved ST elevation in the right-sided precordial leads. Three patterns of ST elevation have been described (Fig. 10.6) [38]. Only the type I pattern is diagnostic of Brugada syndrome. An individual

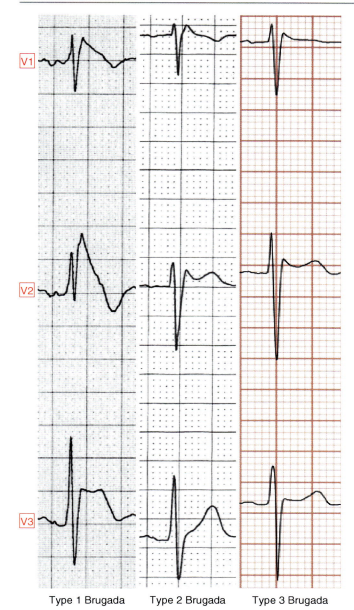

Type 1 Brugada   Type 2 Brugada   Type 3 Brugada

Fig. 10.6 Recognized ECG patterns in the Brugada syndrome. Type I pattern is characterized by coved ST elevation of >2 mm in at least two contiguous precordial leads with associated T wave inversion. Type II pattern has a similar distribution, but is associated with saddle ST elevation of >2 mm and either a positive or biphasic T wave. Type III pattern is characterized by either coved or saddle ST elevation of <1 mm. Only the type I Brugada pattern is considered pathognomonic for the condition. Increased vagal tone, febrile illness, and certain medications (www.brugadadrugs.com), particularly sodium channel blockers, have the potential to unmask a type 1 pattern from the latter 2

bundle branch block, early repolarization pattern, pericarditis, myocardial infarction, pulmonary embolism, and rarely extrinsic compression of the right ventricular outflow tract by a mediastinal tumor. A Brugada-like ECG pattern is occasionally observed transiently following DC cardioversion [40]. The clinical significance of this remains uncertain.

Brugada syndrome typically occurs in the setting of a structurally normal heart. Abnormal late potentials on SAECG have been observed in patients with Brugada syndrome. Ordinarily this reflects intramyocardial conduction delay from structural heart disease. In the case of Brugada syndrome, these late potentials are due to the delayed upstroke of the epicardial action potential or alternatively represent local phase II reentry.

A number of triggers for SCD have been recognized. These include periods of increased vagal tone such as during sleep; medications, particularly class I antiarrhythmics; hypokalemia; hypoglycemia; and fever. These triggers can unmask a type I pattern in those with a normal ECG or type II or III pattern at baseline. Consequently class I antiarrhythmic agents such as procainamide, flecainide, or ajmaline are used as provocation tests to unmask the diagnostic type I Brugada pattern. Administration of class I antiarrhythmic agents should be performed with caution in the elderly or those with evidence of baseline AV conduction disease. In these individuals, testing should be performed in an EP lab, preferably after insertion of a temporary pacing wire. Otherwise healthy individuals can have testing performed in any monitored area with appropriately trained staff and resuscitation equipment. Class I antiarrhythmic infusion should be discontinued once the following are observed: type I Brugada pattern is unmasked, >2 mm of additional ST elevation in type II pattern, ventricular ectopy or other ventricular arrhythmia, QRS widening ≥130 % of baseline, or evidence of heart block. Isoproterenol should reverse the ECG changes induced by class I antiarrhythmics in patients with Brugada syndrome.

Brugada syndrome has an autosomal dominant pattern of inheritance. More than 293 disease-causing mutations have been identified in the SCN5A gene that codes for the alpha subunit of the cardiac Na^+ channel. Despite this, only 21 % of patients with a Brugada phenotype test positive for a known gene mutation [19]. The absence of a known gene mutation therefore does not rule out the diagnosis of Brugada syndrome. Mutations in the SCN5A gene are detected more often in familial than sporadic cases. Current knowledge of the mutations that cause Brugada syndrome is inadequate to determine prognosis associated with specific mutations.

Risk stratification in Brugada syndrome is controversial beyond those with resuscitated SCD and symptomatic patients. The largest prospective study to date carried out by Probst et al. followed 1,029 patients with Brugada syndrome diagnosed on the basis of a spontaneous or drug-induced

who harbors the relevant mutation may exhibit any one of the three patterns or alternatively a normal ECG. The use of high precordial lead position (V_1 and V_2 recorded in the second intercostal rather than the fourth intercostal space) improves the diagnostic yield of the 12-lead ECG [39]. A Brugada ECG pattern needs to be distinguished from atypical right

type 1 ECG pattern [41]. During a median follow-up period of 31.9 months, the cardiac event rate per year was 7.7, 1.9, and 0.5 % in patients enrolled with aborted SCD, syncope, and no symptoms, respectively. A cardiac event was described as SCD, appropriate ICD therapy, or documented sustained ventricular tachyarrhythmia. Only the presence of symptoms (cardiac arrest or syncope) and spontaneous type I ECG pattern were predictive of arrhythmic events [41]. Gender, family history of SCD, inducibility of ventricular tachyarrhythmia at EP study, and the presence of an SCN5A mutation were not associated with an increased arrhythmic risk [41]. Separate multivariate analysis in asymptomatic patients found no predictors for arrhythmic events [41]. Of interest, a family history of SCD did not predict a worse outcome, suggesting that there is no discernible prognostic difference between familial and sporadic forms of the disease. The role for EP study to determine the risk of SCD in asymptomatic patients remains controversial based on conflicting data gathered from separate large registries, but is generally discouraged [41–45].

The only proven effective treatment in Brugada syndrome is an ICD, although quinidine is effective in management of ventricular arrhythmias [46]. Current guidelines recommend ICD implantation in those with resuscitated SCD with either spontaneous or provoked type I Brugada pattern and those with spontaneous type I pattern and symptoms of unexplained syncope, seizures, or nocturnal agonal respiration. Asymptomatic patients with provoked type I pattern should be followed closely with appropriate lifestyle and pharmacological precautions.

Patients are advised to promptly treat febrile illness aggressively with antipyretics and seek medical attention early to determine the need for antibiotics if appropriate. A list of medications to avoid in Brugada syndrome can be found at www.brugadadrugs.org. Patients that are being followed closely should immediately report any syncope, seizure activity, or nocturnal agonal respiration to their physician. Family screening is warranted, particularly among those under the age of ~60–65.

The treatment of electrical VF storm in Brugada syndrome is with isoproterenol and/or quinidine [46]. Quinidine is believed to exert its antiarrhythmic effects by blocking the I_{to} receptor and restoring the balance of currents that are active during the early part of the action potential in the epicardium, reducing the dispersion of refractoriness.

Catecholaminergic Polymorphic VT

Catecholaminergic polymorphic VT (CPVT) is a rare hereditary channelopathy characterized by bidirectional or polymorphic VT triggered by exercise or emotional stress, which is highly malignant if untreated. The prevalence of the condition is approximately 1:10,000 and is responsible for 13 % of cardiac arrests in structurally normal hearts [19, 47]. Mutations in the gene encoding the cardiac ryanodine receptor type 2 (RyR2) are found in 55 % of cases, with a further 1–2 % of cases caused by mutations in the gene encoding cardiac calsequestrin (CASQ2) [47]. The modes of inheritance are autosomal dominant and autosomal recessive, respectively. Mutations in the RyR2 or CASQ2 gene lead to increased cytosolic calcium in response to epinephrine. This, in turn, leads to delayed afterdepolarizations, which are responsible for ventricular ectopy and polymorphic ventricular tachycardia under conditions of beta-adrenergic stimulation. The initiating beat of VT is late coupled and usually has a consistent morphology typically originating from the outflow tracts [47].

Presentation typically occurs in the second decade of life with syncope, seizures, cardiac arrest, or SCD [48]. Up to 60 % of untreated patients develop cardiac symptoms over 8 years while [48] 25 % of untreated patients experience a fatal or near-fatal cardiac event over the same period [48]. In one study, 26 % of patients experienced supraventricular tachycardia including paroxysmal atrial fibrillation [47].

CPVT is diagnosed if ≥3 beats of polymorphic or bidirectional VT are observed during exercise stress testing or epinephrine infusion challenge. The phenotypic diagnosis also requires the absence of structural heart disease and ischemic heart disease. The resting ECG is normal in CPVT. The sensitivity of genetic testing is between 60 and 77 %. [47, 48] It is noteworthy that up to 21 % of genotype-positive family members of probands do not express the phenotype at the time of diagnosis, yet their risk of cardiac events is similar [47, 48].

Independent predictors for cardiac, fatal, and near-fatal events include younger age at diagnosis, the absence of beta-blocker therapy, and resuscitated cardiac arrest [48]. A history of syncope is not predictive of cardiac events.

Once the diagnosis of CPVT has been established, treatment is mandatory even if asymptomatic. Exercise restriction is an important component of treatment. First line therapy consists of beta-blockers. Nadolol has been suggested to be superior to other beta-blockers [48]. Resting bradycardia has been shown to be idiosyncratic to the CPVT genotype and should not dissuade clinicians from initiating beta-blockers [19, 49]. It is paramount that adequate dosing and high compliance rates are achieved with beta-blockers. Serial exercise stress testing can be used to guide efficacy of treatment and to titrate dosing. In spite of beta-blocker therapy, the incidence of fatal and near-fatal cardiac events was 11 % over 8 years of follow-up [48]. Current guidelines recommend implantation of an ICD in patients who have recurrent syncope, resuscitated cardiac arrest, or documented VT while on beta-blocker therapy. ICD implantation in young patients has obvious drawbacks such as the cumulative risk of infection, lead fractures, and the need for multiple generator changes over their lifetime. ICD therapy in CPVT is particularly ill-suited and presents unique challenges. The pain and fear generated from a shock, even if potentially lifesaving, causes greater adrenergic stimulus and could lead to a vicious cycle of arrhythmic storm and multiple shocks. The psychological impact of such an event, especially in children should not be underestimated. There is also a risk that an inappropriate shock due to supraventricular tachycardia including sinus tachycardia could be proarrhythmic and lead to polymorphic VT [47, 50]. Left cardiac sympathetic denervation (LCSD) has been shown in small case series to be very effective in reducing shocks [50]. The procedure is performed within 40 min using a minimally invasive extrapleural approach through an incision at the base of the neck. Current practice is to spare the cranial half of the stellate ganglion thus avoiding ipsilateral Horner's syndrome. LCSD should be strongly advocated as third-line therapy in preference to ICD implantation. Unfortunately it is not widely available. The adjuvant use of flecainide as second-line therapy has been shown to either completely or partially suppress exercise-induced ventricular arrhythmia [49]. Flecainide works in CPVT by directly blocking the abnormal RyR2 channel [49] not through Na^+ channel blockade. Calcium channel blockers can also be added to beta-blocker therapy, although efficacy is limited.

Key Points
- SCD is a major public health issue that ranks among the leading causes of mortality in the developed world. The underlying etiology is primarily ischemic heart disease, although susceptibility to SCD is a complex process with multiple interactions between genes that regulate cardiac and vascular function and other physiological and environmental factors.
- Prevention of SCD is hampered by our inability to predict who is at risk at an individual level, since the majority of cases occur as the index event. The advent of the ICD has been perceived as a panacea for SCD, although in reality the degree of residual risk is significant.
- Ongoing research into genetic susceptibilities and the development of complex computer modeling may provide us with a better understanding of this complex disease process in the future. Until such time, SCD is destined to remain a significant public health threat that requires further study.

References

1. Zipes DP, Camm AJ, Borggrefe M, et al. ACC/AHA/ESC 2006 guidelines for management of patients with ventricular arrhythmias and the prevention of sudden cardiac death: a report of the American College of Cardiology/American Heart Association Task Force and the European Society of Cardiology Committee for Practice Guidelines (writing committee to develop guidelines for management of patients with ventricular arrhythmias and the prevention of sudden cardiac death): developed in collaboration with the European Heart Rhythm Association and the Heart Rhythm Society. Circulation. 2006;114(10):e385–484.
2. Zheng ZJ, Croft JB, Giles WH, Mensah GA. Sudden cardiac death in the United States, 1989 to 1998. Circulation. 2001;104(18):2158–63.
3. Josephson M, Wellens HJ. Implantable defibrillators and sudden cardiac death. Circulation. 2004;109(22):2685–91.
4. Myerburg RJ. Sudden cardiac death: exploring the limits of our knowledge. J Cardiovasc Electrophysiol. 2001;12(3):369–81.
5. Bayes de Luna A, Coumel P, Leclercq JF. Ambulatory sudden cardiac death: mechanisms of production of fatal arrhythmia on the basis of data from 157 cases. Am Heart J. 1989;117(1):151–9.
6. Myerburg RJ, Castellanos A. Cardiac electrophysiology: from cell to bedside, vol. 1. 5th ed. Philadelphia: Saunders Elsevier; 2009.
7. Spector PS. Diagnosis and management of sudden cardiac death. Heart. 2005;91(3):408–13.
8. Bunch TJ, Hohnloser SH, Gersh BJ. Mechanisms of sudden cardiac death in myocardial infarction survivors: insights from the randomized trials of implantable cardioverter-defibrillators. Circulation. 2007;115(18):2451–7.
9. Jouven X, Desnos M, Guerot C, Ducimetiere P. Predicting sudden death in the population: the Paris Prospective Study I. Circulation. 1999;99(15):1978–83.
10. Myerburg RJ. Implantable cardioverter-defibrillators after myocardial infarction. N Engl J Med. 2008;359(21):2245–53.
11. Kaikkonen KS, Kortelainen ML, Linna E, Huikuri HV. Family history and the risk of sudden cardiac death as a manifestation of an acute coronary event. Circulation. 2006;114(14):1462–7.
12. Ford ES, Ajani UA, Croft JB, et al. Explaining the decrease in U.S. deaths from coronary disease, 1980–2000. N Engl J Med. 2007;356(23):2388–98.
13. Echt DS, Liebson PR, Mitchell LB, Peters RW, Obias-Manno D, Barker AH, Arensberg D, Baker A, Friedman L, Greene HL, et al. Mortality and morbidity in patients receiving encainide, flecainide, or placebo. The cardiac arrhythmia suppression trial. N Engl J Med. 1991;324:781–8.
14. Waldo AL, Camm AJ, deRuyter H, et al. Effect of d-sotalol on mortality in patients with left ventricular dysfunction after recent and remote myocardial infarction. The SWORD Investigators. Survival With Oral d-Sotalol. Lancet. 1996;348(9019):7–12.
15. Bardy GH, Lee KL, Mark DB, et al. Amiodarone or an implantable cardioverter-defibrillator for congestive heart failure. N Engl J Med. 2005;352(3):225–37.
16. Alberte C, Zipes DP. Use of nonantiarrhythmic drugs for prevention of sudden cardiac death. J Cardiovasc Electrophysiol. 2003;14(9 Suppl):S87–95.
17. Connolly SJ, Hallstrom AP, Cappato R, et al. Meta-analysis of the implantable cardioverter defibrillator secondary prevention trials. AVID, CASH and CIDS studies. Antiarrhythmics vs Implantable Defibrillator study. Cardiac Arrest Study Hamburg. Canadian Implantable Defibrillator Study. Eur Heart J. 2000;21(24):2071–8.
18. Moss AJ, Zareba W, Hall WJ, et al. Prophylactic implantation of a defibrillator in patients with myocardial infarction and reduced ejection fraction. N Engl J Med. 2002;346(12):877–83.
19. Modi S, Krahn AD. Sudden cardiac arrest without overt heart disease. Circulation. 2011;123(25):2994–3008.

20. White JA, Patel MR. The role of cardiovascular MRI in heart failure and the cardiomyopathies. Cardiol Clin. 2007;25(1):71–95, vi.

21. White JA, Fine NM, Gula L, et al. Utility of cardiovascular magnetic resonance in identifying substrate for malignant ventricular arrhythmias. Circ Cardiovasc Imaging. 2012;5(1):12–20.

22. Wong JA, Gula LJ, Klein GJ, Yee R, Skanes AC, Krahn AD. Utility of treadmill testing in identification and genotype prediction in long-QT syndrome. Circ Arrhythm Electrophysiol. 2010;3(2):120–5.

23. Sy RW, Chattha IS, Klein GJ, et al. Repolarization dynamics during exercise discriminate between LQT1 and LQT2 genotypes. J Cardiovasc Electrophysiol. 2010;21(11):1242–6.

24. Sy RW, van der Werf C, Chattha IS, et al. Derivation and validation of a simple exercise-based algorithm for prediction of genetic testing in relatives of LQTS probands. Circulation. 2011;124(20):2187–94.

25. Chattha IS, Sy RW, Yee R, et al. Utility of the recovery electrocardiogram after exercise: a novel indicator for the diagnosis and genotyping of long QT syndrome? Heart Rhythm. 2010;7(7):906–11.

26. Krahn AD, Healey JS, Chauhan V, et al. Systematic assessment of patients with unexplained cardiac arrest: Cardiac Arrest Survivors With Preserved Ejection Fraction Registry (CASPER). Circulation. 2009;120(4):278–85.

27. Obeyesekere MN, Klein GJ, Modi S, et al. How to perform and interpret provocative testing for the diagnosis of Brugada syndrome, long-QT syndrome, and catecholaminergic polymorphic ventricular tachycardia. Circ Arrhythm Electrophysiol. 2011;4(6):958–64.

28. Priori SG, Schwartz PJ, Napolitano C, et al. Risk stratification in the long-QT syndrome. N Engl J Med. 2003;348(19):1866–74.

29. Johnson JN, Hofman N, Haglund CM, Cascino GD, Wilde AA, Ackerman MJ. Identification of a possible pathogenic link between congenital long QT syndrome and epilepsy. Neurology. 2009;72(3):224–31.

30. Roden DM. Drug-induced prolongation of the QT interval. N Engl J Med. 2004;350(10):1013–22.

31. Goldenberg I, Moss AJ, Zareba W. QT interval: how to measure it and what is "normal". J Cardiovasc Electrophysiol. 2006;17(3):333–6.

32. Napolitano C, Priori SG, Schwartz PJ, et al. Genetic testing in the long QT syndrome: development and validation of an efficient approach to genotyping in clinical practice. JAMA. 2005;294(23):2975–80.

33. Viskin S, Postema PG, Bhuiyan ZA, et al. The response of the QT interval to the brief tachycardia provoked by standing: a bedside test for diagnosing long QT syndrome. J Am Coll Cardiol. 2010;55(18):1955–61.

34. Vyas H, Hejlik J, Ackerman MJ. Epinephrine QT stress testing in the evaluation of congenital long-QT syndrome: diagnostic accuracy of the paradoxical QT response. Circulation. 2006;113(11):1385–92.

35. Moss AJ, Zareba W, Hall WJ, et al. Effectiveness and limitations of beta-blocker therapy in congenital long-QT syndrome. Circulation. 2000;101(6):616–23.

36. Monnig G, Kobe J, Loher A, et al. Implantable cardioverter-defibrillator therapy in patients with congenital long-QT syndrome: a long-term follow-up. Heart Rhythm. 2005;2(5):497–504.

37. Schwartz PJ, Priori SG, Cerrone M, et al. Left cardiac sympathetic denervation in the management of high-risk patients affected by the long-QT syndrome. Circulation. 2004;109(15):1826–33.

38. Antzelevitch C, Brugada P, Borggrefe M, et al. Brugada syndrome: report of the second consensus conference: endorsed by the Heart Rhythm Society and the European Heart Rhythm Association. Circulation. 2005;111(5):659–70.

39. Shimizu W, Matsuo K, Takagi M, et al. Body surface distribution and response to drugs of ST segment elevation in Brugada syndrome: clinical implication of eighty-seven-lead body surface potential mapping and its application to twelve-lead electrocardiograms. J Cardiovasc Electrophysiol. 2000;11(4):396–404.

40. Kok LC, Mitchell MA, Haines DE, Mounsey JP, DiMarco JP. Transient ST elevation after transthoracic cardioversion in patients with hemodynamically unstable ventricular tachyarrhythmia. Am J Cardiol. 2000;85(7):878–81, A879.

41. Probst V, Veltmann C, Eckardt L, et al. Long-term prognosis of patients diagnosed with Brugada syndrome: results from the FINGER Brugada Syndrome Registry. Circulation. 2010;121(5):635–43.

42. Priori SG, Napolitano C. Should patients with an asymptomatic Brugada electrocardiogram undergo pharmacological and electrophysiological testing? Circulation. 2005;112(2):279–92; discussion 279–92.

43. Brugada P, Brugada R, Brugada J. Should patients with an asymptomatic Brugada electrocardiogram undergo pharmacological and electrophysiological testing? Circulation. 2005;112(2):279–92; discussion 279–92.

44. Brugada J, Brugada R, Brugada P. Determinants of sudden cardiac death in individuals with the electrocardiographic pattern of Brugada syndrome and no previous cardiac arrest. Circulation. 2003;108(25):3092–6.

45. Paul M, Gerss J, Schulze-Bahr E, et al. Role of programmed ventricular stimulation in patients with Brugada syndrome: a meta-analysis of worldwide published data. Eur Heart J. 2007;28(17):2126–33.

46. Belhassen B, Glick A, Viskin S. Efficacy of quinidine in high-risk patients with Brugada syndrome. Circulation. 2004;110(13):1731–7.

47. Sy RW, Gollob MH, Klein GJ, et al. Arrhythmia characterization and long-term outcomes in catecholaminergic polymorphic ventricular tachycardia. Heart Rhythm. 2011;8(6):864–71.

48. Hayashi M, Denjoy I, Extramiana F, et al. Incidence and risk factors of arrhythmic events in catecholaminergic polymorphic ventricular tachycardia. Circulation. 2009;119(18):2426–34.

49. van der Werf C, Kannankeril PJ, Sacher F, et al. Flecainide therapy reduces exercise-induced ventricular arrhythmias in patients with catecholaminergic polymorphic ventricular tachycardia. J Am Coll Cardiol. 2011;57(22):2244–54.

50. Wilde AA, Bhuiyan ZA, Crotti L, et al. Left cardiac sympathetic denervation for catecholaminergic polymorphic ventricular tachycardia. N Engl J Med. 2008;358(19):2024–9.

51. Myerburg RJ, Interian Jr A, Mitrani RM, et al. Frequency of sudden cardiac death and profiles or risk. Am J Cardiol. 1997;80:10F–9.

Top Ten Electrocardiographic (ECG) Abnormalities Not to Miss

Lea El Hage, Nitish Badhwar, and Nora Goldschlager

Abstract

This chapter presents ten cases with characteristic electrocardiographic (ECG) findings that should not be missed. The first case demonstrates the chronological ECG changes seen during ST segment elevation myocardial infarction. The case presenting sinus node dysfunction (SND) highlights the various ECG manifestations of SND. The case of atrioventricular (AV) block highlights the approach to the diagnosis of 2:1 AV block. The case of Wolff–Parkinson–White (WPW) syndrome describes the diagnostic ECG criteria for WPW syndrome and the supraventricular tachycardias associated with it. The wide complex tachycardia (WCT) case presents a stepwise algorithmic approach to the diagnosis of WCT. The case of hypertrophic cardiomyopathy focuses on risk stratification for sudden death. We present the characteristic ECG findings in patients with Brugada syndrome, long QT syndrome, and early repolarization syndrome that are causes of sudden death in young patients without structural heart disease. Finally, we present the approach to the diagnosis of artifact on the ECG that is important to prevent expensive workups and unnecessary treatments.

Keywords

Brugada syndrome • Wolff–Parkinson–White • ECG artifacts • Early repolarization • Sinus node dysfunction • Long QT syndrome

L. El Hage, MD • N. Badhwar, MBBS (✉)
Cardiac Electrophysiology,
Department of Medicine/Cardiology,
University of California, San Francisco,
500 Parnassus Ave, MUE-431, San Francisco,
CA 94143, USA
e-mail: l_hage85@hotmail.com;
badhwar@medicine.ucsf.edu

N. Goldschlager, MD
Cardiology Division, Department of Medicine,
University of California, San Francisco,
San Francisco General Hospital,
1001 Potrero Avenue,
San Francisco, CA 94110, USA
e-mail: ngoldschlager@medsfgh.ucsf.edu

ST Elevation Myocardial Infarction

A 64-year-old female with a 40-year history of smoking presented with the acute onset of epigastric pain that was increasing in intensity over the last 4 h. The epigastric pain was associated with nausea, vomiting, and syncope. In the emergency department, she was noted to have the electrocardiogram in Fig. 11.1.

There is normal sinus rhythm at a rate of 94 bpm with normal PR, QT-corrected (QTc), and QRS complex intervals. Leads II, III, and aVF show Q waves associated with ST segment elevations. Serum troponin and creatine kinase-MB (CK-MB) levels were found to be 1.7 and 5.63 ng/ml, respectively. Based on this, acute ST elevation inferior myocardial infarction was diagnosed. Urgent cardiac catheterization revealed 100 % occlusion in the mid-right coronary artery that received primary percutaneous intervention to open the

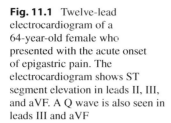
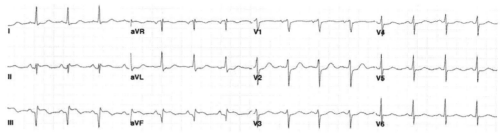

Fig. 11.1 Twelve-lead electrocardiogram of a 64-year-old female who presented with the acute onset of epigastric pain. The electrocardiogram shows ST segment elevation in leads II, III, and aVF. A Q wave is also seen in leads III and aVF

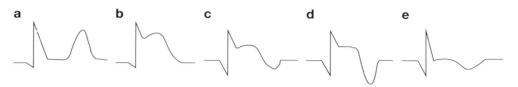

Fig. 11.2 Stages of a transmural infarct. (**a**) Appearance of hyperacute (tall, asymmetrical, and peaked) T waves. (**b**) ST segment elevation. (**c**, **d**) Q wave formation with T wave inversion. (**e**) Decrease in R wave amplitude with return of the ST segment to baseline and decrease in T wave inversion

vessel. Left ventriculography showed inferior basilar wall motion hypokinesis with an ejection fraction of 60 %.

The diagnosis of ST segment elevation myocardial infarction (STEMI) involves the evaluation of the patient's symptoms, ECG findings, and cardiac enzyme changes such as elevations in troponin and CK-MB. Cardiac enzymes begin to rise 4 h after the ischemic event [1]. Patients presenting within this 4-h window will have normal cardiac enzyme levels.

During acute ischemia, a voltage gradient between ischemic and normal cells causes a flow of current between the two regions. This is represented by ST segment changes on the ECG. ECG vectors always point away from the negative zones and towards positive zones. In a transmural (involving the epicardium, myocardium, and endocardium) infarct, the vector is directed towards the outer epicardial layers, resulting in ST segment elevation and hyperacute (tall and asymmetrically peaked) T waves. The T waves are the first to change on the ECG (Fig. 11.2a) [2]. They are then followed by ST segment changes that depend on the location of the infarct (Fig. 11.2b). For the diagnosis of STEMI, the ST segment must be elevated by greater than or equal to 0.2 mV in at least 2 consecutive limb leads and/or greater than or equal to 0.1 mV in at least 2 consecutive precordial leads. A Q wave then forms (Fig. 11.2c, d) that is defined as any Q wave in leads V_1 to V_3 or a Q wave that is greater than or equal to 30 ms in leads I, II, aVL, aVF, or V_4 to V_6. Q waves must be present in at least two contiguous leads and should be ≥ 1 mm in depth [2, 3]. Finally, there is a decrease in the R wave amplitude with return of the ST segment to baseline and T wave inversion (Fig. 11.2e).

It is important to note that patients with conditions that can hinder voltage detection by the ECG machine, such as emphysema, pericardial effusion, and obesity, may have low QRS amplitudes. These patients should be further evaluated with other modalities such as cardiac enzymes,

echocardiography, or left heart catheterization before STEMI can be decisively ruled out.

The location of the infarct can be determined by evaluating the ECG leads. Occlusion of the left anterior descending (LAD) artery produces anterior wall myocardial infarctions (MIs) that are represented by changes in the precordial leads as well as leads I, aVL, and aVR. Anterior MIs can also be divided into anteroseptal (leads V_1–V_2 involved), anterolateral (leads V_3–V_4 involved), and anteroapical (leads V_5–V_6 involved), although correlations with imaging techniques such as magnetic resonance imaging are imperfect. ST segment elevation in lead aVR and V1 can be seen in patients with MI involving the proximal LAD, the proximal right coronary artery (RCA), or the left main coronary artery.

Occlusions in the RCA and left circumflex artery (LCX) produce inferior and posterior wall MIs, reflected by changes in leads II, III, and aVF. ST segment elevation in lead III > II favors RCA occlusion and vice versa. When inferior wall MI is diagnosed, the right-sided precordial leads and posterior leads (V_7–V_9) should also be evaluated for right ventricular and posterior wall MI, respectively. Occlusions of the LCX produce lateral wall MIs with anterior ST segment depressions, which are reciprocal to posterior wall ST segment elevations.

Sinus Node Dysfunction (Sick Sinus Syndrome)

An 84-year-old female nursing home resident with a history of left ventricular systolic dysfunction, previous myocardial infarction, hypertension, and diabetes mellitus type II was admitted to the hospital due to newly altered mental status. Twelve-lead ECG showed the following rhythm in Fig. 11.3a.

Fig. 11.3 (**a**) Twelve-lead electrocardiogram of an 84-year-old female who presented with altered mental status. Atrial flutter with 2:1 atrioventricular conduction is seen. (**b**) 12-lead electrocardiogram showing flutter termination. A 4.9-s period of asystole is noted before ventricular activity resumes. The patient had multiple sinus pauses during sinus rhythm. These rhythms are typical of Tachy–Brady syndrome and are characteristic of sick sinus syndrome

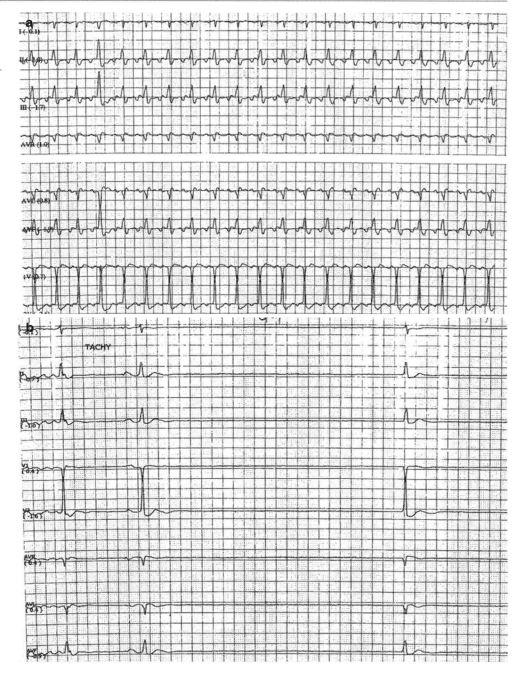

In Fig. 11.3a, there is a narrow QRS complex tachycardia at a rate of 125 bpm. The atrial rhythm is flutter with negatively directed flutter waves in leads II, III, and aVF and positive waves in lead V_1, suggestive of typical flutter. The atrioventricular (AV) conduction ratio is 2:1. When the flutter terminates (Fig. 11.3b), there is a period of asystole lasting 4.9 s before ventricular activity resumes. The asystolic periods are terminated by junctional escape beats. The patient had multiple sinus pauses during sinus rhythm with the longest being at least 4.9 s (Fig. 11.3b). These rhythms

are typical of tachycardia–bradycardia syndrome and are characteristic of sick sinus syndrome.

Sinus node dysfunction, or sick sinus syndrome (SSS), is a degenerative disease of the sinus node that usually affects the elderly, although it can occasionally be seen in infants and adolescents. It is characterized by significant sinus bradycardia (although not always), sinus pauses, sinus arrest, and sinoatrial exit block. Junctional escape rhythms usually, but not always, terminate the pauses in rhythm. The failure of junctional escape rhythms to emerge may lead to symptomatic bradycardia or even asystolic periods. Around 50 % of SSS patients exhibit the tachycardia–bradycardia syndrome, in which atrial tachyarrhythmias, mainly atrial fibrillation and flutter, occur, followed by long pauses on their termination. These atrial arrhythmias seem to develop slowly over time, possibly the result of a progressive pathological process that affects the sinoatrial (SA) node and the atrium. The most common cause of SSS is fibrosis of the sinus node, though narrowing of the SA nodal artery, inferior myocardial infarction, and, rarely, infiltrative myocardial disease, epicardial and pericardial disease, inflammatory conditions, drugs, trauma, and infection may also play a role in specific cases [4].

Symptoms of bradycardia include light-headedness, presyncope or syncope, dyspnea on exertion, and angina, whereas palpitations are felt during the tachycardias. The diagnosis of SSS is based upon the clinical symptoms, the ECG, or more prolonged monitoring (e.g., telemetry, Holter, or implanted loop recorders), and, sometimes, electrophysiology study findings. Prolonged ECG recordings are more sensitive and can show transient changes that are often not documented on a single 12-lead ECG. Chronotropic incompetence, or inability of the heart rate to increase in response to an increase in metabolic need, if seen during exercise testing, can also be helpful in the diagnosis of SSS; due to the SA node dysfunction, patients are unable to achieve at least 80 % of their age-predicted maximum heart rate or have a monotonic heart rate over a 24-h period. Drugs that stimulate the pacemaker cells and increase the heart rate such as atropine and isoproterenol can be used in the diagnosis of SSS. A subnormal response to these medications, defined as an increase in sinus rate by less than 25 % or to a rate of less than 90 bpm, is suggestive of SSS. It is important to know, however, that even if the response is normal, the patient can still have SSS. In patients with deficient chronotropic response to atropine administration, it has been suggested

that the response to isoproterenol may identify individuals with inadequate chronotropic reserve [5–7].

Electrophysiology studies involve measurement of the intrinsic heart rate, sinus node recovery time, SA conduction time, and response to parasympathetic (vagal) stimulation assessed by carotid massage. The intrinsic heart rate (IHR) is the heart rate present when beta-blockers and atropine are given to completely denervate the SA node and is a function of age ($IHR = 117.2 - [0.53 \times age]$). IHR is mainly used to differentiate intrinsic from extrinsic SSS caused by increased parasympathetic tone or drugs. Intrinsic SSS is presumed to be present if the sinus rate does not exceed the predicted IHR after atropine, while a normal IHR suggests extrinsic SSS.

Atrioventricular Block

A 76-year-old female with a history of coronary artery disease and prior coronary artery bypass graft surgery, hypertension, dyslipidemia, and symptomatic premature ventricular complexes presented with complaints of dizziness. A 12-lead ECG was recorded (Fig. 11.4).

There is normal sinus rhythm with 2:1 conduction to the ventricles. Differentiating atrioventricular (AV) nodal from infranodal conduction delay is very important in patients with 2:1 AV block. In this case, evaluation of the PR and QRS durations can be useful. Long PR intervals with narrow QRS complexes usually indicate AV nodal conduction delay, while normal PR intervals with wide QRS complexes suggest an infranodal block. The best method to differentiate the two involves changing the sinus rate through carotid massage (which will also further delay conduction through the AV node through increases in vagal tone), exercise, or atropine administration (which will also enhance conduction

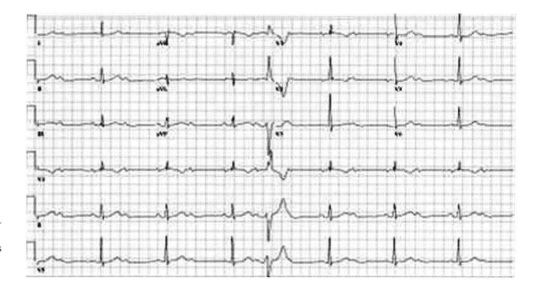

Fig. 11.4 Twelve-lead electrocardiogram of a 76-year-old female who presented with dizziness showing normal sinus rhythm with 2:1 conduction to the ventricles

through the AV node through adrenergic input) [8]. In the presence of AV nodal disease, therefore, slowing the sinus rate may increase the number of non-conducted beats due to vagal influences on the AV node itself. In contrast, in the presence of infranodal conduction disease, slowing the sinus rate can lead to 1:1 AV conduction since the infranodal system is stimulated less rapidly, while increasing the sinus rate can result in a greater number of non-conducted P waves.

The PR interval is measured from the beginning of the P wave to the beginning of the QRS complex and represents the time it takes for the electrical impulse to travel from the sinus node through the AV node and His–Purkinje system. AV block occurs when there is a delay in impulse transmission from the atria to the ventricles. It is due to impaired conduction that can be transient or permanent and can present as presyncope, syncope, or exertional dyspnea.

Wolff–Parkinson–White Syndrome

A 49-year-old male with a history of hypertension presented with palpitations associated with dizziness. He had been having symptoms since the age of 7. He denied syncope or family history of similar problems or sudden death. During an episode of palpitations, the following 12-lead ECG was recorded (Fig. 11.5a).

Figure 11.5a reveals narrow QRS complexes at a rate of 184 bpm. The differential diagnosis for paroxysmal supraventricular tachycardia (PSVT) includes atrioventricular (AV) reentrant tachycardia (AVRT), AV nodal reentrant tachycardia (AVNRT), and atrial tachycardia. These can be distinguished on the ECG based on the relationship of the QRS complex to the P wave (R–P) during tachycardia (see Fig. 11.6). AVRT usually presents as "short R–P" tachycardia (Fig. 11.6a), while atrial tachycardia presents as "long R–P" tachycardia (Fig. 11.6b). In AVNRT, the P wave is usually superimposed on or buried within the QRS complex [9] (Fig. 11.6c). There is a deflection between the QRS complexes and ST segments in the ECG shown in Fig. 11.5a (★) suggestive of P waves, making the rhythm a "short R–P" tachycardia. The most likely diagnosis is therefore AVRT using the AV node as the antegrade limb and accessory pathway as the retrograde limb.

Evaluation of his baseline ECG (Fig. 11.5b) reveals normal and regular QRS complexes at a rate of 84 bpm. Delta waves are seen, indicating Wolff–Parkinson–White (WPW) syndrome. The location of the accessory pathway is determined to be in the left posterior wall based on the positive delta wave in lead V_1 and negative delta wave in the inferior leads [10, 11]. He underwent electrophysiologic study with induction of the tachycardia and mapping of the accessory pathway. Successful catheter ablation of the accessory pathway was performed.

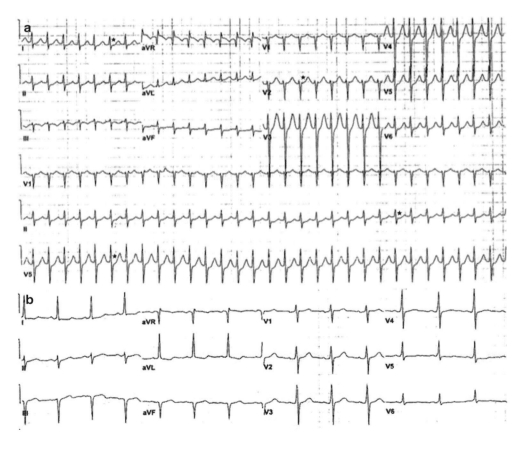

Fig. 11.5 (**a**) Twelve-lead electrocardiogram of a 49-year-old male who presented with palpitations and dizziness. A short RP tachycardia can be seen determined by the location of the P waves (★). (**b**) Baseline electrocardiogram of the patient showing normal sinus rhythm with short PR interval and delta waves (best seen in leads I, V_4, and V_5) that are suggestive of Wolff–Parkinson–White

Fig. 11.6 Distinguishing between atrioventricular (AV) reentrant tachycardia (AVRT), AV nodal reentrant tachycardia (AVNRT), and atrial tachycardia based on the electrocardiogram. AVRT usually presents as short R–P tachycardia (**a**), while atrial tachycardia usually presents as long R–P tachycardia (**b**). In AVNRT, the P wave is usually superimposed on or buried within the QRS complex (**c**)

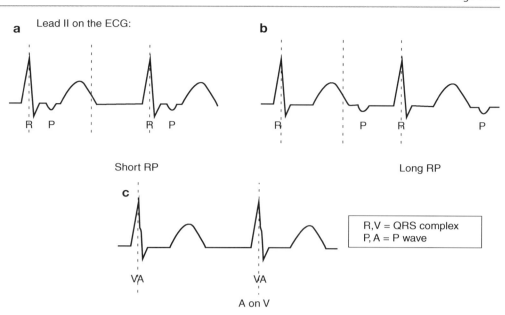

Wide QRS Complex Tachycardia

A 59-year-old female with a history of postpartum dilated cardiomyopathy, coronary artery disease, hypertension, diabetes mellitus, chronic obstructive pulmonary disease, and gout presented with left lower quadrant abdominal pain. She was diagnosed with diverticulitis and appropriate treatment was started. Her left ventricular ejection fraction was found to be 20 % but no wall motion abnormalities were present, and a baseline ECG showed left bundle branch block (LBBB). During telemetry monitoring, the following rhythm was recorded (Fig. 11.7).

The initial rhythm is sinus, which is followed by a wide QRS complex tachycardia (WCT) at a rate of 150 bpm with left axis deviation. The QRS duration is approximately 180 ms. The rate at the beginning of the tachycardia is transiently irregular and is followed by a regular rhythm and rate.

Normal conduction to the ventricles starts from the sinus node in the right atrium and travels to the His–Purkinje system via the AV node where there is normally a delay in conduction. In the presence of an accessory pathway (AP), the ventricles are depolarized via both the AP and the AVN, and the QRS complexes therefore represent fusion complexes. APs lack the rate-slowing properties of the AVN and thus enable faster and earlier depolarization of ventricular myocardium (ventricular preexcitation). The impulse conducted through the AVN then joins the earlier depolarization via the AP, resulting in a shortened PR interval and a wider QRS complex duration with slurring at the beginning of the QRS complex (ventricular preexcitation), known as a delta wave [12].

Analysis of the QRS morphology in V_1 shows typical right bundle branch block (RBBB) morphology with the right "rabbit ear" larger than the left, suggesting that the tachycardia is supraventricular (SVT) in origin, with intraventricular (IV) aberrancy. However, a fusion beat (★), in which the ventricles are depolarized from two sources, is seen at the onset of tachycardia. Further evaluation reveals P waves that are occurring at regular intervals at a rate slower than that of the QRS complexes, indicating atrioventricular (AV) dissociation (◆). The frontal plane QRS axis is pointed in a "northwest" direction (towards aVR). Based on these findings, the cause of the WCT is ventricular tachycardia (VT). This case highlights the lack of specificity of QRS morphology in evaluating patients with WCT to arrive at the correct diagnosis.

When confronted with an ECG with WCT, it is important to be able to differentiate between SVT with aberrancy, WPW conduction with ventricular preexcitation, and VT. Other rare causes include pacemaker-mediated tachycardia (in which ventricular pacing is occurring in response to sensed P waves conducted retrograde) and artifact. We present the following algorithms when evaluating a patient with WCT [4]:

Step 1 – History and physical examination: A detailed history and physical examination is of upmost importance and can often provide clues to the diagnosis of WCT. VT is more likely in patients with a history of myocardial ischemia or infarction. Cannon "a" waves in the neck and variable intensity of S_1 noted on physical examination during WCT suggest AV dissociation, thus favoring a diagnosis of VT. Conversely, SVT with aberrancy is favored when the tachycardia terminates in response to carotid massage or vagal maneuvers. An exception to this

Fig. 11.7 Telemetry monitoring of a 59-year-old female admitted with heart failure exacerbation that shows wide complex tachycardia. Narrow complex beats (★) are seen preceding the onset of the wide complex tachycardia with different QRS morphology than the sinus rhythm. These fusion beats preceded by P waves are diagnostic of ventricular tachycardia. AV dissociation is also seen (◆)

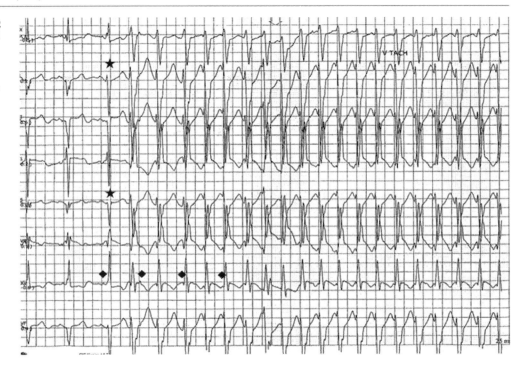

is seen in idiopathic VT arising from the right ventricular outflow tract since that form of VT can also terminate with carotid massage. A comparison of the ECG during WCT to that of a baseline tracing made during sinus rhythm is also crucial. The presence of infarction Q waves on prior ECG in sinus rhythm increases the probability of the WCT being VT. On the other hand, SVT with aberrancy is more likely when the intraventricular conduction pattern seen during the WCT matches that seen during sinus rhythm. Lastly, a WPW pattern that is similar to the WCT ECG pattern points towards preexcited tachycardia. It is important to note that orthodromic SVT is more common than antidromic SVT in WPW patients.

Step 2 – Rhythm and axis: An irregularly irregular rhythm argues against VT. However, a transient irregular rhythm at the onset of tachycardia, followed by a regular rhythm, known as a "warm-up phenomenon," is often indicative of VT, although the same "warm-up" phenomenon can be seen in supraventricular arrhythmias. The mean frontal plane QRS axis is of little diagnostic value unless a right superior axis (from −90 to +/−180°) is present; such an axis is rarely seen in aberrancy unless there is underlying severe right ventricular hypertrophy or lung disease, and hence this axis favors VT. Likewise, patients with VT almost always have a right axis with an LBBB pattern. Also, any shift in axis during the WCT from baseline by greater than 40° is usually indicative of VT.

Step 3 – Atrioventricular (AV) relationship: AV dissociation is one of the most helpful criteria in differentiating SVT from VT in WCT. It is characterized by atrial activity that

is independent of ventricular activity, with atrial rates slower than the tachycardia rate. Although AV dissociation is 100 % specific for VT, the sensitivity is very low (approximately 10 %) [13].

Step 4 – Narrow complex beats (fusion and capture beats) within the WCT: Fusion or capture beats are 100 % specific for the diagnosis of VT. Fusion beats occur when the ventricular tachycardia focus fuses with a sinus beat that conducts to the ventricle through the AV node. Capture beats are narrow beats in the middle of WCT due to complete capture of the ventricle by a sinus beat through the AV node.

Step 5 – Brugada criteria: The Brugada criteria involve evaluation of the R-to-S durations in all the precordial leads. The R–S is measured from the beginning of the QRS complex to the nadir of the S wave. Absence of an R–S complex in all precordial leads (QRS concordance) or an R-to-S duration greater than 100 ms in one precordial lead favors a diagnosis of VT [14].

Step 6 – Specific QRS morphology: Most forms of VT are myocardial in origin so the QRS complex morphology does not look like typical LBBB or RBBB. Hence, certain ECG criteria based on QRS morphology in leads V_1, V_2, and V_6 have used these differences to distinguish VT from SVT with aberrant conduction. Atypical RBBB seen during VT usually appears as monophasic or biphasic R waves with R > R′ in lead V1 and an R:S ratio less than 1 in V_6. The Kindwall criteria suggest an atypical LBBB morphology when any Q wave is seen in lead V_6 and at least one of the following is seen in lead V_1 or V_2: an

R wave >30 ms, a notch in the downstroke of the S wave, and an R–S interval >60 ms [15]. However, morphologic criteria have limitations. Idiopathic VT arising from the conduction system (e.g., bundle branch reentry VT, fascicular VT) will have the same morphology as bundle branch block with aberrancy and hence satisfy morphology criteria for SVT.

Step 7 – Lead II evaluation: Recently, the time to the peak of the R wave in Lead II has been shown to be effective in differentiating VT from aberrancy. The R wave peak time is measured from the onset of QRS to the nadir of the Q or peak of the R wave. VT is strongly suggested when this R wave peak time is ≥50 ms in lead II [16].

Step 8 – Lead aVR evaluation: Investigators have found VT to be the most likely underlying arrhythmia when any of the following are seen in lead aVR: an initial R wave, an initial Q or R wave >40 ms, a notch on the descending limb of a negative QRS complex, and a ventricular activation–velocity ratio (vi/vt) less than or equal to 1. This ratio measures the voltage change between the initial and terminal 40 ms of a QRS complex [13].

Hypertrophic Cardiomyopathy

A 16-year-old boy was referred for management due an abnormal ECG recorded prior to elective oral surgery. The patient was previously healthy and denied any symptoms of palpitations, dizziness, dyspnea, or syncope. He was a member of his school water polo team and had always been physically very active. His ECG is shown in Fig. 11.8.

There is normal sinus rhythm at a rate of 73 bpm with a normal mean frontal plane QRS axis, QRS, and QTc intervals. High-voltage QRS complexes associated with short

PR intervals and inverted T waves in leads II, III, aVF, and V_4–V_6 were noted and were suggestive of left ventricular hypertrophy (LVH). There was no history of hypertrophic cardiomyopathy (HCM) or sudden cardiac death in his family. His echocardiogram, performed because of the abnormal ECG, revealed apical HCM with a septal thickness of 21 mm. A 24-h Holter monitor showed 363 isolated premature ventricular beats (PVCs), but no couplets or episodes of VT. The patient's heart rate increased to 185 bpm during treadmill stress echocardiography, with an appropriate increase in blood pressure during exercise and no postexercise hypotension. The patient was determined to be at low risk of sudden cardiac death (SCD) and implantation of an implantable cardioverter defibrillator (ICD) was not recommended. However, the patient was advised against playing on the school water polo team based on current guidelines that recommend against participation in competitive sports [17]. He was referred for genetic testing.

The most common type of HCM not associated with left ventricular outflow tract (LVOT) obstruction is apical HCM, also known as Yamaguchi syndrome. It is usually associated with negative T waves in the precordial leads (especially in leads V_4–V_6) on the ECG, as was observed in our patient.

Most patients with HCM are asymptomatic. When symptoms are present, they generally include dyspnea, chest pain, palpitations, dizziness, fatigue, syncope, and even sudden cardiac death. Syncope can be due to decreased cardiac output (from an increased LVOT gradient in HOCM), ischemia, arrhythmia, or left ventricular underfilling from any cause, including dehydration.

Electrocardiography will demonstrate LVH in most patients although the ECG can be normal. Some studies have shown the importance of abnormal Q waves [defined as Q waves that are greater than 0.04 s in duration and 3 mm in

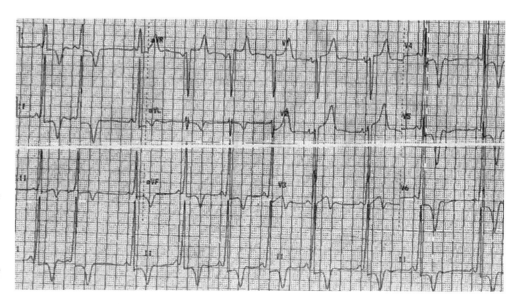

Fig. 11.8 Twelve-lead electrocardiogram of a previously healthy 16-year-old boy recorded prior to elective oral surgery. There is left ventricular hypertrophy by voltage criteria. In the absence of a history of hypertension, this is diagnostic of hypertrophic cardiomyopathy

depth or more than one third of the R wave in at least two consecutive leads (with the exception of aVR)] as an early sign of LVH development in asymptomatic patients [18]. As the patient gets older, these Q waves may disappear as LVH develops. However, Q waves in young athletes can be a normal finding and thus it is recommended that patients with cardiac symptoms or a family history of cardiomyopathy undergo further evaluation for LVH when Q waves are found. A Holter monitor or an event monitor is also recommended to evaluate possible arrhythmias that are not present on the 12-lead ECG. Common arrhythmias associated with HCM include atrial fibrillation, PVCs, and non-sustained VT.

Brugada Syndrome

A 61-year-old male with a history of hypertension, hyperlipidemia, and gout presented with syncope. The patient was sitting at home when he suddenly lost consciousness without any preceding symptoms. In the emergency department, he was found to be in ventricular fibrillation and was successfully defibrillated. His echocardiogram showed normal left ventricular function and coronary angiography did not show significant coronary artery disease (CAD). The 12-lead ECG post-defibrillation is shown in Fig. 11.9.

There is sinus bradycardia at a rate of 54 bpm with a normal mean frontal plane QRS axis. His PR and QTc intervals are 194 and 443 ms, respectively. There are ST segment elevations in leads V_1 and V_2 that, together with the clinical presentation and absence of structural heart disease and CAD, are consistent with a diagnosis of Brugada syndrome. The patient underwent genetic testing that revealed sodium channel (SCN5A) mutation. His two sisters and

son were also found to have the same genetic abnormality. Electrophysiology study resulted in inducible polymorphic VT at a rate of 120 bpm. He was referred for an ICD implant to prevent cardiac arrest due to ventricular arrhythmias.

It is important to recognize the Brugada pattern on ECG since it is associated with an increased risk of SCD. SCD may be the first and only presentation in these patients. Mortality is more common in males (9:1 male to female ratio) and usually occurs in adulthood. SCD in patients with the Brugada syndrome is usually not related to exercise and tends to occur during sleep, suggesting that the arrhythmia trigger could be the result of an imbalance between sympathetic and parasympathetic tone. Patients at highest risk of SCD are those with a previous history of cardiac arrest or syncope. Symptoms include palpitations, dizziness, syncope, and cardiac arrest.

Three types of repolarization patterns in ECG leads V_1–V_3 have been identified and they can be permanent or transient [19, 20]. Brugada type 1 pattern describes the classic or coved ST–T waveform type and is associated with a high incidence of death in structurally normal hearts. It is characterized by ST segment elevation that is greater than or equal to 2 mm seen in more than one of the right precordial leads (V_1–V_3) and followed by an inverted T wave in these leads (Fig. 11.10a).

Brugada syndrome is characterized by the presence of a Brugada type 1 pattern on the ECG in structurally normal hearts or appearance of the pattern after sodium channel blocker administration (e.g., flecainide, procainamide, or ajmaline), in addition to at least one of the following criteria: documented ventricular fibrillation (VF) or VT, a family history of SCD before the age of 45, type 1 coved ST segment elevation in family members, inducible VT/VF during

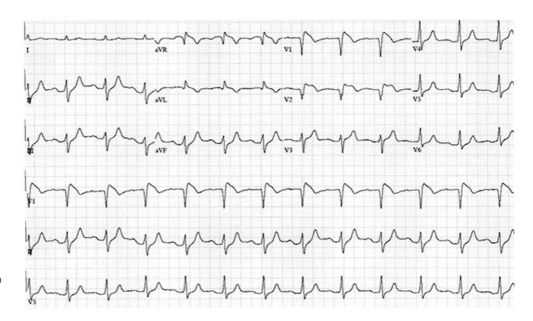

Fig. 11.9 Post-defibrillation 12-lead electrocardiogram of a 61-year-old who presented with syncope. ST segment elevation is seen in leads V_1 and V_2

The three types of Brugada patterns shown in lead V₂

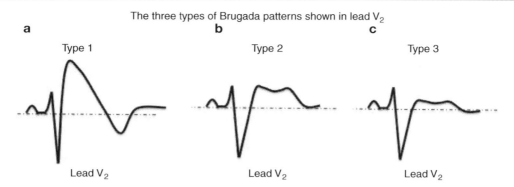

Fig. 11.10 (**a**) Brugada type 1 pattern: ST segment elevation greater than or equal to 2 mm in more than one of the right precordial leads (V₁–V₃) followed by an inverted T wave in these leads. (**b**, **c**) Type 2 and 3 Brugada pattern: "saddleback" ST segment elevation that returns towards baseline before rising to meet an upright or biphasic T wave. In type 2 Brugada pattern (**b**), the ST segment elevation is greater than or equal to 1 mm. In type 3 Brugada pattern (**c**), the ST segment elevation is less than or equal to 1 mm and is less specific for the diagnosis

electrophysiologic study, unexplained syncope, and nocturnal agonal respiration.

Types 2 and 3 Brugada patterns: Although these two patterns are not diagnostic of the Brugada syndrome, they are more frequently encountered than type 1. They are characterized by a "saddleback" ST segment elevation that returns towards baseline before rising to meet an upright or biphasic T wave. In type 2, there is greater than or equal to 1 mm ST segment elevation (Fig. 11.10b), whereas in type 3 there is a less than 1 mm ST elevation (Fig. 11.10c).

Confounding factors that can produce ECG changes similar to the Brugada pattern must be excluded before a diagnosis of Brugada is made. These include atypical RBBB, LVH, early repolarization, acute pericarditis, acute myocardial ischemia or infarction, pulmonary embolism, hyperkalemia, and drugs (such as calcium channel blockers, tricyclic antidepressants, fluoxetine, lithium, trifluoperazine, antihistamines, and cocaine).

Symptomatic Brugada patients carry the highest risk of SCD, especially if they initially present with syncope or SCD. In asymptomatic patients, males with spontaneous type 1 ECG are at highest risk, while those with Brugada-type ECG changes induced by drugs like sodium channel blockers are at low risk of sudden cardiac death [21, 22].

Long QT Syndrome

A 52-year-old previously healthy female was admitted to the hospital for treatment of community-acquired pneumonia. On admission, she was found to be hypoxic and required intubation. Chest x-ray revealed air under the diaphragm, so emergent surgery was carried out for gastric perforation. Her medications consisted of quinapril, furosemide, famotidine, lorazepam, haloperidol, piperacillin/tazobactam, levofloxacin, and vancomycin. During her intensive care unit stay after surgery, this lead II rhythm strip was recorded (Fig. 11.11).

The rhythm is sinus at a rate of 85 bpm with normal PR and QRS durations. However, her QTc interval is prolonged (more than half of the R–R interval) and the T waves are broad and notched. These findings are consistent with long QT syndrome (LQTS). The rhythm degenerated into polymorphic VT (torsades de pointes) within a few hours (Fig. 11.12).

She was cardioverted to normal sinus rhythm and treated with intravenous isoproterenol and lidocaine to shorten the QT interval. Serum calcium, magnesium, and potassium levels were within normal limits. She was diagnosed with haloperidol-induced LQTS. She had dramatic prolongation of her QT interval after stopping the lidocaine infusion that normalized with an additional intravenous bolus (Fig. 11.13a, b) [23]. Based on this response to lidocaine, she was treated with mexiletine (the same antiarrhythmic class as lidocaine) to normalize the QT interval and prevent further long QT-induced ventricular arrhythmias.

LQTS is an inherited channelopathy that is associated with SCD. Mutations in the potassium and sodium ion channels can produce delays in ventricular repolarization, predisposing patients to an increased risk of ventricular arrhythmias and SCD. The repolarization delay is reflected as QTc prolongation on the ECG. The QTc interval is measured by dividing the measured QT duration (measured from the beginning of the QRS complex to the end of the T wave in milliseconds) by the square root of the R–R interval measured in seconds (Bazett's correction). The upper limit of normal of the QTc is 460 ms for women and 440 ms for men. Any QTc measurement above the upper limit is considered abnormal and must be further evaluated, especially if associated with abnormal T waves (inverted, peaked, notched, or widened).

U waves can be seen on the ECG following T waves. They are assumed to represent repolarization of the papillary muscles and His–Purkinje system. The amplitudes of U waves are usually less than 0.2 mV and they are frequently separate from the T waves. Occasionally, a U wave can be

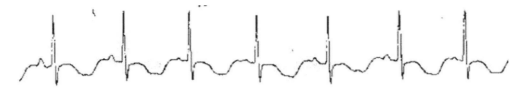

Fig. 11.11   Lead II rhythm strip recorded in the intensive care unit of a 52-year-old female who was admitted to the hospital for treatment of community-acquired pneumonia. The QTc interval is prolonged (greater than half R–R) and is associated with broad and notched T waves

Fig. 11.12 Rhythm strip of lead
II showing polymorphic
ventricular tachycardia (torsades
de pointes) recorded a few hours
after the rhythm strip in
Fig. 11.11

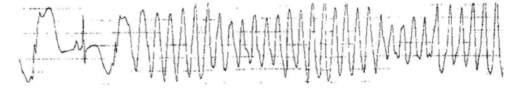

Fig. 11.13   Twelve-lead
electrocardiogram showing
prolongation of the QT interval
after stopping the lidocaine drip
(**a**) that normalized after
intravenous bolus of lidocaine (**b**)

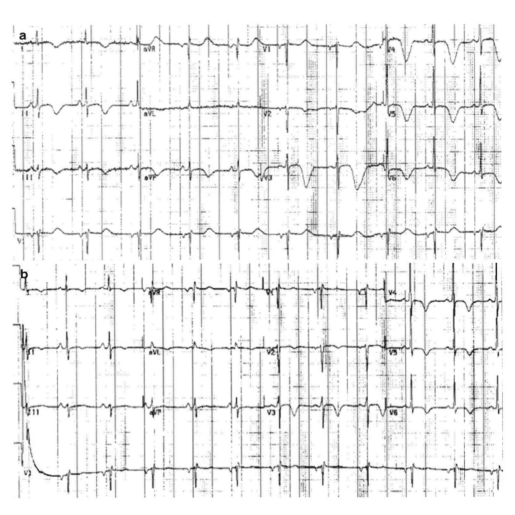

merged with the T wave. In this case, the tangent method has been proposed to determine the end of the T wave [24]. A tangent line is drawn to the steepest part of the descending portion of the T wave. The point where the tangent line intercepts the isoelectric line is considered to be the end of the T wave (Fig. 11.14).

Jervell and Lange-Neilsen were the first to describe autosomal recessive form of long QT syndrome that was associated with congenital deafness. Romano Ward subsequently described autosomal dominant form of LQTS that is not associated with deafness. Acquired LQTS is caused by drugs (such as certain antiarrhythmic agents, erythromycin,

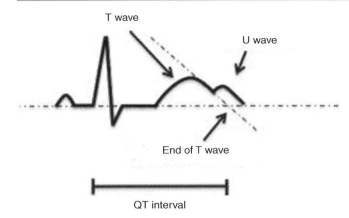

Fig. 11.14 The tangent method can be used for calculating the QT interval in the presence of a merged U wave. Here, a tangent line is drawn to the steepest part of the descending portion of the T wave. The point where the tangent line intercepts the isoelectric line is considered to be the end of the T wave

phenothiazines, antipsychotics) and electrolyte abnormalities (hypokalemia, hypomagnesemia, and hypocalcemia). The most common forms of LQTS are LQT1, LQT2, and LQT3. Patients with LQT1 syndrome have episodes of torsades de pointes VT triggered by exercise, including diving and swimming [25]. Prolongation of the QT interval is pronounced during or after exercise or epinephrine challenge. Torsades de pointes VT can occur in patients with LQT2 syndrome during rest or stress and is usually triggered by sudden loud noises such as that emanating from an alarm clock [25, 26]. Patients with LQT3 develop torsades de pointes VT with slower heart rates, mainly during sleep [25].

Symptoms of LQTS include palpitations, presyncope, syncope, and SCD. LQTS is diagnosed by ECG findings and genetic testing. Prolonged QTc intervals can sometimes be a normal variant. LQTS is suspected if it is associated with abnormal T waves. In patients with high suspicion for LQTS, the diagnosis can be confirmed by prolongation of the QTc interval in response to change in posture, exercise, and epinephrine administration [25]. The risk of SCD is highest with QTc>500 ms in patients with LQT1and LQT2 and in males with LQT3 [27]. Genetic testing is the gold standard for the diagnosis of LQTS and screening of family members. It identifies around 75–80 % of patients with LQTS [28].

Early Repolarization

A 39-year-old male presented with palpitations that were triggered by activity and associated with chest discomfort. He was noted to be in VT in the emergency department, where he was cardioverted to sinus rhythm. Family history was significant for cardiac death in 2 uncles and 2 cousins all before the age of 40 years. A 12-lead ECG taken after cardioversion showed the following (Fig. 11.15).

There is normal sinus rhythm at a rate of 62 bpm with normal mean frontal plane QRS axis, PR, QTc, and QRS intervals. However, in leads II, III, aVF, and V_3–V_6, concave ST segment and J point elevations were noted. The echocardiogram and coronary angiogram were within normal limits.

The differential diagnosis of the J point elevations includes early repolarization, acute pericarditis, ventricular hypertrophy, and myocardial ischemia. On the ECG, acute pericarditis is usually seen as diffuse ST segment elevation (except for ST segment depression in leads V_1 and aVR), not confined to a specific coronary artery distribution of leads. In addition, pericarditis can be differentiated from other causes of ST segment elevation by the presence of PR segment depression (measured from the end of the P wave to the beginning to the QRS complex), usually seen in leads II, III, and aVF, and PR segment elevation in lead aVR ("knuckle sign"). Left ventricular hypertrophy usually presents as ST segment elevation in leads V_1–V_3 with QRS complex voltages that adhere to the criteria for LVH. According to the American College of Cardiology/American Heart Association (ACC/AHA) guidelines, ST elevation reflecting myocardial ischemia or infarction is less likely in the presence of a concave (as is seen on this ECG) rather than a convex ST segment [29]. Thus, this patient was diagnosed with early repolarization syndrome associated with SCD based on his strong family history and presentation with VT. Electrophysiology study showed inducible ventricular tachycardia. An ICD was implanted for primary prevention of sudden death.

Early repolarization is common in the general population, with an incidence of 1–5 % [30]. It is diagnosed on the ECG by evaluation of the J point. The J point reflects the end of depolarization and the beginning of repolarization and is seen as the point where the end of the QRS complex joins the ST segment on the ECG. The diagnosis of early repolarization requires J point elevation of at least 0.1 mV (seen as either a slurring or notching of the downslope of the QRS complex), associated with concave ST segment elevation and, occasionally, notched T waves in at least two contiguous leads. These J point deflections, known as J waves, can be transient or permanent and may disappear during tachycardia. Inferior ST segment elevation is generally seen in the elderly, females, and at high heart rates. Lateral and global ST segment elevation is usually seen in younger individuals, African-Americans, in those with LVH, and at low heart rates.

Early repolarization is generally benign and this benign form is often seen in males, African-Americans (Fig. 11.16), Asians, athletes, patients with LVH, and in those with high vagal tone. As patients age, the early repolarization pattern typically regresses. The pattern is usually normalized with isoproterenol and exercise while beta-blockers enhance it. The ST segment elevation is mainly concave and normal in these patients. Rapidly ascending concave ST segment

Fig. 11.15 Twelve-lead electrocardiogram of a 39-year-old male who presented with palpitations. This ECG was taken after cardioversion from ventricular tachycardia. Leads II, III, aVF, and V_3–V_6 reveal concave ST segment and J point elevations

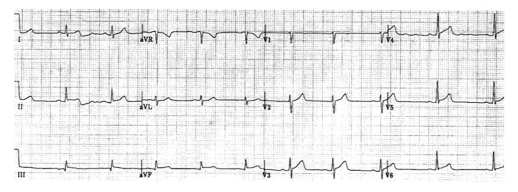

Fig. 11.16 Twelve-lead electrocardiogram showing benign early repolarization pattern in an African-American patient. A rapidly ascending concave ST segment elevation after the J point is shown that is considered to be a benign variant of early repolarization pattern

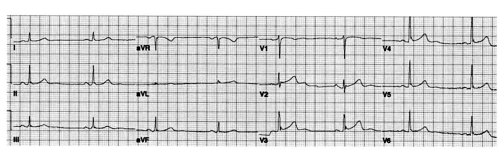

elevation after the J point is considered to be a benign variant and is not associated with an increased risk of SCD [31].

Recent reports have documented a higher incidence of VF and SCD in certain patients with early repolarization [30]. The risk of developing idiopathic VF in the general population is 3:100,000. This risk increases to 11:100,000, in patients with J waves and 30:100,000 in patients with J waves followed by a horizontal ST segment elevation [32]. Early repolarization and Brugada syndrome have recently been categorized as belonging to the "J wave syndromes" [33]. Four types have been described based on the lead location of the early repolarization pattern. Type 1 shows early repolarization in the lateral precordial leads that is seen in healthy male athletes and has the lowest risk of malignant arrhythmias. Type 2 shows early repolarization in the inferior or inferolateral leads and is associated with a greater risk of malignant arrhythmia. Type 3 shows early repolarization pattern in all ECG leads and has the highest risk of malignant arrhythmias. Brugada Syndrome is classified as type 4.

The risk factors for sudden death in patients with early repolarization include those with J point elevations greater than 0.2 mV, extensive distribution on multiple ECG leads, remarkable fluctuation without any apparent cause, pause-dependent augmentation, and J waves associated with horizontal or descending ST segment slopes [31, 34].

Artifact

A 44-year-old male with a history of oral amphetamine abuse and nonischemic cardiomyopathy presented to the emergency department with chest pain. An echocardiogram

revealed a left ventricular ejection fraction of 40 %. The following rhythm strip was recorded from leads II and V_1 (Fig. 11.17).

There is normal sinus rhythm at a rate of 90 bpm with normal PR, QRS, and QTc intervals. The rhythm is interrupted by a run of what appears to be WCT - SVT with intraventricular aberration, preexcited tachycardia such as occurring with WPW syndrome, and artifact. Close examination of the rhythm strip shows notches in the middle of the tachycardia (★) that march through the rhythm strips at the same intervals as those of the sinus rate (Fig. 11.18). This is highly suggestive of artifact, resulting in what appears to be a wide complex tachycardia. This artifact coincided with skin scratching near the electrodes during the recording of the ECG. Further evaluation, including electrophysiology study, was deferred.

The ECG is one of the most widely used modalities in medicine. Thus, improving its sensitivity and specificity in the diagnosis of various medical problems is important. Despite constant improvements in the ECG, artifacts are still seen and can lead to inappropriate and sometimes even harmful management when misdiagnosed. To help differentiate artifacts from true arrhythmias, the use of the "notch sign" has been proposed [35]. If the notch-to-notch intervals during the apparent wide complex tachycardia are equal to or multiples of the RR intervals during sinus rhythm (or preceding rhythm), the diagnosis of artifact is made. In the presence of atrial fibrillation, the notch-to-notch intervals can be irregular.

The ECG records the electrical activity of the heart. However, other signals either from the body or from outside sources can sometimes produce frequencies that can interfere with the ECG recording. Hence, artifact signals can arise from

Fig. 11.17 Rhythm strip (leads II and V₁) showing wide complex tachycardia in a 44-year-old male who presented with chest pain

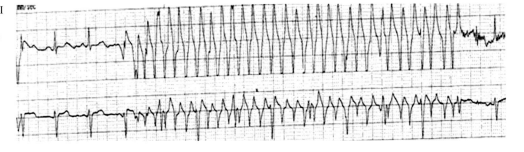

Fig. 11.18 Evaluation of the rhythm strip shows notches in the middle of the wide complex tachycardia (★) that represent sinus QRS complexes. This is diagnostic of recording artifact

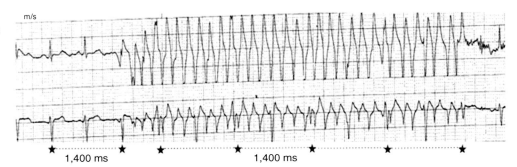

physiologic and/or external sources. Physiologic artifacts are mainly seen with interference from muscle or epidermal signals, while external signals can be generated from electrical outlets, instruments, or connection problems [36–38].

Muscle activity produces electrical signals that can be seen as narrow, rapid spikes that correspond to movement. This is mainly seen in patients with Parkinson's disease and fine tremors, as well as in anxious, shivering, or inadequately relaxed patients. These signals can sometimes be mistaken for P waves or flutter waves and thus can lead to unnecessary treatment unless the observer is aware of their presence. Moving the electrodes to areas of less muscle bulk can reduce electromyographic artifacts. In addition, the skin can also produce electrical signals when the epidermis is stretched, causing motion artifact. This type of artifact is seen as large baseline shifts occurring when the patient changes positions in bed, ambulates, or eats.

Artifacts can also arise when grounding of the electrodes is not properly done. Grounding helps to prevent interference between the leads. In addition, improper calibration of the ECG or telemetry monitoring may result in incorrect reading due to the production of greater or smaller voltage complexes (known as over-damping or under-damping of the ECG) [39]. Low-voltage artifacts can arise from impairments in conduction between the electrodes and electrical activity of the heart such as occurrs in patients with emphysema, obesity, and edematous conditions. On the other hand, high-voltage artifacts can be seen in patients with a thin chest wall, anemia, and hyperthyroidism.

Movement of electrodes during ECG recordings can also produce low-voltage baseline shifts and wandering baselines; thus, proper connection of the electrodes to the skin is essential in decreasing these artifacts. The connection is improved by proper skin preparation such as shaving, cleaning with alcohol to remove body oils, and gentle scrubbing to remove dead skin cells. Proper cleaning of the electrodes to remove any gel coat should also be performed to allow proper contact with the skin. As with the electrodes, movement of the cable connecting the electrodes to the ECG machine's input relative to the body of the patient can also produce artifacts. This is mainly seen when the cables are long as well as by breathing movements, and thus can be avoided by reducing the length of the cables and by asking the patients to hold their breath during the recording.

The 60-Hz pickup refers to the 60-Hz current that supplies power to the electrical wall outlets and can cause interference with the ECG recording whether or not appliances are plugged in. It produces a wide and fuzzy baseline on the ECG that can be minimized by good electrode contact with the skin. Most ECG machines now have a filtering option to block such interference. In addition, high-frequency electromagnetic interference from instruments such as electrocautery can be seen. The electrodes themselves can also store voltage that can interfere with the ECG recording. This stored voltage is known as the offset potential and is influenced by the metal used to make the electrodes and the material used in the gel. Usually, silver–silver chloride produces the least interference and is most widely used in production.

The gel type used mainly affects signal transmission (electrode impedance) with only minimal contribution to motion artifact. Thus, inadequate amounts of electrode gel can enable a 60-Hz pickup interference and thus affect the quality of the ECG recording. Moreover, any break in the wires and connections between the electrode and the monitor can produce artifacts on the ECG in the form of loss of the ECG tracing, 60-Hz pickup, or tracing instability; such artifacts have been mistaken for long pauses or asystole. Recognizing artifacts and taking appropriate measures to minimize interferences with the ECG recording is important and will not only improve the diagnostic value of the ECG but also prevent unnecessary procedures that can cause more complications than benefits.

Key Points

- Sinus node dysfunction (SND), or sick sinus syndrome (SSS), is a degenerative disease of the sinus node characterized by significant sinus bradycardia, sinus pauses, sinus arrest, and sinoatrial exit block.
- When confronted with an ECG with wide complex tachycardia, it is important to be able to differentiate between supraventricular tachycardia with aberrancy, Wolff–Parkinson–White syndrome with ventricular preexcitation and ventricular tachycardia.
- A Brugada pattern on ECG is associated with an increased risk of sudden cardiac death.
- Long QT syndrome is diagnosed by ECG findings and genetic testing.
- The differential diagnosis of J point elevation includes early repolarization, acute pericarditis, ventricular hypertrophy, and myocardial ischemia.
- Recognizing artifacts with the ECG recording improves the diagnostic value of the ECG and prevents unnecessary procedures.

References

1. Wagner GS, Macfarlane P, Wellens H, et al. AHA/ACCF/HRS recommendations for the standardization and interpretation of the electrocardiogram: part VI: acute ischemia/infarction: a scientific statement from the American Heart Association Electrocardiography and Arrhythmias Committee, Council on Clinical Cardiology; the American College of Cardiology Foundation; and the Heart Rhythm Society. Endorsed by the International Society for Computerized Electrocardiology. J Am Coll Cardiol. 2009;53(11):1003–11.
2. Mendis S, Thygesen K, Kuulasmaa K, et al. World Health Organization definition of myocardial infarction: 2008–09 revision. Int J Epidemiol. 2011;40(1):139–46.
3. Huang HD, Birnbaum Y. ST elevation: differentiation between ST elevation myocardial infarction and nonischemic ST elevation. J Electrocardiol. 2011;44(5):494.e491–12.
4. Badhwar N, Kusumoto F, Goldschlager N. Arrhythmias in the coronary care unit. J Intensive Care Med. 2012;27(5):267–89.
5. Adan V, Crown LA. Diagnosis and treatment of sick sinus syndrome. Am Fam Physician. 2003;67(8):1725–32.
6. Brignole M. Sick sinus syndrome. Clin Geriatr Med. 2002;18(2):211–27.
7. Epstein AE, DiMarco JP, Ellenbogen KA, et al. ACC/AHA/HRS 2008 guidelines for device-based therapy of cardiac rhythm abnormalities: a report of the American College of Cardiology/American Heart Association Task Force on Practice Guidelines (writing committee to revise the ACC/AHA/NASPE 2002 guideline update for implantation of cardiac pacemakers and antiarrhythmia devices) developed in collaboration with the American Association for Thoracic Surgery and Society of Thoracic Surgeons. J Am Coll Cardiol. 2008;51(21):e1–62.
8. Barold SS. 2:1 Atrioventricular block: order from chaos. Am J Emerg Med. 2001;19(3):214–7.
9. Maury P, Zimmermann M, Metzger J. Distinction between atrioventricular reciprocating tachycardia and atrioventricular node reentrant tachycardia in the adult population based on P wave location; should we reconsider the value of some ECG criteria according to gender and age? Europace. 2003;5(1):57–64.
10. Arruda MS, McClelland JH, Wang X, et al. Development and validation of an ECG algorithm for identifying accessory pathway ablation site in Wolff-Parkinson-White syndrome. J Cardiovasc Electrophysiol. 1998;9(1):2–12.
11. Fitzpatrick AP, Gonzales RP, Lesh MD, Modin GW, Lee RJ, Scheinman MM. New algorithm for the localization of accessory atrioventricular connections using a baseline electrocardiogram. J Am Coll Cardiol. 1994;23(1):107–16.
12. Keating L, Morris FP, Brady WJ. Electrocardiographic features of Wolff-Parkinson-White syndrome. Emerg Med J. 2003;20(5):491–3.
13. Vereckei A, Duray G, Szenasi G, Altemose GT, Miller JM. Application of a new algorithm in the differential diagnosis of wide QRS complex tachycardia. Eur Heart J. 2007;28(5):589–600.
14. Brugada P, Brugada J, Mont L, Smeets J, Andries EW. A new approach to the differential diagnosis of a regular tachycardia with a wide QRS complex. Circulation. 1991;83(5):1649–59.
15. Kindwall KE, Brown J, Josephson ME. Electrocardiographic criteria for ventricular tachycardia in wide complex left bundle branch block morphology tachycardias. Am J Cardiol. 1988;61(15):1279–83.
16. Pava LF, Perafan P, Badiel M, et al. R-wave peak time at DII: a new criterion for differentiating between wide complex QRS tachycardias. Heart Rhythm. 2010;7(7):922–6.
17. Pelliccia A, Zipes DP, Maron BJ. Bethesda Conference #36 and the European Society of Cardiology Consensus Recommendations revisited a comparison of U.S. and European criteria for eligibility and disqualification of competitive athletes with cardiovascular abnormalities. J Am Coll Cardiol. 2008;52(24):1990–6.
18. Rao U, Agarwal A. Importance of Q waves in early diagnosis of hypertrophic cardiomyopathy. Heart. 2011;97(23):1993–4.
19. Antzelevitch C, Brugada P, Borggrefe M, et al. Brugada syndrome: report of the second consensus conference: endorsed by the Heart Rhythm Society and the European Heart Rhythm Association. Circulation. 2005;111(5):659–70.
20. Antzelevitch C, Brugada P, Brugada J, Brugada R. Brugada syndrome: from cell to bedside. Curr Probl Cardiol. 2005;30(1):9–54.
21. Priori SG, Napolitano C, Gasparini M, et al. Natural history of Brugada syndrome: insights for risk stratification and management. Circulation. 2002;105(11):1342–7.
22. Brugada J, Brugada R, Antzelevitch C, Towbin J, Nademanee K, Brugada P. Long-term follow-up of individuals with the electrocardiographic pattern of right bundle-branch block and ST-segment elevation in precordial leads V1 to V3. Circulation. 2002;105(1):73–8.
23. Viskin S. Torsades de Pointes. Curr Treat Options Cardiovasc Med. 1999;1(2):187–95.
24. Lepeschkin E, Surawicz B. The measurement of the Q-T interval of the electrocardiogram. Circulation. 1952;6(3):378–88.
25. Jackman WM, Friday KJ, Anderson JL, Aliot EM, Clark M, Lazzara R. The long QT syndromes: a critical review, new clinical observations and a unifying hypothesis. Prog Cardiovasc Dis. 1988;31(2):115–72.

26. Schwartz PJ, Priori SG, Spazzolini C, et al. Genotype-phenotype correlation in the long-QT syndrome: gene-specific triggers for life-threatening arrhythmias. Circulation. 2001;103(1):89–95.
27. Priori SG, Schwartz PJ, Napolitano C, et al. Risk stratification in the long-QT syndrome. N Engl J Med. 2003;348(19):1866–74.
28. Schwartz PJ, Crotti L. QTc behavior during exercise and genetic testing for the long-QT syndrome. Circulation. 2011;124(20):2181–4.
29. Antman EM, Anbe DT, Armstrong PW, et al. ACC/AHA guidelines for the management of patients with ST-elevation myocardial infarction; a report of the American College of Cardiology/ American Heart Association Task Force on Practice Guidelines (committee to revise the 1999 guidelines for the management of patients with acute myocardial infarction). J Am Coll Cardiol. 2004;44(3):E1–211.
30. Haissaguerre M, Derval N, Sacher F, et al. Sudden cardiac arrest associated with early repolarization. N Engl J Med. 2008;358(19):2016–23.
31. Tikkanen JT, Junttila MJ, Anttonen O, et al. Early repolarization: electrocardiographic phenotypes associated with favorable long-term outcome. Circulation. 2011;123(23):2666–73.
32. Viskin S, Rosso R, Halkin A. Making sense of early repolarization. Heart Rhythm. 2012;9(4):566–8.
33. Antzelevitch C, Yan GX. J wave syndromes. Heart Rhythm. 2010;7(4):549–58.
34. Aizawa Y, Sato A, Watanabe H, et al. Dynamicity of the J-wave in idiopathic ventricular fibrillation with a special reference to pause-dependent augmentation of the J-wave. J Am Coll Cardiol. 2012;59(22):1948–53.
35. Littmann L, Monroe MH. Electrocardiographic artifact. N Engl J Med. 2000;342(8):590–1; author reply 592.
36. Krasnow AZ, Bloomfield DK. Artifacts in portable electrocardiographic monitoring. Am Heart J. 1976;91(3):349–57.
37. Patel SI, Souter MJ. Equipment-related electrocardiographic artifacts: causes, characteristics, consequences, and correction. Anesthesiology. 2008;108(1):138–48.
38. Adams-Hamoda MG, Caldwell MA, Stotts NA, Drew BJ. Factors to consider when analyzing 12-lead electrocardiograms for evidence of acute myocardial ischemia. Am J Crit Care. 2003;12(1):9–16; quiz 17–8.
39. Mirvis DM, Berson AS, Goldberger AL, et al. Instrumentation and practice standards for electrocardiographic monitoring in special care units. A report for health professionals by a Task Force of the Council on Clinical Cardiology, American Heart Association. Circulation. 1989;79(2):464–71.

Primary Prevention of Cardiovascular Disease

12

Fátima Rodriguez and JoAnne M. Foody

Abstract

Cardiovascular disease (CVD) remains the leading cause of death in the United States and is largely preventable through lifestyle modifications and risk factor control. Primary prevention seeks to prevent disease in otherwise asymptomatic individuals. CVD risk factors may be classified as non-modifiable risk factors (age, gender, and family history) and modifiable risk factors (smoking, hypertension, dyslipidemia, obesity, inactivity, and diabetes). Primary prevention of CVD relies heavily on lifestyle modifications and aggressive treatment of risk factors such as hypertension and dyslipidemia. Global risk score prediction models include the Framingham Risk Score (FRS) that evaluates the 10-year risk of developing coronary heart disease in adults. Limitations of the FRS include underestimation of risk in certain populations and not accounting for lifetime CVD risk. More recently, novel cardiovascular risk factors such as high-sensitivity C-reactive protein (hs-CRP) have been shown to have additional predictive power for CVD events beyond that of traditional risk factors. In addition to targeting high-risk individuals for improved risk factor control, primary prevention relies on population-based approaches to shift the population distribution towards greater CVD health.

Keywords

Primary prevention • Cardiovascular disease • Risk stratification • Lipids • Hypertension • Diabetes • Smoking • Obesity • C-reactive protein

F. Rodriguez, MD, MPH
Department of Medicine,
Resident of Internal Medicine,
Brigham and Woman's Hospital,
75 Francis Street,
Boston, MA 02115, USA
e-mail: farodriguez@partners.org

J.M. Foody, MD, FACC, FAHA (✉)
Cardiovascular Wellness Program,
Department of Medicine,
Brigham and Women's Hospital,
75 Francis Street, Boston, MA 02115, USA
e-mail: jfoody@partners.org

Introduction

Cardiovascular disease (CVD) remains the leading cause of death for adults in the United States and is an increasing problem in developing nations as they experience a demographic transition [1]. Despite advances in treatment strategies and diagnostic technology, death rates for CVD are expected to rise by 2030 [2]. Presently, one in three adults suffers from coronary heart disease and CVD consumes 17 % of the national health expenditures in the United States [1]. Given the increase of cardiovascular risk factors and the aging of the population, the prevalence of CVD and its associated costs are expected to rise without changes in prevention or treatment practices. Importantly, cardiovascular disease is largely preventable through lifestyle modifications, adequate risk factor management, and adjunctive use of novel therapies.

K. Stergiopoulos, D.L. Brown (eds.), *Evidence-Based Cardiology Consult*,
DOI 10.1007/978-1-4471-4441-0_12, © Springer-Verlag London 2014

Table 12.1 Cardiovascular risk factors

Modifiable	Non-modifiable
Smoking	Age
Diabetes	Family history
Hypertension	Gender
Dyslipidemia	
Obesity	
Inactivity	

Primary prevention focuses on delaying or preventing disease in individuals without disease. In recent years, there has been mounting evidence supporting the role of primary prevention as a strategy to combat the growing epidemic of cardiovascular disease. Early identification of cardiovascular risk factors and detection of subclinical cardiovascular disease and modification of risk factors can result in substantial reductions in CVD incidence.

Risk factors that drive the growing rates of CVD can be classified as modifiable and non-modifiable (Table 12.1). Non-modifiable risk factors include age, gender, and family history. Modifiable risk factors, on the other hand, include dyslipidemia, hypertension, obesity, inactivity, diabetes, and smoking. Other biomarkers such as C-reactive protein (CRP) or imaging approaches such as coronary artery calcium (CAC), and carotid intima-media thickness (CIMIT) can further guide in the early detection of cardiovascular risk [3].

The worldwide INTERHEART study, a large prospective study which represented patients from 52 countries, identified nine potentially modifiable risk factors that accounted for over 90 % of the population attributable risk for first myocardial infarction (MI) in men and 94 % of this risk in women [4]. These risk factors include diet, smoking, hypertension, dyslipidemia, physical inactivity, abdominal obesity, psychosocial factors, diabetes mellitus, and alcohol use.

Effective primary prevention requires an assessment of risk to categorize patients for the selection of the most appropriate interventions. Estimating cardiovascular risk over a period of 10 years has often relied on the Framingham Risk Score (FRS). The major independent risk factors for coronary heart disease (CHD) according to this risk score are cigarette smoking, hypertension, hypercholesterolemia, diabetes, and age. The Framingham Heart study and others have convincingly demonstrated the importance of these risk factors to CVD risk [5, 6]. More recently, the lack of global and lifetime risk estimates has proven to be a major limitations of traditional risk scores.

Pathophysiology

Trials of lipid lowering and glucose and hypertension control, as well as recent studies exploring the role of inflammation in heart disease, have added to our understanding of the pathophysiology and prevention of coronary atherosclerosis. Aggressive risk factor control and lifestyle modification serve as the mainstay for the primary prevention of cardiovascular disease [7].

Risk factors drive the pathophysiology of cardiovascular disease. Age is the strongest predictor of CVD risk with over 90 % of all CVD deaths occurring in adults over 65 years of age [8]. However, studies such as the Pathologic Determinants of Atherosclerosis in Youth (PDAY), have shown that atherosclerosis begins as early as in childhood and progresses into adolescents and young adulthood, largely due to underlying risk factors [9]. Similarly, male gender confers an increased risk of CVD prevalence and mortality, namely because CVD typically occurs 10 years later in women, which is thought to be a consequence of the protective effects of estrogen [10]. Family history is also an important independent risk factor for CVD. A recent cohort study of 20,000 adults showed that approximately 15 % of cases of CHD were independently attributable to family history [11].

Hypertension

Hypertension is a very common problem, with over 76 million Americans suffering from the disease, many of whom are unaware of the diagnosis [1]. Hypertension is generally described as a systolic pressure ≥140 mmHg and/or diastolic pressure ≥90 mmHg [12]. However, even patients with systolic blood pressures ≥120 mmHg and/or diastolic blood pressure ≥80 mmHg are at increased cardiovascular risk.

Most adults have essential hypertension with no identifiable cause. Secondary causes of hypertension include sleep apnea, chronic kidney disease, medication-related (particularly steroids), renovascular disease, thyroid disease, pheochromocytoma, primary hyperaldosteronism, and Cushing's syndrome. Hypertension is a well-established risk factor for numerous adverse cardiovascular events including stroke, coronary heart disease, peripheral vascular disease, MI, and congestive heart failure [12].

In the INTERHEART study, hypertension accounted for 18 % of the attributable risk for a first MI, with an even greater impact for women [4].

Dyslipidemia

It is well-established that the higher the level of serum cholesterol, the higher the risk of CVD in both men and women [13]. Elevated serum cholesterol is a crucial factor for the development of atherosclerosis. Epidemiologic investigations have demonstrated a direct relationship between total cholesterol (TC) and low-density lipoprotein cholesterol (LDL-C) in both men and women [1]. Risk of CHD is inversely related to serum high-density lipoprotein cholesterol (HDL-C). The probability of MI rises by 25 % for each 5 mg/dL increase in the mean value of LDL-C for men and women [5, 6, 14]. On the other hand, high serum HDL-C has been shown to be atheroprotective, namely through reverse cholesterol transport via apolipoprotein A-1 and modulation of inflammation [15]. Epidemiological studies link low HDL-C levels with increase risk of incident cardiovascular events [3, 16, 17]. In general, high HDL-C levels (≥60 mg/dL) are protective, whereas low HDL-C levels (≤40 mg/dL in men and ≤50 mg/dL in women) are independent risk factors for CVD.

Evidence of the role of triglycerides (TGs) in CHD is mixed. It is thought that high TGs are a modest independent risk factor for CHD mortality [18, 19]. In women, nonfasting TG levels have are associated with incident cardiovascular events, controlling for other traditional risk factors [20, 21]. Hypertriglyceridemia is also one of the criteria for the diagnosis of the metabolic syndrome.

Smoking

Smoking is one of the strongest risk factors for CVD, resulting in a threefold increase in the risk of MI [22]. Passive or secondhand smoke exposure also increases CHD in a dose-response relationship [23]. Smoking cessation confers a significant reduction in the risk of MI [24, 25]. Despite significant progress in smoking cessation efforts, in 2010 over 21 % of men and 17 % of women over 18 years of age were smokers [1].

Diabetes Mellitus

The entire spectrum of insulin resistance and impaired glucose tolerance is associated with an increased risk of CHD. The metabolic syndrome, which comprises a cluster of risk factors, significantly increases the risk of CHD. In fact, diabetes is considered a CHD-equivalent risk factor, since diabetics have similar risk of subsequent MI as nondiabetics with a prior MI [26, 27]. Diabetes is the strongest cardiovascular risk factor in women [10]. Paralleling the growing burden of obesity, diabetes is becoming an increasingly common problem, with an estimated lifetime risk of 40 % for Americans. Complications from diabetes include both microvascular complications (retinopathy, neuropathy, and nephropathy) and macrovascular complications (CHD, peripheral artery disease, and stroke).

Metabolic syndrome is defined as three or more of the following [28]:
1. Abdominal obesity (waist circumference >40 in. in men and >35 in. in women)
2. TGs ≥150 mg/dL
3. SBP ≥130 or DBP ≥85 (or pharmacologic treatment for hypertension)
4. HDL-C ≤40 mg/dL in men or ≤50 mg/dL in women
5. Fasting glucose ≥110 mg/dL

Obesity

The American Heart Association (AHA) defines obesity as a major risk factor for CVD. Overweight is defined as a total body mass index (BMI) ≥25 kg/m² whereas obesity is defined as a BMI ≥30 kg/m². Obesity is associated with a 50 % increase in CVD mortality [29]. Abdominal adiposity poses a particularly risk as it predisposes to diabetes, elevated triglycerides, and a prothrombotic state. Recent estimates show that at least two-thirds of adults in the United States are overweight or obese (Fig. 12.1) [1].

Diagnosis

Cardiovascular Risk Scores

Preventive efforts should target each major modifiable risk factor discussed above. The Framingham Heart Study established the primary risk factors for CVD, which serve as primary targets for therapeutic agents. The Framingham Risk Score (FRS) is the most widely employed tool to estimate the risk of CHD. It incorporates six traditional risk factors for CVD (age, sex, TC, HDL-C, blood pressure, and cigarette smoking) [5, 6]. The Framingham Risk Calculator can be used to assess a patient's 10-year absolute risk of CHD and, on that basis, to categorize the patient as being at high, intermediate, or low risk.

However, the FRS has several limitations including the absence of consideration of family history and lifetime risk, as well as lack of generalizability to more diverse populations [30–32]. The FRS may underestimate CVD risk, particularly in women who may have nontraditional risk factors. To enhance risk prediction, additional classification schemes include the Reynolds Risk Score (RRS), which has been used to predict the 10-year CHD risk for women using the Women's Health Initiative cohort [33]. It adds family history of heart attack before age 60 and novel biochemical markers.

Screening the Asymptomatic Patient for Cardiovascular Disease

Primary prevention relies on screening for heart disease before disease is present. Patients who are considered high risk by traditional methods benefit from aggressive risk factor control. Many risk scores have not been validated in younger populations and may grossly underestimate risk in certain populations. Although younger adults may have low 10-year CVD risk, their lifetime risk may be quite high.

Current primary prevention guidelines from the American Heart Association (AHA) recommend that, beginning at age 20, all adults should undergo routine screening for

Fig. 12.1 National Obesity Trends, 2010 (Source: Behavioral risk factor surveillance system, CDC)

Obesity trends* among U.S. adults
BRFSS, 2010
(* BMI ≥ 30, or ~30 lb overweight for 5′ 4″ person)

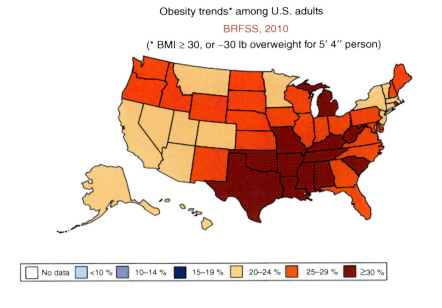

No data | <10 % | 10–14 % | 15–19 % | 20–24 % | 25–29 % | ≥30 %

cardiovascular risk factors including smoking status, diet, physical activity, and alcohol intake [34]. Blood pressure, BMI, and waist circumference should be measured at each visit, occurring at least every 2 years. Screening for hyperglycemia and dyslipidemia should occur according to each patient's risk, at least every 5 years or at 2-year intervals if risk factors are present. These guidelines recommend global risk estimation for CHD risk for all adults over age 40, typically with the FRS.

Novel Risk Factors

Although there are many different markers of inflammation that are associated with CVD risk, high-sensitivity C-reactive Protein (hs-CRP) remains the most powerful predictor of future cardiovascular risk [3, 35–42]. In large prospective cohort studies, higher levels of hs-CRP are associated with increased rates of MI, stroke, and sudden cardiac death [35]. This has led to the recognition that systemic inflammation plays a role in the pathogenesis of cardiovascular disease.

Because of limitations posed by traditional risk prediction models, hs-CRP can be applied for clinical cardiovascular risk assessment in primary prevention. Hs-CRP levels can be categorized into three clinically relevant categories: <1 mg/L as low risk, 1–3 mg/L as intermediate risk, and levels >3 mg/L as high risk for future cardiovascular events. According to a joint statement by the AHA and Centers for Disease Control and Prevention, individuals at intermediate risk by global risk assessment may benefit from measurement of hs-CRP [14]. Measurement of hs-CRP may guide some practitioners to initiate statin therapy after consideration of patient risk. Canadian guidelines similarly recommend screening for hs-CRP measurements for primary prevention of CVD in individuals considered to be of intermediate risk by the FRS [43].

Screening asymptomatic adults for subclinical disease with noninvasive tests such as the ankle-brachial index (ABI), coronary artery calcium (CAC), and carotid artery intima-media thickness (CIMIT) may add incremental value to risk prediction models [32] yet remain controversial as screening tools for asymptomatic adults [44]. According to the American College of Cardiology Foundation (ACCF)/ AHA 2010 guidelines, measurement of CIMIT and ABI may be reasonable for adults at intermediate risk for CHD. Measurement of CAC may be reasonable in intermediate-risk adults and diabetics over 40 years of age [45]. On the other hand, the US Preventive Services Task Force reports insufficient evidence to recommend any of these screening modalities for early identification of atherosclerosis in asymptomatic adults [44].

Management

Ideal Cardiovascular Health

The AHA has defined a goal of "ideal cardiovascular health" that seeks to reduce cardiac and stroke mortality 20 % by 2020 [1]. There are seven health behaviors and factors that define "ideal cardiovascular health"; these include not smoking, BMI <25 kg/m², moderate exercise, a healthy diet, and maintenance of normal values of cholesterol, fasting glucose, and blood pressure (Fig. 12.2). Meeting all seven criteria established by the AHA for optimal CVD health may prevent 59 % of all deaths, 64 % of those from cardiovascular disease, and 63 % of those from ischemic heart disease over a roughly 20-year period [46].

Fig. 12.2 Ideal
cardiovascular health [1]

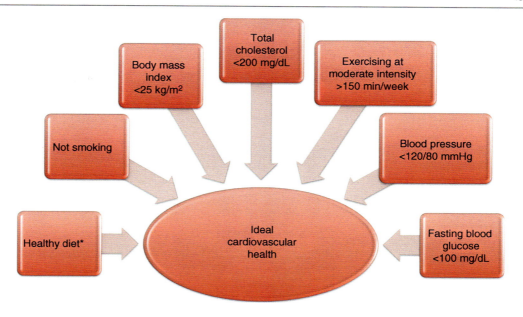

*Healthy diet includes: Sodium <1.5 g/day; sugar sweetened beverages <36 oz/
week; ≥4.5 cups of fruits and vegetables/day; ≥ two 3.5 oz servings of oily fish/week; ≥ three 1 oz
servings of whole grains/day

Risk Factor Management

Smoking

Smoking remains the leading cause of preventable death and disability. All clinicians should regularly screen their patients for smoking status. Based on individual assessment, patients should be given information on smoking cessation services, counseling, and referral to a specialist or pharmacotherapy [34].

Obesity

Obesity portends significant cardiovascular risk both independently and through its effect on several modifiable risk factors including hypertension and the entire spectrum of insulin resistance. Individuals who are overweight should be counseled on physical activity and nutrition programs geared towards caloric restriction. For individuals with morbid obesity (BMI >40 kg/m²), bariatric surgery appears to be a promising solution to reduce overall mortality and concomitant CVD risk factors [47].

Inactivity

The AHA recommends moderate-intensity exercise for 150 min or vigorous-intensity exercise for 75 min a week [1]. Clinicians should counsel their patients on these guidelines and encourage physical activity based on an individual's comorbidities.

Hypertension

The goals of antihypertensive therapy include reducing cardiovascular and renal morbidity and mortality. Most adults with elevated blood pressure benefit from a combination of lifestyle and pharmacologic therapy. The treatment algorithm for the treatment of hypertension according to the Joint National Committee on Prevention, Detection, Evaluation, and Treatment of High Blood Pressure (JNC 7) guidelines is outlined in Table 12.2 [12]. Notably, in the absence of specific indications for other drug classes, thiazide diuretics are recommended as first-line treatment for hypertensive patients. Compelling indications for choosing other drug classes as first-line monotherapy are described in Table 12.3.

Dyslipidemia

A 10 % decrease in total cholesterol is associated with an approximately 10–15 % reduction in CHD mortality [3, 13]. The 3-hydroxy-3-methylglutaryl coenzyme A reductase inhibitors (statins) are the most widely studied lipid-lowering agents and lower LDL cholesterol by approximately 20–50 % while lowering TGs and raising HDL-C to a lesser extent.

Numerous, large, randomized primary prevention trials have shown that statin therapy is effective in lowering CVD events. The West of Scotland Coronary Prevention Study (WOSCOPS) was a randomized, placebo-controlled trial of 6,595 patients with elevated total cholesterol. At 5 years, the pravastatin group had a 29 % reduction in nonfatal MIs

Table 12.2 JNC 7 classification and management of blood pressure

Blood pressure classification	Initial recommended therapy	Second line therapy
Normotensive SBP <120 mmHg DBP <80 mmHg	No therapy	
Prehypertension SBP 130–140 mmHg DBP 80–90 mmHg	Lifestyle modification; consider starting medication if compelling indication	Optimize dosages and/or add additional drug categories Consider consultation with specialist
Stage I hypertension SBP 140–159 mmHg DBP 90–99 mmHg	Thiazide-type diuretics May consider ACE inhibitor, ARB, β(beta)-blocker, and CCB, if compelling indication	

Stage II hypertension
SBP ≥160 mmHg
DBP ≥100 mmHg
	Drug combination
	    Thiazide + ACE inhibitor or ARB
	    Thiazide + β-blocker or CCB	

Adapted from Chobanian et al. [12]

SBP systolic blood pressure, *DBP* diastolic blood pressure, *ACE* angiotensin-converting enzyme, *ARB* angiotensin receptor blocker, *CCB* calcium channel blocker

Table 12.3 Compelling indications for specific antihypertensive drug classes

Indication	Recommended drug classes
Coronary artery disease	Beta-blocker, diuretic, ACE inhibitors, CCB
Diabetes mellitus	Diuretic, B-blocker, ACE inhibitor, ARB, CCB
Chronic kidney disease	ACE inhibitor, ARB
Heart failure	Diuretic, beta-blocker, ACE inhibitor, ARB, aldosterone antagonist
Post-myocardial infarction	Beta-blocker, ACE inhibitor, aldosterone antagonist
Poststroke prevention	Diuretic, ACE inhibitor

ACE angiotensin-converting enzyme, *ARB* angiotensin receptor blocker, *CCB* calcium channel blocker

($p<0.001$) [48]. Similarly, the Air Force/Texas Coronary Atherosclerosis Prevention Study (AFCAPS/TexCAPS) showed that for men and women with below average cholesterol, lovastatin reduced the risk for acute major coronary events by 37 % [49]. The atorvastatin versus placebo arm of the Anglo-Scandinavian Cardiac Outcomes Trial (ASCOT) also showed that the atorvastatin group had a significant reduction in nonfatal MI in hypertensive patients with normal cholesterol levels and was terminated prematurely given this significant benefit [50].

More recently, the Collaborative Atorvastatin Diabetes Study (CARDS) enrolled patients with Type 2 diabetes and randomized them to a low dose of atorvastatin or placebo [51]. The trial was terminated early due to a 37 % reduction in the primary endpoint of cardiovascular events in patients randomized to receive atorvastatin.

Prior studies have demonstrated that pharmacological reduction of TG levels may substantially reduce CVD events [18, 19]. However, the highly publicized AIM-HIGH trial demonstrated the lack of mortality benefit of elevating serum HDL levels and lowering TGs with high-dose niacin for patients already on statin therapy [52].

Statins

The Justification for the Use of Statins in Prevention: An Intervention Evaluating Rosuvastatin (JUPITER) trial investigated the effects of rosuvastatin in primary prevention of CVD [53]. The study enrolled 18,000 adults (men ≥50 years of age and women ≥60) with LDL cholesterol levels <130 mg/dL and high-sensitivity CRP levels >2.0 mg/dL and randomized them to 20 mg of rosuvastatin or placebo. The study found a 44 % reduction in cardiovascular events in the treatment group, independent of effects on LDL-C. Risk reductions with statins have proved similar for members of racial and ethnic minority groups [39]. This suggests that statins have additional benefits, independent of LDL lowering, in reducing CVD risk.

Diabetes Mellitus

In a large randomized multicenter trial, intensive glycemic control (HgA1c <6 %) did not improve mortality, likely due to more episodes of hypoglycemia [54]. Current guidelines suggest targeting glucose levels in diabetics to a HgA1c <7 % with fasting plasma glucose levels <110 mg/dL and more stringent control of concomitant risk factors of hypertension and dyslipidemia. Blood pressure goals for diabetics are <130/80 mmHg and LDL-C goal of <100 mg/dL [34].

Other Pharmacological Agents

Aspirin irreversibly inhibits platelet-dependent enzyme cyclooxygenase (COX), thus inhibiting the synthesis of prostaglandins. Platelet activation and aggregation is thought to play a critical role in onset of MI and stroke. Antiplatelet therapy plays a key role in the treatment and prevention of CVD. Aspirin may be used for primary prevention but the balance between benefits and risks of bleeding must be carefully considered. The Antithrombotic Trialists' (ATT) Collaboration conducted a meta-analysis and found that the use of aspirin resulted in a 12 % reduction in composite vascular events with a concomitant increase in risk of gastrointestinal side effects and extracranial bleeds [55]. Low-dose aspirin is therefore recommended for moderate- and high-risk patients, particularly in those with a 10-year CHD risk ≥10 %, after consideration of bleeding risks.

Individual Versus Population Risk

The Polypill

The current medical paradigm focuses on identifying high-risk individuals and treating their individual risk factors. Population-based approaches, on the other hand, seek to control risk in a large number of people, resulting in an overall larger scale success for society and an overall smaller individual benefit. This approach was popularized by epidemiologist Geoffrey Rose who suggested that a population-based approach might result in the greatest reduction in risk by shifting the population distribution towards greater overall health [56].

Similarly, Wald and colleagues have applied this same reasoning towards the concept of the "polypill," which combines medications to lower lipids and blood pressure, yielding an estimated 80 % reduction in overall CVD risk [57]. Currently, clinical trials with polypills are ongoing in the developing world. The double-blinded Indian Polycap Study (TIPS) showed that a combination pill could significantly reduce blood pressure and LDL-C in middle-aged adults without preexisting CVD [58]. Similarly, a feasibility study of a polypill containing aspirin, simvastatin, lisinopril, and hydrochlorothiazide has already been conducted in Sri Lanka and shows high acceptability among patients and physicians [59].

Population-Based Approach for CVD Prevention

Numerous trials have shown the benefit of pharmacological treatment of CVD risk factors including dyslipidemia and hypertension. However, the majority of CVD events occur in the population with average or mildly elevated risk. Therefore, population strategies are necessary to complement our current medical model of high-risk strategies, which target high-risk individuals, while ignoring most of the truly "at-risk" population [60]. Implementing primordial prevention at the societal level includes policies and regulations that optimize an individual's environment to promote CVD health. For example, raising tobacco excise taxes, reducing sodium in the food supply, and promoting an environment that allows for physical activity throughout the day can all have a remarkable impact on a large segment of the population [52]. National policy initiatives are ongoing to create healthier communities, worksites, and schools [61].

Key Points

- Cardiovascular disease (CVD) represents the number 1 cause of morbidity and mortality in the United States and is largely preventable through lifestyle modification and control of CVD risk factors.
- Risk factors may be used in risk assessment to predict future cardiovascular events and serve as key targets for interventions to lower CVD risk.
- Non-modifiable risk factors include age, gender, and family history. Modifiable risk factors include smoking, obesity, inactivity, dyslipidemia, hypertension, and diabetes.
- The Framingham Risk Score uses age, sex, total cholesterol, high-density lipoprotein, blood pressure, and cigarette smoking to predict the 10-year risk for coronary heart disease.
- Novel cardiovascular risk factors such as high-sensitivity C-reactive protein (hs-CRP) may be used to guide clinical therapy when patients are considered intermediate risk by traditional screening methods.
- In addition to targeting high-risk individuals, population-based approaches targeting healthier choices are essential to shift the population distribution towards greater CVD health.

Summary of AHA Guidelines

See Table 12.4.

Table 12.4 Summary of AHA guidelines for the primary prevention of cardiovascular disease [34]

Risk factor	Recommendations
Smoking	Providers should ask about tobacco use at each visit
	Assist by counseling and developing a plan for quitting
	Urge avoidance of secondhand smoke exposure
Blood pressure control	Recommend lifestyle modifications such as weight reduction and reduction of sodium intake
	Initiate drug therapy for patient with comorbid conditions (i.e., heart failure or diabetes) if BP is ≥130/80 mmHg
	Initiate drug therapy if lifestyle interventions fail after 6–12 months for patients with BP ≥140/90 mmHg
Aspirin therapy	Consider initiation of low-dose aspirin in persons with a 10-year risk of CHD ≥10 % after consideration of bleeding risks
Lipid management	If LDL-C is above goal, initiate dietary modifications
	Emphasize weight reduction and physical activity
	Initiate statin therapy if:
	≥2 CHD risk factors and LDL-C is ≥130 mg/dL or
	≥1 risk factor and LDL-C is 160 mg/dL or
	LDL-C >190 mg/dL without any risk factors
Physical activity	Recommend at least 30 min of moderate-intensity physical activity on most days
Weight management	BMI goal <25 kg/m²
	If the patient is obese, recommend reduction of body weight by 10 % each year
Diabetes management	Initiate appropriate therapy to achieve HgA1c <7 % and fasting glucose <110 mg/dL
	Treat other risk factors aggressively
	BP goal <130/80 mmHg
	LDL-C goal <100 mg/dL

BP blood pressure, *CHD* coronary heart disease, *LDL-C* low-density lipoprotein cholesterol, *BMI* body mass index, *HgA1c* hemoglobin A1c

References

1. Roger VL, Go AS, Lloyd-Jones DM, et al. Heart disease and stroke statistics – 2012 update: a report from the American Heart Association. Circulation. 2012;125(1):e2–220.
2. Weintraub WS, Daniels SR, Burke LE, et al. Value of primordial and primary prevention for cardiovascular disease: a policy statement from the American Heart Association. Circulation. 2011;124(8):967–90.
3. Kones R. Primary prevention of coronary heart disease: integration of new data, evolving views, revised goals, and role of rosuvastatin in management. A comprehensive survey. Drug Des Devel Ther. 2011;5:325–80.
4. Yusuf S, Hawken S, Ounpuu S, et al. Effect of potentially modifiable risk factors associated with myocardial infarction in 52 countries (the interheart study): case-control study. Lancet. 2004;364(9438):937–52.
5. Kannel WB, McGee D, Gordon T. A general cardiovascular risk profile: the Framingham study. Am J Cardiol. 1976;38(1):46–51.
6. Wilson PW, D'Agostino RB, Levy D, et al. Prediction of coronary heart disease using risk factor categories. Circulation. 1998;97(18):1837–47.
7. Kahn R, Robertson RM, Smith R, Eddy D. The impact of prevention on reducing the burden of cardiovascular disease. Circulation. 2008;118(5):576–85.
8. Heron M. Deaths: leading causes for 2007. Natl Vital Stat Rep. 2011;59(8):1–95.
9. Wissler RW. USA multicenter study of the pathobiology of atherosclerosis in youth. Ann N Y Acad Sci. 1991;623:26–39.
10. Jarvie JL, Foody JM. Recognizing and improving health care disparities in the prevention of cardiovascular disease in women. Curr Cardiol Rep. 2010;12(6):488–96.
11. Andresdottir MB, Sigurdsson G, Sigvaldason H, Gudnason V. Fifteen percent of myocardial infarctions and coronary revascularizations explained by family history unrelated to conventional risk factors. The Reykjavik cohort study. Eur Heart J. 2002;23(21):1655–63.
12. Chobanian AV, Bakris GL, Black HR, et al. The seventh report of the joint national committee on prevention, detection, evaluation, and treatment of high blood pressure: the JNC7 report. JAMA. 2003;289(19):2560–72.
13. Mills EJ, Rachlis B, Wu P, et al. Primary prevention of cardiovascular mortality and events with statin treatments: a network meta-analysis involving more than 65,000 patients. J Am Coll Cardiol. 2008;52(22):1769–81.
14. U.S. Preventive Services Task Force. Using nontraditional risk factors in coronary heart disease risk assessment: U.S. preventive services task force recommendation statement. Ann Intern Med. 2009;151(7):474–82.
15. Navab M, Reddy ST, Van Lenten BJ, Fogelman AM. Hdl and cardiovascular disease: atherogenic and atheroprotective mechanisms. Nat Rev Cardiol. 2011;8(4):222–32.
16. Nicholls SJ, Tuzcu EM, Sipahi I, et al. Statins, high-density lipoprotein cholesterol, and regression of coronary atherosclerosis. JAMA. 2007;297(5):499–508.
17. Gordon DJ, Probstfield JL, Garrison RJ, et al. High-density lipoprotein cholesterol and cardiovascular disease. Four prospective American studies. Circulation. 1989;79(1):8–15.
18. Frick MH, Elo O, Haapa K, et al. Helsinki heart study: primary-prevention trial with gemfibrozil in middle-aged men with dyslipidemia. Safety of treatment, changes in risk factors, and incidence of coronary heart disease. N Engl J Med. 1987;317(20):1237–45.
19. Jeppesen J, Hein HO, Suadicani P, Gyntelberg F. Triglyceride concentration and ischemic heart disease: an eight-year follow-up in the Copenhagen male study. Circulation. 1998;97(11):1029–36.
20. Bansal S, Buring JE, Rifai N, et al. Fasting compared with nonfasting triglycerides and risk of cardiovascular events in women. JAMA. 2007;298(3):309–16.
21. Mora S, Rifai N, Buring JE, Ridker PM. Fasting compared with nonfasting lipids and apolipoproteins for predicting incident cardiovascular events. Circulation. 2008;118(10):993–1001.
22. Willett WC, Green A, Stampfer MJ, et al. Relative and absolute excess risks of coronary heart disease among women who smoke cigarettes. N Engl J Med. 1987;317(21):1303–9.
23. He J, Vupputuri S, Allen K, et al. Passive smoking and the risk of coronary heart disease – a meta-analysis of epidemiologic studies. N Engl J Med. 1999;340(12):920–6.

24. Rosenberg L, Kaufman DW, Helmrich SP, Shapiro S. The risk of myocardial infarction after quitting smoking in men under 55 years of age. N Engl J Med. 1985;313(24):1511–4.

25. Kawachi I, Colditz GA, Stampfer MJ, et al. Smoking cessation and time course of decreased risks of coronary heart disease in middle-aged women. Arch Intern Med. 1994;154(2):169–75.

26. Haffner SM, Lehto S, Ronnemaa T, Pyorala K, Laakso M. Mortality from coronary heart disease in subjects with type 2 diabetes and in nondiabetic subjects with and without prior myocardial infarction. N Engl J Med. 1998;339(4):229–34.

27. Almdal T, Scharling H, Jensen JS, Vestergaard H. The independent effect of type 2 diabetes mellitus on ischemic heart disease, stroke, and death: a population-based study of 13,000 men and women with 20 years of follow-up. Arch Intern Med. 2004; 164(13):1422–6.

28. Expert Panel on Detection, Evaluation, and Treatment of High Blood Cholesterol in Adults. Executive summary of the third report of the national cholesterol education program (NCEP) expert panel on detection, evaluation, and treatment of high blood cholesterol in adults (adult treatment panel III). JAMA. 2001;285(19):2486–97.

29. Bogers RP, Bemelmans WJ, Hoogenveen RT, et al. Association of overweight with increased risk of coronary heart disease partly independent of blood pressure and cholesterol levels: a meta-analysis of 21 cohort studies including more than 300,000 persons. Arch Intern Med. 2007;167(16):1720–8.

30. D'Agostino Sr RB, Grundy S, Sullivan LM, Wilson P. Validation of the Framingham coronary heart disease prediction scores: results of a multiple ethnic groups investigation. JAMA. 2001; 286(2):180–7.

31. Hurley LP, Dickinson LM, Estacio RO, Steiner JF, Havranek EP. Prediction of cardiovascular death in racial/ethnic minorities using Framingham risk factors. Circ Cardiovasc Qual Outcomes. 2010; 3(2):181–7.

32. Berger JS, Jordan CO, Lloyd-Jones D, Blumenthal RS. Screening for cardiovascular risk in asymptomatic patients. J Am Coll Cardiol. 2010;55(12):1169–77.

33. Ridker PM, Buring JE, Rifai N, Cook NR. Development and validation of improved algorithms for the assessment of global cardiovascular risk in women: the Reynolds risk score. JAMA. 2007;297(6):611–9.

34. Pearson TA, Blair SN, Daniels SR, et al. Aha guidelines for primary prevention of cardiovascular disease and stroke: 2002 update: consensus panel guide to comprehensive risk reduction for adult patients without coronary or other atherosclerotic vascular diseases. American Heart Association Science Advisory and Coordinating Committee. Circulation. 2002;106(3):388–91.

35. Buckley DI, Fu R, Freeman M, Rogers K, Helfand M. C-reactive protein as a risk factor for coronary heart disease: a systematic review and meta-analyses for the U.S. Preventive Services Task Force. Ann Intern Med. 2009;151(7):483–95.

36. Calabro P, Willerson JT, Yeh ET. Inflammatory cytokines stimulated C-reactive protein production by human coronary artery smooth muscle cells. Circulation. 2003;108(16):1930–2.

37. Ridker PM. C-reactive protein and the prediction of cardiovascular events among those at intermediate risk: moving an inflammatory hypothesis toward consensus. J Am Coll Cardiol. 2007;49(21):2129–38.

38. Ridker PM, MacFadyen J, Libby P, Glynn RJ. Relation of baseline high-sensitivity C-reactive protein level to cardiovascular outcomes with rosuvastatin in the justification for use of statins in prevention: an intervention trial evaluating rosuvastatin (Jupiter). Am J Cardiol. 2010;106(2):204–9.

39. Albert MA, Glynn RJ, Fonseca FA, et al. Race, ethnicity, and the efficacy of rosuvastatin in primary prevention: the justification for the use of statins in prevention: an intervention trial evaluating rosuvastatin (Jupiter) trial. Am Heart J. 2011;162(1):106–14. e102.

40. Ridker PM. Clinical application of C-reactive protein for cardiovascular disease detection and prevention. Circulation. 2003; 107(3):363–9.

41. Ridker PM, Bassuk SS, Toth PP. C-reactive protein and risk of cardiovascular disease: evidence and clinical application. Curr Atheroscler Rep. 2003;5(5):341–9.

42. Ridker PM, Stampfer MJ, Rifai N. Novel risk factors for systemic atherosclerosis: a comparison of C-reactive protein, fibrinogen, homocysteine, lipoprotein(a), and standard cholesterol screening as predictors of peripheral arterial disease. JAMA. 2001; 285(19):2481–5.

43. Genest J, McPherson R, Frohlich J, et al. 2009 Canadian Cardiovascular Society/Canadian guidelines for the diagnosis and treatment of dyslipidemia and prevention of cardiovascular disease in the adult – 2009 recommendations. Can J Cardiol. 2009; 25(10):567–79.

44. Rodondi N, Auer R, de Bosset Sulzer V, Ghali WA, Cornuz J. Atherosclerosis screening by noninvasive imaging for cardiovascular prevention: a systematic review. J Gen Intern Med. 2012; 27(2):220–31.

45. Greenland P, Alpert JS, Beller GA, et al. 2010 ACCF/AHA guideline for assessment of cardiovascular risk in asymptomatic adults: a report of the American College of Cardiology Foundation/American Heart Association Task Force on practice guidelines. Circulation. 2010;122(25):e584–636.

46. Yang Q, Cogswell ME, Flanders WD, et al. Trends in cardiovascular health metrics and associations with all-cause and CVD mortality among US adults. JAMA. 2012;307(12):1273–83.

47. Sjostrom L, Narbro K, Sjostrom CD, et al. Effects of bariatric surgery on mortality in Swedish obese subjects. N Engl J Med. 2007;357(8):741–52.

48. Shepherd J, Cobbe SM, Ford I, et al. Prevention of coronary heart disease with pravastatin in men with hypercholesterolemia. West of Scotland coronary prevention study group. N Engl J Med. 1995;333(20):1301–7.

49. Downs JR, Clearfield M, Weis S, et al. Primary prevention of acute coronary events with lovastatin in men and women with average cholesterol levels: results of AFCAPS/TexCAPS. Air force/Texas coronary atherosclerosis prevention study. JAMA. 1998; 279(20):1615–22.

50. Sever PS, Dahlof B, Poulter NR, et al. Prevention of coronary and stroke events with atorvastatin in hypertensive patients who have average or lower-than-average cholesterol concentrations, in the Anglo-Scandinavian cardiac outcomes trial – lipid lowering arm (ASCOT-LLA): a multicentre randomised controlled trial. Lancet. 2003;361(9364):1149–58.

51. Colhoun HM, Betteridge DJ, Durrington PN, et al. Primary prevention of cardiovascular disease with atorvastatin in type 2 diabetes in the collaborative atorvastatin diabetes study (CARDS): multicentre randomised placebo-controlled trial. Lancet. 2004;364(9435):685–96.

52. Boden WE, Probstfield JL, Anderson T, et al. Niacin in patients with low HDL cholesterol levels receiving intensive statin therapy. N Engl J Med. 2011;365(24):2255–67.

53. Ridker PM, Danielson E, Fonseca FA, et al. Rosuvastatin to prevent vascular events in men and women with elevated C-reactive protein. N Engl J Med. 2008;359(21):2195–207.

54. Gerstein HC, Miller ME, Byington RP, et al. Effects of intensive glucose lowering in type 2 diabetes. N Engl J Med. 2008; 358(24):2545–59.

55. Baigent C, Blackwell L, Collins R, et al. Aspirin in the primary and secondary prevention of vascular disease: collaborative meta-analysis of individual participant data from randomised trials. Lancet. 2009;373(9678):1849–60.

56. Rose G. Sick individuals and sick populations. Int J Epidemiol. 1985;14(1):32–8.

57. Wald NJ, Law MR. A strategy to reduce cardiovascular disease by more than 80%. BMJ. 2003;326(7404):1419.

58. Yusuf S, Pais P, Afzal R, et al. Effects of a polypill (polycap) on risk factors in middle-aged individuals without cardiovascular disease (tips): a phase II, double-blind, randomised trial. Lancet. 2009; 373(9672):1341–51.

59. Soliman EZ, Mendis S, Dissanayake WP, et al. A polypill for primary prevention of cardiovascular disease: a feasibility study of the World Health Organization. Trials. 2011;12:3.

60. Lloyd-Jones DM. Improving the cardiovascular health of the us population. JAMA. 2012;307(12):1314–6.

61. Frieden TR, Berwick DM. The "million hearts" initiative – preventing heart attacks and strokes. N Engl J Med. 2011; 365(13):e27.

The Role of Cardiovascular Nuclear Imaging in Clinical Consultation

Judith L. Meadows and Robert Soufer

Abstract

The ability of nuclear cardiology techniques to assess myocardial perfusion is vital in the cardiology consultants' evaluation of patients with suspected or known coronary artery disease. This chapter will begin with a description of the physiologic principles underlying perfusion imaging. With this intellectual framework, the consultant can employ nuclear cardiology techniques to assist in the diagnosis of coronary artery disease, to assess cardiovascular prognosis and risk stratification, and to guide medical and revascularization strategies in the management of coronary artery disease. This chapter concludes with an overview of the performance of nuclear cardiology tests.

Keywords

Myocardial perfusion imaging (MPI) • Single photon emission computed tomography (SPECT) • Positron emission tomography (PET) • Exercise stress test • Vasodilator stress test • Bayes theorem

Abbreviations

3VD	Three-vessel coronary disease
ACS	Acute coronary syndrome
CAD	Coronary artery disease
CFR	Coronary flow reserve
DSE	Dobutamine stress echocardiogram
FFR	Fractional flow reserve
LAD	Left anterior descending coronary artery
LCx	Left circumflex coronary artery
LHR	Lung-to-heart ratio
LM	Left main
MPI	Myocardial perfusion imaging
MSI	Mental stress ischemia
NPV	Negative predictive value
PET	Positron emission tomography
PPV	Positive predictive value
RCA	Right coronary artery
SPECT	Single photon emission computed tomography
TID	Transient ischemic dilation

J.L. Meadows, MD, MPH (✉) • R. Soufer, MD
Department of Internal Medicine/Cardiology,
Yale School of Medicine, Yale University/VACT
Healthcare System, 111B, 950 Campbell Avenue,
West Haven, CT 06516, USA
e-mail: judith.meadows@yale.edu; robert.soufer@yale.edu

Introduction

In a 1998 American College of Cardiology/American Heart Association (ACC/AHA) meeting on Practice Guidelines and Quality of Care, the task force referred back to Hippocratic writings from 400 B.C.:

> If a physician finds himself in difficulties on occasion over a patient … he should urge the calling in of others, in order to learn by consultation the truth about the case. … For when a diseased condition is stubborn … one must not be self-confident … it is no mistaken idea to call in a consultant [1].

As such, our modern cardiology consultant must assist in the cardiovascular decision making for patients who have multiple comorbidities with competing medical needs.

An effective cardiology consultant employs diagnostic testing to support decision making and to guide management. Each cardiovascular diagnostic test answers particular clinical questions, is associated with a ratio of risks and benefits, and must be interpreted in the context of the consultant's assessment of the likelihood of having disease. This chapter will begin with a description of the physiologic principles underlying perfusion imaging, followed by a discussion of the clinical questions addressed by nuclear cardiology and an overview of the performance of nuclear cardiology tests.

A Brief History of Nuclear Cardiology

Noninvasive cardiovascular imaging began in the 1970s with the advent of thallium (Tl)-201 planar imaging to image resting coronary blood flow [2]. The rapid evolution of modern cardiology has been inspired by a desire to directly visualize disease in the heart. The early nuclear cardiology experiments were performed at the bedside to understand the concepts of resting blood flow and blood flow during chest pain in patients hospitalized in the intensive care unit with chest discomfort [3].

The diagnostic accuracy of nuclear cardiology has advanced with the use of 3-dimensional (3D) single photon emission computed tomography (SPECT) and positron emission tomography (PET) imaging, gated imaging, and the recent introduction of solid-state cameras. In the past few years, solid-state detector cameras using cadmium zinc telluride have been introduced which has improved spatial resolution (4.3–4.9 mm vs. 9–11 mm), increased count detection, and allowed for more rapid imaging acquisition (5–6 min vs. 14–15 min) as compared to traditional SPECT cameras.

In the decade prior to the advent of nuclear cardiology, coronary angiography was developed to visualize coronary anatomy. What followed was the central dogma that (1) more severe stenoses result in worse angina and (2) a higher number of stenoses translate into a greater risk of myocardial damage. While intuitive, this framework cannot explain why there might be asymptomatic patients who have multiple significant stenoses on angiogram and why a patient might present with acute vessel occlusion in the absence of a history of significant angina. These discrepancies make clear that the functional significance of any given coronary stenosis lies in the complementary relationship of anatomy (coronary) with physiology (stress MPI and stress echocardiography). Nuclear cardiology techniques are therefore indispensible for the evaluation of ischemic coronary artery disease (CAD).

Physiology of Stress Myocardial Perfusion Imaging

Myocardial perfusion imaging (MPI) is a powerful noninvasive tool to assess myocardial perfusion and myocardial cell function. In a resting heart without significant

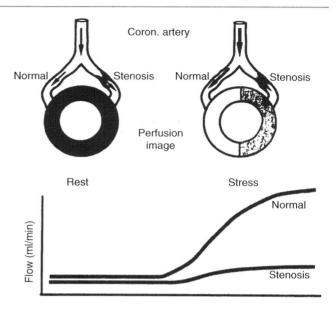

Fig. 13.1 Coronary perfusion. Schematic representation of the principle of rest/stress myocardial perfusion imaging. (*Top*) two branches of a coronary artery are shown; one is normal (*left*) and one has a significant stenosis (*right*). (*Middle*) myocardial perfusion images of the territories supplied by the two branches. (*Bottom*) schematic representation of coronary blood flow in the branches at rest and during stress. At rest, myocardial blood flow is equal in the two branches. When myocardial radiotracer is injected at rest, uptake is homogenous (normal image). During exercise stress, coronary blood flow increases 2.0–2.5 times in the normal branch, but not to the same extent in the stenosed branch, resulting in heterogeneous distribution of blood flow (abnormal image with a myocardial perfusion defect) [3]

coronary stenosis, there is homogenous uptake of the nuclear tracer in all segments of the myocardium, reflective of normal perfusion. Normal coronary perfusion is 1–2 cc/kg/min.

Under stress conditions, normal coronary arteries dilate to accommodate an increase in blood flow. Exercise induces hyperemia and increases coronary blood flow by 2–2.5 times above baseline levels. Under vasodilator stress, with adenosine or dipyridamole, the epicardial coronary vessels dilate to accommodate an increase in flow four to five times above resting values. In the absence of coronary artery stenosis, stressors will increase coronary blood flow equally in all coronary vascular territories. The stress perfusion images of the myocardium will continue to have a homogenous appearance.

This augmented coronary flow in response to a stressor is called coronary flow reserve (CFR) [4]. CFR is defined as the ratio of maximum coronary blood flow under stress conditions to coronary blood flow at rest (Fig. 13.1).

Clinical evaluation of the relevance of a particular coronary artery stenosis deemed to be critical often reflects the competency of autoregulatory mechanisms, which includes post-stenotic dilation of the microvascular system. This results in a lowered distal microvascular resistance in the presence of a severe stenosis, which promotes an increase in regional blood flow and volume. The inability of a particular vascular bed in the presence of a suspected critical epicardial stenosis to increase flow to a myocardial stressor reflects the functional significance of that particular stenosis.

The reduced distal arterial perfusion pressure allows maintenance of normal *resting* blood flow. In the presence of a >50 % luminal narrowing in an epicardial coronary artery, there may be adequate blood flow in resting conditions due to distal microvasculature dilation. Under stress, however, there is a failure to augment coronary flow since the distal vasculature may already be maximally dilated. The myocardium subtended by the stenotic coronary artery may receive relatively less coronary blood flow when compared to a myocardial wall that is supplied by a non-stenotic vessel. Clinically we term the latter as "blunted CFR." The myocardium supplied by the stenotic coronary artery will appear less bright than the myocardium supplied by the normal coronary artery. CFR decreases as severity of stenosis increases.

Ischemia is represented by a decrease in tracer activity under stress conditions, which is seen in a coronary territory that appeared normal under rest conditions. This is called a reversible perfusion defect (Fig. 13.2). On the other hand, a fixed defect represents an infarction or scar. The stress images will demonstrate heterogeneous tracer activity, which will appear unchanged on rest imaging (Fig. 13.3). Resting coronary blood flow is not altered until there is at least an 85 % luminal narrowing [5].

As a corollary to CFR, there are invasive physiologic techniques to measure both (1) blood velocity and (2) pressure drop across a stenosis. In the more common of the two techniques, an intracoronary pressure wire is employed to record the pressure drop across a stenosis. The ratio between the pressures distal to a stenosis in relation to the pressure proximal to a stenosis is expressed as fractional flow reserve (FFR). The FFR is measured at rest and after maximal hyperemia, as induced by adenosine. Studies have demonstrated the CFR reduction and FFR reduction are linearly related to each other, and both are related to the severity of narrowing on conventional angiography [6]. In another study, CFR and FFR measurements were divergent in over 10 % of mid-LAD lesions [7]. It was hypothesized that FFR captured the focal effect of a single stenosis, while CFR was a global assessment of disease along the entire artery.

In the current practice of clinical nuclear cardiology, absolute coronary blood flow is not measured in SPECT studies. Instead, we qualitatively or semiquantitatively assess for heterogeneity in the myocardial images. Regardless, we continue to use CFR as a construct to understand heterogeneity in scintigraphic activity. PET MPI allows for quantification of absolute blood flow and calculation of CFR. The use of CFR in PET is well described in the literature and will likely become a clinical tool in the future [8]. It offers promise for evaluation of microvascular disease and assessment of multivessel CAD.

Image Interpretation

Perfusion images may be interpreted qualitatively, semiquantitatively, or through the use of computer-aided quantitative analysis. All three approaches have been compared to coronary angiography, which is the current gold standard for identification of CAD. One must recognize that coronary angiography is an anatomic assessment of a stenosis. In comparison, MPI offers noninvasive assessment of the physiologic significance of a coronary plaque. MPI can identify perfusion defects, localize the ischemia, and assess the severity in flow limitation and the amount of jeopardized myocardium [9].

Perfusion defects are described in terms of location, size, severity, reversibility, and coronary artery disease pattern [10] (Table 13.1). The location of the defect is described using a standardized 17-segment model, similar to what is used in the other cardiac imaging modalities. In addition, other image features will be described: left ventricular size, right ventricular size, ratio of lung uptake to heart uptake (LHR), transient ischemic dilation (TID), and extra-cardiac tracer uptake.

Semiquantitative scoring of perfusion is expressed as sum stress score (SSS), sum rest score (SRS), and a sum difference score (SDS). In SPECT imaging, the SSS grading system of perfusion defects is normal <4, mildly abnormal 4–8, moderately abnormal 9–13, and severely abnormal ≥14. Automated programs can also score a % stress perfusion defect, % rest perfusion defect, and % reversibility.

In clinical practice, it is not uncommon that coronary angiography fails to identify a significant coronary stenosis to explain heterogeneity in perfusion seen on MPI. This has been described in the literature in settings of endothelial dysfunction, diffuse noncritical disease, and other myopathic processes beyond CAD (Fig. 13.4).

Role of Nuclear Cardiology to Address Clinical Questions

Nuclear cardiology techniques are employed to assess myocardial blood flow, myocardial metabolism, and ventricular function. As such, the cardiology consultant will utilize the tools of nuclear cardiology to aid in answering questions of:
1. Diagnosis
   - To investigate the presence of CAD in a patient suspected of having CAD based upon symptoms and with an intermediate pretest probability of CAD
   - To detect preclinical disease in the asymptomatic patient
   - To evaluate for an underlying ischemic etiology in a patient with systolic dysfunction/cardiomyopathy

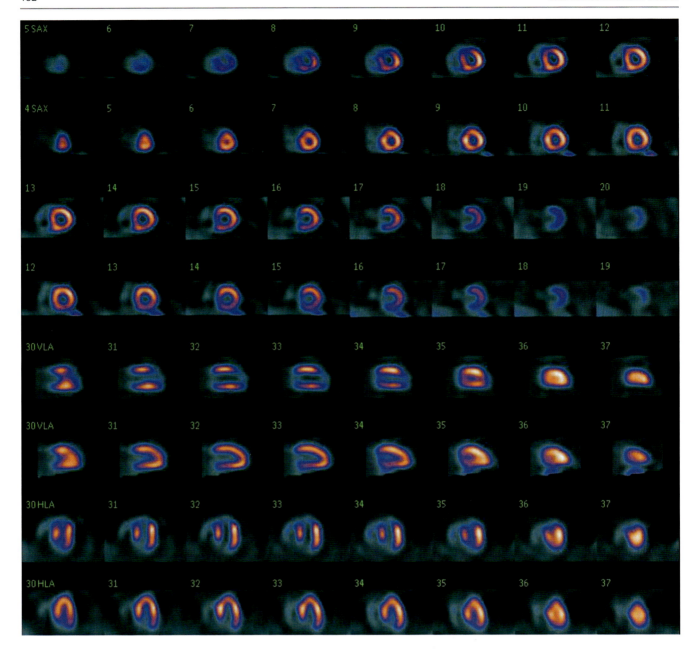

Fig. 13.2 SPECT ischemia, reversible defect. A 61-year-old male with a history of hypertension and dyslipidemia who presented with exertional chest discomfort. He exercised on a modified Bruce protocol for 8 min achieving an estimated workload of 7 METs and a peak heart rate of 101 % of maximum predicted heart rate for age. He had a normal blood pressure response to exercise. His exercise ECG demonstrated 1.5 mm upsloping ST segment depressions in the inferior and lateral leads, along with 1.5 mm ST segment elevation in leads V1 and aVR. He developed chest pain at 4 min into exercise, which resolved by 4 min into recovery. He underwent a same day imaging protocol, with 10.7 mCi of 99m-Tc at rest followed by injection of 29.4 mCi of 99m-Tc at peak stress. Perfusion imaging is displayed in oblique slices. Short axis slices (*rows 1–4*) are displayed from apex to base, with the stress images above and the rest images below. Vertical long axis slices (*rows 5–6*) display the anterior and inferior walls, from the septum to lateral wall. Horizontal long axis slices (*rows 7–8*) display the septal and lateral walls, from inferior to anterior aspects of the left ventricle. There is a large area of severely decreased scintigraphic activity in the mid-anterior wall, all 4 apical segments, and the true apex, which is seen on the stress images and completely improves on the rest images. This is suggestive of ischemia in the left anterior descending coronary artery territory. There is also evidence of transient ischemic dilation (TID ratio 1.24)

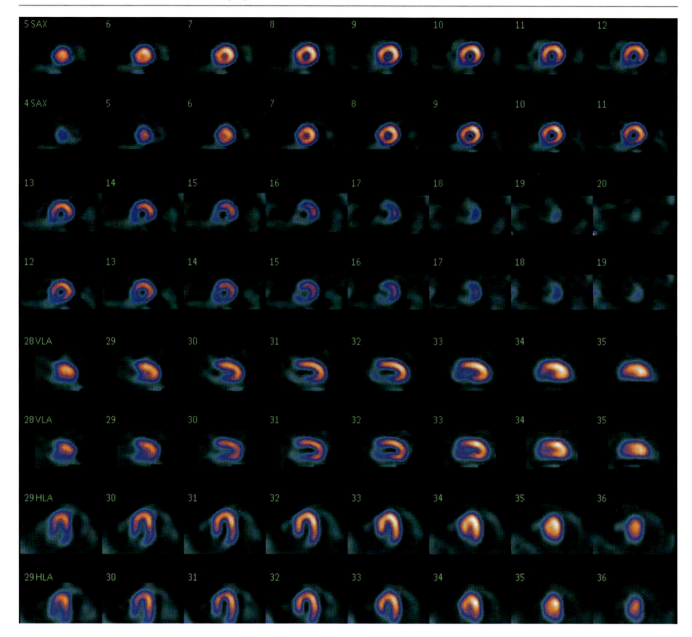

Fig. 13.3 SPECT infarction, fixed defect. A 78-year-old male with abdominal aortic aneurysm, dyslipidemia, and obstructive sleep apnea who presented with complaint of shortness of breath. He exercised on a Bruce protocol for 5 min. He achieved an estimated workload of 6 METs and a peak heart rate of 85 % of maximum predicted heart rate for age. His blood pressure response to exercise was blunted. His exercise ECG demonstrated 2 mm horizontal ST segment depressions in the inferior and lateral leads, along with 1.5 mm ST segment elevation in leads V1 and aVR. Exercise was terminated for shortness of breath. He underwent a same day imaging protocol, with 11.9 mCi of 99m-Tc at rest followed by injection of 32 mCi of 99m-Tc at peak stress. Perfusion imaging is displayed in oblique slices. There is a large area of moderately decreased scintigraphic activity in the entire inferior wall and basal to mid-inferolateral wall, which is seen on stress images and only partially improves on rest images. This is suggestive of infarct in the right coronary artery territory, along with mild peri-infarct ischemia. The gated images demonstrated inferior wall hypokinesis

Table 13.1 Semiquantitative scoring and quantitative scoring. Image interpretation involves a description of (**A**) location of perfusion defect by 17-segment model and coronary artery distribution, (**B**) size of perfusion defect as described quantitatively (% of myocardium) or semiquantitatively (number of myocardial segments), (**C**) severity of perfusion defect, and (**D**) reversibility of the perfusion defect and (**E**) by semiquantitative scoring of perfusion with summation of number of segments and severity score for each segment [10]

A. Location of perfusion defect

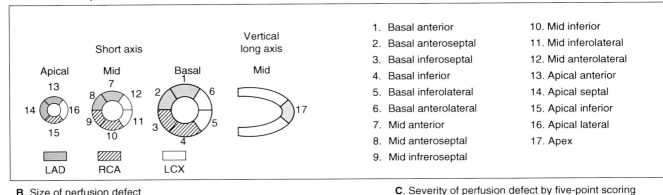

1. Basal anterior
2. Basal anteroseptal
3. Basal inferoseptal
4. Basal inferior
5. Basal inferolateral
6. Basal anterolateral
7. Mid anterior
8. Mid anteroseptal
9. Mid infreroseptal
10. Mid inferior
11. Mid inferolateral
12. Mid anterolateral
13. Apical anterior
14. Apical septal
15. Apical inferior
16. Apical lateral
17. Apex

B. Size of perfusion defect

Small	Medium	Large
< 10 % myocardium	10–20 % myocardium	>20 % myocardium
1–2 segments	3–4 segments	>4 segments

C. Severity of perfusion defect by five-point scoring

Severity	Score
Normal perfusion	0
Mild reduction in counts (not definitely abnormal)	1
Moderate reduction in counts (definitely abnormal)	2
Severe reduction in counts	3
Absent uptake	4

D. Reversibility of perfusion defect and clinical correlate

Reversible	Ischemia
Persistent/fixed	Infarction/scar
Mixed	Scar with peri-infarct ischemia

E. Semi-quantitative scoring of perfusion

Sum rest score (SRS): infarction
Sum stress score (SSS): ischemia + infarction
Sum difference score (SDS) = SRS–SSS = ischemia

2. Prognosis
   - Risk stratification in patients with established CAD (chronic ischemic disease)
   - In the setting of a normal MPI
   - Preoperative risk stratification prior to noncardiac surgery
   - Risk stratification following acute coronary syndrome in a patient with low thrombolysis in myocardial infarction (TIMI) score or in a patient with incomplete revascularization (following myocardial infarction (MI) and following revascularization)
3. Guide Management
   - To guide management in patients with known CAD who has had a change in symptoms (chronic ischemic heart disease)
   - To demonstrate location and extent of perfusion defects to guide medical management and revascularization strategies
   - To assess for viability in myocardial segments with regional wall motion abnormalities and reduced perfusion
   - Future direction: guide invasive heart failure interventions such as CRT
   - Non-CAD: assess for disease activity in sarcoidosis and others. To assess for mental stress ischemia and stress-induced cardiomyopathy

The appropriate use of nuclear cardiology studies has been summarized in guidelines as below:

Diagnosis of CAD: Initial Investigation for the Presence of CAD in a Patient Suspected to Have CAD Based Upon Symptoms and an Intermediate Pretest Probability of CAD

Stress MPI is appropriate as initial investigation for the presence of CAD in a patient suspected to have CAD based upon

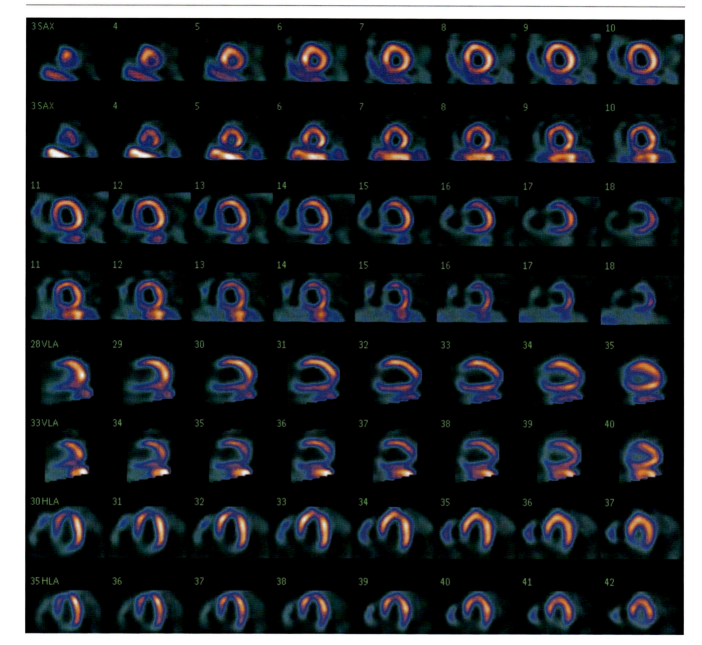

Fig. 13.4 SPECT of cardiomyopathy. A 57-year-old male with hypertension and dyslipidemia who presents for preoperative cardiovascular risk assessment with complaints of dyspnea with minimal exertion. He exercised on a Bruce protocol for 6 min achieving an estimated workload of 6 METs and a peak heart rate of 89 % of maximum predicted heart rate for age. His exercise ECG was nondiagnostic because of baseline ECG abnormalities. Exercise was terminated for shortness of breath. He underwent a same day imaging protocol, with 13 mCi of 99m-Tc at rest followed by injection of 32 mCi of 99m-Tc at peak stress. Perfusion imaging is displayed in oblique slices. The left ventricle is enlarged. There is intense extra-cardiac tracer uptake adjacent to the inferior wall. There is a small area of mildly decreased scintigraphic activity in the true apex, which is fixed. Gated SPECT imaging demonstrated severely reduced left ventricular systolic function with global hypokinesis. A coronary angiogram did not demonstrate coronary artery disease. The presumptive diagnosis is nonischemic cardiomyopathy

symptoms and if the patient has an intermediate pretest probability of CAD [11].

A simplified summary of the Bayes theorem is that an initial belief plus new data results in an improved belief [12] (Fig. 13.5). This is aptly applied to nuclear cardiology stress testing. The consultant defines the initial estimate of the likelihood of CAD based upon the patient's clinical history. This pretest probability determines the need for noninvasive testing or even the need to proceed directly to cardiac catheterization. Given that nuclear cardiology has a certain rate of false-positive and false-negative findings, the interpretation of the test results is strongly influenced by the pretest probability of disease.

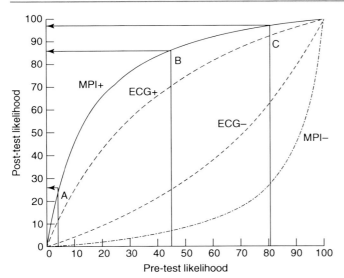

Fig. 13.5 Bayes theorem. Bayes theorem incorporates pretest probability and posttest probability to assess the likelihood of coronary artery disease with ECG and MPS, using sensitivities of 68 and 92 %, respectively, and specificities of 77 and 88 %, respectively. Curved lines from top to bottom represent MPS+, ECG+, ECG–, and MPS– (Adapted from[13]). (*A*) Low risk: 45-year-old female with dyslipidemia who has non-anginal chest pain. Pretest probability of 5 %. (*B*) Intermediate risk: 55-year-old male with tobacco use and family history who has atypical angina. Pretest probability 45 %. (*C*) High risk: 65 year old male with >3 cardiovascular risk factors and typical angina. Pretest probability >80 %

If a patient has a very high pretest likelihood (>90 %), noninvasive testing is only recommended for assessing cardiac prognosis. If the patient's pretest likelihood is very low (<10 %) such as an asymptomatic patient with 1 or no risk factors, diagnostic stress testing is not recommended. In patients whose pretest probability is within a low range (10–20 %), an exercise ECG would be a first step since a negative test would indicate a very low likelihood of CAD. For patients within the intermediate pretest probability range of CAD (20–80 %), a negative exercise ECG alone is unlikely to provide sufficient diagnostic accuracy. Thus, an exercise ECG with stress myocardial perfusion imaging is recommended.

There are a number of algorithms which incorporate age, gender, symptoms, resting ECG findings, and other cardiac risk factors to assess the likelihood of CAD in the symptomatic patient [14–16] (Table 13.2). Determination of pretest probability also aids in understanding the false-positive and false-negative rate for interpretation of the stress test data [18].

Diagnostic Accuracy of Myocardial Perfusion Imaging

The diagnostic accuracy of MPI is determined by how it performs when compared to angiographic detection of a 50–70 % stenosis. The significance of this degree of stenosis

Table 13.2 Estimation of pretest probability. Determination of pretest probability by (**A**) type of chest pain, age, and gender and by (**B**) scoring system to account for cardiovascular risk factors [15, 17]

a

Age, years	Non-anginal CP		Atypical angina		Typical angina	
	Men	Women	Men	Women	Men	Women
30–39	0.05	0.01	0.22	0.04	0.70	0.26
40–49	0.14	0.03	0.46	0.13	0.87	0.55
50–59	0.22	0.08	0.59	0.32	0.92	0.79
60–69	0.28	0.19	0.67	0.54	0.94	0.91

b

Scoring method			
Age and gender			
Men	9 points	6 points	3 points
Women	> 55 years	40–55 years	<40 years
	> 65 years	50–65 years	<50 years
Symptoms	Typical angina	Atypical angina	Nonanginal
	5 points	3 points	1 point
Estrogen status	Positive	Negative	Male/unknown
	– 3 points	+ 3 points	0 point
Diabetes	2 points	Hypertension	1 point each
		Smoking	
		Hyperlipidemia	
		Family history	
		Obesity	
Low probability: 0–8 points	Intermediate probability: 9–15 points	High probability: 16–24 points	

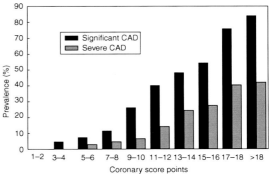

Probability categories: very low risk <10 %, low risk 10–20 %, intermediate risk 20–80 %, and high risk >80 %

is extrapolated from animal models, which demonstrated a blunted CFR at 50 % narrowing. First, we must recall that angiography addresses a question of anatomy, which is distinct from the physiologic answer that is derived from MPI. Second, we use a dichotomous definition of CAD (stenosis >50–70 %) in our discussion of MPI test performance, which then defines CAD pathology as that of plaque encroachment, rather than our modern understanding, which incorporates endothelial dysfunction, and a natural history that is punctuated by plaque instability and rupture.

Test performance is described in relation to a gold standard, which is coronary angiography in the case of CAD:

- *Sensitivity*: test's ability to "rule out" disease if test is negative.
- *Specificity*: test's ability to "rule in" disease if positive.
- *Predictive accuracy*: percentage of test responses (both positive and negative) that are true. This measures test characteristics and disease prevalence.

In a review of 1,441 patients from 6 different studies, exercise 201-Tl SPECT MPI was compared to coronary angiography with a sensitivity of 90 % (82–98 %): single vessel disease 83 %, two-vessel disease 93 %, and three-vessel disease 95 % [19]. The specificity of the MPI was 70 % (43–91 %). This study had a high normalcy rate (89 %), which was defined as the rate of normal perfusion studies in patients with a <5 % likelihood of CAD based on the clinical and ECG stress data.

When 201-Tl MPI is compared to 99m-technetium (Tc), 99m-Tc MPI studies are associated with an increase in sensitivity (90 % vs. 82 %), an increase in specificity (93 % vs. 80 %), and an increase in the normalcy rate (100 % vs. 77 %) [20]. Based on these observations, 99m-Tc perfusion agents are the more commonly used radiotracers. Attenuation correction with transmission or computed tomography (CT) improves specificity and accuracy, but use of attenuation correction does not alter test sensitivity.

To compare the test performance of different stress modalities, Garber et al. performed a meta-analysis to evaluate test performance in patients with an intermediate pretest probability for the presence of CAD (25–75 %) [21] (Table 13.3). In general, SPECT MPI had a higher sensitivity, but a lower specificity than stress echocardiogram. PET MPI demonstrated both a higher sensitivity and a higher specificity compared SPECT MPI, but this was associated with increased cost.

Imaging characteristics that improve test sensitivity include known or extensive CAD, high-grade coronary stenosis, proximal location of stenosis, and the presence of wall motion abnormalities. Factors that diminish the sensitivity for detection of CAD include single vessel disease, left circumflex stenosis, branch vessel stenosis, distal stenosis, mild stenosis (<50 %), inadequate HR response during exercise, and concurrent antianginal therapy. Importantly, the method for inducing ischemia (exercise vs. pharmacologic) *does not* have a large effect on the diagnostic accuracy of the imaging study. Stress test accuracy is dependent on the patient population characteristics and varies by ethnicity, gender, pretest probability of disease, presence of left bundle branch block (LBBB), and presence of left ventricular hypertrophy (LVH) and in diabetes.

Table 13.3 ACC/AHA appropriateness criteria

Diagnostic test	Sensitivity (range)[a]	Specificity (range)[a]	Studies *n*	Patients	Patients with coronary disease %	Sensitivity for left main or three-vessel disease	Studies *n*	Patients
Planar thallium imaging	0.79 (0.70–0.94)	0.73 (0.43–0.97)	6	510	66	0.93	2	72
Single-photon emission computed tomography	0.88 (0.73–0.98)	0.77 (0.53–0.96)	8	628	70	0.98	3	92
Echocardiography[b]	0.76 (0.40–1.00)	0.88 (0.80–0.95)	10	1,174	64	0.94	4	115
Positron emission tomography	0.91 (0.69–1.00)	0.82 (0.73–0.88)	3	206	68	Not available		
Exercise electrocardiography[c]	0.68	0.77	132	24,074	66	0.86	48	

2009 ACC/AHA appropriateness guidelines on radionuclide imaging, appropriate use category *A* appropriate, *U* uncertain, *I* inappropriate, Score (1–9) [22]

[a]Range of sensitivity and specificity reported in individual studies

[b]Test characteristics for echocardiography are based on pooled studies of dobutamine, dipyridamole, and exercise as stressors. Pooling only studies that used dobutamine as a stressor gave similar results, with a sensitivity of 0.76 and a specificity of 0.87 for all coronary disease

[c]Sensitivity of exercise electrocardiography for detection of all coronary artery disease is based on a meta-analysis that included 144 studies for estimates of sensitivity and 132 studies for specificity. Exercise electrocardiography results for sensitivity in left main and three-vessel disease were based on another meta-analysis. No studies of positron emission tomography reported sensitivity for left main and three-vessel disease

Diagnosis: Detection of Preclinical Disease in the Asymptomatic Patient

Asymptomatic patients have a low pretest probably of significant CAD and are generally not screened using stress testing. The risk of developing CAD over the next 10 years can be estimated using the Framingham risk score [23]. Asymptomatic patients with a moderate or high risk of CAD may be considered for stress testing in specific situations, such as airline pilots. Asymptomatic patients can be categorized into risk categories: high risk (>5 % annual mortality), intermediate risk (1–5 % annual mortality), or low risk (<1 % annual mortality).

Diagnosis of CAD: Evaluation of an Underlying Ischemic Etiology in a Patient with Systolic Dysfunction/Cardiomyopathy

Of the five million cases of heart failure, it is estimated that 60–70 % of these patients have CAD [24]. Patients with LV systolic dysfunction, which is attributable to CAD, have a worse prognosis than those with nonischemic cardiomyopathy. It is imperative to distinguish between LV dysfunction, which is causally related to CAD from LV dysfunction, which coexists with CAD. At present, guidelines recommend coronary angiography in patients who present with heart failure and angina.

Interestingly, only a minority of patients with both CAD and LV dysfunction who have residual myocardial viability experience angina [25]. The IMAGINE (Investigation of Myocardial Gated SPECT Imaging) study evaluated 201 patients hospitalized with new-onset heart failure who underwent stress MPI using 99m-Tc. A sum stress score >3 had a sensitivity of 96 % for ischemic cardiomyopathy. The abnormalities on an MPI illustrate the pathology of scar, repetitive stunning, and hibernation, which underlie the myopathy. While a negative study might rule out an ischemic etiology, a small number of false-negative studies can occur in the setting of balanced ischemia [26].

Diagnosis: Stress-Induced Cardiomyopathy and Mental Stress-Induced Ischemia

Reversible myocardial stunning in response to emotional stress, takotsubo cardiomyopathy (TC), represents the extreme in a spectrum of processes by which mental/psychological stress can profoundly and acutely affect myocardial performance and myocardial perfusion.

The clinical presentation of TC is associated with markedly increased serum catecholamine levels accompanying a transient and profound decrease in left ventricular systolic function with no angiographic evidence of significant coronary artery disease [27]. Most of the case series typically describe the absence of significant coronary disease, though TIMI frame counts have demonstrated significant abnormalities in coronary flow as compared to controls [28, 29]. While the pathophysiology of this entity is unknown, mechanisms involving multivessel coronary vasospasm, abnormalities in coronary microvascular function, and/or catecholamine-mediated cardiotoxicity have been proposed.

SPECT myocardial perfusion imaging of these patients [30, 31] consistently shows impairment immediately after hospital admission, with considerable improvement at 3–5 days. PET studies with N-13 and fludeoxyglucose (FDG) have documented a regional transient decrease in myocardial blood flow and coronary flow reserve during the acute phase of TC that completely resolved after 3 months [32].

Prognosis: Risk Stratification in Patients with Established CAD (Chronic Ischemic Disease)

When the stress modality is exercise, exercise variables can help refine the pretest probability of disease but can also aid in risk stratification for prediction of future cardiovascular (CV) events. Exercise predictors of poor prognosis include a poor exercise capacity (<5 metabolic equivalents (METs)), exercise-induced angina especially if it occurs at a low workload, abnormal peak systolic blood pressure (<130 mmHg) or a fall in systolic blood pressure from resting value, and chronotropic incompetence [33, 34].

The Duke Treadmill Score (DTS) is a commonly used tool to assess prognosis. It was derived from a cohort of 2,758 patients with a median age of 49 years who present for an exercise treadmill test (ETT) for evaluation of chest pain and were also referred for angiography. Patients with prior revascularization and recent MI were excluded [35].

$$DTS = (\text{exercise time on Bruce protocol}) - (5 \times \text{max ST segment deviation}) - \left(4 \times \text{angina} \begin{bmatrix} 0 = none, 1 = non-limiting, \\ 2 = exercise\ limiting \end{bmatrix}\right).$$

Low risk >= +5, moderate risk −10 to +4, high risk <= −11

The low-risk group demonstrated a 97 % 5-year survival. On angiogram, 60 % of low-risk patients had no coronary stenosis ≥75 % [36]. On the other hand, the high-risk group demonstrated a 65 % 5-year survival, and 74 % of patients were found to have three-vessel disease or left main disease on angiogram.

MPI performed with exercise stress and with adenosine or dipyridamole stress is comparable in ability to risk stratify patients, but patients that undergo pharmacologic stress are at higher risk for subsequent cardiac events than those patients that are able to exercise [37]. The prognostic value of regadenoson has not been evaluated but is likely similar to that of adenosine.

The presence/extent of perfusion defects on MPI provides additional prognostic information [38]. High-risk features associated with negative prognosis in patients with known CAD:

- Extensive ischemia involving >20 % of the left ventricle
- Defects in more than one coronary territory, suggestive of multivessel disease
- Amount of myocardial scar
- Transient or persistent LV dilation (TID)
- Resting LVEF <40 %
- Increased lung uptake of 201-Tl or 99m-Tc, which is a marker of exercise-induced LV dysfunction

In 5,183 patients with known or suspected CAD who were followed for mean of 1.8 years, there was a graded relationship between the severity of MPI abnormality and survival. Normal, mildly abnormal, moderately abnormal, and severely abnormal MPI results were associated with cardiac death rates of 0.5, 2.7, 2.9, and 4.2 %, respectively [38].

The degree of inducible ischemia may help determine which patients will have a survival benefit from revascularization. In a retrospective study of >10,000 patients without prior MI or revascularization who underwent MPI, powerful predictors of revascularization within 2 months after MPI included inducible ischemia and anginal symptoms. After adjusting for non-randomization, cardiac mortality was lower in patients with moderate to severe ischemia (>10 % of myocardium) who underwent revascularization. Mortality was significantly lower in patients with no or mild ischemia (<10 % of myocardium) who were managed medically [39].

Prognosis: In the Setting of Normal Myocardial Perfusion Imaging

Normal perfusion can identify a group of patients that is at low risk for cardiac events. In patients with suspected CAD, normal perfusion on nuclear imaging is associated with a negative predictive value of cardiac death and MI of 99 % (95 % confidence interval [CI] 98.5–99.0) over 3 years of follow-up. The annualized event rate was 0.45 % per year [40]. In patients with abnormal exercise ECG, a normal MPI is still associated with a benign prognosis. In 156 patients with a positive ETT but normal MPI, there were no deaths or nonfatal MIs at 34 months of follow-up [41].

The prognosis of a normal scan is slightly worse in patients with diabetes, in older patients, and in patients with cardiac enlargement [42]. In a patient population with known CAD by angiography, a normal MPI was associated with an annualized event rate of 0.9 % [43].

Prognosis in Special Populations: Diabetes and Female Gender

Patients with diabetes have a two- to eight-fold increased prevalence of cardiovascular disease as compared to those without diabetes, thus increasing the pretest probability of CAD. In a series of 1,271 diabetics, the annual cardiovascular event rate was 1–2 % in those with a normal MPI, 2–4 % with a mildly abnormal MPI, 7 % in those with a moderate–severely abnormal MPI, and 22 % in those who were unable to exercise and had a large perfusion defect [44]. While there are no evidence-based guidelines to support screening asymptomatic individuals with diabetes, 20–25 % of asymptomatic diabetics will demonstrate perfusion abnormalities on MPI. This must be appreciated in the context that diabetics often have variant presentations of angina and that the presence of silent ischemia is associated with a worse prognosis. Randomized controlled trials of screening in the asymptomatic diabetics have failed to demonstrate a reduction in event rates in those randomized to MPI [45].

Special consideration must also be paid to the assessment of CAD in women. Gender and menopausal status are important considerations for determination of pretest probability of CAD. Several studies have supported improvement in the diagnostic accuracy of stress MPI over ETT without imaging, because of a high false-positive rate of ETT in women as compared to men. Some of the historical limitations that reduced diagnostic accuracy of MPI in women, such as breast attenuation and limited spatial resolution in small hearts, are now less problematic because current nuclear cardiology techniques incorporate attenuation correction, prone imaging, electrocardiogram (ECG) gating, PET imaging, and new solid-state SPECT cameras [46].

Prognosis: Cardiovascular Preoperative Risk Stratification Prior to Noncardiac Surgery

The cardiology consultant is frequently asked to assess cardiovascular risk in the preoperative patient prior to noncardiac surgery. Noninvasive imaging is an adjunctive tool to evaluate patients who are deemed intermediate risk by clinical criteria and by risk indices, such as the revised cardiac risk index (RCRI) [47]. Noninvasive testing is useful in a small segment of preoperative patients who are undergoing elective surgery and have a stable cardiovascular condition. Patients with active conditions (unstable angina, decompensated heart failure, severe valvular stenosis, ventricular arrhythmias) should be managed according to ACC/AHA guidelines.

Overall, stress testing in the preoperative period has a high negative predictive value (80–90 %), but a low positive predictive value (6–67 %) for detection of death and nonfatal

MI [48]. As such, stress testing is useful for identifying low-risk patients but is poor at predicting which high-risk patients will have events.

Exercise stress testing provides important information about functional tolerance. It has been shown that exercise tolerance is a stronger predictor of perioperative outcomes than ischemic ECG changes [49]. The inability to reach >85 % of maximal predicted heart rate (MPHR) is associated with high risk for perioperative CV events, even in the absence of ECG changes [50]. When exercise ECG is performed in the absence of imaging, the sensitivity and specificity are 74 and 69 % for perioperative death and nonfatal MI [51].

The addition of imaging to exercise MPI allows for identification of high-risk imaging features, such as reversible large anterior wall defect, multiple reversible defects, ischemia at a low heart rate, extensive stress-induced wall motion abnormalities, and transient ischemic dilation. In the correct clinical context, these high-risk imaging features may warrant referral to coronary angiography.

In regards to patients referred prior to aortic surgery, exercise has been demonstrated to be safe in patients with abdominal aortic aneurysm (AAA) <6 cm in diameter or if the aneurysm is asymptomatic [52].

Vasodilator stress with imaging is appropriate for patients who cannot exercise or have a LBBB. Selection between dobutamine stress echocardiogram (DSE) and vasodilator MPI may be determined by local expertise. In a meta-analysis of five studies including 1,410 patients referred prior to vascular surgery, the test characteristics of dipyridamole MPI included a sensitivity 85 % and a specificity 60 % with negative predictive value (NPV) of 98 %, but a positive predictive value (PPV) of only 18 % [49]. DSE has a similar efficacy as vasodilator MPI with a sensitivity of 85 % and a specificity of 70 % [51].

Overall, MPI may be considered in intermediate-risk patients who are to undergo intermediate- or high-risk surgery. In patients undergoing vascular surgery, the NPV is 96–100 % for prediction of postoperative cardiac death and MI, but the PPV is only 4–20 %. Although, perfusion markers of high risk include a large area of ischemia, perfusion defects in multiple vascular territories, LV dilation, and increased lung 201-Tl uptake, it has not been conclusively demonstrated that angiography and revascularization improve perioperative outcomes.

Rather than a simplified interpretation of an imaging test as presence/absence of ischemia, there is value in determining the extent of reversible ischemia, also referred to as "jeopardized myocardium." In a meta-analysis of nine studies of preoperative patients, the probability of cardiac death and MI rose in a graded relationship to the amount of jeopardized myocardium: 3–4 % event rate in those with normal imaging or only fixed defects, 9 % event rate in those with

<20 % of myocardium at risk, 18 % event rate in those with 30–49 % of myocardium at risk, and 45 % event rate in those with >50 % of myocardium at risk [53].

Taken together, preoperative stress testing has a high NPV for predicting events following surgery, but has limited PPV.

There has been some published literature that questions the utility of preoperative stress testing. The Dutch Echocardiographic Cardiac Risk Evaluation Applying Stress Echocardiography (DECREASE) II trial enrolled 770 patients scheduled to undergo major vascular surgery awith1-2 RCRI risk factors and randomized subjects to pharmacologic stress testing or no testing. All patients received perioperative beta-blockers for strict heart rate control. A patient was referred for revascularization if there was a moderate amount of ischemia. There was no significant difference in a combined endpoint of cardiac death and nonfatal MI (1.8 % vs. 2.3 %, p 0.78) [54].

Prognosis: Risk Stratification Following Acute Coronary Syndrome in a Patient with Low TIMI Score or in a Patient with Incomplete Revascularization (Following MI and Following Revascularization)

The majority of patients who present with non-ST elevation myocardial infarction or unstable angina (NSTEMI/USA) are referred to the catheterization lab either immediately or within 48 h or presentation. In these patients, predischarge stress testing has a limited role.

Assessment for residual ischemia is performed in patients who did not receive revascularization. In these patients, stress testing is useful (1) to detect amount of residual ischemia and (2) to assess functional tolerance prior to an exercise prescription. In an early series of 158 patients who underwent exercise planar 201-Tl MPI studies within 4 weeks after hospital discharge for chest pain, a reversible perfusion defect was associated with a 21 % risk of death and nonfatal MI within a year, as compared to a 2 % risk associated with normal MPI imaging [55]. In patients who did not undergo revascularization or underwent partial revascularization, exercise testing is safe in the absence of heart failure or anginal symptoms in the 12–24 h preceding the stress test.

Guide Management: In Patients with Known CAD Who Have Had a Change in Symptoms (Chronic Ischemic Disease) with Goals to (1) Ameliorate of Symptoms and (2) Change Natural History of Disease

Nuclear cardiology is often employed in the patient with chronic CAD to assess if a change in symptoms may be attributed to a worsening of coronary perfusion, as demonstrated on MPI. MPI is able to identify the extent, severity, and location of ischemia. As such, MPI results may aid in decision making to refer for possible revascularization as compared to intensification of medical therapy.

When anatomic assessment with angiography demonstrates intermediate lesions or stenoses in multiple vascular territories, MPI may provide a "perfusion road map" to illustrate the physiologic significance of a coronary lesion or may help to identify the culprit stenosis. Several interventional trials of FFR have demonstrated revascularization that is guided by physiologic assessment of coronary stenosis results in improvement in patient outcomes. A similar intellectual framework argues for the use of MPI to direct revascularization strategies, though future studies may help strengthen this connection between CFR-directed revascularization and patient outcomes.

Given that MPI assesses heterogeneity of flow between different vascular territories, identification of left main (LM) disease and 3-vessel disease (3VD) can prove difficult because all 3 coronary territories may have an equal reduction in coronary perfusion. While rare, identification of LM disease or 3VD has important prognostic and management implications because of a demonstrated improvement in survival with revascularization. Although, LM/3VD implies a large extent of jeopardized myocardium, the SPECT images may appear normal in 19 % of cases and demonstrate perfusion abnormalities in all 3coronary territories in only 29 % of scans [56, 57]. Possible explanations for this phenomenon include balanced ischemia throughout the myocardium, plateau of tracer uptake at high flow rates which may mask any disparity in CFR, inability of SPECT to quantify absolute blood flow, and soft tissue attenuation which may produce a false-negative homogenous appearance [58].

Since SPECT underestimates the extent and severity of the perfusion defect, ancillary findings have additive value in predicting the presence of severe CAD and can be used to improve the accurate identification of these patients to 83 % [59]. These findings include:

- Increased pulmonary uptake of tracer, which is expressed as lung-to-heart ratio (LHR), due to stress-induced increase in left ventricular end diastolic pressure (LVEDP) and pulmonary capillary pressure (PCWP)
- Transient ischemic dilation (TID) due to (1) a true physical increase in LV cavity size following stress or (2) apparent LV dilation from diffuse subendocardial hypoperfusion following stress
- Increase in right ventricular tracer uptake following stress
- Exercise-induced systolic dysfunction with a fall in post-stress left ventricular (LV) EF >5 % compared to rest LV EF
- Blood pressure A blunted blood pressure response to exercise or a fall in blood pressure with exercise

- Exercise-induced ST segment changes: ST segment depressions occurring at a low workload, ST depressions which persist for a prolonged duration, or ST segment elevations

Guide Management: Identification of the Location and Extent of Perfusion Defects to Guide Medical Management and Revascularization Strategies

While early noninvasive testing does not play in a high-risk patient, MPI may be helpful in assessing the presence of ischemia and the need for early invasive therapy in patients with less acutely ill patients or those with low TIMI risk scores who present with ACS.

In a patient who presents to the emergency room with chest pain and a nondiagnostic ECG, injection of radioisotope within 2 h of chest pain can demonstrate abnormal rest perfusion. Studies have demonstrated that rest perfusion in this patient population has a high NPV and has been demonstrated to reduce hospitalization rates.

Management of the patient with NSTEMI requires a continuous process of risk stratification to reassess appropriateness of medical management as compared to early revascularization. Vasodilator MPI can provide reliable information about the presence of significant coronary stenosis early in the care of an ACS patient. In 170 patients who were managed medically for NSTEMI and underwent vasodilator MPI after 24 h of resolution of chest pain, the MPI was safe and had a sensitivity and specificity of 91 and 79 % for detection of >70 % coronary stenosis when compared to angiography that was performed within 2 months of the NSTEMI presentation [60]. As opposed to exercise MPI, vasodilator MPI allows for safe and early identification of ischemic burden. Submaximal exercise MPI tends to underestimate the severity and presence of CAD in this patient population. Moderate to large or multiple areas of reversible ischemia serve as an indication for referral to angiography with possible revascularization. Similar to other patient populations, the lack of ischemia on MPI is associated with an excellent long-term prognosis.

In higher risk populations, MPI remains useful in the following circumstances:
- ST elevation myocardial infarction (STEMI): identification of jeopardized myocardium. Repeat studies can demonstrate salvaged myocardium and residual infarct size.
- Post-MI: assessment of infarct size and residual peri-infarct ischemia.
- Following CABG: SPECT MPI retains diagnostic and prognostic accuracy.

Of note, periprocedural perfusion defects can still be visualized on MPI in the first 4–6 weeks following revascularization and as such are considered false-positive studies. In addition, routine testing is not indicated in the first 2 years following revascularization in the asymptomatic patient.

Guide Therapy: Assessment for Viability in Myocardial Segments with Regional Wall Motion Abnormalities and Reduced Perfusion

Left ventricular systolic dysfunction results from a spectrum of pathophysiologies: necrosis/scar, hibernation, and myocardial stunning. Nuclear cardiology and other noninvasive imaging techniques (dobutamine echocardiography, delayed enhancement imaging using cardiac MRI) are used to assess myocardial viability. Viability assessment seeks to identify dysfunctional myocardium that will improve with successful revascularization to achieve (1) improvement in survival, (2) improvement in regional and global systolic function, (3) improvement in functional class and quality of life, and (4) reduction in heart failure admissions and risk of sudden cardiac death.

For detection of viability, nuclear cardiology techniques can demonstrate cell membrane integrity (201-Tl imaging), intact mitochondrial function (99m-Tc), and preserved myocardial metabolism (PET 18-FDG). The 201-Tl technique employs stress-redistribution imaging, with possible late redistribution imaging at 18–24 h. Late redistribution has a high PPV (~95 %) for identification of segments that will improve with revascularization but has a limited ability to demonstrate lack of viability in defects that remain fixed on late redistribution imaging. This can be improved with a reinjection protocol [61].

PET imaging is a more robust nuclear tool for assessment of viability because it is able to assess both perfusion and metabolism simultaneously (Fig. 13.6). Under ischemic/hibernating conditions, myocytes preferentially take up glucose rather than free fatty acids. As such, fluorine-18-labeled FDG acts as a glucose analog and is localized to hibernating myocardium. FDG images are compared to Rb-82 perfusion images. Using PET, we categorize abnormal myocardium as follows:

- Perfusion-metabolism *matched* defect: concordant reduction in both myocardial blood flow and FDG is considered irreversibly injured/nonviable. Associated with a 20 % chance of functional improvement following revascularization.
- Perfusion-metabolism *mismatch*: FDG relatively preserved or increased despite perfusion defect is considered ischemic but viable. Associated with 80–85 % chance of functional improvement following revascularization.
- Perfusion-metabolism *reverse mismatch*: preserved perfusion in the absence of increased FDG uptake. Can either represent poor glucose preparation or represent viable tissue [62, 63].

In a meta-analysis of 24 studies of CAD patients with systolic dysfunction, revascularization in patients with demonstrated viability was associated with an 80 % reduction in annual mortality when compared to medical therapy alone [64].

Nuclear Cardiology in the Matrix of Multimodality Imaging

There are a variety of tests available for the noninvasive diagnosis of CAD: stress echocardiography, myocardial perfusion imaging, coronary artery calcification (CAC), cardiac computed tomography angiography (CCTA), and perfusion MRI.

The detection of CAC has been demonstrated to provide incremental prognostic and diagnostic information to MPI, most notably in patients with severe multivessel CAD and in patients with a higher pretest probability of CAD [65]. SPECT and PET cameras with CT for attenuation correction allow for assessment of a calcium score, but this requires an additional ~1 mSv of radiation exposure. While CAC does not provide information about obstructive stenosis or location of CAD, the CAC-based Agatston score is linearly associated with presence and degree of inducible ischemia. In observational studies, approximately 30 % of patients with CAC scores of ≥400 had inducible ischemia on stress MPI, whereas only 11% of patients with an Agatston score >1,000 demonstrated a normal MPI [66].

In comparison, CCTA has been shown to have a high sensitivity and specificity when compared to angiography, but it is an anatomic study (rather than functional study) and has limited diagnostic accuracy in patients with an Agatston score ≥400. The selection of noninvasive testing for diagnosis and prognosis is dependent on the pretest probability of disease, ability to exercise, patient comorbidities, and the balance of risk and benefit of studies.

Test Performance

An understanding of the performance of MPI informs our clinical use of the test and our appreciation of its limitations. In simplified terms, an MPI is performed by injection of a radioisotope. Delivery of the radioisotope to the myocardium is approximately proportional to coronary blood flow delivery to the myocardium, though this exact relationship varies by tracer. The isotope is extracted from the blood by viable myocytes and retained inside the myocyte for some period of time. Myocyte uptake of the radioisotope depends upon coronary perfusion and the presence of myocardial cells to retain tracer. Depending on the tracer, this is related to membrane integrity and/or the presence of viable myocardial cells.

Photons are emitted from the myocardium in proportion to the magnitude of tracer uptake such that photon emission

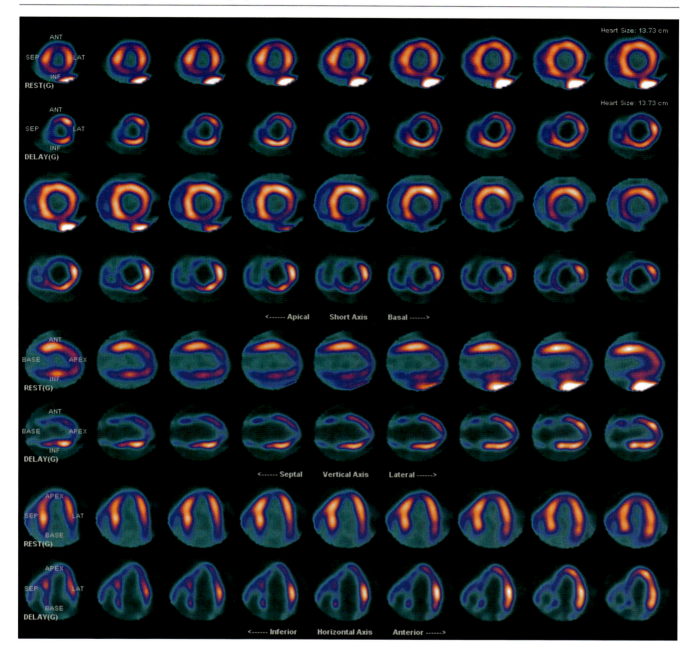

Fig. 13.6 PET FDG to assess viability. A 58-year-old female with multiple cardiac risk factors with new-onset heart failure symptoms. Initial echo demonstrated moderate LV systolic dysfunction and her coronary angiogram demonstrated 3-vessel coronary artery disease. She was referred for PET-FDG to assess for myocardial viability prior to revascularization. She initially underwent rest perfusion with Rb-82 45 mCi, as represented on the top row for each of the cuts. She has perfusion defects in both the LAD and LCx territory. Next, she was given 25 g oral glucose followed by 18 units of regular insulin to optimize myocardial glucose uptake, which allowed stabilization of finger sticks at 150 mg/dl without the need of a euglycemic insulin clamp. She was injected with FDG 10 mCi and imaged after 1 h, as represented on the bottom row for each of the cuts. There is a medium-sized matched severe perfusion defect involving the apical LV segments and LV apex with modestly preserved metabolism, representing a prior MI in the distal left anterior descending (LAD) coronary arteryterritory with significant residual viable myocardium in the rest of the LAD coronary territory. There is a matched large/severe defect involving the mid and basal inferior and inferolateral walls showing concordant reduction in FDG uptake, suggestive of prior MI in the left circumflex or right coronary artery coronary territory with minimal peri-infarct viability

from the myocardium is proportional to perfusion. The gamma photons collide with a detector crystal in the standard gamma camera where they are absorbed and converted into a visible light event, called a scintillation event. Scintillation events are detected by a photomultiplier tube. This information is converted into digital data to represent magnitude and location of uptake. The image is processed and filtered prior to interpretation.

Radionuclide Tracers

There are 3 common tracers used in clinical nuclear cardiology: thallium-201- and 2technetium-99m-labeled tracers, sestamibi (Cardiolite), and tetrofosmin (Myoview).

Thallium-201 (201-Tl) was developed in the 1970s as the first tracer used for clinical MPI. Given that 201-Tl is a potassium analog, the uptake of 201-Tl requires the presence of an intact transport system and electrochemical gradient, along with an intact cell membrane. Redistribution of 201-Tl begins within 10–15 min and is related to the concentration gradient and the presence of functioning myocytes. This property allows 201-Tl to assess for presence of hibernating myocardium.

Since their introduction in the 1990s, the 299m-Tc-labeled perfusion agents, sestamibi and tetrofosmin, are now commonly used in clinical nuclear cardiology. 99m-Tc is a monovalent hydrophilic cation whose uptake depends on coronary blood flow along with plasma and mitochondrial-derived membrane electrochemical gradient. In comparison to 201-Tl, 99m-Tc has a higher photon energy of 140 keV (vs. 201-Tl 70–80 keV), which results in better spatial resolution with less attenuation and scatter. 99m-Tc provides improved image quality in women and obese patients since there is less soft tissue attenuation as compared to 201-Tl. 99m-Tc has a shorter half-life than 201-Tl (6 h vs. 72 h) which permits a higher dose to be administered while maintaining adequate counts in the image, resulting in a lower radiation dose than thallium. The minimal redistribution of 99m-Tc allows greater flexibility when imaging. Imaging can be performed at 10 min but also up to 4 h after injection.

Higher counts and lack of redistribution permits ECG-triggered gated acquisition for assessment of LV systolic function, which is acquired simultaneous with the perfusion information. Unfortunately, 99m-Tc has a lower first-pass extraction (60 %) compared to 201-Tl (85 %), which attenuates a linear relationship of tracer uptake with coronary perfusion. In addition, 99m-Tc is cleared by the liver and concentrated by the gallbladder. After injection, patients are imaged after a time delay (30–60 min following pharmacologic stress and 10–45 min following exercise stress) to reduce GI tracer activity so that the inferior wall can be accurately assessed.

Nuclear Cardiology Imaging Protocols

Selection of a nuclear imaging protocol depends upon patient characteristics, the pretest probability of CAD in that patient, and local variation in practice. Depending on the protocol,

the test takes 2–4 h over 1–2 days. On most SPECT cameras, the imaging component of the test requires that a patient lie flat and still for 15–20 min with arms up. Acquisition time and patient positioning is changing with the introduction of solid-state cardiac-specific cameras.

A one-day split-dose protocol is performed with stress imaging followed by rest or the alternative sequence of rest followed by stress imaging. The first study is performed with administration of low-dose radioisotope at 8–10 mCi. The second study is performed 1.5–2.5 h after the first injection to minimize contamination between the two injections. The second study is performed with high-dose radiotracer at 20–30 mCi.

In obese patients that weigh >250 lb, the single-isotope study is performed over 2 days so that both the first and second studies, regardless of sequence, can be performed with administration of high-dose radioisotope (20–30 mCi). This allows for adequate counts on both the rest and stress images.

As an alternative, stress-only imaging may be appropriate in patients who (1) have no known history of CAD or (2) have a history of CAD but no prior MI or CABG and in patients who are imaged on a system with attenuation correction. If a stress-only perfusion study is completely normal or completely abnormal, no rest imaging may be required. The benefits of stress-only imaging are increased efficiency and reduction in radiation dose. When stress-only imaging is combined with exercise, a normal study is associated with a <1 % annual event rate, which is equivalent to a normal 1-day stress/rest split-dose protocol [67].

The use of single-isotope studies provides flexibility in the nuclear lab for the performance of different protocols depending on lab and patient needs. Single-isotope studies improve the ease of interpretation and evaluation of transient ischemic dilation, allow use of attenuation correction which has been validated in 99m-Tc studies, and reduce the radiation exposure, as compared to a dual-isotope protocol. In comparison, a dual-isotope study is performed with administration of 3 mCi of 201-Tl at rest with imaging after 10 min followed by administration of 25–30 mCi of 99m-Tc at stress with imaging after 30–60 min [68]. The dual-isotope study can take advantage of the redistribution properties of 201-Tl to assess for viability in a region of apparent myocardial scar.

Physicians who order nuclear stress tests must be cognizant of the dosage of radiation and work with specialists in nuclear cardiology to deliver care in accordance with the As Low As Reasonably Achievable (ALARA) philosophy. The estimated doses for nuclear cardiology protocols are as follows:

- Single-isotope rest/stress 99m-Tc: 8–10 mSv
- Stress-only 99m-Tc: 7 mSv
- Single-isotope rest/stress 201-Tl: 18–20 mSv
- Dual-isotope imaging: 25–30 mSv
- PET rest/stress 82-Rb: 4–6 mSv [69]

In comparison, a chest x-ray is 0.1 mSv, a diagnostic coronary angiogram is 4–15 mSv, and environmental exposure for the average American is 3 mSv per year.

Stress Modality

The selection of the stress modality (exercise, vasodilator, inotropic) is based upon a patient's comorbidities and a patient's ability to exercise to a high enough level to produce meaningful results.

Exercise Stress

Treadmill and bicycle stress is the preferred form of stress since exercise provides a link between symptoms and evidence of ischemia. Exercise testing offers information about functional capacity, stress-induced ECG changes, and hemodynamic responses to physical activity, which all shape our understanding of the pretest probability for CAD and inform our interpretation of the nuclear perfusion images.

Exercise is appropriate in patients that have the ability to exercise and achieve an adequate heart rate (defined as ≥85 % of age-predicted MPHR), rate pressure product (RPP) ≥20 K (defined as product of peak systolic blood pressure (SBP) and heart rate (HR)), or workload (defined as ≥80 % functional aerobic capacity). Unfortunately, the sensitivity of the stress study to rule out myocardial ischemia is reduced in patients that are unable to achieve a peak heart rate ≥85 % of MPHR if the test is otherwise negative for chest pain or ECG changes.

Inadequate exercise may lead to an underestimation of the presence and severity of CAD [70]. In patients who fail to achieve adequate exercise levels, there is a significantly lower rate of detection of single vessel coronary disease (35 % vs. 56 %), 2-vessel disease (58 % vs. 80 %), and 3-vessel disease (56 % vs. 88 %) [71]. In addition, the sensitivity for detection of ischemia falls if exercise duration is <6 min (<7 METs) on a Bruce protocol (89 % vs. 66 %, $p < 0.01$) [72].

Importantly, a low functional tolerance (<6 METs) is associated with a fourfold increased risk of cardiac mortality [73]. The inability to exercise, as in an amputee, must be distinguished from a patient that is unable to adequately exercise due to low functional tolerance.

In patients with LBBB on baseline ECG, vasodilator stress may be preferable to exercise because of an increased likelihood of a false-positive perfusion defect in the septum with exercise stress in the absence of LAD disease [74, 75].

Vasodilator Stress Agents

In patients who are unable to perform an exercise stress test, vasodilator stress offers diagnostic accuracy that is comparable to exercise. The vasodilator agents in current clinical use are dipyridamole, adenosine, and regadenoson.

Vasodilators act through adenosine receptors on vascular smooth muscle cells and endothelial cells to enhance arterial dilation and increase coronary blood flow. Unlike exercise, which induces a myocardial oxygen demand-flow mismatch to evaluate for heterogeneous CFR, vasodilators manipulate the homeostatic response to evaluate for heterogeneity in CFR. Importantly, the diagnostic accuracy of vasodilator stress MPI is comparable to exercise MPI and is equivalent among the different vasodilator stress agents [76, 77].

Patients will experience fewer side effects with vasodilator agents that selectively act on the A2A adenosine receptor (regadenoson) and that have a shorter half-life (adenosine and regadenoson). Side effects from vasodilators are common (shortness of breath, dizziness, palpitations, transient heart block, and nausea), but serious complications remain rare. Because of selectivity, tolerability, and ease of use, regadenoson is now becoming the vasodilator stress agent of choice.

Vasodilators may be used along with exercise in patients whom exercise information is additive but are unable to achieve an adequate exercise level [78]. Exercise will improve tolerability of the vasodilator agents and will improve image quality because of reduced GI tracer contamination.

Caffeine and certain medications act as adenosine receptor antagonists and may reduce the hemodynamic response to the vasodilator stress agents and increase the likelihood of a false-negative stress perfusion [79]. Therefore, patients are instructed to refrain from caffeine for 12–24 h and to hold methylxanthines and dipyridamole for the 48 h preceding their stress test. Other studies have demonstrated a less prominent effect of caffeine, though small studies suggest that caffeine may be ingested up to 2 h prior to a regadenoson stress without a reduction in diagnostic accuracy of the MPI [80]. Of note, vasodilator stress agents are contraindicated in patients with resting hypotension, 2nd-degree atrioventricular (AV) block/Mobitz II, or 3rd-degree AV block without pacing. In addition, caution must be exercised with the use of adenosine and dipyridamole in the setting of bronchospastic airway disease. Regadenoson has been shown to be safe in mild–moderate asthma [81].

Inotropic/Adrenergic Stress Agent

In patients in whom exercise and vasodilator stress is not appropriate, a consultant may consider dobutamine stress MPI. Dobutamine is an inotropic and adrenergic stress agent. Similar to exercise, dobutamine increases heart rate, blood pressure, and coronary blood flow. Like exercise, perfusion abnormalities induced by dobutamine are the result of ischemia in contrast to perfusion abnormalities from vasodilators, which are the result of induced flow heterogeneity. Dobutamine is inappropriate in patients with poorly controlled hypertension, significant aortic aneurysm or poorly controlled supraventricular or ventricular arrhythmias.

Choice of Pharmacologic Stress Agent

Exercise is the preferable stress modality for the multiple reasons outlined above. Vasodilator MPI or dobutamine echocardiogram may be appropriate in patients who are unable to walk, have a LBBB, or have a paced rhythm, unless the patient is known to return to native rhythm with exercise. Pharmacologic stress (adenosine MPI, dipyridamole MPI, and dobutamine echo) was evaluated in a meta-analysis of 82 studies enrolling 10,817 patients and demonstrated similar sensitivity and specificity for detection of CAD when compared to the gold standard of coronary angiography [82]. Regadenoson stress MPI correlates well with adenosine MPI [77].

Chest pain and ECG changes occur less often during vasodilator stress than exercise stress. Given that vasodilator MPI studies cannot provide important prognostic indicators such as functional capacity and hemodynamic response to exercise, an increased significance is placed upon superior SPECT image quality, reproducibility, and interpretability. Given the limitations of vasodilator MPI, one might consider the performance of a submaximal treadmill test in conjunction with a vasodilator MPI to minimize vasodilator-associated side effects, to improve image quality, and to provide prognostic exercise information [83, 84].

Medical Management Prior to Stress Myocardial Perfusion Imaging

The decision to withhold cardiovascular medications prior to stress MPI must be individualized to the patient and to the clinical question. When calcium channel blockers, nitrates, and beta-blockers are taken 24–48 h prior to vasodilator MPI, the MPI may underestimate the extent and severity of perfusion defects [85]. If the MPI is for the initial diagnosis of CAD, the consultant might hold antianginal and AV nodal agents. On the other hand, if the MPI is employed to assess new symptoms or burden of ischemia in a patient with known CAD, the consultant might continue all cardiovascular medicines on the morning of the exam.

ECG-Gated Imaging

In patients with a regular heart rhythm, ECG-gated imaging can be performed simultaneous with 99m-Tc SPECT imaging and 82-Rb PET imaging to allow for the assessment of LV systolic function and regional wall motion.

Automated programs calculate LV ejection fraction and are highly reproducible. The normal LVEF by SPECT is ≥45 %. Of note, a normal LVEF is not comparable between different cardiac imaging modalities since they vary in temporal and spatial resolution, nor is it comparable across different processing software. Gated LVEF may be inaccurate in the setting of an arrhythmia or in small-sized hearts. Unfortunately, if a wall has severely reduced or absent counts, the automated LVEF cannot be calculated, and the LV systolic function will be reported by qualitative assessment. In SPECT MPI, post-stress LVEF will typically be equal to or higher than the rest LVEF. In moderate to severe stress-induced ischemia, myocardial stunning may cause a drop in LVEF, and this post-stress LVEF may be more than 5 % lower than resting LVEF [86].

Normal regional systolic function is depicted as brightening of the myocardial walls. Brightness, or count recovery, is a function of radiotracer concentration and wall thickness. Wall motion is helpful adjunctive information in the interpretation of photopenic regions on perfusion images. Semiquantitative programs score wall motion and wall thickening. Myocardial scar may demonstrate reduced wall motion. Normal wall motion will be seen in normal myocardium, ischemic regions, apical thinning, and regions with soft tissue attenuation and scatter.

Comparison to Positron Emission Tomography (PET) Imaging

PET offers an alternative to SPECT, with improved image quality because of greater counts, less attenuation, and improvement in spatial resolution. The growth of PET MPI has been hampered by cost, limited availability of PET scanners, and inability to perform exercise stress.

In a similar fashion to SPECT imaging, the underlying principle of PET is the injection of a radiotracer into the bloodstream, which is extracted from the blood by viable myocytes. A PET radiotracer stabilizes by emission of a positron, called beta decay. The positron travels a few millimeters before it collides with an electron. This collision causes annihilation of the positron and electron and conversion to two gamma rays, which have an energy of 511 keV. At the camera head, the gamma rays create a scintillation event, which is detected by the photomultiplier tube. Localization in the X and Y planes relies upon intrinsic collimation from two gamma rays.

The radiotracer is labeled with a positron-emitting isotope and has characteristics identical to naturally occurring elements, such as oxygen, nitrogen, carbon, and fluoride. Most PET perfusion radiotracers are produced by on-site cyclotrons and have short half-lives, such as N-13 and O-15. The advent of generator-produced PET tracers made the clinical use of PET myocardial imaging more feasible. Rubidium-82 (Rb-82) has become a common clinically used myocardial perfusion agent that is generator-produced. Rb-82 is a cation with similar properties to potassium and thallium. Myocyte uptake of Rb-82 reflects absolute blood flow, but its uptake plateaus under more hyperemic conditions.

Compared to SPECT imaging, PET perfusion studies have a higher spatial resolution that improves the diagnostic accuracy of the study along with improved attenuation and scatter correction [87]. This makes PET perfusion a compelling test in patients that may have limitations with soft tissue attenuation and scatter on SPECT, such as obese patients and women. Rb-82 has a short half-life (72 s), which shortens study duration and limits the need for a delay between injection and imaging, as there is in SPECT imaging. Unfortunately, a short half-life limits the stress modality to only pharmacologic stress. Currently, there are new ^{18}F-flurpiridaz radiotracers in clinical trials, which will expand PET perfusion to include exercise stress as well. While F-18 has a longer half-life when compared to Rb-82, it has much improved spatial resolution and better image quality as compared to Rb-82 [88].

PET perfusion tracers allow quantification of absolute myocardial blood flow and calculation of CFR. It has been demonstrated that estimates of CFR are inversely related to the severity of a coronary stenosis [89]. Small studies have demonstrated that quantification of CFR improves the identification of and the extent of CAD and improves risk stratification, but CFR cannot distinguish between epicardial disease and microvascular dysfunction [90, 91].

In addition to perfusion assessment, nuclear imaging allows for evaluation of cardiac metabolism. The most common application is PET imaging of glucose metabolism using radiotracer 18-F-fluoro-2-deoxyglucose (18-FDG) to assess for myocardial viability. 18-FDG can also be used to assess for evidence of active myocardial inflammation in the setting of cardiac sarcoidosis. Viability assessment will be discussed below. Other metabolic tracers used in clinical research allow for assessment of fatty acid uptake (SPECT 123-1 and BMIPP, PET C11 palmitate), assessment of glucose uptake (PET 11-C glucose), and assessment of oxygen utilization (PET 15-0 and 11-C acetate).

Blood Pool Imaging

Radionuclide ventriculography (RVG) is also called multiple-gated cardiac blood pool imaging (MUGA) and equilibrium radionuclide angiography (ERNA). It is a highly reproducible and accurate method to assess global and regional LV systolic function. RVG is performed either by injection with Tc-ppm pertechnetate or by in vitro labeling of the patient's blood. Imaging is usually performed as equilibrium RVG in which data is accumulated over a 5–10 min period, but imaging can also be performed as first-pass RVG in which case the tracer is imaged during right-sided, pulmonary and left-sided cardiac transit over a small number of cardiac cycles. The primary clinical use of RVG is in serial monitoring of LV systolic function in patients receiving cardiotoxic medications such as anthracyclines for malignancy.

Key Points

In summary, nuclear cardiology techniques to assess coronary perfusion are and will remain integral tools for the cardiology consultant to assess and care for the cardiac patient. Key points in understanding the clinical use of myocardial perfusion include:

MPI provides powerful information for diagnosis, prognosis, and to guide therapy:

- *Diagnosis*: initial investigation for presence coronary artery disease (CAD) in a patient suspected to have CAD or to evaluate for an ischemic etiology for heart failure
- *Prognosis*: risk stratification in patients with established CAD, following myocardial infarction or prior to noncardiac surgery
- *Guide therapy*: demonstrate location and extent of perfusion defects to guide medical management and revascularization strategies

In recommending that a patient undergo a nuclear cardiology test, the cardiology consultant must weigh the benefits and risks of a nuclear cardiology test:

- *Benefit*: the patient's management and outcomes will be altered by the results of the nuclear cardiology test and their risk of adverse cardiovascular events will be reduced.
- *Risk*: the risks of testing include (1) risk of the stress modality, (2) radiation exposure, (3) cost of the nuclear cardiology test and its downstream costs, and (4) risk of a false-positive test.

References

1. Fye WB, et al. 28th Bethesda conference. Task force 4: referral guidelines and the collaborative care of patients with cardiovascular disease. J Am Coll Cardiol. 1997;29(6):1162–70.
2. Strauss HW. Stress myocardial perfusion imaging- the beginning. JACC Cardiovasc Imaging. 2008;1(2):238–40.
3. Wackers FJ. Exercise myocardial perfusion imaging. J Nucl Med. 1994;35(4):726–9.

4. Ganz p and Ganz W, Coronary blood flow and myocardial ischemia. Zipes D, Braunwald E, Libby P, editors. Heart disease. 6th ed. Philadelphia: WB Saunders Company; 2001. 1087–113.
5. Gould KL, Lipscomb K. Effects of coronary stenoses on coronary flow reserve and resistance. Am J Cardiol. 1974;34(1):48–55.
6. Johnson NP, Kirkeeide RL, Gould KL. Is discordance of coronary flow reserve and fractional flow reserve due to methodology or clinically relevant coronary pathophysiology? JACC Cardiovasc Imaging. 2012;5(2):193–202.
7. Meimoun P, et al. Comparison between non-invasive coronary flow reserve and fractional flow reserve to assess the functional significance of left anterior descending artery stenosis of intermediate severity. J Am Soc Echocardiogr. 2011;24(4):374–81.
8. Klein R, Beanlands RS, DeKemp RA. Quantification of myocardial blood flow and flow reserve: technical aspects. J Nucl Cardiol. 2010;17(4):555–70.
9. Michelena HI, VanDecker WA. Radionuclide-based insights into the pathophysiology of ischemic heart disease: beyond diagnosis. J Investig Med. 2005;53(4):176–91.
10. Tilkemeier PL, et al. American society of nuclear cardiology information statement: standardized reporting matrix for radionuclide myocardial perfusion imaging. J Nucl Cardiol. 2006;13(6):e157–71.
11. Fraker Jr TD, et al. 2007 chronic angina focused update of the ACC/AHA 2002 guidelines for the management of patients with chronic stable angina: a report of the American College of Cardiology/American Heart Association Task Force on Practice Guidelines Writing Group to develop the focused update of the 2002 guidelines for the management of patients with chronic stable angina. J Am Coll Cardiol. 2007;50(23):2264–74.
12. Bayes T. An essay toward solving a problem in the doctrine of chance. Philos Trans R Soc Lond. 1763;53:370–418.
13. Underwood SR, et al. Myocardial perfusion scintigraphy: the evidence. Eur J Nucl Med Mol Imaging. 2004;31(2):261–91.
14. Weiner DA, et al. Exercise stress testing. Correlations among history of angina, ST-segment response and prevalence of coronary-artery disease in the Coronary Artery Surgery Study (CASS). N Engl J Med. 1979;301(5):230–5.
15. Morise AP, Haddad WJ, Beckner D. Development and validation of a clinical score to estimate the probability of coronary artery disease in men and women presenting with suspected coronary disease. Am J Med. 1997;102(4):350–6.
16. Pryor DB, et al. Value of the history and physical in identifying patients at increased risk for coronary artery disease. Ann Intern Med. 1993;118(2):81–90.
17. Beller GA, Gibson RS. Sensitivity, specificity, and prognostic significance of noninvasive testing for occult or known coronary disease. Prog Cardiovasc Dis. 1987;29(4):241–70.
18. Gibbons RJ, et al. ACC/AHA 2002 guideline update for exercise testing: summary article: a report of the American College of Cardiology/American Heart Association Task Force on Practice Guidelines (committee to update the 1997 exercise testing guidelines). Circulation. 2002;106(14):1883–92.
19. Mahmarian JJ, Verani MS. Exercise thallium-201 perfusion scintigraphy in the assessment of coronary artery disease. Am J Cardiol. 1991;67(14):2D–11.
20. Maddahi J, Kiat H, Friedman JD, et al. Technetium-99m-sestamibi myocardial perfusion imaging for evaluation of coronary artery disease. In: Beller G, Zaret BL, editors. Nuclear cardiology: state of the art and future directions. 1st ed. St. Louis: Mosby Year Book; 1993.
21. Garber AM, Solomon NA. Cost-effectiveness of alternative test strategies for the diagnosis of coronary artery disease. Ann Intern Med. 1999;130(9):719–28.
22. Hendel RC, et al. ACCF/ASNC/ACR/AHA/ASE/SCCT/SCMR/SNM 2009 appropriate use criteria for cardiac radionuclide imaging: a report of the American College of Cardiology Foundation Appropriate Use Criteria Task Force, the American Society of Nuclear Cardiology, the American College of Radiology, the American Heart Association, the American Society of Echocardiography, the Society of Cardiovascular Computed Tomography, the Society for Cardiovascular Magnetic Resonance, and the Society of Nuclear Medicine. Circulation. 2009;119(22):e561–87.
23. Wilson PW, et al. Prediction of coronary heart disease using risk factor categories. Circulation. 1998;97(18):1837–47.
24. Gheorghiade M, et al. Navigating the crossroads of coronary artery disease and heart failure. Circulation. 2006;114(11):1202–13.
25. Cleland JG, et al. Myocardial viability as a determinant of the ejection fraction response to carvedilol in patients with heart failure (CHRISTMAS trial): randomised controlled trial. Lancet. 2003;362(9377):14–21.
26. Soman P, et al. Etiology and pathophysiology of new-onset heart failure: evaluation by myocardial perfusion imaging. J Nucl Cardiol. 2009;16(1):82–91.
27. Gianni M, et al. Apical ballooning syndrome or takotsubo cardiomyopathy: a systematic review. Eur Heart J. 2006;27(13):1523–9.
28. Kurisu S, et al. Time course of electrocardiographic changes in patients with tako-tsubo syndrome: comparison with acute myocardial infarction with minimal enzymatic release. Circ J. 2004;68(1):77–81.
29. Bybee KA, et al. Clinical characteristics and thrombolysis in myocardial infarction frame counts in women with transient left ventricular apical ballooning syndrome. Am J Cardiol. 2004;94(3):343–6.
30. Akashi YJ, et al. 123I-MIBG myocardial scintigraphy in patients with "takotsubo" cardiomyopathy. J Nucl Med. 2004;45(7):1121–7.
31. Ito K, et al. Assessment of Takotsubo (ampulla) cardiomyopathy using 99mTc-tetrofosmin myocardial SPECT – comparison with acute coronary syndrome. Ann Nucl Med. 2003;17(2):115–22.
32. Alexanderson E, et al. Transient perfusion and motion abnormalities in takotsubo cardiomyopathy. J Nucl Cardiol. 2007;14(1):129–33.
33. Diaz LA, et al. Independent contribution of myocardial perfusion defects to exercise capacity and heart rate recovery for prediction of all-cause mortality in patients with known or suspected coronary heart disease. J Am Coll Cardiol. 2001;37(6):1558–64.
34. Lauer MS, et al. Impaired chronotropic response to exercise stress testing as a predictor of mortality. JAMA. 1999;281(6):524–9.
35. Mark DB, et al. Exercise treadmill score for predicting prognosis in coronary artery disease. Ann Intern Med. 1987;106(6):793–800.
36. Shaw LJ, et al. Use of a prognostic treadmill score in identifying diagnostic coronary disease subgroups. Circulation. 1998;98(16):1622–30.
37. Navare SM, et al. Comparison of risk stratification with pharmacologic and exercise stress myocardial perfusion imaging: a meta-analysis. J Nucl Cardiol. 2004;11(5):551–61.
38. Hachamovitch R, et al. Incremental prognostic value of myocardial perfusion single photon emission computed tomography for the prediction of cardiac death: differential stratification for risk of cardiac death and myocardial infarction. Circulation. 1998;97(6):535–43.
39. Hachamovitch R, et al. Comparison of the short-term survival benefit associated with revascularization compared with medical therapy in patients with no prior coronary artery disease undergoing stress myocardial perfusion single photon emission computed tomography. Circulation. 2003;107(23):2900–7.
40. Metz LD, et al. The prognostic value of normal exercise myocardial perfusion imaging and exercise echocardiography: a meta-analysis. J Am Coll Cardiol. 2007;49(2):227–37.

41. Schalet BD, et al. Prognostic implications of normal exercise SPECT thallium images in patients with strongly positive exercise electrocardiograms. Am J Cardiol. 1993;72(15):1201–3.

42. Gibbons RJ, et al. Long-term outcome of patients with intermediate-risk exercise electrocardiograms who do not have myocardial perfusion defects on radionuclide imaging. Circulation. 1999;100(21):2140–5.

43. Brown KA. Prognostic value of thallium-201 myocardial perfusion imaging. A diagnostic tool comes of age. Circulation. 1991;83(2):363–81.

44. Vanzetto G, et al. Prediction of cardiovascular events in clinically selected high-risk NIDDM patients. Prognostic value of exercise stress test and thallium-201 single-photon emission computed tomography. Diabetes Care. 1999;22(1):19–26.

45. Young LH, et al. Cardiac outcomes after screening for asymptomatic coronary artery disease in patients with type 2 diabetes: the DIAD study: a randomized controlled trial. JAMA. 2009;301(15):1547–55.

46. Mieres JH, Rosman DR, Shaw LJ. The clinical role of stress myocardial perfusion imaging in women with suspected coronary artery disease. Curr Cardiol Rep. 2004;6(1):27–31.

47. Lee TH, et al. Derivation and prospective validation of a simple index for prediction of cardiac risk of major noncardiac surgery. Circulation. 1999;100(10):1043–9.

48. Auerbach A, Goldman L. Assessing and reducing the cardiac risk of noncardiac surgery. Circulation. 2006;113(10):1361–76.

49. Mangano DT, Goldman L. Preoperative assessment of patients with known or suspected coronary disease. N Engl J Med. 1995;333(26):1750–6.

50. McPhail N, et al. The use of preoperative exercise testing to predict cardiac complications after arterial reconstruction. J Vasc Surg. 1988;7(1):60–8.

51. Kertai MD, et al. A meta-analysis comparing the prognostic accuracy of six diagnostic tests for predicting perioperative cardiac risk in patients undergoing major vascular surgery. Heart. 2003;89(11):1327–34.

52. Best PJ, et al. The safety of treadmill exercise stress testing in patients with abdominal aortic aneurysms. Ann Intern Med. 1998;129(8):628–31.

53. Etchells E, et al. Semiquantitative dipyridamole myocardial stress perfusion imaging for cardiac risk assessment before noncardiac vascular surgery: a meta-analysis. J Vasc Surg. 2002;36(3):534–40.

54. Poldermans D, et al. Should major vascular surgery be delayed because of preoperative cardiac testing in intermediate-risk patients receiving beta-blocker therapy with tight heart rate control? J Am Coll Cardiol. 2006;48(5):964–9.

55. Madsen JK, et al. Prognosis and thallium-201 scintigraphy in patients admitted with chest pain without confirmed acute myocardial infarction. Br Heart J. 1988;59(2):184–9.

56. Lima RS, et al. Incremental value of combined perfusion and function over perfusion alone by gated SPECT myocardial perfusion imaging for detection of severe three-vessel coronary artery disease. J Am Coll Cardiol. 2003;42(1):64–70.

57. Afonso L, Mahajan N. Single-photon emission computed tomography myocardial perfusion imaging in the diagnosis of left main disease. Clin Cardiol. 2009;32(12):E11–5.

58. Aarnoudse WH, Botman KJ, Pijls NH. False-negative myocardial scintigraphy in balanced three-vessel disease, revealed by coronary pressure measurement. Int J Cardiovasc Intervent. 2003;5(2):67–71.

59. Berman DS, et al. Underestimation of extent of ischemia by gated SPECT myocardial perfusion imaging in patients with left main coronary artery disease. J Nucl Cardiol. 2007;14(4):521–8.

60. Zhu YY, et al. Dipyridamole perfusion scintigraphy: the experience with its application in one hundred seventy patients with known or suspected unstable angina. Am Heart J. 1991;121(1 Pt 1):33–43.

61. Kiat H, et al. Late reversibility of tomographic myocardial thallium-201 defects: an accurate marker of myocardial viability. J Am Coll Cardiol. 1988;12(6):1456–63.

62. Tillisch J, et al. Reversibility of cardiac wall-motion abnormalities predicted by positron tomography. N Engl J Med. 1986;314(14):884–8.

63. Marwick TH, et al. Metabolic responses of hibernating and infarcted myocardium to revascularization. A follow-up study of regional perfusion, function, and metabolism. Circulation. 1992;85(4):1347–53.

64. Allman KC, et al. Myocardial viability testing and impact of revascularization on prognosis in patients with coronary artery disease and left ventricular dysfunction: a meta-analysis. J Am Coll Cardiol. 2002;39(7):1151–8.

65. Scholte AJ, et al. Different manifestations of coronary artery disease by stress SPECT myocardial perfusion imaging, coronary calcium scoring, and multislice CT coronary angiography in asymptomatic patients with type 2 diabetes mellitus. J Nucl Cardiol. 2008;15(4):503–9.

66. Berman DS, et al. Relationship between stress-induced myocardial ischemia and atherosclerosis measured by coronary calcium tomography. J Am Coll Cardiol. 2004;44(4):923–30.

67. Bhavnani SP, Heller GV. Stress-only myocardial perfusion imaging … it is time for a change! J Nucl Cardiol. 2011;18(5):836–9.

68. Berman DS, et al. Separate acquisition rest thallium-201/stress technetium-99m sestamibi dual-isotope myocardial perfusion single-photon emission computed tomography: a clinical validation study. J Am Coll Cardiol. 1993;22(5):1455–64.

69. Cerqueira MD, et al. Recommendations for reducing radiation exposure in myocardial perfusion imaging. J Nucl Cardiol. 2010;17(4):709–18.

70. Heller GV, et al. Influence of exercise intensity on the presence, distribution, and size of thallium-201 defects. Am Heart J. 1992;123(4 Pt 1):909–16.

71. Iskandrian AS, et al. Effect of exercise level on the ability of thallium-201 tomographic imaging in detecting coronary artery disease: analysis of 461 patients. J Am Coll Cardiol. 1989;14(6):1477–86.

72. Stratmann HG, et al. Effect of the stress level achieved during symptom-limited exercise technetium-99m sestamibi myocardial tomography on the detection of coronary artery disease. Clin Cardiol. 1996;19(10):787–92.

73. Snader CE, et al. Importance of estimated functional capacity as a predictor of all-cause mortality among patients referred for exercise thallium single-photon emission computed tomography: report of 3,400 patients from a single center. J Am Coll Cardiol. 1997;30(3):641–8.

74. Vaduganathan P, et al. Detection of left anterior descending coronary artery stenosis in patients with left bundle branch block: exercise, adenosine or dobutamine imaging? J Am Coll Cardiol. 1996;28(3):543–50.

75. Koepfli P, et al. Left bundle branch block causes relative but not absolute septal underperfusion during exercise. Eur Heart J. 2009;30(24):2993–9.

76. Santos-Ocampo CD, et al. Comparison of exercise, dipyridamole, and adenosine by use of technetium 99m sestamibi tomographic imaging. J Nucl Cardiol. 1994;1(1):57–64.

77. Iskandrian AE, et al. Adenosine versus regadenoson comparative evaluation in myocardial perfusion imaging: results of the ADVANCE phase 3 multicenter international trial. J Nucl Cardiol. 2007;14(5):645–58.

78. Kwon DH, et al. Lessons from regadenoson and low-level treadmill/regadenoson myocardial perfusion imaging: initial clinical experience in 1263 patients. J Nucl Cardiol. 2010;17(5):853–7.

79. Klocke FJ, et al. ACC/AHA/ASNC guidelines for the clinical use of cardiac radionuclide imaging – executive summary: a

report of the American College of Cardiology/American Heart Association Task Force on Practice Guidelines (ACC/AHA/ASNC committee to revise the 1995 guidelines for the clinical use of cardiac radionuclide imaging). J Am Coll Cardiol. 2003;42(7):1318–33.

80. Zoghbi GJ, et al. Effect of caffeine on ischemia detection by adenosine single-photon emission computed tomography perfusion imaging. J Am Coll Cardiol. 2006;47(11):2296–302.

81. Thomas GS, et al. Safety of regadenoson, a selective adenosine A2A agonist, in patients with chronic obstructive pulmonary disease: a randomized, double-blind, placebo-controlled trial (RegCOPD trial). J Nucl Cardiol. 2008;15(3):319–28.

82. Kim C, et al. Pharmacologic stress testing for coronary disease diagnosis: a meta-analysis. Am Heart J. 2001;142(6):934–44.

83. Casale PN, et al. Simultaneous low level treadmill exercise and intravenous dipyridamole stress thallium imaging. Am J Cardiol. 1988;62(10 Pt 1):799–802.

84. Thomas GS, et al. Treadmill exercise during adenosine infusion is safe, results in fewer adverse reactions, and improves myocardial perfusion image quality. J Nucl Cardiol. 2000;7(5):439–46.

85. Taillefer R, et al. Acute beta-blockade reduces the extent and severity of myocardial perfusion defects with dipyridamole Tc-99m sestamibi SPECT imaging. J Am Coll Cardiol. 2003;42(8):1475–83.

86. Johnson LL, et al. Postischemic stunning can affect left ventricular ejection fraction and regional wall motion on post-stress gated sestamibi tomograms. J Am Coll Cardiol. 1997;30(7):1641–8.

87. Bateman TM, et al. Diagnostic accuracy of rest/stress ECG-gated Rb-82 myocardial perfusion PET: comparison with ECG-gated Tc-99m sestamibi SPECT. J Nucl Cardiol. 2006;13(1):24–33.

88. Maddahi J. Properties of an ideal PET perfusion tracer: new PET tracer cases and data. J Nucl Cardiol. 2012;19 Suppl 1:S30–7.

89. Uren NG, et al. Relation between myocardial blood flow and the severity of coronary-artery stenosis. N Engl J Med. 1994;330(25):1782–8.

90. Parkash R, et al. Potential utility of rubidium 82 PET quantification in patients with 3-vessel coronary artery disease. J Nucl Cardiol. 2004;11(4):440–9.

91. Di Carli MF, Murthy VL. Cardiac PET/CT for the evaluation of known or suspected coronary artery disease. Radiographics. 2011;31(5):1239–54.

Role of Echocardiography in Cardiology Consultation

14

Philip G. Haines, Nidhi Mehta, and James N. Kirkpatrick

Abstract

Echocardiography can be used to evaluate almost any cardiovascular disease process and provide structural/anatomical, functional, and hemodynamic information in real time at the patient's bedside. It can be used in both stable and critically ill patients. This chapter discusses important elements and uses of transthoracic, transesophageal, and stress echocardiography that are important to consultative cardiology, including appropriate ordering, echocardiographic techniques, and standard and emerging clinical uses.

Keywords

Echocardiography • Transesophageal echocardiography • Stress echocardiography • Doppler echocardiography • Contrast echocardiography • Appropriateness

Introduction

Noninvasive imaging in cardiology has revolutionized the diagnosis and management of many cardiovascular diseases. It provides useful and often critical diagnostic information to guide management at a fraction of the risk of invasive procedures. Cardiac computed tomography (CT), cardiac magnetic resonance imaging (MRI), nuclear cardiology, and echocardiography all have unique and overlapping advantages and disadvantages in terms of diagnostic potential, practicality, availability, cost, and risk. Echocardiography remains the least expensive, most widely accessible, and most frequently used imaging modality in cardiology with the least risk to the patient. Echocardiography can be used to evaluate almost any cardiovascular disease process and provide structural/anatomical, functional, and hemodynamic information in real time at the patient's bedside. It can be used in both stable and critically ill patients. Two-dimensional (2D) imaging provides thin slice tomographic views of the heart from which anatomy, structure, and function can be determined. Doppler echocardiography provides assessment of function, flow, and pressures. Transesophageal echocardiography (TEE) provides an additional approach for interrogating cardiac structure and function with ultrasound and often provides enhanced resolution of structures in patients who have poor precordial acoustic windows. TEE is also used to guide management in the operating room and cardiac catheterization laboratories [1, 2]. Dynamic testing with stress echocardiography can provide crucial diagnostic and prognostic information in patients with established or suspected coronary artery disease, valvular disease, or symptoms with an unclear etiology. A detailed discussion of

P.G. Haines, BM, BCh, MPH, MRCP (UK) • N. Mehta, MD
J.N. Kirkpatrick, MD (✉)
Department of Cardiology,
Hospital of the University of Pennsylvania,
3400 Spruce Street, Philadelphia,
PA 19104, USA
e-mail: philip.haines@uphs.upenn.edu;
nidhi.mehta@uphs.upenn.edu;
james.kirkpatrick@uphs.upenn.edu

The online version of this chapter (doi:10.1007/978-1-4471-4441-0_14) contains supplementary material, which is available to authorized users.

K. Stergiopoulos, D.L. Brown (eds.), *Evidence-Based Cardiology Consult*,
DOI 10.1007/978-1-4471-4441-0_14, © Springer-Verlag London 2014

echocardiography is beyond the scope of this chapter, which will focus instead on a general overview of echocardiographic techniques important for consultative cardiology. .

Ordering and Interpreting Echocardiograms

There has been a dramatic increase in the use of cardiovascular imaging in health care. This increase is also accompanied by the potential for the inappropriate use and/or overuse of these imaging resources. In addition, it has been recognized that inappropriately ordered nontoxic imaging procedures, such as echocardiography, can lead to other tests or interventions which could harm patients. In response to these concerns, the American College of Cardiology Foundation (ACCF) in partnership with the American Society of Echocardiography (ASE) and other relevant specialty organizations published Appropriate Use Criteria for specific modalities. In 2011, these societies published a comprehensive report on Appropriate Use Criteria (AUC) for echocardiography covering TTE, TEE, and stress echocardiography [3]. The AUC are intended to guide ordering of echocardiograms by medical providers but are also explicitly intended to guide payers in deciding whether to cover echocardiographic procedures. Although exhaustive in scope, the AUC essentially classifies echocardiograms as inappropriate if the results do not have the potential to change clinical management, if the study is performed as a routine follow-up when there are no changes in the clinical condition and for screening purposes in the absence of signs or symptoms of cardiovascular disease. Echocardiography to evaluate signs and symptoms of cardiovascular disease, to detect structural changes in certain disease states, and to establish indications for specific therapies is appropriate. A number of indications are of uncertain or unclassified appropriateness because there is inadequate evidence. Because TEE provides improved spatial resolution (since the TEE probe is located directly behind the left atrium with minimal soft tissue separating the probe from the myocardium), TEE is indicated when TTE views are inadequate or as the first test when TTE is unlikely to be able to answer the clinical question (e.g., excluding left atrial appendage thrombus prior to cardioversion, since TTE does not visualize the left atrial appendage well). TTE and TEE are complimentary. While TEE can provide superior resolution of most cardiac structures, it is sometimes inferior to TTE in visualizing anterior structures such as the LV apex, the RV, and the pulmonic valve. Furthermore, Doppler interrogation of valves is usually superior with TTE. TEE is a semi-invasive procedure which requires conscious sedation in most cases. Complications are rare but include risks of esophageal intubation (dental trauma, esophageal trauma/perforation, bleeding, aspiration) and risks of conscious sedation (hypoxia, hypotension,

arrhythmias). Intracardiac echo (ICE) involves placement of a catheter with an attached miniature echo probe through the venous system into the right heart. ICE is primarily used to guide transseptal puncture during left atrial ablation procedures for atrial fibrillation and to position atrial septal closure devices. However, it can also be used to examine the left atrial appendage for thrombus prior to cardioversion [4].

In addition to appropriately ordering echocardiograms, medical providers should take care to provide accurate and adequate information in the clinical order. Sonographers will often focus on specific structures that are known to be of clinical importance based, in part, on the stated indication for the echocardiogram. If the ordering provider supplies erroneous information, there is a chance that inadequate images will be obtained. Similarly, echocardiographers often rely on the clinical indication to direct specific interpretations.

When reading echocardiogram reports and considering what to do with their findings, it is important for the medical provider to note overall technical quality and statements about the visualization of specific structures of interest. The findings should be compared to prior echo reports and other imaging. If something does not make sense, it is reasonable to personally review images with the echocardiographer. In some cases it is helpful to seek a second opinion.

Echocardiographic Techniques

M-mode imaging sends and receives a single beam of ultrasound. The resulting single scan line is plotted over time to show movement of structures. M-mode has very high temporal and spatial resolution and is useful for tracking fine movements and making measurements. The accuracy of these measurements is frequently compromised when the M-mode interrogation angle is not perpendicular to the imaged structures, leading to an overestimate. In 2D imaging, the transducer sends out and receives a series of scan lines over an arc of 90°. Real-time images constructed from these lines are displayed to make a moving picture of the heart. 2D temporal and spacial resolution has improved to rival that of M-mode but is still compromised when patients have poor acoustic windows (e.g., lung disease, obesity, post-cardiac surgery).

Types of Doppler ultrasound include continuous wave (CW) and pulsed wave (PW) (collectively called "spectral Doppler"), color Doppler, and tissue Doppler. CW Doppler uses two ultrasound crystals—one continuously transmitting and the other continuously receiving. Advantages include the fact that very high velocities can be measured because sampling is continuous. Drawbacks include the fact that signals from the entire length of the ultrasound beam are recorded rendering accurate spatial localization of specific velocities impossible. It is crucial to align

Doppler ultrasound beams as parallel as possible to flow to resolve the peak velocities. In contrast, PW Doppler uses a single crystal to transmit a pulse of ultrasound and, after a specified time interval (determined by depth of interest), the crystal receives the reflected/backscattered signals. The transmit-wait-receive cycle time (pulse repetition frequency (PRF), number of pulses transmitted per second) increases with increasing depths of interest. PW allows one to determine the velocities at a specific location but it cannot resolve high velocity signals. Color Doppler uses PW Doppler techniques. Hence, it has same advantages and disadvantages as PW Doppler. Color Doppler places multiple sample volumes along multiple sampling lines generating a 2D anatomical image of movement, whether of blood or tissue. Velocities are displayed using a set color scale. Spatial pattern of flow is the focus of color Doppler rather than velocities; hence, valuable information can be gained despite imperfect interrogation angles. Color Doppler allows for assessment of spatial/anatomical location, speed, and direction of motion. In general, red color denotes movement towards the transducer, blue denotes movement away from the transducer, and white, yellow, or green signal turbulent flow. Tissue Doppler imaging (TDI) records the motion of tissue rather than blood cells. Therefore, the echo machine settings are changed to allow for the detection of lower velocity signals from tissue movement (usually <30 cm/s) which is in contrast to the velocities measured for blood (up to 800 cm/s). TDI uses the PW Doppler technique to acquire data from specific locations in the myocardium. The common locations sampled clinically include the septal and lateral mitral valve (MV) annulus and the lateral tricuspid valve (TV) annulus for assessment of LV diastolic function and RV systolic function.

Three-dimensional (3D) echocardiography allows the contemporaneous visualization of cardiac structures and their relationship to each other. In general, it provides more accurate measurements of ventricular volumes and mass than 2D echocardiography [5]. 3D TEE is particularly useful in characterizing MV pathology (Fig. 14.1, Video 14.1). Precise definition of the origin and cause of regurgitant jets and accurate planimetry of the MV diastolic orifice are possible. However, since the resolution of current systems is relatively low, fine structures are often seen better with 2D imaging. Suboptimal 2D images generally portend inadequate 3D images. Single beat 3D acquisitions have a limited field of view. The large-field, "full-volume" 3D acquisitions consist of 4–6 pyramids of data acquired in 4–6 separate cardiac cycles which are "stitched" together, leading to artifacts in the setting of arrhythmias, deep breathing, and cardiac translational motion. Acquisition, analysis, and interpretation of 3D datasets require specialized training [6].

Contrast agents used in echocardiography consist of agitated saline and synthetic microbubbles. Both sources of bubbles are good reflectors of ultrasound waves and generate strong signals, leading to bright contrast in the heart

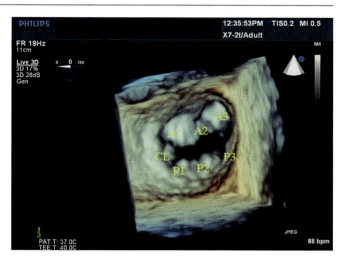

Fig. 14.1 Mitral valve in 3D. Three-dimensional transesophageal echocardiographic images of the mitral valve from the "surgeon's view"—the left atrial perspective. The anterior leaflet is on top and the posterior leaflet is on the bottom. This technique provides a unique perspective from which to evaluate all scallops of the mitral valve leaflets—from left (lateral) to right (medial) aspects of the posterior leaflet, P1, P2, and P3, and the corresponding scallops of the anterior leaflet, A1, A2, and A3. In this patient there is also a medial commissural leaflet (*CL*) which located at the intersection of the anterior and posterior leaflets. The video demonstrates prolapse of the P2 segment (middle portion of the posterior leaflet) and P3 (medial or rightward portion of the posterior leaflet)

chambers. Agitated saline is composed of air mixed with saline, producing bubbles which can be injected into the right side of the heart. These bubbles are trapped in the pulmonary capillaries and will not pass into the left heart unless there is an intracardiac or intrapulmonary shunt. The appearance of bubbles in the left side of the heart within 5 cardiac cycles of right-sided opacification and increase in left-sided bubbles in the release phase of Valsalva suggest intracardiac shunting. Left-sided bubbles appearing after 5 cycles denote intrapulmonary shunting. Synthetic microbubble contrast agents consist of an inert gas inside of a protein or lipid shell. Contrast agents are about the size of red blood cells and therefore traverse the pulmonary capillaries, opacifying the left side of the heart. Contrast agents can improve delineation of wall motion and measurement of LVEF in patients with suboptimal echocardiographic images. Both types of contrast agents can also be used to augment Doppler signals, such as the TV regurgitant jet [7].

Speckle tracking is a new echocardiographic technique that tracks unique patterns of echo-bright speckles in the myocardium. Tracking the displacement and velocity of these speckles over the cardiac cycle allows the calculation of myocardial strain (motion of a myocardial segment relative to its position at rest) and strain rate. The clinical applications of speckle tracking are still under investigation, but it has been used to assess systolic function, wall motion, diastolic function, left atrial function, and dyssynchrony. Speckle tracking requires high-resolution images which are not possible on all patients [8].

Basic TTE and TEE Views

A basic knowledge of what can be visualized in the common TTE and TEE views may help the cardiovascular consultant in ordering, interpreting, and using information from echocardiography (Table 14.1).

Specific Uses of Echocardiography

Chamber Quantification

Left Ventricle

Various types of echocardiographic characteristics of specific disease states have been characterized for the left ventricle (LV) (Fig. 14.2, Videos 14.2a and 14.2b) (Fig. 14.3, Videos 14.3a and 14.3b). Echocardiographic measures of LV chamber size, geometry, wall thickness, and function are strong independent predictors of morbidity and mortality and, as such, play a significant role in cardiovascular

Table 14.1 Main transthoracic and transesophageal echocardiography views and anatomy

View	Left heart anatomy	Right heart anatomy	Extracardiac anatomy
TTE: parasternal long-axis view	Aortic valve right and noncoronary cusps	Muscular RVOT	Aortic root
	MV anterior and posterior leaflets		Sinuses of Valsalva
	Mitral subvalvular structures		Sinotubular junction
	LA		Ascending aorta (proximal 3–4 cm)
	Coronary sinus		RPA
	LV (anterior septum and inferolateral wall)		Descending aorta (short axis)
			Intrapericardial space (fat, fluid)
			Intrapleural space (pleural effusion)
TTE: parasternal RV inflow view		RV	IVC entering RA inferior to coronary sinus
		RA	
		TV anterior and posterior	
		Moderator band	
		Coronary sinus entering RA (near TV annulus)	
		Eustachian valve (junction of IVC and RA)	
TTE: parasternal TV outflow view		RVOT	
		PV	
		Pulmonary artery	
TTE: short-axis view			
Aortic valve level	All three aortic valve leaflets (right, left, and noncoronary cusps)	RVOT	Pulmonary artery
	LA	TV septal and anterior leaflets	
	Interatrial septum	RV inflow	
		RA	
		Interatrial septum	
Mitral valve level	Segments (scallops) of anterior (A1, A2, A3) and posterior (P1, P2, P3) MV leaflets		
	Medial and lateral MV commissures		
Mid-ventricular (papillary muscle) level:	Medial and lateral papillary muscles		Posterior pericardium
Chamber quantification and LV function	LV wall segments (mid): anterior, anterolateral, inferolateral, inferior, inferoseptum, anteroseptum		
Abnormal septal motion (RV volume/pressure overload, conduction disease, prior cardiac surgery, pericardial disease)	Interventricular septum		
Apical level	LV wall apical segments: anterior, lateral, inferior, and septal		

Table 14.1 (continued)

View	Left heart anatomy	Right heart anatomy	Extracardiac anatomy
TTE: apical 4-chamber view	LV wall segments: anterolateral, inferoseptum, apex	RV free wall	Right upper pulmonary vein
	MV anterior and posterior leaflets and annulus	TV septal leaflet (adjacent to septum) and anterior or posterior leaflet	Descending aorta (lateral to LA)
	LA	RA	
	Interatrial septum		
TTE: apical 5-chamber view	Spectral Doppler of aortic valve		
TTE: apical 2-chamber view	LV (anterior and inferior walls)		Long axis of descending aorta (adjacent to posterior wall of LA)
	MV (anterior leaflet)		
	LA		
TTE: apical long-axis view	Identical to PLAX	RVOT	Aortic root
	LV (anteroseptum, inferolateral walls)		
	LVOT		
	Aortic valve		
	Mitral valve		
	LA		
TTE: subcostal view	LV (septum, anterolateral walls)	RV free wall	IVC size and collapsibility (RA pressure)
	LA	RA	Hepatic veins (RA pressure, pericardial diseases, TR)
	Interatrial septum (best TTE view)		
TTE: suprasternal notch view	Superior portion of LA (inferior to pulmonary arteries)		Ascending aorta
			Aortic arch
			Proximal descending aorta
			Origins of brachiocephalic artery
			Left common carotid
			Subclavian artery
			SVC (adjacent to ascending aorta)
			RPA inferior to arch
TEE: mid-esophageal position	LV wall segments	RV free wall	Pulmonary veins
	MV anterior and posterior leaflets and annulus	TV septal leaflet (adjacent to septum) and anterior or posterior leaflet	Aortic root
	LA	RA	Sinus of Valsalva
	Left atrial appendage	RA appendage	Ascending aorta
	Interatrial septum	Coronary sinus	Pulmonary artery
			SVC
			IVC
TEE: transgastric position	LV short axis	RV short axis	IVC
	Sub-mitral apparatus	Spectral Doppler of pulmonic valve	Pericardium
	Spectral Doppler of aortic valve		

TTE transthoracic echocardiogram, *TEE* transesophageal echocardiogram, *RVOT* right ventricular outflow tract, *LV* left ventricle, *RV* right ventricle, *RA* right atrium, *TV* tricuspid valve, *IVC* inferior vena cava, *PV* pulmonic valve, *LA* left atrium, *MV* mitral valve, *PLAX* parasternal long-axis view, *SAX* short-axis view, *TR* tricuspid regurgitation, *RVOT* right ventricular outflow tract, *LVOT* left ventricular outflow tract, *RPA* right pulmonary artery, *SVC* superior vena cava, *IVC* inferior vena cava

disease diagnosis, management, risk stratification, and prognosis [9].

Several different methods are available to quantify the LV. Dimensional measurements using M-mode echocardiography allow calculation of LV internal diameters during systole and diastole, septal and posterior wall thickness, fractional shortening, and ejection fraction. Dimensions are measured in a single plane, leading to inaccuracies in converting linear measurements into 3D volumes. Volumetric measurements rely on high-resolution 2D apical 2-and

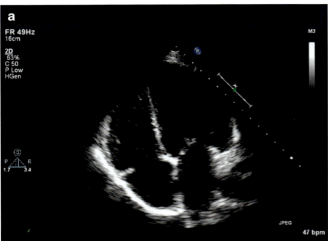

Fig. 14.2 Stress-induced cardiomyopathy. (**a**) Apical 4-chamber view demonstrates akinesis of the mid chamber to the apex, consistent with either multivessel coronary ischemia or stress-induced cardiomyopathy (Takotsubo). (**b**) Several weeks later, repeat echocardiography demonstrates complete resolution of the wall motion abnormalities, consistent with a diagnosis of stress-induced cardiomyopathy

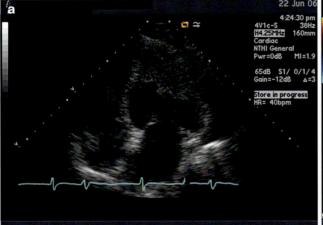
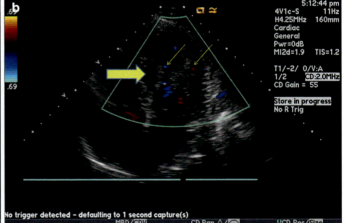

Fig. 14.3 Echodensity filling the left ventricle. (**a**) The left ventricle is filled from the mid wall to the apex with a large echodensity. The differential diagnosis included thrombus and endocardial fibroelastosis. (**b**) However, color Doppler demonstrated flow within the echodensity (*small arrows*) and highlighted deep crypts (*large arrow*). These morphological findings are consistent with non-compaction cardiomyopathy

4-chamber views with good endocardial border definition for tracing the cavity. These measurements can also be made from specific TEE views. End-systolic (ESV) and end-diastolic volumes (EDV) can be calculated using the modified Simpson's rule, which calculates the total LV volume in systole and diastole by dividing them into disks. Each disk has a specific area and height, from which can be calculated the disk volume. The LV volume is the summation of these disks. The area-length method can be used when endocardial definition is inadequate. This method assumed the LV is bullet shaped. The mid-LV cross-sectional area is measured via planimetry and the length of the LV is taken from a line drawn from the MV annulus to the apex in the 4-chamber view. Measurements are performed in end diastole and end systole. EDV and ESV are calculated from both these methods as

$$EF = (EDV - ESV)/EDV$$

Foreshortening of the chambers (failing to obtain an imaging plane that visualizes the true long and short axes of a chamber) is a significant pitfall which can be overcome by using 3D imaging.

LV mass is a strong independent predictor of outcome and response to therapy. LV mass can be calculated using M-mode, 2D, or 3D approaches and is based on the subtraction of the LV cavity volume from the total volume surrounded by the LV epicardium. This technique provides the LV muscle volume. This volume is converted to mass by multiplying by the myocardial density. Although calculations can be based on either linear M-mode or 2D measurements, 3D measurements provide the best accuracy when endocardial definition is adequate.

Chamber remodeling refers to the size, geometry, wall thickness, and functional changes that occur over time in response to various physiological and pathological states. These remodeling processes can occur to any chamber of the heart, though LV remodeling has garnered the most attention. LV remodeling provides diagnostic and prognostic utility in the clinical setting in addition to acting as a surrogate endpoint for animal and human clinical intervention trials. Relative wall thickness (RWT) incorporates measures of wall thickness and chamber diameter. This formula is based on the linear measurements:

$$RWT = (2 \times PWTd / LVIDd)$$

where PWTd = posterior wall thickness in diastole and LVIDd = left ventricular internal diameter in diastole. This formula allows one to classify increases in LV mass.

Concentric hypertrophy is marked by increased LV mass due primarily to increased wall thickness, while eccentric hypertrophy is characterized by increased LV mass from enlargement of the LV chamber. Compensatory remodeling in chronic pressure overload states (e.g., hypertension, aortic stenosis) usually results in concentric hypertrophy (increased wall thickness, normal cavity volume and a preserved EF with an increased RWT and increased LV mass). Compensatory remodeling also occurs in chronic volume overload states (e.g., severe mitral or aortic regurgitation) and usually results in eccentric hypertrophy (increased chamber diameter out of proportion to increased wall thickness).

Concentric remodeling consists of increased wall thickness with normal LV mass and represents physiological remodeling. It is found in athletes' hearts in response to chronic increased levels of activity, but it can also be seen in chronic hypertension associated with high peripheral resistance, increased arterial stiffness, and reduced cardiac index. The transition to pathological remodeling involves progressive dilatation and shape change of the LV resulting in significant changes in chamber geometry and reduced systolic and diastolic function. Pathological LV remodeling represents the final downstream pathway common to pressure overload, volume overload, many cardiomyopathic processes, and myocardial infarction.

Left Atrium

Left atrial (LA) size represents a powerful independent predictor of outcomes and provides essential diagnostic infor-

mation about left-sided filling pressures, LV diastolic function, and MV function [10]. LA size can be measured using linear methods from the parasternal long axis. A more accurate method, however, takes into account the fact that the LA can dilate in multiple different directions. Left atrial volume is measured in ways similar to LV volumes. Wherever possible, LA volume should be indexed to body mass index. Newer techniques such as speckle tracking have been used to quantify left atrial function but require further validation [10].

Right Ventricle, Right Atrium, and Pulmonary Artery

Right ventricular (RV) chamber dilatation and RV systolic dysfunction have been shown to be strong independent predictors of outcome, morbidity, and mortality. RV geometry is complex; it is a crescent-shaped structure which wraps around the LV. 2D visualization of the RV and, therefore, area/length measurements are highly sensitive to probe position with significant inter- and intraobserver variability. Therefore, assessment of RV structure and function requires an integrated approach utilizing several different approaches and multiple views. The important parameters include (1) RV free-wall thickness as a marker of RV hypertrophy, (2) RV chamber dimensions, (3) septal motion (indicative of RV volume and/or pressure overload, constrictive physiology, left bundle branch block (LBBB), pacing), and (4) RV fractional area change and tricuspid annular plane systolic excursion (TAPSE) as markers of systolic function. RV free-wall thickness can be measured from 2D or M-mode in the parasternal long-axis (PLAX) or subcostal views. RV chamber dimensions include the right ventricular outflow tract (RVOT) diameter (short-axis (SAX) view), the RV longitudinal length, and the basal and mid diameters (apical 4-chamber view). RV fractional area change is akin to measurements of the LVEF except that area, rather than volume, is used, with normal values from 32 to 60 %. TAPSE measures RV longitudinal motion during systole (approximately 70 % of RV systolic function occurs in the longitudinal direction) and can be measured in the apical 4-chamber view using M-mode or 2D techniques. Right atrial size is also measured as an area with enlargement defined as area >18 cm². The pulmonary artery dimension is measured in the SAX view at the level of the ascending aorta [11].

Aorta

While echocardiography cannot visualize the entire aorta, many sections of the aorta can be measured and assessed for dissection, calcification, atherosclerotic plaques, and intramural hematomas. Using the TTE PLAX views, the maximal diameter of the aortic root at the sinuses of Valsalva and the sinotubular junction are easily seen. The aortic arch can be visualized by placing the echo transducer in the suprasternal notch. 2D and

Doppler interrogation of the proximal descending aorta can be used to assess for aortic coarctation. Portions of the descending thoracic aorta can be seen posterior to the LA in PLAX and apical 2-chamber views. The proximal portion of the abdominal aorta can be seen in the subcostal view. Aortic root dilatation at the sinus of Valsalva is defined by an echo-derived diameter greater than the 95 % confidence interval of the reference population, indexed to age and body surface area.[2] Aneurysms of other segments can be determined when the segment is larger than contiguous segments of apparently normal size. Enlargement of the root and ascending aorta should trigger careful assessment of the aortic valve, as bicuspid valves are associated with aortopathy. Approximately 3–4 cm of the ascending aorta can also be visualized.

In dissection, echocardiography identifies a flap separating the true from the false lumen (the true lumen expands during systole). Color Doppler can detect differential flow on either side of the flap (or thrombus in the false lumen) and intimal tears with flow from the true into the false lumen. Important other findings include hemopericardium, aortic regurgitation, and ventricular dysfunction (possibly signifying obstruction of coronary arteries). TTE is 77–80 % sensitive and 93–96 % specific for identifying proximal aortic dissection. TEE usually is superior in assessing size and atheromatous disease of every section of the aorta, except the abdominal aorta and a small portion of the superior aspect of the ascending aorta (where the trachea and left mainstem bronchus may interfere with visualization). It is 88–98 % sensitive and 90–95 % specific for identifying proximal aortic dissection [12]. TEE has an advantage over CT and MRI of the aorta in that it can be performed at bedside in unstable patients and is able to determine mobility of atheromatous plaques. TEE can differentiate intramural hematomas (smooth luminal surface crescent-shaped) from dissections with thrombus (intimal flap, non-crescent-shaped) and thrombus or plaque (irregular surface).

Echocardiographic Assessment of Diastolic Function

The clinical importance of identifying and quantifying the severity of diastolic dysfunction and the presence of elevated left heart filling pressures has been demonstrated in many trials. Parameters of diastolic dysfunction are strong independent predictors of morbidity and mortality in heart failure patients and have also been shown to predict the future development of heart failure in asymptomatic patients. Left ventricular hypertrophy (LVH) and increased LV mass are associated with and predictive of diastolic dysfunction and adverse outcomes [13]. The presence of severe diastolic dysfunction correlates more strongly with symptoms in heart failure patients than ejection fraction [14].

Echocardiography plays a central role in assessing diastolic function; methods for evaluating diastolic function and left-sided filling pressures have been standardized [15]. The most important goals when assessing diastolic function are to determine the grade of diastolic dysfunction and whether there are normal or elevated left-sided filling pressures (Table 14.2). Whether the LVEF is preserved or decreased impacts the evaluation of diastolic function. Patients with systolic dysfunction almost always have some degree of diastolic dysfunction. Structural diastolic parameters include LA size/LA volume, LVH, and LV mass. Volumetric measurement of LA size, in particular, should be a standard part of diastolic functional assessment, though it can reflect disease processes besides diastolic dysfunction, such as atrial fibrillation, mitral regurgitation and stenosis, and heart transplantation. Functional measures include mitral valve inflow Doppler parameters. These parameters include the ratio of peak early diastolic filling velocity (E wave) to peak atrial contraction filling velocity (A wave) and deceleration time of the E wave (a short time indicates fast equalization of LA and LV pressures, suggesting high LV filling pressures). Supporting measures of diastolic function are necessary in many cases, because a so-called "pseudonormal" pattern of mitral E velocity and E/A ratio exists, indicative of moderate diastolic dysfunction. These other measures include the ratio of peak systolic to diastolic velocity from spectral Doppler recording in the pulmonary veins, the LA size index, the difference between the duration of mitral inflow and pulmonary vein flow reversal during atrial contraction, flow propagation from the mitral annulus to the LV apex, and the pulmonary artery systolic pressure. MV annular early diastolic relaxation velocity measured from tissue Doppler imaging (e′ or e_a) provides an assessment of diastolic ventricular compliance. Using a combination of these parameters, one can classify patients as having normal diastolic function or mild, moderate, or severe diastolic dysfunction. The ratio of E to e′ can also be used as a measure of left atrial pressure (< or >/= 15 mmHg), in combination with other measurements.

"Echo Swan"

Various echocardiographic techniques have been used to estimate cardiac hemodynamics. The "echo swan" approach can provide estimates of filling pressure which correlate with specific invasive hemodynamic values (pulmonary artery systolic, mean and diastolic pressures, pulmonary vascular resistance) or ranges of pressures (right atrial pressure) or provide an estimate above or below a certain value (pulmonary capillary wedge pressure, LV end-diastolic pressure) (Table 14.3).

Table 14.2 Simplified echocardiographic assessment of diastolic function

	Reference values supporting diastolic dysfunction[a]	
	Females	*Males*
Structural parameters:		
LA volume index (2- or 4-chamber view), ml/m^2	≥34	≥34
LV septal wall thickness, cm	>0.9 cm	>1.0
LV posterior wall thickness, cm	>0.9 cm	>1.0
LV mass index, g/m^2	>95	>102
	Reference values	
	Normal	
Functional parameters:		
Mitral valve E/A ratio	≥1–<2*	
Mitral E wave velocity, cm/s	≤50*	
Mitral valve E wave Deceleration time (DT)	160–200 ms*	
Pulmonary vein systolic/diastolic inflow velocity ratio	>1	
Septal E′	≥8	
Lateral E′	≥10	
Septal E/E′ (left sided filling pressures)	≤8	
Lateral E/E′ (left sided filling pressures)	≤8	
*Also seen in "pseudonormal" pattern		

↑**Left-sided filling pressures** (in patients with normal EF)	**Grade of diastolic dysfunction**		
Likely ↑*Filling pressures*	*Grade 1 (mild)*	*Grade 2 (moderate)*	*Grade 3 (severe)*
E/A ratio ≥1	Septal E′ <8	Septal E′ <8	Septal E′ <8
LAVI ≥34 ml/m^2	Lateral E′ <10	Lateral E′ <10	Lateral E′ <10
Septal E/E′ >15	LAVI ≥34 ml/m^2	LAVI ≥34 ml/m^2	LAVI ≥34 ml/m^2
Lateral E/E′ >12	E/A ratio <0.8	E/A ratio 0.8–1.5	E/A ratio ≥2
Av E/E′ >13	DT >200 ms	DT 160–200 ms	DT <160 ms

↑**Left-sided filling pressures** (in patients with low EF)		
Likely ↑*Filling pressures*	↑ *Filling pressures*	
E/A ratio ≥1 – <2	E/A >2	
E/A <1 and E Vmax >50 ms	DT <150 ms	
E/E′ (avg E′) >15	E/E′ >15	
Pulmonary S/D ratio <1		

LA left atrium, *LV* left ventricle, *LAVI* left atrial volume index, *DT* deceleration time, *EF* ejection fraction, *E* early rapid filling wave, *A* filling wave due to atrial contraction, *E/A ratio* ratio of early rapid to atrial filling, *S/D ratio* pulmonary vein systolic/diastolic peak velocity ratio, *E′* early diastolic tissue Doppler velocity, *Av* average

[a]Nagueh et al. [15]

Echocardiography of Valves

Echocardiographic modalities play an integral role in the identification, structural and functional evaluation, and serial monitoring of patients with valvular heart disease. These modalities establish the presence and etiology of a valve abnormality and estimate the severity of valvular dysfunction. Echocardiography also provides an assessment of the hemodynamic and functional consequences of valvulopathies on cardiac structure and function.

Guidelines on the assessment of valve stenosis [16] and regurgitation [17] emphasize the importance of employing a comprehensive and integrated approach to aim for concordance between the different parameters assessed (Table 14.4). Explanations for discordance should be sought. Echocardiography also plays a central role in the evaluation of prosthetic valve function. Echocardiographic techniques can help detect and distinguish between prosthetic valve obstruction (pannus, thrombosis) and patient-prosthetic valve mismatch and provide a comprehensive

Table 14.3 Echocardiographic hemodynamics

Hemodynamic parameter	Echocardiographic equivalent
RA pressure (RAP)	2D subcostal view of IVC in long axis
	Based on size of IVC and degree of collapse with inspiration, pressure estimated as 0–5, 6–10, or 10–20 mmHg
	For simplicity, use 3, 8, and 15 mmHg
Pulmonary artery systolic pressure (PASP)[a]	CW spectral Doppler of TR velocity used to calculate peak TR pressure gradient ($4v^2$)
	$RVSP = TR\ pressure\ gradient + RA\ pressure$
Pulmonary artery diastolic pressure (PADP)	CW spectral Doppler of PR velocity (measurement taken at end diastole) used to calculate PR end-diastolic pressure gradient ($4v^2$)
	$PADP = PR\ end\text{-}diastolic\ pressure\ gradient + RAP$
Mean pulmonary artery pressure	CW of spectral Doppler of TR velocity envelope (VTI of TR envelope) to measure mean TR pressure gradient
	$PA\ mean\ pressure = mean\ TR\ gradient + RAP$
Pulmonary vascular resistance (PVR)	Measure TR Vmax and PW spectral Doppler of RVOT flow (velocity time integral)
	$PVR = TR\ Vmax/(RVOT\ VTI \times 10 + 0.16)$
Pulmonary capillary wedge pressure (PCWP)	Mitral valve inflow E wave Vmax/ tissue Doppler of septal annulus E' Vmax
Left atrial pressure (LAP)	E/E' < 8 → PCWP 5–12 mmHg
	E/E' > 15 → PCWP > 20 mmHg
	CW spectral Doppler of AR (Vmax) to calculate AR pressure gradient ($4v^2$)
	$LA\ pressure = diastolic\ BP - AR\ pressure\ gradient$
Stroke volume (SV), cardiac output, and cardiac index (CO/CI)	PW spectral Doppler of LVOT flow (VTI of LVOT)
	$LVOT\ area = \pi\ (LVOT\ diameter/2)^2$
	$SV = LVOT\ VTI \times LVOT\ area$
	$SV \times HR = CO$
	$CO/BSA - CI$

[a]Subtract pulmonic valve gradient if pulmonic valve stenosis present

RAP right atrial pressure, *PASP* pulmonary artery systolic pressure, *PADP* pulmonary artery diastolic pressure, *2D* 2 dimensional, *IVC* inferior vena cava, *TR* tricuspid regurgitation, *RA* right atrial, *PR* pulmonic regurgitation, *CW* continuous wave Doppler, *VTI* velocity time integral, *v* velocity, *RVSP* right ventricular systolic pressure, *PA* pulmonary artery, *Vmax* maximal velocity, *E wave* early diastolic filling, *PCWP* pulmonary capillary wedge pressure, *AR* aortic regurgitation, *LA* left atrial, *LAP* left atrial pressure, *BP* blood pressure, *PW* pulse wave Doppler, *LVOT* left ventricular outflow tract, *SV* stroke volume, *CO* cardiac output, *CI* cardiac index, *HR* heart rate, *BSA* body surface area

assessment of regurgitation (valvular vs. perivalvular, detection and characterization of valve dehiscence). 3D TEE has proven particularly helpful for characterization of MV prosthetic dysfunction.

Valvular Stenosis

Assessing the severity of valvular stenosis by echocardiography involves the measurement of peak and mean gradients and valve areas. A detailed description of echo calculations is beyond the scope of this chapter, but there are two important simple equations that should be understood. From the modified Bernoulli equation (pressure = $4 \times$ velocity^2), pressure gradients across an orifice can be estimated. Thus, spectral Doppler velocities can be used to measure diastolic, systolic, and mean pressures across an orifice. Mean and peak pressure gradients are useful for assessing the severity of stenotic lesions (particularly aortic, mitral, pulmonic, and tricuspid valve stenosis and LV/LV outflow tract (OT) obstruction). The flow volume equation (Fig. 14.4) can be used to measure stenotic valve areas because the flow volume through an area proximal to the valve must equal the flow volume through the valve.

Aortic stenosis severity is based on three parameters: aortic stenosis jet velocity, mean transaortic gradient, and aortic valve area (AVA) by continuity equation. Aortic jet velocity is measured by CW Doppler (apical, suprasternal, right upper sternal border) to obtain the highest velocity that is parallel to the ultrasound beam. The velocity profile should have a triangular shape with the peak in early systole with mild AS. As the stenosis worsens, the profile becomes rounded with the peak occurring at mid-systole.

The main limitations in the calculation of aortic gradients are misalignment of the aortic jet, inclusion of the mitral regurgitant jet and pressure recovery. Pressure recovery needs to be considered when the ascending aorta is <30 mm in diameter. As the aortic jet ejects through a narrow orifice, the flow decreases, and the kinetic energy is converted to potential energy and heat loss. The conversion to potential

Table 14.4 Echocardiographic assessment of valves

Aortic stenosis

Parameter	Mild	Moderate	Severe
AVA (cm^2)	>1.5 cm	1.0–1.5	<1.0
Mean gradient mm Hg	<20	20–40	>40
Aortic jet velocity (m/s)	2.6–2.9	3.0–4.0	>4.0
Indexed AVA (cm^2/m^2)			<0.6

Mitral stenosis

Specific findings	Mild	Moderate	Severe
MVA (cm^2)	>1.5	1.0–1.5	<1.0
Supportive findings			
Mean gradient (mmHg)	<5	5–10	>10
PASP (mmHg)	<30	30–50	>50

Aortic regurgitation

Specific signs	Mild	Moderate	Severe
	Central jet width <25 % of LVOT	Signs of AR > mild but no criteria for severe AR	Central jet width ≥65 % of LVOT
	Vena contracta <0.3 cm^2		Vena contracta >0.6 cm^2
Supportive signs	Deceleration slope >500 ms	Holodiastolic flow reversal in descending aorta	Deceleration slope <200 ms; ≥ moderate LV enlargement (except acute AR); Holodiastolic aortic flow reversal in abdominal aorta
	Normal LV size (except acute AR)		
	No or brief early diastolic flow reversal in descending aorta		
Quantitative			
Regurgitant volume, ml/beat	<30 ml	30–59 ml	>60 ml
Effective regurgitant orifice area, cm^2	<0.10 cm^2	0.10–0.29 cm^2	≥0.30 cm^2

Mitral regurgitation

Specific	Mild	Moderate	Severe
	Small central jet (<20 % LA area)	Signs of MR > mild present, no features of severe MR	Vena contracta width >0.7 cm
	Vena contracta width <0.3 cm		Large central jet (>40 % of LA area) or swirling
			Pulmonary vein S wave reversal
			Flail leaflet/ruptured papillary muscle
Supportive	Pulmonary vein S > D		Dense, triangular spectral Doppler MR signal
	Soft density, parabolic spectral Doppler MR signal		E wave dominance (>1.2 m/s)
	Normal LA/LV size		Dilated LA/LV (except acute MR)
Quantitative			
Regurgitant volume (ml/beat)	<30 ml	30–59 ml	≥60 ml
Effective regurgitant orifice area, EROA (cm^2)	<0.20 cm^2	0.20–0.39 cm^2	≥0.40 cm^2

Tricuspid regurgitation

Parameter	Mild	Moderate	Severe
Morphology of valve	Normal		Flail leaflet/poor coaptation
RV/RA/IVC size	Normal	Dense, variable contour	Dilated (except acute TR)
Jet density and contour	Soft and parabolic		Dense, triangular, early peaking
Jet area-central jets (cm^2)	<5	5–10	>10
Hepatic vein flow	S > D	S wave velocity	S reversal

Tricuspid stenosis[a]

Specific findings	Significant stenosis
Mean gradient (mmHg)	≥5

Table 14.4 (continued)

Inflow VTI (cm)	>60		
PHT (ms)	$\geq$190		
Valve area	$\leq$1 cm^2		
Supportive findings			
RA size	$\geq$ moderate		
Dilated IVC			
Pulmonary stenosis[b]			
Parameter	*Mild*	*Moderate*	*Severe*
Peak velocity (m/s)	<3	3–4	4
Peak gradient (mmHg)	<36	36–64	>64
Pulmonary regurgitation[c]			
Parameter	*Mild*	*Moderate*	*Severe*
Morphology	Normal	Normal	Normal or abnormal
Jet size (color Doppler)	Thin (<10 mm) with narrow origin	Intermediate	Large with wide origin
Jet density and deceleration rate (CW)	Soft, slow deceleration	Dense, variable deceleration	Dense, steep deceleration early termination of diastolic flow

[a]In presence of > mild TR, estimated valve area will be underestimated. However, valve $\leq$1 cm^2 suggests significant hemodynamic impact on the right heart
[b]Pressure gradients are used to estimate severity due to the challenge in obtaining accurate pulmonary valve areas
[c]Parameters not well validated
AVA aortic valve area, *Indexed AVA* indexed AVA to body surface area, *MVA* mitral valve area, *PASP* pulmonary artery systolic pressure, *LVOT* left ventricular outflow tract, *AR* aortic regurgitation, *MR* mitral regurgitation, *LA* left atrium, *LV* left ventricle, *S* pulmonary or hepatic vein systolic wave, *D* pulmonary or hepatic vein diastolic wave, *PHT* pressure halftime, *IVC* inferior vena cava, *CW* continuous wave Doppler, *TR* tricuspid regurgitation, *RA* right atrium, *RV* right ventricle, *VTI* velocity time integral, *EROA* effective regurgitant orifice area

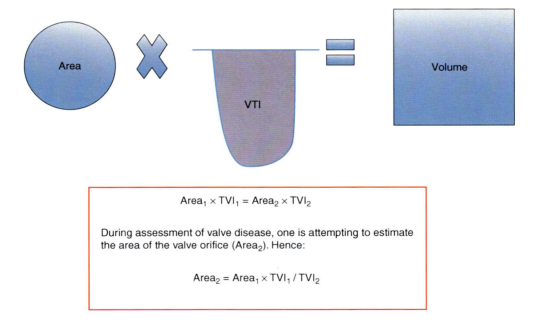

$$Area_1 \times TVI_1 = Area_2 \times TVI_2$$

During assessment of valve disease, one is attempting to estimate the area of the valve orifice (Area$_2$). Hence:

$$Area_2 = Area_1 \times TVI_1 / TVI_2$$

Fig. 14.4 The flow volume equation. Volumes of blood can be calculated by multiplying area (cm^2) × integral of the Doppler velocity profile (time velocity integral, TVI), in cm (integral of flow over time = distance traveled by all the blood cells in a specific area over a specific time period). The area of a circle ($\pi \times r^2 = D^2 \times 0.785$, where r is the radius and D the diameter of the area) is multiplied by the TVI of the Doppler velocity profile to calculate stroke volume at that site.
Example: calculation of aortic valve area

stroke volume through aortic valve = stroke volume through LVOT

volume = area × TVI

$$AVA \times AV_{TVI} = LVOT\ area \times LVOT_{TVI}$$

$$AVA = LVOT\ diameter^2 \times 0.785 \times LVOT_{TVI} / AV_{TVI}$$

where AVA = aortic valve area, AVTVI = time velocity integral through the aortic valve, and LVOTTVI = time velocity integral of the left ventricular outflow tract

energy raises pressure differential across the valve, which is measured by echocardiography. This pressure "recovers" in the narrow ascending aorta when some of the kinetic energy is converted back to pressure, leading to a reduction in the pressure gradient. Echocardiography thus measures a higher pressure gradient than is measured invasively. Other limitations of measuring the aortic valve area by echocardiography are the LVOT diameter, which is squared in the continuity equation; measurement of effective valve area rather than anatomic flow area, due to contraction of flow at the narrowed orifice; and the changes in valve area due to flow rates ("pseudostenosis" in the setting of low output, in which the flow generated by the dysfunctional LV is unable to push open the aortic valve to its full extent).

In patients with LVH, especially elderly women, the aortic valve area may be small due to low gradients from a small left ventricle and reduced stroke volume. Concurrent severe aortic regurgitation can increase the mean gradient and maximum velocity since there is increased flow across the aortic valve. Severe mitral regurgitation can cause reduced aortic flow and, therefore, reduced transaortic gradients; however, the valve area calculation is accurate. Mitral stenosis can reduce cardiac output and therefore mimic low-flow/low-gradient AS.

Pressure halftime (PHT) is the time it takes for the pressure gradient (not the velocity) between two chambers to fall to half of its peak value. PHT measured from CW across the MV can be used to calculate MV area = 220/PHT. This technique can be fraught with error since the pressure drop can be significantly affected by LA pressures and LV compliance and pressures. Pathologic states such as LVH and aortic regurgitation can decrease pressure halftime, whereas mitral regurgitation can increase pressure halftime. Exercise testing can help determine the clinical significance of mitral stenosis. Additional parameters that are considered when assessing severity are LA size, LA thrombus formation, and pulmonary hypertension. Mitral stenotic area may be best calculated by 3D-guided planimetry.

Valvular Regurgitation

Assessment of valvular regurgitation is often done by examining the size of the regurgitant color jet and assigning a semiquantitative score (e.g., mild, moderate, severe, or 1+, 2+, 3+, 4+). Jet area in the receiving chamber is influenced by the morphology of the jet (central vs. wall impinging), as well as flow rate and velocity. Jet area is sometimes not correlated with severity since it is influenced by afterload, jet direction, and size of the receiving chamber.

There are quantitative means of assessing the effective regurgitant orifice area (EROA) and the regurgitant volume using the flow volume equation (see Table 14.4). Proximal isovelocity surface area (PISA), or flow convergence, is based on the principle that velocity of blood increases as it approaches an orifice, therefore forming concentric, hemi-spheric shells. The flow through these shells is the same as flow through the effective orifice, the area of which can be solved if flow and hemispheric area are measured. Accuracy of the PISA technique is better for central jets as opposed to wall-impinging jets. It is important to obtain an accurate hemispheric shell to apply the equation for calculating the EROA. The vena contracta is the narrowest diameter of the color flow profile near the valve and approximates the diameter of the regurgitant orifice. Vena contracta is not affected by flow rate or blood pressure for a fixed orifice, but the orifice size may change with hemodynamics. The slope of the decay of pressure differential between the 2 chambers can also be used to assess severity of regurgitation. The greater the degree or regurgitation, the faster the pressure rises in the receiving chamber and the faster the pressure gradient will decay, yielding a steep slope. This method is limited by receiving chamber compliance and pressure.

Mitral regurgitation assessment involves jet area, PISA, and vena contracta. The density of CWD signal, mitral inflow E velocity and pulmonary vein flow reversal are additional parameters used to assess severity. Because the imaging transducer is closer to the mitral valve, TEE generally provides better resolution of the mitral valve and the direction and degree of mitral regurgitation.

The parameters that are used to assess the severity of aortic regurgitation (AR) include PISA, regurgitant jet size, vena contracta, and pressure halftime. Regurgitant jet size is assessed in the PLAX view by taking the ratio of the jet width immediately below the aortic valve to the LVOT diameter. The measurement is limited by jet direction and jet shape. The vena contracta, also measured in the PLAX view, is more robust that the jet width. PISA is limited by image resolution in the apical views, by ascending aortic aneurysms, which distort the valve plane and by early diastolic timing for peak AR velocity. Aortic diastolic flow reversal in the upper descending aorta or lower descending aorta is an additional parameter used to evaluate AR severity. Holodiastolic reversal is a sign of at least moderate AR.

Tricuspid stenosis and pulmonic stenosis are assessed similarly to the left-sided lesions. Significant tricuspid regurgitation is usually due to RV or tricuspid annular dilatation secondary to pulmonary hypertension or RV dysfunction. PW Doppler of the hepatic veins shows blunting of systolic flow with moderate TR and systolic flow reversal with severe TR. Pathologic pulmonic regurgitation is usually observed in patients with structural right heart disease.

Echocardiography is the primary modality for the evaluation of prosthetic valve stenosis and regurgitation. Although Doppler gradients and other measures of valve function are easily obtained by TTE, diagnostic 2D and 3D visualization of prosthetic valves often requires TEE (especially when valvular vegetations and paravalvular abscesses are suspected).

Mechanical valves cause artifacts which obscure structures which lie beyond the valve relative to the ultrasound transducer [18].

Pericardial Disease and Masses

Echocardiography can be helpful in the evaluation of the etiology and hemodynamic consequences of pericardial disease and cardiac masses and should be involved early in the diagnostic workup of these conditions. Cardiac masses are often first found on echocardiography performed for some other reason or for nonspecific symptoms. Certain echocardiographic features such as location, size, shape, and associated

cardiac findings can help identify the likely etiology of cardiac masses (Fig. 14.5, Video 14.4) (Fig. 14.6, Videos 14.5a and 14.5b). Echocardiographic contrast plays a role in detecting cardiac masses in patients with difficult echocardiographic windows and differentiating true masses from artifacts [10]. Because contrast microbubbles go wherever red blood cells go, contrast perfusion of masses may play a role in determining the etiology of masses. A "dark" mass without microbubbles suggests thrombus, whereas a "bright" mass signals a vascular mass (malignancy or highly vascular tumor) [19]. Echocardiography plays a significant role in diagnosing pericardial effusion in the setting of LV rupture postinfarction, chest trauma, post-catheter procedures, aortic dissection, Dressler's syndrome, uremia, collagen vascular disease, post-cardiac surgery, radiation, cancer, and infectious pericarditis. Echocardiography is very useful for differentiating between constrictive disease, restrictive disease, and tamponade (Table 14.5).

Stress Echocardiography

Stress echocardiography can be used in the assessment of ischemia, valvular disease, dyspnea, and pulmonary hypertension. For the evaluation of coronary artery disease (CAD), exercise echo is recommended over pharmacologic stress because exercise capacity is a predictor of cardiovascular outcomes. Dobutamine stress echo is safe for patients with LV dysfunction, aortic and cerebral aneurysms, and implantable defibrillators. To evaluate for ischemia, LV wall thickening and motion is measured at rest and with stress and is described as normal or hyperdynamic, hypokinetic, akinetic, dyskinetic, or aneurysmal. In addition, LV shape, cavity size, and global contractility should be evaluated (Fig. 14.7, Video 14.6). Contrast

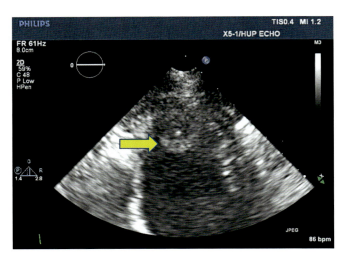

Fig. 14.5 Apical mass. Zoomed view of the apex in the apical 2-chamber view, demonstrating a large mass (*arrow*). It is well circumscribed with smooth borders and has an echotexture similar to that of the adjacent myocardium. As seen in the video, there is anterior apical and inferior hypokinesis. These findings suggest the mass is a thrombus

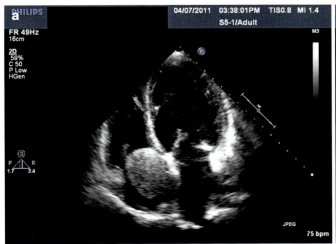
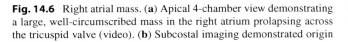
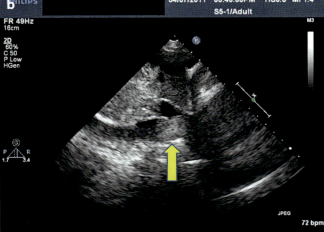

Fig. 14.6 Right atrial mass. (**a**) Apical 4-chamber view demonstrating a large, well-circumscribed mass in the right atrium prolapsing across the tricuspid valve (video). (**b**) Subcostal imaging demonstrated origin of the mass in the inferior vena cava (*arrow*). Pathology was consistent with carcinoid tumor

Table 14.5 Echocardiography in pericardial diseases

Pericardial effusions and tamponade	Pericardial constriction
Confirmation of location fluid	Assessment of diastolic dysfunction and restrictive physiology
Assessment of etiology of effusion	Assessment of ventricular hemodynamics specific to constriction
Evaluation of hemodynamic impact of effusion	Dissociation of intrathoracic and intracardiac pressure
Determination of safety for percutaneous drainage	Increased LV-RV interdependence
Assistance with the safe percutaneous drainage of the effusion	
Assessment of post-drainage complications (e.g., RV perforation)	
Findings	**Findings**
Right- or left-sided chamber collapse (pulmonary hypertension can prevent chamber collapse in the presence of tamponade)	Right-sided volume overload (nonspecific sign)
IVC dilatation and lack of respiratory collapse signifying right-sided volume overload	Thick, echodense pericardium (note: CT/MRI is the gold standard for assessing the pericardial tissue)
Significant respirophasic variation in tricuspid and mitral valve inflow Doppler velocity profiles	Abnormal septal motion (2D and M-mode)
	Associated pericardial effusion

Respiratory changes in inflow velocities:

Inspiration:	*Expiration:*
LA/LV	LA/LV
↓ Mitral valve inflow velocities	↑ Mitral valve inflow velocities
↓ Pulmonary vein inflow velocities	↑ Pulmonary vein inflow velocities
RA/RV	*RA/RV*
↑ Tricuspid valve inflow velocities	↓ Tricuspid valve inflow velocities
↑ Hepatic vein inflow velocities	↓ Hepatic vein inflow velocities, prominent diastolic expiratory prominent atrial reversal

Restrictive mitral valve inflow filling patters
   Increased E wave peak velocity (E/A ratio often >2)
   Decreased E wave deceleration time (DT often <160 ms)
   Preserved/elevated E′ and abnormal septal E′/lateral E′ ratio (usually >1)

Abbreviations as in Tables 14.1 and 14.2. *CT* computed tomography, *MRI* magnetic resonance imaging

agents for LV opacification are used when greater than 2 segments are not visualized on baseline echocardiography [8]. Stress echocardiography is approximately 80 % sensitive and 86 % specific for the detection of CAD. False negative results are found in patients with valvular regurgitation due to hyperdynamic states and in patients with thick walls and small cavities, since the LV volumes are small and there tends to be global hyperkinesis. Rapid declines in heart rate after treadmill exercise and before echo imaging, as well as difficulty in achieving an adequate stress workload (common in bicycle exercise) also reduce the sensitivity of stress echocardiography. False positive results are observed in patients with hypertension and abnormal septal motion from LBBB and RV pacing. Post-sternotomy patients also often have abnormal septal motion. Although quantitative methods have been tested, wall motion analysis in stress echo is most often assessed subjectively, and the expertise of the sonographer and interpreter can affect accuracy.

Stress echo can be helpful in the evaluation of viability prior to revascularization. Hibernating myocardium represents reversible myocardial dysfunction. Dobutamine echo is utilized to evaluate contractile reserve. If any segments are thin (<0.5–0.6 cm) and bright, they are probably scarred and the chance of recovery is minimal. Improvement in the grade of dysfunction in two or more segments with dobutamine is considered evidence of viability. The test is most sensitive if improvement is observed with low-dose dobutamine. For patients who have >25 % viable myocardium, there is a high likelihood of improvement in function after revascularization. Patients with CAD and resting wall motion abnormalities amenable to revascularization will usually demonstrate wall motion improvement with low-dose dobutamine and re-worsening of wall motion with high-dose dobutamine [20].

Stress echo can be used to assess diastolic function. Abnormalities in diastolic function appear early in the ischemic process; demonstration of stress-induced diastolic dysfunction may uncover the etiology of dyspnea on exertion.

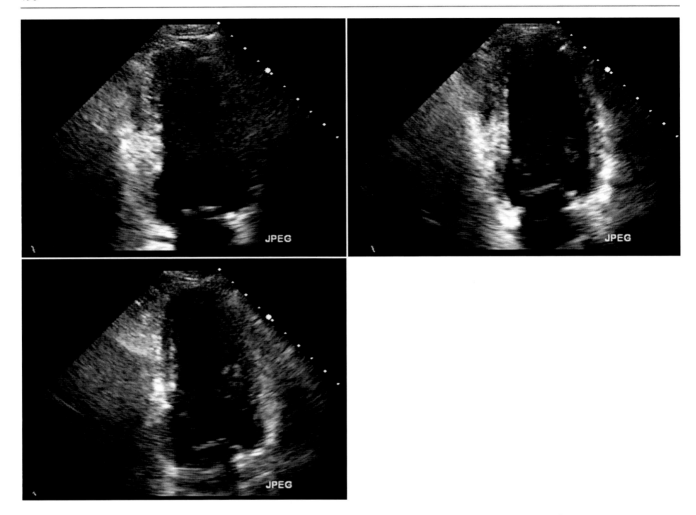

Fig. 14.7 Stress echocardiogram demonstrating ischemia. Comparison rest (*upper left*), stress (*upper right*), and recovery (*lower left*) 2-chamber views during exercise stress echocardiography. The stress images demonstrate reduced ejection fraction with a mid to distal inferior wall motion abnormality, consistent with a significant right coronary artery stenosis. Recovery images demonstrate resolution of the wall motion abnormality

Speckle tracking or tissue Doppler is used to measure delay in relaxation with stress and demonstrate elevation of LV filling pressures. During exercise, the ratio of mitral inflow velocity (E) to mitral annulus velocity (e′) is increased in patients with elevated LV filling pressures due to impaired relaxation.

Pulmonary artery pressures can be measured during exercise to provide information about LV diastolic function, RV systolic function and severity of mitral regurgitation and mitral stenosis. Pulmonary systolic pressure greater than 60 mmHg during exercise is a class IIa indication for mitral valve surgery. For patients with mitral stenosis, stress echocardiography is indicated in asymptomatic patients with significant lesions based on hemodynamics obtained at rest and symptomatic patients with fairly normal resting hemodynamics. Exercise-induced dyspnea, transmitral gradient >15 mmHg with exercise and PASP >60 mmHg with exercise, is suggestive of hemodynamically significant mitral stenosis which may be amenable to percutaneous valvulotomy.

Low-flow/low-gradient aortic stenosis is defined as LVEF <40 %, effective orifice area <1 cm², and mean aortic gradient <30–40 mmHg. A dobutamine stress echocardiogram may help determine if the reduced valve area is secondary to a stenotic aortic valve or to reduced LV stroke volumes preventing aortic valve opening. A patient with reduced EF but an AV velocity >4 m/s and mean aortic valve gradient >40 mmHg does not usually need a dobutamine stress echocardiogram since these measurements are makers of severe aortic stenosis.

Device Evaluation

Echocardiography is increasingly being used in patients with cardiac devices, including cardiac implantable electrical devices (such as pacemaker and defibrillators) and ventricular assist devices (VADs). Echocardiography establishes

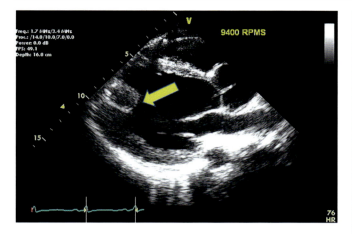

Fig. 14.8 LVAD imaging. Parasternal long-axis view of a patient with a left ventricular assist device (LVAD) set at 9,400 rpm. The video demonstrates that the left ventricular (LV) ejection fraction is severely decreased (~10 %) and that there is no aortic valve opening. The inflow cannula of the LVAD is seen near the LV apex (*arrow*). It is normally positioned and is unlikely to be subject to any suction events, in which portions of the ventricle or the mitral apparatus are drawn into the opening of the cannula, obstructing flow. The septum is neutral between the LV and right ventricle (RV), indicating adequate LV decompression from LVAD function and suggesting that there is no RV volume or pressure overload

LVEF, a key criterion for implantation of these devices, and can identify pathologies that can complicate device placement. In the immediate post-implant period, echocardiography is used to assess for procedural complications, particularly pericardial effusion and tamponade. In the long term, echocardiography has been used to assess how a device affects the heart, including remodeling induced by cardiac resynchronization therapy (CRT) [21] and VADs, and ventricular failure from chronic right ventricular pacing. Echocardiographic measurements are used in some centers to guide optimization of CRT devices and VADs [22] (Fig. 14.8, Video 14.7). Investigation of suspected infection of device components (leads, cannulae) often requires TEE.

Key Points

- Echocardiography can be used to evaluate almost any cardiovascular disease process and provide structural/anatomical, functional, and hemodynamic information in real time.
- Echocardiography for signs and symptoms of cardiovascular disease, for the purpose of detecting structural changes in certain disease states, and for the purpose of establishing indications for specific therapies is appropriate.
- Take care to provide accurate and adequate indications when ordering an echocardiogram as this

---

information has the potential to impact the performance and interpretation.
- Echocardiogram findings should be compared to prior echo reports and other imaging reports and the clinical circumstances to put the findings into proper context.
- Echocardiographic measures of LV chamber size, geometry, wall thickness, and function are strong independent predictors of morbidity and mortality and, as such, play a significant role in cardiovascular disease diagnosis, management, risk stratification, and prognosis.
- Echocardiographic assessment of LA size, RV size and function, aortic size, and aortic plaques provides important clinical information.
- Echocardiography is the primary modality for evaluating cardiac valve structure and function. Assessment of valvular function, especially regurgitation, should involve integration of multiple echocardiographic parameters. 3D TEE is particularly useful in the assessment of mitral valve pathology.
- Stress echocardiography can be used in the assessment of ischemia, valvular disease, dyspnea, and pulmonary hypertension.
- Echocardiography is increasingly being used in patients with cardiac devices, including cardiac implantable electrical devices (such as pacemaker and defibrillators) and ventricular assist devices (VADs).

Summary of Guidelines

There are many statements and guidelines produced by the ASE that provide technical guidance for echocardiographers and sonographers, but there are only a few guidelines and other documents addressing the use of echocardiography that are pertinent to cardiovascular consultation.

In 2003, the ACC/AHA/ASE produced a guideline update to the 1997 guideline for the clinical application of echocardiography [23]. Class I indications included TTE for first-degree relatives of patients with dilated cardiomyopathy and dobutamine stress echocardiography for assessment of myocardial viability when required to guide revascularization. Class IIa indications included echocardiography for assessment of LV function in postinfarction patients to guide ICD therapy, evaluation of patients after MAZE procedures to monitor LA function, and assessment of pulmonary emboli and suspected clots in the right atrium. Class IIb recommendations included echocardiography in patients with MV disease or hypertrophic cardiomyopathy who have been on long-term anticoagulation at therapeutic levels before cardioversion and assessment of late prognosis after myocardial infarction (≥ 2 years).

Echocardiography was not recommended (class III) in patients without MV disease or hypertrophic cardiomyopathy who have been on therapeutic long-term anticoagulation prior to cardioversion; routine screening prior to sports participation in patients with normal cardiovascular history, electrocardiogram (ECG), and examination; and suspected myocardial contusion in the hemodynamically stable patient with a normal ECG and no abnormal cardiovascular findings.

Other recommendations, particularly those pertaining to valve disease, are either mirrored or superseded by later guidelines.

Heart Failure

The 2005 Guidelines for the Diagnosis and Management of Heart Failure in Adults (focused update in 2009) [24] recommends (class I) that echocardiography be performed during initial evaluation of patients presenting with heart failure symptoms for LVEF, LV size, wall thickness, and valve function (Level of Evidence: C). A class IIa recommendation was given for the indication of repeat measurement of EF and evaluation of severity of structural remodeling in patients with heart failure who have had a change in clinical status or experienced or recovered from a clinical event or received treatment that might have affect cardiac function (Level of Evidence: C).

Valves

The 2008 focused update of the ACC/AHA 2006 Guidelines for the Management of Patients with Valvular Heart Disease [25] gives multiple indications for echocardiography. In evaluating murmurs, the guidelines state that echocardiography is indicated in the following cases: (1) asymptomatic patients with certain murmurs (grade 3 or louder, mid-peaking systolic, diastolic, continuous, holosystolic, late systolic, associated with ejection clicks, radiate to the neck or back) or with murmurs and signs or symptoms of heart failure, ischemia/infarction, syncope, thrombotic events, endocarditis, or evidence of structural heart disease (class I, Level of Evidence: C); (2) asymptomatic patients with murmurs and other abnormal cardiac physical findings or abnormal ECG or chest X-ray (class IIa, Level of Evidence: C); and (3) patients with noncardiac signs or symptoms but in whom a cardiac basis cannot be excluded (class IIa, Level of Evidence: C). These guidelines recommend against echocardiography for patients who have a grade 2 or softer mid-systolic murmur identified as innocent or functional by an experienced observer (Level of Evidence: C).

In addressing specific valvulopathies, the guidelines give class I indications for detection and evaluation of stenosis and regurgitation severity and secondary effects of valve dysfunction (such as LV mass, size, and function in left-sided lesions), the reevaluation of patient with changing signs or symptoms, and the evaluation of hemodynamic changes during pregnancy (Level of Evidence: B). The recommended follow-up of asymptomatic patients is yearly for severe disease, 1–2 years for moderate disease, and 3–5 years for mild disease (Level of Evidence: B), except in moderate to severe mitral regurgitation, in which the recommended follow-up is 6 months to 1 year (Level of Evidence: C). Echocardiography to reevaluate pulmonary artery pressures in asymptomatic patients with mitral stenosis received a class IIa indication (Level of Evidence: C).

For mitral stenosis, echocardiography is specifically recommended as a class I indication to assess valve morphology to determine suitability for percutaneous mitral valvotomy (Level of Evidence: B). TEE is indicated in mitral stenosis to evaluate for LA thrombus and to grade the severity of concomitant mitral regurgitation (Level of Evidence: C).

TTE or TEE is recommended (class I) in mitral regurgitation to discern whether the morphology is amenable to repair or replacement (Level of Evidence: B). Echocardiography is indicated to evaluate LV size and function and valve hemodynamics after MV replacement or repair (Level of Evidence: C). In contrast to the AUC, the valve guidelines recommend transthoracic echocardiography to detect valvular vegetations with or without positive blood cultures (Level of Evidence: B). Echocardiography is also recommended to define the hemodynamic severity of valvular lesions and other complications of endocarditis (Level of Evidence: B) and for reassessment of high-risk patients (Level of Evidence: C) (Fig. 14.9, Video 14.8). The reevaluation of prosthetic valve endocarditis by TTE, even in the absence of clinical change, was given a class IIb indication (Level of Evidence: C).

Class I indications for TEE include evaluating endocarditis in patients with nondiagnostic TTE (Level of Evidence: C) and as a first-line imaging modality in patients with prosthetic valve endocarditis (Level of Evidence: C) or prosthetic valve thrombosis, to assess valve motion and clot burden (Level of Evidence: B).

Exercise echocardiography for assessment of mean MV gradient and pulmonary artery systolic pressure to evaluate discrepancies between resting gradients and clinical signs received a class I indications (Level of Evidence: C). Exercise echocardiography for asymptomatic patients with severe mitral regurgitation to measure pulmonary artery pressure and regurgitation severity with exercise was considered class IIa (Level of Evidence: C). Dobutamine stress echocardiography for low-flow/low-gradient aortic stenosis in the setting of LV dysfunction is a class IIa recommendation (Level of Evidence: B).

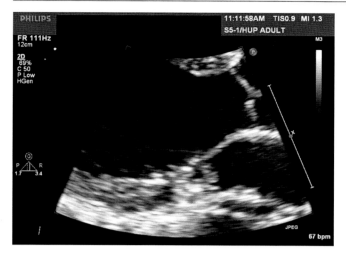

Fig. 14.9 Endocarditis. Parasternal long-axis zoomed view of the mitral valve demonstrating a very large, multilobulated and highly mobile echodensity on both sides and both leaflets of the mitral valve, consistent with endocarditis lesion

Class III indications include exclusion of MV prolapse in patients without specific signs or symptoms of MV prolapse (Level of Evidence: B), routine evaluation of asymptomatic patients with MV prolapse and mild regurgitation (Level of Evidence: C), routine follow-up of patients with mild mitral regurgitation (Level of Evidence: C), and routine evaluation of native valve endocarditis without clinical change (Level of Evidence: C).

Aorta

The 2010 ACCF/AHA Guidelines for the Diagnosis and Management of Patients with Thoracic Aortic Disease includes only a formal recommendation on technical aspects of aortic imaging by echocardiography but does mention that the primary role of TTE in following patients with aortopathy is in imaging disorders confined to the root, such as Marfan syndrome and in assessing other associated pathology such as bicuspid aortic valve and mitral valve prolapse [26].

Appropriate Use Criteria

The 2011 AUC for echocardiography, described above, rates 202 indications for transthoracic, transesophageal, and stress echocardiography as appropriate, inappropriate, and of uncertain appropriateness (not enough evidence to rate). Table 14.6 provides a sample of the most important indications for transthoracic, transesophageal, and stress echocardiography encountered in typical cardiology consultative practice and their appropriateness rating. Appropriate indications for stress echocardiography to evaluate ischemic disease generally mirror those for stress testing in general.

Acknowledgements The authors would like to thank Carol Dennis for her assistance with formatting of the manuscript.

Table 14.6 Selected indications for echocardiography

Transthoracic echocardiography indications	
General evaluation of cardiac structure and function	
Symptoms or results from prior testing with suspected cardiac etiology	Appropriate
Arrhythmias (excluding isolated premature beats)	Appropriate
Signs or symptoms with history of cardiac diagnosis known to cause these symptoms (e.g., presyncope/syncope with history of aortic stenosis, hypertrophic cardiomyopathy, heart failure)	Appropriate
Routine general or perioperative evaluation of LV function in the absence of new or changing cardiac symptoms/signs	Inappropriate
Evaluation of suspected pulmonary hypertension or routine surveillance ≥1 year of known pulmonary hypertension	Appropriate
Cardiac evaluation in acute setting	
Hemodynamic or respiratory instability of unclear etiology	Appropriate
Evaluation of patient with chest pain, ischemic equivalent, or suspected complication of myocardial infarction	Appropriate
Assessment of volume status in critically ill patient	Uncertain
Evaluation of LV following acute coronary syndrome	Appropriate
Suspected pulmonary embolism to establish diagnosis	Inappropriate
Known acute pulmonary embolism to guide therapy	Appropriate
Severe decoration injury or chest trauma	Appropriate
Evaluation of valvular function	
Murmur or click when there is a reasonable suspicion of valvular or structural heart disease	Appropriate
Reevaluation of known native or prosthetic valvular disease when there has been change in clinical status	Appropriate
Routine surveillance (≥3 year) of mild valvular *stenosis* without change in clinical status	Appropriate
Routine surveillance (≥3 year) of mild valvular *regurgitation* without a change in clinical status or cardiac exam	Uncertain
Routine surveillance (≥1 year) of moderate or severe valvular *stenosis* or *regurgitation* without change in clinical status	Appropriate

(continued)

Table 14.6 (continued)

Initial postoperative evaluation of prosthetic valve for establishment of baseline	Appropriate
Routine surveillance (≥3 year) after valve implantation if no known or suspected valve dysfunction	Appropriate
Infective endocarditis (native or prosthetic valves)	
Initial evaluation of suspected infective endocarditis with positive blood cultures or new murmur	Appropriate
Transient fever without evidence of bacteremia or a new murmur and/or documented nonendovascular source of infection	Inappropriate
Evaluation for intracardiac and extracardiac structures and aortic disease	
Suspected cardiac mass, source of embolus, pericardial disease	Appropriate
Evaluation of ascending aorta in patient with history of conditions known to cause aneurysms and dissection	Appropriate
Reevaluation of known ascending aortic aneurysm to assess rate of progression or reevaluation of patient with history of aneurysm/dissection and change clinical status	Appropriate
Routine surveillance of implanted device without a change in clinical status or cardiac exam	Inappropriate
Evaluation of cardiac structure and function in patients with hypertension and heart failure	
Initial evaluation of suspected hypertensive heart disease or heart failure	Appropriate
Routine evaluation of systemic hypertension without signs or symptoms of hypertensive heart disease	Inappropriate
Reevaluation of heart failure with change in clinical status (without clear change in medication or diet)	Appropriate
Reevaluation of heart failure to guide pharmacological, device, mechanical therapy	Appropriate
Monitoring for rejection in cardiac transplant patient	Appropriate
Screening evaluation for structure and function in first-degree relatives of a patient with an inherited cardiomyopathy	Appropriate
Baseline and serial reevaluations in a patient undergoing therapy with cardiotoxic agents	Appropriate
Transesophageal echocardiography indications	
High likelihood of nondiagnostic TTE	Appropriate
Reevaluation of prior TEE for interval change for guidance of therapy	Appropriate
Suspected acute aortic pathology, including dissection	Appropriate
Evaluation of valve for type of intervention required	Appropriate
Diagnose infective endocarditis with moderate or high pretest probability	Appropriate
Evaluation for cardiac source of embolus with no identified noncardiac source	Appropriate
To aid clinical decision making for anticoagulation, cardioversion, and/or RF ablation	Appropriate
Stress echocardiography indications	
Severe asymptomatic chronic mitral stenosis or regurgitation	Appropriate
Severe asymptomatic chronic aortic regurgitation	Appropriate
Moderate symptomatic chronic mitral stenosis or regurgitation	Appropriate
Equivocal symptomatic chronic aortic stenosis (low flow or pseudostenosis)	Appropriate
Acute moderate or severe aortic or mitral regurgitation	Inappropriate
Suspected pulmonary artery hypertension	Uncertain
Normal or borderline elevated estimated right ventricular systolic pressure on resting echocardiographic study	
Microbubble contrast	
Selective use of contrast	Appropriate
≥2 contiguous LV segments are not seen on noncontrast images	

American College of Cardiology Foundation Appropriate Use Criteria Task Force et al. [3]

LV left ventricle, *TEE* transesophageal echocardiography, *TTE* transthoracic echocardiography

References

1. Silvestry FE, Kerber RE, Brook MM, Carroll JD, Eberman KM, Goldstein SA, Herrmann HC, Homma S, Mehran R, Packer DL, Parisi AF, Pulerwitz T, Seward JB, Tsang TS, Wood MA. Echocardiography-guided interventions. J Am Soc Echocardiogr. 2009;22(3):213–31.
2. Zamorano JL, Badano LP, Bruce C, Chan KL, Gonçalves A, Hahn RT, Keane MG, La Canna G, Monaghan MJ, Nihoyannopoulos P, Silvestry FE, Vanoverschelde JL, Gillam LD. EAE/ASE recommendations for the use of echocardiography in new transcatheter interventions for valvular heart disease. J Am Soc Echocardiogr. 2011;24(9):937–65.
3. American College of Cardiology Foundation Appropriate Use Criteria Task Force; American Society of Echocardiography; American Heart Association; American Society of Nuclear Cardiology; Heart Failure Society of America; Heart Rhythm Society; Society for Cardiovascular Angiography and Interventions; Society of Critical Care Medicine; Society of Cardiovascular Computed Tomography; Society for Cardiovascular Magnetic Resonance, Douglas PS, Garcia MJ, Haines DE, Lai WW, Manning WJ, Patel AR, Picard MH, Polk DM, Ragosta M, Ward RP, Weiner RB. ACCF/ASE/AHA/ASNC/HFSA/HRS/SCAI/SCCM/SCCT/SCMR 2011 Appropriate Use Criteria for Echocardiography. A Report of the American College of Cardiology Foundation Appropriate Use Criteria Task Force, American Society of Echocardiography, American Heart Association, American Society of Nuclear Cardiology, Heart Failure Society of America, Heart Rhythm Society, Society for Cardiovascular Angiography and Interventions, Society of Critical Care Medicine, Society of Cardiovascular Computed Tomography, and Society for Cardiovascular Magnetic Resonance Endorsed by the American College of Chest Physicians. J Am Coll Cardiol. 2011;57(9):1126–66.

4. Saksena S, Sra J, Jordaens L, Kusumoto F, Knight B, Natale A, Kocheril A, Nanda NC, Nagarakanti R, Simon AM, Viggiano MA, Lokhandwala T, Chandler ML; ICE-CHIP Investigator Study Group. A prospective comparison of cardiac imaging using intracardiac echocardiography with transesophageal echocardiography in patients with atrial fibrillation: the intracardiac echocardiography guided cardioversion helps interventional procedures study. Circ Arrhythm Electrophysiol. 2010;3(6):571–7.

5. Lang RM, Mor-Avi V, Sugeng L, et al. Three dimensional echocardiography: the benefits of the addition dimension. J Am Coll Cardiol. 2006;48:2053–69.

6. Lang RM, Badano LP, Tsang W, Adams DH, Agricola E, Buck T, Faletra FF, Franke A, Hung J, de Isla LP, Kamp O, Kasprzak JD, Lancellotti P, Marwick TH, McCulloch ML, Monaghan MJ, Nihoyannopoulos P, Pandian NG, Pellikka PA, Pepi M, Roberson DA, Shernan SK, Shirali GS, Sugeng L, Ten Cate FJ, Vannan MA, Zamorano JL, Zoghbi WA, American Society of Echocardiography; European Association of Echocardiography. EAE/ASE recommendations for image acquisition and display using three-dimensional echocardiography. J Am Soc Echocardiogr. 2012;25(1):3–46.

7. Mulvagh SL, Rakowski H, Vannan MA, Abdelmoneim SS, Becher H, Bierig SM, Burns PN, Castello R, Coon PD, Hagen ME, Jollis JG, Kimball TR, Kitzman DW, Kronzon I, Labovitz AJ, Lang RM, Mathew J, Moir WS, Nagueh SF, Pearlman AS, Perez JE, Porter TR, Rosenbloom J, Strachan GM, Thanigaraj S, Wei K, Woo A, Yu EH, Zoghbi WA, American Society of Echocardiography. American Society of Echocardiography Consensus statement on the clinical applications of ultrasonic contrast agents in echocardiography. J Am Soc Echocardiogr. 2008;21(11):1179–201.

8. Mor-Avi V, Lang RM, Badano LP, Belohlavek M, Cardim NM, Derumeaux G, Galderisi M, Marwick T, Nagueh SF, Sengupta PP, Sicari R, Smiseth OA, Smulevitz B, Takeuchi M, Thomas JD, Vannan M, Voigt JU, Zamorano JL. Current and evolving echocardiographic techniques for the quantitative evaluation of cardiac mechanics: ASE/EAE consensus statement on methodology and indications endorsed by the Japanese Society of Echocardiography. J Am Soc Echocardiogr. 2011;24(3):277–313.

9. Lang RM, Bierig M, Devereux RB, et al. Recommendations for chamber quantification: a report from the American Society of Echocardiography's guidelines and standards committee and the chamber quantification writing group, developed in conjunction with the European association of echocardiography, a branch of the European Society of Cardiology. J Am Soc Echocardiogr. 2005;18(12):1440–63.

10. Tsang MY, Barnes ME, Tsang TS. Left atrial volume: clinical value revisited. Curr Cardiol Rep. 2012;14(3):374–80.

11. Rudski LG, Lai WW, Afilalo J, Hua L, Handschumacher MD, Chandrasekaran K, Solomon SD, Louie EK, Schiller NB. Guidelines for the echocardiographic assessment of the right heart in adults: a report from the American Society of Echocardiography endorsed by the European Association of Echocardiography, a registered branch of the European Society of Cardiology, and the Canadian Society of Echocardiography. J Am Soc Echocardiogr. 2010;23(7):685–713.

12. Shiga T, Wajima Z, Apfel CC, et al. Diagnostic accuracy of transesophageal echocardiography, helical computed tomography, and magnetic resonance imaging for suspected thoracic aortic dissection: systematic review and meta-analysis. Arch Intern Med. 2006;166:1350–6.

13. Barbieri A, Bursi F, Mantovani F, Valenti C, Quaglia M, Berti E, Marino M, Modena MG. Prognostic impact of left ventricular mass severity according to the classification proposed by the American Society of Echocardiography/European Association of Echocardiography. J Am Soc Echocardiogr. 2011;24(12):1383–91.

14. Hayley BD, Burwash IG. Heart failure with normal left ventricular ejection fraction: role of echocardiography. Curr Opin Cardiol. 2012;27(2):169–80.

15. Nagueh SF, Appleton CP, Gillebert TC, Marino PN, Oh JK, Smiseth OA, Waggoner AD, Flachskampf FA, Pellikka PA, Evangelista A. Recommendations for the evaluation of left ventricular diastolic function by echocardiography. J Am Soc Echocardiogr. 2009;22(2):107–33.

16. Baumgartner H, Hung J, Bermejo J, Chambers JB, Evangelista A, Griffin BP, Iung B, Otto CM, Pellikka PA, Quiñones M, American Society of Echocardiography; European Association of Echocardiography. Echocardiographic assessment of valve stenosis: EAE/ASE recommendations for clinical practice. J Am Soc Echocardiogr. 2009;22(1):1–23.

17. Zoghbi WA, Enriquez-Sarano M, Foster E, Grayburn PA, Kraft CD, Levine RA, Nihoyannopoulos P, Otto CM, Quinones MA, Rakowski H, Stewart WJ, Waggoner A, Weissman NJ, American Society of Echocardiography. Recommendations for evaluation of the severity of native valvular regurgitation with two-dimensional and Doppler echocardiography. J Am Soc Echocardiogr. 2003;16(7):777–802.

18. Zoghbi WA, Chambers JB, Dumesnil JG, Foster E, Gottdiener JS, Grayburn PA, Khandheria BK, Levine RA, Marx GR, Miller Jr FA, Nakatani S, Quiñones MA, Rakowski H, Rodriguez LL, Swaminathan M, Waggoner AD, Weissman NJ, Zabalgoitia M, American Society of Echocardiography's Guidelines and Standards Committee; Task Force on Prosthetic Valves; American College of Cardiology Cardiovascular Imaging Committee; Cardiac Imaging Committee of the American Heart Association; European Association of Echocardiography; European Society of Cardiology; Japanese Society of Echocardiography; Canadian Society of Echocardiography; American College of Cardiology Foundation; American Heart Association; European Association of Echocardiography; European Society of Cardiology; Japanese Society of Echocardiography; Canadian Society of Echocardiography. Recommendations for evaluation of prosthetic valves with echocardiography and Doppler ultrasound: a report from the American Society of Echocardiography's Guidelines and Standards Committee and the Task Force on prosthetic valves, developed in conjunction with the American College of Cardiology Cardiovascular Imaging Committee, Cardiac Imaging Committee of the American Heart Association, the European Association of Echocardiography, a registered branch of the European Society of Cardiology, the Japanese Society of Echocardiography and the Canadian Society of Echocardiography, endorsed by the American College of Cardiology Foundation, American Heart Association, European Association of Echocardiography, a registered branch of the European Society of Cardiology, the Japanese Society of Echocardiography, and Canadian Society of Echocardiography. J Am Soc Echocardiogr. 2009;22(9):975–1014.

19. Kirkpatrick JN, Wong T, Bednarz JE, Spencer KT, Sugeng L, Ward RP, DeCara JM, Weinert L, Krausz T, Lang RM. Differential diagnosis of cardiac masses using contrast echocardiographic perfusion imaging. J Am Coll Cardiol. 2004;43(8):1412–9.

20. Pellikka PA, Nagueh SF, Elhendy AA, Kuehl CA, Sawada SG, American Society of Echocardiography. American Society of Echocardiography recommendations for performance, interpretation, and application of stress echocardiography. J Am Soc Echocardiogr. 2007;20(9):1021–41.

21. Gorcsan 3rd J, Abraham T, Agler DA, Bax JJ, Derumeaux G, Grimm RA, Martin R, Steinberg JS, Sutton MS, Yu CM, American Society of Echocardiography Dyssynchrony Writing Group. Echocardiography for cardiac resynchronization therapy: recommendations for performance and reporting – a report from the American Society of Echocardiography Dyssynchrony Writing Group endorsed by the Heart Rhythm Society. J Am Soc Echocardiogr. 2008;21(3):191–213.

22. Kirkpatrick JN, Wiegers SE, Rame JE, Lang RM. Use of echocardiography to optimize left ventricular assist devices. U S Cardiology. 2010;7(2):11–5.

23. Cheitlin MD, Armstrong WF, Aurigemma GP, Beller GA, Bierman FZ, Davis JL, Douglas PS, Faxon DP, Gillam LD, Kimball TR, Kussmaul WG, Pearlman AS, Philbrick JT, Rakowski H, Thys DM, Antman EM, Smith Jr SC, Alpert JS, Gregoratos G, Anderson JL, Hiratzka LF, Hunt SA, Fuster V, Jacobs AK, Gibbons RJ, Russell RO. American College of Cardiology; American Heart Association; American Society of Echocardiography. ACC/AHA/ASE 2003 guideline update for the clinical application of echocardiography: summary article: a report of the American College of Cardiology/American Heart Association Task Force on Practice Guidelines (ACC/AHA/ASE committee to update the 1997 guidelines for the clinical application of echocardiography). Circulation. 2003;108(9):1146–62.

24. Jessup M, Abraham WT, Casey DE, Feldman AM, Francis GS, Ganiats TG, Konstam MA, Mancini DM, Rahko PS, Silver MA, Stevenson LW, Yancy CW. 2009 focused update: ACCF/AHA guidelines for the diagnosis and management of heart failure in adults: a report of the American College of Cardiology Foundation/American Heart Association Task Force on practice guidelines: developed in collaboration with the International Society for Heart and Lung Transplantation. Circulation. 2009;119(14):1977–2016. Epub 2009 Mar 26.

25. Bonow RO, Carabello BA, Chatterjee K, de Leon AC, Jr FDP, Freed MD, Gaasch WH, Lytle BW, Nishimura RA, O'Gara PT, O'Rourke RA, Otto CM, Shah PM, Shanewise JS, American College of Cardiology/American Heart Association Task Force on Practice Guidelines. 2008 focused update incorporated into the ACC/AHA 2006 guidelines for the management of patients with valvular heart disease: a report of the American College of Cardiology/American Heart Association Task Force on Practice Guidelines (writing committee to revise the 1998 guidelines for the management of patients with valvular heart disease). Endorsed by the Society of Cardiovascular Anesthesiologists, Society for Cardiovascular Angiography and Interventions, and Society of Thoracic Surgeons. J Am Coll Cardiol. 2008;52(13):e1–142.

26. Hiratzka LF, Bakris GL, Beckman JA, Bersin RM, Carr VF, Casey Jr DE, Eagle KA, Hermann LK, Isselbacher EM, Kazerooni EA, Kouchoukos NT, Lytle BW, Milewicz DM, Reich DL, Sen S, Shinn JA, Svensson LG, Williams DM, American College of Cardiology Foundation/American Heart Association Task Force on Practice Guidelines; American Association for Thoracic Surgery; American College of Radiology; American Stroke Association; Society of Cardiovascular Anesthesiologists; Society for Cardiovascular Angiography and Interventions; Society of Interventional Radiology; Society of Thoracic Surgeons; Society for Vascular Medicine. 2010 ACCF/AHA/AATS/ACR/ASA/SCA/SCAI/SIR/STS/SVM guidelines for the diagnosis and management of patients with thoracic aortic disease. A report of the American College of Cardiology Foundation/American Heart Association Task Force on Practice Guidelines, American Association for Thoracic Surgery, American College of Radiology, American Stroke Association, Society of Cardiovascular Anesthesiologists, Society for Cardiovascular Angiography and Interventions, Society of Interventional Radiology, Society of Thoracic Surgeons, and Society for Vascular Medicine. J Am Coll Cardiol. 2010;55(14):e27–129.

The Role of Coronary Computed Tomography Angiography in Cardiology Consultation

Cheng Ting Lin, Alexander J. Abramowicz, and Michael Poon

Abstract

Cardiac computed tomography (CCT) has rapidly become an integral part of noninvasive diagnostic cardiovascular imaging. Coronary artery calcium scoring using either electronic beam computed tomography (CT) or multidetector row CT is useful in the reclassification of coronary artery disease (CAD) risk when combined with the clinical CAD risk scoring in asymptomatic individuals. Coronary computed tomography angiography (CCTA) has a very high negative predictive value for ruling out the presence of significant obstructive CAD in symptomatic patients with either chronic or acute chest pain. Newer generation of scanners and software algorithms allows CCT studies to be performed easily in more patients with much lower effective radiation exposure. CCTA allows infinite viewing angle of the heart and its associated vascular structure retrospectively and is thus an invaluable and unique diagnostic tool for the assessment of cardiac structure and morphology prior to invasive procedures. Moreover, CCT aids in the diagnosis and management of patients with complex congenital heart disease and suspected coronary anomalies. It often obviates the need for invasive coronary angiography prior to noncoronary cardiac surgery and early post-coronary artery bypass grafting or coronary stenting for evaluation of the patency of native, grafted, or stented coronary vessels. Novel research applications of CCTA in the assessment of stress and rest myocardial perfusion, cardiac viability, and atherosclerotic plaque imaging may further open the window of opportunity for CCT to be the ultimate multipurpose diagnostic imaging modality of the future.

Keywords

Cardiac computed tomography • Angiography • Coronary • Imaging • Calcium • Plaque • Congenital heart • Chest pain

C.T. Lin, MD • A.J. Abramowicz, BS
Department of Radiology,
Stony Brook University Medical Center,
100 Nicolls Rd, Stony Brook,
NY 11794-8460, USA
e-mail: cheng.t.lin@gmail.com;
alexander.abramowicz@stonybrookmedicine.edu

M. Poon, MD (✉)
Advanced Cardiovascular Imaging,
Department of Radiology,
Stony Brook University Medical Center,
100 Nicolls Rd, Stony Brook,
NY 11794-8460, USA
e-mail: michael.poon@stonybrook.edu

Introduction

Rapid development of multidetector computed tomography (MDCT) now enables noninvasive imaging of the fast-beating heart with concomitant accurate depiction of small coronary anatomy. Significant research efforts focused on the appearance of coronary artery disease (CAD) and other cardiac structures on cardiac CT (CCT). Coronary CT angiography (CCTA) characterizes the location and extent of CAD with high negative predictive value (NPV), allowing clinicians to exclude CAD with confidence. The multiple practical applications for CCTA range from CAD risk

K. Stergiopoulos, D.L. Brown (eds.), *Evidence-Based Cardiology Consult*,
DOI 10.1007/978-1-4471-4441-0_15, © Springer-Verlag London 2014

stratification in asymptomatic individuals to the evaluation of emergency department (ED) patients with acute chest pain. MDCT features a very rapid acquisition time and is a suitable alternative to magnetic resonance imaging (MRI) in depiction of cardiac structures and surveillance of congenital heart disease. Extensive comparison studies are under way to assess the complementary role of CT alongside other established modalities such as echocardiography, cardiac scintigraphy, and conventional angiography.

Coding and Indications

CPT Codes

As of 2010, four permanent category I Current Procedural Terminology (CPT) codes encompass the appropriate uses of CCT:

- 75571 – Noncontrast CT for coronary calcium measurement
- 75572 – Contrast CT imaging of cardiac structure and morphology
- 75573 – Contrast CT evaluation for congenital heart disease
- 75574 – CCTA with evaluation of coronary arteries in patients with or without bypass grafts

Training

A CCT reader with sufficient level of expertise is a requirement for any practice offering cardiac imaging. The American College of Cardiology Foundation (ACCF) and American Heart Association (AHA) defined three levels of training:

- Level 1 – Introductory training to CCT
- Level 2 – Required for independent performance and interpretation of CCT. Requires interpretation of 150 CCTs
- Level 3 – Highest level of training suitable for the director of a CCT section with the ability to manage both the technical and personnel aspects of image acquisition. Requires interpretation of 300 contrast and 100 noncontrast CCTs

Guidelines

The ACCF/AHA along with other key specialty societies created consensus statements outlining the appropriate use criteria for coronary artery calcium (CAC) scans in 2007 and CCTA in 2010 [1, 2]. For each of the numerous clinical indications examined, the documents assigned one of 3 ratings for the appropriateness of CAC or CCTA: inappropriate, uncertain, and appropriate. CAC scans are appropriate in the evaluation of

low-risk patients presenting with atypical cardiac symptoms and asymptomatic intermediate-risk patients (low risk, <10 % 10-year risk of cardiac events; intermediate risk, 10–20 %; high risk, >20 %). There are 35 clinical indications in which CCTA is an appropriate modality (along with 29 uncertain and 29 inappropriate), and several representative clinical applications are listed below. The European Society of Cardiology (ESC) has also supported the use of CCTA to exclude acute coronary syndromes (ACS) or other causes of chest pain in select scenarios. The American College of Radiology (ACR) has compared CCT to competing imaging modalities in several clinical situations with similar conclusions.

Common Clinical Applications of CCTA

1. Acute Chest Pain
   CCTA can reliably exclude CAD in low- or intermediate-risk patients (NPV 99 %) and facilitate triage of ED patients with acute chest pain when initial cardiac biomarkers and ECG are negative or nondiagnostic for acute myocardial injury. Patients with suspected pulmonary embolism or aortic dissection can alternatively undergo a "triple rule-out" protocol for additional coverage of the pulmonary arteries and thoracic aorta.
2. Chronic Stable Chest Pain with Inconclusive Stress Test
   Low- or intermediate-risk patients with equivocal stress test results can undergo CCTA for evaluation of CAD as the high NPV of CCTA makes it an ideal follow-up diagnostic test to avoid the procedural risk of invasive coronary angiography.
3. Congestive Heart Failure (CHF)
   MDCT enables exclusion of ischemic heart disease as a potentially reversible cause of CHF. It also allows the measurement of ejection fraction and analysis of regional left ventricular wall motion function.
4. Preoperative Assessment
   CCTA is an acceptable alternative to stress test or myocardial perfusion single-photon emission computed tomography (SPECT) for preoperative assessment of low- to intermediate-risk patients prior to noncoronary cardiac surgery.
5. Bypass Graft Assessment
   CCTA is useful to demonstrate patency of bypass grafts and can potentially diagnose graft stenoses in selected patients.
6. Coronary Stent Assessment
   In a symptomatic patient, CCTA may be useful in the evaluation of stent patency with stents of certain types and a stent diameter of at least 3 mm.
7. Evaluation of Cardiac Structures
   Pre-procedure planning, e.g., atrial fibrillation ablation, and delineation of the course of coronary arteries can be reasonably achieved with CCT.

Multidetector Row CT (MDCT)

Scanner Technology

While historical data on coronary calcium scoring and CCTA have been obtained using electron beam CT (EBCT), MDCT technology continued to evolve and now represents the state-of-the-art noninvasive imaging modality of the coronary arteries. MDCT scanners are characterized primarily by the number of slices, also known as the number of detectors or channels on which CT attenuation data is gathered. The thickness of each detector determines the intrinsic spatial resolution of the scanner along the z-axis. Typical CCT studies are obtained on a 64- to 320-slice scanner with submillimeter spatial resolution of 0.5–0.75 mm, while the *x-y* or "in-plane" resolution is usually 0.4–0.5 mm. A scan time of 10 s on a 64-slice scanner covers a 10–12 cm field of view; less than 0.5 s on a 320-slice scanner allows up to 16 cm coverage. Low gantry rotation time of at most 330–500 ms (64-slice to 320-slice MDCT) is necessary to minimize cardiac motion artifact. The baseline temporal resolution is equal to about one-half the gantry rotation time. Dual-source CT, with two x-ray tubes and two corresponding detectors mounted onto the rotating gantry with an angular offset of 90°, offers a theoretical temporal resolution of 83 ms.

Two types of scanning modes are used in CCT: axial and helical (spiral). In the axial scanning mode, the table moves in a stepwise fashion with data acquisition occurring only when the table is stationary. No interpolation of imaging data is necessary. In contrast, with helical scanning the CT tube is on during continuous table movement, generating source data along a spiral path around the patient. Since detector channels receive projection data from multiple contiguous slices of the patient, an algorithm is required that uses interpolation to recreate data in axial slices. Pitch refers to the degree of overlap of the x-ray beam as it rotates around the moving patient and is defined as the amount of table feed per beam width. While standard CT uses a pitch of around 1, a low pitch of 0.15–0.3 (high overlap) is required for electrocardiogram (ECG)-gated CCT. The evolution of MDCT technology led to an increase in the number of slices (64-slice scanner in 2004, 320-slices scanner in 2008) as well as the introduction of dual-source CT and high-definition CT. Modern CT scanning techniques aim to strike a balance between diagnostic image quality and limiting radiation exposure to patients.

Radiation Dose and Safety

From 1980 to 2006, medical radiation dose to the US population increased sixfold (0.53–3.0 mSv per capita per year) as reported by the National Council on Radiation Protection and Measurements (NCRP). Nuclear cardiology accounted for 56 % and CCT accounted for 15 % of the effective dose from diagnostic and interventional sources. Rising utilization of cardiac imaging led to concerns about the carcinogenic risks of ionizing radiation. The Biological Effects of Ionizing Radiation (BEIR) VII report states that current evidence best supports a linear no-threshold (LNT) between radiation dose and cancer risk, suggesting that any exposure to ionizing radiation presents a risk [3]. Physicians who order CCT must be aware of the effects of radiation in the body and the potential ramifications.

Absorbed radiation is directly related to both deterministic and stochastic effects. Deterministic effects are predictable outcomes that occur once a threshold dose is met. Significant deterministic effects occur at high radiation doses (e.g., skin erythema at 3–6 Gy) which are well above doses typical for noninvasive CCT. In comparison, an individual's risk for stochastic effects are random and cannot be predicted. With increasing dose, the probability of these effects increases while the severity remains unchanged. Stochastic effects can be further divided into genetic and carcinogenic effects. A relationship has not been found between radiation exposures of parents and the potential genetic effects in their children.

The principal concern with diagnostic doses of radiation is increased risk of malignancy. Radiation protection is based on the assumption that there is no radiation dose at which stochastic effects do not occur (i.e., LNT model). The onset of cancer after radiation exposure has long latency periods of 5–15 years for leukemia and 20–60 years for solid tumors, which makes it difficult to establish a direct relationship. Organs with high cellular turnover are particularly susceptible, i.e., bone marrow, colon, lung, female breast, stomach, and children's thyroid gland. Radiation-induced cancers pose a greater concern for young and female patients, whereas the benefit/risk ratio of CCT is greater for older and male patients.

Absorbed doses that cause stochastic and deterministic effects are influenced by the type of radiation and the sensitivity of tissue to radiation. Equivalent dose (H) takes into account the type of radiation by multiplying the absorbed dose (D) by a radiation weighting factor (W_R) to give a unit in Sieverts (Sv). Gamma rays and x-rays, utilized by nuclear cardiology and CCT respectively, both have a W_R equal to 1. To adjust for nonuniform radiation exposure, effective dose (E) incorporates the radiosensitivity of each organ by multiplying the equivalent dose by an organ weighting factor *w*, summed over all exposed organs. Lung and breast are among the most radiosensitive organs ($w = 0.12$) within the irradiated region during a CCT, while the thyroid is moderately sensitive ($w = 0.04$).

CCTA and CAC scans generate dose information in the form of $CTDI_{vol}$ and DLP, which are dose estimates derived from phantom simulation. $CTDI_{vol}$ quantifies the amount of radiation for a standardized volume of the scan without

Table 15.1 Comparison of radiation doses in select cardiac imaging procedures

Source	Typical dose (mSv)	Cardiac CT
Annual background radiation	3	
Chest radiograph (PA)	0.02	
$^{13}NH_3$ rest-stress	2	Calcium score CT
	4.4	CCTA (320-slice volume scan)
Invasive coronary angiography	7	
^{99m}Tc Sestamibi SPECT	11	
	12	CCTA typical dose [4, 5]
^{82}Rb myocardial PET	13	
	18	CCTA (64-slice retrospective scan)
Dual isotope ^{201}Tl and ^{99m}Tc study	24	

Adapted from Einstein et al. [6, 7]

factoring scan length, whereas DLP is the product of $CTDI_{vol}$ and scan length. DLP (in units mGy·cm) can be converted to effective dose by applying a E/DLP conversion factor for the type of CT examination performed, which is 0.014 mSv·mGy^{-1}·cm^{-1} for CCT.

Effective dose allows comparison of stochastic risk between exams of varying nonuniform exposures. An excess relative risk of stochastic effects at 5 ± 1 %/Sv was reported by the International Commission of Radiological Protection (ICRP). Risk calculations are averaged over both gender and age, making such estimates appropriate for assessing risk to a population but not to a specific patient. On an average-sized patient, the radiation dosage from coronary calcium scoring is 1–1.4 mSv. One multicenter study (PROTECTION I) demonstrated that the standard CCTA radiation dose to a typical-sized patient with BMI of 20–30 is ~12 mSv [4, 5].

Representative effective doses to adult patients undergoing several sources of cardiac imaging are shown in Table 15.1. The effective dose for cardiac scintigraphy varies greatly with the choice of radionuclide and protocol. Since diagnostic nuclear cardiology doses are calculated from dosimetry data from an anatomical model of a typical patient, care must be taken when assessing risk for an individual patient. Likewise, CCT dose can vary markedly as a function of patient habitus and heart rate, underlying the importance of minimizing radiation dose through technique optimization.

Several techniques to minimize CCTA dose have been explored and validated. Prospective-triggering and tube current modulation protocols effectively lower radiation in patients with optimum heart rate control ($\leq$55 bpm) [8]. Pre-patient filters (e.g., bow-tie filter) can be applied to reduce dose by attenuating x-ray beams at the periphery of the scan.

Adjustments in tube voltage and current should be made according to the patient's size, aiming for the settings yielding the lowest dose while providing acceptable image quality. As the computational capabilities of scanners improve, the noise reduction achievable with iterative reconstruction over traditional filtered back projection allows for improved lesion conspicuity at a reduced radiation dose. For example, a recently published multicenter, multivendor trial has demonstrated radiation dosages as low as ~2 mSv [9].

Clinicians choosing CT or scintigraphic cardiac examinations must weigh their utility against the potential harm of ionizing radiation. Carcinogenic effects remain a concern regardless of the dosage level. The United States Environmental Protection Agency (EPA) requires that all exposure situations to individuals and populations be maintained as low as reasonably achievable (ALARA). A thorough understanding of the risks and benefits of cardiac imaging aids the clinician and patient in making a well-informed decision.

Patient Preparation

Each patient must be individually optimized for CCT. When coronary imaging is a priority, minimizing cardiac motion is critical to prospective-triggered synchronization of image acquisition and cardiac phase. Barring any contraindication, the patient is given an oral dose of beta-blocker (e.g., 50–100 mg metoprolol) 1 h before the exam. A regular heart rate below 65 bpm produces motion-free cardiac images. Patients with arrhythmias such as atrial fibrillation or high heart rates (greater than 70 bpm) not amenable to beta-blockade are more suited for a retrospective-gated scan.

An 18- or 20-gauge intravenous line typically placed in the antecubital vein is needed to accommodate a flow rate of at least 4–6 mL/s. A higher iodine concentration of 370 mg I/mL is preferred to optimize contrast opacification and homogeneity of coronary arteries. Experienced support staff should explain the potential complications of contrast media and address any concerns from the patient prior to the scan to minimize anxiety-related motion artifact. The patient is routinely given 0.4–0.8 mg nitroglycerin sublingually approximately 5 min prior to the contrast administration to take advantage of its fast-acting vasodilating effects on the coronary arteries to maximally dilate the coronary arteries while minimizing the chance of vasospasm at the time of the scan.

Scanning Protocol

At the start of each scan, low-dose frontal and lateral scout tomograms are acquired with the patient at end inspiration. From these films, the technologist then selects an appropriate field of view and scan range that extends from the carina to 2 cm below the diaphragm for a CAC scan or coronary protocol angiogram. Examinations for post-CABG evaluation or "triple rule-out" protocol require expanded scan ranges that include the top of the aortic arch and entire thorax, respectively.

ECG synchronization is the cornerstone of modern cardiac CT imaging and enables data acquisition at a predefined phase of the cardiac cycle. Two methods of synchronization are available: retrospective gating and prospective triggering. In retrospective-gated scans the CT tube is continuously active throughout the entire cardiac cycle. The computer then reconstructs CT data to their corresponding phase of the cycle, with the 0 % phase defined as the start of R-R interval and the mid-diastolic phase typically at the 70–75 % phase. We routinely reconstruct retrospective CT data in phase increments of 10 %. Advantages of retrospective gating include functional information such as left ventricular ejection fraction (LVEF) calculation and wall motion assessment. The retrospective technique is also appropriate in patients with arrhythmia or tachycardia, as the imaging window for these patients is not suitable for the prospective technique. CT dose modulation reserves the full tube current output for the diastolic phase and thereby reduces radiation dose by 30–40 % in retrospective-gated scans.

Prospective triggering takes advantage of the relative lack of coronary motion during mid-diastole. While this imaging window increases as the heart rate slows, the cardiac rhythm must be free of abnormal beats (e.g., premature ventricular contractions, atrial fibrillation). A 64-slice scanner with 4 cm of coverage requires 5–7 cardiac cycles to image the heart (3–4 cycles to acquire data and 2–3 cycles in between for table movement). In contrast, true volume CT of the heart (e.g., 320-slice scanner) completes a scan in the duration of one heartbeat without table movement. Since the total scan time is lower with the prospective technique, prospective-triggered scans led to nearly 90 % reduction in radiation dose compared to retrospective-gated scans [10]. Radiation exposure is minimized when the scan is limited to a preset phase of the cardiac cycle, typically 65–81 %. Widening of the imaged phases (or "padding") generates additional data for reconstruction at the expense of higher radiation dose. Therefore, one key disadvantage of prospective scans is the limited reconstruction options to correct imaging artifacts, emphasizing the need for patient optimization.

The patient first undergoes a noncontrast scan to calculate the calcium score (CAC scan) in several clinical scenarios. Exceptions include patients with prior bypass, stent, known severe CAD, or recent CAC (<6 months ago). CAC scans are performed at 120 kVp, slice thickness of 2.5–3 mm, and ECG synchronization with either retrospective or prospective techniques. The superior and inferior extents of the coronaries can then be localized on the CAC scan in order to further refine the scan range for dedicated coronary scans that also helps to minimize the radiation dose exposure.

The peak tube voltage for CCTA is chosen among three common values: 80, 100, or 120 kVp. A patient with high BMI (e.g., >30) will require a more penetrating beam at 120 kVp in order to limit image noise. On the other hand, tube voltage should be lowered in thin to average-sized patients as doing so substantially lowers radiation dose at essentially no cost to image quality (radiation dose is proportional to the square of the tube voltage).

The scan delay or time between the start of contrast injection and the start of the scan is determined either by administering a test bolus or bolus tracking, depending on the imager's preference. A test bolus is a small amount of contrast injected followed by a saline bolus at the same rate as the primary bolus. The transit time to peak enhancement within an assigned vessel is determined by repeated imaging of the timing vessel. Diagnostic injection then proceeds using the derived contrast transit time. With bolus tracking, the entire contrast bolus and saline bolus chaser are administered in one run. The scanner then monitors the Hounsfield unit (HU) within an assigned region of interest (ROI) such as the thoracic aorta when left heart opacification is desired. Intermittent single-slice scans are performed and the scanner automatically prompts the start of a scan when the threshold HU value has been exceeded. At our institution, the threshold for the descending aorta ROI is set at 180 HU for a routine coronary protocol. For a "triple rule-out" protocol, we place an additional ROI in the pulmonary artery with a threshold of 90 HU and lower the descending aortic ROI to 140 HU (Fig. 15.1). Scan timing is further calibrated with a breath-hold exercise and a delay chosen to minimize heart rate variability during breath holding. A breath hold of 10–15 s corresponds to the average scan time on a 64-slice scanner.

Upon completion of scan, CT data is transferred from the gantry to the control computer to be processed using reconstruction algorithms called kernels or "filters." The choice of kernel depends on the clinical task and the acceptable tradeoff between spatial resolution and relative noise. For instance, evaluation of coronary plaques is optimal with a smooth kernel, whereas a sharp kernel improves visualization of coronary stents at the expense of increasing noise. While modern CT scanners can generate reconstructions expeditiously with filtered back projection algorithms, there is much interest in the more computationally intensive iterative reconstruction algorithm as a mean of minimizing CT artifacts and reducing radiation dose.

Image Post-processing, Pitfalls and Artifacts

The axial source data sent from the scanner can be further manipulated by advanced imaging workstations that are capable of 3-dimensional (3D) post-processing techniques. Standard axial, coronal, and sagittal projections are insufficient for detailed evaluation of the coronary arteries and cardiac structures. Several 3D reconstruction methods are utilized in the routine analysis of CCTA: volume rendering

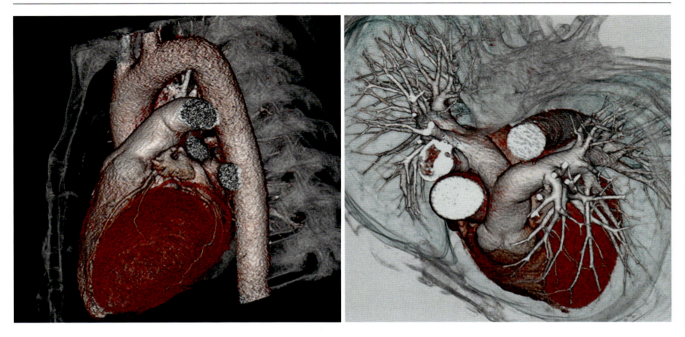

Fig. 15.1 Coronary computed tomography angiography – triple rule-out protocol. *Left panel*: volume rendering technique (VRT) image of the thoracic aorta and coronary arteries. *Right panel*: VRT image of the pulmonary arteries and coronary arteries

(VR), maximum intensity projection (MIP), and multiplanar reconstruction (MPR). Many workstations incorporate templates that enable rapid demonstration of coronary anatomy with these key post-processing techniques.

VR reconstructions display the entire of volume of data from a defined camera in space relative to the object of interest. Each voxel is assigned a value for opacity according to its CT density such that lower-intensity voxels (lung, fat) are more translucent, whereas higher-intensity voxels are more opaque (due to contrast in coronaries and aorta). VR is useful for evaluating complex coronary anatomy and bypass grafts along with soft tissue, muscle, and bone, which may contribute to a more comprehensive understanding of pathologic processes. Patients and referring physicians may find abnormalities demonstrated on VR images to be easier to comprehend.

MIP are 2-dimensional (2D) projections through a chosen slab of the imaged volume displaying only the highest-intensity pixels. It provides good anatomical overview when contrast-opacified coronaries comprise the bulk of maximum intensity pixels. A weakness of MIP is the loss of 3D orientation among structures and obscuration of lower-intensity voxels (e.g., noncalcified plaque) by higher-intensity voxels (e.g., calcified plaque). As a result, stenosis detection using MIP is only appropriate in the absence of calcifications that cause blooming artifacts. A similar reconstruction called minimum intensity projection (MinIP) chooses lower-intensity pixels which may highlight myocardial perfusion defects.

MPR produces 2D grayscale images that display the mean attenuation value of all pixels in a plane through the imaged

volume. Orthogonal planes and even curved MPR (cMPR) can be reconstructed. Accurate depiction of a coronary stenosis requires short-axis MPR images which can be created manually or with software assistance (e.g., automatic centerline extraction). MPR also produces long- and short-axis views of cardiac structures analogous to the standard views of echocardiography and cardiac magnetic resonance imaging.

CT attenuation data is organized by a 3D array of HU that corresponds to the attenuation value of the tissue within each voxel. The standard 8-bit grayscale display maps a selected range of HU onto 256 shades of gray. The window center defines the attenuation value that is medium in brightness on the grayscale. The window width determines the range of HU with the mean at the window center that is displayed within the grayscale. Voxels above or below this range are assigned the maximum and minimum values, respectively. A low window width or narrow window is useful for evaluating myocardium, while a wider window may be useful for calcified lesions and coronary stents.

The diagnostic accuracy of CCTA studies can be reduced as a result of several possible pitfalls and artifacts which are generally minimized with optimal patient preparation. Heart rate control with beta-blockers and coronary arterial dilation with nitroglycerin both contribute to improved image quality by reducing cardiac motion and improving signal-to-noise ratio (SNR), respectively. Cardiac motion causes blurring of cardiac structures and coronaries, and in severe cases, the coronary arteries can appear duplicated. One remedy for cardiac motion is to select the cardiac phase with the best image quality for the structure of interest. The most motion-free phase can occasionally be found at end systole or the 30–40 % phase. Therefore, one potential drawback to CT dose modulation is the increased noise during systole, limiting interpretation of systolic phase images for cardiac wall motion only. Evaluation of cardiac phases in increments of 5 % rather than 10 % may be helpful for clarifying suspected lesions [11]. It is not unusual to repeatedly change phases when evaluating the segments of a coronary artery affected by cardiac motion. When cardiac motion is due to premature ventricular contractions, ECG editing can correct for any ectopic beat by removing the affected cycle from the dataset.

Slice misregistration artifact occurs from motion during axial acquisition, resulting in a straight plane of discontinuity between two different slices separated in time. Such artifacts frequently interrupt the path of the coronaries and possibly creating false-positive lesions. Respiratory motion causes misregistration of chest wall or diaphragmatic structures, as well as blurring of pulmonary vasculature. Centerline analysis is often susceptible to creating "pseudo-lesion" at the discontinuity caused by misregistration.

Patient cooperation is crucial for a properly controlled contrast injection and subsequent diagnostic image quality. For instance, patient motion can displace the preset ROI during the intermittent scans of bolus tracking, leading to a suboptimal scan delay time and poor opacification of cardiac structures. The patient's elbow must stay immobile during contrast injection to prevent kinking and obstruction of the IV flow. Suboptimal contrast opacification of the coronaries results in low SNR and compromises the accuracy of the exam, often requiring follow-up with a repeat exam or a different modality.

Dense objects preferentially absorb low-energy x-rays, a phenomenon called beam hardening, leading to streak artifacts and areas of signal loss on CT images. Reconstructions created from a filtered back projection algorithm are particularly prone to beam hardening, while iterative reconstruction is effective at reducing streak artifact. Calcifications, coronary stents, surgical clips and wires, and pacemaker leads all cause beam hardening to varying degrees on CCTA. Careful scrutiny of the systolic and diastolic phases can allow the cardiac position to move relative to the affected area of signal loss.

Coronary stents and calcifications have an apparent expansion in size on CT due to blooming artifacts, which causes overestimation of the severity of luminal stenoses. On smooth kernel and standard window settings, blooming artifacts exaggerate the size of calcified plaques and obscure the lumen, leading to uninterpretable lesions. Techniques to reduce blooming artifact and improve luminal visualization include widening the window width, application of a sharp kernel, avoidance of MIP, and using thin slice MPR to minimize partial volume effects.

Contraindications

Beta-blockers should be withheld in patients with significant bradycardia (<60 bpm), atrioventricular heart block (greater than Mobitz type I block), hypotension (mean BP of less than 60 mmHg), decompensated heart failure, and asthma (except mild intermittent asthma). In patients with contraindications to beta-blockers, IV diltiazem is the preferred calcium channel blocker (CCB) for rate control as other CCBs have greater negative inotropic effects. Contraindications to nitroglycerin include hypotension, recent usage of phosphodiesterase (PDE-V) inhibitors (treatment for erectile dysfunction and pulmonary hypertension) and severe aortic stenosis.

Before administration of CT contrast media, the patient should be screened for renal insufficiency (minimum glomerular filtration rate of 50 mL/min at our institution) or prior allergy to iodinated contrast. The exams of apprehensive or uncooperative patients will frequently be of poor quality or nondiagnostic since the patient will be required to breath hold and remain motion-free for approximately 10–20 s. Efforts should be made to alleviate anxiety and only rarely should conscious sedation be needed. An alternative modality should be considered in morbidly obese patients (BMI >40) due to a high likelihood of poor-quality scan due to underpenetration of photons.

Asymptomatic Indications

Coronary Arterial Calcium (CAC) (CPT: 75571)

Coronary arterial calcification represents an integral and active stage of atherosclerosis. Calcium hydroxyapatite deposition in the coronary intima, driven by growth factors, indicates chronic plaque inflammation. The degree of calcification correlates moderately well with overall plaque area, but not with severity of luminal stenosis for an individual plaque. Also, culprit lesions in ACS are generally noncalcified plaques that comprise 80 % of all plaques [12]. However, a highly calcified plaque burden portends a higher overall risk of an obstructive lesion (>50 % stenosis).

In 1990, Agatston developed a scoring system for coronary calcium quantification with noncontrast CT scans [13]. Determining the CAC score first involves highlighting of coronary calcifications using computer software on a dedicated workstation (Fig. 15.2). Noncoronary calcifications such as aortic annular calcification and CT densities less than 1 mm^2 in area are excluded from the analysis. The area of each plaque is multiplied by a density coefficient that is determined by the maximum HU value within that region (1 for 130–199 HU, 2 for 200–299 HU, 3 for 300–399 HU, and 4 for 400 HU and above). The calcium score is derived from the summation of area/density coefficient products.

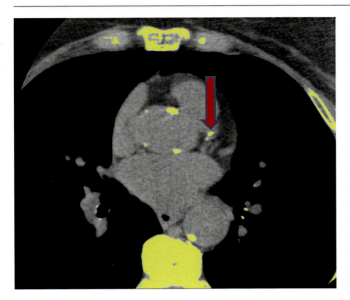

Fig. 15.2 Calcium score software. *Red arrow* pointing to calcified plaques colored in yellow in the proximal left anterior descending (LAD) artery

A standardized protocol historically based on EBCT and adapted for MDCT was devised to calculate calcium scores with high reproducibility. In the past, CAC scans performed on EBCT achieved sub-mSv doses. While radiation exposure is higher on MDCT, the use of a prospective-triggering technique decreases the radiation dose to 1–1.4 mSv [14]. Calcium scores generated from both types of CT are highly correlated, leading to the preferential usage of MDCT for its faster acquisition time and better spatial resolution [15].

Calcium scores are usually divided into the following disease classes: no plaque burden for score of 0, minimal plaque burden for 1–10, mild plaque burden for 11–100, moderate plaque burden for 101–400, and extensive plaque burden for >400 [13]. A zero calcium score is associated with a very low probability of unstable plaque and obstructive lesions. Patients with scores less than 100 likely have minimal or mild luminal stenosis and a low likelihood of abnormal functional exams [16]. On the other hand, scores above 400 indicate that a significant coronary stenosis is highly probable and should be further evaluated if clinically indicated.

Calcium scoring provides incremental and independent prognostic information over traditional risk stratification strategies based on Framingham risk scores. The pretest probabilities are divided into three categories: low (10-year risk of coronary event <10 %), intermediate (10–20 % risk), and high (>20 % risk) [17]. The intermediate-risk group represents about 25–40 % of the population. This population experiences the greatest therapeutic impact, or a change in treatment class, from CAC testing. Additionally, multiple prospective studies demonstrate the independent predictive value of calcium scores in predicting coronary events [18, 19]. Coronary

calcium is also a valuable surrogate marker for CAD in patients presenting with ACS and ischemic cardiomyopathy [20–23].

Results from CAC scans should be individualized beyond a simple score-risk relationship. The number of involved vessels provides incremental prognostic value and is associated with overall mortality. Data from the Multi-Ethnic Study of Atherosclerosis (MESA) showed that Caucasians have the greatest frequency and quantity of coronary arterial calcium, followed by Chinese, Hispanic, and African-Americans [24]. In a comparison of outcomes, African-Americans experienced the highest mortality for a given calcium score [25]. Serial CAC scans are not recommended for monitoring CAD, even in patients at high risk of worsening disease. Interscan variability for the same patient on the same day can be over 20 %, making repeat scans unreliable for detecting actual disease progression [26].

The AHA and ACC support the use of calcium score CT for asymptomatic intermediate-risk patients to determine their risk of developing coronary disease beyond that predicted by standard risk factor models. CAC scan is also appropriate in low-risk patients with a family history of premature coronary heart disease. Calcium scoring is a valuable adjunct to CCTA by identifying patients at risk for obstructive disease and quantifying their plaque burden. Incorporating calcium CT into the diagnostic arsenal for the management of CAD helps ensure the proper initiation of evidence-based therapy [27].

Emergent Clinical Indications

Acute Chest Pain (CPT: 75574)

CCTA is considered appropriate in the assessment of CAD in low- to intermediate-risk patients presenting with acute chest pain and possible ACS. These patients must also have normal/uninterpretable ECGs and normal/equivocal serum troponin levels. In cases where a hypercoagulable state is suspected (e.g., elevated D-dimers), a "triple rule-out" can be performed to additionally evaluate for the possibility of pulmonary embolism and aortic dissection. In the acute setting, CT angiography is most appropriately used to exclude CAD, and the need for invasive angiograms in patients whose likelihood of disease is not high [28–30].

Hoffmann et al. demonstrated that MDCT accurately excludes ACS (high NPV) in the prospective evaluation of acute chest pain patients [28]. In patients who underwent invasive coronary angiography for non-ST elevation ACS, MDCT detected coronary stenosis at a high accuracy (sensitivity 100 %, specificity 75 %, PPV 96 %, NPV 100 %) [29]. Rubinshtein found no major adverse cardiac event within 1 year for 58 patients prospectively evaluated with CCTA for acute chest pain [30]. An observational study by Hollander similarly showed a very low (<1 %) rate of cardiovascular events within 1 year among 481 ED patients with negative CCTA results [31].

In a randomized study comparing CCTA and standard of care, Goldstein et al. demonstrated a shorter time to diagnosis with CT (3.4 vs. 15 h) at a lower hospital cost ($1,586 vs. $1,872) and that both approaches were 100 % safe [32]. In the CT-STAT (Coronary Computed Tomographic Angiography for Systematic Triage of Acute Chest Pain Patients to Treatment) trial, CCTA-based strategies and standard of care were compared for 750 ED patients presenting with acute chest pain, leading to an earlier time to diagnosis (3 vs. 7 h) and a lower cost of CAD diagnosis ($2,000 vs. $3,500) [33]. Recently published ACRIN/PA (Pennsylvania Department of Health and the American College of Radiology Imaging Network) and ROMICAT-II (Rule Out Myocardial Infarction Using Computer Assisted Tomography II) trials both affirmed the clinical efficacy of CCTA in the evaluation of ED patients with acute chest pain particularly in decreasing the unnecessary hospital admission rate and ED length of stay [34, 35].

Evidence firmly supports the role of CCTA in the assessment of low- to intermediate-risk ED patients with suspicion of ACS. CT angiography both excludes CAD with a high NPV and detects significant stenosis at a modest PPV in this population. Advantages in patient throughput and cost reduction strongly encourage the use of CCTA in the initial workup of acute chest pain.

Triage Algorithm for Acute Chest Pain Patients Evaluated with CCTA

The high NPV of CCTA permits exclusion of CAD in patients with normal coronary arteries (no plaque burden or visible stenosis) or nonobstructive CAD (<50 % stenosis). In light of the clinical significance of noncalcified plaque, CT angiography should be performed in addition to a CAC scan in the assessment of emergency department (ED) patients with acute chest pain. CCTA should not be performed in patients at high pretest probability of CAD (uncertain indication), with persistent ST-segment elevation (uncertain indication) or with definite myocardial infarction (inappropriate indication). Normal results allow patients to be discharged from the ED without increased risk of major adverse cardiac events (MACE) [36]. Mild nonobstructive CAD initially diagnosed on CT angiography should be managed with outpatient cardiology follow-up for risk factor modification and initiation of medical therapy, if applicable.

Patients with obstructive CAD (>50 % stenosis) may require additional functional testing such as provocative testing with stress myocardial perfusion imaging or diagnostic

conventional angiography with fractional flow reserve. Blooming artifact from calcified plaques frequently precludes accurate luminal assessment and results in false-positive or uninterpretable lesions. Potential solutions include using sharp kernel and thinner MPR slices to reduce artifact. Obstructive lesions with >70 % stenosis or >50 % in the left main artery in the setting of acute chest pain may need to be interrogated with cardiac catheterization for further diagnosis and potential intervention (Fig. 15.3).

While careful attention is paid to coronary assessment, a number of noncoronary pathologies can present in acutely symptomatic patients. Other causes of chest pain include, but are not limited to, pneumonia, pulmonary embolism, rib fracture, pneumothorax, aortic dissection, and pericardial disease. Therefore, reconstructions with full field of view to include the lung fields should be routinely assessed for any disease that may influence patient management.

Nonemergent Clinical Indications

Pulmonary Vein Morphology (CPT: 75572)

Noninvasive cardiac imaging is essential for visualizing pulmonary veins (PV) and guiding electrophysiological procedures in patients with atrial fibrillation. Advantages of CCTA for this indication include accurate and reproducible delineation of the left atrium, pulmonary venous anatomy, and adjacent structures (Fig. 15.4). Quantitative measurements of the pulmonary ostia and branching distances are reliably calculated on MPR images. Pre-procedural CT also provides a baseline comparison in the assessment for posttreatment complications.

The underlying cause of atrial fibrillation is the presence of ectopic electrical foci, frequently originating in the PV [37]. A detailed analysis of PV on MDCT includes the number of PV, the presence of supernumerary PV or common pulmonary trunk, distance to first-order branch point, and PV ostial measurements. Relevant information regarding left atrium (LA) includes LA size, presence or absence of left atrial appendage thrombus, and configuration of the interatrial septum. When a left atrial appendage thrombus is suspected, a short delayed scan (1–2 min) should be performed to distinguish between mixing artifact and actual thrombus.

The presence of any anomalous venous drainage, such as partial anomalous pulmonary venous return and persistent left superior vena cava, should be reported. The anatomic locations of the esophagus and descending aorta with respect to the LA should be discussed to minimize post-ablation complications such as atrioesophageal fistula. In the postoperative CT, evaluation for pulmonary vein thrombosis and stenosis is greatly aided by a pre-ablation CT for direct comparison.

3D VRT   2D MIP   2D MPR cross section

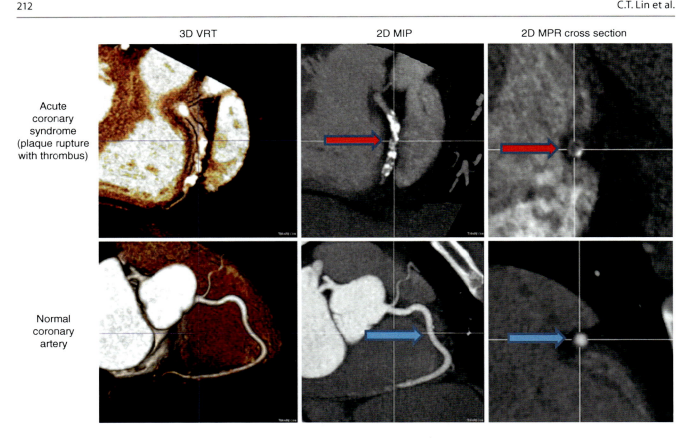

Acute
coronary
syndrome
(plaque rupture
with thrombus)

Normal
coronary
artery

Fig. 15.3 CCTA – post-processing methods. The use of all three post-processing techniques, e.g., volume rendering technique (*VRT*), maximum intensity projection (*MIP*), and multiplanar reformatting (*MPR*), in the assessment of a patient with normal coronaries (*blue arrows*) and a patient with acute coronary syndrome with plaque rupture and thrombosis (*red arrows*)

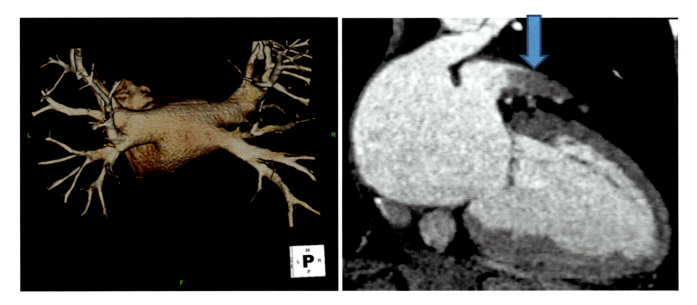

Fig. 15.4 CCTA in the evaluation of pulmonary veins. *Left panel*: volume rendering technique (VRT) image of the left atrium and pulmonary veins. *Right panel*: multiplanar reformatting (MPR) image of a large left atrium and left atrial appendage thrombus (*blue arrow*) – a contraindication for atrial fibrillation ablation

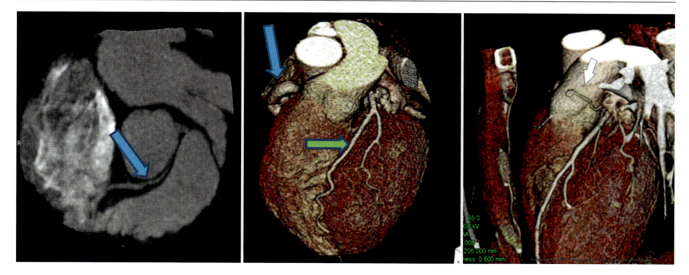

Fig. 15.5 Coronary anomalies. *Left panel*: maximum intensity projection (MIP) image of anomalous right coronary artery (RCA) (*blue arrow*) from left coronary sinus with slit-like opening of the origin of the RCA. *Middle panel*: volume rendering technique (VRT) image of a large RCA coronary aneurysm (*blue arrow*) – unusually large RCA compared to left anterior descending (LAD) (*green arrow*) in VRT. *Right panel*: VRT image of a small left main to main pulmonary artery fistula (*white arrow*)

The scan protocol for atrial fibrillation pre-ablation is adjusted for pulmonary vein opacification by timing the contrast for peak enhancement of the left atrium. Cardiac CT for pulmonary vein mapping can be performed at a lower tube current and higher slice thickness to reduce radiation exposure. CT images can also be fused with electroanatomic maps to be used by the electrophysiologist during procedures [38, 39]. The resultant savings in fluoroscopic time, in addition to steady improvements in dose-lowering CT technology, further supports the use of CCTA for PV mapping.

Coronary Anomalies (CPT: 75574 or 75573)

Congenital anomalies of a coronary artery occur at an incidence of 0.6–1.3 % in invasive coronary angiography series [40]. The majority of coronary variants are benign, hemodynamically stable incidental findings on CCTA performed for other indications. Nevertheless, malignant coronary variants need to be recognized as they are thought to be the second most common cause of sudden cardiac death in young athletes [41, 42]. CCTA has the ability to depict coronary anatomy at high spatial resolution and distinguish between benign and malignant morphology [43–45].

The left and right sinuses of Valsalva give rise to the left main (LCA) and right coronary (RCA) arteries, respectively. The LCA or RCA ostium can have unusually high or low takeoffs of more than 1 cm from the sinotubular junction. Another anomaly occurs when the LCA is absent, leading to the left anterior descending (LAD) and left circumflex (LCX) arteries having separate ostia from the left sinus of Valsalva. Rarely, the RCA origin is absent and results in a condition called single coronary artery syndrome. Precise anatomic description of these variations can often facilitate cannulation on coronary angiography.

Coronary arteries with origins at an abnormal aortic sinus will adopt an anomalous course. Left-sided arteries (LCA, LAD, LCX) can have an aberrant origin from the right sinus, and, likewise, the RCA can arise from the left sinus (Fig. 15.5). Several courses can follow from the aberrant origin, including posteroinferior to the aortic root (retroaortic), between the aorta and pulmonary artery (interarterial) and anterior to the pulmonary trunk (prepulmonic). A retroaortic anomalous course of the LCX or RCA occupies the normally vessel-free space between the noncoronary sinus and the atria. An interarterial course is a malignant variant that poses a risk of exertion-related sudden cardiac death, thought to be due to compression of the coronary artery by the great vessels during a high-output state. Coronary arteries with retroaortic or prepulmonic course do not have this risk and are considered benign entities [46]. The proximal portion of an anomalous coronary should be examined carefully for any kinking or intramural segments, which may affect surgical approach.

A pulmonary arterial origin of the LCA, otherwise known as an anomalous LCA from the pulmonary artery (ALCAPA) or Bland-White-Garland syndrome, most commonly presents in infancy with volume overload and heart failure. ALCAPA patients rarely survive to adulthood and can present with ACS, heart failure, or coronary steal phenomenon [47, 48]. In contrast, a pulmonary arterial origin of the RCA, LAD, and LCX may be clinically silent [49, 50]. Variations of coronary arteries originating from other abnormal locations, such as the "noncoronary" sinus, thoracic aorta, or aortic arch vessels have been described.

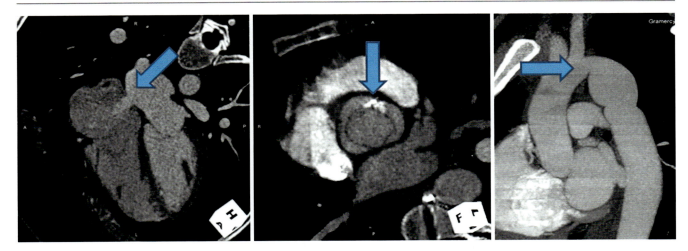

Fig. 15.6 Congenital heart disease. *Left panel*: multiplanar reformatting (MPR) image of a large secundum atrial septal defect (*blue arrow*) with contrast crossing the defect between the left and right atrium indicating left-to-right shunt. *Middle panel*: MPR image of a unicuspid aortic valve with calcification of the aortic commissure (*blue arrow*). *Right panel*: maximum intensity projection (MIP) image of coarctation of the aorta with poststenotic dilatation (*blue arrow*)

A myocardial bridge is a common coronary anomaly defined by an intramyocardial course of a normally epicardial coronary artery segment. This most commonly occurs at the mid-segment of the LAD, followed by the LCX and RCA. The bridging can be superficial where the artery contacts the myocardium or deep where the coronary segment is completely encased by the myocardium. While a myocardial bridge in isolation is not thought to be clinically significant, its potential role in causing coronary ischemia is under debate [51]. Luminal stenosis of the intramyocardial segment may be observed on CCTA and confirmed on invasive angiography, although diastolic coronary blood flow is infrequently compromised. An intraluminal or intracavitary course is comparatively rare and can complicate cardiac surgical procedures.

Coronary artery aneurysms are characterized by dilation of the coronary diameter to greater than 1.5 times the normal adjacent segments (Fig. 15.5). Coronary artery fistulas occur from an abnormal termination of coronary arteries into cardiac chambers, pulmonary vessels, or the coronary sinus. Smaller fistulas are rarely hemodynamically significant (Fig. 15.5), whereas coronary steal phenomenon and myocardial ischemia may manifest in larger fistulas that warrant endovascular or surgical intervention [52, 53].

CCTA is a rapid, noninvasive exam capable of defining coronary anatomy and adjacent cardiac structures. High spatial and contrast resolution make MDCT the modality of choice for characterizing abnormal coronary arteries. In patients for whom x-ray exposure is a concern, radiation dose can be lowered by decreasing tube settings and increasing slice thickness without loss of diagnostic accuracy. The clinical value of CCTA in evaluating coronary anomalies lies in its ability to distinguish between benign variants and abnormalities that require aggressive intervention.

Congenital Heart Disease (CPT: 75573)

The assessment of congenital heart disease (CHD) requires a multimodality approach that can include cardiac CT. While MRI and echocardiography offer functional and dynamic information about the cardiac defect without the use of ionizing radiation, CT provides superior spatial resolution in return for radiation exposure [54].

Understanding the clinical objective and type of CHD being evaluated is critical to choosing the proper CT scan protocol. One determinant for contrast timing is the anticipated shunt physiology. For example, left heart opacification demonstrates left-to-right shunts and right heart opacification shows right-to-left shunts. Right-to-left shunts in cyanotic CHD are seen in tetralogy of Fallot (TOF), transposition of the great arteries (TGA), and Eisenmenger syndrome. Acyanotic CHD in the setting of increased pulmonary vascularity raises the possibility of a left-to-right shunt, including ventricular septal defect (VSD), patent ductus arteriosus (PDA), atrioventricular septal defect (AVSD), partial anomalous pulmonary venous return (PAPVR), and atrial septal defect (ASD) (Fig. 15.6). Significant left-to-right shunt physiology often manifests with CT evidence of volume overload, such as pulmonary arterial enlargement, flattening or leftward bowing of the interventricular septum, and enlargement of the right heart chambers. Arterial phase imaging is appropriate for assessing abnormal vessels in the systemic circulation, e.g., coronary anomaly, major aortopulmonary collateral arteries, and coarctation of the aorta (CoA).

When CHD is suspected, an appropriate imaging range that fully covers the involved anatomy should be chosen (e.g., aortic arch to diaphragm for evaluation of CoA and PDA). Restriction of the scan length to only what is necessary

Fig. 15.7 CCTA of bypass grafts. *Left panel*: volume rendering technique (VRT) of left internal mammary artery (*LIMA*) (*blue arrow*) to distal left anterior descending (LAD) (*yellow arrow*). *Right panel*: VRT of saphenous vein graft (*SVG*) (*white arrow*) to obtuse marginal (OM) traversing across the main pulmonary artery

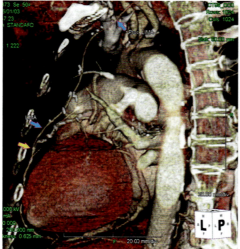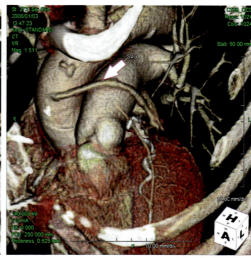

for diagnosis is important for radiation dose consideration. Other strategies to reduce CT dose include using non-gated CT for pediatric patients, ECG-tube current modulation and lowering tube potential to 80 kVp for pediatric patients and 100 kVp for adult patients of average BMI [55]. On occasion, CHD is incidentally discovered on a cardiac CT performed for other indications. Lesions such as ASD, mitral valve prolapse, aortic valvular anomalies (bicuspid or unicuspid aortic valve), and, less commonly, CoA and PDA can be initially diagnosed during a routine CCTA evaluation (Fig. 15.6). A fundamental understanding CT protocols and congenital cardiac abnormalities is essential to optimize the complementary role of cardiac CT in the diagnosis and long-term evaluation of CHD.

Coronary Artery Bypass Graft Assessment (CPT: 75574)

The use of CCTA in the setting of prior bypass grafting is considered appropriate in symptomatic patients with typical angina and for localization of bypass grafts prior to redo surgery. Bypass graft patency and occlusion are diagnosed on CCTA with very high accuracy (above 95 % sensitivity and specificity in most studies) [56–58]. Note that the use of CT angiography in asymptomatic patients with prior CABG is considered uncertain (CABG over 5 years ago) or inappropriate (CABG less than 5 years ago).

The scan range is extended to include the entire course of bypass grafts, their origin from the aortic arch (venous grafts) or subclavian arteries (internal mammary grafts). Beta-blockade and a prospective-triggered scan are recommended to decrease radiation dose. Sharp kernel can improve visualization of heavily calcified vessels. If available, the use of iterative reconstruction improves SNR and reduces metallic artifact.

On CCTA images, coronary bypass graft patency is confirmed by direct visualization of intravascular contrast. Arterial grafts generally have higher patency rates compared to venous grafts [59]. The presence of internal mammary artery (IMA) grafts can be quickly verified by noting the absence of a normally located IMA within the chest wall adjacent to the lateral borders of the sternum. A thorough analysis of bypass grafts should include MPR to evaluate the graft and anastomosis for stenosis/occlusion. Curved MPR with centerline analysis is helpful to show the entire course of the graft in a single plane [60]. Volume rendered images are useful for provide a broad overview of the bypass graft course (Fig. 15.7). The order of venous graft implantation along the ascending aorta is such that the bypass graft to the RCA territory is earliest and most inferior, followed by grafts to the LAD territory and then LCX. Occasionally, a vein graft may be a "jump" graft with both a side-to-side anastomosis at its midcourse and an end-to-side anastomosis.

Potential diagnostic difficulty lies in obscuration of the lumen by streak artifacts caused by ostial markers, surgical clips, and sternotomy wires. Metal artifacts cause beam hardening that may possibly be misinterpreted as luminal disease. Evaluating the affected region in different cardiac phases may show the graft moving away from the metallic density. Contrast opacification of native coronaries near the anastomotic site is also a sign of graft patency, although it can alternatively represent collateral flow. Assessment of the native coronary arteries is usually limited due to severe plaque burden and small vessel diameters contributing to a high false-positive rate [61]. An occluded graft can sometimes be directly visualized or assumed by the configuration of residual surgical clips, while invasive angiography simply shows nonopacification of the graft [62]. Aneurysms and pseudoaneurysms of the saphenous vein graft are rare and potentially lethal complications well depicted on CT.

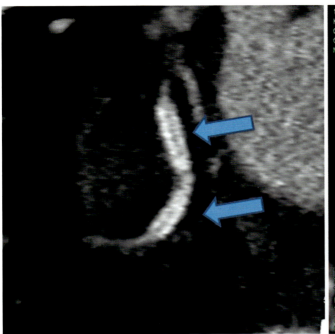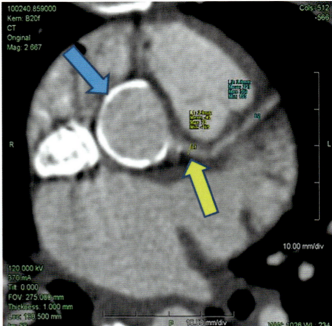

Fig. 15.8 CCTA of coronary stents and calcified aortic annulus. *Left panel*: multiplanar reformatting (MPR) image of 2 patent stents (*blue arrows*) in a large obtuse marginal (OM) branch. *Right panel*: maxi- mum intensity projection (MIP) image of densely calcified aortic annulus (*blue arrow*) and left main (LM) (*yellow arrow*)

Evaluation of bypass grafts is highly accurate on MDCT, despite potential problems from metal artifact. Invasive coronary angiography remains the traditional gold standard for graft assessment with CCTA serving as a valuable noninvasive alternative.

Coronary Stent and Left Main Patency (CPT: 75574)

Coronary stents are the mainstay of current revascularization therapy. With invasive angiography as the gold standard, CCTA plays a complementary role in the assessment of in-stent restenosis. However, the varying types and sizes of coronary stents result in inconsistent diagnostic accuracy of CCTA with a high rate of false positives. According to the 2010 Appropriateness Criteria, the only appropriate indication for CCTA is in an asymptomatic patient with LCA stents of at least 3.0 mm diameter. Evaluation of symptomatic patients and patients with a stent diameter of less than 3.0 mm is considered uncertain and inappropriate indications, respectively.

A number of technical limitations can affect the evaluation of coronary stents including motion, metallic blooming, and beam hardening artifacts [63]. The patient's heart rate should be controlled in order to minimize motion artifacts. Metallic blooming artifact causes the stent walls to appear thicker and limits assessment of the lumen. Beam hardening artifacts increase intraluminal noise and further impair diagnostic accuracy. Depending on stent material and size, these artifacts may prevent the direct visualization of intraluminal contrast needed to confirm stent patency [64, 65].

Several techniques are available to optimize stent visualization on CCTA. The stent is placed in the imaging plane using thin MPR to reduce volume averaging and maximize spatial resolution at the cost of increased noise (Fig. 15.8). The minimum slice thickness available should be selected. Sharp kernel and widened window width both reduce blooming artifacts and improve luminal examination. Decreasing slice increment or spacing (increasing slice overlap) may also be beneficial.

Indirect evidence of stent filling may be present. Intracoronary opacification immediately distal to the stent is associated with stent patency, but is also observed in retrograde filling via collateral flow [66]. Whereas dense circumferential aortic annular calcifications and porcelain aorta pose a challenge for invasive angiography, LCA ostial patency can be readily confirmed on CCTA (Fig. 15.8). The absence of intraluminal stent opacification and distal flow is diagnostic of in-stent restenosis. Additionally, the native coronary arteries should be routinely assessed for disease progression.

With proper patient selection and imaging techniques, CCTA is a powerful noninvasive tool in the management of asymptomatic patients with certain coronary stents.

Appropriateness ratings of other clinical scenarios may change as CT technology continues to develop.

Future CT Applications

CT Perfusion (CTP)

CTP is an exciting new development in advanced CCT imaging. The concept is based on calculations of myocardial blood flow and myocardial blood volume before and after pharmacological stress, typically using a vasodilator [67–69]. The most intriguing aspect of CTP is the ability to combine both an anatomical test (CCTA) and a functional test (i.e., stress and rest perfusion) in one exam versus the current requirement of two diagnostic exams to determine anatomy and function. Currently, a major weakness of CCTA is its inability to accurately diagnose patients with known CAD or significant coronary artery lesions; it is hopeful that the addition of a functional exam such as CTP will help improve the diagnostic accuracy of coronary CTA in patients with obstructive disease. At this moment, this imaging technique is still considered an investigative tool and more large-scale clinical trial data on outcomes and clinical effectiveness are needed to justify its use in everyday clinical practice.

Plaque Analysis

While CCTA readily distinguishes between noncalcified and calcified plaques, efforts to further characterize noncalcified plaque yielded mixed results. Comparison with intravascular ultrasound showed that CCTA underestimates noncalcified and mixed plaque volume and overestimates calcified plaque volume [70]. Another study found good concordance between IVUS and dual-source CT noncalcified plaque quantification when an automated wall segmentation algorithm was applied to the CCTA data [71]. Development of an accurate approach to noncalcified plaque quantification with MDCT will potentially lead to an improved risk stratification model based on the noncalcified plaque volume [72, 73].

Plaque characterization using CCTA attempts to identify vulnerable plaques that are at higher risk of rupturing. Culprit lesions in ACS tend to be lipid-rich plaques as opposed to fibrous plaques. Lipid-rich plaques generally demonstrate lower attenuation values than fibrous plaques. However, there is substantial overlap between the HU measurements for the two types of plaques [74]. Other plaque characteristics associated with ACS include greater remodeling and larger plaque size [75].

Quantification, characterization, and prognostication based on CCTA appearance of noncalcified plaques are currently limited. While the presence of nonobstructive noncalcified plaque is predictive of all-cause mortality, at present CCTA for the purpose of risk stratification is not justified. Ongoing investigative efforts strive to more accurately delineate the coronary arterial wall and assess plaque burden.

Summary

CAD is the leading cause of death in the United States. Early detection and treatment of patients with vulnerable atherosclerotic plaques remain the holy grail of modern day medicine. CAC and CCTA are the one-two punch of diagnostic cardiac imaging. On one hand, CAC provides important information on CAD risk stratification and prognosis in asymptomatic individuals. On the other hand, the extremely high NPV of CCTA allows rapid exclusion of significant obstructive CAD in symptomatic individuals. CCTA is also a versatile noninvasive diagnostic imaging tool for the evaluation of native coronary arteries and bypass graft. Patients with atrial fibrillation routinely undergo CCT for pre- or post-ablation evaluation of cardiac structure. CCTA is also the imaging modality of choice for the initial evaluation of a suspected coronary anomaly or coronary fistula. The major Achilles' heel of CCTA includes radiation exposure, the need for a contrast agent, and the lack of functional and dynamic information. Further improvements in scanner design and detector technology directly address these drawbacks and are likely to significantly lower the radiation exposure, ultimately allowing for more creative applications of CCTA such as for CTP and plaque analysis. Slowly but surely, CCTA has become an integral part of the diagnostic tools commonly used by cardiology consultant.

Key Points
- Coronary computed tomography angiography (CCTA) is the most accurate noninvasive imaging modality for ruling out obstructive coronary artery disease.
- Coronary artery calcium score is useful in the reclassification of coronary artery disease risk in asymptomatic individuals.
- CCTA is safe and cost-effective in the emergency department triage of acute chest pain.
- CCTA is valuable for the pre- and post-procedure evaluation of cardiac structure and morphology as well as native, bypassed, or stented coronary arteries.
- CCTA is indicated for the evaluation of complex congenital heart disease and coronary anomalies.

References

1. Greenland P, Bonow RO, Brundage BH, et al. ACCF/AHA 2007 clinical expert consensus document on coronary artery calcium scoring by computed tomography in global cardiovascular risk assessment and in evaluation of patients with chest pain: a report of the American College of Cardiology Foundation Clinical Expert Consensus Task Force (ACCF/AHA writing committee to update the 2000 expert consensus document on electron beam computed tomography) developed in collaboration with the Society of Atherosclerosis Imaging and Prevention and the Society of Cardiovascular Computed Tomography. J Am Coll Cardiol. 2007; 49(3):378–402.

2. Taylor AJ, Cerqueira M, Hodgson JM, et al. ACCF/SCCT/ ACR/AHA/ASE/ASNC/NASCI/SCAI/SCMR 2010 appropriate use criteria for cardiac computed tomography: a report of the American College of Cardiology Foundation Appropriate Use Criteria Task Force, the Society of Cardiovascular Computed Tomography, the American College of Radiology, the American Heart Association, the American Society of Echocardiography, the American Society of Nuclear Cardiology, the North American Society for Cardiovascular Imaging, the Society for Cardiovascular Angiography and Interventions, and the Society for Cardiovascular Magnetic Resonance. J Am Coll Cardiol. 2010;56(22): 1864–94.

3. Committee to Assess Health Risks from Exposure to Low Levels of Ionizing Radiation, National Research Council. Health risks from exposure to low levels of ionizing radiation: BEIR VII phase 2. Washington, DC: The National Academies Press; 2006.

4. Bischoff B, Hein F, Meyer T, et al. Impact of a reduced tube voltage on CT angiography and radiation dose: results of the PROTECTION I study. JACC Cardiovasc Imaging. 2009;2(8): 940–6.

5. Hausleiter J, Meyer T, Hermann F, et al. Estimated radiation dose associated with cardiac CT angiography. JAMA. 2009;301(5): 500–7.

6. Einstein AJ, Moser KW, Thompson RC, Cerqueira MD, Henzlova MJ. Radiation dose to patients from cardiac diagnostic imaging. Circulation. 2007;116(11):1290–305.

7. Einstein AJ, Elliston CD, Arai AE, Chen MY, Mather R, Pearson GD, Delapaz RL, Nickoloff E, Dutta A, Brenner DJ. Radiation dose from single-heartbeat coronary CT angiography performed with a 320-detector row volume scanner. Radiology. 2010;254(3): 698–706.

8. Raff GI Chinnaiyan KM, Share DA, et al. Radiation dose from cardiac computed tomography before and after implementation of radiation dose–reduction techniques. JAMA. 2009;301(22): 2340–8.

9. Hausleiter J, Meyer TS, Martuscelli E, et al. Image quality and radiation exposure with prospectively ECG-triggered axial scanning for coronary CT angiography: the multicenter, multivendor. Randomized PROTECTION-III study. JACC Cardiovasc Imaging. 2012;5(5):484–93.

10. Husmann L, Herzog BA, Gaemperli O, Tatsugami F, Burkhard N, Valenta I, Veit-Haibach P, Wyss CA, Landmesser U, Kaufmann PA. Diagnostic accuracy of computed tomography coronary angiography and evaluation of stress-only single-photon emission computed tomography/computed tomography hybrid imaging: comparison of prospective electrocardiogram-triggering vs. retrospective gating. Eur Heart J. 2009;30(5):600–7.

11. Mayo JR, Leipsic JA. Radiation dose in cardiac CT. AJR Am J Roentgenol. 2009;192(3):646–53.

12. Rumberger JA, Brundage BH, Rader DJ, Kondos G. Electron beam computed tomographic coronary calcium scanning: a review and guidelines for use in asymptomatic persons. Mayo Clin Proc. 1999;74(3):243–52.

13. Agatston AS, Janowitz WR, Hildner FJ, Zusmer NR, Viamonte Jr M, Detrano R. Quantification of coronary artery calcium using ultrafast computed tomography. J Am Coll Cardiol. 1990; 15(4):827–32.

14. Morin RL, Gerber TC, McCollough CH. Radiation dose in computed tomography of the heart. Circulation. 2003;107(6):917–22.

15. Horiguchi J, Yamamoto H, Akiyama Y, Marukawa K, Hirai N, Ito K. Coronary artery calcium scoring using 16-MDCT and a retrospective ECG-gating reconstruction algorithm. AJR Am J Roentgenol. 2004;183(1):103–8.

16. Berman DS, Wong ND, Gransar H, et al. Relationship between stress-induced myocardial ischemia and atherosclerosis measured by coronary calcium tomography. J Am Coll Cardiol. 2004;44(4): 923–30.

17. Wilson PW, D'Agostino RB, Levy D, Belanger AM, Silbershatz H, Kannel WB. Prediction of coronary heart disease using risk factor categories. Circulation. 1998;97(18):1837–47.

18. Vliegenhart R, Oudkerk M, Hofman A, Oei HH, van Dijck W, van Rooij FJ, Witteman JC. Coronary calcification improves cardiovascular risk prediction in the elderly. Circulation. 2005;112(4): 572–7.

19. Detrano R, Guerci AD, Carr JJ, Bild DE, Burke G, Folsom AR, Liu K, Shea S, Szklo M, Bluemke DA, O'Leary DH, Tracy R, Watson K, Wong ND, Kronmal RA. Coronary calcium as a predictor of coronary events in four racial or ethnic groups. N Engl J Med. 2008;358(13):1336–45.

20. Schmermund A, Baumgart D, Gorge G, et al. Coronary artery calcium in acute coronary syndromes: a comparative study of electron-beam computed tomography, coronary angiography, and intracoronary ultrasound in survivors of acute myocardial infarction and unstable angina. Circulation. 1997;96(5):1461–9.

21. Budoff MJ, Shavelle DM, Lamont DH, et al. Usefulness of electron beam computed tomography scanning for distinguishing ischemic from nonischemic cardiomyopathy. J Am Coll Cardiol. 1998;32(5): 1173–8.

22. Le T, Ko JY, Kim HT, Akinwale P, Budoff MJ. Comparison of echocardiography and electron beam tomography in differentiating the etiology of heart failure. Clin Cardiol. 2000;23(6):417–20.

23. Budoff MJ, Achenbach S, Blumenthal RS, et al. Assessment of coronary artery disease by cardiac computed tomography: a scientific statement from the American Heart Association Committee on Cardiovascular Imaging and Intervention, Council on Cardiovascular Radiology and Intervention, and Committee on Cardiac Imaging, Council on Clinical Cardiology. Circulation. 2006;114(16):1761–91.

24. McClelland RL, Chung H, Detrano R, Post W, Kronmal RA. Distribution of coronary artery calcium by race, gender, and age: results from the Multi-Ethnic Study of Atherosclerosis (MESA). Circulation. 2006;113(1):30–7.

25. Nasir K, Shaw LJ, Liu ST, Weinstein SR, Mosler TR, Flores PR, Flores FR, Raggi P, Berman DS, Blumenthal RS, Budoff MJ. Ethnic differences in the prognostic value of coronary artery calcification for all-cause mortality. J Am Coll Cardiol. 2007;50(10): 953–60.

26. Lu B, Budoff MJ, Zhuang N, Child J, Bakhsheshi H, Carson S, Mao SS. Causes of interscan variability of coronary artery calcium measurements at electron-beam CT. Acad Radiol. 2002;9(6):654–61.

27. Waugh N, Black C, Walker S, McIntyre L, Cummins E, Hillis G. The effectiveness and cost-effectiveness of computed tomography screening for coronary artery disease: systematic review. Health Technol Assess. 2006;10(39):iii–iv, ix–x, 1–41.

28. Hoffmann U, Nagurney JT, Moselewski F, Pena A, Ferencik M, Chae CU, Cury RC, Butler J, Abbara S, Brown DF, Manini A, Nichols JH, Achenbach S, Brady TJ. Coronary multidetector computed tomography in the assessment of patients with acute chest pain. Circulation. 2006;114(21):2251–60.

29. Meijboom WB, Mollet NR, Van Mieghem CA, Weustink AC, Pugliese F, van Pelt N, Cademartiri F, Vourvouri E, de Jaegere P, Krestin GP, de Feyter PJ. 64-Slice CT coronary angiography in patients with non-ST elevation acute coronary syndrome. Heart. 2007;93(11):1386–92.

30. Rubinshtein R, Halon DA, Gaspar T, Jaffe R, Goldstein J, Karkabi B, Flugelman MY, Kogan A, Shapira R, Peled N, Lewis BS. Impact of 64-slice cardiac computed tomographic angiography on clinical decision-making in emergency department patients with chest pain of possible myocardial ischemic origin. Am J Cardiol. 2007; 100(10):1522–6.

31. Hollander JE, Chang AM, Shofer FS, Collin MJ, Walsh KM, McCusker CM, Baxt WG, Litt HI. One-year outcomes following coronary computerized tomographic angiography for evaluation of emergency department patients with potential acute coronary syndrome. Acad Emerg Med. 2009;16(8):693–8.

32. Goldstein JA, Gallagher MJ, O'Neill WW, Ross MA, O'Neil BJ, Raff GL. A randomized controlled trial of multi-slice coronary computed tomography for evaluation of acute chest pain. J Am Coll Cardiol. 2007;49(8):863–71.

33. Goldstein JA, Chinnaiyan KM, Abidov A, Achenbach S, Berman DS, Hayes SW, Hoffmann U, Lesser JR, Mikati IA, O'Neil BJ, Shaw LJ, Shen MY, Valeti US, Raff GL. The CT-STAT (coronary computed tomographic angiography for systematic triage of acute chest pain patients to treatment) trial. J Am Coll Cardiol. 2011;58(14):1414–22.

34. Hoffmann U, Truong QA, Schoenfeld DA, et al. Coronary CT angiography versus standard evaluation in acute chest pain. N Engl J Med. 2012;367(4):299–308.

35. Litt HI, Gatsonis C, Snyder B, et al. CT angiography for safe discharge of patients with possible acute coronary syndromes. N Engl J Med. 2012;366(15):1393–403.

36. Gruettner J, Fink C, Walter T, Meyer M, Apfaltrer P, Schoepf UJ, Saur J, Sueselbeck T, Traunwieser D, Takx R, Kralev S, Borggrefe M, Schoenberg SO, Henzler T. Coronary computed tomography and triple rule out CT in patients with acute chest pain and an intermediate cardiac risk profile. Part 1: impact on patient management. Eur J Radiol. 2013;82:100–5.

37. Haïssaguerre M, Jaïs P, Shah DC, et al. Spontaneous initiation of atrial fibrillation by ectopic beats originating in the pulmonary veins. N Engl J Med. 1998;339(10):659–66.

38. Kistler PM, Rajappan KIM, Jahngir M, et al. The impact of CT image integration into an electroanatomic mapping system on clinical outcomes of catheter ablation of atrial fibrillation. J Cardiovasc Electrophysiol. 2006;17(10):1093–101.

39. Kistler PM, Earley MJ, Harris S, et al. Validation of three-dimensional cardiac image integration: use of integrated CT image into electroanatomic mapping system to perform catheter ablation of atrial fibrillation. J Cardiovasc Electrophysiol. 2006;17(4):341–8.

40. Angelini P, Velasco JA, Flamm S. Coronary anomalies: incidence, pathophysiology, and clinical relevance. Circulation. 2002; 105(20):2449–54.

41. Frescura C, Basso C, Thiene G, et al. Anomalous origin of coronary arteries and risk of sudden death: a study based on an autopsy population of congenital heart disease. Hum Pathol. 1998;29(7): 689–95.

42. Eckart RE, Scoville SL, Campbell CL, et al. Sudden death in young adults: a 25-year review of autopsies in military recruits. Ann Intern Med. 2004;141(11):829–34.

43. Tariq R, Kureshi SB, Siddiqui UT, Ahmed R. Congenital anomalies of coronary arteries: diagnosis with 64 slice multidetector CT. Eur J Radiol. 2012;81(8):1790–7.

44. Datta J, White CS, Gilkeson RC, et al. Anomalous coronary arteries in adults: depiction at multi–detector row CT angiography. Radiology. 2005;235(3):812–8.

45. Schmitt R, Froehner S, Brunn J, et al. Congenital anomalies of the coronary arteries: imaging with contrast-enhanced, multidetector computed tomography. Eur Radiol. 2005;15(6): 1110–21.

46. Angelini P. Coronary artery anomalies: an entity in search of an identity. Circulation. 2007;115(10):1296–305.

47. Ihekwaba FN, Davidson KG, Ogilvie B, Caves PK. Anomalous origin of the left coronary artery from the pulmonary artery with coronary artery steal in adults. Report of two cases and review of the literature. Thorax. 1976;31(3):337–45.

48. Werner B, Wróblewska-Kałuzewska M, Pleskot M, Tarnowska A, Potocka K. Anomalies of the coronary arteries in children. Med Sci Monit. 2001;7(6):1285–91.

49. Ayalp R, Mavi A, Serçelik A, Batyraliev T, Gümüsburun E. Frequency in the anomalous origin of the right coronary artery with angiography in a Turkish population. Int J Cardiol. 2002;82(3): 253–7.

50. Cieslinski G, Rapprich B, Kober G. Coronary anomalies: incidence and importance. Clin Cardiol. 1993;16(10):711–5.

51. Thej MJ, Kalyani R, Kiran J. Atherosclerosis and myocardial bridging: not a benign combination. An autopsy case report. J Cardiovasc Dis Res. 2012;3(2):176–8.

52. Gupta NC, Beauvais J. Physiologic assessment of coronary artery fistula. Clin Nucl Med. 1991;16(1):40–2.

53. Ata Y, Turk T, Bicer M, Yalcin M, Ata F, Yavuz S. Coronary arteriovenous fistulas in the adults: natural history and management strategies. J Cardiothorac Surg. 2009;4:62.

54. Kilner PJ. Imaging congenital heart disease in adults. Br J Radiol. 2011;84(Spec no 3):S258–68.

55. Stinn B, Stolzmann P, Fornaro J, Hibbeln D, Alkadhi H, Wildermuth S, Leschka S. Technical principles of computed tomography in patients with congenital heart disease. Insights Imaging. 2011;2(3):349–56.

56. Anand DV, Lim E, Lipkin D, Lahiri A. Evaluation of graft patency by computed tomographic angiography in symptom-free post-coronary artery bypass surgery patients. J Nucl Cardiol. 2008;15(2): 201–8.

57. Meyer TS, Martinoff S, Hadamitzky M, et al. Improved noninvasive assessment of coronary artery bypass grafts with 64-slice computed tomographic angiography in an unselected patient population. J Am Coll Cardiol. 2007;49(9):946–50.

58. Ropers D, Pohle FK, Kuettner A, et al. Diagnostic accuracy of non-invasive coronary angiography in patients after bypass surgery using 64-slice spiral computed tomography with 330-ms gantry rotation. Circulation. 2006;114(22):2334–41; quiz 2334.

59. Gaudino M, Cellini C, Pragliola C, et al. Arterial versus venous bypass grafts in patients with in-stent restenosis. Circulation. 2005;112(9 Suppl):I265–9.

60. Cai W. 3D planar reformation of vascular central axis surface with biconvex slab. Comput Med Imaging Graph. 2007; 31(7):570–6.

61. Onuma Y, Tanabe K, Chihara R, et al. Evaluation of coronary artery bypass grafts and native coronary arteries using 64-slice multidetector computed tomography. Am Heart J. 2007;154(3): 519–26.

62. Weustink AC, Nieman K, Pugliese F, et al. Diagnostic accuracy of computed tomography angiography in patients after bypass grafting: comparison with invasive coronary angiography. JACC Cardiovasc Imaging. 2009;2(7):816–24.

63. Chung SH, Kim YJ, Hur J, et al. Evaluation of coronary artery in-stent restenosis by 64-section computed tomography: factors affecting assessment and accurate diagnosis. J Thorac Imaging. 2010;25(1):57–63.

64. Schuijf JD, Pundziute G, Jukema JW, et al. Evaluation of patients with previous coronary stent implantation with 64-section CT. Radiology. 2007;245(2):416–23.

65. de Graaf FR, Schuijf JD, van Velzen JE, et al. Diagnostic accuracy of 320-row multidetector computed tomography coronary angiography to noninvasively assess in-stent restenosis. Invest Radiol. 2010;45(6):331–40.

66. Maintz D, Grude M, Fallenberg EM, Heindel W, Fischbach R. Assessment of coronary arterial stents by multislice-CT angiography. Acta Radiol. 2003;44(6):597–603.

67. Blankstein R, Shturman LD, Rogers IS, et al. Adenosine-induced stress myocardial perfusion imaging using dual-source cardiac computed tomography. J Am Coll Cardiol. 2009;54(12):1072–84.

68. George RT, Arbab-Zadeh A, Miller JM, et al. Computed tomography myocardial perfusion imaging with 320-row detector computed tomography accurately detects myocardial ischemia in patients with obstructive coronary artery disease. Circ Cardiovasc Imaging. 2012;5(3):333–40.

69. George RT, Arbab-Zadeh A, Miller JM, et al. Adenosine stress 64- and 256-row detector computed tomography angiography and perfusion imaging: a pilot study evaluating the transmural extent of perfusion abnormalities to predict atherosclerosis causing myocardial ischemia. Circ Cardiovasc Imaging. 2009;2(3):174–82.

70. Leber AW, Becker A, Knez A, von Ziegler F, Sirol M, Nikolaou K, Ohnesorge B, Fayad ZA, Becker CR, Reiser M, Steinbeck G, Boekstegers P. Accuracy of 64-slice computed tomography to classify and quantify plaque volumes in the proximal coronary system: a comparative study using intravascular ultrasound. J Am Coll Cardiol. 2006;47(3):672–7.

71. Brodoefel H, Burgstahler C, Heuschmid M, Reimann A, Khosa F, Kopp A, Schroeder S, Claussen CD, Clouse ME. Accuracy of dual-source CT in the characterisation of non-calcified plaque: use of a

colour-coded analysis compared with virtual histology intravascular ultrasound. Br J Radiol. 2009;82(982):805–12.

72. Hausleiter J, Meyer T, Hadamitzky M, Kastrati A, Martinoff S, Schomig A. Prevalence of noncalcified coronary plaques by 64-slice computed tomography in patients with an intermediate risk for significant coronary artery disease. J Am Coll Cardiol. 2006;48(2):312–8.

73. Voros S, Rinehart S, Qian Z, et al. Prospective validation of standardized, 3-dimensional, quantitative coronary computed tomographic plaque measurements using radiofrequency backscatter intravascular ultrasound as reference standard in intermediate coronary arterial lesions: results from the ATLANTA (assessment of tissue characteristics, lesion morphology, and hemodynamics by angiography with fractional flow reserve, intravascular ultrasound and virtual histology, and noninvasive computed tomography in atherosclerotic plaques) I study. JACC Cardiovasc Interv. 2011;4(2):198–208.

74. Pohle K, Achenbach S, Macneill B, Ropers D, Ferencik M, Moselewski F, Hoffmann U, Brady TJ, Jang IK, Daniel WG. Characterization of non-calcified coronary atherosclerotic plaque by multi-detector row CT: comparison to IVUS. Atherosclerosis. 2007;190(1):174–80.

75. Hoffmann U, Moselewski F, Nieman K, Jang IK, Ferencik M, Rahman AM, Cury RC, Abbara S, Joneidi-Jafari H, Achenbach S, Brady TJ. Noninvasive assessment of plaque morphology and composition in culprit and stable lesions in acute coronary syndrome and stable lesions in stable angina by multi-detector computed tomography. J Am Coll Cardiol. 2006;47(8):1655–62.

The Role of Cardiac Magnetic Resonance Imaging in Cardiology Consultation

Muzammil H. Musani, Ammar Chaudhry, Szilard Voros, and Michael Poon

Abstract

Cardiovascular magnetic resonance imaging (CMR) has emerged as a powerful, multipurpose, noninvasive imaging modality of great value to cardiac consultants who are asked increasingly to evaluate increasingly complex cases of cardiac anatomy and pathophysiology. CMR, unlike other imaging modalities that require ionizing radiation, is extremely safe and suited for the evaluation of both congenital and acquired cardiac diseases. CMR is the gold standard for the evaluation of global systolic function, abnormal tissue characteristics, and myocardial viability. This chapter will review key fundamental principles in MR physics that form the basis of MR imaging followed by a brief discussion of image acquisition and signal processing that are unique for CMR. Basic CMR pulse sequences and common clinical applications of these sequences will be discussed including the use of flow/velocity encoding sequences in the quantitative analysis of flow and myocardial stress imaging. The chapter will also touch on the common roles of CMR in the assessment of restrictive, dilated, and hypertrophic cardiomyopathies, valvular heart disease, congestive heart failure, myocarditis, cardiac neoplasms, pericardial disease, and congenital heart disease. Technical and patient safety issues will also be reviewed. To date, CMR remains a relatively time-consuming and technically difficult imaging modality and is not commonly available. Future improvement in hardware and software as well as simplifying image post-processing will improve the availability of CMR and allow it to be performed on even more challenging patients.

Keywords

Cardiac magnetic resonance imaging • Physics • Safety • Cardiac function • Viability • Cardiac masses

M.H. Musani, MD
Department of Radiology, Stony Brook University,
100 Nicholls Road, HSC4, Room 120, Stony Brook,
NY 11794-8460, USA
e-mail: muzammil.musani@stonybrookmedicine.edu

A. Chaudhry
Department of Diagnostic Radiology,
Stony Brook University Medical Center,
101 Nicholls Road, LVL 4, Stony Brook, NY 11794, USA
e-mail: ammar84@aol.com

S. Voros, MD
Department of Radiology, Stony Brook Medicine,
100 Nicholls Rd, HSC Level 4, Room 120,
Stony Brook, NY 11794-8460, USA
e-mail: szilard.voros@stonybrookmedicine.edu

M. Poon, MD (✉)
Department of Radiology,
Stony Brook University Medical Center,
100 Nicolls Rd, Stony Brook, NY 11794-8460, USA
e-mail: michael.poon@stonybrook.edu

K. Stergiopoulos, D.L. Brown (eds.), *Evidence-Based Cardiology Consult*,
DOI 10.1007/978-1-4471-4441-0_16, © Springer-Verlag London 2014

Introduction

In 1945, Bloch and Purcell separately developed the technique of nuclear magnetic resonance (NMR) spectroscopy to analyze the composition of different chemical compounds [1]. This Nobel prize-winning concept was introduced into the medical and pharmaceutical communities during the 1960s and 1970s through the contributions of Damadian, Lauterbur, and other investigators [2]. The transition from the single dimension of NMR spectroscopy to the second dimension of spatial orientation formed the foundation of today's magnetic resonance imaging (MRI).

Cardiovascular magnetic resonance imaging (CMR) has emerged as a robust noninvasive technique for the assessment of global systolic function, myocardial viability, valvular pathology, and congenital heart diseases. Although CMR is performed using the same basic concepts of a regular MRI, one of the biggest differences is the challenge of overcoming cardiac and respiratory motion to acquire high-quality images. A complete review of CMR physics is beyond the scope of this chapter. Therefore, this chapter focuses mainly on the clinical applications of CMR in a tertiary cardiac referral environment while offering a brief review of the basic principles of MR physics, image acquisition, and common CMR pulse sequences. In addition, this chapter touches on the practical aspects of patient care, including gating techniques, patient comfort, and contraindications to MRI.

Basic Principles of MRI: MRI Physics

The physics of generating MRI is based on the random distribution of water and fat protons (^{1}H) within the body and the spin of those protons. Hydrogen is the most prevalent charged element in living tissues. The magnetic field created by a spinning proton is known as the magnetic dipole moment and is in the direction perpendicular to the rotation of the spin (Fig. 16.1). In the body, all the hydrogen protons normally spin in a random fashion, and the sum of all the magnetic dipole moments cancel each other out. When an external magnetic field (Bo) is applied, the axes of the magnetic dipole moments will align in one of two energy states based on quantum mechanics. A dipole moment is considered parallel if it is aligned along the direction of Bo and antiparallel if opposite to the direction of Bo (Fig. 16.2). The longitudinal magnetization created by placing protons in an external magnetic field cannot be detected by the receiving MR coils. In order to detect the physical presence of the protons in a given body of tissue, the longitudinal magnetization (aligned along the z-axis) of the protons must be forced into the x-y plane. This is accomplished by the introduction of a weak electromagnetic wave or radiofrequency (RF) pulse. The frequency of the RF pulse must match the precise frequency of the spinning protons (i.e., Larmor frequency), in

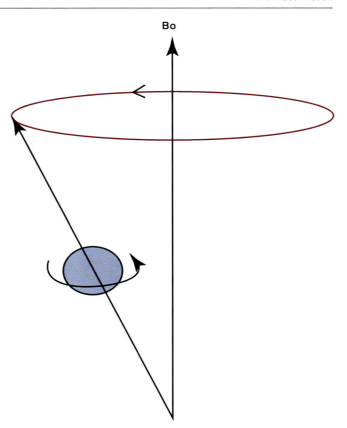

Fig. 16.1 A spinning proton with its own magnetic dipole moment circling around an external magnetic field (B0)

order for the longitudinal magnetization to be "flipped." The flip angle (θ), an MRI parameter, is the degree from the z-axis that the longitudinal magnetization has been tipped. Its magnitude is dependent on both the frequency and duration of the RF pulse and typically ranges between <90° and 180°, depending on the clinical application [2]. After the RF pulse is applied, the longitudinal magnetization is diminished and a new magnetization, called *transverse magnetization*, is generated by the precession of the protons in the x-y plane. Immediately after the transient RF pulse is turned off, exponential recovery and decay of the longitudinal and transverse magnetizations, respectively, occurs. The precession of protons in the x-y plane produces an MR signal, known as the *free induction decay* (FID), which also decomposes exponentially. The frequency of these signals is then determined using a Fourier transform and the amplitude in relation with time is calculated. MRI pulse sequences are programmed to sample, store, and process the FID signal so as to eventually reconstruct the MR image.

Relaxation Time and MR Contrast

The recovery of the longitudinal magnetization and the decay of transverse magnetization after the application of the RF pulse are commonly referred to as "relaxation" times – i.e.,

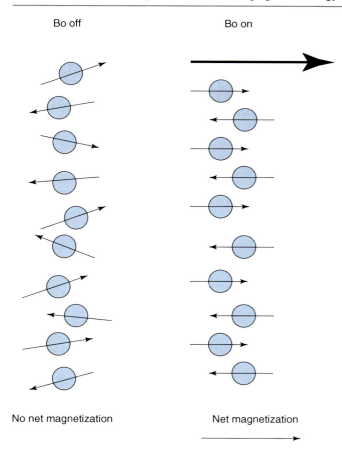

Bo off   Bo on

No net magnetization   Net magnetization

Fig. 16.2 In the body, all the hydrogen protons are normally spinning in a random fashion, and all the magnetic dipole moments, in sum, cancel each other out, resulting in no net magnetization (B0 off). When an external magnetic field (B0 on) is applied, the axes of the magnetic dipole moments will align in one of two energy states, either parallel or antiparallel, based on quantum mechanics

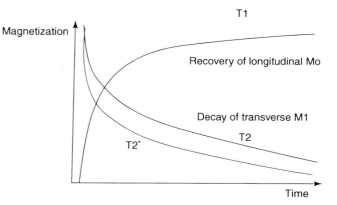

Fig. 16.3 Three types of relaxation time (T1, T2, and T2*). T1 relaxation is the time it takes for spins to realign along the z-axis (recovery of the longitudinal magnetization, Mo) or to give up the energy gained from the RF pulse excitation to the surrounding environment. T2 relaxation is an exponential decay process caused by dephasing of spins in the x-y plane or the randomization of the phase of the spinning protons. T2* relaxation is the relaxation time that takes into account both the T2 effect, the field inhomogeneity, and other environment factors

the time it takes for spins to return to their lowest energy states. The longitudinal relaxation time (T1) is the time it takes for spins to realign along the z-axis (recovery of the longitudinal magnetization) or to give up the energy gained from the RF pulse excitation to the surrounding environment. T1 is thus dependent on interactions between the spins and the surrounding environment and is also known as the lattice relaxation. For myocardium, the T1 is approximately 900 ms at 1.5-T field strength (and is less in a weaker magnetic field). The time it takes for the decay of the transverse magnetization is denoted by T2 relaxation (transverse relaxation). T2 relaxation is an exponential decay process caused by the dephasing of spins in the x-y plane or the randomization of the phase of the spinning protons. This is secondary to the interactions between neighboring spins themselves (also known as spin–spin relaxation). The T2 for myocardium is about 80 ms. In reality, the FID (decay of the transverse magnetization) occurs at a much faster rate than that represented by the T2 time. This is the result of additional factors contributing to dephasing of the spins – namely, the fixed inhomogeneity of the external magnetic field and

cardiac respiratory motions. Therefore, T2* (T2 "star") is the relaxation time that takes into account the T2 effect, the field inhomogeneity, and other environment factors, representing a more accurate measure of the FID. Different tissues have unique T1, T2, and T2* relaxations (Fig. 16.3). These unique physical properties of various tissues are used by the MRI technology to generate image contrasts, and the various pulse sequences are optimized to aid tissue characterization by focusing on the specific relaxation property of the tissue of interest, giving rise to the terms "T1 or T2 weighting."

Image Acquisition and Signal Processing

The sampled FID is the electromagnetic signal emanating from the entire body while in the magnet and does not contain any information regarding the specific position in the body from which the signal is coming. For an image to be created, signals must go through a series of complicated spatial encoding steps and signal processing. The first important step is the use of gradients to encode MR signals spatially. A *gradient* is a magnetic field that has a nonuniform distribution and shows a linear increase in field strength from one end to the other. The gradient is generated by gradient coils embedded in the main magnet bore. Typically, three gradients are created in the x, y, and z directions; they are referred to as Gx, Gy, and Gz (Fig. 16.4). Gz, which runs in the craniocaudal direction, is referred to as the *slice-select gradient*, as MRI slices are based on the selection of the appropriate bandwidth that correlates to the frequency associated along the Gz gradient. Gx, which runs in the left-right direction, is known as the *frequency-encoding gradient* and is usually turned on during the readout of the echo. For this reason, it is sometimes referred to as the readout gradient. Gy, which

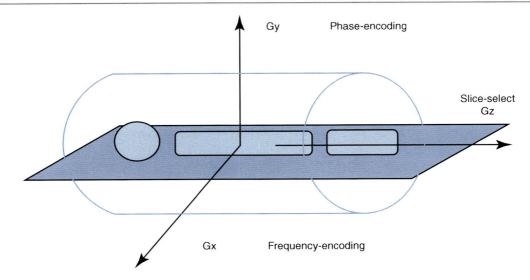

Fig. 16.4 Three gradients are created by embedding the gradient coils in the main magnet bore. The gradients are arranged in the x, y, and z directions and are referred to as Gx, Gy, and Gz. Gz, which runs in the craniocaudal direction, is referred to as the slice-select gradient, as MRI slices are based on the selection of the appropriate bandwidth that cor- relates to the frequency associated along the Gz gradient. Gx, which runs in the left-right direction, is known as the frequency-encoding gra- dient and is usually turned on during the readout of the echo (also known as "readout" gradient). Gy, which runs in the anteroposterior direction, is known as the phase-encoding gradient

runs in the anteroposterior direction, is known as the phase-encoding gradient. The three gradients are turned on and off at specific times to properly encode MR signals spatially. The assignments above are commonly used today, but in reality they are arbitrary and may be altered depending on the patient's orientation.

Once the MR signals are read, they are placed in a data matrix known as k-space. The stored data or signals are in the frequency domain and, thus, they do not correlate with the actual MR image itself. In order to reconstruct the actual image, the Fourier transformation is applied to data in k-space to form the resultant MR image for clinical use.

Basic Cardiac Sequences

A pulse sequence is a series of computer instructions and algorithms that prepare and generate a MR signal. Pulse sequences utilize a series of RF pulses and various magnetic gradients to enhance or suppress tissue signals in order to obtain images with the desired contrast. There are many pulse sequences, of which spin-echo (SE) and gradient-recalled echo (GRE) sequences are the most commonly uti- lized in cardiac imaging.

Spin-Echo ("Dark Blood" Sequence)

The basic SE pulse sequence consists of a 90° excitation RF pulse followed by one or more 180° refocusing pulses. Recall that after the RF pulse is turned off, the FID (the MR signal)

rapidly decomposes due to T2* effects (Fig. 16.5). The purpose of the 180° pulse is to allow the spins in the transverse plane (which are actively dephasing) to rephrase and reform the signal, thus the term *echo*. The time between the 90° excitation RF pulse and the echo is denoted as *time of echo* (TE). This dual pair of excitation and rephasing pulses may be repeated as further spatial encoding is applied (via gradients). The time between one 90° RF pulse to the next 90° RF pulse is known as the *time to repetition* (TR). TE and TR times may be set by the computer and enhance important contrast characteristics between tissues being imaged based on the tissue's T1 and T2 characteristics (i.e., T1 and T2 weighting). In general, in SE sequences, short TE and TR times favor T1 weighting, whereas long TE and TR times favor T2 weighting.

SE sequences are also referred to as "dark blood" imaging because rapidly flowing blood moves out of the slice being excited and thus does not receive the 180° refocusing pulse. Therefore, no echo is formed and the moving-blood signal void is represented as a dark image. In that regard, SE sequences provide great contrast between the blood pool and the surrounding tissues; as a result, they are commonly used in assessing cardiovascular morphology such as the pericar- dium, mediastinum, myocardium, and great vessels.

Gradient-Recalled Echo ("Bright Blood" Sequence)

GRE sequences utilize a series of slice-selective RF pulses that have flip angles α (usually much less than the 90° used

Fig. 16.5 Diagram of a typical spin-echo (SE) pulse sequence with its 90° excitation RF pulse followed by one or more 180° refocusing pulses. The time between the 90° excitation RF pulse and the echo is denoted as *TE* (time of echo). The time between one 90° RF to the next 90° RF is known as the *TR* (time to repetition)

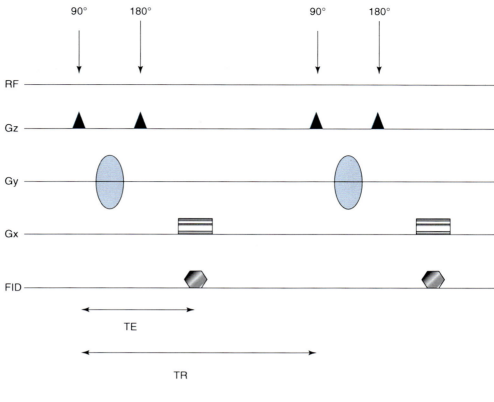

Fig. 16.6 Diagram of a typical GRE pulse sequence utilizing a series of slice-selective RF pulses that have a flip angle of **α**-degrees (usually much less than the 90° used in spin-echo sequences)

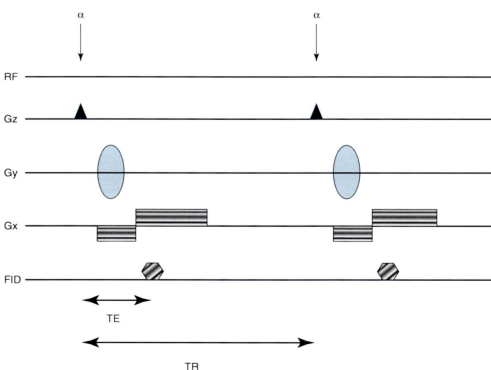

in SE sequences) (Fig. 16.6). Because of the smaller flip angles, the recovery of longitudinal magnetization is faster and thus allows for much shorter TR and scanning times. In addition, no 180° refocusing pulses are used; instead,

active dephasing and rephasing of the transverse magnetization are accomplished by the use of dual-polarity readout gradients to regenerate the FID. Because of the repeated use of multiple small flip-angled RF pulses that are slice selective, flowing blood, which was initially outside of the imaging plane and thus has not been affected by the excitation, will have a higher longitudinal magnetization component to be flipped in the subsequent RF pulse. Compared to the stationary surrounding environment, which has been experiencing multiple flip-angle excitations, blood will carry higher signal intensity; thus, GRE sequences produce images that display flowing blood as bright.

The shorter scanning time afforded by the GRE sequences makes them ideal for imaging protocols where temporal resolution is of paramount importance. A variant of the basic GRE sequence is known as *echo-planar imaging* (EPI). In this sequence, instead of just one echo being recalled, a full set of rapid phase-encoded GREs are recalled through the use of a series of oscillating frequency-encoding gradients. EPI allows for a greater signal-to-noise ratio (SNR) and can dramatically reduce the imaging time (or increase temporal resolution) depending on the length of the echo train. Currently, GRE sequences are utilized routinely in assessing ventricular function, cardiac perfusion, coronary artery imaging, valvular motion, and turbulent flow.

Other pulse sequences that are employed in cardiac imaging are not discussed in this chapter. Suffice to say that a good number of these sequences are simply variations of the SE and GRE sequences that allow for a greater reduction in scan time or that selectively enhance or null specific tissues of interest in order to achieve better contrast.

Technical Issues and Patient Safety

Unlike other organs in the body, the heart is constantly in motion due to a combination of its own pulsation and the patient's respiratory activity. Cardiac motion can be "frozen" in time by using electrocardiographic (ECG) gating. The acquisition of data for a specific image spans many cardiac cycles. The most commonly used method is known as ECG-gated k-space segmentation. The limitations of ECG gating may be related to arrhythmia and artifacts (magneto-hydrodynamic effects). In these situations, vector ECG or peripheral pulse gating may be used. In peripheral pulse gating, the images are not acquired at the same time in the cardiac cycle as in ECG gating because of the delay between the R wave and the transmitted pulse.

Various methods are used to suppress respiratory motion artifacts. Of these, the most commonly used is breath holding, which usually occurs at end-expiration and can take 30 s or longer. Many patients with respiratory conditions, pulmonary hypertension, or heart failure may find it difficult to hold their breath long enough for the image to be acquired;

in such cases, respiratory bellows gating may be used. This technique involves placement of air-filled bellows between the chest wall and a rigid structure. A circumferential belt detects pressure changes due to chest wall movement, enabling acquisitions to be timed to a specific part of the pressure curve. A more advanced respiratory gating system involves navigator echoes. In this technique, RF excitations in high-contrast interfaces, such as the liver/lung or cardiac/lung borders, are used to gauge respiratory motion. Acquisition of images is then timed to a specific reference value in a manner similar to the technique of respiratory bellows gating.

As the clinical use of cardiovascular imaging is increasing, issues of patient safety should be highlighted. Safe MRI practice involves performing tests for the appropriate indication, detailed patient screening for absolute and relative contraindications, and common and fatal adverse reactions. Powerful magnetic fields can be hazardous due to their potential to move and/or dislodge metallic objects. RF fields can generate heat in metallic electrodes, wires, or devices. Cardiac patients with cardiac pacemakers, thermodilution catheters, and/or automatic implantable cardioverter defibrillators (AICDs) cannot be exposed to an MR environment without detailed pre-assessment. These devices may contain ferromagnetic material that can react to the magnetic field generated by the scanner which can alter the device settings. Sternal wires, modern mechanical prosthetic heart valves, and coronary stents are not contraindications for MR. Table 16.1 summarizes the recommendations for the performance of MR in patients with implantable devices, and Table 16.2 summarizes the absolute and relative contraindications to MR [3–5].

Physicians should also be aware of the possibility of adverse reactions to contrast medium that may be used for the procedure. MRI contrast medium is based on gadolinium chelates which are very well tolerated by most patients with a reported frequency of acute adverse events after appropriate intravenous injection as 0.07–2.4 % [3]. Table 16.3 lists the acute events, and Table 16.4 summarizes the risk factors for adverse reactions to gadolinium. Adverse reactions considered "allergic" are rare with a reported frequency ranging from 0.004 to 0.7 %. The most common symptoms of these reactions include rash, hives, urticaria, and, more rarely, bronchospasm. The incidence of critical life-threatening anaphylactoid or nonallergic anaphylactic reactions is 0.001–0.01 % [3]. There were five cases of critical adverse reactions to gadolinium in a case series of 687,000 patients studied. The American College of Radiology Manual on Contrast Media [3] recommends patients with previous reactions who require future gadolinium-based contrast material to be premedicated similarly to the protocol used for iodinated contrast media. This includes

Table 16.1 Recommendations for the performance of magnetic resonance imaging (MR) examinations in patients with pacemakers or implantable cardiac defibrillators (ICDs)

General recommendations:

Advanced Cardiac Life Support (ACLS) support available

MR examination of non-pacemaker-dependent patients is discouraged and should be considered only in cases in which there is a strong clinical indication and the benefits clearly outweigh the risks

MR examination of pacemaker-dependent patients should not be performed unless there are highly compelling circumstances and the benefits clearly outweigh the risks

MR examination of patients with ICDs should not be performed unless there are highly compelling circumstances and the benefits clearly outweigh the risks

Scanning should only be performed at extremely experienced centers with expertise in MR imaging and electrophysiology

Establish and document the risk-benefit ratio for the patient

Obtain written and verbal informed consent. Written informed consent should specifically list the possibilities of (1) pacemaker/ICD dysfunction, (2) pacemaker/ICD damage, (3) arrhythmia, and (4) death

A physician with ACLS and pacemaker/ICD expertise should decide whether it is necessary to reprogram the pacemaker/ICD before the MR examination and should be in attendance for the entire study

A person with expertise in MR physics and safety should be involved with the scan to optimally plan to minimize risk. Consideration should be given to using scanning parameters (e.g., lowest radio frequency power levels, weakest/slowest necessary gradient magnetic fields) that are believed to minimize study risk

Pre-scanning steps outside the MR environment:

For non-pacemaker-dependent patients, pretest pacemaker functions

For pacemaker-dependent patients, pretest pacemaker functions and reprogram to asynchronous mode

For patients with ICDs, pretest ICD functions and disable therapy and detection for tachycardia/bradycardia modes

The patient's heart rhythm and vital signs should be monitored throughout the MR procedure

Appropriate personnel and a code cart including a defibrillator must be available throughout the procedure to address an adverse event

Maintain visual and voice contact with the patient throughout the procedure

Instruct the patient to alert the MR system operator to any unusual sensations or problems

After the examination:

For non-pacemaker-dependent patients, a physician with electrophysiological expertise should interrogate the pacemaker and reprogram as needed

For pacemaker-dependent patients, a physician with electrophysiological expertise should interrogate the pacemaker function and reprogram the pacemaker

For patients with ICDs, a physician with electrophysiological expertise should perform post-scan device reprogramming and defibrillation threshold testing

Adapted from Levin et al. [4]

premedication with antihistamines and corticosteroids 12–24 h before administration of gadolinium. Fatal reactions have occurred following gadolinium but are exceedingly rare [3].

Table 16.2 Safety concerns with magnetic resonance imaging

Caution and/or contraindications

Central nervous system aneurysm clips

Cochlear implant

Implanted neural stimulator

Implanted cardiac pacemaker or defibrillator

Insulin pump

Ocular foreign body (e.g., metal shavings)

Metal shrapnel or bullet

Other implanted medical devices (e.g., drug infusion ports)

Pregnant women (patients who are uncertain as to whether they are pregnant will be required to have a screening urine or blood pregnancy test)

Adapted from Levin et al. [4]
Note: Cardiac MR is safe with atrial septal defect/patent foramen ovale closure devices, coronary stents, most prosthetic heart valves, joint replacements and sternal wires

Table 16.3 Common acute adverse events following use of intravenous gadolinium

Coldness/warmth/pain at injection site

Nausea and/or vomiting

Headache

Paraesthesias

Dizziness

Itching

Table 16.4 Risk factors for adverse reactions to gadolinium

Previous reaction to gadolinium

Frequency of acute adverse reactions is approximately eight times higher, and second reactions can be more severe than the previous reaction

History of asthma and various other allergies, including to other medications or foods are also at greater risk, with reports of adverse reaction rates as high as 3.7 %

Non-acute adverse reactions to gadolinium include nephrogenic systemic fibrosis (NSF) which is a sclerosing disease that most commonly involves the skin but can involve other organs including the esophagus, heart, skeletal muscles, and lungs. The most common initial reaction includes pruritis with or without skin thickening. The symptoms can develop acutely and progress rapidly resulting in contractures and immobility. NSF is rare in an otherwise healthy patient. The strongest association and the highest number of reported cases are in patients with acute, acute-on-chronic, or chronic severe (GFR <30 ml/min/1.73 m^2) to end-stage kidney disease (GFR <15 ml/min/1.73 m^2). Other risk factors for NSF include high doses of gadolinium, metabolic acidosis, medications that increase the risk for metabolic acidosis, hypercalcemia, hyperphosphatemia, elevated serum iron levels, immunosuppression, high-dose erythropoietin therapy, vasculopathy, and infection [3].

Common Clinical Consultative Roles of Cardiac MRI

Following is a list of Current Procedural Terminology (CPT) codes to encompass the appropriate use of cardiac MRI in clinical practice:

75557 = Cardiac magnetic resonance imaging for morphology and function without contrast material(s) and further sequences
75558 = 75557 + flow/velocity quantification
75559 = 75557 + stress imaging
75560 = 75557 + flow/velocity quantification and stress imaging
75561 = Cardiac magnetic resonance imaging for morphology and function without contrast material(s) followed by contrast material(s) and further sequences
75562 = 75561 + flow/velocity quantification
75563 = 75561 + stress imaging
75564 = 75561 + flow/velocity quantification and stress imaging

Heart Failure

The assessment of cardiac function is essential in the diagnosis, follow-up, and management of heart disease in patients with left ventricular and right ventricular (RV) dysfunction [6]. Moreover, the accurate assessment of RV functional parameters are important in the long-term follow-up of many congenital heart diseases (CHD) [7], arrhythmogenic right ventricular cardiomyopathy (ARVC), and primary pulmonary hypertension [6]. As CMR provides more accurate determination of parameters of cardiac function compared to planar imaging methods (e.g., echocardiography and ventriculography) due to its superior spatial and temporal resolution as well as signal-to-noise (SNR) and contrast-to-noise ratios (CNR) [8], it is currently accepted as the "gold standard technique" for the quantification of ventricular volumes and ejection fraction [9].

Pulse sequences commonly used for acquisition of volume datasets are segmented k-space turbo gradient echo (TGE) and the newer steady-state free precession techniques (SSFP). Measurements of ventricular volumes between TGE and SSFP pulse sequences have been compared in several studies [10, 11]. These comparisons demonstrated a systematic difference between the two techniques, with SSFP yielding larger end-diastolic volumes (EDV) and end-systolic volumes (ESV) and smaller LV mass measurements than TGE [6]. The difference between these techniques is a result of the improved contrast and hence border definition at the endocardial border in SSFP imaging. As a result, SSFP has become the pulse sequence of choice for cine CMR [6].

Reduced cardiac function leads to decreased blood velocity and increased blood transit times. Dynamic imaging by first-pass perfusion (FPP) using CMR is able to visualize and record the transit time of gadolinium from the RV to the LV cavity [12]. Prolonged blood flow between cardiac cavities may indicate impaired cardiac function and is inversely related to cardiac output. Peak ventricular transit time measured with CMR is an easy tool for functional description of cardiac function in subjects with normal cardiac functional parameters and in patients with impaired cardiac pump function using CMR first-pass perfusion imaging. Peak ventricular transit time (PVTT) is significantly prolonged in patients with heart failure, and the degree of prolongation shows a strong association to EDV, ESV, and left ventricular ejection fraction (LVEF). Consequently, the right-to-left PVTT is a valuable tool for assessment of cardiac function using CMR. The automated curve analysis facilitates a high reproducibility of measurements and, possibly, more precise interpretation of overall heart function [12].

Evaluation of Cardiomyopathy

Restrictive Cardiomyopathy

Restrictive cardiomyopathy is characterized by abnormal diastolic function of the ventricles with relatively intact and in some cases hyperdynamic systolic function. The restrictive abnormality of ventricular function can result from myocardial or endomyocardial disease [13], due to amyloidosis, hemochromatosis, glycogen deposition, and fibrosis of diverse etiologies [14]. Restrictive cardiomyopathy frequently is complicated by mitral and tricuspid regurgitation and biatrial enlargement which can be demonstrated and quantified by using cine CMR (Fig. 16.7) [15].

Amyloidosis is a common cause of restrictive cardiomyopathy associated with a poor prognosis [16]. In cardiac amyloidosis, CMR shows a characteristic pattern of abnormal myocardial and blood-pool gadolinium kinetics coupled with global subendocardial late enhancement [17]. CMR demonstrates high myocardial gadolinium concentrations early after injection and global subendocardial late gadolinium enhancement. These findings are of diagnostic value in this relatively rare condition [17].

Sarcoidosis is a multisystem granulomatous disorder of unknown etiology. Myocardial lesions of sarcoidosis are found in 20–60 % of autopsies [18]. However, the diagnostic yield of endomyocardial biopsy for cardiac sarcoidosis using myocardial biopsy is less than 50 % due to the nonuniform distribution of the sarcoid granulomas. Delayed Enhancement Cardiac Magnetic Resonance (DE-CMR) is more than twice as sensitive for detecting cardiac involvement in sarcoidosis (Fig. 16.8) [18].

In patients with known or suspected *hemochromatosis* with iron deposition in the myocardium, T2* mapping may be performed to exclude the presence of cardiac siderosis. In addition, the T2* CMR technique is also valuable for the estimation of myocardial iron deposition [19].

Dilated Cardiomyopathy

Dilated cardiomyopathy (DC) is characterized by abnormal dilatation of all four chambers of the heart in association with systolic dysfunction (Fig. 16.9). CMR is particularly useful for the quantitative evaluation of RV and LV volumes,

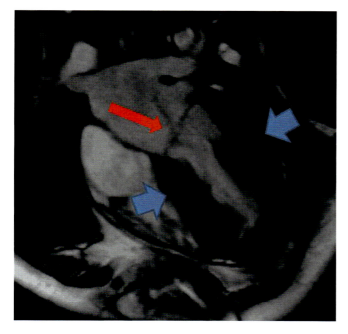

Fig. 16.7 Restrictive cardiomyopathy. Significant concentric myocardial thickening throughout the left ventricle (*blue arrows*) and associated mitral regurgitation (*red arrow* pointing to the jet)

RV and LVEF, and mass and wall stress as well as for monitoring functional status of the LV over time in patients with DC [20–22]. Short-axis CMR also has been used to define the 3-dimensional functional geometry of the LV by determining systolic wall thickening at multiple levels from base to apex. In the normal left ventricle, an increasing gradient in wall thickening from apex to base is present, whereas in patients with DC, this gradient is absent [20–23]. Furthermore, CMR may provide important insight into the potential cause of the DC by defining cardiac tissue characteristics, e.g., the presence of myocardial edema in T2-weighted images, the presence of abnormal tissue or fatty infiltration of the myocardium in T1- and T2-weighted dark blood images with and without fat saturation, the presence and pattern of myocardial scar or fibrosis in delayed hyperenhancement images, and abnormal myocardial uptake of contrast during first-pass perfusion study (Fig. 16.9).

Hypertrophic Cardiomyopathy

Hypertrophic cardiomyopathy (HCM) is most commonly characterized by asymmetrical thickening of the septal myocardium (ASH) often creating an outflow obstruction (Fig. 16.10). CMR allows a better morphological assessment of the degree and extent of LV hypertrophy than echocardiography in HCM due to its superior CNR and SNR in spite of its relatively inferior temporal resolution compared to echocardiography. Functional assessment of HCM can be

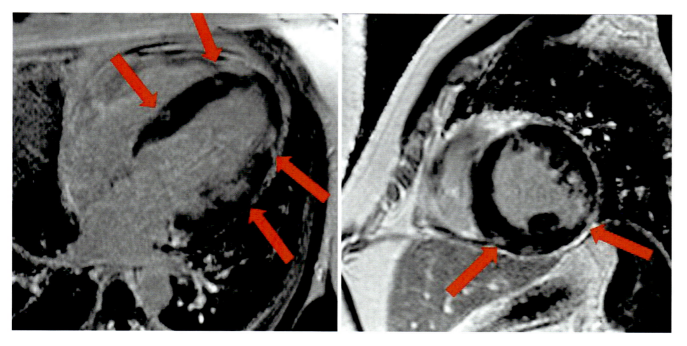

Fig. 16.8 Cardiac sarcoidosis. The presence of diffuse sarcoid granulomatous nodules in the left ventricular septum and lateral wall (*red arrows*) on delayed hyperenhancement imaging

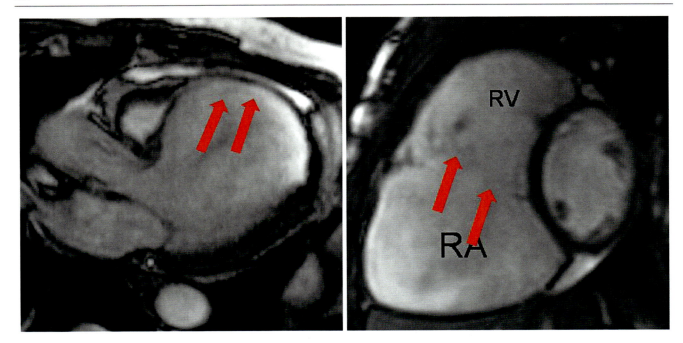

Fig. 16.9 (*Left panel*) Dilated cardiomyopathy. Bright blood image of a dilated left ventricle due to coronary artery disease. Anterior wall (*red arrows*) is thin and aneurysmal resulting from previous infarction. (*Right panel*) Dilated right ventricle due to atrialization of the right ventricle in Ebstein's anomaly). Red arrow points to the abnormal displacement of the tricuspid valve toward the right ventricular (*RV*) apex. *RA* right atrium

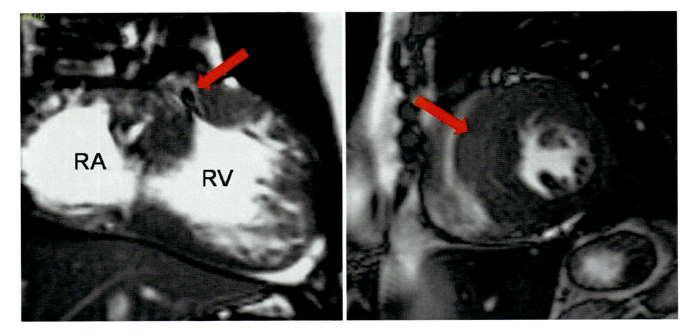

Fig. 16.10 Right ventricular (*RV*) infundibular stenosis (*left panel*) with high-velocity jet in the RV outflow tract (*red arrow*). Hypertrophic cardiomyopathy (HCM, *right panel*) with abnormal thickening of the LV septum (*red arrow*)

performed by using CMR to demonstrate characteristics of the left ventricle, such as outflow tract obstruction and systolic anterior motion of the mitral valve (SAM), and to assess the severity of mitral regurgitation [24]. CMR allows reliable and reproducible quantification of LV mass, wall stress, ventricular volumes, and EF in these patients [24] instantaneously and longitudinally. Similar to its LV counterpart, RV outflow tract hypertrophy can also lead to outflow tract obstruction in the case of the RV infundibular stenosis (Fig. 16.10).

Myocarditis

Several CMR pulses sequences have been used to evaluate patients with suspected acute myocarditis [16]. Friedrich et al. [25] demonstrated that early in the time course of the disease, the site and extent of inflammation within the myocardium can be defined by contrast-enhanced T1-weighted MR images [15]. Newer DE-MRI techniques provide an order of magnitude improvement in both SNR and CNR for detecting acutely and chronically injured myocardium compared with older spin-echo techniques.

Cardiac Tumors and Masses

CMR is particularly suited for the assessment of cardiac masses. In addition to having a large field of view that allows imaging of the paracardiac space and the great vessels, CMR, because of its multiplanar capability, is able to assess tissue characteristics, blood flow, and contrast enhancement of masses [26]. In addition, ECG gating allows for freezing of heart motion and permits high-quality and accurate imaging of tumor morphology and composition [27]. Typical CMR features of cardiac masses are presented on Table 16.5. CMR has higher sensitivity and specificity (88 and 99 %, respectively) than transthoracic echocardiography (23 and 96 %) and transesophageal echocardiography (40 and 96 %), respectively, for the diagnosis of LV thrombus (Fig. 16.11) [33].

Pericardial Diseases

Normal pericardial thickness is 2 mm or less. A thickness of greater than 4 mm suggests pericardial constriction, and a thickness of greater than 6 mm has a high specificity for constriction [34]. Computed tomography (CT), especially ultrafast and cine-gated CT, and CMR are the imaging

Table 16.5 Typical CMR features of common benign and malignant cardiac masses

Myxomas	Most commonly atrial septal origin, pedunculated, hypointense signal intensity in gradient-recalled echo images, contrast enhancement, no effusion, or infiltration
Fibromas	Left heart location
	Homogenous tissue, composition, hypointense signal intensity in T1- and T2-weighted images, no contrast enhancement, caval, infiltration in 50 %
Lipomas	Hyperintense signal intensity in T1- and T2-weighted images
Thrombi	Typical location left atrial appendage, especially with dilated atrium, atrial fibrillation, no effusion, or infiltration
	No contrast enhancement, hypointense on gradient-recalled echo images [28–32]

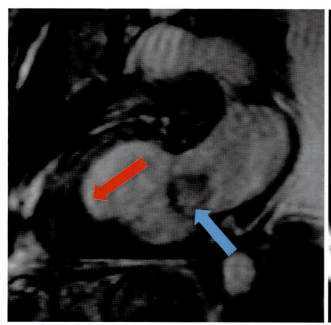
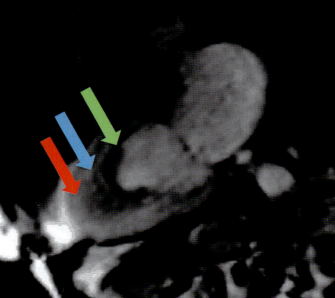

Fig. 16.11 Eosinophilic endomyocarditis. The left ventricular apex is covered with eosinophils and mural thrombi. Bright blood image of the left ventricle (LV) (*left panel*) showing apical thickening of the LV (*red arrow*) and mitral regurgitation (*blue arrow*). First-pass myocardial perfusion image (*right panel*) showing 3 layers, normal myocardium (*red arrow*), eosinophlic infiltration of the myocardium (*blue arrow*), and mural thrombus (*green arrow*)

modalities most commonly used to assess pericardial thickness [35]. The choice of CT or CMR depends on the clinical question, the age of the patient and local expertise, and availability of the advanced imaging equipment. In general, a particular advantage of CT imaging is the ability to delineate pericardial calcification accurately and comprehensively [36], while CMR is free of ionizing radiation but takes significantly longer time to acquire the images and requires more cooperation of the subject during a rather lengthy examination.

Constrictive Pericarditis

Pericardial constriction is best assessed using a combination of turbo spin-echo (TSE) morphology and steady-state free precession (SSFP) cine imaging [16]. The key advantage of TSE over conventional SE sequences is that acquisition time is substantially shorter, allowing an image to be acquired during a single breath hold. SSFP cine is also useful in evaluating the pericardium because it can provide both high spatial resolution and dynamic functional information. Real-time CMR can be used to demonstrate ventricular interdependence, a hemodynamic hallmark of pericardial constriction. Abnormal ventricular septal wall motion during inspiration appears to be helpful in distinguishing between constrictive pericarditis and restrictive cardiomyopathy [37].

Pericardial Effusion

The MR technique is very sensitive for identifying generalized or localized pericardial effusions and appears to be superior to echocardiography in defining the nature and extent of pericardial effusion (Fig. 16.12) [38]. A nonhemorrhagic effusion has low intensity on T1-weighted spin-echo images and high intensity on T2-weighted spin-echo and gradient-echo images [38]. Complex effusions may appear heterogeneous and darker on T2 and SSFP imaging [16].

Valvular Heart Diseases (Structure and Flow Analysis)

Cine balanced steady-state free precession (b-SSFP) images can visualize changes in valvular anatomy as well as valvular motion and alterations in ventricular function. Masses on valves such as vegetations, thrombi, or tumors may be further characterized by additional T1-weighted (T1w) or T2w sequences if their size is sufficiently large [39]. Non-cine, T1w, and T2w sequences based on gradient-recalled echo (GRE) or turbospin-echo (TSE) techniques with or without fat suppression are also beneficial for the assessment of extracardiac anatomy and the thoracic vasculature [39].

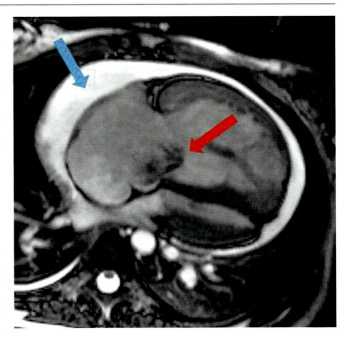

Fig. 16.12 Pericardial effusion. Large right ventricle and atrium due to severe primary pulmonary hypertension. Significant tricuspid regurgitation (*red arrow*) and circumferential mild to moderate pericardial effusion (*blue arrow*)

Dephasing of moving spins under a magnetic field gradient can also be used for quantification of flow [39].

Valvular Stenosis

CMR provides a good visual tool for the qualitative assessment of valvular stenosis (Fig. 16.13). Valve area, transvalvular pressure gradient, and peak antegrade velocity are standard measures in CMR used to describe the severity of valvular stenosis. Narrowing of the valvular orifice leads to an increased pressure gradient and, thus, increased flow velocities across the stenotic valve [39]. Data from flow velocity measurements can therefore be used for calculation of the transvalvular pressure gradient and the effective opening of the valve also referred to as physiological valve area [39]. Calculated values for physiological aortic valve area are typically smaller than the anatomic valve area due to contraction of flow in the narrowed orifice [40]. It is important to image the aortic valve in the correct short-axis plane across the valve leaflet tips for planimetric measurements on cine MRI and velocity measurements on velocity-encoded MRI (VENC-MRI) [41].

Valvular Regurgitation

Regurgitant jet area, regurgitant volume, and regurgitant fraction are the most important parameters used to describe

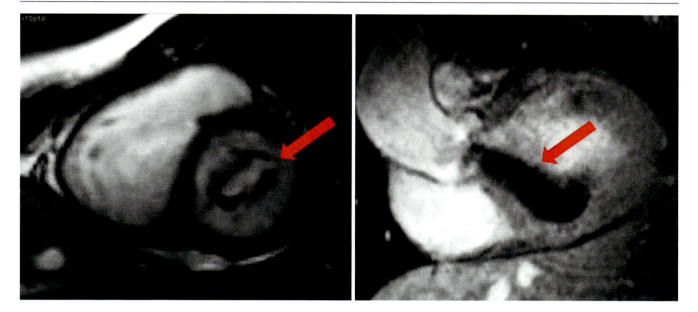

Fig. 16.13 Valvular heart disease. Rheumatic mitral stenosis (*left panel*) with thickening of the mitral valve leaflets (*red arrow*). Significant aortic regurgitation (*right panel*) with a large regurgitant jet appears as a large jet of signal drop-off returning to the left ventricular cavity (*red arrow*)

the severity of valvular regurgitation (Fig. 16.13) [39]. Visualization of flow disturbances by signal void is useful for detecting valvular regurgitation and assessing the direction and origin of jets [39]. With this technique, sensitivities of 90 % and specificities of almost 100 % are reported for detection of aortic [42–44] and mitral regurgitation [42, 44–46] in comparison to color Doppler echocardiography and cardiac catheterization. Velocity mapping and flow quantification by phase-contrast MRI allow for a direct measurement of regurgitant flow. The method has been successfully applied to quantify antegrade and retrograde flow volumes in the aorta and pulmonary artery and is considered the procedure of choice for quantifying valve regurgitation. Reported accuracy rates are 84 and 89 % for regurgitant volume and regurgitant fraction in aortic regurgitation [47–50] and 78 and 76 % in pulmonary regurgitation, respectively [51].

Congenital Heart Diseases

Cardiac MR imaging is an essential modality for the evaluation of many patients with congenital heart disease because of *(a)* its proven quantitative accuracy and reproducibility in the evaluation of ventricular size and blood flow [52–55] and *(b)* its ability to delineate extracardiac structures without ionizing radiation [56]. At present, this is usually accomplished by using a series of predominantly planar pulse sequences, including 2-dimensional (2D) cine phase-contrast and 2-D cine balanced steady-state free precession sequences [56] (Fig. 16.14).

Cardiac MRI aids in evaluation of the severity of intracardiac shunts by measuring flow across the pulmonic

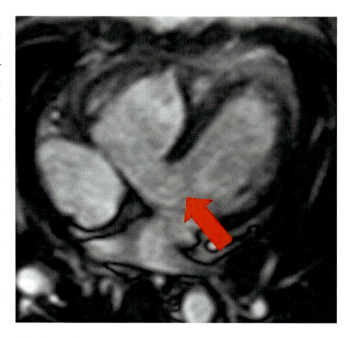

Fig. 16.14 Congenital heart disease. Large ventricular septal defect (*red arrow*) in a patient with Eisenmenger syndrome

and aortic valves (Qp/Qs). While quantitative analysis is used to characterize these lesions, direct visualization of the morphology of shunts and valvular leaks can be difficult with the planar pulse sequences that are typically used [56].

Future advances such as 4-dimensional (4-D) phase-contrast MR imaging has the potential to address some of the limitations of conventional cardiac MR imaging by simultaneously capturing a volume of time-varying anatomic data and a vector field of motion, which can be used to evaluate blood flow [57]. In addition to its quantitative value, with velocity-fusion visualization, the compressed-sensing parallel-imaging 4-D phase-contrast sequence can augment conventional CMR imaging by improving sensitivity for and depiction of hemodynamically significant shunts and valvular regurgitation [56].

Viability of Myocardium

Identifying viable myocardium in a patient with congestive heart failure related to coronary artery disease or after myocardial infarction (MI) is of utmost clinical importance. CMR has been an important diagnostic tool in assessing myocardial viability. The following CMR methods are used to assess myocardial viability: (a) resting assessment of left ventricular (LV) end-diastolic wall thickness (EDWT), (b) low-dose dobutamine (LDD) stress assessment of contractile reserve, and (c) delayed contrast enhancement (DE) to assess for scar tissue [58–60]. DE MRI provides the highest sensitivity and NPV (95 and 90 %) for predicting functional improvement after revascularization of hibernating myocardium of any technique in clinical practice (i.e., positron emission tomography (PET) (92 and 87 %), rest-redistribution thallium-201-SPECT (87 and 79 %), technetium-99 m sestamibi-SPECT (83 and 76 %), and dobutamine stress echocardiography (DSE) (80 and 83 %)). Similarly, LDD CMR provides the highest specificity and positive predictive value (91 and 93 %) compared to other modalities, including PET (63 and 74 %), rest-redistribution thallium-201-SPECT (54 and 67 %), technetium-99 m sestamibi-SPECT (65 and 74 %), and DSE (78 and 75 %) [61].

DE MRI is used to create images with high contrast between abnormal myocardial tissue, which generally accumulates excess gadolinium, and normal tissue in which gadolinium concentration is low (Fig. 16.15). This is currently best achieved using a segmented, gradient-refocused echo (GRE) imaging engine with inversion recovery pre-pulse modifier to provide very strong T1 weighting [60, 62–64].

Stress Testing

MR imaging is being increasingly used to assess myocardial perfusion [65, 66]. Recent studies [67, 68] suggest that the diagnostic accuracy of this method is comparable to, or even better than, that of SPECT. One advantage of contrast material-enhanced cardiac MR imaging over SPECT is that it lends itself to quantitative measurement of first-pass myocardial perfusion [69–71]. Tarroni et al. [72] demonstrated that despite the extreme dynamic nature of contrast-enhanced CMR image sequences and respiratory motion, near-automated frame-by-frame detection of myocardial segments and high-quality quantification of myocardial contrast is feasible both at rest and during vasodilator stress.

First-pass perfusion (FFP) MRI during adenosine vasodilatation is rapidly becoming the stress test of choice in clinical CMR centers [16]. FFP was introduced in 1991 [73] and is now widely accepted as a part of routine clinical CMR examinations [74–77]. FPP increases the myocardium signal intensity, allowing a better visualization of impaired myocardial blood flow in patients with vascular disease [74–77]. Perfusion MRI has excellent spatial resolution, lack of ionizing radiation, and a shorter test time which makes it a

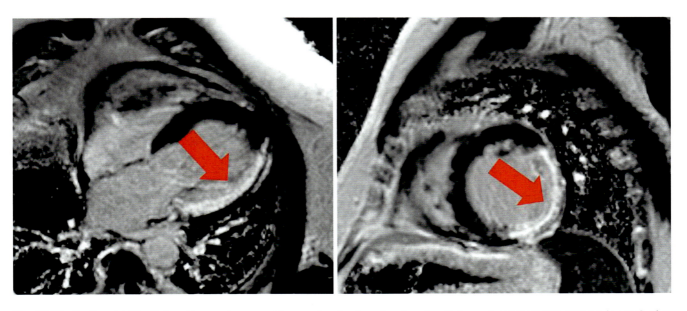

Fig. 16.15 Cardiac viability. Delayed hyperenhancement images showing four-chamber view (*left panel*) and short-axis view (*right panel*) of an extensive lateral wall transmural myocardial infarction with nonviable scar (*red arrow*)

valuable test for assessment of the myocardium. Stress perfusion MRI has shown good correlation with radionuclide imaging and coronary angiography [16]. High-dose dobutamine stress MRI is superior to DSE [78].

Coronary Artery Evaluation

Although published data support the ability of CMR to directly visualize a coronary artery stenosis [79], this capability is not currently being used in most centers. Currently, CMR evaluation of the coronary arteries is generally limited to the evaluation of anomalous origins of coronary arteries in children or young adults. Because of its high temporal resolution, CMR does not require oral or intravenous β-blockade for coronary imaging.

Key Points

- Cardiac magnetic resonance (CMR) is considered the gold standard for the evaluation of cardiac function and viability. It is also widely accepted as the imaging modality of choice for tissue characterization and evaluation of cardiac masses and pericardial disease.
- Phase-contrast and time-resolved magnetic resonance angiography (MRA) are extremely valuable in the assessment of cardiac and valvular flow, transit time, and shunts.
- Stress CMR using either vasodilator or dobutamine offers important functional information for the assessment of obstructive coronary artery disease.

References

1. Sem DS, Pellecchia M. NMR in the acceleration of drug discovery. Curr Opin Drug Discov Devel. 2001;4:479.
2. Damadian R. Field focusing NMR (FONAR) and the formation of chemical images in man. Philos Trans R Soc Lond B Biol Sci. 1980;289:489.
3. Cohan RH, Dillman JR, Hartman RP, et al. ACR manual on contrast media. Am Coll Radiol. 2012;Version 8:59–63.
4. Levine GN, Gomes AS, Arai AE, et al. Safety of magnetic resonance imaging in patients with cardiovascular devices. Circulation. 2007;116:2878–91.
5. Brown JJ. ACR practice guideline for performing and interpreting magnetic resonance imaging. Am Coll Radiol. 2011; Resolution 19:1–6.
6. Alfakih K, Reid S, Jones T, et al. Assessment of ventricular function and mass by cardiac magnetic resonance imaging. Eur Radiol. 2004;14:1813–22.
7. Lorenz CH, Walker ES, Graham Jr TP, et al. Right ventricular performance and mass by use of cine MRI late after atrial repair of transposition of the great arteries. Circulation. 1995;92:233–9.
8. Marcu CB, Beek AM, van Rossum AC. Clinical applications of cardiovascular magnetic resonance imaging. CMAJ. 2006;175:911–7.
9. Pennell DJ, Sechtem UP, Higgins CB, et al. Clinical indications for cardiovascular magnetic resonance (CMR): consensus panel report. Eur Heart J. 2004;25:1940–65.
10. Plein S, Bloomer TN, Ridgway JP, et al. Steady-state free precession magnetic resonance imaging of the heart: comparison with segmented k-space gradient-echo imaging. J Magn Reson Imaging. 2001;14:230–6.
11. Alfakih K, Thiele H, Plein S, et al. Comparison of right ventricular volume measurement between segmented k-space gradient-echo and steady-state free precession magnetic resonance imaging. J Magn Reson Imaging. 2002;16:253–8.
12. Hansch A, Heyne JP, Jung C, et al. Quantitativefirstpassperfusion in cardiovascularmagnetic resonance for determination of peak ventricular transit time-A technique for evaluation of heart function. Eur J Radiol. 2012;81:e996–1001.
13. Child JS, Perloff JK. The restrictive cardiomyopathies. Cardiol Clin. 1988;6:289–316.
14. Benotti JR, Grossman W, Cohn PF. Clinical profile of restrictive cardiomyopathy. Circulation. 1980;61:1206–12.
15. Frank H, Globits S. Magnetic resonance imaging evaluation of myocardial and pericardial disease. J Magn Reson Imaging. 1999;10:617–26.
16. Hurst JW, Fuster V, et al. Hurst's the heart. 13th ed. New York: McGraw-Hill Medical; 2011.
17. Maceira AM, Joshi J, Prasad SK, et al. Cardiovascular magnetic resonance in cardiac amyloidosis. Circulation. 2005;111:186–93.
18. Patel MR, Cawley PJ, Heitner JF, et al. Detection of myocardial damage in patients with sarcoidosis. Circulation. 2009;120:1969–77.
19. Anderson LJ, Holden S, Davis B, et al. Cardiovascular T2-star (T2*) magnetic resonance for the early diagnosis of myocardial iron overload. Eur Heart J. 2001;22:2171–9.
20. Semelka RC, Tomei E, Wagner S, et al. Interstudy reproducibility of dimensional and functional measurements between cine magnetic resonance studies in the morphologically abnormal left ventricle. Am Heart J. 1990;119:1367–73.
21. Wagner S, Auffermann W, Buser P, et al. Functional description of the left ventricle in patients with volume overload, pressure overload, and myocardial disease using cine magnetic resonance imaging. Am J Card Imaging. 1991;5:87–97.
22. Fujita N, Hartiala J, O'Sullivan M, et al. Assessment of left ventricular diastolic function in dilated cardiomyopathy with cine magnetic resonance imaging: effect of an angiotensin converting enzyme inhibitor, benazepril. Am Heart J. 1993;125:171–8.
23. Semelka RC, Tomei E, Wagner S, et al. Normal left ventricular dimensions and function: interstudy reproducibility of measurements with cine MR imaging. Radiology. 1990;174:763–8.
24. Pattynama PM, Lamb HJ, van der Velde EA, et al. Left ventricular measurements with cine and spin-echo MR imaging: a study of reproducibility with variance component analysis. Radiology. 1993;187:261–8.
25. Friedrich MG, Strohm O, Schulz-Menger J, et al. Contrast media-enhanced magnetic resonance imaging visualizes myocardial changes in the course of viral myocarditis. Circulation. 1998;97:1802–9.
26. Hoffmann U, Globits S, Schima W, et al. Usefulness of magnetic resonance imaging of cardiac and paracardiac masses. Am J Cardiol. 2003;92:890–5.
27. Task Force of the European Society of Cardiology, in association with the Association of European Paediatric Cardiologists. Task Force Report. The clinical role of magnetic resonance in cardiovascular disease. Eur Heart J. 1998;19:19–39.
28. Araoz PA, Mulvagh SL, Tazelaar HD, et al. CT and MR imaging of benign primary cardiac neoplasms with echocardiographic correlation. Radiographics. 2000;20:1303–19.
29. Kiaffas MG, Powell AJ, Geva T. Magnetic resonance imaging evaluation ofcardiac tumor characteristics in infants and children. Am J Cardiol. 2002;89:1229–33.

30. Burke AP, Virmani R. Cardiac myxoma. A clinicopathologic study. Am J Clin Pathol. 1993;100:671–80.
31. Grebenc ML, Rosado-de-Christenson ML, Green CE, et al. Cardiac myxoma: imaging features in 83 patients. Radiographics. 2002;22:673–89.
32. Matsuoka H, Hamada M, Honda T, et al. Morphologic and histologic characterization of cardiac myxomas by magnetic resonance imaging. Angiology. 1996;47:693–8.
33. Srichai MB, Junor C, Rodriguez LL, et al. Clinical, imaging, and pathological characteristics of left ventricular thrombus: a comparison of contrast-enhanced magnetic resonance imaging, transthoracic echocardiography, and transesophageal echocardiography with surgical or pathological validation. Am Heart J. 2006;152:75–84.
34. Spodick DH. The pericardium: a comprehensive textbook. New York: M. Dekker; 1997. p. 233, 464.
35. Talreja DR, Edwards WD, Danielson GK, et al. Constrictive pericarditis in 26 patients with histologically normal pericardial thickness. Circulation. 2003;108:1852–7.
36. Alter P, Figiel JH, Rupp TP, et al. MR, CT, and PET imaging in pericardial disease. Heart Fail Rev. 2013;18:289–306.
37. Francone M, Dymarkowski S, Kalantzi M, et al. Assessment of ventricular coupling with real-time cine MRI and its value to differentiate constrictive pericarditis from restrictive cardiomyopathy. Eur Radiol. 2006;16(4):944–51.
38. White CS. MR evaluation of the pericardium. Top Magn Reson Imaging. 1995 Fall;7:258–66.
39. Sommer G, Bremerich J, Lund G. Magnetic resonance imaging in valvular heart disease: clinical application and current role for patient management. J Magn Reson Imaging. 2012;35:1241–52.
40. Otto CM. Valvular aortic stenosis: disease severity and timing of intervention. J Am Coll Cardiol. 2006;47:2141–51.
41. Caruthers SD, Lin SJ, Brown P, et al. Practical value of cardiac magnetic resonance imaging for clinical quantification of aortic valve stenosis: comparison with echocardiography. Circulation. 2003;108:2236–43.
42. Utz JA, Herfkens RJ, Heinsimer JA, et al. Valvular regurgitation: dynamic MR imaging. Radiology. 1988;168:91–4.
43. Mitchell L, Jenkins JPR, Watson Y, et al. Diagnosis and assessment of mitral and aortic valve disease by cine-flow magnetic resonance imaging. Magn Reson Med. 1989;12:181–97.
44. Wagner S, Auffermann W, Buser P, et al. Diagnostic accuracy and estimation of the severity of valvular regurgitation from the signal void on cine magnetic resonance images. Am Heart J. 1989;118:760–7.
45. Aurigemma G, Reichek N, Schiebler M, et al. Evaluation of aortic regurgitation by cardiac cine magnetic resonance imaging: planar analysis and comparison to Doppler echocardiography. Cardiology. 1991;78:340–7.
46. Nishimura T, Yamada N, Itoh A, et al. Cine MR imaging in mitral regurgitation: comparison with color Doppler flow imaging. AJR Am J Roentgenol. 1989;153:721–4.
47. Dulce MC, Mostbeck GH, O'Sullivan M, et al. Severity of aortic regurgitation: interstudy reproducibility of measurements with velocity-encoded cine MR imaging. Radiology. 1992;185:235–40.
48. Honda N, Machida K, Hashimoto M, et al. Aortic regurgitation: quantitation with MR imaging velocity mapping. Radiology. 1993;186:189–94.
49. Sondergaard L, Lindvig K, Hildebrandt P, et al. Quantification of aortic regurgitation by magnetic resonance velocity mapping. Am Heart J. 1993;125:1081–90.
50. Ley S, Eichhorn J, Ley-Zaporozhan J, et al. Evaluation of aortic regurgitation in congenital heart disease: value of MR imaging in comparison to echocardiography. Pediatr Radiol. 2007;37:426–36.
51. Rebergen SA, Chin JG, Ottenkamp J, et al. Pulmonary regurgitation in the late postoperative follow-up of tetralogy of Fallot: volumetric quantitation by nuclear magnetic resonance velocity mapping. Circulation. 1993;88:2257–66.
52. Luijnenburg SE, Robbers-Visser D, Moelker A, et al. Intra-observer and inter-observer variability of biventricular function, volumes and mass in patients with congenital heart disease measured by CMR imaging. Int J Cardiovasc Imaging. 2010;26:57–64.
53. Powell AJ, Maier SE, Chung T, et al. Phase-velocity cine magnetic resonance imaging measurement of pulsatile blood flow in children and young adults: in vitro and in vivo validation. Pediatr Cardiol. 2000;21:104–10.
54. Buonocore MH, Bogren H. Factors influencing the accuracy and precision of velocity-encoded phase imaging. Magn Reson Med. 1992;26:141–54.
55. Pelc NJ, Bernstein MA, Shimakawa A, et al. Encoding strategies for three-direction phase-contrast MR imaging of flow. J Magn Reson Imaging. 1991;1:405–13.
56. Hsiao A, Lustig M, Alley MT, et al. Evaluation of valvular insufficiency and shunts with parallel-imaging compressed-sensing 4D phase-contrast MR imaging with stereoscopic 3D velocity-fusion volume-rendered visualization. Radiology. 2012;265:87–95.
57. Pelc NJ, Herfkens RJ, Shimakawa A, et al. Phase contrast cine magnetic resonance imaging. Magn Reson Q. 1991;7:229–54.
58. Perrone-Filardi P, Bacharach SL, Dilsizian V, et al. Metabolic evidence of viable myocardium in regions with reduced wall thickness and absent wall thickening in patients with chronic ischemic left ventricular dysfunction. J Am Coll Cardiol. 1992;20:161–8.
59. Baer FM, Voth E, LaRosee K, et al. Comparison of dobutamine transesophageal echocardiography and dobutamine magnetic resonance imaging for detection of residual myocardial viability. Am J Cardiol. 1996;78:415–9.
60. Simonetti OP, Kim RJ, Fieno DS, et al. An improved MR imaging technique for the visualization of myocardial infarction. Radiology. 2001;218:215–23.
61. Schinkel AF, Bax JJ, Poldermans D, et al. Hibernating myocardium: diagnosis and patient outcomes. Curr Probl Cardiol. 2007;32:375–410.
62. Fieno DS, Kim RJ, Chen EL, et al. Contrast-enhanced magnetic resonance imaging of myocardium at risk: distinction between reversible and irreversible injury throughout infarct healing. J Am Coll Cardiol. 2000;36:1985–91.
63. Kim RJ, Fieno DS, Parrish TB, et al. Relationship of MRI delayed contrast enhancement to irreversible injury, infarct age, and contractile function. Circulation. 1999;100:1992–2002.
64. Wagner A, Mahrholdt H, Holly TA, et al. Contrast-enhanced MRI and routine single photon emission computed tomography (SPECT) perfusion imaging for detection of subendocardial myocardial infarcts: an imaging study. Lancet. 2003;361:374–9.
65. Klem I, Heitner JF, Shah DJ, et al. Improved detection of coronary artery disease by stress perfusion cardiovascular magnetic resonance with the use of delayed enhancement infarction imaging. J Am Coll Cardiol. 2006;47:1630–48.
66. Nandalur KR, Dwamena BA, Choudhri AF, et al. Diagnostic performance of stress cardiac magnetic resonance imaging in the detection of coronary artery disease: a meta-analysis. J Am Coll Cardiol. 2007;50:1343–53.
67. Schwitter J, Wacker CM, van Rossum AC, et al. MR-IMPACT: comparison of perfusion-cardiac magnetic resonance with single-photon emission computed tomography for the detection of coronary artery disease in a multicentre, multivendor, randomized trial. Eur Heart J. 2008;29:480–9.
68. Greenwood JP, Maredia N, Younger JF, et al. Cardiovascular magnetic resonance and single-photon emission computed tomography for diagnosis of coronary heart disease (CE-MARC): a prospective trial. Lancet. 2012;379:453–60.
69. Jerosch-Herold M, Wilke N, Stillman AE. Magnetic resonance quantification of the myocardial perfusion reserve with a Fermi function model for constrained deconvolution. Med Phys. 1998;25:73–84.

70. Al-Saadi N, Nagel E, Gross M, et al. Improvement of myocardial perfusion reserve early after coronary intervention: assessment with cardiac magnetic resonance imaging. J Am Coll Cardiol. 2000;36:1557–64.

71. Rieber J, Huber A, Erhard I, et al. Cardiac magnetic resonance perfusion imaging for the functional assessment of coronary artery disease: a comparison with coronary angiography and fractional flow reserve. Eur Heart J. 2006;27:1465–71.

72. Tarroni G, Corsi C, Antkowiak PF, et al. Myocardial perfusion: near-automated evaluation from contrast-enhanced MR images obtained at rest and during vasodilator stress. Radiology. 2012;265(2):576–83.

73. Manning WJ, Atkinson DJ, Grossman W, et al. First-pass nuclear magnetic resonance imaging studies using gadolinium-DTPA in patients with coronary artery disease. J Am Coll Cardiol. 1991;18: 959–65.

74. Barmeyer AA, Stork A, Muellerleile K, et al. Comparison of quantitative coronary angiography and first-pass perfusion magnetic resonance imaging for the detection of an impaired coronary perfusion in non-severe coronary stenosis. J Magn Reson Imaging. 2008;27:1005–11.

75. Canyigit M, Turkbey B, Hazirolan T, et al. Magnetic resonance imaging firstpass myocardial perfusion in evaluation of hemodynamic effects of myocardial bridging. J Comput Assist Tomogr. 2008;32:274–5.

76. Su MY, Yang KC, Wu CC, et al. First-pass myocardial perfusion cardiovascular magnetic resonance at 3 Tesla. J Cardiovasc Magn Reson. 2007;9:633–44.

77. Arai AE. Magnetic resonance first-pass myocardial perfusion imaging. Top Magn Reson Imaging. 2000;11:383–98.

78. Nagel E, Lehmkuhl HB, Klein C, et al. Influence of image quality on the diagnostic accuracy of dobutamine stress magnetic resonance imaging in comparison with dobutamine stress echocardiography for the noninvasive detection of myocardial ischemia. Z Kardiol. 1999;88:622–30.

79. Schuetz GM, Zacharopoulou NM, Schlattmann P, et al. Meta-analysis: non-invasive coronary angiography usingcomputed tomography versus magnetic resonance imaging. Ann Intern Med. 2010;152:167–77.

Implantable Cardioverter and Defibrillator Therapy

17

Ahsanuddin Ahmad, Ania Garlitski, Mark Link, Munther K. Homoud, and N.A. Mark Estes III

Abstract

Internal cardioverter defibrillator (ICD) therapy is extremely effective in terminating ventricular tachycardia or ventricular fibrillation (VT/VF) and reducing total mortality in select populations. Common indications for ICDs include survival of prior cardiac arrest, unexplained syncope with inducible VT/VF on electrophysiology study, ischemic cardiomyopathy with EF ≤30 % in patients who are more than 40 days post-myocardial infarction, and cardiomyopathy (ischemic or nonischemic) with EF ≤35 % and New York Heart Association (NYHA) Class II–III heart failure symptoms. ICDs may also be indicated in certain individuals from special populations who suffer from inherited conditions which predispose to sudden cardiac death such as hypertrophic cardiomyopathy, long QT syndrome, Brugada syndrome, arrhythmogenic right ventricular dysplasia, catecholaminergic polymorphic ventricular tachycardia, and cardiac sarcoidosis.

Keywords

Internal cardioverter defibrillator (ICD) therapy • Ventricular tachycardia • Ventricular fibrillation • Internal cardioverter defibrillator (ICD) indications • Cardiac resynchronization therapy (CRT) • Brugada syndrome • Arrhythmogenic right ventricular dysplasia • Catecholaminergic polymorphic ventricular tachycardia • Cardiac sarcoidosis

Sudden cardiac death (SCD) is the most common cause of death worldwide, accounting for approximately 250,000–300,000 deaths annually in the United States [1]. Robust clinical evidence supports the use of implantable cardiac defibrillators (ICDs) in multiple well-defined patient populations. The recent decline in the incidence of SCD is partially due to the use of the ICD in primary and secondary prevention of SCD [1, 2]. As ICD therapy has become a vital aspect of cardiac care, it is now increasingly important for the general cardiologist to fully appreciate its clinical role in preventing SCD, as well as to recognize its potential limitations. This chapter will attempt to provide the reader with a practical understanding of ICD indications, outcomes, complications, and limitations within a framework of the latest clinical evidence and guidelines.

A. Ahmad, MD
Division of Cardiology, Tufts Medical Center,
750 Washington St, Boston, MA 02111, USA
e-mail: aahmad1@tuftsmedicalcenter.org

A. Garlitski, MD • M. Link, MD • M.K. Homoud, MD
N.A.M. Estes III, MD (✉)
Division of Cardiology, Tufts University School of Medicine,
800 Washington St, Suite 197, Boston, MA 02111, USA
e-mail: agarlitski@tuftsmedicalcenter.org;
mlink@tuftsmedicalcenter.org; mhomoud@tuftsmedicalcenter.org;
nestes@tuftsmedicalcenter.org

Evidence-Based Guidelines

The randomized clinical trials showing ICD benefit are classified into two categories: primary and secondary prevention of SCD. There are numerous studies to support the guidelines for ICD therapy in common conditions, such as ischemic and nonischemic dilated cardiomyopathy (NIDCM).

K. Stergiopoulos, D.L. Brown (eds.), *Evidence-Based Cardiology Consult*,
DOI 10.1007/978-1-4471-4441-0_17, © Springer-Verlag London 2014

Table 17.1 Primary prevention ICD trials

Trial (year published)	Follow-up analysis (years)	Patients (n)	LVEF (%)	Study population	All-cause mortality		Benefit		Hazard ratio	P-value
					Control (%)	ICD (%)	RelRR	AbsRR		
MADIT (1996)	2	196	≤35	Prior MI, NSVT, positive EPS	32	13	−59 %	19 %	0.46	0.009
MADIT II (2002)	2	1,232	≤30	Prior MI (>1 month)	22	16	−28 %	−6 %	0.69	0.016
MUSTT (1999)	5	1,397	≤40 %	Prior MI, NSVT, positive EPS	55	24	−58 %	−31 %	0.77	0.005
SCD-HeFT (2,005))	5	1,676	≤35	Prior MI (52 %) or NICM (48 %)	36	29	−23 %	−7 %	0.77	0.007
DEFINITE (2004)	2.5	485	≤35	NICM, NSVT, PVC's	14	8	−44 %	−6 %	0.65	0.08
CABG-Patch (1997)	2.5	900	≤36	CABG, positive SAECG	18	18	N/A	N/A	1.07	0.63
DINAMIT (2004)	2.5	674	≤35	Recent MI (6–40 days, mean 18 days), abnormal HRV	17	19	N/A	N/A	1.08	0.66
IRIS (2009)	2.5	898	≤40	Recent MI (<30 days, mean 13 days), HR >90, or NSVT	25	26	N/A	N/A	0.82	0.78

Obtained, with permission, from Estes [3] and publisher

CABG indicates coronary artery bypass grafting, *CABG-Patch* coronary artery bypass graft-patch *CI* confidence interval, *DEFINITE* defibrillators in nonischemic cardiomyopathy treatment evaluation *DINAMIT* defibrillator in acute myocardial infarction trial, *EP* electrophysiological study, *HR* heart rate, *HRV* heart rate variability, *LVEF* left ventricular ejection fraction, *MADIT I* multicenter automatic defibrillator implantation trial I, *MADIT II* multicenter automatic defibrillator implantation trial II, *MI* myocardial infarction, *MUSTT* multicenter unsustained tachycardia trial, *NICM* nonischemic cardiomyopathy, *NSVT* nonsustained ventricular tachycardia, *PVCs* premature ventricular complexes, *SAECG* signal-averaged electrocardiogram, *SCD-HeFT* sudden cardiac death in heart failure trial, and *VT* ventricular tachycardia, *RelRR* relative risk reduction, *AbsRR* absolute risk reduction

The results of these clinical trials are summarized in Tables 17.1 and 17.2. However, for less common cardiovascular conditions, such as the inherited sudden death syndromes, ICD indications are based largely on observational data and/or expert opinion as randomized controlled trials have not been performed.

Guideline documents in general list indications for treatments as Class I, Class IIA, Class IIB, and Class III [4]. Class I is defined as the treatment being useful that the benefit greatly outweighs the risk and the treatment should be administered. Class IIA indicates that the benefit outweighs the risk and it is reasonable to administer the treatment. Class IIB means that the benefit probably outweighs the risk and that the treatment may be considered. Class III specifies that the risk outweighs the benefit and the treatment should not be performed.

Secondary Prevention Guidelines

It has long been observed that survivors of sudden cardiac arrest (with documented VT or VF) are at significantly greater risk of future SCD [5, 6]. The results of three seminal trials have confirmed these original observations and have led to the acceptance of ICD therapy as definitive therapy for survivors of SCD in the absence of reversible factors [7–9]. The AVID trial (antiarrhythmics vs. implantable defibrillators), which is the largest of these studies, showed a 7 % reduction in the absolute risk of total mortality with ICDs compared to antiarrhythmic drug therapy at 2 years of follow-up [7]. This study has resulted in a Class I recommendation for ICD with Level of evidence A in survivors of cardiac arrest due to VT/VF without any reversible causes [4]. Importantly, VT/VF that occurs within 48 h of an acute myocardial infarction (AMI) is not an indication for an ICD for secondary prevention, since this is thought to be a reversible condition due to acute ischemia [4]. However, if VT/VF occurs after 48 h of an AMI, an ICD may be considered if a cardiac catheterization does not reveal a significant culprit vessel occlusion [4]. ICDs are also indicated for individuals with sustained VT in the setting of structural heart disease (Class I, Level of evidence B), as well as for patients with sustained VT with normal or near-normal LVEF (Class IIA, Level of evidence C) [4].

ICD therapy is also appropriate in selected patients with unexplained syncope. The CIDS trial (Canadian Implantable Defibrillator Study) included patients with unexplained syncope and showed that a positive electrophysiology (EP)

Table 17.2 Secondary prevention ICD Trials

Trial (year published)	Follow-up analysis (years)	Patients (n)	Study population	LVEF (%)	All-cause mortality		Benefit			
					Control (%)	ICD (%)	RelRR (%)	AbsRR (%)	Hazard ratio	P-value
AVID (1997)	2	1,016	VF, VT with syncope, or VT with EF ≤40 %	32 ± 13	25	18	−27	−7	0.62	0.012
CASH (2000)	9	191	VF, VT	46 ± 18	44	36	−23	−8	0.76	0.081 (1-sided analysis)
CIDS (2000)	2	659	VF, VT with syncope, VT with symptoms and EF ≤ 35 %, unmonitored syncope with subsequent inducible VT on EP study	34 ± 14	21	15	−30	−6	0.82	0.142

Obtained, with permission, from Estes [3] and publisher
AVID indicates antiarrhythmics vs. implantable defibrillators, *CASH* cardiac arrest study Hamburg, *CIDS* Canadian implantable defibrillator study, *VT* ventricular tachycardia, *VF* ventricular fibrillation, *EF* ejection fraction, *EP* electrophysiology, *LVEF* left ventricular ejection fraction, *RelRR* relative risk reduction, *AbsRR* absolute risk reduction

study in this group predicted future ventricular tachyarrhythmic events; furthermore, these patients attained mortality benefit from an ICD placement if they had a positive EP study [8]. As such, an ICD is recommended in survivors of unexplained syncope with inducible VT/VF during an EP study (Class I, Level of evidence B) [4]. In addition, ICD therapy is considered reasonable for NIDCM patients with unexplained syncope (Class IIA, Level of evidence C) [4].

Primary Prevention Guidelines

ICD therapy for a primary prevention strategy is typically differentiated by an ischemic or nonischemic cause of cardiomyopathy. Further risk stratification is primarily dependent on left ventricular ejection fraction (LVEF) and New York Heart Association (NYHA) functional class. Of note, the recommendations for ICD therapy for either of these etiologies requires the patient to be on optimal medical therapy with a life expectancy of at least 1 year [4].

Ischemic Cardiomyopathy

ICD guidelines for the ischemic cardiomyopathy (ICM) patient population are based on the results of a multitude of large randomized trials (see Table 17.1). The landmark MADIT II (Multicenter Automatic Defibrillator Implantation Trial) showed a 30 % relative risk reduction in mortality in ICM patients with an LVEF ≤30 % who had an ICD compared to patients without an ICD [10]. Based on this, an

ICD is recommended for ICM patients with an LVEF ≤30 % and NYHA functional Class I heart failure (Class I indication, Level of evidence A) [4]. For patients with ICM and LVEF ≤35 %, an ICD is recommended only if their NYHA functional class is II–III (Class I indication, Level of evidence A) [4]. However, if the LVEF is ≤40 % in the ischemic patient population, then further risk stratification with an electrophysiology (EP) study has been shown to predict SCD in the MUST (Multicenter Unsustained Tachycardia) trial [11]. As such, for ischemic patients with an LVEF ≤40 %, the guidelines provide a Class I (Level of evidence B) recommendation for ICD therapy if the patient has inducible VT or VF during an EP study, as well as documented nonsustained ventricular tachycardia (NSVT) [4].

The ICD indications for primary prevention for ischemic cardiomyopathy (ICM) patients require the patient to be at least 40 days post-myocardial infarction [4]. This is because a low LVEF alone within 40 days of myocardial infarction (MI) has not been shown to identify patients at risk of SCD in excess of their total mortality [12, 13]. Furthermore, the ICD has not been demonstrated to confer a mortality benefit in patients immediately after a transmural MI. This observation is also in agreement with subgroup analyses of larger ICD trials, which show that the benefit of an ICD increases as time from MI to ICD implant increases [14]. The DINAMIT study (Defibrillator in Acute Myocardial Infarction Trial) and IRIS trial (Immediate Risk-Stratification Improves Survival) randomized high-risk patients immediately after an MI to guideline-based medical therapy with or without an ICD [12, 13]. Neither trial demonstrated survival benefit with ICD placement in patients with depressed LVEF up to 40 days after an acute MI [12, 13]. Interestingly, the ICD patients of both of these trials demonstrated a significant reduction in arrhythmic death within the first 40 days post-MI [12, 13]. However, this was offset by an increase in non-arrhythmic mortality [12, 13]. The VALIANT (Valsartan in Acute Myocardial Infarction Trial) study also demonstrated that the highest risk of SCD is in the first 30 days after an acute MI [15].

The reasons for the lack of survival benefit with early risk stratification and ICD intervention in post-MI patients in both the DINAMIT and IRIS trials remain unknown [3]. However, recent autopsy observations of patients experiencing sudden cardiac arrest in the immediate post-MI period indicate that there is a high frequency of cardiac rupture or recurrent MI in the first month after the index MI, whereas arrhythmic deaths become more likely subsequently [16]. This may help to explain the lack of benefit of early ICD therapy after MI.

Another possible strategy to prevent SCD in patients with LV dysfunction due to an acute MI may be via wearable cardiac defibrillators. Analysis of clinical registries demonstrates that therapy from noninvasive vest defibrillators is efficacious in the detection and termination of VT/VF [17]. The potential benefit of this strategy is further highlighted by the results of the HAT (Home Automated External Defibrillator Trial), which demonstrated no survival benefit from home automated external defibrillators (AEDs) in high-risk post-MI patients compared to conventional resuscitation methods [18]. While there is a reasonable rationale for a strategy of short-term use of noninvasive vest defibrillation in high-risk post-MI patients, this approach remains to be evaluated in appropriately designed prospective trials. The VEST (Vest Prevention of Early Sudden Death Trial) is a multicenter, randomized, controlled study that is currently under way to determine whether a wearable defibrillator vest reduces death in the first 2 months following an acute MI [19].

Nonischemic Dilated Cardiomyopathy

Unlike ICM, the clinical trial data to support ICD therapy for NIDCM is less robust mainly due to the relatively smaller study populations. As such, the ICD guideline recommendations for NIDCM patients are based on a lower level of evidence. The SCD-HeFT (Sudden Cardiac Death-Heart Failure Trial) studied both ICM and NIDCM patients with an LVEF ≤35 % and showed a relative risk reduction of 23 % in the ICD group vs. placebo [20]. Although the relative risk reduction for death was similar in both ICM and NIDCM groups, the absolute mortality benefit was greater in the NIDCM population [20]. The DEFINITE trial (Defibrillator Implantation in Patients with Nonischemic Dilated Cardiomyopathy) was a relatively small study, but the only

one to evaluate a pure NIDCM cohort in a prospective randomized fashion [21]. The DEFINITE trial showed that ICDs significantly reduced the risk of sudden death from arrhythmia in NIDCM patients and was associated with a nonsignificant reduction in all-cause mortality [21]. These trials served as the basis for a recommendation for ICD therapy for primary prevention in the NIDCM population with an LVEF ≤35 % and NYHA functional Class II–III (Class I indication, Level of evidence B) [4]. Clinical evidence for ICD therapy is weaker for NYHA functional Class I patients in this NIDCM cohort with an LVEF ≤35 %; as such, a Class IIB (Level of evidence C) indication for ICD implant is given for this patient group [4]. Importantly, ICD therapy for primary prevention is not recommended in NIDCM patients with an LVEF of >35 %.

Other Populations

Several less common diseases are known to increase the risk of SCD. These include acquired, congenital, and inherited conditions. However, due to the low incidence of these diseases, there are no randomized clinical trials large enough to effectively study these high-risk groups. As such, the ICD indications for this cohort in the practice guidelines are derived from registries and expert opinion. For secondary prevention, there is strong agreement that these high-risk patients who survive cardiac arrest should receive an ICD (Class I, Level of evidence A) [4]. However, the role of ICD therapy for primary prevention of SCD in these patients is less clear. The following discussion will focus on primary prevention strategies for hypertrophic cardiomyopathy (HCM), arrhythmogenic right ventricular dysplasia (ARVD), Brugada syndrome, long QT syndrome (LQTS), catecholaminergic polymorphic ventricular tachycardia (CPVT), and cardiac sarcoidosis.

Hypertrophic Cardiomyopathy

Hypertrophic cardiomyopathy is one of the most well-known inheritable causes of SCD. However, not all patients with HCM are at risk of sudden death. Further risk stratification for primary prevention of SCD in the HCM population is based on the following five risk factors: (1) family history of SCD, (2) maximum LV wall thickness >30 mm, (3) history of unexplained syncope, (4) nonsustained ventricular tachycardia (NSVT), and (5) decrease in blood pressure during exercise [22]. The first three of these risk factors are considered more significant than the latter two [22]. Accordingly, the most recent HCM expert consensus statement recommends an ICD for HCM patients with either a family history of SCD, LV wall thickness of 30 mm or more, or a history of unexplained syncope (Class IIA, Level of evidence C) [22]. For HCM patients with isolated NSVT or decrease in BP during exercise, it is considered reasonable to implant an ICD for primary prevention (Class IIB, Level of evidence C) [22]. Importantly, the degree of left ventricular outflow tract (LVOT) obstruction is not considered a risk factor for SCD and, as such, should not be used in isolation as a reason to implant an ICD for primary prevention [4, 22].

Arrhythmogenic Right Ventricular Dysplasia

Arrhythmogenic right ventricular dysplasia (ARVD) is a rare inheritable disorder that results in fibrofatty deposition in the RV and, possibly, the LV. It is characterized by ventricular arrhythmias and SCD in young patients with few or no prior symptoms. Clinical registries have shown the following risk factors to predict SCD: (1) syncope due to VT, (2) evidence of extensive RV disease, (3) LV involvement, and (4) polymorphic VT and RV apical aneurysm [4]. ICD implantation for primary prevention of SCD is reasonable in ARVD if one or more of the aforementioned risk factors are present (Class IIA, Level of evidence C) [4]. Interestingly, family history of ARVD was not found to increase the risk of SCD and, therefore, is not an indication for ICD implantation [22–24].

Brugada Syndrome

Brugada syndrome has received much publicity since its original description from Spain in 1992 [25]. When to implant an ICD in an asymptomatic patient with Brugada syndrome remains a challenge, as the low prevalence of this disease precludes studying the survival benefit of ICDs in a randomized fashion. Nonetheless, there have been a series of case cohorts that serve as the basis for the management strategies provided in the guideline documents regarding the primary prevention of sudden death in Brugada syndrome [26, 27]. According to the ACC/AHA 2008 guidelines, an ICD is recommended for primary prevention with a Class IIA indication (Level of evidence C) if the patient has one of the following risk factors: (1) symptomatic VT or (2) unexplained syncope (Table 17.3) [4]. Of note, family history of Brugada syndrome is not considered an indication for ICD placement [4].

Further risk stratification of Brugada syndrome with an EP study remains an area of much debate. According to European guidelines, an EP study is recommended for further risk stratification in asymptomatic patients with Brugada syndrome; [28] if the EP study demonstrates the patient is inducible for VT/VF, then a Class IIA recommendation is provided for placement of an ICD [28]. In contrast, the 2008 ACC/AHA guidelines do not recommend an EP study to predict SCD in asymptomatic patients with Brugada syndrome [4]. This suggestion has been supported by several subsequent studies that show a very poor positive predictive value of VT/VF inducibility during an EP study in identifying patients at risk of SCD [29–31].

Congenital Long QT Syndrome

Congenital long QT syndrome (LQTS) is another inheritable condition that increases the risk of sudden death. Beta-blockers are generally recommended as first-line

Table 17.3 ICD indications for common conditions based on 2008 ACC/AHA/HRS guidelines [4]

Indication	Classification	Level of evidence	Supporting studies
Survivors of cardiac arrest due to VT or VF without reversible causes	Class I	A	AVID, CASH, CIDS
Structural heart disease and sustained VT	Class I	B	AVID, CASH, CIDS
Syncope of undetermined origin with inducible VT/VF during EP study	Class I	B	CIDS
Unexplained syncope with significant LV dysfunction and NICM	Class IIa	C	Expert opinion
Syncope with structural heart disease and negative invasive and noninvasive studies	Class IIb	C	Expert opinion
ICM with LVEF ≤30 %, at least 40 days post-MI regardless of NYHA functional class	Class I	A	MADIT II
ICM with LVEF ≤35 %, at least 40 days post-MI with NYHA Class II–III symptoms	Class I	A	SCD-HeFT
ICM with LVEF ≤40 % with NSVT and inducible VT/VF at EP study	Class I	B	MADIT, MUSTT
NICM with LVEF ≤35 % and NYHA Class II–III symptoms	Class I	A	SCD-HeFT
NICM with LVEF ≤35 % and NYHA Class I symptoms	Class IIb	C	Expert opinion
Sustained VT with normal or near-normal LV function	Class IIa	C	Expert opinion

VT indicates ventricular tachycardia, *VF* ventricular fibrillation, *AVID* antiarrhythmics vs. implantable defibrillators, *CASH* cardiac arrest study Hamburg, *CIDS* Canadian implantable defibrillator study, *MADIT* multicenter automatic defibrillator implantation trial, *MADIT II* multicenter automatic defibrillator implantation trial II, *SCD-HeFT* sudden cardiac death in heart failure trial, *MUSTT* multicenter unsustained tachycardia trial, *NSVT* nonsustained VT, *NYHA* New York Heart Association, *EP* electrophysiology, *NICM* nonischemic cardiomyopathy, *MI* myocardial infarction

therapy for patients who are asymptomatic or those with syncope not on beta-blockers [4]. However, for congenital LQTS patients who experience syncope and/or VT while on beta-blockers, the guidelines provide a Class IIA recommendation (Level of evidence B) for ICD implantation for primary prevention [4]. For LQTS types 2 and 3 (which are associated with a greater risk of SCD than LQTS type 1), it is considered reasonable to implant an ICD for primary prevention regardless of beta-blocker therapy (Class IIB, Level of evidence B) [4]. ICD therapy is not indicated for patients with only a family history of LQTS or SCD, or for those with a LQTS genotype without a prolonged QT interval.

Catecholaminergic Polymorphic Ventricular Tachycardia

Catecholaminergic polymorphic ventricular tachycardia (CPVT) is another rare genetic condition that increases the risk of SCD via triggered activity from delayed afterdepolarization, similar to the pathophysiology of digoxin toxicity [32]. Beta-blockers are considered first-line therapy for asymptomatic individuals diagnosed with CPVT [4]. However, if a patient with CPVT develops unexplained syncope or sustained VT while on beta-blockers, then an ICD is indicated for primary prevention (Class IIA, Level of evidence C) [4]. ICD therapy is not indicated for primary prevention for patients who develop symptoms without prior beta-blocker treatment [4].

Cardiac Sarcoidosis

Cardiac sarcoidosis can result in SCD, as sarcoid granulomas in the ventricular myocardium can lead to abnormal automaticity or cause reentrant ventricular arrhythmias [33]. These granulomas may be identified as scars on cardiac magnetic resonance imaging (MRI) via late gadolinium enhancement [34]. No specific ICD indications exist for cardiac sarcoidosis. However, the 2006 ACC/AHA practice guidelines state that "spontaneous VT, severe LV dysfunction, and severe intraventricular conduction disturbance warrant ICD and/or pacemaker therapy as appropriate." [35] In the 2008 ACC/AHA guideline update, a Class IIB (Level of evidence C) recommendation was given for ICD placement for cardiac sarcoidosis regardless of the presence of VT or heart failure [4]. Although no guidelines exist for risk stratification of cardiac sarcoidosis via cardiac MRI, one promising study has shown late gadolinium enhancement on cardiac MRI to be strongly predictive of SCD [34]. Larger randomized trials are needed to determine if cardiac MRI should be used to guide ICD therapy in this population.

Cardiac Resynchronization Therapy Guidelines

Cardiac resynchronization therapy (CRT) is defined as biventricular pacing in patients with interventricular dyssynchrony, which can be caused by bundle branch block or interventricular conduction delay. The LV is usually paced by placing a pacing lead into a branch vessel of the coronary sinus. The seminal trials studied CRT in patients with LVEF ≤35 % with NYHA functional Class III or IV and a QRS duration of ≥120 ms [36–38]. These studies demonstrated CRT to improve heart failure symptoms, increase LVEF, reduce heart failure hospitalizations, and improve survival [36–38]. As such, CRT with or without an ICD is recommended for patients with an LVEF ≤35 % with NYHA functional Class III or IV and a QRS duration of ≥120 ms (Class I, Level of evidence A) [4]. Based on evidence that chronic right ventricular pacing can also cause interventricular dyssynchrony [39] and exacerbate heart failure [40], CRT is also indicated in individuals with an LVEF ≤35 % who require frequent ventricular pacing in the setting of NYHA Class III–IV heart failure (Class IIA indication, Level of evidence C) or NYHA Class I–II heart failure (Class IIB indication, Level of evidence C) [4].

More recently, trials have demonstrated CRT benefit in even milder degrees of heart failure. Specifically, data from the REVERSE trial (Resynchronization Reverses Remodeling in Systolic Left Ventricular Dysfunction) [41], MADIT-CRT (Multicenter Automatic Defibrillator Implantation Trial with Cardiac Resynchronization Therapy) [42], and RAFT (Resynchronization Defibrillation for Ambulatory Heart Failure Trial) [43] have demonstrated that CRT therapy in patients with NYHA functional Class I or II symptoms can improve LVEF [41], reduce hospitalizations [42], and improve mortality [43]. A meta-analysis of these studies has confirmed these findings [44]. Importantly, the majority of CRT benefit in these studies was in patients with QRS durations ≥150 ms and those with LBBB [41–43]. These trials were published after the last ACC/AHA ICD guideline update in 2008 and, as such, are not included in this document. However, the European guideline update in 2010 recommended CRT therapy for patients with an LVEF ≤35 % with NYHA Class II heart failure and a QRS duration of ≥150 ms (Class I, Level of evidence A) [45]. Note that the European guidelines do not recommend CRT therapy in NYHA Class I heart failure patients, since this population was not well represented in the trials [41–43]. Further guidance on CRT therapy in NYHA Class I and II heart failure patients will be provided by the ACC/AHA ICD guideline update to be released in 2012.

Approximately one-third of patients do not derive benefit from biventricular pacing [46]. Initially smaller studies suggested that interventricular dyssynchrony diagnosed by echocardiography would identify potential responders to

CRT. However, a more recent large multicenter study failed to show the benefit of any echocardiographic measure of dyssynchrony in predicting response to CRT [47]. As such, it is currently unclear if the presence of dyssynchrony on echocardiogram is useful in identifying patients who will benefit from CRT. Nevertheless, a sub-study of the MADIT-CRT demonstrated the predictive power of the combined assessment of the following factors in identifying CRT responders: (1) female sex, (2) nonischemic origin, (3) left bundle branch block, (4) QRS $\geq$150 ms, (5) prior heart failure hospitalization, (6) left ventricular end-diastolic volume $\geq$125 mL/m^2, and (7) left atrial volume <40 mL/m^2 [46]. More studies are needed to establish predictors of CRT response.

ICD Implantation Outcomes

Incidence of Complications

Although ICDs have been shown to effectively prevent SCD, there are a variety of complications that may occur after ICD placement. ICD-related adverse events may be defined as major or minor. Major complications include death, cardiac arrest, cardiac perforation, pericardial tamponade, stroke, MI, valve injury, coronary venous dissection, hemothorax, and pneumothorax. Minor complications include conduction block, pocket hematoma, lead dislodgement, peripheral nerve injury, and infection related to the device. Data from national registries has demonstrated the periprocedural incidence of any complication (major or minor) to be approximately 2–3 % after ICD placement [48]. The majority of these complications are minor and tend to be pocket hematomas (~ 0.7 %), lead dislodgements (~0.5 %), and infections (0.1–0.5 %) [48–50]. The incidence of major periprocedural complications is very low (<1 %) [48, 49], with pneumothorax, death of any cause, cardiac arrest, stroke, and MI being the main contributors, accounting for approximately 0.36, 0.2, 0.3, 0.05, and 0.02 % of the major periprocedural complications, respectively [48, 49].

Of note, these complication rates are derived from national registries, which are limited by the assessment of only in-hospital outcomes. When analysis is extended to include long-term follow-up, studies show an increase in complication rates that is comprised mainly of mechanical issues with the lead; [50] this includes lead dislodgement, lead malfunction, or device protrusion which has a 7–8 % incidence at 90 days [50]. An incremental increase in infection is also seen with longer follow-up, with an incidence of approximately 2 % at 90 days [50]. Despite this increase in long-term complication rate, the majority of postoperative complications continue to occur during the index hospital stay [50].

ICD-Related Infections

With the recent rise in ICD implantation rates, there has been a concomitant increase in ICD-related infections [50, 51]. As such, this specific ICD complication deserves special attention. Device infections are generally categorized as pocket infections or deeper infections. Pocket infections involve the subcutaneous tissues containing the pulse generator and leads, but not the transvenous segment of the leads. In some pocket infections, a portion of the device or leads may erode through the overlying skin. Deeper infections involve the transvenous portion of the lead, which is usually associated with bacteremia and/or endocarditis due to vegetations on the lead or a valve. Coagulase negative staphylococci and staphylococcus aureus account for the majority of these infections [52]. Diagnosis requires a transesophageal echocardiogram regardless of the results of transthoracic echocardiography (Class I, Level of evidence B) [53], 2 sets of blood cultures drawn prior to starting antimicrobial therapy (Class I, Level of evidence C) [53], as well as Gram stain and culture of the pocket tissue and lead tip at the time of explant (Class I, Level of evidence C) [53]. Importantly, percutaneous aspiration of the generator pocket is not recommended for diagnostic evaluation as it may result in infection of the ICD pocket (Class III, Level of evidence C) [53].

Treatment of device-related infections begins in the preoperative period, as prophylactic antibiotics have been shown to reduce the risk of potentially serious infections [54]. A single dose of antibiotics with staphylococcal coverage is recommended to be administered 1 h prior to the procedure (Class I indication, Level of evidence A) [53]. Currently, there are no data to support the use of postoperative antibiotics for prevention of infection after device implantation so this strategy is not recommended [53].

In patients who develop superficial or incisional infection at the pocket site with no involvement of the device, hardware extraction is not required and 7–10 days of antibiotics with staphylococcal coverage is considered sufficient [53]. In contrast, in addition to antibiotic therapy, complete removal of all hardware is strongly recommended for pocket infections (as evidenced by abscess formation, device erosion, or chronically draining sinus), endocarditis with or without lead involvement, or occult staphylococcal bacteremia (Class I, Level of evidence A) [53]. Complete device and lead removal is also reasonable in occult Gram-negative bacteremia despite appropriate antibiotic therapy (Class II, Level of evidence A) [53]. The duration of antibiotics should be 10–14 days for pocket site infections and 4–6 weeks for more complicated infections (i.e., endocarditis, septic thrombophlebitis, osteomyelitis, or persistent blood stream infections despite device removal) [53]. For patients who are not candidates for complete device removal, long-term suppressive antibiotics are reasonable (Class IIB, Level of evidence C) [53].

Predictors of Outcomes

In addition to appreciating potential ICD-related complications, it may be even more prudent for the clinician to recognize elements in a patient's profile that may predict adverse events after ICD implantation. Several studies have determined risk factors for infectious complications after device placement [55–57]. These include (1) recent manipulation of the device, (2) temporary pacing prior to permanent device placement, (3) generator replacement, (4) diabetes mellitus, (5) prior treatment with anticoagulation or glucocorticoids, (6) heart failure, (7) renal dysfunction (GFR < 60 mL/min), and (8) operator inexperience [55–57]. Furthermore, studies have shown that noninfectious complications are higher with (1) placement of dual chamber ICDs compared to single chamber devices; [46] (2) non-electrophysiologist operators, especially cardiothoracic surgeons; [49, 50] (3) operator inexperience; [58] (4) female patients; [50] (5) chronic lung disease; [50] (6) dementia; [50] and (7) renal disease [50].

A recent study has developed a point score to more objectively determine the risk associated with ICD implantation [59]. The following are risk factors established by this risk score model: age >70 years (1 point), female (2 points), NYHA Class III (1 point), NYHA Class IV (3 points), atrial fibrillation (1 point), prior valve surgery (3 points), chronic lung disease (2 points), BUN >30 (2 points), reimplantation for reasons other than battery change (6 points), dual chamber ICD type (2 points), biventricular ICD type (4 points), and nonelective ICD implant (3 points) [59]. The risk of any in-hospital complication increased from 0.6 % among patients with a score of less than 5–8.4 % among the patients with greater than 19 risk points [59]. Recognition of these predictors of complications is crucial for minimizing postoperative complications.

ICD Shocks and Therapy

Prognostic Impact of ICD Shocks

Despite the proven survival benefits of ICDs in patients at risk of SCD, ICD therapy comes at a cost. Recent studies have demonstrated that ICD shocks, whether appropriate or inappropriate, can increase heart failure events and worsen mortality [60, 61]. It was initially felt that the deleterious effects of ICD discharges were a reflection of a sicker patient population who has a higher baseline risk of death. However, a recent study has revealed that the mortality risk associated with ICD shocks is independent of the patient's baseline risk of death as estimated by the Seattle Heart Failure Model [62]. The underlying mechanism to explain why an ICD shock would increase the risk of death is unclear, but may be related to myocardial damage induced by ICD shocks [63]. Certainly, older literature has described adverse cellular, tissue, and cardiac mechanical responses to large electric

currents during defibrillation shocks in animals and humans [64–66]. Since ICD discharges are associated with worsened heart failure outcomes, an ICD shock should serve as an opportunity for clinicians to intensify and optimize heart failure therapy [63]. In addition to causing increased mortality and heart failure, ICD shocks are also perceived as exquisitely painful, resulting in serious psychological sequelae (such as depression, anxiety, anger and post-traumatic stress disorder) which may also worsen quality of life [63].

Antitachycardia Pacing

Given the harmful effects of ICD shocks, it is paramount to implement device programming to minimize ICD shocks. One approach to achieve this goal is via anti-tachycardia pacing (ATP). ATP therapies have been shown to terminate reentrant ventricular arrhythmias using short, rapid bursts of pacing [67, 68]. It is important to note that ATP is not effective in treating VF as this is not a reentrant rhythm. Based on the results of two large trials [67, 68], ATP is now routinely used to terminate VT (<188 beats/min) with an efficacy of >90 % and a minimal risk (<5 %) of accelerating VT to a more unstable rhythm requiring a shock [69]. Due to the painless nature of ATP therapy, studies have shown that patients undergoing ATP therapy have less physical and emotional trauma compared to shock therapy [69]. In addition to reducing the burden of ICD shocks [68], ATP has also recently been demonstrated to reduce total mortality compared to shock therapy [70]. This adds further evidence to the detrimental effects of ICD shocks and brings ATP therapy to the forefront for minimizing ICD discharges for ventricular arrhythmias.

Inappropriate Shocks

Inappropriate shocks comprise 10–25 % of ICD discharges [69]. The vast majority of inappropriate ICD therapy is due to atrial fibrillation (AF) and supraventricular tachycardia (SVT), as inappropriate shocks may be delivered if AF or an SVT with rapid ventricular rate falls into a device's programmed VT or VF heart rate zone [69]. To avoid this problem, newer device algorithms have implemented SVT discriminators based on QRS morphology, heart rate stability, and onset of tachycardia to distinguish between VT and SVT. Inappropriate ICD therapy may also be delivered due to oversensing resulting in QRS and T-wave double counting. This issue can usually be corrected with device reprogramming in which T waves are "blinded" by the device; if this is done, then defibrillation testing is often performed to ensure the device is not also accidentally "blinded" to low amplitude ventricular fibrillation waves. Other possible causes of inappropriate ICD therapy are mechanical problems such as lead fracture, insulation break, and lead dislodgement. This should be suspected in patients presenting with multiple shocks in rapid succession and can be confirmed by device interrogation demonstrating a change in lead impedance and often a failure to sense or capture appropriately.

Remote Monitoring

According to the most recent expert consensus statement from the ACC/AHA/HRS [71], patients should be followed every 3–5 months after ICD implantation and more frequently as battery approaches elective replacement. This results in numerous patient visits and can place significant strain to the workflow in an outpatient clinic. Although transtelephonic monitoring has been present for many years, its utility has been limited by its ability to provide only basic information on battery status and capture thresholds. More recently, home transmitters have been developed by most device manufacturers that allow full interrogation of the ICD, either manually by the patient waving a telemetry wand or automatically on a predefined periodic basis via a wireless Internet-based telemetry system [72]. This information is then sent by the transmitter to the physician via e-mail, fax, text message, or phone. In addition, the data is stored in a central server where it can be accessed by the physician via the Internet. This is referred to as remote monitoring. The data available from these remote monitoring systems is detailed and equivalent to the level of information that could be obtained manually from the device at the outpatient clinic [72]. Two recent trials have demonstrated that not only is remote monitoring safe and effective, but it also results in (1) less frequent office visits, (2) more rapid recognition of

clinical events, and (3) decreased time to clinical action of an arrhythmia event or issue with ICD lead or generator [73, 74]. Although the use of remote monitoring is not discussed in the 2008 ACC/AHA guideline update [4], remote monitoring of ICDs and pacemakers may become an important element of device management in the future.

Limitations of Current Risk Stratification Techniques for SCD

Although ICDs are extremely effective at detecting and terminating VT/VF, identifying individuals who should receive this therapy remains challenging. Impaired LVEF and heart failure are certainly sensitive indices of SCD risk [10, 20] and serve as a guide for current ICD indications. However, these parameters identify populations in whom absolute arrhythmic events are low [2]. Herein lies the dilemma: the absolute number of SCDs is highest in patients who have unrecognized CAD with normal LVEF or are at low risk of CAD or heart failure based on conventional risk markers [2], yet the cumulative incidence of SCD in this population is very low [2]. Prophylactic ICD placement in this very large population is precluded by the inability to accurately identify these individuals [2]. In contrast, the presence of LV dysfunction and heart failure identifies patients with highest incidence of SCD, but misses the majority of patients who will suffer SCD, since most individuals who experience cardiac arrest have a normal LVEF [2]. This concept is illustrated in Fig. 17.1. The failure of LV dysfunction to predict SCD in the vast majority of patients who will suffer this

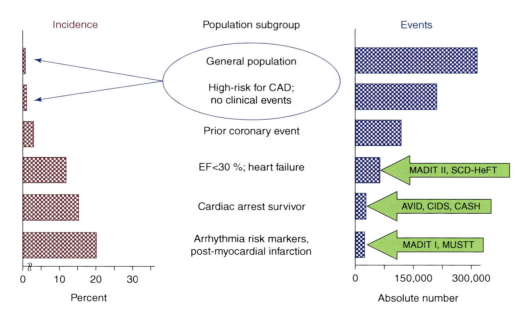

Fig. 17.1 Comparison of incidence and absolute number of SCD anually within different populations. Obtained, with permission, from Myeburg et al. [2]. With recognition of increasingly improved risk factors, the incidence of SCD increases, but is accompanied by a progressive decrease in total events in each group. This occurs because each risk

factors identifies a smaller population subgroup and, therefore, a smaller number of events; it also lowers the denominator pool and results in a higher SCD incidence. In contrast, the highest number of SCD events occur in the lower risk population. Since this population is very large, there is a higher denominator pool producing a lower incidence of SCD

event highlights the weakness of LVEF as a marker of SCD. Newer methods of risk stratification are sorely needed to identify people in the general population at risk of SCD who have a normal LVEF and are at low risk of CAD. Such a paradigm shift would impact the public health issue of SCD in a much greater fashion than does the current emphasis given to the small, very high-risk patient population studied in the randomized clinical trials to date.

Key Points

- ICD therapy is extremely effective in terminating VT/VF and reducing total mortality in select populations.
- Common indications for ICDs include survival of prior cardiac arrest, unexplained syncope with inducible VT/VF on EPS, ICM with EF ≤30 % who are more than 40 days post-MI, and cardiomyopathy (ICM or NIDCM) with EF ≤35 % and NYHA Class II–III heart failure symptoms.
- ICDs may also be indicated in certain individuals from special populations who suffer from inherited conditions which predispose to SCD, such as HCM, long QT syndrome, Brugada syndrome, ARVD, CPVT, and cardiac sarcoidosis (Table 17.4).
- CRT devices have also been shown to improve mortality, reduce heart failure hospitalizations, and improve quality of life in selected individuals with cardiomyopathy and interventricular dyssynchrony, even with only mild symptoms of heart failure.
- Despite its effectiveness in terminating VT/VF, ICDs are limited by potential procedural complications, the risk of psychological trauma, heart failure, and death associated with ICD shocks.
- Efficient use of ICDs is further limited by the lack of reliable markers to predict cardiac arrest in the large majority of patients who suffer SCD with a normal LVEF.

Table 17.4 ICD indications in special populations

Indication	Classification	Level of evidence	Supporting studies
Congenital heart disease with prior cardiac arrest without a reversible cause	Class I[a]	B	Expert opinion
Congenital heart disease with symptomatic sustained VT with normal invasive hemodynamics and negative EP study	Class I[a]	C	Expert opinion
Congenital heart disease and unexplained syncope with either impaired ventricular function or inducible VT/VF on EP study	Class IIa[a]	C	Expert opinion
Congenital heart disease with recurrent syncope and systemic ventricular dysfunction when invasive and noninvasive studies fail to identify a cause	Class IIb[a]	C	Expert opinion
HCM with >1 of the following risks: family history of SCD, LV wall thickness ≥30 mm, unexplained syncope	Class IIa[b]	C	Expert opinion
HCM with ≥1 of the following risks: isolated NSVT, decrease in BP during exercise	Class IIb[b]	C	Expert opinion
ARVD with ≥1 of the following risk factors: syncope due to VT, extensive RV disease, LV involvement, polymorphic VT, RV apical aneurysm	Class IIa[a]	C	Expert opinion
Long QT syndrome with syncope or VT while on beta-blockers	Class IIa[a]	B	Expert opinion
Brugada syndrome with unexplained syncope or VT	Class IIa[a]	C	Expert opinion
CPVT with syncope or VT while on beta-blockers	Class IIa[a]	C	Expert opinion
Cardiac sarcoidosis, giant cell myocarditis, or Chagas disease	Class IIa[a]	C	Expert opinion
Nonhospitalized patient awaiting cardiac transplantation	Class IIa[a]	C	Expert opinion
Familial cardiomyopathy associated with SCD	Class IIb[a]	C	Expert opinion
LV noncompaction	Class IIb[a]	C	Expert opinion

[a]Based on 2008 ACC/AHA/HRS Guidelines [4]
[b]Based on 2011 ACC/AHA Guidelines [22]
EP indicates electrophysiology, *SCD* sudden cardiac death, *HCM* hypertrophic cardiomyopathy, *ARVD* arrhythmogenic right ventricular dysplasia

References

1. Adabag AS, Luepker RV, Roger VL, et al. Sudden cardiac death: epidemiology and risk factors. Nat Rev Cardiol. 2010;7: 216–25.

2. Myerburg RJ, Reddy V, Castellanos A. Indications for implantable cardioverter-defibrillators based on evidence and judgment. J Am Coll Cardiol. 2009;54:747–63.

3. Estes 3rd NA. The challenge of predicting and preventing sudden cardiac death immediately after myocardial infarction. Circulation. 2009;120:185–7.

4. Epstein AE, DiMarco JP, Ellenbogen KA, et al. ACC/AHA/HRS 2008 guidelines for device-based therapy of cardiac rhythm abnormalities: a report of the American College of Cardiology/American Heart Association Task Force on Practice Guidelines (Writing Committee to Revise the ACC/AHA/NASPE 2002 Guideline Update for Implantation of Cardiac Pacemakers and Antiarrhythmia Devices): developed in collaboration with the American Association for Thoracic Surgery and Society of Thoracic Surgeons. Circulation. 2008;117:e350–408.

5. Schaffer WA, Cobb LA. Recurrent ventricular fibrillation and modes of death in survivors of out-of-hospital ventricular fibrillation. N Engl J Med. 1975;293:259–62.

6. Cobbe SM, Dalziel K, Ford I, et al. Survival of 1476 patients initially resuscitated from out of hospital cardiac arrest. BMJ. 1996;312:1633–7.

7. The Antiarrhythmics versus Implantable Defibrillators (AVID) Investigators. A comparison of antiarrhythmic-drug therapy with implantable defibrillators in patients resuscitated from near-fatal ventricular arrhythmias. N Engl J Med. 1997;337:1576–83.

8. Connolly SJ, Gent M, Roberts RS, et al. Canadian implantable defibrillator study (CIDS): a randomized trial of the implantable cardioverter defibrillator against amiodarone. Circulation. 2000; 101:1297–302.

9. Kuck KH, Cappato R, Siebels J, et al. Randomized comparison of antiarrhythmic drug therapy with implantable defibrillators in patients resuscitated from cardiac arrest: the Cardiac Arrest Study Hamburg (CASH). Circulation. 2000;102:748–54.

10. Moss AJ, Zareba W, Hall WJ, et al. Prophylactic implantation of a defibrillator in patients with myocardial infarction and reduced ejection fraction. N Engl J Med. 2002;346:877–83.

11. Buxton AE, Lee KL, Fisher JD, et al. A randomized study of the prevention of sudden death in patients with coronary artery disease. Multicenter Unsustained Tachycardia Trial Investigators. N Engl J Med. 1999;341:1882–90.

12. Hohnloser SH, Kuck KH, Dorian P, et al. Prophylactic use of an implantable cardioverter-defibrillator after acute myocardial infarction. N Engl J Med. 2004;351:2481–8.

13. Steinbeck G, Andresen D, Seidl K, et al. Defibrillator implantation early after myocardial infarction. N Engl J Med. 2009;361: 1427–36.

14. Wilber DJ, Zareba W, Hall WJ, et al. Time dependence of mortality risk and defibrillator benefit after myocardial infarction. Circulation. 2004;109:1082–4.

15. Pfeffer MA, McMurray JJ, Velazquez EJ, et al. Valsartan, captopril, or both in myocardial infarction complicated by heart failure, left ventricular dysfunction, or both. N Engl J Med. 2003;349: 1893–906.

16. Pouleur AC, Barkoudah E, Uno H, et al. Pathogenesis of sudden unexpected death in a clinical trial of patients with myocardial infarction and left ventricular dysfunction, heart failure, or both. Circulation. 2010;122:597–602.

17. Chung MK, Szymkiewicz SJ, Shao M, et al. Aggregate national experience with the wearable cardioverter-defibrillator: event rates, compliance, and survival. J Am Coll Cardiol. 2010;56:194–203.

18. Bardy GH, Lee KL, Mark DB, et al. Home use of automated external defibrillators for sudden cardiac arrest. N Engl J Med. 2008;358:1793–804.

19. Vest Prevention of Early Sudden Death Trial (VEST). http://clinicaltrials.gov/ct2/show/NCT01446965. Accessed 18 Mar 2012.

20. Bardy GH, Lee KL, Mark DB, et al. Amiodarone or an implantable cardioverter-defibrillator for congestive heart failure. N Engl J Med. 2005;352:225–37.

21. Kadish A, Dyer A, Daubert JP, et al. Prophylactic defibrillator implantation in patients with nonischemic dilated cardiomyopathy. N Engl J Med. 2004;350:2151–8.

22. Gersh BJ, Maron BJ, Bonow RO, et al. 2011 ACCF/AHA guideline for the diagnosis and treatment of hypertrophic cardiomyopathy: a report of the American College of Cardiology Foundation/ American Heart Association Task Force on Practice Guidelines. Circulation. 2011;124:e783–831.

23. Corrado D, Calkins H, Link MS, et al. Prophylactic implantable defibrillator in patients with arrhythmogenic right ventricular cardiomyopathy/dysplasia and no prior ventricular fibrillation or sustained ventricular tachycardia. Circulation. 2010;122:1144–52.

24. Bhonsale A, James CA, Tichnell C, et al. Incidence and predictors of implantable cardioverter-defibrillator therapy in patients with arrhythmogenic right ventricular dysplasia/cardiomyopathy undergoing implantable cardioverter-defibrillator implantation for primary prevention. J Am Coll Cardiol. 2011;58:1485–96.

25. Brugada P, Brugada J. Right bundle branch block, persistent ST segment elevation and sudden cardiac death: a distinct clinical and electrocardiographic syndrome. A multicenter report. J Am Coll Cardiol. 1992;20:1391–6.

26. Priori SG, Napolitano C, Gasparini M, et al. Natural history of Brugada syndrome: insights for risk stratification and management. Circulation. 2002;105:1342–7.

27. Brugada J, Brugada R, Antzelevitch C, et al. Long-term follow-up of individuals with the electrocardiographic pattern of right bundle-branch block and ST-segment elevation in precordial leads V1 to V3. Circulation. 2002;105:73–8.

28. Antzelevitch C, Brugada P, Borggrefe M, et al. Brugada syndrome: report of the second consensus conference: endorsed by the Heart Rhythm Society and the European Heart Rhythm Association. Circulation. 2005;111:659–70.

29. Priori SG, Gasparini M, Napolitano C, Bella PD, Ottonelli AG, Sassone B, Giordano U, Pappone C, Mascioli G, Rossetti G, De Nardis R, Colombu M. Risk stratification in Brugada syndrome: results of the PRELUDE (PRogrammed ELectrical stimUlation preDictive valuE) registry. J Am Coll Cardiol. 2012;59:37–45.

30. Probst V, Veltmann C, Eckardt L, et al. Long-term prognosis of patients diagnosed with Brugada syndrome: results from the FINGER Brugada Syndrome Registry. Circulation. 2010;121:635–43.

31. Delise P, Allocca G, Marras E, et al. Risk stratification in individuals with the Brugada type 1 ECG pattern without previous cardiac arrest: usefulness of a combined clinical and electrophysiologic approach. Eur Heart J. 2011;32:169–76.

32. Kontula K, Laitinen PJ, Lehtonen A, et al. Catecholaminergic polymorphic ventricular tachycardia: recent mechanistic insights. Cardiovasc Res. 2005;67:379–87.

33. Sekiguchi M, Numao Y, Imai M, et al. Clinical and histopathological profile of sarcoidosis of the heart and acute idiopathic myocarditis. Concepts through a study employing endomyocardial biopsy. I. Sarcoidosis. Jpn Circ J. 1980;44:249–63.

34. Patel MR, Cawley PJ, Heitner JF, et al. Detection of myocardial damage in patients with sarcoidosis. Circulation. 2009;120: 1969–77.

35. Zipes DP, Camm AJ, Borggrefe M, et al. ACC/AHA/ESC 2006 guidelines for management of patients with ventricular arrhythmias and the prevention of sudden cardiac death: a report of the American College of Cardiology/American Heart Association Task Force and the European Society of Cardiology Committee for Practice Guidelines (writing committee to develop Guidelines for Management of Patients With Ventricular Arrhythmias and the Prevention of Sudden Cardiac Death): developed in collaboration with the European Heart Rhythm Association and the Heart Rhythm Society. Circulation. 2006;114:e385–484.

36. Abraham WT, Fisher WG, Smith AL, et al. Cardiac resynchronization in chronic heart failure. N Engl J Med. 2002;346:1845–53.

37. Bristow MR, Saxon LA, Boehmer J, et al. Cardiac-resynchronization therapy with or without an implantable defibrillator in advanced chronic heart failure. N Engl J Med. 2004;350:2140–50.

38. Cleland JG, Daubert JC, Erdmann E, et al. The effect of cardiac resynchronization on morbidity and mortality in heart failure. N Engl J Med. 2005;352:1539–49.

39. Lee MA, Dae MW, Langberg JJ, et al. Effects of long-term right ventricular apical pacing on left ventricular perfusion, innervation, function and histology. J Am Coll Cardiol. 1994;24:225–32.

40. Wilkoff BL, Cook JR, Epstein AE, et al. Dual-chamber pacing or ventricular backup pacing in patients with an implantable defibrillator: the Dual Chamber and VVI Implantable Defibrillator (DAVID) Trial. JAMA. 2002;288:3115–23.

41. Linde C, Abraham WT, Gold MR, et al. Randomized trial of cardiac resynchronization in mildly symptomatic heart failure patients and in asymptomatic patients with left ventricular dysfunction and previous heart failure symptoms. J Am Coll Cardiol. 2008;52:1834–43.

42. Moss AJ, Hall WJ, Cannom DS, et al. Cardiac-resynchronization therapy for the prevention of heart-failure events. N Engl J Med. 2009;361:1329–38.

43. Tang AS, Wells GA, Talajic M, et al. Cardiac-resynchronization therapy for mild-to-moderate heart failure. N Engl J Med. 2010;363:2385–95.

44. Al-Majed NS, McAlister FA, Bakal JA, et al. Meta-analysis: cardiac resynchronization therapy for patients with less symptomatic heart failure. Ann Intern Med. 2011;154:401–12.

45. Dickstein K, Vardas PE, Auricchio A, et al. 2010 Focused Update of ESC Guidelines on device therapy in heart failure: an update of the 2008 ESC Guidelines for the diagnosis and treatment of acute and chronic heart failure and the 2007 ESC Guidelines for cardiac and resynchronization therapy. Developed with the special contribution of the Heart Failure Association and the European Heart Rhythm Association. Europace. 2010;12:1526–36.

46. Goldenberg I, Moss AJ, Hall WJ, et al. Predictors of response to cardiac resynchronization therapy in the Multicenter Automatic Defibrillator Implantation Trial with Cardiac Resynchronization Therapy (MADIT-CRT). Circulation. 2011;124:1527–36.

47. Chung ES, Leon AR, Tavazzi L, et al. Results of the Predictors of Response to CRT (PROSPECT) trial. Circulation. 2008; 117:2608–16.

48. Dewland TA, Pellegrini CN, Wang Y, et al. Dual-chamber implantable cardioverter-defibrillator selection is associated with increased complication rates and mortality among patients enrolled in the NCDR implantable cardioverter-defibrillator registry. J Am Coll Cardiol. 2011;58:1007–13.

49. Curtis JP, Luebbert JJ, Wang Y, et al. Association of physician certification and outcomes among patients receiving an implantable cardioverter-defibrillator. JAMA. 2009;301:1661–70.

50. Al-Khatib SM, Greiner MA, Peterson ED, et al. Patient and implanting physician factors associated with mortality and complications after implantable cardioverter-defibrillator implantation, 2002–2005. Circ Arrhythm Electrophysiol. 2008;1:240–9.

51. Cabell CH, Heidenreich PA, Chu VH, et al. Increasing rates of cardiac device infections among Medicare beneficiaries: 1990–1999. Am Heart J. 2004;147:582–6.

52. Sohail MR, Uslan DZ, Khan AH, et al. Management and outcome of permanent pacemaker and implantable cardioverter-defibrillator infections. J Am Coll Cardiol. 2007;49:1851–9.

53. Baddour LM, Epstein AE, Erickson CC, et al. Update on cardiovascular implantable electronic device infections and their management: a scientific statement from the American Heart Association. Circulation. 2010;121:458–77.

54. Da Costa A, Kirkorian G, Cucherat M, et al. Antibiotic prophylaxis for permanent pacemaker implantation: a meta-analysis. Circulation. 1998;97:1796–801.

55. Klug D, Balde M, Pavin D, et al. Risk factors related to infections of implanted pacemakers and cardioverter-defibrillators: results of a large prospective study. Circulation. 2007;116:1349–55.

56. Bloom H, Heeke B, Leon A, et al. Renal insufficiency and the risk of infection from pacemaker or defibrillator surgery. Pacing Clin Electrophysiol. 2006;29:142–5.

57. Lekkerkerker JC, van Nieuwkoop C, Trines SA, et al. Risk factors and time delay associated with cardiac device infections: Leiden device registry. Heart. 2009;95:715–20.

58. Al-Khatib SM, Lucas FL, Jollis JG, et al. The relation between patients' outcomes and the volume of cardioverter-defibrillator implantation procedures performed by physicians treating Medicare beneficiaries. J Am Coll Cardiol. 2005;46:1536–40.

59. Haines DE, Wang Y, Curtis J. Implantable cardioverter-defibrillator registry risk score models for acute procedural complications or death after implantable cardioverter-defibrillator implantation. Circulation. 2011;123:2069–76.

60. Daubert JP, Zareba W, Cannom DS, et al. Inappropriate implantable cardioverter-defibrillator shocks in MADIT II: frequency, mechanisms, predictors, and survival impact. J Am Coll Cardiol. 2008;51:1357–65.

61. Poole JE, Johnson GW, Hellkamp AS, et al. Prognostic importance of defibrillator shocks in patients with heart failure. N Engl J Med. 2008;359:1009–17.

62. Larsen GK, Evans J, Lambert WE, et al. Shocks burden and increased mortality in implantable cardioverter-defibrillator patients. Heart Rhythm. 2011;8:1881–6.

63. Raitt MH. Implantable cardioverter-defibrillator shocks: a double-edged sword? J Am Coll Cardiol. 2008;51:1366–8.

64. Dahl CF, Ewy GA, Warner ED, et al. Myocardial necrosis from direct current countershock. Effect of paddle electrode size and time interval between discharges. Circulation. 1974;50:956–61.

65. Barker-Voelz MA, Van Vleet JF, Tacker Jr WA, et al. Alterations induced by a single defibrillating shock applied through a chronically implanted catheter electrode. J Electrocardiol. 1983;16: 167–79.

66. Epstein AE, Kay GN, Plumb VJ, et al. Gross and microscopic pathological changes associated with nonthoracotomy implantable defibrillator leads. Circulation. 1998;98:1517–24.

67. Wathen MS, DeGroot PJ, Sweeney MO, et al. Prospective randomized multicenter trial of empirical antitachycardia pacing versus shocks for spontaneous rapid ventricular tachycardia in patients with implantable cardioverter-defibrillators: Pacing Fast Ventricular Tachycardia Reduces Shock Therapies (PainFREE Rx II) trial results. Circulation. 2004;110:2591–6.

68. Wilkoff BL, Williamson BD, Stern RS, et al. Strategic programming of detection and therapy parameters in implantable cardioverter-defibrillators reduces shocks in primary prevention patients: results from the PREPARE (Primary Prevention Parameters Evaluation) study. J Am Coll Cardiol. 2008;52: 541–50.

69. Mishkin JD, Saxonhouse SJ, Woo GW, et al. Appropriate evaluation and treatment of heart failure patients after implantable cardioverter-defibrillator discharge: time to go beyond the initial shock. J Am Coll Cardiol. 2009;54:1993–2000.

70. Sweeney MO, Sherfesee L, DeGroot PJ, et al. Differences in effects of electrical therapy type for ventricular arrhythmias on mortality in implantable cardioverter-defibrillator patients. Heart Rhythm. 2010;7:353–60.

71. Wilkoff BL, Auricchio A, Brugada J, et al. HRS/EHRA expert consensus on the monitoring of cardiovascular implantable electronic devices (CIEDs): description of techniques, indications, personnel, frequency and ethical considerations. Heart Rhythm. 2008;5: 907–25.

72. Jung W, Rillig A, Birkemeyer R, et al. Advances in remote monitoring of implantable pacemakers, cardioverter defibrillators and cardiac resynchronization therapy systems. J Interv Card Electrophysiol. 2008;23:73–85.

73. Crossley GH, Boyle A, Vitense H, et al. The CONNECT (Clinical Evaluation of Remote Notification to Reduce Time to Clinical Decision) trial: the value of wireless remote monitoring with automatic clinician alerts. J Am Coll Cardiol. 2011;57:1181–9.

74. Varma N, Epstein AE, Irimpen A, et al. Efficacy and safety of automatic remote monitoring for implantable cardioverter-defibrillator follow-up: the Lumos-T Safely Reduces Routine Office Device Follow-up (TRUST) trial. Circulation. 2010;122:325–32.

Part II

Cardiac Problems in Specific Populations

Cardiovascular Disease in Women

18

Lisa Rosenbaum, Shimoli V. Shah, and Malissa J. Wood

Abstract

Cardiovascular disease (CVD) is the leading cause of death among women, causing more annual deaths than cancer, accidents, Alzheimer's disease, and respiratory diseases combined. Recent data suggest that CVD causes approximately one death per minute among women living in the United States. Somewhat surprisingly, although cardiovascular disease claims more women's lives each year than it does for men, women actually have lower rates of both obstructive coronary disease and depressed left ventricular function. Though great strides have been made in reducing the overall burden of cardiovascular disease, the improvement among women has lagged behind that of men, and the prevalence of cardiovascular disease in young women is actually on the rise. A number of differences exist in the effects of risk factors for and the presentation of cardiovascular disease in women. Overall, women are more likely to present without chest pain than men, and mortality in the setting of myocardial infarction is higher among women than similarly aged men, a difference that is particularly pronounced among young women. Despite a lesser burden of obstructive coronary disease, however, women have worse outcomes than men. Women face higher myocardial infarction-related mortality and are more frequently hospitalized for heart failure exacerbations. This disconnect between the burden of obstructive coronary disease and outcomes has led to the recognition that the pathophysiology of coronary disease among women is quite heterogeneous with microvascular dysfunction, a more common explanation than previously recognized. Additional cardiovascular conditions unique to or more common in women include stress cardiomyopathy and cardiovascular disease associated with rheumatologic conditions.

Keywords

Women and heart disease • Takotsubo cardiomyopathy • Stress cardiomyopathy • Autoimmune disorders and cardiovascular disease • Cardiac syndrome X • Microvascular disease • Ischemic heart disease

L. Rosenbaum, MD
Division of Cardiology, University of Pennsylvania,
1200 Walnut Street, Apt 403, Philadelphia, PA 19107, USA
e-mail: lisarose@med.upenn.edu

S.V. Shah, MD
Department of Cardiology,
Washington University School of Medicine – St. Louis/Barnes
Jewish Hospital, 660 S. Euclid Avenue, Campus Box 8086,
St. Louis, MO 63110, USA
e-mail: svshah@dom.wustl.edu

M.J. Wood, MD, FACC, FASE, FAHA (✉)
Department of Medicine/Cardiology,
Harvard/Massachusetts General Hospital,
55 Fruit Street Blake 256, Boston, MA 02114, USA
e-mail: mjwood@partners.org

K. Stergiopoulos, D.L. Brown (eds.), *Evidence-Based Cardiology Consult*,
DOI 10.1007/978-1-4471-4441-0_18, © Springer-Verlag London 2014

Introduction

Cardiovascular disease (CVD) is the leading cause of death among women, causing more deaths each year than cancer, accidents, Alzheimer's disease, and respiratory diseases combined [1]. Indeed, data from 2007 suggest that CVD causes approximately one death per minute among women living in the United States [2]. One in 30 deaths among females is due to breast cancer, whereas 1 in 6.4 is due to heart disease [2].

Though great strides have been made in reducing the overall burden of cardiovascular disease, the improved prognosis among women has lagged behind that of men. Indeed, cardiovascular disease is actually becoming more prevalent among younger women [3]. Overall, women are more likely to present without chest pain than men, and mortality in the setting of myocardial infarction is higher among women than similarly aged men, a difference that is particularly pronounced among young women [4].

Somewhat surprisingly, although cardiovascular disease claims more women's lives each year than it does men's, women actually have lower rates of both obstructive coronary disease and depressed left ventricular (LV) function [5]. Up to 50 % of women who present with chest pain and undergo coronary angiography have normal or only slightly abnormal, coronary arteries, compared to only 17 % of men [6]. Despite a lesser burden of obstructive coronary disease, however, women have worse outcomes than men [7]. Women face higher myocardial infarction (MI)-related mortality and are more frequently hospitalized for heart failure exacerbations [5, 8]. This disconnect, between the burden of obstructive coronary disease and adverse events, has led to the recognition that the pathophysiology of coronary disease among women is quite heterogeneous, with microvascular dysfunction a contributing factor for many.

Ischemic Heart Disease in Women

Epidemiology of Ischemic Heart Disease Among Women

Ischemic heart disease (IHD) affects men and women differently. Though women have a lower burden of obstructive coronary disease than men, women experience greater ischemia-related morbidity and mortality than men. Indeed, women present more frequently with chest pain, are more persistently symptomatic, are more often hospitalized, consume greater healthcare resources, and have higher MI-related mortality and greater rates of heart failure [5, 8]. Given this ostensible disconnect between the burden of obstructive coronary disease and ischemia-related morbidity and mortality, the Women's Ischemia Syndrome Evaluation

(WISE) investigators have proposed the term "Ischemic Heart Disease," rather than "Coronary Heart Disease," to describe the nature of ischemia among women [5]. IHD is inclusive of women with classic obstructive epicardial disease, as well as the subset with ischemia and nonobstructive disease [5].

Risk Factors for Ischemic Heart Disease Among Women

Women's cardiac risk stems from both traditional risk factors, as well as well as gender-specific factors. After their fifth decade, women tend to have higher cholesterol levels than men, and high-density lipoprotein (HDL) tends to drop after menopause [5]. Obesity also affects women disproportionately [9] and is a trend that is still on the rise, with nearly 2 out of 3 women over age 20 overweight or obese [2]. Increasing obesity is also contributing to the growing epidemic of diabetes among women. Diabetes increases women's risk for IHD more than threefold, [10] and, interestingly, diabetic women have higher rates of ischemic heart disease mortality than diabetic men.

Many have also investigated how nontraditional risk factors may affect women. For instance, women have higher levels of the inflammatory marker, C-reactive protein (CRP). Higher levels of high-sensitivity CRP correlate with increasing cardiovascular risk [11]. The WISE investigators also noted the association of altered endogenous hormones with the cardiometabolic syndrome, which includes at least three of the following risk factors: insulin resistance, dyslipidemia (increased triglycerides, low HDL), hypertension, or abdominal obesity [12]. They suggest that risk-factor clustering, in conjunction with higher levels of inflammatory markers, such as CRP, may predispose women to more vascular dysfunction, both in the setting of obstructive and nonobstructive coronary artery disease, creating a distinct IHD phenotype among women [12]. However, these hypotheses warrant further investigation (Fig. 18.1).

Treatment and Outcomes

In current practice, women with IHD are treated the same as men. Nevertheless, given the suggestion of a gender-specific pathophysiology of IHD among women, as well as continued evidence that women experience worse ischemia-related outcomes, novel treatment approaches are clearly needed for women. Indeed, even though it is now widely understood that coronary artery disease (CAD) is not just a man's disease, recent data suggest that women with "stable" CAD have more MIs than men and women with acute coronary syndromes (ACS) have higher mortality than males [13, 14].

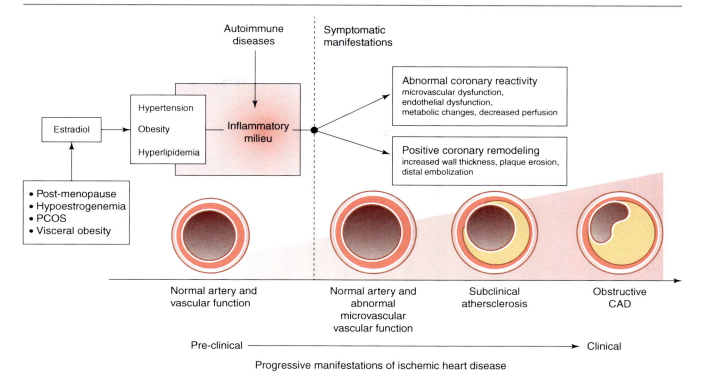

Fig. 18.1 Spectrum of ischemic heart disease in women ranging from normal arterial structure and vascular function to obstructive coronary artery disease (CAD) (Reproduced with permission Shaw et al. [5])

Though there are some data to suggest that evidence-based therapies are underutilized among women with obstructive CAD, this discrepancy alone does not seem to explain the persistent gap in ischemia-related outcomes among women [15]. More likely, the distinct pattern of IHD among women, which remains incompletely understood, requires a different treatment paradigm than the one proven effective for obstructive CAD among men [13].

Cardiac Syndrome X

The term "Cardiac Syndrome X" was coined in 1973 to describe the triad of persistent angina, ischemia on stress-testing, and the absence of obstructive CAD on angiography [16]. Since then, it has become widely recognized that coronary heart disease varies between men and women, both in its underlying pathophysiology, as well as its clinical manifestations. Indeed, one of the most salient differences is that Cardiac Syndrome X (CSX), often now referred to as "microvascular disease," occurs far more commonly among women. The following section will discuss the key features of microvascular disease as it pertains to women, with particular focus upon basic epidemiology, possible etiologies, diagnostic approaches, and treatment paradigms associated with this syndrome.

Epidemiology

Women present frequently with chest pain, but up to 50 % of women who undergo coronary angiography have normal or only slightly abnormal coronary arteries compared to only 17 % of men [6]. Importantly, more than half of women without obstructive CAD continue to have chest pain after coronary angiography [5]. These women were, for many years, assumed to have "noncardiac," chest pain. However it is increasingly recognized that these women likely have true ischemia related to impairment in the coronary microcirculation [17]. Compared to asymptomatic women, women with persistent chest pain in the absence of obstructive disease have a fourfold higher cardiovascular event rate at 5 years than women who remain asymptomatic [18]. These women thus consume more healthcare resources than men owing to more frequent office visits, diagnostic procedures, and therapeutic interventions and hospitalizations [8].

The WISE study was a 3-phase trial initiated in 1996 to broadly investigate IHD among women. Much of the growing understanding of microvascular disease stems from this effort. Women who had undergone coronary angiography as part of their work-up for chest pain syndrome were enrolled; substudies looked particularly at women without obstructive coronary disease to better understand their underlying pathophysiology, as well as to track outcomes over time [6].

It is critical to note that microvascular disease is a heterogeneous disease state whose possible etiologies include abnormal coronary reactivity, altered pain perception, and plaque erosion/distal microembolization [5]. Understandably, women with microvascular disease pose a unique challenge to clinicians, as despite growing knowledge of the potential pathophysiology, little is known about optimal diagnostic and therapeutic strategies.

Pathophysiology of Microvascular Disease

Several studies have examined the role of endothelial dysfunction among women with microvascular disease and suggest that its presence is a marker of increased risk [12]. One study, for instance, studied vasomotor reactivity among women in the WISE study and found that impaired vasomotor response to acetylcholine was associated with adverse cardiovascular outcomes, independent of the degree of CAD [19]. Another study found that patients with CSX also had impaired vasodilatory response, primarily in the microvasculature rather than the epicardial arteries [20].

Several studies have noted [21] endothelium-independent vasoconstriction among women with CSX induced by vasodilators such as adenosine or dipyridamole, suggesting that an impairment in smooth muscle cell relaxation may be contributory. Importantly for these women, many of whom are symptomatic with exercise, some studies have noted that exercise induces vasoconstriction rather than vasodilation. One study, for instance, measured coronary flow ratios among women with both exercise and dipyridamole and noted a subgroup of women with CSX in whom exercise induced distal coronary vasoconstriction and dipyridamole failed to elicit vasodilation [22].

Microvascular dysfunction is thought to contribute to the distinct phenotype of IHD among women. Using intravascular ultrasound (IVUS) to measure plaque burden among both men and women with early CAD, it has been demonstrated that men have significantly greater epicardial atheroma while women exhibit more diffuse disease of the microcirculation [23].

Some have also suggested the role of altered pain perception among women with CSX. Overall, these patients demonstrate greater sensitivity to pain when presented with a number of different stimuli [17]. One group, for instance, assessed stimuli such as cardiac manipulation, pacing, and contrast medium among patients with CSX. They found that CSX patients responded to various stimuli with a much higher rate of their typical chest pain than other patients with chest pain secondary to other forms of CVD [24]. Another study found that 75 % of patients with CSX had abnormal adrenergic cardiac nerve function, suggesting a cardiac origin of chest pain among these patients [25].

The WISE authors emphasize the role of sex-hormone variability, particularly the hypoestrogenemic state, in creating a predisposition to IHD among women [5]. It is thought that estrogen may be cardioprotective, which is thought to explain why women typically develop cardiovascular disease later in life. Estrogen stimulates production of HDL and decreases low-density lipoprotein (LDL) by stimulating reverse cholesterol transport [17]. Menopause thus induces a state of risk-factor clustering in which many women develop obesity, hyperlipidemia, and hypertension [7].

This hypoestrogenemic state has also been directly linked to the abnormal vasoreactivity seen in some women with microvascular angina. One study, for instance, demonstrated that among 15 postmenopausal women with CSX, 14 exhibited vasoconstriction upon receiving acetylcholine. After 24 h of an estrogen patch, coronary reactivity testing was again preformed and 12 women then demonstrated a vasodilatory response [26]. The WISE investigators suggest that vascular dysfunction, in the absence of obstructive disease, is more common in women than among men, secondary to this sex-hormone variability [12]. The investigators also postulate that this vascular dysfunction confers a greater risk even among women with obstructive CAD, who have more persistent symptoms post-revascularization [12].

Presentation

Although much effort has been expended to differentiate the angina of CSX from the chest pain of an obstructive stenosis, there are no convincing data to suggest a difference exists. One recent study, for instance, recruited 305 patients who had been referred for non-emergent percutaneous coronary intervention (PCI) and used balloon inflation to induce symptoms of ischemia. There were no sex differences in rates of chest pain or typical ischemic discomfort, though women did note a higher rate of jaw pain. Some have also observed that women with CSX with effort angina have symptoms that persist several minutes beyond the cessation of exercise and are less likely to respond to nitroglycerin [21, 27].

Diagnosis

Microvascular disease is a diagnosis of exclusion. Only after coronary angiography has been performed to rule out obstructive CAD should the diagnosis of CSX be given to patients with ischemia and persistent angina. WISE study investigators noted that the paradigm of using diagnostic tools to seek the "culprit" lesion among women with microvascular disease is misguided. They advocate an approach that uses noninvasive testing to provide independent prognostic information [12]. Accurate risk assessment is possible within our existing armamentarium, but distinct attention must be paid to functional capacity, plaque burden, extent and severity of perfusion abnormalities, global ventricular function measurements, and inflammatory markers [12]. They also note that prediction models may additionally be strengthened by the inclusion of left ventricular hypertrophy because it confers a greater mortality risk among women than among men [28]. However, there are no data at this juncture to support the use of any of these markers as a means to improve outcomes.

Regarding diagnostic testing, it is critical to note that what we have long referred to as "false-positive" tests among women with chest pain and ischemic findings on exercise testing, but no obstructive coronary disease, may indeed be true myocardial ischemia [29]. Though breast artifact is often given as an explanation for false-positive results among women, it is not appropriate to label perfusion abnormalities in the setting of nonobstructive CAD as false positives in women if accompanied by objective signs of ischemia, such as chest pain, electrocardiographic abnormalities, or reduced functional capacity [5].

Existing imaging modalities can also be falsely negative among women with CSX [17]. For instance, wall motion abnormalities are often absent among women with chest pain and normal coronary arteries who have demonstrated ischemia on exercise treadmill testing [30]. Dobutamine stress echo has also been observed to be normal among women with microvascular or endothelial dysfunction [31–33]. Some have thus suggested that either ischemia is not operative in CSX or that our current methods of detection are not sensitive enough to detect smaller perfusion abnormalities that may exist [17].

Although the optimal stress imaging method among women with microvascular disease is unknown, much prognostic information can be gleaned from exercise testing. The Duke Treadmill score, which incorporates exercise capacity and degree of ST-segment depression, accurately predicts IHD-related morality among women [5]. One study of over 5,000 asymptomatic women found that for every unit increase in the Duke Treadmill score, mortality rate increased by 9 %, whereas every additional metabolic equivalent (MET) of exercise capacity decreased mortality by 17 % [18].

Treatment

In the absence of a data-driven treatment paradigm and because CSX appears to be a heterogeneous disease state, risk-factor modification and symptom control are the mainstays of therapy. All women should receive typical risk-factor management with attention paid to blood pressure, body mass index, lipids, diabetes, diet, exercise, and smoking cessation in accordance with the recommendations of the ACC/AHA

guidelines for prevention of cardiovascular disease in women. The recommended goals for ideal cardiovascular health in women include blood pressure <120/80 mmHg, body mass index <25 kg/m^2, fasting total cholesterol <200 mg/dL, fasting blood glucose <100 mg/dL, adherence to the Dietary Approaches to Stop Hypertension – like eating pattern – participation in physical activity at recommended levels (150 min per week), and abstinence from smoking.

Symptom management often proves challenging. Calcium channel blockers have not consistently proven effective in reducing symptoms, and there are no data to suggest that they improve coronary flow reserve [5, 17]. Nitrates, the mainstay of therapy for classic angina, seem less effective in this cohort [27]. Beta-blockers have the most demonstrated efficacy for the relief of chest pain among these patients and are recommended as first line therapy [5, 34]. Notably, no large randomized trials have been conducted among patients with CSX to demonstrate the ideal therapy for either optimal symptom management or improving long-term outcomes.

Some authors recommend the addition of imipramine to address the component of abnormal nocioception [17]. One study found that imipramine reduced angina without improving quality of life among 18 women with CSX who had failed conventional antianginal therapies [35]. Some also recommend therapies such as angiotensin-converting enzyme (ACE) inhibitors and statins which can improve exercise duration via nitric oxide-mediated improvements in coronary flow reserve [17, 36, 37]. Finally, although estrogen improves endothelial function, given the increased risk for cardiovascular events conferred by hormone replacement therapy (HRT), as well as a paucity of data on HRT among women with CSX, HRT is not recommended [17].

Heart Failure in Women

Heart failure (HF) is a major cause of cardiovascular morbidity and mortality. Women affected by heart failure demonstrate distinct differences compared to men. Women are more likely to have nonischemic cardiomyopathies, valvular heart disease, hypertension, and left bundle branch block [38]. Women are also more likely than men to present at an older age, to have heart failure with preserved ejection fraction (HFPEF) [39], and less likely to die from heart failure compared to men [39, 40]. Women appear to respond more favorably to treatment with beta-blockers and cardiac resynchronization than men but have a worse prognosis with digoxin therapy and lower survival with implantable defibrillators. Women with symptomatic systolic heart failure derive a significant mortality benefit from spironolactone or eplerenone [41, 42]. While women with systolic dysfunction appear to derive a mortality benefit from ACE inhibitors, there is a greater mortality reduction in men. Since women were not included in the early studies of ACE-inhibition in systolic dysfunction, this attenuated benefit may partially reflect the smaller numbers of women studied [43].

While men and women with New York Heart Association (NYHA) class III and IV heart failure, LV systolic dysfunction, and a wide QRS interval derive similar benefits from cardiac resynchronization therapy (CRT) in reduction in hospitalization and all-cause mortality, the Providing Regional Observations to Study Predictors of Events in the Coronary Tree (PROSPECT) study found that women had a greater reduction in LV volumes than men [44]. In the Multicenter Autonomic Defibrillator Implantation Trial – Cardiac Resynchronization Therapy (MADIT-CRT) study, women with nonischemic cardiomyopathy experienced a reduction in risk of heart failure, death, or both and fewer heart failure events than do men following CRT [45]. Gender-specific forms of systolic dysfunction include Takotsubo cardiomyopathy and peripartum cardiomyopathy.

Takostubo Cardiomyopathy

Takotsubo cardiomyopathy (TC) was first reported in Japan [46]. It is named after the Japanese octopus fishing pot or "tako-tsubo," which has a characteristic narrow neck and wide bottom. In its classic form, TC is associated with regional systolic dysfunction of the mid- and apical LV and hyperkinesis of the basal segments. It is also known as stress cardiomyopathy (SC) or apical ballooning syndrome (ABS). The clinical features, which strongly mimic an acute MI but without evidence of obstructive coronary disease, include evidence of chest pain, ST-segment elevation, cardiac biomarker release, and LV dysfunction [47, 48]. TC is more prevalent in postmenopausal women following a period of extreme emotional or physical stress.

Pathophysiology

Proposed mechanisms underlying TC include catecholamine-mediated cardiotoxicity, coronary vasospasm, and coronary microvascular dysfunction. In one of the largest prospective cohort studies to date ($n = 130$), 89 % of cases of TC were precipitated by intensely stressful emotional or physical events [49]. Elevated plasma catecholamine levels have been invoked as a cause of TC. One prospective study of 19

patients presenting with TC due to emotional stress found elevated plasma catecholamine and metanephrine levels compared to controls presenting with an acute MI.

Increased sympathetic tone with transient epicardial or microvascular vasospasm has been proposed as a mechanism for TC [50]. However, the data is limited. Several small studies have shown evidence of coronary artery spasm occurring spontaneously or after provocative testing with acetylcholine or ergonovine in patients with TC [50–52]. Thrombolysis in Myocardial Infarction (TIMI) frame counts on coronary angiography in 16 women with TC were significantly higher than in control patients which suggests increased coronary microvascular resistance in patients with TC [53]. Further studies are needed to delineate whether epicardial or microvascular coronary alterations play a role in the pathogenesis of TC.

Direct catecholamine-induced myocyte injury has also been suggested as an underlying mechanism of TC. Endomyocardial biopsy specimens examined by light and electron microscopy and immunohistochemistry show evidence of reversible changes which include hypertrophied, glycogen-rich myocytes filled with cellular debris with increased areas of fibrosis and accumulation of mononuclear lymphocytes [54]. Several other studies have reported similar findings [55, 56].

Diagnosis

There is no general consensus on the diagnostic criteria for TC. A systematic review of 7 case series showed a higher incidence in postmenopausal (mean age 62–75) females (range 82–100 %) [47]. Symptoms can be difficult to distinguish from an ACS and include chest pain at rest, dyspnea, ST-segment elevation on electrocardiogram (ECG), and a rise in cardiac biomarkers [49]. An emotional or physical stressful event precedes the onset of TC in a majority of patients [57] (Table 18.1).

A prospective study of 59 women with TC found that anterior ST-segment elevation (STE) is the most common acute abnormality on ECG (56 %) and is often accompanied by pathologic Q waves. The amplitude of STE is less than in those with acute anterior MI and reciprocal changes may be absent [57, 58]. In those without STE, diffuse T-wave inversions (TWI) are the next most common finding on presentation [49, 58]. ECG changes during the recovery phase of TC

Table 18.1 Clinical features distinguishing Takotsubo cardiomyopathy (TC) from acute myocardial infarction (AMI) and myocarditis

	Chest pan	Troponin	Wall motion	Recovery
TC	+	+	Hypokinesis to akinesis involving multiple coronary territories (Predilection for mid- and apical segments)	Usually complete within weeks to months
AMI	+	+	Distinct wall motion abnormalities confined to specific coronary artery distributions	Unlikely to occur in the absence of coronary revascularization
Myocarditis	+/–	+/–	Subtle or diffuse	Possible

(i.e., the period in which LV function normalizes) can include diffuse TWI (regardless of presenting ECG) and prolongation of the QT_c [58].

A rise in cardiac troponins is seen in most patients with TC and can occur within 24 h of symptom onset. Biomarker elevation is typically less than patients with acute MI [59–61].

The Mayo Clinic has proposed criteria for the diagnosis of TC: (1) transient hypokinesis, akinesis, or dyskinesis of the LV extending beyond a single epicardial vascular distribution; (2) no evidence of obstructive coronary disease or an acute plaque rupture; (3) new ECG abnormalities or modest elevation in cardiac troponin; and (4) no evidence of pheochromocytoma or myocarditis [56, 60]. The absence of obstructive coronary disease on cardiac catheterization is a hallmark feature of TC [60]. Left ventriculography shows wall motion abnormalities that do not correspond to a single major epicardial coronary distribution. The most common pattern is systolic dysfunction of the mid-ventricle and apex with sparing of the base (Figs. 18.2 and 18.3). However, additional patterns have also been described [56].Two studies of cardiac magnetic resonance imaging in patients with TC have shown mid- and apical LV involvement as well as cases of isolated apical, mid-, or basal ballooning. Biventricular involvement has also been reported [49, 62, 63].

Most cases of LV dysfunction associated with TC are reversible. However, a retrospective study of 100 patients with TC followed for 4.4 years demonstrated a recurrence rate of 11.4 %. Four-year survival was no different in patients with TC compared to an age- and gender-matched population [64]. Short- and long-term follow-up of patients with TC should include surveillance echocardiography to assess LV function.

Cardiovascular Risk in Women with Autoimmune Disease

In 1976, a seminal study was published describing the bimodal distribution of death among patients with systemic lupus erythematosus (SLE). Those who die early after diagnosis typically die of active SLE and its associated complications; those who died later in the course of their disease died of cardiovascular disease [65]. This observation paved the way for the now widespread recognition of the increased risk of cardiovascular disease conferred by autoimmune diseases such as SLE and rheumatoid arthritis (RA). The following section will describe the general epidemiology of cardiovascular risk among patients with SLE and RA, possible pathophysiology, and existing diagnostic and treatment recommendations. For the purposes of discussion, the diseases will be considered simultaneously unless explicitly stated otherwise.

Epidemiology

Though the treatment of autoimmune disease has substantially improved in the last several decades, the mortality associated with cardiovascular risk has persisted. In contrast to earlier studies, contemporary studies suggest that cardiovascular disease now accounts for a substantial portion of the

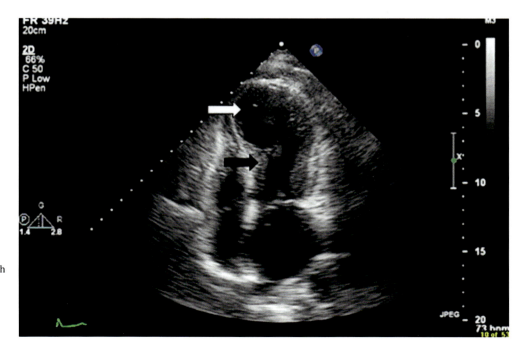

Fig. 18.2 Transthoracic echocardiogram with apical four-chamber view of patient with Takotsubo at end-systole demonstrating apical ballooning (*white arrow* with preserved contractility of the base of the heart (*black arrow*)

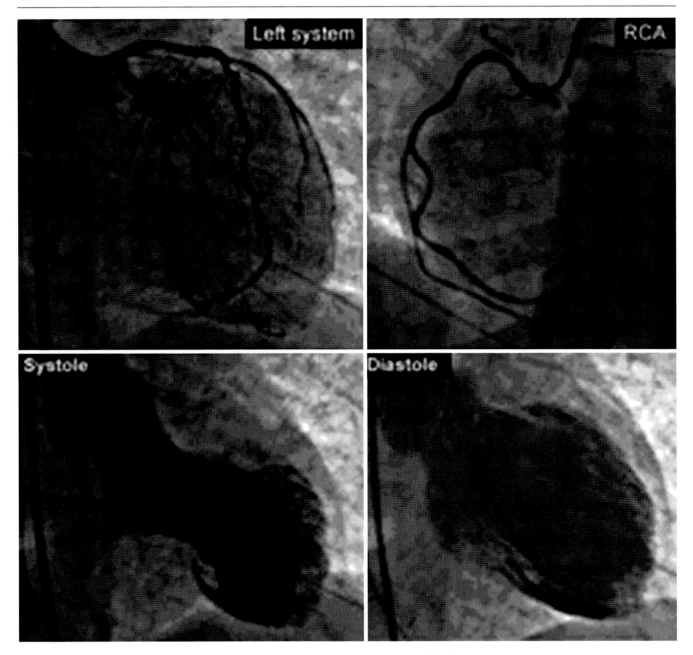

Fig. 18.3 Normal coronary angiography and apical ballooning with hypercontractile basal myocardium on left ventriculography (Reproduced with permission, Bybee and Prasad [56])

early mortality associated with these diseases [66–68]. Patients with lupus are five times more likely to have an MI than the general population [69]. Furthermore, cardiovascular risk exists even among patients with subclinical autoimmune disease, such as those with only a positive rheumatoid factor [66].

Estimates of the excess cardiovascular risk conferred by autoimmune disease differ. Recent prospective data from the Nurses Health Study suggests that women with SLE have a greater than twofold increased risk of cardiovascular disease [70]. One study, for example, looked at a cohort of women with lupus and compared them to age-matched controls and found that women between the ages of 35 and 44 with lupus were more than 50 times more likely to have an MI [69].

Patients with RA are also at increased risk of cardiovascular events. Data from the Nurses Health Study suggest that the risk of cardiovascular disease among women with RA is twice that of those without RA. Moreover, women who had had RA for at least 10 years had a threefold higher rate of MI [71]. This observation is consistent with the general finding from several studies that the longer the duration of disease, the greater the cardiovascular risk.

Pathophysiology

Historically it was believed that the increased cardiovascular risk seen in autoimmune disease was due to an increased prevalence of traditional risk factors, which were all exacerbated by corticosteroid therapy. Indeed, data suggest that SLE patients have higher rates of traditional cardiovascular risk factors, such as hyperlipidemia and hypertension, at a younger age [72, 73]. However, epidemiologic data also suggest that the associated risk exceeds that conferred by the burden of traditional risk factors alone [74]. Moreover, it has become clear that the more active the disease, the higher the cardiovascular risk [75]. Thus, although corticosteroids exacerbate insulin resistance, data suggest that active disease is more deleterious to patients' cardiovascular risk than corticosteroids themselves [76].

Given that traditional risk factors do not fully account for the degree of cardiovascular risk conferred by both SLE and RA, many have investigated the role of inflammation in accelerating the development of atherosclerosis. The coronary calcium score, a marker for atherosclerosis, is increased at a younger age in asymptomatic lupus patients [77]. On carotid ultrasound, patients with lupus are more likely to have atherosclerosis. This risk did not appear to be associated with corticosteroid therapy, as those with less aggressive treatment actually had a higher risk of carotid atherosclerosis [76]. Both studies suggest a prevalence of atherosclerosis around 33 % among women under 50 with SLE. These studies lend credence to the hypothesis that some of the additional risk associated with these diseases stems from accelerated atherosclerosis.

Diagnosis

Despite the recognition that women with both SLE and RA have a higher prevalence and early onset of atherosclerosis, there is no evidence to suggest that screening these patients with coronary calcium scoring or carotid ultrasound improves outcomes. Thus, screening asymptomatic patients for subclinical atherosclerosis is not recommended at this time. For patients with symptoms, the diagnostic approach and the use of imaging should mirror that of patients without autoimmune disease. However, physicians should retain a high index of suspicion for coronary disease among these patients who often have many other reasons to have shortness of breath or chest pain.

Management

Tremendous controversy exists regarding the optimal approach to cardiovascular risk reduction among patients with RA and SLE. In the absence of robust outcomes data, the cornerstone of prevention and treatment is aggressive risk factor modification, as well as treatment of the underlying autoimmune disease.

Both statins and ACE inhibitors have known anti-inflammatory properties. Treatment of RA patients with atorvastatin results in reduced disease activity, as well as a decrease in CRP, which is a cardiovascular risk marker [78–80]. In SLE patients, atorvastatin improves endothelin-dependent vasodilation in the brachial artery [81]. Given that risk factor control is often predicated upon scoring models that do not take these diseases into account, some experts suggest that risk assessment incorporate markers of risk specific to these diseases. For instance, the European League Against Rheumatism (EULAR) recommends multiplying risk by 1.5 for RA patients who have at least two of the following: disease duration of more than 10 years, rheumatoid factor or anti-CCP positivity, or the presence of certain extra-articular manifestations which typify more severe disease [82, 83]. For patients who are hypertensive with RA, EULAR recommends the use of ACE inhibitors or angiotensin-receptor blockers given their anti-inflammatory activity [82].

In both SLE and RA, it is now clear that it is the disease itself, rather than the treatment, that contributes to premature atherosclerosis. For instance, among patients with SLE, those treated with lower doses of steroids, cyclophosphamide, or azathioprine have accelerated atherosclerosis progression [84, 85]. Although antimalarial agents, which have a favorable effect on risk factors such as glucose tolerance and lipid profiles, should theoretically mitigate cardiovascular risk, this benefit has not been demonstrated in randomized trials [84].

The emphasis upon treatment of disease activity to prevent cardiovascular disease is similar for RA. EULAR emphasizes the importance of early treatment and suggests that both methotrexate and antitumor necrosis factor agents are independently associated with a decreased cardiovascular risk. One issue of particular importance for patients with RA is the safety of nonsteroidal anti-inflammatory drugs (NSAIDs), particularly the use of selective (cyclo-oxygenase) COX-2 inhibitors, such as celecoxib, which have been shown to increase the risk of cardiovascular disease [86]. There is no consensus regarding the use of NSAIDs or selective COX-2 inhibitors. Nevertheless, it is clear that as a class COX-2 inhibitors increase cardiovascular risk [87].

Key Points

- Coronary heart disease affects men and women differently with women being more likely to have ischemia, persistent chest pain, and nonobstructive coronary disease.

- Women are more likely than men to present *without* chest pain, and mortality in the setting of MI is higher among women than similarly aged men, a difference that is particularly pronounced among young women.

- Cardiac syndrome X, or microvascular disease, presents unique diagnostic and management challenges for clinicians with possible etiologies including endothelial dysfunction and abnormal coronary reactivity which are likely potentiated by the female hormonal milieu. Therapy focuses on risk-factor modification and symptom management.

- Both SLE and RA confer a markedly increased risk of cardiovascular disease.

- The risk is related to an increased prevalence of traditional risk factors as well as a distinct predisposition to premature atherosclerosis conferred by the disease itself.

- The cornerstone of management is aggressive treatment of risk factors and the underlying disease.

References

1. Lloyd-Jones D, Adams RJ, Brown TM, et al. Heart disease and stroke statistics–2010 update: a report from the American Heart Association. Circulation. 2010;121(7):e46–215.
2. Roger VL, Go AS, Lloyd-Jones DM, et al. Heart disease and stroke statistics–2011 update: a report from the American Heart Association. Circulation. 2011;123(4):e18–209.
3. Ford ES, Capewell S. Coronary heart disease mortality among young adults in the U.S. from 1980 through 2002: concealed leveling of mortality rates. J Am Coll Cardiol. 2007;50(22):2128–32.
4. Canto JG, Rogers WJ, Goldberg RJ, et al. Association of age and sex with myocardial infarction symptom presentation and in-hospital mortality. JAMA. 2012;307(8):813–22.
5. Shaw LJ, Bugiardini R, Merz CN. Women and ischemic heart disease: evolving knowledge. J Am Coll Cardiol. 2009;54(17):1561–75.
6. Merz CN, Kelsey SF, Pepine CJ, et al. The Women's Ischemia Syndrome Evaluation (WISE) study: protocol design, methodology and feasibility report. J Am Coll Cardiol. 1999;33(6):1453–61.
7. Shaw LJ, Bairey Merz CN, Pepine CJ, et al. Insights from the NHLBI-Sponsored Women's Ischemia Syndrome Evaluation (WISE) Study: part I: gender differences in traditional and novel risk factors, symptom evaluation, and gender-optimized diagnostic strategies. J Am Coll Cardiol. 2006;47(3 Suppl):S4–20.
8. Shaw LJ, Merz CN, Pepine CJ, et al. The economic burden of angina in women with suspected ischemic heart disease: results from the National Institutes of Health–National Heart, Lung, and Blood Institute–sponsored Women's Ischemia Syndrome Evaluation. Circulation. 2006;114(9):894–904.
9. Mokdad AH, Bowman BA, Ford ES, Vinicor F, Marks JS, Koplan JP. The continuing epidemics of obesity and diabetes in the United States. JAMA. 2001;286(10):1195–200.
10. Spencer EA, Pirie KL, Stevens RJ, et al. Diabetes and modifiable risk factors for cardiovascular disease: the prospective Million Women Study. Eur J Epidemiol. 2008;23(12):793–9.
11. Ridker PM, Buring JE, Shih J, Matias M, Hennekens CH. Prospective study of C-reactive protein and the risk of future cardiovascular events among apparently healthy women. Circulation. 1998;98(8):731–3.
12. Bairey Merz CN, Shaw LJ, Reis SE, et al. Insights from the NHLBI-Sponsored Women's Ischemia Syndrome Evaluation (WISE) Study: part II: gender differences in presentation, diagnosis, and outcome with regard to gender-based pathophysiology of atherosclerosis and macrovascular and microvascular coronary disease. J Am Coll Cardiol. 2006;47(3 Suppl):S21–9.
13. Merz CN. The Yentl syndrome is alive and well. Eur Heart J. 2011;32(11):1313–5.
14. Bugiardini R, Yan AT, Yan RT, et al. Factors influencing underutilization of evidence-based therapies in women. Eur Heart J. 2011;32(11):1337–44.
15. Blomkalns AL, Chen AY, Hochman JS, et al. Gender disparities in the diagnosis and treatment of non-ST-segment elevation acute coronary syndromes: large-scale observations from the CRUSADE (Can Rapid Risk Stratification of Unstable Angina Patients Suppress Adverse Outcomes with Early Implementation of the American College of Cardiology/American Heart Association Guidelines) National Quality Improvement Initiative. J Am Coll Cardiol. 2005;45(6):832–7.
16. Kemp Jr HG. Left ventricular function in patients with the anginal syndrome and normal coronary arteriograms. Am J Cardiol. 1973;32(3):375–6.
17. Nugent L, Mehta PK, Bairey Merz CN. Gender and microvascular angina. J Thromb Thrombolysis. 2011;31(1):37–46.
18. Gulati M, Cooper-DeHoff RM, McClure C, et al. Adverse cardiovascular outcomes in women with nonobstructive coronary artery disease: a report from the Women's Ischemia Syndrome Evaluation Study and the St James Women Take Heart Project. Arch Intern Med. 2009;169(9):843–50.
19. von Mering GO, Arant CB, Wessel TR, et al. Abnormal coronary vasomotion as a prognostic indicator of cardiovascular events in women: results from the National Heart, Lung, and Blood Institute-Sponsored Women's Ischemia Syndrome Evaluation (WISE). Circulation. 2004;109(6):722–5.
20. Egashira K, Inou T, Hirooka Y, Yamada A, Urabe Y, Takeshita A. Evidence of impaired endothelium-dependent coronary vasodilatation in patients with angina pectoris and normal coronary angiograms. N Engl J Med. 1993;328(23):1659–64.
21. Lanza GA, Crea F. Primary coronary microvascular dysfunction: clinical presentation, pathophysiology, and management. Circulation. 2010;121(21):2317–25.
22. Bortone AS, Hess OM, Eberli FR, et al. Abnormal coronary vasomotion during exercise in patients with normal coronary arteries and reduced coronary flow reserve. Circulation. 1989;79(3):516–27.
23. Han SH, Bae JH, Holmes Jr DR, et al. Sex differences in atheroma burden and endothelial function in patients with early coronary atherosclerosis. Eur Heart J. 2008;29(11):1359–69.
24. Cannon RO 3rd, Quyyumi AA, Schenke WH, Fananapazir L, Tucker EE, Gaughan AM, Gracely RH, et al. Abnormal cardiac sensitivity in patients with chest pain and normal coronary arteries. Pain. 1990;16:1359–66.
25. Lanza GA, Giordano A, Pristipino C, et al. Abnormal cardiac adrenergic nerve function in patients with syndrome X detected by [123I] metaiodobenzylguanidine myocardial scintigraphy. Circulation. 1997;96(3):821–6.

26. Roque M, Heras M, Roig E, et al. Short-term effects of transdermal estrogen replacement therapy on coronary vascular reactivity in postmenopausal women with angina pectoris and normal results on coronary angiograms. J Am Coll Cardiol. 1998;31(1):139–43.

27. Kaski JC, Rosano GM, Collins P, Nihoyannopoulos P, Maseri A, Poole-Wilson PA. Cardiac syndrome X: clinical characteristics and left ventricular function. Long-term follow-up study. J Am Coll Cardiol. 1995;25(4):807–14.

28. East MA, Jollis JG, Nelson CL, Marks D, Peterson ED. The influence of left ventricular hypertrophy on survival in patients with coronary artery disease: do race and gender matter? J Am Coll Cardiol. 2003;41(6):949–54.

29. Bugiardini R, Bairey Merz CN. Angina with "normal" coronary arteries: a changing philosophy. JAMA. 2005;293(4):477–84.

30. Nihoyannopoulos P, Kaski JC, Crake T, Maseri A. Absence of myocardial dysfunction during stress in patients with syndrome X. J Am Coll Cardiol. 1991;18(6):1463–70.

31. Lewis JF, Lin L, McGorray S, et al. Dobutamine stress echocardiography in women with chest pain. Pilot phase data from the National Heart, Lung and Blood Institute Women's Ischemia Syndrome Evaluation (WISE). J Am Coll Cardiol. 1999;33(6):1462–8.

32. Panting JR, Gatehouse PD, Yang GZ, et al. Abnormal subendocardial perfusion in cardiac syndrome X detected by cardiovascular magnetic resonance imaging. N Engl J Med. 2002;346(25):1948–53.

33. Vermeltfoort IA, Bondarenko O, Raijmakers PG, et al. Is subendocardial ischaemia present in patients with chest pain and normal coronary angiograms? A cardiovascular MR study. Eur Heart J. 2007;28(13):1554–8.

34. Lanza GA, Colonna G, Pasceri V, Maseri A. Atenolol versus amlodipine versus isosorbide-5-mononitrate on anginal symptoms in syndrome X. Am J Cardiol. 1999;84(7):854–6, A8.

35. Cox ID, Hann CM, Kaski JC. Low dose imipramine improves chest pain but not quality of life in patients with angina and normal coronary angiograms. Eur Heart J. 1998;19(2):250–4.

36. Pizzi C, Manfrini O, Fontana F, Bugiardini R. Angiotensin-converting enzyme inhibitors and 3-hydroxy-3-methylglutaryl coenzyme A reductase in cardiac Syndrome X: role of superoxide dismutase activity. Circulation. 2004;109(1):53–8.

37. Kayikcioglu M, Payzin S, Yavuzgil O, Kultursay H, Can LH, Soydan I. Benefits of statin treatment in cardiac syndrome-X1. Eur Heart J. 2003;24(22):1999–2005.

38. Barsheshet A, Brenyo A, Goldenberg I, Moss AJ. Sex-related differences in patients' responses to heart failure therapy. Nat Rev Cardiol. 2012;9(4):234–42.

39. Levy D, Kenchaiah S, Larson MG, et al. Long-term trends in the incidence of and survival with heart failure. N Engl J Med. 2002;347(18):1397–402.

40. Redfield MM, Jacobsen SJ, Burnett Jr JC, Mahoney DW, Bailey KR, Rodeheffer RJ. Burden of systolic and diastolic ventricular dysfunction in the community: appreciating the scope of the heart failure epidemic. JAMA. 2003;289(2):194–202.

41. Pitt B, Remme W, Zannad F, et al. Eplerenone, a selective aldosterone blocker, in patients with left ventricular dysfunction after myocardial infarction. N Engl J Med. 2003;348(14):1309–21.

42. Pitt B, Zannad F, Remme WJ, et al. The effect of spironolactone on morbidity and mortality in patients with severe heart failure. Randomized Aldactone Evaluation Study Investigators. N Engl J Med. 1999;341(10):709–17.

43. Shekelle PG, Rich MW, Morton SC, et al. Efficacy of angiotensin-converting enzyme inhibitors and beta-blockers in the management of left ventricular systolic dysfunction according to race, gender, and diabetic status: a meta-analysis of major clinical trials. J Am Coll Cardiol. 2003;41(9):1529–38.

44. Chung ES, Leon AR, Tavazzi L, et al. Results of the Predictors of Response to CRT (PROSPECT) trial. Circulation. 2008;117(20):2608–16.

45. Arshad A, Moss AJ, Foster E, et al. Cardiac resynchronization therapy is more effective in women than in men: the MADIT-CRT (Multicenter Automatic Defibrillator Implantation Trial with Cardiac Resynchronization Therapy) trial. J Am Coll Cardiol. 2011;57(7):813–20.

46. Dote K, Sato H, Tateishi H, Uchida T, Ishihara M. [Myocardial stunning due to simultaneous multivessel coronary spasms: a review of 5 cases]. J Cardiol. 1991;21(2):203–14.

47. Bybee KA, Kara T, Prasad A, et al. Systematic review: transient left ventricular apical ballooning: a syndrome that mimics ST-segment elevation myocardial infarction. Ann Intern Med. 2004;141(11):858–65.

48. Akashi YJ, Goldstein DS, Barbaro G, Ueyama T. Takotsubo cardiomyopathy: a new form of acute, reversible heart failure. Circulation. 2008;118(25):2754–62.

49. Sharkey SW, Windenburg DC, Lesser JR, et al. Natural history and expansive clinical profile of stress (tako-tsubo) cardiomyopathy. J Am Coll Cardiol. 2010;55(4):333–41.

50. Lacy CR, Contrada RJ, Robbins ML, et al. Coronary vasoconstriction induced by mental stress (simulated public speaking). Am J Cardiol. 1995;75(7):503–5.

51. Kurisu S, Sato H, Kawagoe T, et al. Tako-tsubo-like left ventricular dysfunction with ST-segment elevation: a novel cardiac syndrome mimicking acute myocardial infarction. Am Heart J. 2002;143(3):448–55.

52. Abe Y, Kondo M, Matsuoka R, Araki M, Dohyama K, Tanio H. Assessment of clinical features in transient left ventricular apical ballooning. J Am Coll Cardiol. 2003;41(5):737–42.

53. Bybee KA, Prasad A, Barsness GW, et al. Clinical characteristics and thrombolysis in myocardial infarction frame counts in women with transient left ventricular apical ballooning syndrome. Am J Cardiol. 2004;94(3):343–6.

54. Nef HM, Mollmann H, Kostin S, et al. Tako-Tsubo cardiomyopathy: intraindividual structural analysis in the acute phase and after functional recovery. Eur Heart J. 2007;28(20):2456–64.

55. Wittstein IS, Thiemann DR, Lima JA, et al. Neurohumoral features of myocardial stunning due to sudden emotional stress. N Engl J Med. 2005;352(6):539–48.

56. Bybee KA, Prasad A. Stress-related cardiomyopathy syndromes. Circulation. 2008;118(4):397–409.

57. Ogura R, Hiasa Y, Takahashi T, et al. Specific findings of the standard 12-lead ECG in patients with 'Takotsubo' cardiomyopathy: comparison with the findings of acute anterior myocardial infarction. Circ J. 2003;67(8):687–90.

58. Sharkey SW, Lesser JR, Menon M, Parpart M, Maron MS, Maron BJ. Spectrum and significance of electrocardiographic patterns, troponin levels, and thrombolysis in myocardial infarction frame count in patients with stress (tako-tsubo) cardiomyopathy and comparison to those in patients with ST-elevation anterior wall myocardial infarction. Am J Cardiol. 2008;101(12):1723–8.

59. Madhavan M, Borlaug BA, Lerman A, Rihal CS, Prasad A. Stress hormone and circulating biomarker profile of apical ballooning syndrome (Takotsubo cardiomyopathy): insights into the clinical significance of B-type natriuretic peptide and troponin levels. Heart (British Cardiac Society). 2009;95(17):1436–41.

60. Prasad A, Lerman A, Rihal CS. Apical ballooning syndrome (Tako-Tsubo or stress cardiomyopathy): a mimic of acute myocardial infarction. Am Heart J. 2008;155(3):408–17.

61. Sharkey SW, Lesser JR, Zenovich AG, et al. Acute and reversible cardiomyopathy provoked by stress in women from the United States. Circulation. 2005;111(4):472–9.

62. Eitel I, von Knobelsdorff-Brenkenhoff F, Bernhardt P, et al. Clinical characteristics and cardiovascular magnetic resonance findings in stress (takotsubo) cardiomyopathy. JAMA. 2011;306(3):277–86.

63. Haghi D, Roehm S, Hamm K, et al. Takotsubo cardiomyopathy is not due to plaque rupture: an intravascular ultrasound study. Clin Cardiol. 2010;33(5):307–10.

64. Elesber AA, Prasad A, Lennon RJ, Wright RS, Lerman A, Rihal CS. Four-year recurrence rate and prognosis of the apical ballooning syndrome. J Am Coll Cardiol. 2007;50(5):448–52.

65. Urowitz MB, Bookman AA, Koehler BE, Gordon DA, Smythe HA, Ogryzlo MA. The bimodal mortality pattern of systemic lupus erythematosus. Am J Med. 1976;60(2):221–5.

66. Goodson N, Symmons D. Rheumatoid arthritis in women: still associated with an increased mortality. Ann Rheum Dis. 2002;61(11):955–6.

67. Kaplan MJ. Cardiovascular complications of rheumatoid arthritis: assessment, prevention, and treatment. Rheum Dis Clin North Am. 2010;36(2):405–26.

68. Bernatsky S, Boivin JF, Joseph L, et al. Mortality in systemic lupus erythematosus. Arthritis Rheum. 2006;54(8):2550–7.

69. Manzi S, Meilahn EN, Rairie JE, et al. Age-specific incidence rates of myocardial infarction and angina in women with systemic lupus erythematosus: comparison with the Framingham Study. Am J Epidemiol. 1997;145(5):408–15.

70. Hak AE, Karlson EW, Feskanich D, Stampfer MJ, Costenbader KH. Systemic lupus erythematosus and the risk of cardiovascular disease: results from the nurses' health study. Arthritis Rheum. 2009;61(10):1396–402.

71. Solomon DH, Karlson EW, Rimm EB, et al. Cardiovascular morbidity and mortality in women diagnosed with rheumatoid arthritis. Circulation. 2003;107(9):1303–7.

72. Skamra C, Ramsey-Goldman R. Management of cardiovascular complications in systemic lupus erythematosus. Int J Clin Rheumtol. 2010;5(1):75–100.

73. Bruce IN, Urowitz MB, Gladman DD, Hallett DC. Natural history of hypercholesterolemia in systemic lupus erythematosus. J Rheumatol. 1999;26(10):2137–43.

74. Esdaile JM, Abrahamowicz M, Grodzicky T, et al. Traditional Framingham risk factors fail to fully account for accelerated atherosclerosis in systemic lupus erythematosus. Arthritis Rheum. 2001;44(10):2331–7.

75. Haque S, Gordon C, Isenberg D, et al. Risk factors for clinical coronary heart disease in systemic lupus erythematosus: the lupus and atherosclerosis evaluation of risk (LASER) study. J Rheumatol. 2010;37(2):322–9.

76. Roman MJ, Shanker BA, Davis A, et al. Prevalence and correlates of accelerated atherosclerosis in systemic lupus erythematosus. N Engl J Med. 2003;349(25):2399–406.

77. Asanuma Y, Oeser A, Shintani AK, et al. Premature coronary-artery atherosclerosis in systemic lupus erythematosus. N Engl J Med. 2003;349(25):2407–15.

78. Sherer Y, Shoenfeld Y. Mechanisms of disease: atherosclerosis in autoimmune diseases. Nat Clin Pract Rheumatol. 2006;2(2):99–106.

79. Recio-Mayoral A, Mason JC, Kaski JC, Rubens MB, Harari OA, Camici PG. Chronic inflammation and coronary microvascular dysfunction in patients without risk factors for coronary artery disease. Eur Heart J. 2009;30(15):1837–43.

80. McCarey DW, McInnes IB, Madhok R, et al. Trial of Atorvastatin in Rheumatoid Arthritis (TARA): double-blind, randomised placebo-controlled trial. Lancet. 2004;363(9426):2015–21.

81. Ferreira GA, Navarro TP, Telles RW, Andrade LE, Sato EI. Atorvastatin therapy improves endothelial-dependent vasodilation in patients with systemic lupus erythematosus: an 8 weeks controlled trial. Rheumatology (Oxford). 2007;46(10):1560–5.

82. Peters MJ, Symmons DP, McCarey D, et al. EULAR evidence-based recommendations for cardiovascular risk management in patients with rheumatoid arthritis and other forms of inflammatory arthritis. Ann Rheum Dis. 2009;69(2):325–31.

83. Bruce IN. Cardiovascular disease in lupus patients: should all patients be treated with statins and aspirin? Best Pract Res Clin Rheumatol. 2005;19(5):823–38.

84. Kahlenberg JM, Kaplan MJ. The interplay of inflammation and cardiovascular disease in systemic lupus erythematosus. Arthritis Res Ther. 2011;13(1):203.

85. Roman MJ, Crow MK, Lockshin MD, et al. Rate and determinants of progression of atherosclerosis in systemic lupus erythematosus. Arthritis Rheum. 2007;56(10):3412–9.

86. Solomon SD, McMurray JJ, Pfeffer MA, et al. Cardiovascular risk associated with celecoxib in a clinical trial for colorectal adenoma prevention. N Engl J Med. 2005;352(11):1071–80.

87. Drazen JM. COX-2 inhibitors–a lesson in unexpected problems. N Engl J Med. 2005;352(11):1131–2.

Cardiovascular Problems in the Elderly

Michael W. Rich

Abstract

Aging is associated with diffuse changes throughout the cardiovascular system that significantly impact the clinical features, management, and prognosis of older patients with cardiovascular disease. As a result of these changes, cardiovascular reserve capacity declines progressively with age, while the incidence and prevalence of cardiovascular diseases increase with age in both men and women. In addition, age-related changes predispose older individuals to specific cardiovascular disorders, including systolic hypertension, non-ST-segment elevation myocardial infarction, heart failure with preserved ejection fraction, aortic stenosis, syncope, atrial fibrillation, and sinoatrial dysfunction. While the management of older patients with cardiovascular disease is generally similar to that in younger patients, prevalent comorbid conditions, quality of life considerations, and personal preferences become increasingly important for ensuring patient-centered care in older adults. This chapter provides an overview of clinically relevant effects of cardiovascular aging and discusses the pathophysiology, diagnosis, and management of cardiovascular conditions commonly encountered in older adults.

Keywords

Aging • Arrhythmias • Coronary artery disease • Elderly • Heart failure • Myocardial infarction • Risk factors • Valve disease

Introduction

The prevalence of cardiovascular disease (CVD) increases progressively with age, exceeding 80 % in both men and women 80 years of age or older (Fig. 19.1) [1]. As a result, although individuals ≥65 years of age comprise only 13 % of the population in the USA, they account for over 60 % of all hospitalizations and over 50 % of all procedures for cardiovascular disorders (Table 19.1) [1, 2]. In addition, over 80 % of deaths attributable to CVD occur in persons over 65 years of age, and two-thirds occur in the 6 % of the population over 75 years of age [1]. Indeed, cancer is the leading cause of mortality among Americans up to age 75, and it is only after age 75 that CVD becomes the dominant cause of death (Fig. 19.2) [1]. Moreover, with the progressive aging of the population over the next several decades, it is anticipated that older adults will represent an increasing proportion of patients with CVD and a steadily increasing segment of the inpatient and outpatient populations for whom cardiology consultation is requested. In this regard, consultation in the geriatric patient is often complicated by the high prevalence of coexisting illnesses and the paucity of definitive age-specific practice guidelines. It is therefore important for the consultant to have an appreciation of the effects of age on cardiovascular structure and function and of the interactions between age, CVD, and common age-associated comorbid conditions.

M.W. Rich, MD
Department of Internal Medicine/Cardiology,
Washington University, 660 S. Euclid Ave,
Campus Box 8086, St. Louis, MO 63110, USA
e-mail: mrich@wustl.edu

K. Stergiopoulos, D.L. Brown (eds.), *Evidence-Based Cardiology Consult*,
DOI 10.1007/978-1-4471-4441-0_19, © Springer-Verlag London 2014

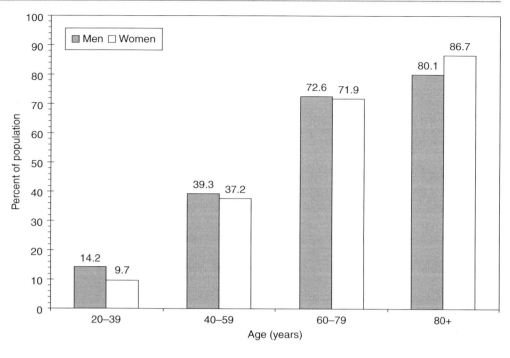

Fig. 19.1 Prevalence of cardiovascular disease in adults ≥20 years of age by age and sex[a] (National Health and Nutrition Examination Survey: 2005–2008; [a]Data include coronary heart disease, heart failure, stroke, and hypertension; Source: National Heart, Lung, and Blood Institute)

Table 19.1 Major cardiovascular procedures by age

	<45		45–64		≥65	
	No.[a]	%	No.[a]	%	No.[a]	%
Cardiac catheterization	91	(8.6)	453	(42.7)	517	(48.7)
Percutaneous coronary revascularization	67	(5.7)	501	(42.5)	610	(51.8)
Coronary bypass surgery	9	(2.2)	165	(40.7)	231	(57.0)
Valve procedures	15	(10.9)	34	(24.6)	89	(64.5)
Permanent pacemaker	11	(3.1)	59	(16.5)	288	(80.4)
Implanted cardioverter-defibrillator	8	(6.9)	43	(37.1)	65	(56.0)
Carotid endarterectomy	–	(NA)	21	(22.6)	72	(77.4)

Adapted from: Roger et al. [1]
[a]In thousands

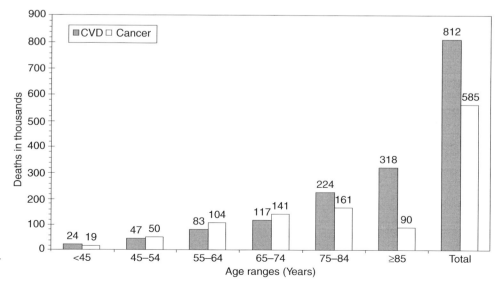

Fig. 19.2 Cardiovascular deaths versus cancer deaths by age in the USA: 2008 (Source: National Center for Health Statistics)

Table 19.2 Principal effects of aging on cardiovascular structure and function

Increased vascular "stiffness," impedance to left ventricular ejection and pulse wave velocity

Impaired left ventricular early diastolic relaxation and mid-to-late diastolic compliance

Diminished responsiveness to neurohumoral stimuli, especially β_1- and β_2-adrenergic stimulation

Altered myocardial energy metabolism and reduced mitochondrial ATP production capacity

Reduced number of sinus node pacemaker cells and impaired sinoatrial function

Endothelial dysfunction and vasomotor dysregulation

Impaired baroreceptor responsiveness

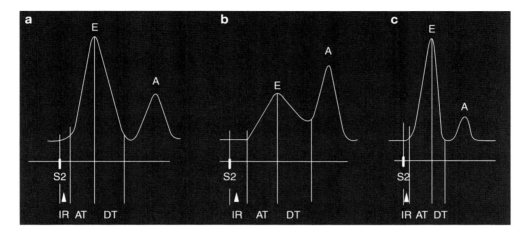

Fig. 19.3 Patterns of left ventricular diastolic filling. In healthy young adults (**a**), left ventricular diastolic filling is characterized by a brief period of isovolumic relaxation (*IR*) following closure of the aortic valve (*S2*), a prominent early filling wave (*E*) with rapid acceleration time (*AT*) and deceleration time (*DT*), and a relatively small atrial contraction wave (*A*). In older adults with impaired relaxation and increased myocardial stiffness (**b**), the IR period is prolonged, the AT and DT slopes are diminished giving rise to a lower amplitude E wave, and there is an augmented atrial contraction wave (*A*) with reversal of the ratio of E:A wave amplitudes. (**c**) Indicates more severe diastolic dysfunction with restrictive filling of the ventricle associated with very short IR interval, narrow E-wave, and small A-wave; this pattern is not seen with normal aging and implies advanced cardiac disease

Pathophysiology

Normal aging is associated with diffuse changes in the heart and vasculature that significantly impact the incidence, clinical manifestations, response to therapeutic interventions, and prognosis of CVD [3, 4]. Major clinically relevant effects of aging are summarized in Table 19.2 and briefly discussed below.

A hallmark of aging is an increase in stiffness and loss of elasticity of the major arteries, including the aorta and great vessels. This results in a gradually progressive increase in systolic blood pressure with age [5]. Conversely, the diastolic blood pressure tends to plateau in late middle age and declines slightly thereafter. The rise in systolic blood pressure leads to an increase in impedance to left ventricular ejection (i.e., afterload), while the decline in diastolic pressure results in a reduction in coronary artery perfusion pressure. Thus, the older heart has to work harder to achieve the same stroke volume as a younger heart despite the potential reduction in coronary blood flow.

Aging is also associated with impaired early diastolic relaxation due to alterations in myocardial calcium metabolism and transport and increased passive myocardial stiffness

related, in part, to compensatory hypertrophy in response to increased afterload [4]. These changes result in characteristic alterations in the pattern of left ventricular diastolic filling (Fig. 19.3), with a decline in early filling coupled with augmentation of atrial contraction ("atrial kick") to maintain left ventricular end-diastolic volume and cardiac output. Age-associated changes in diastolic function result in a shift to the left of the normal left ventricular pressure-volume relationship, such that a small increase in left ventricular diastolic volume (as, e.g., following a high salt meal) leads to a greater increase in left ventricular diastolic pressure than in younger individuals. These effects, in turn, predispose older patients to the development of heart failure with preserved ejection fraction (HFPEF) and atrial fibrillation (AF).

A third effect of aging is a progressive decline in responsiveness to beta-adrenergic stimulation [3, 4]. This results in an almost linear decline in maximum attainable sinus heart rate, often approximated by the formula: peak heart rate = 220 – age. Because cardiac output is the product of heart rate and stroke volume, the effect of age on heart rate also means that peak cardiac output (e.g., in response to exercise) also declines progressively with age. Further, impaired beta-adrenergic responsiveness also contributes to

Table 19.3 Effects of aging on other organ systems

Kidneys
  Gradual decline in glomerular filtration rate, ~8 cc/min/decade
  Impaired fluid and electrolyte homeostasis
Lungs
  Reduced ventilatory capacity
  Increased ventilation/perfusion mismatching
Neurohumoral system
  Reduced cerebral perfusion autoregulatory capacity
  Diminished reflex responsiveness
  Impaired thirst mechanism
Musculoskeletal system
  Decreased muscle mass and strength (sarcopenia)
  Decreased bone density (osteopenia)
Hemostatic system
  Increased levels of coagulation factors
  Increased platelet activity and aggregability
  Increased inflammatory cytokines and C-reactive protein
  Increased inhibitors of fibrinolysis and angiogenesis

an age-related decline in peak contractility, and older adults are less able to increase ejection fraction as a mechanism to increase stroke volume. An age-related decline in the capacity of the mitochondria to upregulate ATP production in response to increased demands further limits peak myocardial contractility. In addition, decreased peripheral responsiveness to beta$_2$-adrenergic stimulation results in a decline in peak blood flow to exercising muscles and to the skin. The latter effect reduces the older person's capacity to eliminate excess heat and predisposes to heat-related disorders such as heat stroke.

Aging is associated with diffuse changes in the cardiac conduction system that result in a modest slowing of impulse conduction [4]. There is also progressive degeneration of sinus node pacemaker cells, such that by age 75 only about 10 % of spontaneously depolarizing cells within the node retain capacity to initiate a heartbeat. Conduction of the impulse to atrial tissue may also be delayed by fibrosis surrounding the node resulting in sinus node exit block. Taken together, these alterations in sinus node function contribute to the increasing prevalence of "sick sinus syndrome" with advancing age, which is the most common indication for pacemaker implantation in older adults [6]. In addition, myocardial fibrosis in the atria and ventricles together with alterations in conduction predisposes older adults to both supraventricular and ventricular arrhythmias, especially atrial fibrillation.

Alterations in endothelial function are another hallmark of vascular aging [3]. Increasing age is associated with a gradually progressive decline in endothelium-dependent vasodilation mediated primarily through diminished nitric oxide synthase activity and altered nitric oxide metabolism. Endothelial dysfunction contributes to the pathogenesis and progression of atherosclerosis. In addition, maximum coronary blood flow, which is dependent, in part, on nitric oxide

production and activity, declines with age. As a result, older patients have impaired capacity to augment oxygen and nutrient delivery to the myocardium in the setting of increased demands (e.g., strenuous exercise, atrial fibrillation with rapid ventricular response, or a systemic illness such as pneumonia). The consequent imbalance between oxygen supply and demand places older patients at risk for developing ischemia even in the absence of obstructive coronary artery disease (CAD), i.e., demand ischemia.

Increasing age is also associated with altered autonomic function and reflex responsiveness. In particular, baroreceptor responsiveness is impaired, as a result of which older adults are less able to maintain effective cerebral blood flow in response to positional changes, such as standing up quickly [7]. This predisposes older patients to dizziness, light-headedness, falls, and syncope. Furthermore, this propensity to falls and syncope is often exacerbated by many of the medications commonly used to treat cardiovascular conditions, including diuretics, beta-blockers, and vasodilators.

In addition to age-related cardiovascular changes, aging is associated with important alterations in other organ systems that impact the clinical manifestations and management of older patients with CVD. Table 19.3 summarizes key changes in other organ systems and their potential implications for older cardiac patients.

Cardiovascular Risk Factors

Hypertension

The prevalence of hypertension in Americans 75 years of age or older is approximately 67 % in men and 78 % in women. Isolated systolic hypertension accounts for over 90 % of all hypertension in persons ≥70 years of age [1, 5]. In addition, systolic blood pressure is the most potent risk factor for CVD and stroke in older adults.

Numerous prospective randomized clinical trials have demonstrated that treatment of systolic and/or diastolic hypertension substantially reduces cardiovascular risk in older adults, including persons ≥80 years of age [8, 9]. Treatment of hypertension is generally similar in older and younger patients. However, a recent consensus document on hypertension in the elderly concluded that a systolic blood pressure treatment threshold of ≥150 mmHg is reasonable in patients 80 years of age or older and that a target systolic blood pressure of 140–145 mmHg is also reasonable for this age group [8].

Hyperlipidemia

In men, total cholesterol and LDL-cholesterol levels increase until late middle age and then tend to level off [10]. In women, total cholesterol and LDL-cholesterol levels rise rapidly after menopause and average 15–20 mg/dl higher than those in men after age 60. HDL-cholesterol levels average about 10 mg/dl higher in women than in men throughout adult life. While the strength of association between total cholesterol and CAD declines with age, low HDL-cholesterol levels and elevated total cholesterol to HDL-cholesterol ratios remain independent risk factors for CAD at older age [11].

Data from multiple primary and secondary prevention studies have shown that statins reduce cardiovascular risk in patients up to 80 years of age [12–14]. However, few patients over age 80 have been enrolled in these trials, and the benefits of statin therapy, especially for primary prevention, remain unproven in this age group. Moreover, epidemiologic studies demonstrate an inverse relationship between total cholesterol and all-cause mortality in persons ≥85 years of age, a phenomenon referred to as "reverse epidemiology" [15, 16]. In addition, recent studies suggest that statins may be associated with memory loss and impaired quality of life in some individuals [17]. Therefore, use of statins in the very elderly should be individualized, and patients treated with statins should be informed about the potential for adverse effects.

Diabetes Mellitus

The prevalence of diabetes increases with age and approaches 30 % in persons over age 65 [1]. The prevalence is higher in men than in women and higher in blacks and Hispanics than in whites. Diabetes is an independent risk factor for CVD in both older men and older women, but the relative risk associated with diabetes is higher in women than in men. The management of diabetes is similar in older and younger adults, except that metformin must be used more cautiously in elderly patients due to the age-related decline in renal function [18].

Tobacco

Smoking prevalence declines with age due to survival bias and successful smoking cessation. However, smoking remains an important risk factor for CAD and stroke in older adults, and smoking cessation is associated with a marked reduction in risk in people of all ages [19]. Therefore, older patients who smoke should be strongly encouraged to quit. Support through counseling and pharmacological interventions should be offered to all individuals who indicate a desire to quit.

Physical Activity

The frequency, duration, and intensity of physical activity correlate inversely with the incidence and prevalence of CVD in older as well as younger adults [20]. In addition, recent studies indicate that slow gait speed (<0.8 m/s in men, <0.7 m/s in women), as assessed using a standard 5 or 6 m walk test, is a strong independent predictor for adverse outcomes in older patients following acute myocardial infarction (MI) or coronary bypass surgery [21, 22]. In the absence of contraindications, regular physical activity, including both aerobic and resistance exercises, is recommended for individuals of all ages [20]. Appropriate precautions should be taken to avoid falls and injuries in elderly patients participating in structured or unstructured exercise programs.

Obesity

Obesity is common among older adults; moderate or severe obesity adversely affects functional capacity, independence, and quality of life at advanced age [23].However, the relationship between obesity and CVD at very elderly age is uncertain, as epidemiologic studies indicate that mild to moderately overweight and obese individuals over 80 years of age have improved survival relative to persons of normal weight, as defined by a body mass index (BMI) of 18.5–25 kg/m^2 (i.e., reverse epidemiology) [23]. There is also no evidence that weight loss leads to improved cardiovascular outcomes or all-cause mortality in the elderly. Thus, although it is reasonable to recommend weight loss in elderly patients with BMIs ≥40 kg/m^2 and in less obese individuals with significant obesity-related disabilities, the value of weight loss in other settings requires further study before it can be routinely recommended.

Coronary Artery Disease

Pathophysiology

Older adults are predisposed to the development of CAD due to age-related arterial changes, especially increased arterial stiffness and impaired endothelial function, coupled with the rising prevalence and longer duration of hypertension, diabetes, and hyperlipidemia. As a result, the incidence and prevalence of CAD increase progressively with age in both men and women. Indeed, autopsy studies in older decedents indicate that up to 75 % of older adults have significant CAD [24]. Further, older patients tend to have more diffuse and more severe disease than younger patients, including a significantly higher prevalence of left main and triple-vessel CAD [25].

In addition to higher CAD prevalence, several factors place older adults at increased risk for myocardial ischemia and acute MI. The age-related decline in diastolic blood pressure in conjunction with alterations in left ventricular (LV) diastolic function leads to a reduction in coronary artery perfusion pressure, further reducing coronary blood flow and predisposing to demand ischemia. Alterations in the hemostatic system (see Table 19.3) shift the intrinsic balance between thrombosis and fibrinolysis in favor of thrombosis [26]. Thus, older individuals are at increased risk for thrombus formation throughout both the arterial and venous circulations, predisposing not only to acute MI, but also to stroke, atrial appendage thrombus, deep venous thrombosis, and pulmonary embolism.

Diagnosis

Compared to younger patients, older patients with acute or chronic CAD are more likely to present with atypical symptomatology, such as shortness of breath without chest discomfort, exertional fatigue, altered sensorium or confusion, neurological symptoms (e.g., dizziness or syncope), abdominal discomfort, or malaise [27, 28]. Indeed, after age 85, fewer than 50 % of patients with severe CAD or acute MI present with chest discomfort; the most common symptom in this age group is shortness of breath. In addition, older CAD patients are more likely than younger patients to have "silent" or asymptomatic ischemia, in part due to their more sedentary lifestyle [29].

Older patients are also more likely than younger patients to have a nondiagnostic 12-lead electrocardiogram (ECG) at the time of presentation due to higher prevalence of preexisting ECG abnormalities, such as bundle branch block, left ventricular hypertrophy, paced rhythm, and nonspecific ST-T abnormalities. Older patients with acute MI are less likely to present with ST-segment elevation (STEMI) than younger patients [27].The higher proportion of non-ST-segment elevation MIs (NSTEMI) in older patients contributes to diagnostic delays and reduced implementation of evidence-based therapies.

Indications for stress testing are similar in older and younger patients [30]. However, older patients are less likely to be able to perform an exercise test, and it is often necessary to conduct a pharmacological study to determine the presence and severity of CAD. The stress ECG is less likely to be diagnostic due to the increased prevalence of resting ECG abnormalities as described above. In addition, since the prevalence and severity of CAD increase with age, the pretest probability of significant CAD is higher in older adults. As a result, the positive predictive value of stress testing is higher and the negative predictive value is lower (i.e., increased likelihood of a false negative test) in older compared to younger patients (Bayes Theorem).

Coronary calcium scans and coronary computed tomography (CT) angiography provide alternatives to stress testing for the noninvasive diagnosis of CAD. Coronary calcium scores increase with age but the correlation between calcium scores and hemodynamically significant coronary stenoses

declines with age [31]. Nonetheless, higher calcium scores are associated with increased risk of coronary events in older adults [32]. CT coronary angiograms may be difficult to interpret in older adults with extensively calcified arteries. In addition, such scans entail a significant intravenous contrast load with potential nephrotoxicity. In part, for these reasons, the role of CT angiography to evaluate older adults for CAD is evolving. The choice of initial noninvasive diagnostic test must be individualized based on the overall clinical context.

The indications for invasive coronary angiography are similar in older and younger patients. However, the risks of bleeding complications and contrast nephropathy increase with age. It is therefore essential to assess the risks and potential benefits of coronary angiography in older adults on an individualized basis, incorporating symptom severity, prognosis, goals of care, quality of life considerations, and personal preferences into the decision-making process. In general, coronary angiography is inappropriate in elderly individuals who are not candidates for revascularization, either due to prevalent comorbidities (e.g., dementia) or patient refusal.

Management

Elderly patients with acute coronary syndrome (ACS), including unstable angina, NSTEMI, and STEMI, comprise a high-risk subgroup as mortality rates for ACS increase in a curvilinear fashion with advancing age [27, 28]. Therefore, the potential benefits of therapeutic interventions are greater in older than in younger individuals. Conversely, the potential risks, especially of invasive procedures, are also higher in the elderly. It is therefore essential to weigh the risks and benefits before embarking on a course of treatment.

For patients with STEMI, fibrinolytic therapy administered within 6–12 h of symptom onset reduces mortality at least up to age 85 [28]. However, the risk of intracranial hemorrhage (ICH) also increases with age, exceeding 1 % in patients 75 years of age or older [28]. In addition, the risk of ICH is higher with fibrin-specific agents (alteplase, reteplase) than with streptokinase [28]. Data on the use of fibrinolytic agents in patients ≥85 years of age are very limited.

Percutaneous coronary intervention (PCI) performed within 90–120 min of hospital arrival is more effective than fibrinolytic therapy in achieving reperfusion in patients with STEMI, although once again data are limited in patients over age 85 [28]. PCI is also associated with a lower risk of ICH but higher risk of bleeding at the arteriotomy site compared with fibrinolytic therapy. In patients with NSTEMI, several randomized trials have shown that a strategy of early intervention with PCI is associated with improved outcomes relative to medical therapy, and the absolute benefit tends to be greater in older patients due to higher baseline risk [27].

Nonetheless, the potential benefits and risks of invasive management vary widely in patients over 75–80 years of age, depending on infarct size, hemodynamic stability, left ventricular function, baseline functional status, and prevalent comorbidities, especially renal insufficiency, cognitive impairment, and frailty. These factors, along with overall goals of care and personal preferences, must therefore be taken into consideration in the decision-making process.

Pharmacological therapy for older patients with ACS is generally similar to that in younger patients, but there are some notable exceptions. Aspirin is of proven benefit in patients ≥70 years of age [33], and the addition of clopidogrel reduces the risk of major cardiovascular events during the 12-month period following hospitalization for NSTEMI, whether or not PCI is performed, with similar benefits in older and younger patients [34]. Prasugrel is associated with improved outcomes relative to clopidogrel in patients with ACS undergoing PCI, but the benefits are limited to patients <75 years of age and those weighing ≥60 kg; [35] therefore, prasugrel is not recommended for patients ≥75 years of age, and the dose should be reduced in patients weighing <60 kg. Ticagrelor is more effective than clopidogrel in patients with ACS with or without STEMI [36]. However, data on ticagrelor are limited in patients ≥75 years of age, among whom the benefits compared to clopidogrel may be attenuated. Glycoprotein IIb/III inhibitors improve clinical outcomes in selected patients with ACS up to the age of 75, but the value of these agents in older patients receiving dual antiplatelet therapy in conjunction with systemic anticoagulation is uncertain, whereas the risk of major bleeding is increased [37]. Therefore, judicious use of these agents in elderly patients is warranted.

Systemic anticoagulation with intravenous unfractionated heparin (UFH) is often administered to older patients with ACS, although the value of such therapy is unproven [38]. Low-molecular-weight heparins (LMWH), such as enoxaparin and dalteparin, are associated with improved clinical outcomes in older patients compared to UFH and may be considered the preferred therapy in the absence of contraindications [39]. However, enoxaparin is not recommended in patients with creatinine clearance <30 cc/min, and caution is also advised when using dalteparin in patients with renal insufficiency or low body weight. Bivalirudin and fondaparinux are associated with improved clinical outcomes and fewer major bleeding complications than either UFH or LMWH in older patients with ACS [40–42]. Bivalirudin is approved for patients undergoing PCI, but dosage reduction is required for patients with renal insufficiency. Fondaparinux is not approved for ACS and it is contraindicated in patients weighing <50 kg and in those with creatinine clearance <30 cc/min. The roles of rivaroxaban and apixaban for treatment of ACS are currently under investigation.

Indications for the use of beta-blockers, nitrates, angiotensin-converting enzyme inhibitors (ACEI), angiotensin-receptor blockers (ARB), aldosterone antagonists, and statins for the treatment of ACS or chronic CAD are generally similar in older and younger patients [27, 28]. However, older patients are at increased risk for adverse events with all of these agents, in part due to age-related changes in pharmacokinetics and pharmacodynamics and in part due to increased risk for drug interactions as a result of polypharmacy. Therefore, it is prudent to start with lower doses and to titrate more gradually than in younger patients while monitoring closely for the appearance of adverse effects. In many cases, older patients may not tolerate guideline-recommended target drug dosages, which are based on clinical trials performed in younger and healthier patients.

In older patients with chronic stable CAD, elective PCI or coronary artery bypass graft (CABG) surgery should be considered in selected patients with persistent symptoms despite optimal medical therapy and in those with high-risk coronary anatomy (e.g., ≥70 % left main stenosis) who are otherwise suitable candidates for revascularization. However, mortality and major complication rates for both PCI and CABG increase with age, especially after age 80 [43]. For example, hospital mortality following elective PCI in octogenarians ranges from 1 to 7 % (vs. <1 % in patients <65 years), and perioperative mortality for isolated elective CABG ranges from 5 to 10 % in patients over age 80 (vs. 1–2 % in patients <65 years). The risk of major bleeding with both procedures is also higher in the very elderly. Older patients are also at increased risk for atrial fibrillation, heart failure, stroke, respiratory disorders, renal insufficiency, and delirium following CABG. As a result, length of stay is longer, fewer patients are discharged home, convalescence is prolonged, and the likelihood of full recovery of independence and functional capacity is reduced. Nonetheless, long-term results following both PCI and CABG in older patients are excellent, with up to 90 % experiencing sustained symptomatic improvement and the majority reporting improved quality of life [43]. In addition, a recent meta-analysis of octogenarians undergoing CABG reported 1-, 3-, and 5-year survival rates of 86, 78, and 68 %, respectively [43]. Similar long-term survival rates have been reported following PCI in this age group.

Valvular Heart Disease

Pathophysiology

The prevalence of clinically significant aortic, mitral, and tricuspid valve disorders increases with age, in part, due to age-related changes in valve structure and, in part, due to the rising prevalence of cardiovascular and systemic diseases that contribute to valve dysfunction (e.g., CAD, chronic kidney disease, pulmonary hypertension). Aging is associated with fibrotic changes in the valve leaflets and valve apparati that predispose to both stenotic and regurgitant valve disorders. Aortic stenosis (AS) severe enough to warrant intervention occurs in 2–3 % of adults over 75 years of age and is the second most common indication for major cardiac surgery in this age group (after CABG). The prevalence of aortic regurgitation (AR) also increases with age, in part, due to dilatation of the ascending aorta related to age-related degenerative changes in the aortic wall. Similarly, degenerative changes in the mitral valve and mitral valve annulus predispose to non-rheumatic calcific mitral stenosis (MS) and to mitral regurgitation (MR). The pulmonic and tricuspid valves are less susceptible to clinically important age-related changes, but the prevalence of pulmonic and tricuspid regurgitation increases with age primarily due to pulmonary hypertension and associated right ventricular (RV) dilatation and dysfunction attributable to an array of age-associated disorders involving the heart, lungs, and pulmonary vasculature.

Diagnosis

Older patients with chronic valvular heart disease are often asymptomatic until the disorder is at an advanced stage. In addition, symptoms are usually nonspecific and may include fatigue, exercise intolerance, and shortness of breath, all of which have a broad differential diagnosis in older individuals. Signs of valvular heart disease are generally similar in older and younger individuals with some notable exceptions. Carotid upstrokes are often well preserved in older adults with severe AS due to reduced vascular compliance and accelerated pulse wave velocity. An opening snap is rarely appreciated in older adults with non-rheumatic calcific MS. In addition, the intensity of all valvular murmurs may be diminished in older adults with reduced cardiac output. For these reasons, the clinician must maintain a high index of suspicion for valvular heart disease in older patients with unexplained symptoms or physical findings suggestive of a valve disorder.

As in younger patients, transthoracic echocardiography is the initial diagnostic procedure of choice in older patients with suspected valvular heart disease [44]. In most cases, the transthoracic echocardiogram is sufficient to evaluate the presence and severity of all valvular lesions, as well as to assess LV and RV size and function. In cases where additional information is required, transesophageal echocardiography, magnetic resonance imaging, and cardiac catheterization provide complementary anatomical and hemodynamic information to aid clinical decision-making. In older patients with valvular heart disease for whom intervention is being considered, coronary angiography is usually indicated to assess the presence and severity of CAD.

Management

The role of medical therapy in the prevention and treatment of valvular heart disease is limited. Afterload-reducing agents, such as ACE inhibitors, may provide palliation in patients with AS, AR, and possibly MR. The value of other agents, such as digoxin, beta-blockers, and aldosterone antagonists, is unproven in the absence of specific indications for their use (e.g., heart failure, atrial fibrillation).

The rate of progression of most chronic valvular heart disorders is relatively slow; therefore, patients with mild to moderate disease can be managed conservatively, especially in the absence of symptoms. Older patients with more severe disease should be managed in accordance with current guidelines [44], with the caveat that consideration of valve repair or replacement must be undertaken in the context of the older patient's overall health, relevant comorbid conditions, life expectancy, goals of care, and personal preferences. In patients for whom intervention is deemed appropriate, surgical valve repair (if feasible) or replacement with a bioprosthetic valve remains the procedure of choice in most cases. Importantly, the risk of valve surgery increases with age, especially after age 80. Perioperative mortality for isolated elective aortic valve replacement ranges from 4 to 7 % in octogenarians, while mortality for mitral valve surgery ranges from 5 to 15 % in this age group. In addition, older adults are at increased risk for heart failure, atrial fibrillation, stroke, cognitive dysfunction, infections, and pulmonary and renal complications following valve surgery.

Recently, both transcutaneous and transapical aortic valve replacement (TAVR) have been shown to provide excellent short- and intermediate-term results, including acceptable mortality and significantly improved quality of life in older patients with severe AS who are judged to be at high risk for surgery [45, 46]. Additional studies of TAVR are ongoing, and the role of this procedure in the management of older patients with aortic valve disease is evolving. Similarly, transcutaneous mitral valve repair is an option for highly selected patients with severe MR [47].

Infective Endocarditis

Age-related changes in valve structure in combination with a rise in prevalence of conditions and procedures associated with bacteremia (e.g., poor dentition, respiratory and urinary tract infections, cystoscopy, and colonoscopy) result in a progressive increase in the incidence of infective endocarditis with advancing age [48]. The diagnosis of endocarditis is often difficult in older adults due to nonspecific clinical manifestations. In addition, blood cultures may be negative, often due to prior treatment with antibiotics. The causative organisms of endocarditis are similar in older and younger patients, with streptococci, staphylococci, and enterococci being the most common agents, followed by gram-negative bacilli and other less common pathogens. Transthoracic echocardiography is diagnostic for vegetations in less than 50 % of cases, but the yield of transesophageal echocardiography approaches 90 %. Treatment of endocarditis is similar in older and younger patients, but mortality is higher in the elderly. For this reason, advanced age per se should not be considered a contraindication to surgical therapy for endocarditis in appropriately selected patients [49].

Heart Failure

Pathophysiology

The net effect of cardiovascular aging is a marked reduction in cardiovascular reserve (Fig. 19.4) [50]. Thus, although cardiovascular performance at rest is generally well preserved in healthy older adults, there is a progressive decline in the capacity to augment cardiac output in response to increased demands. As a result, healthy octogenarians typically have a maximum oxygen consumption (VO_2max) of <20 ml O_2/min/kg, which roughly corresponds to that of a middle-aged person with New York Heart Association class II heart failure (HF). From the clinical perspective, this means that elderly individuals are at markedly increased risk

for developing HF in response to stressors that are usually well-tolerated in younger persons, e.g., non-ST-elevation ACS, atrial fibrillation, cardiac and noncardiac surgery, poorly controlled hypertension, anemia, pneumonia, and many other conditions. In addition, the prevalence rates of hypertension and CAD, which account for 70–80 % of HF cases in the USA, also increase progressively with age. It is therefore not surprising that the incidence and prevalence of HF increase exponentially with age, doubling with each decade after age 50 [51]. Indeed, patients ≥75 years of age account for approximately 50 % of all HF cases and more than two-thirds of all HF deaths. Moreover, HF is the most common cause of both hospitalization and rehospitalization in the Medicare age group, and it is by far the most costly diagnosis-related group [52]. HF is also a leading cause of chronic disability and loss of independence in older adults, and there is a strong association between HF and cognitive impairment [53]. Of particular note, the proportion of HF patients with preserved LV ejection fraction (HFPEF) increases strikingly with age, especially in women [54]. Thus, while HFPEF accounts for only about 10 % of HF cases in patients <65 years of age, it accounts for at least 50 % of cases in patients ≥65 years of age, including about 40 % of men and two-thirds of women. The dominance of HFPEF in women compared to men in part reflects the fact that hypertension is the leading cause of HF in older women, whereas in older men the etiology is more balanced between hypertension and CAD. Also, although the incidence of HF is higher in men than in women at all ages, the greater longevity of women leads to an increase in the proportion of HF cases occurring in women with increasing age, which exceeds 50 % after age 80.

Diagnosis

HF in older adults is both overdiagnosed and underdiagnosed. The cardinal symptoms of HF – effort intolerance, fatigue, shortness of breath, and edema – are common in the elderly, and these symptoms are often attributed to HF even when caused by other disorders. Conversely, sedentary older adults may not report exertional symptoms, leading patients and physicians alike to ascribe effort intolerance or fatigue to noncardiac disorders, deconditioning, or even "normal aging." Further, older HF patients, especially those over 80–85 years of age, often present with atypical symptoms, such as altered sensorium, irritability, or gastrointestinal disturbances, such as anorexia or bloating [52]. Similarly, the physical findings associated with HF in older adults are often nonspecific or atypical. For example, pulmonary crackles may be due to chronic lung disease or atelectasis, and lower extremity edema may be due to venous stasis or medications (e.g., calcium channel blockers).

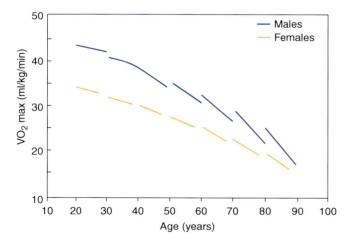

Fig. 19.4 Age and VO_2max in healthy subjects [86]. Increasing age is associated with an accelerating decline in VO_2max in healthy men and women

As with symptoms and signs, findings from diagnostic tests are less reliable in older adults. The chest radiograph may be difficult to interpret in older adults with chronic lung disease, marked kyphosis or inadequate inspiratory expansion. Plasma B-type natriuretic peptide (BNP) and n-terminal pro-BNP (nt-pro-BNP) levels increase with age, especially in women, as well as in the presence of impaired renal function [55]. As a result, the specificity and predictive accuracy of these neurohormones for diagnosing HF decline with age. Nonetheless, in cases of diagnostic uncertainty, a normal BNP or nt-pro-BNP level effectively excludes active HF, whereas markedly elevated levels provide strong support for the diagnosis.

As in younger patients, older patients with suspected HF should undergo routine laboratory studies, including blood tests, an electrocardiogram, and an echocardiogram to rule out potentially treatable disorders and to evaluate LV and RV systolic and diastolic function [56]. Additional evaluation, such as stress testing, magnetic resonance imaging, and cardiac catheterization, should be performed on an individualized basis and in accordance with existing guidelines.

Management

The principal goals of HF management in elderly patients are to maximize quality of life, preserve independence, reduce resource utilization (esp. hospitalizations), and extend functional survival. Basic management should include appropriate control of risk factors, especially hypertension, as well as other coexisting conditions, such as CAD, atrial fibrillation, thyroid disorders, and anemia. Patients should receive dietary counseling, including limitation of sodium intake to no more than 1.5–2 g/day, as well as avoidance of excess fluid intake (i.e., patients with HF, renal insufficiency, or other fluid-retaining states should not drink "8–10 glasses of water" everyday, as is often suggested for healthy individuals). Patients should be advised to weigh themselves on a daily basis and to either contact their health provider or self-adjust their diuretic dosages (if appropriate) if the weight is outside a specified range. Patients should also be encouraged to engage in regular physical activity at a level consistent with their overall health and functional capacity. Older HF patients in particular benefit from resistance training in addition to aerobic exercise [57].

Management of older HF patients is often complicated by the presence of multiple comorbidities, polypharmacy, cognitive impairment, and socioeconomic factors that contribute to repetitive hospitalizations and poor clinical outcomes. Such patients require close follow-up, especially during periods of transition (e.g., hospital to home), and this is best accomplished through the use of a multidisciplinary team approach, most commonly coordinated by a nurse or nurse practitioner. Multiple studies and systematic reviews have confirmed the value of multidisciplinary care in reducing hospitalizations and improving quality of life without increasing cost of care in older HF patients, especially those at increased risk for recurrent hospital admissions [58].

Medical therapy for HF with reduced ejection fraction (HFREF) is generally similar in older and younger patients [56]. However, it should be recognized that older patients were markedly underrepresented in most of the large randomized HF trials. Moreover, patients with major comorbidities (especially, advanced renal insufficiency) as well as nursing home residents were systematically excluded. Therefore, the generalizability of study findings to patients of very advanced age is uncertain. This problem is further complicated by the fact that older patients are at increased risk for serious adverse effects from HF medications due to age-related changes in renal and hepatic function, alterations in drug absorption and distribution, and the potential for drug-drug interactions related to polypharmacy. Therefore, selection of HF medications for older patients must be individualized; therapy should be initiated at low dosages and up-titrated very gradually, and patients should be carefully monitored for potential adverse events. Specific concerns related to the use of HF medications in older patients include increased risks for electrolyte disturbances with diuretics; worsening renal function and hyperkalemia with ACEIs, ARBs, and aldosterone antagonists (especially if used in combination); bradyarrhythmias with beta-blockers; and digitalis intoxication.

Device therapies, including implantable cardioverter-defibrillators (ICDs), cardiac resynchronization therapy (CRT), and ventricular assist devices (VADs), are playing an increasingly important role in the management of patients with HFREF. As a general principle, advanced age per se is not a contraindication to use of these procedures in appropriately selected patients. However, it should be recognized that data on the value of ICDs, CRT, and especially VADs in patients ≥80 years of age is quite sparse. With respect to ICDs, very elderly patients have a shorter life expectancy, lower likelihood of dying from a ventricular tachyarrhythmia, higher likelihood of dying from noncardiac causes (e.g., pneumonia, hip fracture), and increased risk for experiencing "inappropriate" ICD shocks (i.e., shocks in the absence of a life-threatening ventricular tachyarrhythmia) due to the higher incidence of AF with rapid ventricular rate relative to younger patients with HFREF [59]. Therefore, the benefit-to-risk ratio of ICDs is shifted towards the null in this age group. ICD implantation for primary prevention of sudden cardiac death in elderly patients should only be undertaken after a frank discussion with the patient and family about the potential benefits and risks. Limited data on CRT in patients over 80 years of age indicate that quality of life and exercise tolerance may be significantly improved in carefully selected patients and that benefits persist for at least 2 years [60]. Although procedural complication rates are higher in this age group, CRT is a reasonable therapeutic option in patients with advanced HF symptoms despite optimal medical therapy. With advances in technology, VADs are increasingly being considered as "destination therapy" in older patients with refractory HFREF [61]. Additional data are needed on outcomes, including quality of life and survival, as well as complication rates in older patients, especially those over 75–80 years of age, before VADs can be considered a standard component of the therapeutic armamentarium.

Medical therapy for HFPEF remains undefined, in part because the pathophysiology of this disorder has not been well characterized and in part because to date no therapeutic interventions have been shown to reduce mortality. As a result, treatment of HFPEF should be directed at controlling hypertension and other risk factors, optimization of therapy for CAD and AF (if applicable), and judicious use of diuretics to relieve congestion and minimize volume overload. However, since patients with HFPEF are often preload dependent, over-diuresis can lead to reduced cardiac output with resultant prerenal azotemia and worsening renal function. Use of other therapies in older patients with HFPEF, including ACEIs, ARBs, beta-blockers, and digoxin, should be individualized based on comorbidities and symptomatic response.

Prevention

HF in older adults is associated with poor prognosis and substantial morbidity. Therefore, aggressive interventions aimed at preventing HF are warranted. At the present time, the most effective preventive measures include controlling blood pressure and reducing the risk of MI. Numerous studies in older patients with hypertension have demonstrated a marked reduction in incident HF with antihypertensive therapy. In the Hypertension in the Very Elderly Trial, for example, among patients 80 years of age or older, diuretic-based treatment with indapamide led to a 21 % reduction in all-cause mortality, 30 % reduction in stroke, and 64 % reduction in incident HF [9]. Similarly, aspirin, statins, beta-blockers, and smoking cessation all reduce the risk of MI and subsequent HF in appropriately selected patients of all ages.

Arrhythmias and Conduction Disorders

Pathophysiology

As previously described, aging is associated with diffuse changes in the cardiac conduction system and myocardium that predispose older adults to the development of a wide range of bradyarrhythmias and conduction disorders, as well as both supraventricular and ventricular premature beats and tachyarrhythmias. Specifically, sinus node dysfunction, AV conduction disorders, and infranodal conduction blocks

(i.e., bundle branch block, left anterior hemiblock) all increase in prevalence with age. In addition, the prevalence and frequency of atrial and ventricular premature depolarizations, as well as short runs of supraventricular tachycardia (SVT), increase with age in both men and women, even in the absence of manifest structural heart disease. In contrast, ventricular tachycardia (five or more beats) is rare in healthy older adults without demonstrable cardiac disease. From the prognostic perspective, the increasing prevalence and complexity of ambient supraventricular and ventricular ectopic activity is generally benign. However, runs of SVT, especially during exertion, are a marker for increased risk of atrial fibrillation, and frequent ventricular premature beats are a harbinger of more serious ventricular arrhythmias in patients with underlying heart disease, especially CAD with ischemic cardiomyopathy. Finally, age-related changes in the sinoatrial conduction system and atrial myocardium, coupled with alterations in left ventricular diastolic function, greatly increase the propensity of older adults to develop atrial fibrillation, the incidence and prevalence of which increase exponentially with age.

Diagnosis

As with other cardiac disorders, symptoms attributable to arrhythmias are highly variable in older adults. Patients with significant bradyarrhythmias, whether due to sinus node dysfunction ("sick sinus syndrome") or AV block, are often asymptomatic if the effective heart rate is 40 beats/min or higher. Alternatively, patients may report nonspecific symptoms, such as fatigue or effort intolerance, that may be attributed to age or other factors. In more severe cases, dizziness, light-headedness, falls, or syncope may be the presenting manifestation. Similarly, patients with supraventricular or ventricular tachyarrhythmias may be asymptomatic or complain of fatigue, palpitations, shortness of breath, light-headedness, falls, or syncope.

The diagnostic evaluation for a suspected heart rhythm disorder is similar in older and younger adults and should include a detailed physical examination, basic laboratory studies, and, in most cases, a 12-lead ECG. Additional evaluation, determined on an individualized basis, may include an assessment of thyroid function, ambulatory monitoring, an echocardiogram, and other procedures as dictated by the clinical context.

Management

Initial management of older patients with symptomatic or otherwise clinically significant bradyarrhythmias includes correction of any potentially reversible contributory factors, such as hypothyroidism or electrolyte disorders. If feasible, heart-rate-lowering medications, such as beta-blockers, non-dihydropyridine calcium channel antagonists, and amiodarone, should be discontinued or the dosage should be reduced. Implantation of a permanent pacemaker is indicated in patients with symptoms directly attributable to a nonreversible bradyarrhythmia as well as in patients with potentially life-threatening bradyarrhythmias (e.g., Mobitz type II 2° AV block with wide QRS) even in the absence of symptoms [62]. Because of the rising prevalence of bradyarrhythmias with age, in the USA persons over 65 years of age account for more than 80 % of all pacemaker implantations, and over 50 % occur in patients 75 years of age or older [63]. For patients in sinus rhythm, dual-chamber pacemakers are associated with lower risk for developing AF, fewer HF hospitalizations, and improved quality of life compared to single-chamber ventricular pacemakers [64].

Atrial fibrillation is the most common and clinically important sustained arrhythmia in older adults. The prevalence of AF increases steeply with age, from <1 % in individuals under age 40 to more than 10 % in those over age 80; the median age of AF patients in the USA is about 75 years [65]. AF is more common in men than in women at all ages, but the proportion of women increases with age. The proportion of strokes attributable to AF also increases with age; in the Framingham Heart Study, AF accounted for 1.5 % of strokes in persons 50–59 years of age but 23.5 % of strokes in persons over 80 years of age [66]. Indeed, increasing age is a powerful independent risk factor for stroke in patients with AF, as indicated by the CHADS$_2$ and CHA$_2$DS$_2$-VASc stroke risk stratification schemes [67, 68].

Management of AF is generally similar in younger and older patients up to age 75 [69]. However, optimal management of patients ≥75 years of age remains challenging. Based on the CHA$_2$DS$_2$-VASc score, which assigns 2 points for age 75 or older, all patients in this age group are at moderate to high risk for stroke and are therefore candidates for systemic anticoagulation. In addition, the greatest benefit of warfarin in reducing the absolute risk of stroke occurs in patients over age 75. Conversely, age is also a potent risk factor for bleeding complications, and the risk of major bleeding, including intracranial hemorrhage (ICH), is highest in patients of advanced age. Bleeding risk is further increased in older patients receiving concomitant antiplatelet therapy (e.g., aspirin and clopidogrel for CAD) or nonsteroidal anti-inflammatory drugs (e.g., for arthritis or chronic pain). Polypharmacy with frequent medication changes also increases the risk for drug-drug interactions with warfarin, thereby reducing the proportion of time that the international normalized ratio (INR) is maintained within the therapeutic range of 2.0–3.0. These concerns have led to consistently low warfarin utilization rates in AF patients ≥75 years of age, which range from 40 to 60 % in most studies [70, 71]. Nonetheless, due to the clear benefits

of warfarin in high-risk AF patients, current guidelines advocate systemic anticoagulation in elderly patients in the absence of compelling contraindications [69]. In this regard, high fall risk, which is the most common reason cited for withholding warfarin therapy in the elderly, should not be considered a contraindication to warfarin unless there is a definite history of significant head trauma or ICH [72].

Recently, dabigatran, a direct thrombin inhibitor, and rivaroxaban and apixaban, both of which are coagulation factor Xa inhibitors, have demonstrated promise as alternatives to warfarin in patients with AF [73–75]. All three agents have been shown to be non-inferior to warfarin with respect to stroke prevention and major bleeding complications and superior to warfarin with respect to the risk for ICH. Additional advantages include ease of use (lack of need to monitor INR or adjust dose) and markedly fewer interactions with other drugs and food. Important disadvantages include inability to monitor efficacy or adherence, lack of reversibility in the event that serious bleeding occurs, and substantially higher cost. In addition, data on all three of these agents are sparse in patients over 75–80 years of age, who may be at increased risk for bleeding complications due to alterations in metabolism, volume of distribution, and elimination. Indeed, post-marketing data on dabigatran suggest increased risk for life-threatening hemorrhage in the very elderly and in patients weighing less than 60 kg [76]. Therefore, dabigatran should be used with caution in these populations. Similarly, additional data are needed on the benefits and risks of rivaroxaban and apixaban in patients over75–80 years of age. In summary, the role of these new agents as alternatives to warfarin in the very elderly is evolving but has not yet been fully defined.

In older patients with AF who are not deemed to be suitable candidates for systemic anticoagulation, aspirin with or without clopidogrel may be considered as an alternative. However, aspirin alone or in combination with clopidogrel is clearly inferior to warfarin for stroke prevention, and the risk of major hemorrhage is similar with dual antiplatelet therapy compared to warfarin (although somewhat lower with aspirin alone) [77]. In addition, there is no convincing evidence that either aspirin alone or aspirin plus clopidogrel is more effective than placebo in reducing stroke risk in AF patients 75 years of age or older [78].

Several randomized trials have shown that in patients with AF who are minimally symptomatic on appropriate medications, there is no utility of using anti-arrhythmic drugs in an attempt to maintain sinus rhythm, in part because the toxicity of currently available agents offsets any potential benefits [79]. In addition, a recent study showed that lenient rate control (resting heart rate <110/min) was associated with similar outcomes during relatively short-term follow-up compared to more strict rate control (resting heart rate <80/min) and required less medication [80]. However, in patients who remain significantly symptomatic despite adequate rate control, efforts to maintain sinus rhythm using anti-arrhythmic medications, direct-current cardioversion, catheter ablation (pulmonary vein isolation), or the surgical maze procedure are appropriate therapeutic options [81, 82]. AV-node ablation with pacemaker implantation is also an option in selected patients. The role of left atrial appendage occlusive devices for management of AF is currently under investigation. Additional studies are needed on the long-term safety and efficacy of all of these procedures in elderly patients.

The management of other supraventricular arrhythmias, including atrial flutter, as well as ventricular arrhythmias, is generally similar in older and younger patients, but the risk of anti-arrhythmic drug toxicity is higher in the elderly. In addition, as discussed above, the use of ICDs in patients over 80 years of age requires careful consideration of the benefits and risks, incorporating goals of care, and personal preferences into the decision-making process.

End-of-Life Care

Older patients with CVD are at increased risk for a multitude of complications, both cardiac and noncardiac, including death. Elderly individuals maintain widely divergent views about the use of life-sustaining interventions and other invasive procedures, as well as what constitutes an acceptable quality of life in the context of chronic or terminal illness [83]. Moreover, patient surrogates, including spouses and physicians, are often unable to reliably predict a patient's preferences under specific end-of-life conditions. Therefore, it is essential to address these issues while the patient is competent and lucid. Health-care providers should be proactive in encouraging patients of all ages to communicate their end-of-life preferences, to develop a living will, and to designate a durable power of attorney. Among other issues, these discussions should delineate preferences for discontinuing or disabling devices (i.e., ICDs, VADs, ventilators, feeding tubes) in the event that the patient is no longer able to make such decisions as the end of life approaches [84]. Palliative care and hospice services should be offered to patients with advanced CVD and limited life expectancy [85].

Key Points
- Aging is associated with extensive changes throughout the cardiovascular system that markedly limit cardiovascular reserve and significantly impact the presentation, diagnosis, management, and prognosis of older patients with or without clinically manifest cardiovascular disease.

- Age is a potent risk factor for cardiovascular disease in both men and women, and there is a progressive rise in the incidence and prevalence of certain cardiovascular diseases with advancing age, including systolic hypertension, coronary artery disease and acute coronary syndromes (esp. non-ST-elevation acute coronary syndromes), aortic stenosis, heart failure (esp. HFPEF), sinus node dysfunction, and atrial fibrillation.

- While the management of cardiovascular disorders is generally similar in older and younger patients, with increasing age there is a progressively greater need to individualize care based on overall health status and prognosis, prevalent comorbidities, quality of life considerations, goals of care, and personal preferences.

- Since the course of cardiovascular disease is unpredictable, end-of-life care planning should be initiated early after presentation, and goals of care and personal preferences should be reassessed periodically as the patient's clinical condition and overall health status evolve.

References

1. Roger VL, Go AS, Lloyd-Jones DM, et al. Heart disease and stroke statistics – 2012 update: a report from the American Heart Association. Circulation. 2012;125:e2–220.
2. Hall MJ, DeFrances CJ, Williams SN, Golosinskiy A, Schwartzman A. National hospital discharge survey: 2007 summary. National health statistics reports; no 29. Hyattsville: National Center for Health Statistics; 2010.
3. Lakatta EG, Levy D. Arterial and cardiac aging: major shareholders in cardiovascular disease enterprises: part I: aging arteries: a "set up" for vascular disease. Circulation. 2003;107:139–46.
4. Lakatta EG, Levy D. Arterial and cardiac aging: major shareholders in cardiovascular disease enterprises: part II: the aging heart in health: links to heart disease. Circulation. 2003;107:346–54.
5. Chobanian AV. Clinical practice. Isolated systolic hypertension in the elderly. N Engl J Med. 2007;357:789–96.
6. Dobrzynski H, Boyett MR, Anderson RH. New insights into pacemaker activity: promoting understanding of sick sinus syndrome. Circulation. 2007;115:1921–32.
7. Monahan KD. Effect of aging on baroreflex function in humans. Am J Physiol. 2007;293:R3–12.
8. Aronow WS, Fleg JL, Pepine CJ, et al. ACCF/AHA 2011 expert consensus document on hypertension in the elderly. J Am Coll Cardiol. 2011;57:2037–114.
9. Beckett NS, Peters R, Fletcher AE, et al. Treatment of hypertension in patients 80 years of age or older. N Engl J Med. 2008;358:1887–98.
10. Ghandehari H, Kamal-Bahl S, Wong ND. Prevalence and extent of dyslipidemia and recommended lipid levels in US adults with and without cardiovascular comorbidities: the National Health and Nutrition Examination Survey 2003–2004. Am Heart J. 2008;156:112–9.

11. Kannel WB, Wilson PWF. An update on coronary risk factors. Med Clin North Am. 1995;79:951–71.
12. Heart Protection Study Collaborative Group. MRC/BHF Heart Protection Study of cholesterol lowering with simvastatin in 20,536 high-risk individuals: a randomised placebo-controlled trial. Lancet. 2002;360:7–22.
13. Shepherd J, Blauw GJ, Murphy MB, et al. Pravastatin in elderly individuals at risk of vascular disease (PROSPER): a randomised controlled trial. Lancet. 2002;360:1623–30.
14. Glynn RJ, Koenig W, Nordestgaard BG, Shepherd J, Ridker PM. Rosuvastatin for primary prevention in older persons with elevated C-reactive protein and low to average low-density lipoprotein cholesterol levels: exploratory analysis of a randomized trial. Ann Intern Med. 2010;152:488–96.
15. Weverling-Rijnsburger AW, Blauw GJ, Lagaay AM, Knook DL, Meinders AE, Westendorp RG. Total cholesterol and risk of mortality in the oldest old. Lancet. 1997;350:1119–23.
16. Newson RS, Felix JF, Heeringa J, Hofman A, Witterman JC, Tiemeier H. Association between serum cholesterol and noncardiovascular mortality in older age. J Am Geriatr Soc. 2011;59:1779–85.
17. Evans MA, Golomb BA. Statin-associated adverse cognitive effects: survey results from 171 patients. Pharmacotherapy. 2009;29:800–11.
18. American Diabetes Association. Standards of medical care in diabetes – 2011. Diabetes Care. 2011;34 Suppl 1:S11–61.
19. Gellert C, Schottker B, Brenner H. Smoking and all-cause mortality in older people. Systematic review and meta-analysis. Arch Intern Med. 2012;172:837–44.
20. Chodzko-Zajko WJ, Proctor DN, Fiatarone Singh MA, et al. American College of Sports Medicine position stand. Exercise and physical activity for older adults. Med Sci Sports Exerc. 2009;41:1510–30.
21. Dodson JA, Reid KJ, Gill TM, et al. Slow gait among older adults post-AMI and risk for hospital readmission. J Am Coll Cardiol. 2012;59(Suppl A):A470.
22. Afilalo J, Eisenberg MJ, Morin JF, et al. Gait speed as an incremental predictor of mortality and major morbidity in elderly patients undergoing cardiac surgery. J Am Coll Cardiol. 2010;56:1668–76.
23. Oreopoulos A, Kalantar-Zadeh K, Sharma AM, Fonarow GC. The obesity paradox in the elderly: potential mechanisms and clinical implications. Clin Geriatr Med. 2009;25:643–59.
24. Elveback L, Lie JT. Continued high prevalence of coronary artery disease at autopsy in Olmstead County, Minnesota, 1950 to 1970. Circulation. 1984;70:345–9.
25. Gersh BJ, Kronmal RA, Frye RL, et al. Coronary arteriography and coronary artery bypass surgery: morbidity and mortality in patients ages 65 or older. A report from the Coronary Artery Surgery Study. Circulation. 1983;67:483–91.
26. Gharacholou SM, Becker RC. Hemostasis and thrombosis in older adults. J Thromb Thrombolysis. 2009;27:249–51.
27. Alexander KP, Newby LK, Cannon CP, et al. Acute coronary care in the elderly, part I: non-ST-segment-elevation acute coronary syndromes. Circulation. 2007;115:2549–69.
28. Alexander KP, Newby LK, Armstrong PW, et al. Acute coronary care in the elderly, part II: ST-segment-elevation myocardial infarction. Circulation. 2007;115:2570–89.
29. Fleg JL, Gerstenblith G, Zonderman AB, et al. Prevalence and prognostic significance of exercise-induced silent myocardial ischemia detected by thallium scintigraphy and electrocardiography in asymptomatic volunteers. Circulation. 1990;81:428–36.
30. Gibbons RJ, Balady GJ, Bricker JT, et al. ACC/AHA 2002 guideline update for exercise testing: summary article. J Am Coll Cardiol. 2002;40:1531–40.
31. Greenland P, Bonow RO, Brundage BH, et al. ACCF/AHA 2007 clinical expert consensus document on coronary artery calcium scoring by computed tomography in global cardiovascular risk assessment and in evaluation of patients with chest pain. J Am Coll Cardiol. 2007;49:378–402.
32. Vliegenthart R, Oudkerk M, Hofman A, et al. Coronary calcification improves cardiovascular risk prediction in the elderly. Circulation. 2005;112:572–7.
33. ISIS-2 (Second International Study of Infarct Survival) Collaborative Group. Randomised trial of intravenous streptokinase, oral aspirin, both, or neither among 17187 cases of suspected acute myocardial infarction: ISIS-2. Lancet. 1988;II:349–60.
34. The Clopidogrel in Unstable Angina to Prevent Recurrent Events Trial Investigators. Effects of clopidogrel in addition to aspirin in patients with acute coronary syndromes without ST-segment elevation. N Engl J Med. 2001;345:494–502.
35. Wiviott SD, Braunwald E, McCabe CH, et al. Prasugrel versus clopidogrel in patients with acute coronary syndrome. N Engl J Med. 2007;357:2001–15.
36. Wallentin L, Becker RC, Budaj A, et al. Ticagrelor versus clopidogrel in patients with acute coronary syndromes. N Engl J Med. 2009;361:1045–57.
37. The PURSUIT Investigators. Inhibition of platelet glycoprotein IIb/IIIa with eptifibatide in patients with acute coronary syndromes. N Engl J Med. 1998;339:436–43.
38. Krumholz HM, Hennen J, Ridker PM, et al. Use and effectiveness of intravenous heparin therapy for treatment of acute myocardial infarction in the elderly. J Am Coll Cardiol. 1998;31:973–9.
39. Cohen M, Demers C, Gurfinkel EP, et al. A comparison of low molecular weight heparin with unfractionated heparin for unstable coronary artery disease. Efficacy and Safety of Subcutaneous Enoxaparin in Non-Q-Wave Coronary Events Study Group. N Engl J Med. 1997;337:447–52.
40. Stone GW, Witzenbichler B, Guagliumi G, et al. Bivalirudin during primary PCI in acute myocardial infarction. N Engl J Med. 2008;358:2218–30.
41. Jolly SS, Faxon DP, Fox KA, et al. Efficacy and safety of fondaparinux versus enoxaparin in patients with acute coronary syndromes treated with glycoprotein IIb/IIIa inhibitors or thienopyridines: results from the OASIS 5 (Fifth Organization to Assess Strategies in Ischemic Syndromes) trial. J Am Coll Cardiol. 2009;54:468–76.
42. Joyner CD, Peters RJ, Afzal R, et al. Fondaparinux compared to enoxaparin in patients with acute coronary syndromes without ST-segment elevation: outcomes and treatment effect across different levels of risk. Am Heart J. 2009;157:502–8.
43. McKellar SH, Brown ML, Frye RL, Schaff HV, Sundt TM. Comparison of coronary revascularization procedures in octogenarians: a systematic review and meta-analysis. Nat Clin Prac Cardiovasc Med. 2008;5:738–46.
44. Bonow RO, Carabello BA, Chatterjee K, et al. 2008 focused update incorporated into the ACC/AHA 2006 guidelines for the management of patients with valvular heart disease. J Am Coll Cardiol. 2008;52:e1–142.
45. Leon MB, Smith CR, Mack M, et al. Transcatheter aortic-valve implantation for aortic stenosis in patients who cannot undergo surgery. N Engl J Med. 2010;363:1597–607.
46. Smith CR, Leon MB, Mack MJ, et al. Transcatheter versus surgical aortic-valve replacement in high-risk patients. N Engl J Med. 2011;364:2187–98.
47. Rudolph V, Knap M, Franzen O, et al. Echocardiographic and clinical outcomes of MitraClip therapy in patients not amenable to surgery. J Am Coll Cardiol. 2011;58:2190–5.
48. Durante-Mangoni E, Bradley S, Selton-Suty C, et al. Current features of infective endocarditis in elderly patients: results of the International Collaboration on Endocarditis Prospective Cohort Study. Arch Intern Med. 2008;168:2095–103.

49. Kiefer T, Park L, Tribouilloy C, et al. Association between valvular surgery and mortality among patients with infective endocarditis complicated by heart failure. JAMA. 2011;306:2239–47.

50. Fleg JL, Morrell CH, Box AG, et al. Accelerated longitudinal decline of aerobic capacity in healthy older adults. Circulation. 2005;112:674–82.

51. Jugdutt BI. Aging and heart failure: changing demographics and implications for therapy in the elderly. Heart Fail Rev. 2010;15:401–5.

52. Rich MW. Heart failure in the 21st century: a cardiogeriatric syndrome. J Gerontol A Biol Sci Med Sci. 2001;56:M88–96.

53. Harkness K, Demers C, Heckman GA, McKelvie RS. Screening for cognitive deficits using the Montreal cognitive assessment tool in outpatients ≥ 65 years of age with heart failure. Am J Cardiol. 2011;107:1203–7.

54. Kitzman DW, Gardin JM, Gottdiener JS, et al. Importance of heart failure with preserved systolic function in patients ≥ 65 years of age. Am J Cardiol. 2001;87:413–9.

55. Redfield MM, Rodeheffer RJ, Jacobsen SJ, Mahoney DW, Bailey KR, Burnett Jr JC. Plasma brain natriuretic peptide concentration: impact of age and gender. J Am Coll Cardiol. 2002;40:976–82.

56. Hunt SA, Abraham WT, Chin MH, et al. 2009 focused update incorporated into the ACC/AHA 2005 guidelines for the diagnosis and management of heart failure in adults. J Am Coll Cardiol. 2009;53:e1–90.

57. Savage PA, Shaw AO, Miller MS, et al. Effect of resistance training on physical disability in chronic heart failure. Med Sci Sports Exerc. 2011;43:1379–86.

58. Roccaforte R, Demers C, Baldassarre F, Teo KK, Yusuf S. Effectiveness of comprehensive disease management programmes in improving clinical outcomes in heart failure patients. A meta-analysis. Eur J Heart Fail. 2005;7:1133–44.

59. Rich MW. Device therapy in the elderly heart failure patient: what is the evidence? Expert Rev Cardiovasc Ther. 2010;8:1203–5.

60. Delnoy PP, Ottervanger JP, Luttikhuis HO, et al. Clinical response of cardiac resynchronization therapy in the elderly. Am Heart J. 2008;155:746–51.

61. Vitale CA, Chandekar R, Rodgers PE, Pagani FD, Malani PN. A call for guidance in the use of left ventricular assist devices in older adults. J Am Geriatr Soc. 2012;60:145–50.

62. Epstein AE, DiMarco JP, Ellengoben KA, et al. ACC/AHA/HRS 2008 guidelines for device-based therapy of cardiac rhythm abnormalities. J Am Coll Cardiol. 2008;51:e1–62.

63. Kozak LJ, DeFrances CJ, Hall MJ. National hospital discharge survey: 2004 annual summary with detailed diagnosis and procedure data. National Center for Health Statistics. Vital Health Stat. 2006;13(162):1–209.

64. Dretzke J, Toff WE, Lip GY, Raftery J, Fry-Smith A, Taylor R. Dual chamber versus single chamber ventricular pacemakers for sick sinus syndrome and atrioventricular block. Cochrane Database Syst Rev. 2004;2, CD003710.

65. Go AS, Hylek EM, Phillips KA, et al. Prevalence of diagnosed atrial fibrillation in adults: national implications for rhythm management and stroke prevention: the AnTicoagulation and Risk Factors in Atrial Fibrillation (ATRIA) Study. JAMA. 2001;285:2370–5.

66. Wolf PA, Abbott RD, Kannel WB. Atrial fibrillation as an independent risk factor for stroke: the Framingham Study. Stroke. 1991;22:983–8.

67. Gage BF, Waterman AD, Shannon W, Boechler M, Rich MW, Radford MJ. Validation of clinical classification schemes for predicting stroke: results from the National Registry of Atrial Fibrillation. JAMA. 2001;285:2864–70.

68. Lip GY, Halperin JL. Improving stroke risk stratification in atrial fibrillation. Am J Med. 2010;123:484–8.

69. Fuster V, Ryden LE, Cannom DS, et al. 2011 ACCF/AHA/HRS focused updates incorporated into the ACC/AHA/ESC 2006 guidelines for the management of patients with atrial fibrillation. J Am Coll Cardiol. 2011;57:e101–98.

70. Piccini JP, Hernandez AF, Zhao X, et al. Quality of care for atrial fibrillation among patients hospitalized for heart failure. J Am Coll Cardiol. 2009;54:1280–9.

71. McCormick D, Gurwitz JH, Goldberg RJ, et al. Prevalence and quality of warfarin use for patients with atrial fibrillation in the long-term care setting. Arch Intern Med. 2001;161:2458–63.

72. Garwood CL, Corbett TL. Use of anticoagulation in elderly patients with atrial fibrillation who are at risk for falls. Ann Pharmacother. 2008;42:523–32.

73. Connolly SJ, Ezekowitz MD, Yusuf S, et al. Dabigatran versus warfarin in patients with atrial fibrillation. N Engl J Med. 2009;361:1139–51.

74. Patel MR, Mahaffey KW, Garg J, et al. Rivaroxaban versus warfarin in nonvalvular atrial fibrillation. N Engl J Med. 2011;365:883–91.

75. Granger CB, Alexander JH, McMurray JJ, et al. Apixaban versus warfarin in patients with atrial fibrillation. N Engl J Med. 2011;365:981–92.

76. Harper P, Young L, Merriman E. Bleeding risk with dabigatran in the frail elderly. N Engl J Med. 2012;366:864–6.

77. Connolly S, Pogue J, Hart R, et al. Clopidogrel plus aspirin versus oral anticoagulation for atrial fibrillation in the Atrial fibrillation Clopidogrel Trial with Irbesartan for prevention of Vascular Events (ACTIVE W): a randomised controlled trial. Lancet. 2006;367:1903–12.

78. Connolly SJ, Pogue J, Hart RG, et al. Effect of clopidogrel added to aspirin in patients with atrial fibrillation. N Engl J Med. 2009;360:2066–78.

79. DeDenus S, Sanoski CA, Carlsson J, Opolski G, Spinler SA. Rate vs. rhythm control in patients with atrial fibrillation: a meta-analysis. Arch Intern Med. 2005;165:258–62.

80. Van Gelder IC, Groenveld HF, Crijns HJ, et al. Lenient versus strict rate control in patients with atrial fibrillation. N Engl J Med. 2010;362:1363–73.

81. Yamada T, Kay GN. Catheter ablation of atrial fibrillation in the elderly. Pacing Clin Electrophysiol. 2009;32:1085–91.

82. Lee AM, Melby SJ, Damiano Jr RJ. The surgical treatment of atrial fibrillation. Surg Clin North Am. 2009;89:1001–20.

83. Hofmann JC, Wenger NS, Davis RB, et al. Patient preferences for communication with physicians about end-of-life decisions. SUPPORT Investigators. Study to understand prognoses and preference for outcomes and risks of treatment. Ann Intern Med. 1997;127:1–12.

84. Lampert R, Hayes DL, Annas GJ, et al. HRS expert consensus statement on the management of cardiovascular implantable electronic devices (CIEDs) in patients nearing end of life or requesting withdrawal of therapy. Heart Rhythm. 2010;7:1008–26.

85. Goodlin SJ. Palliative care in congestive heart failure. J Am Coll Cardiol. 2009;54:386–96.

86. Fleg JL, Bos AG, Brant LH, O'Connor FC. Longitudinal decline of aerobic capacity accelerates with age. Circulation. 2000;102 (Suppl II):II-602.

The Athlete's Heart: Cardiovascular Disease in the Athlete

Jodi L. Zilinski and Aaron L. Baggish

Abstract

With the rising popularity of recreational and competitive athletics, clinicians will benefit from an understanding of the unique physiology, clinical presentations, and management of highly trained athletes. Cardiac enlargement in athletes has been documented since the late 1800s and our understanding of the "athlete's heart" continues to advance as cardiovascular diagnostic technology improves. The term exercise-induced cardiac remodeling has been used to describe the significant changes in myocardial structure and function that result from repeated exposure to vigorous physical exercise. In clinical practice, these adaptations can be encountered during the physical examination and are clearly manifest on the electrocardiogram and during echocardiography of trained athletes. The approach to the athlete with symptoms including chest pain, syncope, or palpitation, all common in this population, requires a careful medical history with thorough assessment of athlete-specific topics including training regimen, competition history, and inquiry about performance-enhancing agents. This review provides an up-to-date summary of the science of cardiac remodeling in athletes as well as an overview of common clinical issues that are encountered in the cardiovascular care of the athlete.

Keywords
Athletes • Exercise-induced cardiac remodeling • Syncope • Chest pain • Palpitations

Introduction

Vigorous exercise can transform an athlete's entire body including the heart. Cardiac adaptations in athletes have fascinated clinicians and scientists for over a century. Our understanding of the "athlete's heart" and the key clinical issues relevant to the care of the athletic patient have paralleled advances in cardiovascular diagnostic technology since initial descriptions of cardiac enlargement in trained skiers in the late 1800s. Contemporary concepts of the athletic heart include numerous distinct morphologic, functional, and electrophysiologic changes that occur in response to training. While exercise promotes good health, athletes and physically active patients are not immune to cardiovascular disease. With the increasing popularity of both recreational exercise and competitive athletics, the need for specialized cardiovascular care for athletes has become increasingly recognized.

J.L. Zilinski, MD • A.L. Baggish, MD (✉)
Department of Cardiology, Massachusetts General Hospital,
55 Fruit St., Boston, MA 02114, USA
e-mail: jzilinski@partners.org, abaggish@partners.org

K. Stergiopoulos, D.L. Brown (eds.), *Evidence-Based Cardiology Consult*,
DOI 10.1007/978-1-4471-4441-0_20, © Springer-Verlag London 2014

Historical Overview

Since the late nineteenth century, there have been multiple descriptions of cardiac enlargement in athletes. The "father of modern medicine," Sir William Osler, observed that individuals who underwent training had "a gradual increase in the capability of the heart … the large heart of athletes may be due to the prolonged use of their muscles, but no man becomes a great runner or oarsman who has not naturally a capable if not large heart" [1]. Many physicians in the late nineteenth and early twentieth centuries harbored the belief that athletic activity had deleterious effects on the heart based on calculations by a German cardiologist, Beneke, in 1879 describing disproportionate growth of the left ventricle relative to the ascending aortic diameter in pediatric athletes [2]. Early reports describing the enlarged cardiac dimensions of athletes based on detailed physical examination were conducted in 1899 as Eugene Darling studied Harvard rowers [3] and Henschen compared Nordic skiers to sedentary individuals [4]. Both of these early investigators speculated that cardiac enlargement in athletes may reflect acquired pathology, not benign or beneficial adaptation. Importantly, early outcomes data in athletes published in 1927 by Felix Deutsch and Emil Kauf at the Vienna Heart Station appeared to refute this notion [5]. These investigators used roentgenographic orthodiagraphy to demonstrate that although the transverse diameter of the heart was enlarged in male and female athletes compared to the normal population, clinical follow-up of these athletes revealed no serious complications [5]. The introduction of newer technologies including electrocardiography (ECG), echocardiography, and magnetic resonance imaging have enhanced the ability of scientists and clinicians to assess the structural and functional adaptations to exercise.

Overview of Exercise Physiology

Successful performance of vigorous exercise requires the integrated coordination of multiple organ systems including the following: (1) uptake of oxygen in the lungs and pulmonary vasculature, (2) transport of oxygen and energy substrate by heart and systemic vasculature, and (3) oxygen utilization and force generation by skeletal muscle. The interplay of these systems in exercise physiology has been reviewed previously, so this discussion will be limited to the key aspects of exercise physiology relevant to cardiac remodeling [6–8].

As exercise intensity increases, oxygen demand increases in both the myocardium and skeletal muscle. The ability to sustain muscular work primarily depends on the cardiovascular system supplying oxygen to exercising muscle, or cardiac output. The Fick equation (cardiac output = oxygen consumption/arteriovenous oxygen difference) quantifies the

Table 20.1 Factors affecting cardiac work efficiency

Five factors modulating cardiac work efficiency	Effect at maximum workloads
Given stroke volume ejects with minimum myocardial shortening if contraction starts at larger volume	Increase
Dilated hearts lose less energy in heart wall friction and tension	Increase
Stretched muscle fiber can provide higher tension than unstretched	Increase
Loss of energy when rapid contraction, i.e., higher heart rate	Increase
Greater heart volume higher myocardial fiber tension needed to sustain intraventricular pressure (LaPlace's law)	Decrease

direct relationship between cardiac output and oxygen consumption, with both central and peripheral mechanisms involved. During strenuous exercise, cardiac output, the product of heart rate and stroke volume, can be amplified fivefold over resting levels.

While cardiac output determines the peak exercise level an athlete can attain, five factors detailed by Astrand and Rodahl [9] (Table 20.1) also influence cardiac work efficiency and thus impact athletic performance. Cardiac work becomes more efficient as chamber size increases (within limits) for three reasons: initiation of contraction at larger volume requires minimal myocardial shortening to eject a given stroke volume, less energy is lost in form of friction and tension in a dilated heart wall, and a stretched muscle fiber can provide higher tension than an unstretched one. This increased efficiency is tempered by another factor (LaPlace's law) because a higher myocardial fiber tension is needed to sustain intraventricular pressure in an enlarged cardiac chamber. LaPlace's law (wall tension = [intraventricular pressure × ventricle radius]/wall thickness) demonstrates that increases in chamber size can be modulated by concomitant increases in wall thickness. The last factor impacting work efficiency is that larger energy losses occur with rapid contraction, i.e., higher heart rate. Taken together these cardinal features theoretically predict an athlete would benefit most from a heart capable of producing a large stroke volume with a hypertrophied ventricular wall operating at a slow heart rate. The mechanical advantage a heart gains by remodeling to optimize work efficiency during stress of exercise training is the foundation of exercise-induced cardiac remodeling.

Exercise-Induced Cardiac Remodeling

As discussed above, to meet the demands of cardiovascular hemodynamics during exercise, the heart remodels to maximize cardiac output. As heart rate, one of the primary determinants of cardiac output, is variable, decreases with age, and cannot be raised with exercise training [10, 11], changes in stroke volume account for the augmentation of cardiac output during demands of strenuous exercise. With exercise the left ventricular (LV) end-diastolic volume can increase and the LV end-systolic volume can decrease resulting in an amplification of stroke volume. Sympathetic nervous stimulation mediates a reduction in LV end-systolic volume (especially in upright exercise), and multiple factors (heart rate, intrinsic myocardial relaxation, ventricular compliance, ventricular filling pressures, atrial contraction, and extracardiac factors) determine diastolic filling and thus LV end-diastolic volume [6, 12].

Left ventricular remodeling in response to exercise training has been well studied, from the increased voltage observed on ECG [13] to the left ventricular hypertrophy and LV dilation seen on echocardiography [14]. Due to an extensive preparticipation screening program, many of the published reference values for LV remodeling have been established in Italian athletes. Pelliccia et al. [15] studied 1,309 athletes from 38 different sports and found left ventricular end-diastolic diameter (LVEDD) ranged from 38 to 66 mm in women and 43–70 mm in men. Markedly dilated LV chambers (>60 mm) were observed in 14 % of the cohort and were more common in endurance athletes with nearly half the athletes having an LVEDD above the upper limit of normal. In addition, Pelliccia et al. [16] studied LV wall thickness in 947 elite athletes, but only a small percentage (1.7 %) had LV wall thickness ≥13 mm (and all athletes had concomitant LV dilation). Similar percentages have been seen in other studies of athletes and the most marked LV hypertrophy is seen more commonly in athletes at highest levels of exercise training, large body size, and Afro-Caribbean descent [17]. An LV wall thickness greater than 13 mm, which is rare even in athletes, should prompt further assessment to delineate adaptive from pathologic hypertrophy with consideration given to training status, body size, and ethnicity.

Various sport disciplines produce different hemodynamic loading conditions and thus impact exercise-induced cardiac remodeling differently. By altering the requirements of cardiac output and change in peripheral vascular resistance (PVR), exercise can be broadly divided into two types [6, 12]. Isotonic exercise, or endurance activities (e.g., running, cycling, swimming), involves sustained elevations in cardiac output with normal or reduced PVR, which acts as a volume challenge on all chambers of the heart. Isometric exercise, or strength training activities (e.g., weight lifting, throwing events), primarily involves increased PVR and normal or only slightly elevated cardiac output. While brief, the increased PVR causes transient systolic hypertension and LV afterload. Many other sports, including soccer, basketball, and hockey, are a mixture of endurance and strength exercise. Figure 20.1 [12] depicts the major training-specific changes in LV hypertrophy, ejection

fraction, diastolic function, and torsion that have been observed. In general, strength-trained athletes develop concentric hypertrophy, whereas endurance-trained athletes develop eccentric hypertrophy [18]. Enhanced early diastolic LV filling has been extensively evaluated using 2D and tissue Doppler echocardiography in endurance athletes [17, 19–21], while one study in strength athletes has suggested impaired LV relaxation in American football players [18]. Functional echocardiography has also been used to assess the mechanics of LV systolic function [22] demonstrating that endurance athletes have increased apical rotation, LV torsion, and peak early diastolic untwisting rate [23].

The adaptations to exercise seen in the left ventricle do not occur in isolation. As previously described, endurance exercise requires a larger volume of blood in both the left and right ventricle (RV), thus the RV must also remodel to accommodate the volume load experienced during endurance training. As compared to sedentary controls, larger RV cavities and a trend toward thicker RV walls have been observed in endurance athletes on echocardiogram [24, 25] and have been confirmed on MRI studies [26], which suggest that RV enlargement parallels LV enlargement. Strength training appears to minimally impact RV architecture. Multiple comparisons of RV parameters in endurance and strength athletes have demonstrated no significant RV dilation in strength athletes [18, 24]. The relative immunity from RV remodeling in strength-trained athletes may be explained by the mitral valve shielding the pulmonary circulation and right side of the heart from the stress of systemic hypertension during isometric exercise.

Left atrial remodeling has also been observed in several echocardiographic studies. The largest study, conducted in 1,777 Italian athletes, demonstrated left atrial enlargement (anterior/posterior diameter >40 mm) in 20 % of athletes [27]. D'Andrea et al. [28] confirmed a high prevalence of left atrial enlargement in endurance-trained athletes. Left atrial enlargement has also been associated with the cumulative lifetime exercise training hours [29]. The clinical implications of left atrial enlargement have been one mechanism postulated for the increased prevalence of atrial fibrillation observed in older endurance athletes.

Diagnosis and Management of Athlete-Specific Cardiovascular Issues

While trained athletes are traditionally viewed as the standard bearers of health, they are not fully protected from cardiovascular disease. Athletes typically present to medical attention either as asymptomatic individuals with structural or functional abnormalities or after development of symptoms suggestive of cardiovascular disease during sport participation. While general fundamentals of patient care

Fig. 20.1 Summary of
ventricular remodeling during
sustained exercise training
highlighting the sport-specific
nature of exercise-induced cardiac
remodeling (Reprinted with
permission from Prog Cardiovasc
Dis 2012;54:382)

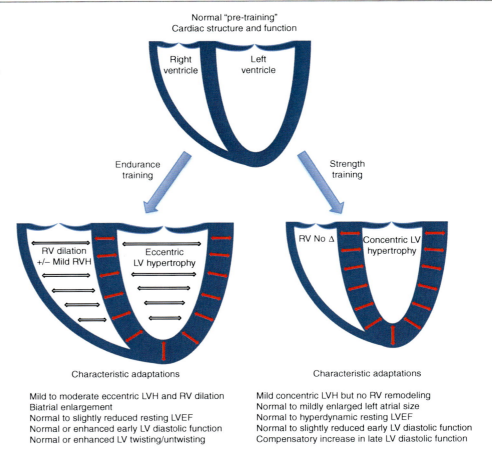

should still apply to athletes, there exist unique aspects to the care of the athletic population.

Additional components to a standard medical history are critical to a complete history in an athlete. The athlete's prior and current training history should be obtained including (1) characterization of prior athletic achievements that can be useful in assessing the athlete's competitive caliber as well as current fitness level, (2) recent training regimen, and (3) plans for future competitions. The physiologic adaptations involved in the "athlete's heart" do not occur immediately and require a certain degree of training frequency and intensity, thus an exercise training history is critical in evaluating whether the cardiovascular structural findings are adaptive or pathologic. If the athlete is presenting with new or recent symptoms, it is important to assess for any changes in the athlete's training habits, diet, or substance use that may correlate with the development of symptoms.

With a recent heightened awareness of sudden cardiac death in athletes after several highly publicized events, athletes presenting for cardiology evaluation should be screened for diseases that increase the risk of sudden cardiac death. A family history of sudden cardiac death is a major risk factor, and a detailed family history is essential. Specific components of the family history include any sudden or unexplained accidents in family members especially at a young age, a history of syncope, and/or any family members with implanted devices (e.g., pacemaker or implantable cardioverter-defibrillator).

In modern competitive athletics, pressure from media, sponsors, and fans for record-breaking performances has resulted in need to push the boundaries of athletic performance. This has led to marked increases in the use of cutting edge pharmacology including the use of illicit substances. Thus, a comprehensive medical history in the athletic patient includes questions focused on drug or supplement use. As with all patients, athletes of all ages should be routinely questioned about use of illicit drugs including traditional drugs of abuse (marijuana, cocaine, alcohol, etc.) as well as use of any performance-enhancing agents (PEAs). In addition to intentional use of PEAs, it is also important to evaluate the ingredient list of any supplement an athlete may be consuming. There is a comprehensive list of medications and substances banned in athletes published by The World Anti-Doping Agency [30], and athletes may be unintentionally using a banned substance in a supplement or over-the-counter medication. Anabolic steroids are the most widely used PEAs and previously have been shown to have deleterious cardiovascular effects such as dyslipidemia, exaggerated blood pressure response, and myocardial dysfunction [31–33]. Sport-specific considerations regarding PEA use should also be considered, for example, power sports, such as weight lifting or bodybuilding, tend to have higher use of anabolic steroids or nonsteroidal muscle mass growth stimulators such as human growth hormone and creatine. Long-term effects of the nonsteroidal muscle mass growth stimulators have been less studied. Athletes in endurance sports such as cycling have a greater likelihood of using erythropoietic stimulants that have been linked to complications such as microvascular myocardial infarction from excessive red cell mass. Stimulant use from prescription medications, such as methylphenidate, as well as over-the-counter use of caffeine or herbal stimulants has been increasing in competitive athletes and should also be specifically questioned, especially in athletes presenting with complaints such as palpitations.

Chest Pain

Within the younger population (<35 years) of highly trained athletes, cardiac causes of chest pain are relatively uncommon (<6 %) but can be life-threatening when present [34]. Table 20.1 lists clinical features that should raise concern for a cardiac cause of chest pain, and Table 20.2 lists cardiac causes of chest pain in athletes. When evaluating a population of athletes over age 35, these cardiovascular causes should be at the forefront of consideration. While regular physical exertion has been linked to decreased incidence of athlerosclerotic coronary artery disease (CAD) [35–37], athletic individuals are still at risk of cardiac events. Indeed, CAD is a leading cause of exercise-related cardiac events in adults over age 30, with an absolute risk of sudden cardiac death associated with vigorous physical exertion of approximately 1 per 200,000–250,000 healthy young individuals [38, 39]. A recent review of cardiac arrests in long-distance runners demonstrated a low overall risk of cardiac arrest (incidence rate, 0.54 per 100,000 participants) with the highest risk group comprised of male marathon runners [38]. Optimal care of the athletic patient with CAD is still being defined primarily based upon extrapolation from guidelines for care of the general population [40, 41] as well as participation guidelines for athletes such as the thirty seventh Bethesda Conference [42].

In general, the care of athletes presenting with symptoms of potential cardiac cause, such as chest discomfort, dyspnea, or decreased exercise tolerance, should be evaluated according to contemporary guidelines [40, 41]. As previously described, a thorough initial evaluation of athletes presenting with symptoms of chest pain should include a detailed history, especially a training history, family history of sudden death, medication, supplement, and/or PEA use history. It is important to note that athletes may minimize their symptoms to avoid being restricted from competition and that many athletes and medical personnel ignore exertion-related complaints such as chest discomfort or dyspnea within the first 5 min of exercise ("warm-up" angina),

Table 20.1 Concerning features in medical history for athlete presenting with chest pain

Concerning clinical features in athlete with chest pain
Syncope or near syncope with chest pain (especially in setting of exercise)
Family history of sudden cardiac death
Electrocardiographic abnormalities not consistent with exercise-induced cardiac remodeling
Murmur on exam consistent with aortic stenosis or hypertrophic cardiomyopathy
Personal or family history of congenital abnormalities such as anomalous coronary arteries

Table 20.2 Cardiac causes of exertional chest pain in athletes

Cardiac causes of chest pain in athletes
Coronary artery disorders
Atherosclerosis
Anomalous origin of coronary artery
Coronary artery dissection
Myocardial bridging
Valvular disorders
Aortic stenosis
Mitral stenosis
Mitral valve prolapse
Myocardial disorders
Hypertrophic cardiomyopathy
Myocarditis
Aortic disorders
Aortic dissection
Electrophysiologic disorders
Supraventricular arrhythmias (atrial fibrillation, Wolff-Parkinson-White syndrome, AVNRT)

AVNRT atrioventricular reentrant nodal tachycardia

exertion-related heartburn, and backache. Other key components of the chest pain history include characterization, timing, relation to exertion, alleviating/exacerbating factors, and any associated symptoms.

Aside from atherosclerotic coronary disease, the differential diagnosis of chest pain in an athlete includes other coronary artery pathologies as listed in Table 20.2. It is important to have a high index of suspicion for congenital coronary artery anomalies because, although rare in the general population (detected in <1 % of individuals at coronary angiography) [43], they have been shown to account for 15–20 % of sudden death events in athletes [44–46]. There are multiple other potential etiologies aside from coronary pathology for chest pain in an athlete, and it is important to consider other organ systems as well as the athlete's particular sport during the evaluation. Common noncardiac causes of chest pain include musculoskeletal disease, trauma, infectious/inflammatory processes, and gastroesophageal reflux disease (GERD) [34, 47]. Table 20.3 details clinical features and specific athletes at risk for noncardiac causes of chest pain. Other miscellaneous and infrequent causes include sickle

Table 20.3 Noncardiac causes of chest pain

Diagnosis	History	Physical exam	Diagnosis	Treatment	Athletes at risk	Return to competition
Musculoskeletal						
Rib fracture	Direct blunt trauma, pleuritic pain	Splinting, tenderness to palpation, bony crepitus, muscle spasm, ecchymosis	CXR to assess for associated injury (PTX, hemothorax, liver laceration), rib detail radiograph	Pain control, intercostal nerve blocks acutely, incentive spirometry	Contact sports (e.g., football, boxing, hockey)	When pain controlled, contact sports should wear flak jacket for 4–6 weeks
Rib stress fracture	Vague chest wall pain progresses to point tenderness	Splinting, tenderness to palpation	Bone scan more sensitive than CXR	Rest and analgesia, encourage deep breaths to avoid atelectasis	Rowers (incidence 12 %), throwing sports, weight lifting	When pain controlled
Costochondritis	Rib pain 2–5 at junction of rib and sternum, provoked by movement	Reproducible pain with direct pressure over costochondral junction	History and exam	Reassurance, NSAIDs	Any, usually younger	When pain controlled
Rib subluxation	Increased mobility of posterior articulation, rib may slip off transverse process, pleuritic posterior pain	Posterior pain, radiates along rib, tender over affected area	History and exam, may consider rib films	Rest and analgesia, may require physical manipulation	Rowers, butterfly swimmers, gymnasts	When rib no longer subluxed and pain adequately controlled
Slipping rib syndrome	Pain from increased mobility of anterior ribs 8–10, irritation of intercostal nerve, refers to abdomen or ant chest wall	Sharp pain for seconds, followed by aching pain for days	"Hooking maneuver" – fingers are hooked under the ribs at the costal margin and the ribs are gently pulled forward	Rest and analgesia	Women > men, mean age 40	When pain controlled
Pulmonary						
Asthma	Exertional chest tightness, shortness of breath, cough, wheezing, start minutes after exercise or in recovery	Prolonged expiratory phase, +/– wheezing	Clinical history, negative cardiac workup, spirometry (possibly pre and post exercise) +/– bronchodilator trial	Inhaled bronchodilator	Cold environment sports (ice hockey, figure skating), endurance athletes	After negative cardiac workup, after inhaled bronchodilator prophylactic trial
Pneumothorax	Spontaneous (tall, thin body habitus, + family hx) or post trauma	Decreased or absent breath sounds, hyperresonance to percussion (tension PTX = absent breath sounds, elevated JVP, hypotension)	Clinical history, exam, AP inspiratory film, expiratory film if not seen	Small apical can be observed or catheter aspiration. Moderate to large require chest tube or those causing symptoms or increasing size	Weight lifting, running, scuba. Risk factors: smoking, substance abuse	Suggested time frame 4–6 weeks prior to contact sports, some case series football players returned within 2 weeks [48]
Pulmonary embolus	Acute chest pain, new wheeze, pleuritic pain, hemoptysis, dyspnea,	Wheeze, evidence of DVT on exam, tachycardia, tachypnea	Contrast chest CT, ventilation perfusion scan	Anticoagulation, consider fibrinolysis if hemodynamically significant	Athletes at risk for thrombosis – recent surgery or injury (leg trauma), family clotting history, women on OCPs	No specific guidelines, contact sports usually prohibited while on anticoagulation

Gastrointestinal

GERD	Heartburn, chest/epigastric pain, belching, nausea, vomiting (50 % during heavy exercise, 90 % of fed runners during and postexercise)	Symptoms may only occur with exercise	History, can consider endoscopy or exercise test with pH probe to demonstrate reflux with exertion	Changes in training or diet habits. Avoid exercise after meals. Avoid high-calorie meals 3 h prior to exercise. Protein supplements decrease gastric emptying and caffeine lowers LES tone, may need to avoid. Trial of anti-reflux medication (PPI)	Runners, jumpers, weight lifters. NSAIDs can worsen	No restrictions but may need alteration in training method

Trauma

Pulmonary contusion	Blunt injury to thorax. Dyspnea, hemoptysis in 50 %	Tachypnea, tachycardia, cyanosis, chest wall bruising, rales, decreased breath sounds	CXR findings variable: patchy infiltrates to consolidation 4–6 h post injury, CT more sensitive at early phase	Assess for associated morbidity, hospitalize, pulmonary toilet, pain management, may need mechanical ventilation (mortality 5–15 %)	Usually great force causing injury, fall from height or high velocity (cycling, motor sports)	No specific guidelines, consider when symptoms and imaging demonstrate resolution. Symptom guided return to activity
Cardiac contusion	Blunt chest trauma. Assoc complications: arrhythmia, CHF, shock, hemopericardium, tamponade. May be asymptomatic	Sinus tachycardia (70 %), hypotension. Varied presentation	ECG shows sinus tachycardia, PAC or PVC, AF, NSVT, RBBB, LBBB, IVCD. Cardiac biomarkers, echocardiography and radionuclide studies not helpful	Admit symptomatic patients and those with ECG changes for monitoring (arrhythmia within 12 h post injury)	Contact sports, any significant blunt trauma (fall/accident while cycling, motor sports)	Sport-specific guidelines do not exist. Depend on extent of cardiac injury

CXR chest radiograph, *PTX* pneumothorax, *NSAIDs* Nonsteroidal anti-inflammatory drugs, *JVP* jugular venous pressure, *DVT* deep vein thrombosis, *CT* computed tomography, *OCPs* oral contraceptive pills, *LES* lower esophageal sphincter, *PPI* proton pump inhibitor, *ECG* electrocardiograph, *PAC* premature atrial contraction, *PVC* premature ventricular contraction, *AF* atrial fibrillation, *NSVT* nonsustained ventricular tachycardia, *RBBB* right bundle-branch block, *LBBB* left bundle-branch block, *IVCD* intraventricular conduction delay

cell disease with chest pain resulting from decreased carrying capacity of erythrocytes in high-output states, pregnancy in the female athlete with new onset chest pain and exercise intolerance, use of drugs of abuse (cocaine, anabolic steroids, and stimulants) [47], and eating disorders involving purging that can cause conditions such as esophagitis and Mallory-Weiss tears.

As part of the initial diagnostic evaluation in athletes presenting with chest pain, an electrocardiogram (ECG) should be obtained. It is important to note that athletes, especially endurance-trained athletes, may demonstrate more ECG abnormalities than are observed in more sedentary individuals. These features include resting sinus bradycardia, mild enlargement of cardiac chambers, early repolarization pattern (presence of a "J wave" at the junction of the QRS and ST segment [49] that has been associated with increased prevalence after intense physical training) [50], or increased voltage suggestive of left ventricular hypertrophy (LVH) [51, 52]. Further workup based on history and physical may include exercise testing, especially if exertional symptoms are described. As some of the characteristic ECG findings in athletes (e.g., LVH) can lead to false-positive results during exercise ECG testing, the addition of an imaging modality such as echocardiography or nuclear scintigraphy may be required [40]. Exercise stress testing in athletes should be performed to maximal exercise capacity and not terminated prematurely due to heart rate. While the Bruce protocol is easily performed and well tolerated by most athletes, athletes who experience symptoms only during their particular activity may need specialized exercise testing designed to simulate their primary sporting activity. Further diagnostic evaluation of suspected CAD after initial history, examination, ECG, and exercise testing may require definition of coronary anatomy by cardiac computed tomography (CT) or coronary angiography. Detection of coronary anomalies and determination of their physiologic relevance requires the use of coronary imaging studies including cardiac CT, cardiac magnetic resonance (CMR), or conventional coronary angiography coupled with exercise stress testing.

The diagnosis of atherosclerotic CAD is defined as follows: (1) history of myocardial infarction (MI); (2) history suggesting angina pectoris, with objective evidence of inducible ischemia; or (3) coronary atherosclerosis demonstrated on imaging (coronary angiogram, CMR, cardiac CT) [42]. Once an athlete has been diagnosed with CAD, management consists of aggressive risk factor modification and risk stratification to guide exercise advice. Secondary prevention of an atherosclerotic event involves antiplatelet therapy, antihypertensive therapy, and lipid-lowering therapy [42, 43, 53]. As with the general population, the mainstay of antiplatelet therapy is aspirin with addition of thienopyridines in patients who have experienced an acute coronary syndrome (ACS) or coronary revascularization [54–56]. In athletes participating in contact sports, the potential risk of hemorrhage on dual antiplatelet therapy should be discussed but is not an absolute contraindication to participation in certain types of sports [53]. For antihypertensive therapy in athletes, vasodilators including angiotensin-converting enzyme inhibitors (ACE-I) and calcium channel blockers are the primary initial medications as they are usually well tolerated. Adjunctive diuretic therapy may be useful but should be administered with caution in endurance athletes prone to exertional dehydration. While β (beta)-blockers have been shown to reduce recurrent events in patients with CAD (especially in setting of reduced left ventricular [LV] ejection fraction [EF]), they are less effective antihypertensive agents and may decrease athletic performance in endurance athletes. However, in athletes with impaired left ventricular function, β (beta)-blockers may be a reasonable strategy [54]. For all patients following ACS, guidelines recommend β (beta)-blockers [57], but for athletes with preserved EF, the negative performance effects may result in decreased adherence. Thus, use of β (beta)-blockers should be tailored on an individualized basis [53]. Lipid-lowering therapy is another core tenant of risk factor modification and primarily involves the use of statins. Recommendations for goal LDL levels in athletic populations are the same as the general population (LDL <70 mg/dL following ACS or 25 % reduction from baseline) [54]. It must be noted that statins commonly cause myalgias, with an increased prevalence in physically active individuals [58] and athletes [59, 60], potentially resulting from augmentation of exercise-related muscle injury. Thus, statin use as a maintenance medication in athletes may be difficult requiring multiple trials, different potency statins, or alternative dosing regimens. Reducing the lipid content of atherosclerotic plaques may help stabilize lipid-rich plaques at risk for exercise-induced rupture. A demonstrated benefit has been shown for early aggressive statin treatment following an ACS event even if statin therapy later needs to be discontinued [61], which has resulted in some experts recommending restriction from aggressive training and competition for 2 years following an ACS event with reduction of LDL to lowest level tolerated [53].

For the athletic patient with CAD as previously defined, comprehensive risk stratification should be performed prior to returning to training or competition. Patients are determined to be at mildly increased risk if they demonstrate the following: (1) preserved LV EF, (2) normal exercise tolerance for age, (3) absence of exercise-induced ischemia or complex ventricular arrhythmia, (4) absence of hemodynamically significant stenosis (>50 % luminal narrowing), and (5) successful revascularization [42]. Such patients can participate in most sports at a moderate to high-intensity level. In contrast, patients with high-risk features may require restriction to low dynamic and low/moderate static competitive sports and should be counseled to avoid intensely competitive situations. Patients at substantially increased risk (those with impaired LV EF, evidence of exercise-induced ischemia or complex ventricular arrhythmia, or hemodynamically significant stenosis [luminal narrowing >50 %]) should be restricted to low-intensity competitive sports [42]. Athletes with a coronary anomaly and inducible myocardial ischemia should be restricted from activity until surgical correction [43].

Arrhythmia/Palpitations

Palpitations, the awareness of forceful, rapid, or irregular heartbeats, are common among trained athletes. Palpitations and benign arrhythmias can be found in younger (school-age) athletic populations and when noted are unlikely to require restriction from activity [62]. In contrast, the complaint of palpitations in older and highly trained athletes is more common [63]. While the majority of palpitations are considered benign, certain conditions such as high premature ventricular contraction (PVC) burden (>2,000 PVCs in 24 h), atrial fibrillation, and exercise-induced palpitations may reflect underlying heart disease or an arrhythmia/conduction abnormality and should be evaluated [64]. The differential diagnosis of possible medical conditions contributing to palpitations and arrhythmias in athletes (Table 20.4) is broad, and diagnosis usually relies on ECG documentation of arrhythmia via either long-term ambulatory monitoring or exercise testing. Diagnosis can be complicated by the fact that both bradyarrhythmias and tachyarrhythmias have been documented in trained athletes.

Athletes often demonstrate bradyarrhythmias, including resting sinus bradycardia (which may reflect cardiovascular fitness), junctional bradycardia, first-degree atrioventricular (AV) block, and Mobitz type I AV block. Resting heart rates (HRs) during sleep may demonstrate profound bradycardia, which reflects heightened parasympathetic activity or increased vagal tone and are not considered pathologic. It has also been suggested that intrinsic sinoatrial slowing may be a result of repeated exercise training [65, 66] and former endurance athletes may demonstrate intrinsic sinus node disease years after their peak training performances.

Tachyarrhythmias, particularly atrial fibrillation, can be the source of arrhythmia-related complaints in athletes. In one study of Italian elite athletes with a history of palpitations, atrial fibrillation was the cause in 40 % of patients [67]. Multiple studies have suggested that athletes, especially older endurance sport athletes, are at increased risk of developing atrial fibrillation both during their periods of active training as well as years after their high-intensity training [67–71]. Multiple potential mechanisms have been postulated to account for the observed increased frequency of atrial fibrillation in athletes including the following:

Table 20.4 Medical conditions contributing to arrhythmias

Medical conditions contributing to arrhythmia
Coronary artery disease
Valvular heart disease
Cardiomyopathy (including HCM, ARVC)
Pericarditis/myocarditis
Long QT syndrome
Brugada syndrome
Anemia
Electrolyte abnormalities
Fever
Thyroid abnormalities
Hypo- or hyperglycemia
Pheochromocytoma
Pulmonary disease (contributes to multifocal atrial tachycardia)
Autonomic neuropathies (e.g., postural orthostatic tachycardia syndrome)

HCM hypertrophic cardiomyopathy, *ARVC* arrhythmogenic right ventricular cardiomyopathy

exercise-induced LA remodeling [27, 72], systemic inflammation [70, 73], augmentation of vagal tone which shortens atrial refractory period facilitating reentry [70], and increased sympathetic activity during exercise. Other supraventricular arrhythmias such as AV nodal reentrant tachycardia, AV reciprocating tachycardia, and atrial tachycardias are not more common in athletes.

Premature atrial contractions (PACs) and PVCs as well as nonsustained ventricular tachycardia (NSVT), a burst of ventricular activity less than 30 s with spontaneous return to sinus rhythm, have all been observed in trained athletes. Premature beats are another common reason for athletes to present with palpitations. As athletes are usually lean and felt to be "in tune" with their bodies, they may have a heightened sensitivity to premature beats. It is important to assess the frequency of PVCs on Holter monitor as well as exclude structural heart disease and evaluate the impact of exercise. The presence of structural heart disease or frequent complex ventricular arrhythmias during exercise in structurally normal hearts may require further testing to exclude conditions such as CAD, arrhythmogenic right ventricular cardiomyopathy (ARVC), or catecholaminergic polymorphic ventricular tachycardia (CPVT) [74]. However, most patients with PVCs have a benign prognosis. In one study of trained Italian athletes, 30 % of the athletes noted to have more than 2,000 PVCs in 24 h were found to have underlying heart disease [63]. In athletes without structural heart disease, especially those with PVCs suppressed by exercise, premature beats have not been related to sudden cardiac death. The frequency of PVCs in both the population of athletes with and without structural heart disease has decreased after deconditioning, which may be useful in treating symptomatic athletes [75]. Reassuring data have also been published regarding the

Table 20.5 Drugs contributing to arrhythmias

Drugs contributing to arrhythmia
QT prolonging agents (antipsychotics, antibiotics, etc.)
Caffeine
Alcohol
Over-the-counter drugs (e.g., pseudoephedrine)
Supplements with stimulants (ephedra, bitter orange, guarana)
Anabolic steroids
Illicit drugs (e.g., cocaine)

benign nature of NSVT in athletes without structural heart disease [66]. US guidelines recommend no restriction on activity in athletes without structural heart disease or symptoms [74].

While no specific recommendations for the evaluation and management of palpitations in an athlete exist, guidelines have focused on recommendations for specific arrhythmias [74, 76]. Athletes presenting with palpitations should have a thorough history and physical focused on timing of palpitations, relation to exertion, associated symptoms, family history of sudden death, and dietary/supplement intake (e.g., caffeine). Table 20.5 lists the drugs and medications that can contribute to palpitations and/or arrhythmias in athletes. Further diagnostic evaluation of the athlete with symptomatic palpitations, tachyarrhythmias, or frequent PVCs should include an assessment for structural and valvular heart disease as well as exclusion of metabolic causes such as hyperthyroidism or hypoglycemia. With frequent or easily reproducible symptoms, a Holter monitor during the athlete's specific exercise may be useful in diagnosis. Exercise testing may need to be adapted to the athlete's specific activity in order to simulate the conditions in which the arrhythmia is experienced, for instance, mode of activity or rate of workload intensity may need to be altered from conventional exercise testing.

Management of athletes with arrhythmias depends on the underlying etiology of the arrhythmia and whether it occurs in fast heart rate conditions (i.e., exercise) or slow heart rate conditions (i.e., sleep, exercise recovery). The management of bradyarrhythmias in the athlete primarily consists of reassurance and documentation of an adequate chronotropic response to exercise. Higher-grade AV block such as Mobitz II or complete heart block is unusual in athletes and should be considered pathologic, likely requiring a pacemaker [74, 77].

The management of tachyarrhythmias in athletes varies with specific etiology and encompasses education, medication, and invasive treatment (catheter ablation). Athletes should be educated on avoidance of drugs that can precipitate tachyarrhythmias (e.g., cocaine, pseudoephedrine). In athletes with supraventricular arrhythmias such as atrial fibrillation, management with nodal agents such as β (beta)-blockers (BB) and calcium channel blockers (CCB) may minimize symptoms but does not affect the frequency of atrial fibrillation episodes. As these agents affect the heart rate both at rest and during exercise, they may reduce exercise capacity in some individuals. In some competitive athletes, it should be noted that agents such as BB may be banned [30]. Class Ic antiarrhythmic agents, such as flecainide or propafenone, may be effective methods of maintaining sinus rhythm. These agents increase AV conduction, thus they usually require a nodal agent to counteract potential accelerated ventricular response in setting of atrial flutter. A "pill in the pocket" strategy using either flecainide or propafenone to abort an episode of symptomatic atrial fibrillation may be an attractive option for athletes who do not wish to take a medication daily [64]. Catheter ablation of some arrhythmias may be preferable to drug treatment in some athletes, although this has only been studied in small populations of athletes with atrial fibrillation [73, 78, 79]. In the setting of Wolff-Parkinson-White (WPW) syndrome, if the conduction through the accessory pathway is very rapid (able to conduct at heart rates greater than 240), patients are felt to be at risk of sudden death and curative ablation is recommended [80, 81]. In some cases, athletes whose arrhythmia has been successfully ablated can return to athletics within days if an easily inducible arrhythmia prior to ablation is unable to be induced post-ablation during isoproterenol administration. Consensus opinions regarding return to play for various arrhythmias have been established [74].

Syncope

In both the athletic and general population, syncope is a common complaint. Syncope is defined as the transient loss of consciousness accompanied by loss of postural tone with spontaneous recovery. Whereas "benign" forms of syncope, including neurally mediated syncope (NMS), often require no evaluation in the general population, syncope in an athlete should always raise concern, especially when syncope occurs during exertion. Determining the specific cause of syncope is not possible in up to ~35 % of cases [82]. Thus, the most important aspect of evaluating a syncopal episode in an athlete is to rule out underlying cardiac etiologies that can cause sudden cardiac death, and athletes may need to be withheld from athletic participation until cardiac pathology has been excluded [74, 76].

The majority of syncope in athletes is unrelated to exercise or occurs postexercise. As seen in one cohort of 7,568 athletes undergoing pre-participation screening, 6.2 % of patients reported a syncopal episode within the last 5 years. In this series, most episodes were not related to exertion, 12 % occurred post-exertion, and 1.3 % were during exercise [83]. The most common cause of syncope in athletes is NMS, and the vast majority of post-exertional syncope is neurally mediated. In normal physiology, venous pooling (from standing, exercise, etc.) causes decreased venous return to the right ventricle, and the body compensates by increasing heart rate, contractility, and peripheral vascular resistance to augment cardiac output, thereby increasing preload and venous return [84, 85]. During exercise, increased sympathetic stimulation raises heart rate and diastolic blood pressure increasing cardiac output, which is distributed to skeletal muscle. This preload-dependent increase in cardiac output is maintained by peripheral muscle activity returning volume to the heart, functioning in effect as a "muscle pump." With abrupt cessation of exercise, the muscle pump ceases and the resulting sudden fall in venous return produces a vigorous contraction in a relatively empty right ventricle stimulating mechanoreceptors that trigger a cardiac depressor reflex resulting in bradycardia and hypotension [80]. Reductions in heart rate and blood pressure combined with decreased venous return ultimately cause decreased cerebral perfusion and syncope.

The history and physical examination are the most essential part of the syncope evaluation and can identify the etiology in about 45 % of cases in which a cause is found [82]. Syncope during exertion has many potential causes (Table 20.6). History taking in syncope can be difficult because the patient often has some degree of amnesia for the event. In athletes this may be even more challenging as symptoms may be withheld due to fear of being removed from competition. Thus, it is important to question bystanders and witnesses and/or obtain any medical records from emergency personnel. The salient historical features of a syncopal episode include the following: any prodrome, inciting factors and the activity being undertaken prior to the episode, duration of syncope, any muscular movements during LOC and their initiation, and post-syncope symptoms such as confusion or bowel/bladder incontinence [86–90]. In addition to a detailed description of the event, a thorough patient history should also be obtained with particular attention to any prior history of syncope, any personal or family history of cardiac problems or sudden death, risk factors for cardiac disease, and a detailed medication list including any over-the-counter supplements, illicit drugs, or PEAs. Important factors in the physical examination of the athlete with syncope include complete vital signs, including orthostatic vital signs as well as blood pressure in both upper extremities and one lower extremity [76]. Careful vascular and neurologic exams may reveal findings suggestive of particular causes of syncope. Cardiac auscultation should include positional maneuvers such as standing, squatting, postexercise, and Valsalva to elicit dynamic changes seen in cardiomyopathies such as hypertrophic cardiomyopathy (HCM) or valve disease such as aortic stenosis or mitral stenosis. Table 20.7 describes clinical features that may suggest a specific etiology.

Table 20.6 Differential diagnosis of exertional syncope

Potential causes of exercise-induced syncope
Aortic stenosis
Hypertrophic cardiomyopathy
Mitral stenosis
Pulmonary hypertension
Ischemia from coronary artery disease
Ischemia from anomalous coronary artery disease
Anaphylaxis
Brugada syndrome
Cardiac dilatation or depressed cardiac function
Catecholamine-dependent polymorphic ventricular tachycardia
Commotio cordis
Dehydration
Eating disorders
Hypoglycemia
Sick sinus syndrome
Ventricular tachycardia/ventricular fibrillation
Ventricular preexcitation (Wolff-Parkinson-White)
Vasodepressor reflex

The initial evaluation of athletes with syncope always includes an ECG to exclude arrhythmias and cardiomyopathy. Careful examination of the ECG in an athletic patient (Table 20.8) is important because several ECG findings can be suggestive of a cardiac cause. Many features that could be considered abnormal in the general population are commonly observed in highly trained athletes and should not be considered as a cause of syncope [50, 91, 92].

After the initial evaluation of history, physical, and ECG, there should be a low threshold for obtaining an echocardiogram and in the case of exertional syncope, an exercise test (after echocardiography) [76]. The leading causes of death in American athletes under age 35 include conditions that may present with syncope such as HCM, anomalous coronary arteries, myocarditis, and ARVC. An echocardiogram may be useful in detecting these conditions or other structural cardiac problems [44, 45, 93]. A detailed assessment including left ventricular and right ventricular size and function, wall thickness, valve lesions, aortic root dilation, elevated right ventricular systolic pressure, and coronary ostia should be conducted. As discussed previously, exercise testing protocols should simulate athlete's training conditions to maximize likelihood of eliciting symptoms [80, 94].

If exercise testing does not reveal any symptoms or reproduce syncope, long-term ambulatory ECG monitoring may be needed. For patients with frequent and easily reproducible symptoms, a Holter monitor worn for 24–48 h may be useful in capturing the episode. However, Holter monitoring is generally low yield when symptoms are intermittent and either an external event monitor or implantable loop recorder (ILR) is recommended. Noncompliance can be an issue with external monitors, especially in athletes in whom the electrodes

Table 20.7 Clinical features suggestive of etiology of syncope

Finding on history or exam	Suggested diagnoses
Occurs with micturition, defecation, cough, deglutition, playing brass instrument, weight lifting	Neurally mediated syncope/situational syncope
Associated with throat or facial pain (glossopharyngeal or trigeminal neuralgia)	Neurally mediated syncope/neuralgia
Occurs within an hour after eating	Neurally mediated syncope/postprandial hypotension
Occurred with prolonged standing	Neurally mediated syncope/vasovagal syncope
Associated with pain, fear, and unpleasant sight, smell, or sound	Neurally mediated syncope/vasovagal syncope
Occur in warm or crowded environment	Neurally mediated syncope/vasovagal syncope
Well-trained athlete with structurally normal heart after exertion	Neurally mediated syncope/vasovagal syncope
Tonic-clonic movements short (<15 s) and occur after loss of consciousness	Neurally mediated syncope/vasovagal syncope
Tonic-clonic movements prolonged and initiates during or prior to loss of consciousness	Seizure
Syncope associated with tongue biting, aching muscles, and prolonged confusion	Seizure
Occurs upon standing	Orthostatic hypotension
Taking one or more antihypertensive medications (especially polypharmacy in elderly)	Drug-induced syncope
Multiple medications prolonging QT or causing bradycardia	Drug-induced syncope
Associated with vertigo, dysarthria, diplopia	TIA, stroke, vertebrobasilar insufficiency
Blood pressure difference between arms	Subclavian steal or aortic dissection
Syncope during arm exercise (e.g., painting a fence)	Subclavian steal
Occurs with change in position (upright to supine, bending over) +/− murmur that also varies with position	Atrial myxoma, thrombus
Family history of sudden cardiac death	Long QT, Brugada, HCM
Deaf patient who experiences syncope after effort or strong emotion	Long QT syndrome
Triggered by laughter or strong emotions with normal cardiac evaluation	Cataplexy
Child <5 years old after frustrating episode or injury	Breath holding spell
Diabetic who skipped meals	Hypoglycemia

TIA transient ischemic attack, *HCM* hypertrophic cardiomyopathy

Table 20.8 Athlete ECG abnormalities and relation to syncope

Observed in trained athletes/ related to training	Suggestive of arrhythmogenic syncope	Unrelated to training	Suggestive of arrhythmogenic syncope
Sinus bradycardia	Rare cause in athlete	Second (Mobitz II) or third-degree AV block	Yes
First-degree AV block	No	T-wave inversion	No
Incomplete right bundle-branch block	No	Pathological Q waves	Possible
Early repolarization	No	Left atrial enlargement	No
Isolated LVH criteria by QRS voltage	No	Left-axis deviation/left anterior hemiblock	Possible
		Right-axis deviation/left posterior hemiblock	Possible
		Right ventricular hypertrophy	Possible
		Preexcitation (i.e., WPW syndrome)	Yes
		Complete left bundle-branch block or right bundle-branch block	Possible
		Abnormal QT interval	Yes
		Brugada pattern	Yes
		T-wave inversion V1–V3, epsilon waves, and ventricular late potentials (i.e., ARVC)	Yes

AV atrioventricular, *LVH* left ventricular hypertrophy, *WPW* Wolff-Parkinson-White, *ARVC* arrhythmogenic right ventricular cardiomyopathy

and monitor may interfere with a training regimen [76]. Therefore, in athletes the placement of an ILR, which is a subcutaneous monitor that automatically records arrhythmias, may be advantageous [80].

Additional diagnostic testing modalities such as tilt-table testing, electrophysiologic (EP) study, and advanced imaging have limited roles in the evaluation of unexplained syncope in athletes due to poor sensitivity and specificity as well as potential for identifying abnormalities unrelated to presenting symptoms. Athletes have a high rate of positive tilt tests, and the reproducibility of tilt tests has been markedly variable [80, 87] such that widespread use is not recommended. The diagnostic utility of EP studies for evaluation of bradyarrhythmias is limited in athletes due to their high vagal tone. In tachyarrhythmias, the role of EP studies is for the confirmation and treatment (via catheter ablation) of specific suspected etiologies [81]. The role of advanced imaging in syncope should likewise be limited to evaluation of specific suspected etiologies, such as cardiac CT to evaluate for anomalous origin of the coronary arteries or aortic pathologies [80] or CMR for enhanced definition of cardiomyopathies, such as HCM or ARVC [95].

Management of syncope should be tailored to the specific etiology found on diagnostic testing. The focus of treatment in NMS involves recognition of pre-syncopal symptoms, avoidance of triggers, and instruction on counterpressure maneuvers (e.g., squatting, arm tensing, leg crossing) to abort orthostatic intolerance [81, 94, 96, 97]. In athletes with structurally normal hearts and NMS, volume and/or salt loading coupled with lower-extremity compression stockings is recommended. The role of pharmacologic therapy in NMS is limited; the best data from randomized controlled trials supports the use of midodrine [96]. Due to the potential for devastating consequences of even benign etiologies of syncope, such as NMS, in athletes participating in high-risk activities (e.g., diving, cycling) or those with minimal prodrome, these athletes may require more intense therapies or restriction from play. According to the thirty sixth Bethesda Conference, athletes with syncope attributed to arrhythmias may return to competition after they have been asymptomatic for 2–3 months following treatment and evaluation by a physician [74]. In patients with ventricular arrhythmia where ablation is not curative or an ICD is placed, moderate- and high-intensity sports as well as contact sports are not recommended [74]. However, there is variation in practice and some cardiologists allow sports participation for athletes with ICDs [98], and a large registry is currently following athletes with implantable devices [99]. Athletes with potentially life-threatening etiologies of syncope should be restricted from play. While the safe return to physical activity is paramount, it is important to consider the emotional, social, and/or financial ramifications from activity restriction in athletes.

Key Points
- Athlete heart – distinct structural entity with sport-type/training-type specific changes:
  - Need to differentiate from pathologic causes of cardiac enlargement
- Historical features:
  - Need to discuss training regimen and/or changes in athlete presenting with new symptoms
  - Need to routinely inquire about performance-enhancing agents
- Chest pain, palpitations, or syncope with exertion are common in athletes and should be evaluated to exclude underlying cardiac disease.
- Athletes should be restricted from training and competition during evaluation until the cardiac diseases associated with increased risk of sudden death are ruled out.
- Management of cardiac conditions in athletes may require individualized treatment regimens as core medical therapies (e.g., statin or β (beta)-blockers) may have negative effects on performance resulting in decreased adherence.

References

1. Osler W. The principles and practice of medicine. New York: Appleton and Company; 1892.
2. Karpovich PV. Textbook fallacies regarding child's heart. Res Quart. 1937;8:33.
3. Darling E. The effects of training: a study of the Harvard University crews. Boston Med Surg J. 1899;161:229–33.
4. Henschen S. Skilauf und Skiwettlauf. Eine medizinische Sportstudie. Mitt Med Klinik Upsala. 1899;2:15–8.
5. Deutsch F, Kauf E. Heart and athletics. St. Louis: CV Mosby Company; 1927.
6. Baggish AL, Wood MJ. Athlete's heart and cardiovascular care of the athlete: scientific and clinical update. Circulation. 2011;123:2723–35.
7. Thompson PD, editor. Exercise and sports cardiology. New York: McGraw-Hill; 2001.
8. Thompson PD. Exercise prescription and proscription for patients with coronary artery disease. Circulation. 2005;112:2354–63.
9. Astrand P, Rodahl K. Textbook of work physiology. New York: McGraw-Hill Book Company; 1977.

10. Jose AD, Collison D. The normal range and determinants of the intrinsic heart rate in man. Cardiovasc Res. 1970;4:160–7.

11. Uusitalo AL, Uusitalo AJ, Rusko HK. Exhaustive endurance training for 6–9 weeks did not induce changes in intrinsic heart rate and cardiac autonomic modulation in female athletes. Int J Sports Med. 1998;19:532–40.

12. Weiner RB, Baggish AL. Exercise-induced cardiac remodeling. Prog Cardiovasc Dis. 2012;54:380–6.

13. Venerando A, Rulli V. Frequency morphology and meaning of the electrocardiographic anomalies found in Olympic marathon runners and walkers. J Sports Med Phys Fitness. 1964;50:135–41.

14. Roeske WR, O'Rourke RA, Klein A, Leopold G, Karliner JS. Noninvasive evaluation of ventricular hypertrophy in professional athletes. Circulation. 1976;53:286–91.

15. Pelliccia A, Culasso F, Di Paolo FM, Maron BJ. Physiologic left ventricular cavity dilatation in elite athletes. Ann Intern Med. 1999;130:23–31.

16. Pelliccia A, Maron BJ, Spataro A, Proschan MA, Spirito P. The upper limit of physiologic cardiac hypertrophy in highly trained elite athletes. N Engl J Med. 1991;324:295–301.

17. Baggish AL, Yared K, Weiner RB, et al. Differences in cardiac parameters among elite rowers and subelite rowers. Med Sci Sports Exerc. 2010;42:1215–20.

18. Baggish AL, Wang F, Weiner RB, et al. Training-specific changes in cardiac structure and function: a prospective and longitudinal assessment of competitive athletes. J Appl Physiol. 2008;104:1121–8.

19. Caso P, D'Andrea A, Galderisi M, et al. Pulsed Doppler tissue imaging in endurance athletes: relation between left ventricular preload and myocardial regional diastolic function. Am J Cardiol. 2000;85:1131–6.

20. D'Andrea A, Cocchia R, Riegler L, et al. Left ventricular myocardial velocities and deformation indexes in top-level athletes. J Am Soc Echocardiogr. 2010;23:1281–8.

21. Prasad A, Popovic ZB, Arbab-Zadeh A, et al. The effects of aging and physical activity on Doppler measures of diastolic function. Am J Cardiol. 2007;99:1629–36.

22. Baggish AL, Yared K, Wang F, et al. The impact of endurance exercise training on left ventricular systolic mechanics. Am J Physiol Heart Circ Physiol. 2008;295:H1109–16.

23. Weiner RB, Hutter Jr AM, Wang F, et al. The impact of endurance exercise training on left ventricular torsion. JACC Cardiovasc Imaging. 2010;3:1001–9.

24. D'Andrea A, Riegler L, Golia E, et al. Range of right heart measurements in top-level athletes: the training impact. Int J Cardiol. 2013;164(1):48–57.

25. Oxborough D, Sharma S, Shave R, et al. The right ventricle of the endurance athlete: the relationship between morphology and deformation. J Am Soc Echocardiogr. 2012;25:263–71.

26. Scharhag J, Schneider G, Urhausen A, Rochette V, Kramann B, Kindermann W. Athlete's heart: right and left ventricular mass and function in male endurance athletes and untrained individuals determined by magnetic resonance imaging. J Am Coll Cardiol. 2002;40:1856–63.

27. Pelliccia A, Maron BJ, Di Paolo FM, et al. Prevalence and clinical significance of left atrial remodeling in competitive athletes. J Am Coll Cardiol. 2005;46:690–6.

28. D'Andrea A, Riegler L, Cocchia R, et al. Left atrial volume index in highly trained athletes. Am Heart J. 2010;159:1155–61.

29. Wilhelm M, Roten L, Tanner H, Wilhelm I, Schmid JP, Saner H. Atrial remodeling, autonomic tone, and lifetime training hours in nonelite athletes. Am J Cardiol. 2011;108:580–5.

30. World Anti-doping agency. The World Anti-Doping Code: The 2013 Prohibited List. 2013; http://www.wada-ama.org/Documents/World_Anti-Doping_Program/WADP-Prohibited-list/2013/WADA-Prohibited-List-2013-EN.pdf (accessed October 9, 2013).

31. Kiraly CL. Androgenic-anabolic steroid effects on serum and skin surface lipids, on red cells, and on liver enzymes. Int J Sports Med. 1988;9:249–52.

32. Riebe D, Fernhall B, Thompson PD. The blood pressure response to exercise in anabolic steroid users. Med Sci Sports Exerc. 1992;24:633–7.

33. Baggish AL, Weiner RB, Kanayama G, et al. Long-term anabolic-androgenic steroid use is associated with left ventricular dysfunction. Circ Heart Fail. 2010;3:472–6.

34. Perron AD. Chest pain in athletes. Clin Sports Med. 2003;22:37–50.

35. Leon AS, Connett J, Jacobs Jr DR, Rauramaa R. Leisure-time physical activity levels and risk of coronary heart disease and death. The multiple risk factor intervention trial. JAMA. 1987;258:2388–95.

36. Blair SN, Kohl 3rd HW, Paffenbarger Jr RS, Clark DG, Cooper KH, Gibbons LW. Physical fitness and all-cause mortality. A prospective study of healthy men and women. JAMA. 1989;262:2395–401.

37. Kannel WB, Wilson P, Blair SN. Epidemiological assessment of the role of physical activity and fitness in development of cardiovascular disease. Am Heart J. 1985;109:876–85.

38. Kim JH, Malhotra R, Chiampas G, et al. Cardiac arrest during long-distance running races. N Engl J Med. 2012;366:130–40.

39. Engelstein ED, Zipes DP. Sudden cardiac death. In: Alexander RW, Schlant RC, Fuster V, editors. The heart, arteries, and veins. New York: McGraw-Hill; 1998. p. 1081–112.

40. Gibbons RJ, Balady GJ, Bricker JT, et al. ACC/AHA 2002 guideline update for exercise testing: summary article: a report of the American College of Cardiology/American Heart Association Task Force on Practice Guidelines (Committee to update the 1997 exercise testing guidelines). Circulation. 2002;106:1883–92.

41. Medicine. ACoS. Guidelines for exercise testing and prescription. 7th ed. Baltimore: Lippincott Williams & Wilkins; 2005.

42. Thompson PD, Balady GJ, Chaitman BR, Clark LT, Levine BD, Myerburg RJ. Task force 6: coronary artery disease. J Am Coll Cardiol. 2005;45:1348–53.

43. Baggish AL, Thompson PD. The Athlete's heart 2007: diseases of the coronary circulation. Cardiol Clin. 2007;25:431–40, vi.

44. Maron BJ, Epstein SE, Roberts WC. Causes of sudden death in competitive athletes. J Am Coll Cardiol. 1986;7:204–14.

45. Maron BJ, Shirani J, Poliac LC, Mathenge R, Roberts WC, Mueller FO. Sudden death in young competitive athletes. Clinical, demographic, and pathological profiles. JAMA. 1996;276:199–204.

46. Corrado D, Thiene G, Nava A, Rossi L, Pennelli N. Sudden death in young competitive athletes: clinicopathologic correlations in 22 cases. Am J Med. 1990;89:588–96.

47. Singh AM, McGregor RS. Differential diagnosis of chest symptoms in the athlete. Clin Rev Allergy Immunol. 2005;29:87–96.

48. Levy AS, Bassett F, Lintner S, Speer K. Pulmonary barotrauma: diagnosis in American football players. Three cases in three years. Am J Sports Med. 1996;24:227–9.

49. Wellens HJ. Early repolarization revisited. N Engl J Med. 2008;358:2063–5.

50. Noseworthy PA, Weiner R, Kim J, et al. Early repolarization pattern in competitive athletes: clinical correlates and the effects of exercise training. Circ Arrhythm Electrophysiol. 2011;4:432–40.

51. Hanne-Paparo N, Drory Y, Schoenfeld Y, Shapira Y, Kellermann JJ. Common ECG changes in athletes. Cardiology. 1976;61:267–78.

52. Huston TP, Puffer JC, Rodney WM. The athletic heart syndrome. N Engl J Med. 1985;313:24–32.

53. Parker MW, Thompson PD. Assessment and management of atherosclerosis in the athletic patient. Prog Cardiovasc Dis. 2012;54:416–22.

54. Kushner FG, Hand M, Smith Jr SC, et al. Focused updates: ACC/AHA guidelines for the management of patients with ST-elevation myocardial infarction (updating the 2004 guideline and 2007

focused update) and ACC/AHA/SCAI guidelines on percutaneous coronary intervention (updating the 2005 guideline and 2007 focused update): a report of the American College of Cardiology Foundation/American Heart Association Task Force on Practice Guidelines. Circulation. 2009;2009(120):2271–306.

55. Wright RS, Anderson JL, Adams CD, et al. ACCF/AHA focused update of the guidelines for the management of patients with unstable angina/non-ST-elevation myocardial infarction (updating the 2007 guideline): a report of the American College of Cardiology Foundation/American Heart Association Task Force on Practice Guidelines. Circulation. 2011;2011(123):2022–60.

56. Gibbons RJ, Abrams J, Chatterjee K, et al. ACC/AHA 2002 guideline update for the management of patients with chronic stable angina – summary article: a report of the American College of Cardiology/American Heart Association Task Force on Practice Guidelines (committee on the management of patients with chronic stable angina). Circulation. 2003;107:149–58.

57. Smith Jr SC, Benjamin EJ, Bonow RO, et al. AHA/ACCF secondary prevention and risk reduction therapy for patients with coronary and other atherosclerotic vascular disease: 2011 update: a guideline from the American Heart Association and American College of Cardiology Foundation. Circulation. 2011;124:2458–73.

58. Bruckert E, Hayem G, Dejager S, Yau C, Begaud B. Mild to moderate muscular symptoms with high-dosage statin therapy in hyperlipidemic patients – the PRIMO study. Cardiovasc Drugs Ther. 2005;19:403–14.

59. Sinzinger H, O'Grady J. Professional athletes suffering from familial hypercholesterolaemia rarely tolerate statin treatment because of muscular problems. Br J Clin Pharmacol. 2004;57:525–8.

60. Meador BM, Huey KA. Statin-associated myopathy and its exacerbation with exercise. Muscle Nerve. 2010;42:469–79.

61. Ford I, Murray H, Packard CJ, Shepherd J, Macfarlane PW, Cobbe SM. Long-term follow-up of the West of Scotland coronary prevention study. N Engl J Med. 2007;357:1477–86.

62. Fuller CM, McNulty CM, Spring DA, et al. Prospective screening of 5,615 high school athletes for risk of sudden cardiac death. Med Sci Sports Exerc. 1997;29:1131–8.

63. Biffi A, Pelliccia A, Verdile L, et al. Long-term clinical significance of frequent and complex ventricular tachyarrhythmias in trained athletes. J Am Coll Cardiol. 2002;40:446–52.

64. Lawless CE, Briner W. Palpitations in athletes. Sports Med. 2008;38:687–702.

65. Stein R, Medeiros CM, Rosito GA, Zimerman LI, Ribeiro JP. Intrinsic sinus and atrioventricular node electrophysiologic adaptations in endurance athletes. J Am Coll Cardiol. 2002;39:1033–8.

66. Baldesberger S, Bauersfeld U, Candinas R, et al. Sinus node disease and arrhythmias in the long-term follow-up of former professional cyclists. Eur Heart J. 2008;29:71–8.

67. Furlanello F, Bertoldi A, Dallago M, et al. Atrial fibrillation in elite athletes. J Cardiovasc Electrophysiol. 1998;9:S63–8.

68. Abdulla J, Nielsen JR. Is the risk of atrial fibrillation higher in athletes than in the general population? A systematic review and meta-analysis. Europace. 2009;11:1156–9.

69. Molina L, Mont L, Marrugat J, et al. Long-term endurance sport practice increases the incidence of lone atrial fibrillation in men: a follow-up study. Europace. 2008;10:618–23.

70. Sorokin AV, Araujo CG, Zweibel S, Thompson PD. Atrial fibrillation in endurance-trained athletes. Br J Sports Med. 2011;45:185–8.

71. Mont L, Elosua R, Brugada J. Endurance sport practice as a risk factor for atrial fibrillation and atrial flutter. Europace. 2009;11:11–7.

72. Wilhelm M, Roten L, Tanner H, Schmid JP, Wilhelm I, Saner H. Long-term cardiac remodeling and arrhythmias in nonelite marathon runners. Am J Cardiol. 2012;110:129–35.

73. Turagam MK, Velagapudi P, Kocheril AG. Atrial fibrillation in athletes. Am J Cardiol. 2012;109:296–302.

74. Zipes DP, Ackerman MJ, Estes 3rd NA, Grant AO, Myerburg RJ, Van Hare G. Task force 7: arrhythmias. J Am Coll Cardiol. 2005;45:1354–63.

75. Biffi A, Maron BJ, Verdile L, et al. Impact of physical deconditioning on ventricular tachyarrhythmias in trained athletes. J Am Coll Cardiol. 2004;44:1053–8.

76. Brignole M, Alboni P, Benditt DG, et al. Guidelines on management (diagnosis and treatment) of syncope – update 2004. Europace. 2004;6:467–537.

77. Barold SS, Padeletti L. Mobitz type II second-degree atrioventricular block in athletes: true or false? Br J Sports Med. 2011;45:687–90.

78. Koopman P, Nuyens D, Garweg C, et al. Efficacy of radiofrequency catheter ablation in athletes with atrial fibrillation. Europace. 2011;13:1386–93.

79. Kelly J, Kenny D, Martin RP, Stuart AG. Diagnosis and management of elite young athletes undergoing arrhythmia intervention. Arch Dis Child. 2011;96:21–4.

80. Hastings JL, Levine BD. Syncope in the athletic patient. Prog Cardiovasc Dis. 2012;54:438–44.

81. Link MS, Estes 3rd NA. How to manage athletes with syncope. Cardiol Clin. 2007;25:457–66, vii.

82. Linzer M, Yang EH, Estes 3rd NA, Wang P, Vorperian VR, Kapoor WN. Diagnosing syncope. Part 1: value of history, physical examination, and electrocardiography. Clinical Efficacy Assessment Project of the American College of Physicians. Ann Intern Med. 1997;126:989–96.

83. Colivicchi F, Ammirati F, Santini M. Epidemiology and prognostic implications of syncope in young competing athletes. Eur Heart J. 2004;25:1749–53.

84. Freeman R. Clinical practice. Neurogenic orthostatic hypotension. N Engl J Med. 2008;358:615–24.

85. Goldschlager N, Epstein AE, Grubb BP, et al. Etiologic considerations in the patient with syncope and an apparently normal heart. Arch Intern Med. 2003;163:151–62.

86. Benditt DG, Remole S, Milstein S, Bailin S. Syncope: causes, clinical evaluation, and current therapy. Annu Rev Med. 1992;43:283–300.

87. Calkins H, Seifert M, Morady F. Clinical presentation and long-term follow-up of athletes with exercise-induced vasodepressor syncope. Am Heart J. 1995;129:1159–64.

88. Calkins H, Shyr Y, Frumin H, Schork A, Morady F. The value of the clinical history in the differentiation of syncope due to ventricular tachycardia, atrioventricular block, and neurocardiogenic syncope. Am J Med. 1995;98:365–73.

89. Kapoor WN. Current evaluation and management of syncope. Circulation. 2002;106:1606–9.

90. Sheldon R, Rose S, Ritchie D, et al. Historical criteria that distinguish syncope from seizures. J Am Coll Cardiol. 2002;40:142–8.

91. Pelliccia A, Maron BJ, Culasso F, et al. Clinical significance of abnormal electrocardiographic patterns in trained athletes. Circulation. 2000;102:278–84.

92. Lawless CE, Best TM. Electrocardiograms in athletes: interpretation and diagnostic accuracy. Med Sci Sports Exerc. 2008;40:787–98.

93. Maron BJ, Doerer JJ, Haas TS, Tierney DM, Mueller FO. Sudden deaths in young competitive athletes: analysis of 1866 deaths in the United States, 1980–2006. Circulation. 2009;119:1085–92.

94. Verma S, Hackel JG, Torrisi DJ, Nguyen T. Syncope in athletes: a guide to getting them back on their feet. J Fam Pract. 2007;56:545–50.

95. Prakken NH, Velthuis BK, Cramer MJ, Mosterd A. Advances in cardiac imaging: the role of magnetic resonance imaging and computed tomography in identifying athletes at risk. Br J Sports Med. 2009;43:677–84.

96. Romme JJ, Reitsma JB, Black CN, et al. Drugs and pacemakers for vasovagal, carotid sinus and situational syncope. Cochrane Database Syst Rev. 2011:CD004194.

97. Benditt DG, Nguyen JT. Syncope: therapeutic approaches. J Am Coll Cardiol. 2009;53:1741–51.

98. Heidbuchel H. Implantable cardioverter defibrillator therapy in athletes. Cardiol Clin. 2007;25:467–82, vii.

99. Lampert R, Olshansky B, Heidbuchel H, et al. Safety of sports for athletes with implantable cardioverter-defibrillators: results of a prospective, multinational registry. Circulation. 2013;127:2021–2030.

Acute Pulmonary Embolism

21

Stavros Z. Apostolakis and Stavros V. Konstantinides

Abstract

Pulmonary embolism (PE) is a common and life-threatening cardiovascular emergency. It is a major cause of morbidity and mortality associated with surgery, injury, and medical illnesses. However, PE may occur in patients without any identifiable predisposing factors. The first and most crucial step in the diagnosis of PE is evaluating the likelihood of the disease based on clinical presentation. The appropriate diagnostic algorithm and the interpretation of diagnostic tests will depend on clinical probability of PE. For normotensive patients with clinically suspected PE, multidetector CT pulmonary angiography is currently the most frequently performed imaging test. Current guidelines emphasize the need to combine this test with assessment of clinical probability and D-dimer testing. As a general rule, anticoagulation with heparin should be initiated without delay in all patients with confirmed PE and should be considered in patients with an intermediate or high clinical probability while awaiting the results of further diagnostic confirmation. Thrombolytic agents rapidly resolve thrombus-related vascular obstruction providing instant hemodynamic relief in the majority of patients with massive PE. For patients with massive PE, in whom thrombolysis has failed or is absolutely contraindicated, surgical embolectomy or alternatively percutaneous catheter thrombectomy is recommended as a lifesaving treatment option. Oral anticoagulants (vitamin K antagonists) should be initiated as soon as possible in all hemodynamically stable patients, preferably on the same day as heparin. New oral anticoagulants seem to be as effective as vitamin K antagonists for the treatment and prevention of venous thromboembolism and PE with possibly improved safety profiles.

Keywords

Pulmonary embolism • Diagnostic algorithms • Multidetector CT pulmonary angiography • D-dimers • Heparin • Oral anticoagulation

Introduction

Pulmonary embolism (PE) is a common and life-threatening cardiovascular emergency. The incidence of venous thromboembolism (VTE) is increasing as the global population ages [1]. Pulmonary embolism and deep vein thrombosis (DVT) are two clinical manifestations of VTE and share the same predisposing factors. In most cases, PE can be considered as a consequence of DVT, since approximately 50 % of patients with proximal DVT have an associated, usually asymptomatic, PE on lung scan, while DVT can be found in more than 70 % of patients with PE if a sensitive diagnostic method is utilized [2]. On the other hand, despite the fact that DVT and PE are manifestations of the same disease, their impact on short- and long-term outcome is different. For example, the risk of death related to recurrent VTE

S.Z. Apostolakis, MD, PhD
S.V. Konstantinides, MD, PhD, FESC (✉)
Department of Cardiology, Democritus University of Thrace,
Alexandroupolis 68100, Greece
e-mail: skonst@med.duth.gr

K. Stergiopoulos, D.L. Brown (eds.), *Evidence-Based Cardiology Consult*,
DOI 10.1007/978-1-4471-4441-0_21, © Springer-Verlag London 2014

is significantly greater in patients who initially present with PE than in those who present with DVT [3].

Epidemiology

Venous thromboembolism remains a major cause of morbidity and mortality associated with surgery, injury, and medical illnesses. Hospitalized patients and nursing home residents account for half of all cases of VTE. In these settings, VTE is responsible for up to 15 % of in-hospital deaths. Pulmonary embolism also remains the leading direct cause of maternal mortality, as it accounts for up to 30 % of deaths associated with pregnancy and delivery. The majority of VTE-related in-hospital deaths are potentially preventable [1, 2].

Overall, 23–69 cases of PE are diagnosed in the United States per 100,000 population-years [1, 2]. These figures probably underestimate the actual incidence which may be as high as 600,000 cases annually [2]. Moreover, these rates mask a considerable variation according to specific populations such as the elderly. Incidence rises from fewer than 5 cases per 100,000 children aged <15 years to 450–600 cases per 100,000 adults aged >80 [4]. In Europe, an epidemiological model derived from 6 countries with a total population of 310.4 million yielded a PE incidence rate of 98 cases per 100,000 person-years. The estimated number of fatalities related to (although not necessarily caused by) VTE amounted to 370,000, or 12 % of all deaths, which corresponds to more than one million annual deaths in the European continent [5]. According to prospective registries, the acute case mortality rate for PE ranges from 7 to 11 %. Outcome is also significantly affected by age; for those aged 65 and older, in-hospital mortality and 1-year mortality due to PE are 21 % and 39 %, respectively [4].

Pathophysiology

Pulmonary artery embolism is defined as a partial or complete mechanical obstruction of a pulmonary arterial branch. Pulmonary embolism can occur in patients without any identifiable predisposing factors; nevertheless, in up to 80 % of cases, at least one predisposing factor can be identified. A variety of acquired and hereditary disorders have been implicated in the pathogenesis of VTE. These disorders can be classified as patient-related and setting-related (environmental); VTE is currently regarded as the result of the interaction between patient-related and setting-related risk factors [2]. All prothrombotic risk factors, either patient- or setting-related, affect one or more of the mechanisms included in the classic triad proposed by Virchow in 1856: venous stasis, increased blood coagulability, and endothelial injury or dysfunction.

Specific Risk Factors

Acquired risk factors for VTE include venous stasis due to external compression, prolonged immobilization, or incompetent venous valves. In addition, several acquired disorders including cancer and the antiphospholipid antibody syndrome are associated with a systemic prothrombotic tendency. Temporary conditions associated with acquired thrombophilia include pregnancy and the use of oral contraceptives or postmenopausal hormone replacement therapy [6].

Inherited predisposing factors consist of "thrombophilias" related to abnormal levels or quality of elements of the coagulation cascade. Genetic alterations related to thrombophilia can be identified in up to 30 % of unselected patients with VTE and at least 50 % of those with familial thrombosis [7]. Most of them affect steps of the activated protein C pathway. Resistance to activated protein C is almost exclusively caused by a single point mutation in the factor V gene. The latter polymorphism has 3–5 % prevalence in the general white population. Relative risk for VTE is increased between five- and ten-fold in heterozygotes. Polymorphisms of the prothrombin gene and genetic deficiency of protein C, protein S, or antithrombin are less frequent disorders and lead to a variety of genotype–phenotype interactions. Importantly, hereditary prothrombotic abnormalities tend to coexist with unpredictable but often multiplicative effect on thromboembolic risk [6, 7].

Inflammation in the form of local injury to the vessel wall or cytokines released from tumors, or from injured or infarcted tissue, is required to trigger thrombus formation. Inflammatory cytokines and platelet products stabilize thrombi by stimulating the synthesis of antifibrinolytic factors (plasminogen activator inhibitors) by the cells of the vessel wall. At the same time, however, upregulated plasminogen activators control and contain the thrombotic response, facilitating clot dissolution or organization [6]. Therefore, the formation of vascular thrombi and their fate are determined by the continuous and complex interplay between thrombogenic and fibrinolytic mechanisms both locally and systemically.

Origin of Thrombi in Pulmonary Embolism

Evidence derived from surgical and autopsy studies revealed that almost 90 % of pulmonary emboli originate in the lower extremity veins. However, intravenous substance abuse and the frequent use of central venous catheters in medicine have resulted in a significant increase in the incidence of upper extremity venous thrombosis. Thrombi originating in the right atrium or ventricle are rarely the cause of PE. Finally, disseminated peripheral thrombosis within the small muscular pulmonary arteries may occur. It is however

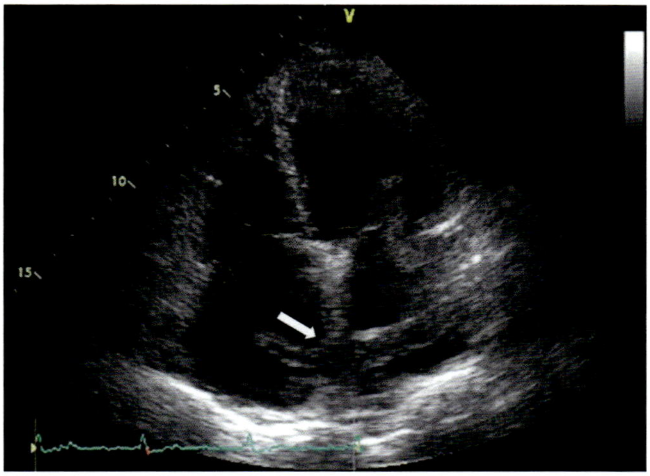

Fig. 21.1 Echocardiographic apical four-chamber view revealing a thrombus of lower-extremity origin trapped in a patent foramen ovale (*white arrow*)

considered a secondary phenomenon, and not the cause of chronic thromboembolic disease [8].

Lower extremity thrombi have been shown to originate in the venous sinuses and valve cusp pockets of the calf, in areas of slow or turbulent flow. Locally disturbed flow predisposes to thrombosis by impairing the clearance of coagulation factors. Thrombi from the veins appear macroscopically as long, thin, friable structures with a shape corresponding to the lumen of the vessel in which they were formed. Pale layers of platelets and fibrin alternating with dark red erythrocyte layers can be seen on their surface corresponding to different stages of in situ development [6, 8]. In vivo, venous thrombi in transit can occasionally be detected by echocardiography. They appear as highly mobile, relatively large twisting masses floating in the right side of the heart or occasionally caught in a patent foramen ovale before causing paradoxical embolism (Fig. 21.1).

Natural History of Pulmonary Emboli

Following PE, the endogenous fibrinolytic mechanisms of the lung are capable of dissolving most thromboemboli, regardless of their size. If the patient survives the acute hemodynamic consequences, progression to chronic thrombotic arteriopathy and chronic thromboembolic pulmonary hypertension is infrequent [9].

An acute increase in pulmonary artery pressure is quite common, occurring in 60–70 % of patients with PE. The most detrimental consequence of PE is related to acute increase of right ventricular afterload which depends on the extent and localization of pulmonary clots. Multiple or large thrombi that obstruct a significant proportion of the pulmonary

vasculature disturb right ventricular performance. Right ventricular dilatation and hypokinesia initiate a vicious cycle of increased myocardial oxygen demand, myocardial ischemia or infarction, and left ventricular preload reduction. Eventually, inability to maintain adequate cardiac output leads to cardiogenic shock. Low systemic output and shock are the underlying mechanism leading to death after an acute massive PE. Thus, right ventricular dysfunction is the critical hemodynamic event and an important determinant of the clinical presentation, course, and prognosis of PE. Respiratory failure is a common finding but is considered less relevant with respect to prognosis compared to hemodynamic instability [10].

Pulmonary infarction is an uncommon complication of PE since the lung normally receives somewhat redundant blood supply from the bronchial arteries. Radiologically, pulmonary infarctions typically present as peripheral wedge-shaped parenchymal opacities and occur in 10–15 % of patients with PE.

Diagnosis

Clinical Presentation

The first and most crucial step in the diagnosis of PE is evaluating the likelihood of the disease based on clinical presentation. Further selection of the appropriate diagnostic algorithm and the interpretation of diagnostic tests will depend on clinical probability of PE. In 90 % of cases, suspicion of PE is raised by symptoms including shortness of breath, chest pain, and syncope. One or more of these symptoms are present in more than 90 % of patients with PE [2, 11]. Chest pain, whether or not combined with dyspnea, is one of the most frequent presentations of PE. The pain is usually caused by pleural irritation due to distal emboli causing pulmonary infarction. Chest pain may also be retrosternal angina-like pain, which may reflect right ventricular ischemia.

Dyspnea of rapid onset is a common symptom, especially in central PE. However, the onset of dyspnea may also be progressive over several days. In patients with preexisting heart failure or pulmonary disease, worsening dyspnea may be the only symptom suggestive of PE. Syncope is a less common but important presentation of PE since it may indicate a severely reduced hemodynamic reserve. In the most severe cases, shock and arterial hypotension may be the presenting syndrome. Pulmonary infarction may be associated with alveolar hemorrhage, sometimes accompanied by hemoptysis [3, 11].

Identification of predisposing factors for VTE is essential in the evaluation of the likelihood of PE. However, in approximately 20 % of cases, PE occurs in the absence of

Table 21.1 Prediction schemes currently used to stratify suspected pulmonary embolism patients into categories of clinical probability

Revised Geneva score [13]		Wells score [12]	
Predisposing factors	Points	*Predisposing factors*	Points
Age >65 years	1	Previous DVT or PE	1.5
Previous DVT or PE	3	Surgery or immobilization the last 4 weeks	1.5
Surgery (under general anesthesia) or fracture (of the lower limbs) within 1 month	2	Malignancy (on treatment, treated in the last 6 months or palliative)	1
Active malignancy (solid or hematologic malignant condition, currently active or considered cured <1 year)	2		
Symptoms		*Symptoms*	
Unilateral lower-limb pain	3	Hemoptysis	1
Hemoptysis	2		
Clinical signs		*Clinical signs*	
Heart rate		Heart rate >100 min^{-1}	1.5
75–94 min^{-1}	3	Clinical signs of DVT (minimum of leg swelling and pain with palpation of the deep veins)	3
≥95 min^{-1}	5	*Clinical judgment*	
Pain on lower-limb deep venous palpation and unilateral edema	4	Alternative diagnosis is less likely than PE	3
Interpretation			
Clinical probability		*Clinical probability (three levels)*	
Low	0–3	Low	0–1
Intermediate	4–10	Intermediate	2–6
High	≥11	High	≥7
		Clinical probability (two levels)	
		PE unlikely	0–4
		PE likely	>4

DVT deep venous thrombosis, *PE* pulmonary embolism

any identifiable predisposing factors. Individual clinical findings and common diagnostic tests are neither sensitive nor specific for the diagnosis of PE. The chest X-ray is usually abnormal, but the most frequently encountered findings are nonspecific. Hypoxemia is a common finding in PE. Nevertheless, up to 20 % of patients with PE have a normal arterial oxygen pressure and a normal alveolar–arterial oxygen gradient. Electrocardiographic (ECG) signs of RV strain, such as inversion of T waves in leads V1–V4, a QR pattern in lead V1, the classic S1Q3T3 type, and incomplete or complete right bundle-branch block, may be helpful, but they lack both sensitivity and specificity. Moreover, such changes are generally associated with the more severe forms of PE [6].

Risk Stratification

Despite the limited sensitivity and specificity of individual symptoms, signs, and common tests, the combination of these variables, either by implicit clinical judgment or by the use of risk prediction schemes, makes it possible to stratify suspected PE patients into categories of clinical

probability. Each stratum corresponds to an increasing prevalence of PE. The posttest probability of PE depends not only on the characteristics of the test used but also on pretest probability [2].

The value of implicit clinical judgment has been shown in several large prospective series. Nevertheless, implicit judgment depends on individual physician's experience and lacks standardization. Explicit clinical prediction rules have been developed and validated in the last years to avoid the limitations of implicit clinical judgment. Explicit prediction rules which combine the clinical findings at presentation with predisposing factors have proven particularly useful in determining the clinical or pretest probability of PE. Thus use of these scores has been strongly recommended by medical societies as they may guide further diagnostic workup and also improve the interpretation of diagnostic procedures [3].

The prediction rule developed by Wells et al. is the most widely used clinical diagnostic score for PE at present (Table 21.1) [12]. It has been validated extensively as a categorical (low, moderate, or high clinical probability) or dichotomous score (PE likely or unlikely). It is simple and based on easily collected information. The revised Geneva rule is also widely utilized in Europe (see Table 21.1) [13].

Both prediction schemes have been included in the latest European guidelines on the diagnosis and management of acute PE [2]. In most validation studies, the proportion of patients with eventually confirmed PE was around 10 % in the low probability category, 30 % in the moderate probability category, and 65 % in the high clinical probability category, regardless of the prediction rule used. Thus, classification of patients into "pretest" probability categories either by implicit clinical judgment or by a validated prediction rule is capable of further determining the choice of the appropriate laboratory and imaging tests to confirm or exclude PE.

Diagnostic Algorithms

D-dimer testing is recommended as the initial diagnostic step for patients with low or moderate pretest probability. High-sensitivity enzyme-linked immunoabsorbent assay (ELISA) assays have a sensitivity of 95 %. A negative D-dimer result (plasma concentration <0.5 mg/L) excludes the presence of circulating fibrin and, consequently, the diagnosis of VTE. Thus, in almost 30 % of the patients with suspected PE, the diagnosis can be excluded without further testing [2]. It must be noted however that D-dimer tests have a low negative predictive value for patients with high clinical probability of PE.

Multidetector CT is recommended as the next step in patients with low or intermediate pretest probability and a positive D-dimer test or as the initial step in patients with high pretest probability. Multidetector CT can safely be used as a single imaging test to diagnose or exclude PE in the majority of cases [14, 15]. Multidetector CT also provides potentially useful prognostic information by permitting assessment of the size and thus the function of the right ventricle [16]. Combining CT pulmonary angiography and CT venography in a single procedure is not recommended, since it increases exposure to radiation without significantly enhancing the predictive performance of the CT angiogram [17].

Ventilation–perfusion lung scanning is still an alternative to CT angiography. It can be useful when contrast media is contraindicated. A normal scan safely excludes the disease. However, in several cases the test may yield inconclusive findings and further testing will be required to safely exclude or confirm PE. A recent randomized trial that involved 1,417 patients randomized to CT pulmonary angiography or ventilation–perfusion lung scanning reported that 99 % of patients with suspected PE could be diagnostically managed safely and effectively with ventilation–perfusion scan [18].

Compression ultrasonography can detect proximal DVT in about 20 % of patients with PE, and the yield is twice as

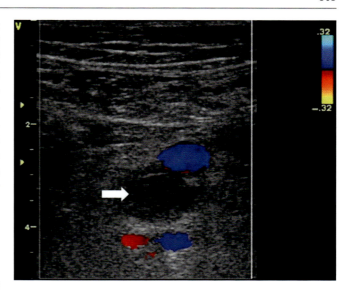

Fig. 21.2 Compression US of the right common femoral vein (*white arrow*). Thrombus is detected by lack of compression. Flow criteria derived by Doppler ultrasonography are unreliable

high when the distal veins are also examined. The only validated diagnostic criterion for DVT is incomplete compressibility of the vein, which indicates the presence of a clot (Fig. 21.2). Flow criteria derived by Doppler ultrasonography are unreliable. A positive result essentially establishes the diagnosis of VTE. Compression ultrasonography when performed in combination with single-detector CT angiography enhances the sensitivity of the latter procedure.

Selective pulmonary angiography is only rarely necessary to confirm or exclude PE unless catheter-based treatment is planned. There are no data to support the use of magnetic resonance imaging of the pulmonary arteries for the diagnosis of PE.

For *normotensive* patients with clinically suspected PE, multidetector CT pulmonary angiography is currently the most frequently performed imaging test. CT-based algorithms which have been validated in prospective management trials emphasize the need to combine this test with assessment of clinical probability and D-dimer testing (Fig. 21.3). If properly followed, the strategy illustrated in Fig. 21.3 permits management decisions in almost 98 % of the cases. The 3-month risk of recurrent VTE in patients left untreated after exclusion of the disease based on the above algorithm is as low as 1 % [2].

Patients with suspected PE who present with arterial hypotension or shock constitute a medical emergency. Multidetector CT is the preferred diagnostic test in most institutions; however, bedside echocardiography demonstrating right ventricular dysfunction may be a valuable alternative if CT is not immediately available or the patient is too unstable to be transferred to the radiology department.

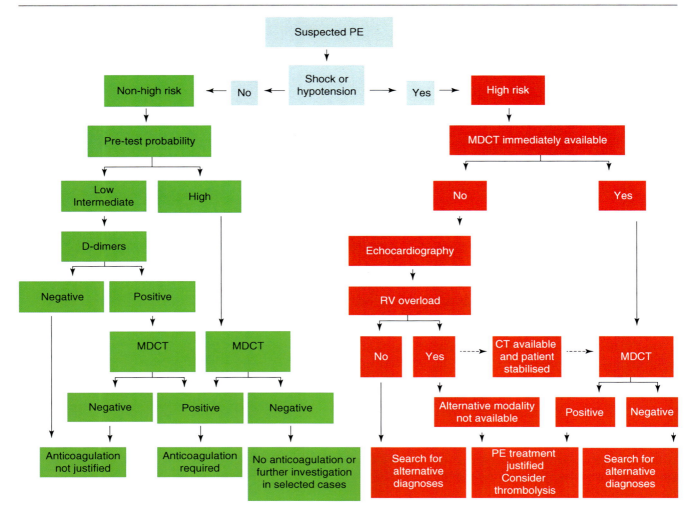

Fig. 21.3 Proposed diagnostic algorithm for patients with suspected pulmonary embolism. *PE* pulmonary embolism, *MDCT* multidetector computed tomography, *RV* right ventricle

Treatment

Acute PE covers a wide spectrum of clinical severity and death risk. In various studies, 30-day mortality rates for patients with confirmed PE vary widely from <1 to >50 % [19]. Accordingly, the recently updated guidelines of the European Society of Cardiology have introduced the terms high-risk and non-high-risk PE in an attempt to further guide treatment based on the individual's estimated risk of adverse outcome (death or recurrent PE). High-risk PE is defined by the presence of hemodynamic instability clinically defined as persistent arterial hypotension (systolic blood pressure <90 mmHg or a systolic blood pressure drop by ≥40 mmHg for at least 15 min) or shock. Five percent of patients with PE present with high-risk features. Nevertheless, in-hospital mortality of high-risk PE patients exceeds 15 %.

Anticoagulation

As a general rule, anticoagulation with heparin should be initiated without delay in all patients with confirmed PE [20]. Due to the high mortality rates associated with untreated PE/VTE, anticoagulant treatment should be considered in patients with an intermediate or high clinical probability while awaiting the results of further diagnostic confirmation [2]. Several major trials have shown that low-molecular-weight heparins or the pentasaccharide fondaparinux is at least as effective and safe compared to unfractionated heparin. Therefore, low-molecular-weight heparins are currently the preferred anticoagulants. Route of administration, recommended dosing, and special considerations with respect to heparins currently approved for treatment of PE are summarized in Table 21.2 [21]. Parenteral anticoagulants are

Table 21.2 Anticoagulant drugs for initial treatment of pulmonary embolism

	Dosage	Route and interval	Comments
Unfractionated heparin	80 IU/kg of body weight as an intravenous bolus, followed by infusion at the rate of 18 IU/kg/h	Continuous intravenous infusion	Adjust infusion rate to maintain aPTT between 1.5 and 2.5 times control, corresponding to therapeutic heparin levels (0.3–0.7 IU/mL by factor Xa inhibition)[a]
Low-molecular-weight heparins[b]			
Enoxaparin	1.0 mg/kg or	Subcutaneously every 12 h	If creatinine clearance <30 mL/min, reduce enoxaparin dosage to 1 mg/kg once daily; consider unfractionated heparin infusion as an alternative
	1.5 mg/kg	Subcutaneously once daily[c]	
Tinzaparin	175 U/kg	Subcutaneously once daily	
Fondaparinux	5 mg (body weight <50 kg); 7.5 mg (body weight 50–100 kg); 10 mg (body weight >100 kg)	Subcutaneously once daily	Contraindicated if creatinine clearance <20 mL/min

Adapted from Konstantinides [21]

aPTT partial thromboplastin time, *LMWH* low-molecular-weight heparin

[a]It is recommended to adjust the treatment dosage based on standardized nomograms such as that proposed by Raschke et al.

[b]Tinzaparin and fondaparinux are explicitly approved for treatment of acute pulmonary embolism. Enoxaparin is approved for treatment of deep vein thrombosis with or without pulmonary embolism

[c]Once-daily injection of enoxaparin at the dosage of 1.5 mg/kg is approved for inpatient (hospital) treatment of pulmonary embolism in the United States and in some, but not all, European countries

usually followed by the administration of oral anticoagulation with vitamin K antagonists. Heparin treatment should be continued for at least 5–6 days with overlapping oral anticoagulation until the international normalized ratio has been within the therapeutic range (2.0–3.0) on 2 consecutive days. At present, low-molecular-weight heparin or fondaparinux is considered adequate treatment for most normotensive patients with low- or intermediate-risk (non-high-risk) PE. Low-molecular-weight heparins have not been tested and thus are not recommended for patients with arterial hypotension or shock. In patients with renal failure, it is recommended that the dose of low-molecular-weight heparins be adjusted according to anti-Xa levels [2]. In the subgroup of patients with severe renal dysfunction (defined as creatinine clearance <30 mL/min), unfractionated heparin is preferred as it is not eliminated by the kidneys, and in those with an increased risk of bleeding (congenital or acquired bleeding diathesis; active ulcerative or angiodysplastic gastrointestinal disease; recent hemorrhagic stroke; recent brain, spinal, or ophthalmological surgery; diabetic retinopathy; or bacterial endocarditis) due to its short half-life and reversible anticoagulant effects.

Due to the risk of heparin-induced thrombocytopenia (HIT), monitoring of the platelet count is recommended during treatment with unfractionated or low-molecular-weight heparins. For unfractionated heparin, monitoring of the platelet count is recommended at baseline and every other day from days 4 to 14 or until heparin is stopped. For low-molecular-weight heparins, monitoring is recommended at baseline and every 2–4 days from days 4 to 14 or until heparin is stopped. The risk of heparin-induced thrombocytopenia depends both on the type of heparin used and the clinical setting. The highest incidence has been reported (3–5 %) in patients following orthopedic surgery that received unfractionated heparin. Medical or surgical patients receiving low-molecular-weight heparin have a reported incidence of less than 1 %. For patients receiving fondaparinux, the risk is probably negligible [22].

Thrombolysis

Thrombolytic agents rapidly resolve thrombus-related vascular obstruction providing instant hemodynamic relief in the majority of patients with high-risk PE. The greatest benefit is observed when treatment is provided within 48 h of symptom onset, but thrombolysis can still be effective in patients who have had symptoms for up to 14 days. Thrombolytic therapy carries a significant bleeding risk. Pooled data from studies assessing various thrombolytic regimens indicated a 13 % cumulative rate of major bleeding and a 1.8 % rate of intracranial/fatal hemorrhage. Thus, the decision to treat a patient with thrombolysis should be based on balancing the risk of death from thromboembolism if the patient is left untreated against the risk of death from bleeding if the patient is treated. In balancing the clinical benefits against the risks of thrombolysis, the presence and severity of right ventricular failure appears to be a critical factor. A meta-analysis of studies which included patients with arterial hypotension or shock due to acute right ventricular failure suggested that thrombolysis effectively reduces the risk of death or recurrent PE in this high-risk patient group [23].

Massive (high-risk) PE with cardiogenic shock or persistent arterial hypotension accounts for 5 % of all cases and is associated with a high risk of in-hospital death, particularly during the first hours after admission. Patients with suspected massive

Table 21.3 Thrombolysis: agents and regimens

Streptokinase[a]	250,000 U as a loading dose over 30 min, followed by 100,000 U/h over 12–24 h
	Accelerated regimen: 1.5 million IU over 2 h[b]
Urokinase[a,c]	4,400 U/kg of body weight as a loading dose over 10 min, followed by 4,400 U/kg/h over 12–24 h
	Accelerated regimen: three million U over 2 h[b]
Alteplase[a]	100 mg over 2 h[d]
	Accelerated regimen: 0.6 mg/kg over 15 min
Reteplase[a,e]	Two bolus injections of 10 U 30 min apart
Tenecteplase[f]	30–50 mg bolus over 5–10 s adjusted for body weight

[a]Unfractionated heparin should not be infused concurrently with streptokinase or urokinase; it can be given during alteplase or reteplase administration. Low-molecular-weight heparins have not been tested in combination with thrombolysis in patients with pulmonary embolism
[b]Short (2 h) infusion periods are generally recommended
[c]Urokinase available in some European countries, not in the United States
[d]FDA-approved regimen
[e]Off-label use
[f]Off-label use. This is the regimen recommended for acute myocardial infarction. Preliminary evidence suggests that it is safe and effective in pulmonary embolism as well

PE should immediately receive a weight-adjusted bolus of unfractionated heparin while awaiting the results of further diagnostic workup. If massive PE is confirmed based on the diagnostic algorithms, thrombolysis should be administered without delay. If thrombolysis is absolutely contraindicated or has failed, surgical embolectomy or catheter-based thrombus fragmentation or suction may be a valuable alternative.

Use of thrombolysis in normotensive patients with PE is less well established. A randomized trial suggested that selected patients with evidence of right ventricular dysfunction and low risk of bleeding may benefit from early thrombolysis [24]. The balance between benefits and risks of thrombolysis in normotensive patients with intermediate-risk PE, that is with right ventricular dysfunction on echocardiography (or CT scan) plus a positive troponin test, is being addressed by the ongoing Pulmonary Embolism Thrombolysis (PEITHO) trial [25]. The results of this study will be available early 2013.

Several approved thrombolytic agents can be used for the management of acute PE (Table 21.3). Existing evidence indicates that the approved thrombolytic agents are equivalent with respect to clinical outcome. It is nevertheless sensible to prefer regimens with shorter infusion periods. Direct infusion of thrombolytic agents via a catheter in the pulmonary artery has not been shown to offer any advantages over systemic intravenous with respect to both safety and efficacy thrombolysis and is therefore not recommended [2]. In addition to a specific therapy, hemodynamic and respiratory support is necessary in patients with suspected or confirmed PE presenting with shock or hypotension.

Surgical and Interventional Management

In a prospective single-center registry of PE patients who underwent thrombolysis, lack of response to thrombolysis—defined as both persistent clinical instability and residual echocardiographic right ventricular dysfunction within the first 36 h—was demonstrated in 8 % of the patients [26]. For patients with massive PE, in whom thrombolysis has failed or is absolutely contraindicated, surgical embolectomy—if available—is recommended as a lifesaving treatment option [2]. Alternatively, selected patients with hemodynamic compromise who cannot receive thrombolytic therapy may be candidates for percutaneous catheter thrombectomy.

Inferior vena cava filters as a means of protection against recurrent VTE have been available the last four decades. Permanent filters are associated with long-term complications such as DVT and the post-thrombotic syndrome. Thus, their use in patients with PE is generally discouraged. Retrievable venous filters may be considered when both the risk of PE recurrence and the expected bleeding risk of anticoagulation are very high. Such situations include, for example, extensive thrombosis in the early postoperative period after neurosurgery or in pregnant women just prior to delivery [2].

Oral Anticoagulation and Secondary Prophylaxis

Anticoagulation with unfractionated heparin or low-molecular-weight heparin should be continued for at least 5 days. Oral anticoagulants (vitamin K antagonists) should be initiated as soon as possible in all hemodynamically stable patients, preferably on the same day as heparin. Parenteral anticoagulation can be stopped as soon as the international normalized ratio (INR) has been in the therapeutic range (between 2.0 and 3.0) on 2 consecutive days. After a first episode of "unprovoked" PE (i.e., in the absence of transient, reversible risk factors), treatment with vitamin K antagonists should be continued for at least 3 months; long-term treatment may be considered in patients with a favorable risk-to-benefit ratio [27].

Dabigatran, a direct oral thrombin inhibitor, has been compared with warfarin in patients with acute symptomatic VTE. The RE-COVER study was a double-blind, double-dummy, noninferiority, randomized trial, comparing 6 months of treatment with dabigatran, at a fixed dose of 150 mg twice daily, with dose-adjusted warfarin therapy, after initial parenteral anticoagulation in patients with symptomatic venous thromboembolism. Recurrent VTE occurred in 30 patients (2.4 %) given dabigatran during the treatment period, as compared to 27 patients (2.1 %) given warfarin ($P < 0.001$ for noninferiority). Major bleeding was reported in 20 patients (1.6 %) allocated to the dabigatran group compared to 24 patients (1.9 %) allocated to the control group. The RE-COVER study thus showed that dabigatran, given after a "not-so-brief" period (mean, 11 days) of parenteral anticoagulation, was as effective and as safe as warfarin for the treatment of VTE [28].

Rivaroxaban, an oral factor Xa inhibitor, has been compared with standard treatment in patients with acute VTE. The arm of the study including patients with acute deep vein thrombosis, EINSTEIN-DVT, was an open-label, randomized, event-driven, noninferiority study that compared oral rivaroxaban alone with subcutaneous enoxaparin followed by a vitamin K antagonist for 3, 6, or 12 months [29]. Recurrent VTE occurred in 36 patients (2.1 %) given rivaroxaban as compared to 51 (3.0 %) given standard therapy ($P < 0.001$ for noninferiority). In the recently published EINSTEIN-PE study which enrolled 4,832 patients, a fixed-dose regimen of rivaroxaban alone was also noninferior ($P = 0.003$) to standard therapy for the initial and long-term treatment of PE, and it showed a potentially improved benefit–risk profile [30]. More specifically, recurrent venous thromboembolism occurred in 2.1 % of patients receiving rivaroxaban compared with 1.8 % of those on standard enoxaparin/warfarin therapy. Major or clinically relevant non-major bleeding occurred in 10.3 % of rivaroxaban patients compared with 11.4 % standard therapy patients ($P = 0.32$); however, major bleeding was observed in only 1.1 % of patients taking rivaroxaban compared with 2.2 % of those on enoxaparin/warfarin ($P = 0.003$). In particular, intracranial bleeding occurred in one rivaroxaban patient compared with ten patients receiving standard therapy. The single oral drug approach has also been evaluated in a trial testing the factor Xa Inhibitor apixaban (AMPLIFY). In this recently published trial, a fixed-dose regimen of apixaban alone was noninferior to conventional therapy (low molecular weight heparin followed by a vitamin K antagonist) for the treatment of acute venous thromboembolism and was associated with significantly less bleeding [31].

Key Points
- Pulmonary embolism (PE) and deep vein thrombosis (DVT) are two clinical presentations of venous thromboembolism (VTE) and share the same risk factors and predisposing conditions but not the same prognosis.

- Pulmonary embolism is a relatively common and potentially life-threatening disease if left untreated.
- Clinical presentation of PE is nonspecific and may include a wide range of symptoms from dyspnea, pleuritic chest pain, and hemoptysis to hypotension and shock.
- Individual symptoms and routine laboratory findings have low diagnostic sensitivity and specificity.
- Patients with suggestive history, symptoms, or signs require prompt clinical evaluation of the probability of PE. This will determine further diagnostic strategy.
- Estimation of pretest probability of PE can be assisted by risk estimation schemes.
- Computerized tomography angiography has become the mainstay of diagnosis.
- Depending on the clinical presentation, definitive treatment decisions can also be made based on other tests, which may be particularly useful under specific circumstances.
- Patients with diagnosed PE require risk stratification, to high risk or non-high risk, based on the presence or absence of hemodynamic compromise secondary to RV failure.
- Patients with PE and shock or hypotension require intensive monitoring and aggressive treatment aiming at recanalization of the pulmonary arterial bed.
- Such management may be also considered in normotensive patients who present with objective signs of RV dysfunction and/or myocardial injury.

Summary of the Key Guidelines

Adopted by the ESC guidelines on the diagnosis and management of acute pulmonary embolism [2]

Key Recommendations on Diagnosis

Suspected High-Risk PE
- In high-risk PE, as indicated by the presence of shock or hypotension, emergency CT or bedside echocardiography (depending on availability and clinical circumstances) is recommended for diagnostic purposes (Class I, level of evidence C).

Suspected Non-High-Risk PE
- In non-high-risk PE, basing the diagnostic strategy on clinical probability assessed either implicitly or using a validated prediction rule is recommended (IA).
- Plasma D-dimer measurement is recommended in emergency department patients to reduce the need for

unnecessary imaging and irradiation, preferably using a highly sensitive assay (IA).

- Pulmonary angiography should be considered when there is discrepancy between clinical evaluation and results of noninvasive imaging tests (IIaC).
- The use of validated criteria for diagnosing PE is recommended (IB).

Suspected Non-High-Risk PE

Low Clinical Probability

- Normal D-dimer level using either a highly or moderately sensitive assay excludes PE (IA).
- Normal perfusion lung scintigraphy excludes PE (IA).
- Nondiagnostic (low or intermediate probability) V/Q scan may exclude PE (IIaB) particularly when combined with negative proximal compression ultrasound (CUS) (IA).
- Negative multidetector computed tomography (MDCT) safely excludes PE (IA).
- Negative single-detector computed tomography (SDCT) only excludes PE when combined with negative proximal CUS (IA).
- High-probability V/Q scan may confirm PE (IIaB), but further testing may be considered in selected patients to confirm PE (IIbB).
- CUS showing a proximal DVT confirms PE (IB).
- SDCT or MDCT showing a segmental or more proximal thrombus confirms PE (IA).

Intermediate Clinical Probability

- Normal D-dimer level using a highly sensitive assay excludes PE (IA).
- Normal perfusion lung scintigraphy excludes PE (IA).
- Negative MDCT excludes PE (IA).
- Negative SDCT only excludes PE when combined with negative proximal CUS (IA).
- High-probability ventilation–perfusion lung scintigraphy confirms PE (IA).
- CUS showing a proximal DVT confirms PE (IB).
- SDCT or MDCT showing a segmental or more proximal thrombus confirms PE (IA).

High Clinical Probability

- In patients with a negative CT, further tests should be considered in selected patients to exclude PE (IIaB).
- High-probability ventilation–perfusion lung scintigraphy confirms PE (IA).
- CUS showing a proximal DVT confirms PE (IB).
- SDCT or MDCT showing a segmental or more proximal thrombus confirms PE (IA).

Key Recommendations for Initial Treatment

High Risk

- Anticoagulation with unfractionated heparin should be initiated without delay in patients with high-risk PE (IA).

- Thrombolytic therapy should be used in patients with high-risk PE presenting with cardiogenic shock and/or persistent arterial hypotension (IA).
- Surgical pulmonary embolectomy is a recommended therapeutic alternative in patients with high-risk PE in whom thrombolysis is absolutely contraindicated or has failed (IC).
- Catheter embolectomy or fragmentation of proximal pulmonary arterial clots may be considered as an alternative to surgical treatment in high-risk patients when thrombolysis is absolutely contraindicated or has failed (IIbC).

Non-High Risk

- Anticoagulation should be initiated without delay in patients with high or intermediate clinical probability of PE while diagnostic workup is still ongoing (IC).
- Use of LMWH or fondaparinux is the recommended form of initial treatment for most patients with non-high-risk PE (IA).
- In patients at high risk of bleeding and in those with severe renal dysfunction, unfractionated heparin with an aPTT target range of 1.5–2.5 times normal is a recommended form of initial treatment (IC).
- Initial treatment with unfractionated heparin, LMWH, or fondaparinux should be continued for at least 5 days and (IA) may be replaced by vitamin K antagonists only after achieving target INR levels for at least 2 consecutive days (IC).

References

1. White RH. The epidemiology of venous thromboembolism. Circulation. 2003;107:I4–8.
2. Torbicki A, Perrier A, Konstantinides S, et al.; ESC Committee for Practice Guidelines (CPG). Guidelines on the diagnosis and management of acute pulmonary embolism: the Task Force for the diagnosis and management of acute pulmonary embolism of the European Society of Cardiology (ESC). Eur Heart J. 2008;29: 2276–315.
3. Carrier M, Le Gal G, Wells PS, Rodger MA. Systematic review: case-fatality rates of recurrent venous thromboembolism and major bleeding events among patients treated for venous thromboembolism. Ann Intern Med. 2010;152:578–89.
4. Blann AD, Lip GY. Venous thromboembolism. BMJ. 2006;332: 215–9.
5. Cohen AT, Agnelli G, Anderson FA et al.; VTE Impact Assessment Group in Europe (VITAE). Venous thromboembolism (VTE) in Europe. The number of VTE events and associated morbidity and mortality. Thromb Haemost. 2007;98:756–64.
6. Konstantinides S, Kasper W. Pulmonary embolism. In: Crawford MH, DiMarco JP, Paulus WJ, editors. Cardiology. 3rd ed. London: Elsevier; 2011.
7. Murin S, Marelich GP, Arroliga AC, Matthay RA. Hereditary thrombophilia and venous thromboembolism. Am J Respir Crit Care Med. 1998;158:1369–73.
8. Wagenvoort CA. Pathology of pulmonary thromboembolism. Chest. 1995;107:10S–7.

9. Becattini C, Agnelli G, Pesavento R, et al. Incidence of chronic thromboembolic pulmonary hypertension after a first episode of pulmonary embolism. Chest. 2006;130:172–5.

10. Lankeit M, Konstantinides S. Mortality risk assessment and the role of thrombolysis in pulmonary embolism. Crit Care Clin. 2011;27: 953–67, vii–viii.

11. Miniati M, Prediletto R, Formichi B, et al. Accuracy of clinical assessment in the diagnosis of pulmonary embolism. Am J Respir Crit Care Med. 1999;159:864–71.

12. Wells PS, Anderson DR, Rodger M, et al. Derivation of a simple clinical model to categorize patients probability of pulmonary embolism: increasing the models utility with the SimpliRED D-dimer. Thromb Haemost. 2000;83:416–20.

13. Le Gal G, Righini M, Roy PM, Sanchez O, Aujesky D, Bounameaux H, et al. Prediction of pulmonary embolism in the emergency department: the revised Geneva score. Ann Intern Med. 2006;144:165–71.

14. Perrier A, Roy PM, Sanchez O, et al. Multidetector-row computed tomography insuspected pulmonary embolism. N Engl J Med. 2005;352:1760–8.

15. van Belle A, Büller HR, Huisman MV et al.; Christopher Study Investigators. Effectiveness of managing suspected pulmonary embolism using an algorithm combining clinical probability, D-dimer testing, and computed tomography. JAMA. 2006;295:172–9.

16. Becattini C, Agnelli G, Vedovati MC, et al. Multidetector computed tomography for acute pulmonary embolism: diagnosis and risk stratification in a single test. Eur Heart J. 2011;32:1657–63.

17. Stein PD, Fowler SE, Goodman LR, et al. Multidetector computed tomography for acute pulmonary embolism. N Engl J Med. 2006; 354:2317–27.

18. Anderson DR, Kahn SR, Rodger MA, et al. Computed tomographic pulmonary angiography vs ventilation-perfusion lung scanning in patients with suspected pulmonary embolism: a randomized controlled trial. JAMA. 2007;298:2743–53.

19. Wicki J, Perrier A, Perneger TV, Bounameaux H, Junod AF. Predicting adverse outcome in patients with acute pulmonary embolism: a risk score. Thromb Haemost. 2000;84:548–52.

20. Barrit DW, Jordan SC. Anticoagulant treatment of pulmonary embolism: a case controlled study. Lancet. 1960;1:1309–12.

21. Konstantinides S. Clinical practice. Acute pulmonary embolism. N Engl J Med. 2008;359:2804–13.

22. Arepally GM, Ortel TL. Clinical practice. Heparin-induced thrombocytopenia. N Engl J Med. 2006;355:809–17.

23. Wan S, Quinlan DJ, Agnelli G, Eikelboom JW. Thrombolysis compared with heparin for the initial treatment of pulmonary embolism: a meta-analysis of the randomized controlled trials. Circulation. 2004;110:744–9.

24. Konstantinides S, Geibel A, Heusel G, Heinrich F, Kasper W, Management Strategies and Prognosis of Pulmonary Embolism-3 Trial Investigators. Heparin plus alteplase compared with heparin alone in patients with submassive pulmonary embolism. N Engl J Med. 2002;347:1143–50.

25. The PEITHO Steering Committee. Single-bolus tenecteplase plus heparin compared with heparin alone for normotensive patients with acute pulmonary embolism who have evidence of right ventricular dysfunction and myocardial injury: rationale and design of the Pulmonary Embolism Thrombolysis (PEITHO) trial. Am Heart J. 2012;163:33–38.e1.

26. Meneveau N, Séronde MF, Blonde MC, et al. Management of unsuccessful thrombolysis in acute massive pulmonary embolism. Chest. 2006;129:1043–50.

27. Lankeit M, Konstantinides S. Is it time for home treatment of pulmonary embolism ? Eur Respir J. 2012;40(3):742–9.

28. Schulman S, Kearon C, Kakkar AK et al.; RE-COVER Study Group. Dabigatran versus warfarin in the treatment of acute venous thromboembolism. N Engl J Med. 2009;361:2342–52.

29. EINSTEIN–PE Investigators, Büller HR, Prins MH, Lensin AW, et al. Oral rivaroxaban for the treatment of symptomatic pulmonary embolism. N Engl J Med. 2012;366:1287–97.

30. EINSTEIN Investigators, Bauersachs R, Berkowitz SD, Brenner B, et al. Oral rivaroxaban for symptomatic venous thromboembolism. N Engl J Med. 2010;363:2499–510.

31. Agnelli G, Buller HR, Cohen A, Curto M, Gallus AS, Johnson M, Masiukiewicz U, Pak R, Thompson J, Raskob GE, Weitz JI. Oral apixaban for the treatment of acute venous thromboembolism. N Engl J Med. 2013. [Epub ahead of print].

Anthony R. Cucci, M. Azam Hadi, and Tim Lahm

Abstract

Right ventricular failure (RVF) is a frequent and formidable clinical challenge in the intensive care unit, the operating room, the general ward, and the outpatient setting. The presence of RVF (1) carries substantial morbidity and mortality and (2) complicates the use of commonly employed treatment strategies in both inpatients and outpatients. In contrast to the left ventricle (LV), the right ventricle (RV) remains relatively understudied, and none of the major professional societies have published any guidelines on how to approach patients with RVF. Due to embryological, anatomical, physiological, biochemical, and electrophysiological differences between the RV and LV, paradigms that are important for the treatment of the failing LV cannot be extrapolated to RVF. However, with pulmonary hypertension (PH) having become a major area of scientific and clinical interest, recent studies have shed more light on the physiology of the normal RV and the pathophysiology of its failure. Using a comprehensive and evidence-based approach, this chapter will (1) highlight the pathophysiology of the failing RV; (2) discuss the etiologies of acute, chronic, and acute-on-chronic RVF; (3) describe invasive and noninvasive approaches that assist in diagnosis and risk stratification; and (4) emphasize treatment strategies for stable (chronic) and decompensated (acute) RVF.

Keywords

Preload • Afterload • Contractility • Inotropic therapy • Pulmonary vasodilators • Diuretics • Pulmonary hypertension • Pulmonary embolism • Heart failure • Cardiogenic shock

A.R. Cucci, MD (✉)
Pulmonary Fellow, Indiana University, Pulmonary/Critical Care,
8355 Codesa Way, Indianapolis, IN 46278, USA
e-mail: acucci@iupui.edu

M.A. Hadi, MD
Department of Cardiology, Indiana University,
1801 N Capitol, Indianapolis, IN 46202, USA
e-mail: mazhadi@iupui.edu

T. Lahm, MD
Division of Pulmonary, Allergy, Critical Care, Occupational,
and Sleep Medicine, Department of Medicine, Indiana University
School of Medicine and Richard L. Roudebush VA Medical
Center, Indianapolis, IN, USA

Introduction

Right ventricular failure (RVF) is a frequent and formidable clinical challenge in both the inpatient and outpatient setting that carries substantial morbidity and mortality. In contrast to the left ventricle (LV), the right ventricle (RV) remains relatively understudied and no treatment guidelines by any of the major professional societies exist. However, with pulmonary hypertension (PH) having become a major area of scientific and clinical interest [1, 2], recent studies have shed more light on RV function and dysfunction.

Pathophysiology

The Normal and the Failing Right Ventricle

Significant anatomical and functional differences exist between the RV and LV, reflecting different embryological origins and different roles in the cardiovascular system (reviewed in [2–4]). The RV is derived from cells from the secondary heart field, while the LV is comprised of progenitors from the primary heart field [5, 6]. As a consequence, RV development, but also adaptive and maladaptive remodeling in adulthood, is regulated by different transcription factors and molecular processes than those in the LV [2, 5, 6]. On an anatomic level, the RV free wall is triangular in shape, while the LV is elliptoid. When cross-sectioning the heart, the RV has a crescentic shape; the LV is circular. Normal RV wall thickness is 2–5 mm (8–11 mm in the LV); RV muscle mass and stroke work are 1/6 of that of the LV, reflecting the fact that the RV pumps blood into a low-pressure system. Two muscle layers are present in the RV: a superficial circumferential layer and a deeper longitudinal layer. The latter significantly contributes to RV contraction, which occurs in a longitudinal manner [7]. In contrast, the LV has three muscle layers, allowing for a more complex contraction involving torsion and rotation. The RV and LV superficial layers are connected in the ventricular grove; this is one of the components responsible for ventricular interdependence.

RV perfusion mainly occurs through the right coronary artery (RCA) and, under normal conditions, is characterized by coronary flow during both systole and diastole. Furthermore, the RV has a lower oxygen demand, higher coronary reserve, and more collaterals than the LV. These features result in higher ischemia tolerance of the normal RV as compared to the LV. RV contraction starts at the apex and advances in a peristaltic, bellows-like fashion toward the infundibulum, thereby bringing the tricuspid annulus and apex closer together. This is accompanied by an inward motion of the RV free wall. The interventricular septum (IVS) contributes 20–40 % to RV ejection fraction (RVEF) [8]. The RV is primarily designed to move volume into the pulmonary circulation and, ultimately, into the LV and systemic vasculature. Since the RV needs to rapidly adapt to changes in preload, it is much more compliant than the LV. As a consequence, it adapts much better to volume overload states. Because of RV geometry, in the normal RV, the Frank-Starling mechanism plays a less prominent role than in the LV. However, any pathologic process that impedes RV filling, such as mechanical ventilation, pericardial constraint, or change in heart rate/atrioventricular (AV) synchrony, may negatively affect RV function. In addition, and very importantly, the RV adapts very poorly to increases in afterload [9]. This is very pertinent, as pressures in the pulmonary

vascular system can rise up to fivefold, while in pathologic states LV afterload increases less than twofold.

Biochemically, the normal RV exhibits a higher content of alpha-myosin heavy chains; these are characterized by high ATPase activity and high contraction velocity, but low force generation, making them ideally suited for a low-pressure system. In contrast, beta-myosin heavy chains (which exhibit low ATPase activity and low contraction velocity, but high force generation) are more prominent in the high-pressure system serving LV, but also in the fetal RV and RV of PAH patients [10–12].

Lastly, differences exist in RV and LV autonomic regulation. While LV myocytes exhibit increased force after alpha1-adrenoceptor stimulation, RV myocytes respond with a decrease in force [13]. In contrast, beta1-adrenergic stimulation increases inotropy in either ventricle. However, beta1-receptor density in the normal RV is higher than in the LV (but decreases with pressure overload) [14]. The RV outflow tract (OFT) and infundibulum may have a higher inotropic response than the inflow region, therefore explaining the dynamic OFT obstruction sometimes seen in cardiac surgery or in children with tetralogy of Fallot [15].

While the pathophysiology of RVF is complex, three key principles need to be emphasized: afterload sensitivity, ventricular interdependence, and RV ischemia. As mentioned, the RV is not designed to overcome significant increases in afterload [13]. As a consequence, the *acutely* failing RV cannot generate a pulmonary artery pressure (PAP) of more than 50–60 mmHg before it decompensates [16, 17]. On the other hand, a chronically volume- or pressure-overloaded RV with an adequate degree of RV hypertrophy can generate higher PAPs. Ventricular interdependence is a term used to describe the dysfunction of one ventricle secondary to a disorder of the other. This is mediated by (1) the connection of RV and LV superficial muscle layers in the ventricular grove, (2) the common pericardial sac that does not allow for expansion of one ventricle without compromising the expansion of its counterpart, and (3) the shared IVS [3, 4, 17]. The latter is particularly important, since flattening of the IVS due to RV pressure and volume overload causes LV diastolic dysfunction and eventually LV underfilling, with subsequent compromise in cardiac output (CO) and resulting hypotension [17]. Lastly, RV ischemia plays a critical role in RVF. With increasing pressure overload and a subsequent increase in transmural pressure, diastolic RV coronary perfusion ceases, leading to a decrease in oxygen delivery in the setting of increase oxygen demand (due to increased RV wall stress and increased workload) [18]. Even though adaptive RV remodeling during stable RVF promotes RV capillarization, in acute or advanced stages of RVF, capillarization cannot "keep up," thereby adding a component of microvascular ischemia to the already existing macrovascular ischemia [19]. Ischemia results in decreased RV contractility and decreased cardiac output (CO), hypotension, and further decreases in coronary perfusion pressure, resulting in a vicious cycle of RV ischemia and dysfunction (Fig. 22.1).

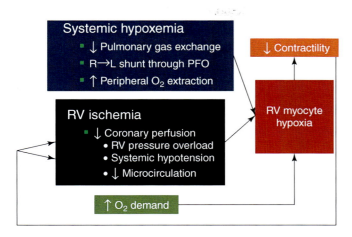

Fig. 22.1 Vicious cycle of pathophysiological alterations in right ventricular failure (RVF). Both global hypoxemia and local RV ischemia lead to RV myocyte hypoxia with subsequent decreases in contractility. Myocyte hypoxia is further exacerbated by the increased oxygen demand of the failing RV. Decreased RV contractility results in worsening cardiac output, with further decreases in RV perfusion and worsening RV ischemia. Systemic hypoxia is usually caused by underlying primary lung disease with reduction of pulmonary gas exchange, right-to-left (R → L) shunting through opening of a patent foramen ovale (PFO) secondary to RV pressure overload, and/or increases in peripheral O₂ extraction. RV ischemia results from decreased macro- and microvascular perfusion due to pressure overload and altered angiogenesis, respectively, and/or systemic hypotension

On a cellular level, these changes are accompanied by mitochondrial dysfunction, proinflammatory cytokine activation, and myocyte apoptosis [20, 21]. Compensatory mechanisms include pressure overload-induced rapid increases in contractility (mediated by rapid alterations in Ca^{2+} sensitivity; known as Anrep effect) [22], neurohormonal activation with catecholamine and endothelin release [23], and (when the RV takes on the more rounded shape of the LV) further increases in contractility through the Frank-Starling mechanism [4]. Once these compensatory processes become insufficient, clinical RVF ensues.

Causes of RVF

In general, RVF is caused by alterations in preload, afterload, or RV contractility/mechanics (Fig. 22.2). Common etiologies are listed in Table 22.1. In general, the most common etiology of RVF is left ventricular failure (LVF). RV dysfunction appears more common in nonischemic than ischemic cardiomyopathy [3]. The development of RVF in LVF is multifactorial, including pulmonary venous congestion, ventricular interdependence, left-sided arrhythmias, neurohormonal interactions, and/or myocardial ischemia [17, 20]. Pulmonary arterial hypertension (PAH; WHO group 1 PH) and secondary forms of pulmonary hypertension (WHO groups 2–5 PH), congenital heart disease (CHD), valvulopathies, and lung disease or hypoxia may also cause RVF [17]. RV ischemia (either occurring as a primary event or

Fig. 22.2 Pathophysiological classification of common etiologies of right ventricular failure (RVF). RVF is caused by alterations in preload, contractility/cardiac mechanics, and/or increases in afterload. *ALI* acute lung injury, *ARVD* arrhythmogenic right ventricular dysplasia, *CHD* congenital heart disease, *LTPx* lung transplantation, *PAH* pulmonary arterial hypertension (WHO group 1 PH), *PH* pulmonary hypertension (WHO group 2–5 PH), *SVC* superior vena cava, *LV* left ventricle, *VHD* valvular heart disease

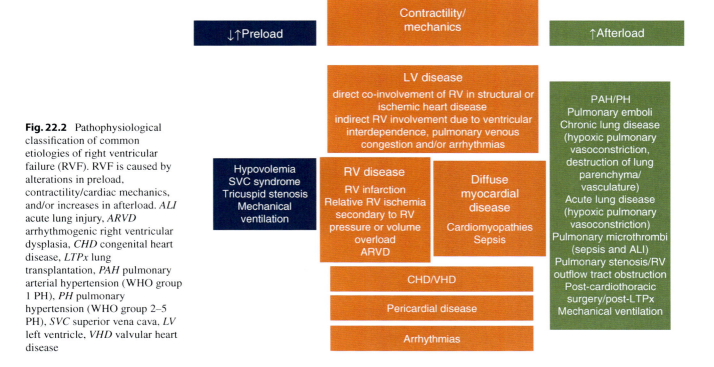

Table 22.1 Causes of right ventricular failure (RVF)

Primary left ventricular dysfunction
- Pulmonary venous congestion (LV systolic/diastolic impairment from any type of LV disease)
- Ventricular interdependence
- LV arrhythmias

Valvular heart disease
- Tricuspid regurgitation
- Pulmonary regurgitation
- Pulmonary stenosis
- Mitral valve disease

Congenital heart disease
- Atrial/ventricular septal defects
- Ebstein's anomaly
- Tetralogy of Fallot
- Transposition of the great arteries
- Anomalous pulmonary venous return
- Uhl's anomaly

Inotropy impairment
- RV ischemia/myocardial infarction*
- Cardiomyopathies
- Acute myocarditis*
- Arrythmogenic RV dysplasia
- Sepsis (proinflammatory cytokine induced)*

Afterload increase
- Pulmonary arterial hypertension (PAH; WHO group 1 pulmonary hypertension)
- WHO group 2–5 pulmonary hypertension
  - Left heart disease
  - Lung disease and/or hypoxemia
  - Chronic thromboemboli
  - Miscellaneous causes (e.g., myeloproliferative disorders, metabolic disorders, sarcoid)
- Acute pulmonary embolism*
- Hypoxic pulmonary vasoconstriction (ALI/ARDS)*
- Mechanical ventilation*
- Pulmonary vein stenosis/RV outflow tract obstruction
- Post-cardiothoracic surgery (CABG/heart or lung transplant/corrective surgery for CHD)*
- Pulmonary microthrombi (sepsis/DIC)*

Preload decrease
- Hypovolemia/acute systemic vasodilatation (sepsis)*
- Tricuspid stenosis
- Mechanical ventilation*
- SVC syndrome

Restrictive cardiomyopathies (diastolic impairment)
- Amyloidosis
- Sarcoidosis
- Idiopathic

Pericardial disease (RVF physiology rather than "true" RVF)
- Constrictive pericarditis
- Cardiac tamponade

Arrhythmias

Conditions marked with an asterisk typically cause acute RVF. Conditions like sepsis and interventions like mechanical ventilation may affect RV performance on multiple levels
ALI acute lung injury. *ARDS* acute respiratory distress syndrome, *CABG* coronary artery bypass grafting, *CHD* congenital heart disease, *DIC* disseminated intravascular coagulation, *LV* left ventricle, *SVC* superior vena cava, *WHO* World Health Organization

Table 22.2 Common causes of acute-on-chronic right ventricular failure

Myocardial ischemia/acute coronary syndrome

Atrial/ventricular arrhythmias

Acute pulmonary embolism

Progression of PAH/PH

Anemia

Acute hypoxia (hypoxic pulmonary vasoconstriction)

COPD/IPF exacerbation
- ALI/ARDS
- High altitude

Untreated sleep disorders
- Obstructive sleep apnea
- Obesity hypoventilation syndrome
- Nocturnal hypoxemia

Infection

Sepsis
- Catheter-related bloodstream infection in PAH patients on chronic epoprostenol therapy

Iatrogenic

Mechanical ventilation
- Excessive diuresis
- Aggressive fluid resuscitation

Medications

NSAIDs
- Nondihydropyridine calcium channel blockers

Behavioral

Medication nonadherence
- Dietary nonadherence

ALI acute lung injury, *ARDS* acute respiratory distress syndrome, *COPD* chronic obstructive pulmonary disease, *IPF* idiopathic pulmonary fibrosis, *NSAIDs* nonsteroidal anti-inflammatory drugs

secondary to another underlying condition) is a common cause of myocardial impairment. Hypotensive states (e.g., sepsis, decompensated LVF) may cause RV coronary hypoperfusion with deterioration in function [16, 17].

Not infrequently, patients present with acute-on-chronic RVF or with decompensated RVF as a de novo manifestation of previously unrecognized chronic RVF. Physicians should be aware of common underlying conditions (Table 22.2). In particular, cardiovascular disorders such as myocardial ischemia, worsening LV function, arrhythmias, and poorly controlled hypertension need to be considered. Hypoxemia and/or hypercarbia from parenchymal or obstructive lung disease, pulmonary vascular disease, sleep-disordered breathing, or hypoxia exposure may acutely worsen RV function by increasing afterload through hypoxic pulmonary vasoconstriction (HPV) or pulmonary vascular obstruction. Non-cardiopulmonary causes (e.g., anemia, volume overload, preload impairment, and dietary or medication noncompliance) always need to be considered. Any hypotensive disorder (e.g., sepsis) in the setting of underlying RV dysfunction can be detrimental. Systemic inflammatory states or sepsis represent a particular problem, as proinflammatory cytokines, endotoxins, endothelial dysfunction, capillary leak, and systemic hypoperfusion all contribute to worsening of an already impaired RV, sometimes leading to cardiogenic shock [16]. Along those lines, mechanical ventilation may worsen RVF by decreasing preload and increasing afterload [16].

Diagnosis

History and Examination

Both acute and chronic RVF share similar signs and symptoms, but can differ in their initial presentation. Since the RV responds poorly to sudden increases in afterload [4, 17], acute RVF more often presents with abrupt symptom onset and hemodynamic instability. Chronic RVF may be more indolent. For both acute and chronic RVF, history and physical examination are important in making a confident diagnosis [24–26].

Early RVF symptoms are nonspecific and include exertional dyspnea, fatigue, weakness, abdominal discomfort, and lower extremity edema [26, 27]. As RVF progresses, dyspnea at rest, lightheadedness, and syncope may occur. Lightheadedness, syncope, and chest pain represent advanced disease with significant reduction in CO and RV ischemia [24, 26]. In patients with PAH, syncope correlates closely with impaired RV function and is associated with increased mortality [24].

Symptoms can also assist in determining the etiology behind RVF. In the acute setting, chest pain and unilateral lower extremity edema may point to underlying acute venous thromboembolism. Orthopnea and paroxysmal nocturnal dyspnea may suggest underlying pulmonary congestion due to LVF [26]. Wheezing may indicate obstructive lung disease. Raynaud's phenomenon may be suggestive of connective tissue disease (CTD)-associated PAH. Daytime somnolence and morning headaches may suggest untreated sleep-disordered breathing.

Symptoms tend to correlate with findings such as hepatomegaly, abdominal distension, and pedal edema. Other findings include prominent jugular venous distension, parasternal heave, right-sided gallop, tricuspid regurgitation murmur, and accentuated pulmonic valve closure sound (P2) [27]. It is important to differentiate these findings from volume overload from liver cirrhosis, end-stage renal disease, fluid resuscitation, or critical illness. Though no studies have specifically evaluated specificity or sensitivity of physical examination findings in RVF, findings of irregular pulse, displaced apical beat, and elevated jugular veins are independently associated with the presence of LVF[26]. Other findings suggest more advanced RVF; these include hypotension, cool extremities, cyanosis, and absence of a pulmonic valve closure sound, the latter being suggestive of worsening RV function [26, 27]. The "classical" RVF patient will exhibit these symptoms in the presence of clear lungs. However, this picture is often clouded if RVF occurs in the setting of preexisting LV or lung disease. On the other hand,

RVF may be the initial sign of a systemic process, such as CTD, sarcoidosis, or myeloproliferative disease, and specific examination findings may assist in elucidating the potential RVF etiology. Digital clubbing may indicate underlying CHD, pulmonary fibrosis, or pulmonary veno-occlusive disease[265]. Alopecia, arthritis, rashes, and digit discoloration suggest underlying CTD. Stigmata of chronic liver disease, though sometimes difficult to differentiate from cardiac cirrhosis, may indicate RVF from porto-pulmonary hypertension. Obesity and oropharyngeal narrowing may indicate obstructive sleep apnea. A finding that is rare yet pathognomonic for chronic thromboembolic pulmonary hypertension (CTEPH) is the presence of bruits over the peripheral lung fields, resulting from turbulent blood flow in partially occluded areas [28]. Though not sensitive (observed in 10 % of CTEPH cases), this finding is highly specific for CTEPH [29].

Invasive and Noninvasive Studies for Diagnosis and Risk Stratification

Direct hemodynamic assessment via right heart catheterization remains the gold standard for RVF diagnosis. This is complimented by important noninvasive tests including biomarkers, echocardiography, and radiographic imaging (Table 22.3).

Biomarkers

Serum biomarkers are increasingly used in the management of RVF. Though nonspecific and potentially confounded by other disease states (e.g., LV disease, renal failure), in the absence of these conditions, increased biomarker levels can point toward RV disease. Biomarkers also help in assessing disease severity and guiding therapy. A major contribution lies in their high negative predictive value (NPV); biomarkers in the normal range essentially rule out RVF.

B-type natriuretic peptide (BNP) and N-terminal fragment pro-BNP (NT-proBNP) are well established in LVF. Their role in RVF is increasingly recognized as elevated levels are closely associated with RV dysfunction [31, 32, 51]. For example, elevated NT-proBNP has strong prognostic value in patients with RVF secondary to PAH. Levels >1,400 pg/ml have 88 % sensitivity, 53 % specificity, and an NPV of 91 % for predicting fatal outcomes [30]. Increased BNP or NT-proBNP also predicts adverse clinical events and increased mortality in patients with RVF secondary to acute pulmonary embolism (PE) [31]. However, a caveat may be spuriously low BNP levels in obese patients. The recent *AHA Statement on Massive and Submassive Pulmonary Embolism* considers BNP >100 pg/ml or pro-BNP >900 pg/ml as markers of moderate-to-severe RV strain [52].

Cardiac troponins are sensitive markers of myocardial injury. Similar to BNP/NT-proBNP, elevated troponin levels predict mortality in PAH [53, 54]. Elevated troponins are also associated with increased mortality and adverse

Table 22.3 Diagnostic testing and risk stratification in right ventricular failure (RVF)

Serum biomarkers	
B-type natriuretic peptide (BNP), NT-proBNP	NT-proBNP >1,400 pg/ml associated with increased mortality in RVF in PAH [30]; BNP >90–100 pg/ml associated with increased mortality and adverse clinical events in RVF in acute PE [31]; BNP >168 pg/ml associated with RV dysfunction in patients with CTEPH [32]; BNP >180 pg/ml associated with significant increase risk of death in PAH [33]
Cardiac troponins	Elevated levels associated with increase in short-term mortality, death secondary to PE, and adverse outcomes in RVF in acute PE [34] and in PAH [30]
Growth differentiation factor (GDF)-15	Increased levels associated with increased risk of death or lung transplantation in RVF in PAH population [35]; levels >4,600 ng/l associated with increased 30-day mortality in RVF in acute PE (GDF-PE) and increased long-term mortality [36]
Sodium, creatinine, glomerular filtration rate (GFR)	Na <136 mmol/l predicts RVF and increased risk of death in PAH patients [37]; predicts survival in PAH patients with acute RVF [38]; Na <135 mmol/l associated with increased 30-day mortality and an independent predictor for hospital readmission in acute PE [39]; GFR <45 ml/min per 1.73 m^2 associated with increased likelihood of death or urgent transplantation in acute PAH-induced RVF [40]
C-reactive protein (CRP)	Predicts survival in PAH patients with acute RVF secondary to CTEPH and PAH [38, 41]; CRP >5 mg/dl associated with decreased survival and event-free survival in patients with PAH [41]; correlates with severity of PAH [41]
Echocardiographic parameters	Several findings associated with poor prognosis in multiple studies; reviewed in [3]
Pericardial effusion	If present, predicts poor outcomes in PAH [33]
RA, RV enlargement	
Septal displacement	
RV hypokinesis	
RV diameter/LV diameter	Can also be measured on chest CT or cardiac MRI; poor prognosis in acute PE if >1 [42]
Tricuspid annular plane systolic excursion (TAPSE)	TAPSE <1.8 cm reflects more severe RV dysfunction and poorer prognosis in PAH [43]
Presence of RV notching (especially if mid-systolic)	Mid-systolic notching predicts increased PVR and more severe RV dysfunction [44]
Severe tricuspid regurgitation	
Tissue Doppler, Tei index, RV myocardial performance index (RVMPI)	Reliable in assessing RVF; less preload dependent [3]
Hemodynamic parameters	
Right atrial pressure (RAP)	Increase associated with poor prognosis [45]; RAP >15 mmHg indication for transplant referral for PAH [46]; RAP >20 mmHg associated with significant increased risk of death in PAH [33]
Pulmonary vascular resistance (PVR)	PVR >1,000–1,200 dyn×s×cm^{-5} contraindication for balloon atrial septostomy in PAH [46]; PVR >32 Wood units associated with decreased survival in PAH [33]
Cardiac output (CO)/cardiac index (CI)	CI <2 l/min/m^2 associated with decreased survival [47]
RV stroke work index (RVSWI)	RVSWI ≤0.25 mmHg×ml/m^2 is strong predictor of RVF after LVAD placement [48]
Functional/clinical parameters	
NYHA functional class	Class III or IV predict of poor prognosis in PAH [33]
6-min walk distance (6MWD)	6MWD <300 m portends to poor outcomes and decreased survival in PAH [49]; 6MWD <165 m associated with significant increased risk of death in PAH [33]; heart rate recovery 1 min after 6-min walk ≤16 beats/min enhances prognostic value of 6MWD [50]
Cardiopulmonary exercise testing (CPET)	Peak exercise systolic blood pressure ≤120 mmHg or VO$_2$max <10.4 ml/kg/min predicts decreased survival in PAH [49]
Respiratory rate (RR)	RR >20/min associated with increased likelihood of death or urgent transplantation in acute PAH-induced RVF [40]

CT computer tomography, *LVAD* left ventricular assist device, *MRI* magnetic resonance imaging, *PAH* pulmonary arterial hypertension, *PE* pulmonary embolism, *VO$_2$max* maximal oxygen uptake during exercise

outcomes in hemodynamically stable patients with RV dysfunction from acute PE [34].

Growth differentiation factor-15 (GDF-15) is a member of the transforming growth factor-β cytokine family that is produced by pressure-overloaded or ischemic myocardial tissue [36, 55, 56]. GDF-15 >1,200 ng/l is strongly associated with increased risk of death or lung transplantation in RVF secondary to PAH [35]. Interestingly, GDF-15 levels >1,200 ng/l were also associated with higher New York Heart Association (NYHA) class, lower 6-min walk distance, elevated NT-proBNP, higher mean right atrial and pulmonary capillary wedge pressures, and lower mixed venous oxygen saturation [35]. Its role in acute PE is also being explored. Concentrations >4,600 ng/l have a prognostic sensitivity of 71 %, a specificity of 90 %, and NPV of 95 % for complicated 30-day clinical outcome [36]. Levels >4,600 ng/l are also associated with increased long-term mortality [36].

Other biomarkers were recently established as prognostic markers in PAH patients with acute RVF admitted to the ICU [38]. These include increased liver function tests (LFTs), increased creatinine, and elevated C-reactive protein. Increased LFTs in RVF may indicate congestive hepatopathy and/or shock liver from forward failure. Similar to LVF, increases in creatinine in RVF are associated with poor outcomes [38, 40]. Hyponatremia, a purported marker of neurohormonal activation, is associated with poor outcomes in acute PE as well as acute RVF in PAH and predicts RVF and poor survival in PAH [37–40].

Electrocardiography and Radiographic Studies

The electrocardiogram (ECG) may point toward an RV etiology of symptoms if it demonstrates right axis deviation, RV hypertrophy, right-sided conduction delay, or RV strain pattern (e.g., SIQIII pattern or T wave inversion in the precordial leads). However, its use is limited by lack of sensitivity [16]. Similarly, *plain chest radiography* lacks sensitivity but may have some utility in determining the etiology of RVF. For example, increased basilar interstitial opacities may be suggestive of underlying interstitial lung disease-associated RVF. Cardiomegaly, pleural effusions, and pulmonary edema on the other hand can be suggestive of LVF as the cause of RVF. Findings of RV dysfunction on chest computed tomography (*CT*), such as right atrial (RA) and RV dilatation, leftward IVS deviation, or reflux of intravenous contrast into the hepatic veins, are often late findings of disease and are associated with increased mortality (Fig. 22.3) [16]. Chest CT

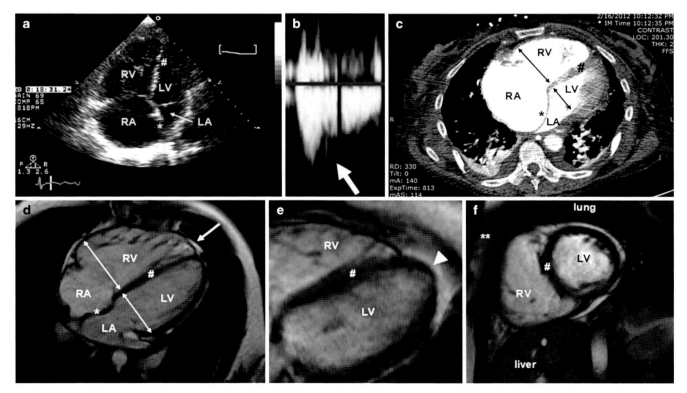

Fig. 22.3 Echocardiographic and radiographic imaging of the failing right ventricle (*RV*). (**a**) Apical four-chamber view of a 41-year-old male patient with pulmonary arterial hypertension indicating severe dilation of the right atrium (*RA*) and RV with leftward displacement of the interventricular septum (IVS; #) and interatrial septum (IAS; *). Note underfilling of left ventricle (*LV*) and left atrium (*LA*). RA and RV diameter should be no greater than the LA or LV diameter. (**b**) Representative image of flow velocity envelope obtained from pulsed-wave Doppler examination of the RV outflow tract from the same patient. *Arrow* indicates mid-systolic notching. (**c**) Chest CT of a 62-year-old female patient with acute-on-chronic RVF due to idiopathic pulmonary arterial hypertension (IPAH). Note severe RA and RV enlargement with massive shift of IAS to the left. IVS is also displaced. LA and LV are severely underfilled. RA pressure was 33 mmHg.

RV/LV diameter ratio is 1.5 (normal ratio is 0.67). Chest CT also shows bilateral atelectasis and small pleural effusions. (**d**) Single cardiac MRI image from a cine steady state free precision (SSFP) series in the 4-chamber plane of a 53-year-old male patient with a dilated heart on chest x-ray. The right heart was difficult to visualize on echocardiogram. MRI revealed moderate-to-severe tricuspid regurgitation. Image demonstrates enlarged RA and RV. RV/LV ratio is 1.1. Also, note significant contribution of the RV to the apex of the heart (*arrow*; also seen in (a) and (c)), a finding that is not observed in the normal heart (**e**), where the apex of the heart is formed by the LV (*arrowhead*). (**f**) Single image from a cine SSFP series in the short-axis plane (same patient as in (d)) again demonstrates RV enlargement. ** indicates anterior chest wall. MRI images were contributed by Dr. Shawn Teague (Dept. of Radiology, Indiana University)

with intravenous contrast is frequently used in the initial evaluation of acute PE. In this setting, an increase in the RV-to-LV diameter was identified as a predictor of PE-related death [42]. However, for the evaluation of CTEPH as a cause of RVF, chest CT with intravenous contrast lacks sensitivity and ventilation/perfusion scanning appears more sensitive [57]. Like chest x-ray, chest CT may point toward pulmonary or left-sided causes of RVF. Cardiac magnetic resonance imaging (cMRI; see Fig. 22.3) is increasingly used in the evaluation of RV and LV function and structure [3]. Even though limited by availability, high cost, and practicality, it currently is considered as the most accurate imaging method for assessment of RV volume, valvular flow, CO, and shunt fraction [3]. cMRI also assesses myocardial perfusion (via gadolinium infusion) and pulmonary artery structure and blood flow [58].

Echocardiography

Echocardiography is essential in the initial diagnosis as well as follow-up management of both acute and chronic RVF. Its availability, noninvasive nature, and ability to be performed at the bedside or in the office make it a critical tool in (1) detection of RVF, (2) identification of underlying causes, and (3) prognostication. The following traditional parameters indicate RV dysfunction: RA enlargement, RV dilation, RV hypokinesis, leftward shift of the IVS, pericardial effusion, significant tricuspid regurgitation, and dilation of the inferior vena cava with lack of respiratory variation. If present in conditions like PH, these findings predict poor outcomes [45, 59, 60].

In the presence of tricuspid regurgitation, echocardiography may allow for estimation of RV systolic pressure (RVSP, a correlate of PA systolic pressure [PASP]) using the modified Bernoulli equation. However, recent data demonstrate echocardiographically estimated RVSP over- or understimates PASP by >10 mmHg in almost 50 % of cases [61]. Both over- and underestimation are equally common. In addition, it is important to recognize that decreases in RVSP in PH may indicate RV forward failure with decreased CO [9]. Therefore, RVSP values should always be used in conjunction with additional markers of RV performance.

Certain echocardiographic parameters are of particular importance in RVF. Injection of *agitated saline* allows for detection of intracardiac shunts as a cause or consequence of RVF. The *McConnell sign* refers to a distinct pattern of RV mid-free-wall hypokinesis with preserved contraction of the apical segments. Initially described in acute PE, this may also be seen in RV infarction or other causes of RVF [62–64]. Findings of left atrial dilatation and LV hypertrophy are suggestive of underlying LV disease as the cause of RVF.

Assessment of RV contractility remains challenging due to RV shape and preload dependency [3]. *Newer indices*, such as tricuspid annular plane systolic excursion (TAPSE),

tissue Doppler, Tei index, and RV myocardial performance index (RVMPI), accurately assess RVF and are less preload dependent [3].

TAPSE measures tricuspid annular systolic displacement toward the apex. It is a simple and reproducible index that correlates closely with RVEF [43, 65]. TAPSE <1.8 cm reflects more severe RV dysfunction and poorer prognosis in PAH [43]. One-year survival for patients with TAPSE <1.8 cm compared to those with values >1.8 cm was 60 % versus 94 % [43]. TAPSE may also indicate RV dysfunction from acute PE and correlates with RV pressure increases [66]. Similarly, tissue Doppler, Tei index, and RVMPI are now being evaluated in PH and/or acute PE [67–69].

A recent study identified systolic deceleration or "notching" of the RV outflow tract Doppler flow velocity envelope (FVE_{RVOT}) as a predictor of severe pulmonary vascular disease and RV dysfunction. The presence of RV notching (identifying exaggerated pulse wave reflection in the RVOT due to increased pulmonary vascular resistance [PVR]) was found to be associated with more severe RV dysfunction, reduced TAPSE, and increased interventricular displacement [44]. Interestingly, the presence of mid-systolic notching (MSN) indicated higher PVR and more severe RV dysfunction than the presence of late-systolic notching (LSN). Both MSN and LSN were associated with a PVR >3 Wood units (WU), while absence of notching predicted PVR <3 WU. Importantly, despite the presence of PH, notching was absent if the pulmonary capillary wedge pressure (PCWP) was >15 mmHg, suggesting that FVE_{RVOT} may also help differentiate pulmonary venous hypertension from primary forms of the disease.

Right Heart Catheterization (RHC)

RHC remains the gold standard for diagnosing RVF and determining its etiology. It also provides significant insight into both disease severity and prognosis [45]. Parameters obtained help guide treatment regimens and facilitate decision making with regard to invasive or surgical treatment options. In acute RVF, RHC often guides complex therapies including inotropes, pulmonary vasodilators, and diuretics. In addition to directly measuring PAP and PCWP, RHC allows for measurement and/or calculation of additional parameters such as right atrial pressure (RAP), CO/cardiac index (CO/CI), mixed venous oxygen saturation, PVR, and RV stroke work index [46, 48, 70–73]. Assessing the acute response to pulmonary vasodilators helps guide treatment regimens for PAH. Venous oxygen saturation step-ups of >7 % between right-sided compartments (e.g., RA and RV) indicate left-to-right shunting. Combination with left heart catheterization allows for assessment of coronary artery disease or structural abnormalities that may contribute to RVF. RAP, CO/CI, and PVR predict survival in PAH [33, 47]. Elevated mPAP and increased PVR in the absence of elevated PCWP is the classic finding of PH. Even though this constellation is commonly seen in "secondary" PH associated with chronic lung disease, sleep-disordered breathing, or chronic hypoxia exposure (WHO group 3 PH) [49, 70], PH in these settings is usually associated with normal or only mildly elevated PVR and rarely requires treatment. PAH (WHO group 1 PH) however, is usually characterized by a marked increase in PVR (>3 WU) in the absence of lung disease and is treated with PAH-specific drugs [49, 74]. Determining the PCWP is fundamental in differentiating pulmonary venous hypertension (WHO group 2 PH) from other forms of PH. However, in a large retrospective analysis, PCWP correlated with left ventricular end-diastolic pressure (LVEDP) in only about 50 % of cases [75]. LVEDP should therefore be measured if the correct diagnosis is in doubt. Some authors suggest a fluid challenge or exercise maneuver in cases of borderline elevation of PCWP, in order to unmask the potential presence of LV diastolic dysfunction [49]. The presence of an elevated transpulmonary gradient (mPAP-PCWP) >12–15 mmHg in the setting of an elevated PCWP is suggestive of increased PVR in addition to elevated pulmonary venous pressures, a scenario sometimes referred to as "out-of-proportion PH" [49, 70]. Similar to RVSP, any PAP value should only be evaluated in conjunction with other parameters of RV function, as a decrease in PAP may reflect decreasing RVEF and worsening RVF [9].

PVR is not the sole component of RV afterload, and several new methods for assessment of additional afterload components have recently gained interest. For example, PA compliance, elastance, and capacitance assess PA stiffness and RV pulsatile load [76, 77]. PA impedance, which evaluates and integrates PVR and PA elastance, flow, pulsatile pressure, and wave reflection, is a superior and more complete method of RV afterload assessment than PVR alone [77]. However, accurate impedance measurement requires use of a dedicated RV catheter for instantaneous flow measurement. Similarly, measurement of RV-PA coupling, an effective method of assessing changes in RV contractility in response to increases in afterload, requires an invasive approach [77].

New noninvasive surrogates of CO (e.g., variations in pulse pressure, systolic blood pressure, or stroke volume) have gained interest in the critical care setting [78]. However, they have mainly been evaluated in sedated, ventilated patients without significant arrhythmias; their role in acute RVF needs further study.

Exercise Parameters

Though not having a significant role in the initial diagnosis of RVF, results of 6-min walk testing and cardiopulmonary exercise testing correlate closely with the degree of RV dysfunction [79–82]. Both modalities are predictors of outcomes in RVF secondary to LVF or PAH and can help guide treatment strategies [79]. For example, 6-min walk distance <300 m, VO$_2$max <10.4 ml/kg/min, or peak exercise systolic arterial pressure ≤120 mmHg predict poor outcomes and decreased survival in PAH [49]. Heart rate recovery <16 beats/min 1 min after 6-min walk correlates with markers of RV dysfunction and enhances prognostic value of the 6-min walk distance in PAH [50].

Management

RVF management focuses on determination of the underlying cause. Additional RV-directed therapies focus on improving RV function by optimizing preload, afterload, and/or contractility (Fig. 22.4). Unfortunately, no RV-specific therapies exist, and most interventions concomitantly target the pulmonary and/or systemic vasculature, as well as the LV. All interventions should be accompanied by general measures and aggressive volume management.

Chronic RVF

General Measures

Treatment strategies for chronic RVF include appropriate immunizations, weight monitoring, salt restriction, graded aerobic exercise, and – in case of daytime or nocturnal hypoxemia – oxygen to avoid HPV [17]. In PAH-induced RVF, physical training improves functional and quality of life (QoL) endpoints [83]. However, isometric activities may provoke syncope and should be avoided [84, 85]. Along those lines, experimental data demonstrate that exercise in *severe* RVF may be detrimental and increase RV inflammation [86]. NSAIDs and nondihydropyridine calcium channel blockers should be avoided [17]. Exacerbating factors (e.g., anemia, sleep apnea, thyroid disease) should be appropriately treated. Finally, due to negative effects on preload and afterload during the second trimester and peripartum period, avoidance of pregnancy should be addressed in female patients with RVF [87].

Neurohormonal Modulators and Diuretics

Beta-blockers, angiotensin converting enzyme (ACE) inhibitors, and diuretics are the mainstay of treatment for chronic LVF. However, their role in isolated RVF is less clear. Beta-blockers reduce mortality in patients with LVF, decrease remodeling, prevent arrhythmias, and improve cardiac function [88–92]. Since neurohormonal activation, remodeling, and supraventricular arrhythmias are common in RVF [20, 88], beta-blockade is conceptually appealing. However, concerns exist about decreased exercise capacity and negative inotropic effects [93]. Recent data demonstrated impressive protective effects of carvedilol on RV function in a rat model

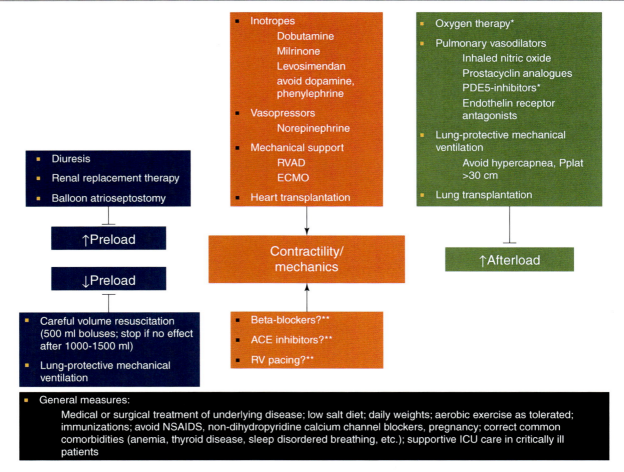

Fig. 22.4 Sensitive cardiac troponin I predicts poor outcomes in pulmonary arterial hypertension. Commonly used therapeutic interventions in right ventricular failure (RVF) and their pathophysiological targets. Note that these treatments should not replace the primary medical and/or surgical strategies directed at correcting the underlying etiology of RVF. Rather, the outlined strategies are used (1) in addition to the primary treatment, (2) as a bridge to primary treatment, or (3) if primary treatments are not available or successful. All interventions listed should be used in conjunction with general measures (see box at bottom). Italicized items are primarily used in acute/decompensated RVF. Afterload-reducing interventions marked with * also directly target the RV through inotropic/lusitropic properties (PDE5 inhibitors) or by attenuating myocyte hypoxia (oxygen). Interventions marked with ** are conceptually appealing but not yet fully established due to lack of high-quality evidence in isolated RVF. *ECMO* extracorporeal membrane oxygenation, *ICU* intensive care unit, *PDE* phosphodiesterase, *Pplat* plateau pressure, *RVAD* right ventricular assist device

of RVF [88], but it remains to be proven whether those translate into human RVF. Carvedilol also improves RVEF in patients with biventricular failure [94]. Likewise, captopril improves RV function in biventricular failure [95]. ACE inhibitors may also protect against HPV [96], but more studies are needed to dissect their potential benefit in isolated RVF. Digoxin leads to moderate short-term improvement in CO in PAH and decreases circulating norepinephrine levels [97]. However, due to its limited therapeutic window and the availability of better alternatives for supraventricular tachyarrhythmias, routine use is not recommended [16, 98].

Diuretics are crucial for RV volume and/or pressure overload, especially if the patient exhibits symptoms of increased RAP (i.e., lower extremity edema, weight gain). However, close monitoring is recommended as RV function is largely preload dependent, and overdiuresis may result in reduced CO/CI and kidney injury. Hemodynamic, echocardiographic, radiographic, and laboratory studies as well as physical examination help guide treatment decisions.

Pulmonary Vasodilators

Pulmonary vasodilators (prostacyclin analogues, endothelin-receptor antagonists (ETRAs), phosphodiesterase [PDE]5 inhibitors) are frequently used in RV dysfunction from PAH. Recent studies have also evaluated their role in RVF associated with secondary forms of PH. Continuous intravenous prostacyclin analogues (*epoprostenol or treprostinil*) improve exercise capacity, QoL, and hemodynamics; however, their use is complicated by the need for continuous intravenous access, complexity of administration, and expense [87, 99–101]. Treprostinil can also be administered subcutaneously [102]. Importantly, epoprostenol is the only intervention proven to improve survival in PAH in a prospective, randomized, controlled trial [99] and represents the most potent treatment for PAH-induced RVF. Inhaled iloprost and treprostinil also improve PAH outcomes and RV function but are less potent than intravenous or subcutaneous therapies [87]. *ETRAs* (*bosentan, ambrisentan*) and *PDE5 inhibitors* (*sildenafil, tadalafil*) improve exercise capacity and CO/CI in PAH-RVF [103–106]. Nevertheless, use of oral agents alone for significant RV dysfunction in PAH is considered insufficient and not recommended [49]. Along those lines, calcium channel blockers, though indicated for PAH patients with a positive vasodilator challenge on RHC, are not considered potent enough for PAH with RVF [49, 87]. Due to potentially favorable effects on the pulmonary vasculature and myocardium, epoprostenol and bosentan have also been evaluated in LV dysfunction. However, their use was associated with increased mortality or fluid retention [107, 108]; prostacyclin or ETRA use is discouraged in LVF-induced RVF.

Effects of PDE5 inhibitors in non-PAH-RVF appear more favorable. PDE5 is highly expressed in the hypertrophied RV and LV, and sildenafil increases contractility in the hypertrophied RV [109]. The drug also attenuates lung endothelial dysfunction and pulmonary vascular remodeling in models of heart failure with preserved EF (HFpEF) [109, 110]. In addition to RV inotropic effects, sildenafil also enhances lusitropy [111]. Based on these promising data, PDE5 inhibitors have been explored in systolic and diastolic dysfunction. Interestingly, in patients with systolic LVF and pulmonary venous hypertension, sildenafil improved exercise capacity, QoL, functional class, and CO and reduced hospitalizations [79]. In HFpEF with associated PH and RV dysfunction, sildenafil improved QoL, RV function and dimensions, LV relaxation, and distensibility; decreased lung water and PCWP; and attenuated cardiac remodeling [112]. In light of other studies demonstrating beneficial sildenafil effects on LV systolic and diastolic function [113], its use for RVF or biventricular failure appears appealing, but long-term studies with dedicated RV and mortality endpoints are needed.

PDE5 inhibitors are also evaluated in RVF from chronic lung disease (cor pulmonale). In idiopathic pulmonary fibrosis (IPF), sildenafil decreased PVR while preserving shunt perfusion, leading to overall improvement in oxygenation [114]. In a larger IPF study, sildenafil treatment was associated with small but significant improvements in oxygenation, diffusion capacity, dyspnea, and QoL [115]. While data supporting beneficial effects on exercise capacity in IPF are mixed [115, 116], a subgroup analysis of IPF patients with echocardiographic evidence of RV dysfunction suggests more pronounced sildenafil effects in this population [117]. Data supporting pulmonary vasodilator use in COPD-induced PH have been disappointing [118, 119]. A recent trial of sildenafil in patients with PH due to COPD showed that PDE5 inhibition improved mPAP and PVR, but worsened oxygenation at rest due to worsening of ventilation/perfusion mismatch [118]. Until more data are available, sildenafil use for COPD-induced cor pulmonale is not recommended. Currently, only long-term oxygen therapy improves survival in this population [120]. Epoprostenol and bosentan worsen ventilation/perfusion mismatch or QoL, respectively, in chronic lung disease [114, 121] and are not recommended for cor pulmonale. Pending further data, oxygen therapy, general measures, and diuretics remain the mainstay of care for this condition.

Interventional and Surgical Therapies

Surgical and interventional approaches are indicated in potentially reversible RVF unresponsive to or intolerant of medical therapy. Surgical or percutaneous correction often is the treatment of choice in RVF secondary to congenital or valvular heart disease. Preoperative optimization of RV filling pressures is critical. Frequently, periprocedural inotropic support is required. Ideally, these interventions should be performed before development of irreversible end-organ injury. Furthermore, surgical or mechanical support is unlikely to benefit patients with advanced RVF and/or massively elevated PVR. For example, pulmonary thrombendarterectomy for CTEPH is not recommended if the PVR is >1,000–1,200 dyn × s × cm^{-5} [46]. Balloon atrial septostomy (BAS) is contraindicated in severe RVF and should not be offered to patients with RAP ≥20 mmHg, significant hypoxemia (<90 % on room air), and/or PVR index ≥4,400 dyn × s × cm^{-5}/m^2 [46, 98, 122–125]. Caution is indicated in ASD repair if RV dysfunction is present [71]. PVR >1,200 dyn × s × cm^{-5} used to prohibit surgical closure. However, preoperative pulmonary vasodilator therapy may improve hemodynamics enough to allow for surgical correction [126].

Pulmonary thrombendarterectomy in CTEPH-RVF improves functional endpoints and survival [46]. Patients with proximal angiographic pulmonary artery obstruction and absent or minimal small vessel disease experience the most significant benefit, especially if the postoperative PVR is reduced to <500 dyn × s × cm^{-5} [127].

In *BAS*, a surgical right-to-left-shunt is created to decompress the RV. The associated decrease in oxygenation is outweighed by increased oxygen delivery due to increased CO [123, 128]. Mortality of the procedure is high (approximately 16 %), but if successful, BAS improves exercise capacity and reduces syncopal events. BAS is offered as a bridge to lung transplantation or as a palliative measure in refractory RVF but is contraindicated with concomitant LV failure [46]. Repeat BAS may be required if the orifice size decreases [128].

Heart, lung, or combined heart-lung transplantation is the last resort for end-stage RVF. In patients with PH, RVF with RAP >15 mmHg and/or CI < 2.0 l/min/m² indicates poor prognosis and warrants transplant referral [46]. However, due to the resilient nature of the RV, even patients with severe RVF from PH can be considered for isolated lung transplantation, with successful outcomes (65–75 % 1-year survival) [17, 129]. BAS, ventricular assist devices (VADs), and extracorporeal membrane oxygenation (ECMO) are sometimes used to help bridge patients to transplantation (see section "Acute/Decompensated RVF").

PH results in prolonged RV contraction due to the significant elevation in RV afterload [130]. This results in prolonged RV systole beyond the point of pulmonic valve closure, thereby reducing RVEF [131–133] and impairing LV filling due to ventricular interdependence [134]. *Cardiac resynchronization therapy* improves LV dyssynchrony in LVF [135], and preclinical data of RV pacing demonstrated restoration of RV and LV synchrony with improved RV systolic and LV diastolic function [131]. A pilot study of RV pacing in CTEPH-RVF demonstrated enhanced RV contractility, LV diastolic filling, and LV stroke volume [136]. Further studies in larger cohorts are needed to confirm these encouraging results.

Acute/Decompensated RVF

General Management

Patients with acute RVF frequently exhibit hemodynamic instability and/or respiratory failure. End-organ failure may be present, and common therapeutic interventions may have deleterious hemodynamic effects. Thus, management of this population can differ significantly compared to their more stable counterparts and typically takes place in the ICU. Management principles are similar and focus on medically or surgically treating the underlying etiology while optimizing preload, afterload, and contractility.

Immediate recognition and treatment of the causative factors leading to RV deterioration are key (see "Causes" section and Table 22.2). Infection is one of the strongest predictors of mortality in patients with RVF secondary to PAH. Thus, the importance of aggressive monitoring, preventive precautions, and management with antibiotics in this population cannot be overemphasized [98]. Supraventricular arrhythmias are common and reflect the important role of atrial contraction in active RV diastolic filling. Development of atrial fibrillation/flutter may result in decompensated RVF. Rate control may be difficult to achieve and immediate cardioversion should be considered [16, 98, 137]. The optimal hemoglobin level for patients with acute RVF is not well defined. While ICU patients usually benefit from a conservative transfusion strategy [138], patients with shock or heart failure may require higher hemoglobin levels in order to maintain oxygen delivery [139, 140]. Measurement of central or mixed venous oxygen saturation ($ScvO_2/SvO_2$) and lactate helps guide treatment decisions regarding transfusion strategies. We aim for $ScvO_2/SvO_2 \geq 65$ % and evidence of lactate clearance.

Volume management is fundamental in acute RVF. Typically, patients with RVF present with volume overload and thus require diuresis. Continuously infused diuretics, ultrafiltration, or renal replacement therapy may be required. However, overdiuresis can reduce preload and decrease CO, leading to systemic hypotension and kidney injury. On the other hand, too much preload will cause forward failure by limiting LV filling due to ventricular interdependence [16]. In hypotensive patients, careful fluid boluses of 500–1,000 ml are recommended, but should be discontinued if no improvement in blood pressure or CO is seen after 1,000–1,500 ml [16]. Pulmonary arterial catheters (PACs) are valuable in guiding volume therapy. However, PACs are more difficult to float and are associated with a higher rate of arrhythmias in decompensated RVF [98], emphasizing the value of bedside echocardiography and biomarkers.

Maintaining oxygen saturation >90–92 % is crucial to avoid HPV. However, due to potential adverse hemodynamic effects, *mechanical ventilation* – if at all possible – should be avoided. Positive pressure ventilation reduces venous return to the RA, thereby decreasing RV preload. Furthermore, increased intrathoracic pressure, by converting West zone 3 to zone 1 or 2 conditions, increases PAP and RV afterload and worsens tricuspid regurgitation. The lowest possible positive end-expiratory pressure (PEEP) and tidal volume (V_T) required to provide adequate oxygenation and ventilation, respectively, should therefore be applied [16, 141, 142]. ARDSNet strategies with limitation of plateau pressures <30 cm H_2O are recommended [16, 17, 98]. However, limitation of V_T may lead to hypercapnia with subsequent pulmonary vasoconstriction and increased afterload. Excessive hypercapnia should therefore be avoided [143, 144]. Hyperventilation, on the other hand, attenuates acidosis-induced vasoconstriction [145]; this can be used to lower PAP quickly, but should not be performed at the expense of a high V_T or excessive respiratory rate (the latter may cause dynamic hyperinflation and auto-PEEP). These complex interactions indicate why mechanical ventilation, if unavoidable, needs to be applied with caution and expertise.

Inotropes and Vasopressors

Patients with significantly decreased CO/CI require inotropic therapy. *Dobutamine*, a β1/β2-receptor agonist, augments ventricular contractility and promotes pulmonary and systemic vasodilatation, thus reducing both RV and LV afterload. These characteristics make dobutamine a valuable agent for decompensated RVF. Preclinical trials demonstrated better improvement in RVEF with dobutamine than norepinephrine [146]. Doses >5 μg/kg/min should be avoided in order to prevent tachyarrhythmias and increased myocardial oxygen consumption [16, 98, 147]. Due to its vasodilator effects, dobutamine may induce systemic hypotension; in those cases, coadministration of norepinephrine may be needed [16].

Milrinone, a PDE3 inhibitor that prevents breakdown of cyclic AMP, also has inotropic and vasodilatory properties. Similar to dobutamine, systemic vasodilatation may limit its use [148]. This is minimized by inhaled milrinone, which maintains its beneficial effects on PVR and RVEF [149]. Due to the lack of beta-receptor effects, milrinone is the preferred inotrope for patients on beta-blockers. Both milrinone and dobutamine can be used in conjunction with inhaled pulmonary vasodilators, such as inhaled nitric oxide [150]. This combination provides additive effects on pulmonary vasodilatation while allowing for lower inotrope doses, thus minimizing the risk of hypotension [151].

Dopamine should be avoided due to concerns for inducing tachyarrhythmias and increasing mortality in cardiogenic shock [152]. *Levosimendan*, a calcium sensitizer, increases RV contractility without increasing oxygen consumption. Preclinical trials showed more significant improvements in RV contractility and afterload reduction compared to dobutamine [153, 154]. Though approved in Europe, levosimendan currently is not available in the USA.

Norepinephrine, via α1-receptor effects, serves two major purposes in decompensated RVF [16, 137]: (1) it may allow for treatment with inotropes in the setting of hypotension, and (2) by increasing arterial blood pressure, it allows for enhanced coronary perfusion pressure and subsequent increases in RVEF and CO [155]. The latter is of particular importance, since increased RV transmural pressure frequently compromises perfusion. Norepinephrine can therefore help break the vicious cycle of RVF (see Fig. 22.1). Importantly, the drug does not appear to increase PAP or PVR [155]. Through β1-receptor agonistic effects, norepinephrine also increases inotropy [155].

Pulmonary Vasodilators

Inhaled nitric oxide (iNO) increases cyclic GMP, thereby mediating pulmonary vasodilation. Rapid hemoglobin-mediated inactivation in the pulmonary capillaries prevents systemic vasodilation. Effects are limited to ventilated lung areas, therefore attenuating HPV, decreasing PAP and PVR, and improving oxygenation without increasing intrapulmonary shunt fraction [156, 157]. In addition, iNO has purported anti-inflammatory effects [98, 158]. Responses to iNO are mixed; in 26 ICU patients with acute RVF, 14 patients exhibited improved CO, PVR, and oxygenation with iNO (35 ppm) [159]. In patients undergoing heart or lung transplantation, iNO use for PH and/or RVF was associated

with lower mortality, while effects were less pronounced in cardiac surgery or hypoxemic medical patients [160]. Improvements in PVR and RV dysfunction were confirmed in heart transplant patients [161] and in PH after mitral valve replacement [162]. Use of iNO is limited by potential methemoglobinemia, production of reactive nitrogen species, acute kidney injury, and rebound PH after rapid discontinuation [98, 163]. As mentioned, iNO is of particular benefit when combined with dobutamine or milrinone [150].

Primarily evaluated in cardiac surgery or transplant patients, PAH-specific medications are also used as afterload reducers in acute/decompensated RVF. Due to its short half-life (3–6 min) and potent vasodilator effects, *epoprostenol* is the preferred agent [16, 137]. However systemic hypotension and increased ventilation/perfusion mismatch may limit its use, and the agent should be avoided in patients with respiratory failure, shock, or LV dysfunction [16]. Epoprostenol is initiated at 1–2 ng/kg/min and increased by 0.5–1 ng/kg/min every 15–30 min. A more cautious approach is recommended in patients with significant comorbidities, hypoxemia, and/or labile hemodynamics. As with iNO, abrupt discontinuation may lead to rebound PH and even death [99, 164]. *Treprostinil* decreases PAP and PVR [165], but has a longer half-life than epoprostenol. In unstable patients, intravenous is preferred over subcutaneous administration, in order to avoid problems with unpredictable absorption. Inhaled prostacyclins avoid systemic side effects and represent a less costly alternative to iNO. In heart or lung transplant recipients with PH, refractory hypoxemia, and RV dysfunction, *inhaled prostacyclin* reduced PAP and improved CI and ScvO$_2$ similar to iNO [166]. *Inhaled iloprost* improves PH and RV function during/after mitral valve surgery, cardiopulmonary bypass, or heart transplantation [167–169] and may be more potent than iNO [170]. In a recent open-label trial of PH patients, *inhaled treprostinil* (15–30 μg) additively decreased PVR and PAP and increased CO when added to sildenafil [171]. No matter the formulation used, management of these agents requires close monitoring of cardiopulmonary hemodynamics (usually by PAC and echocardiography).

Due to concerns about unreliable absorption in decompensated RVF, *oral vasodilators* are less frequently used. However, they are useful for (1) less severe forms of RVF and (2) patients that have become more hemodynamically stable, with plans to either continue or remove the parenteral agent [137]. ETRA use in the ICU is limited by relatively long half-lives and potential hepatotoxicity [87, 103]. In general, more data are available for PDE5 inhibitors. In patients undergoing mitral valve repair or LV assist device (LVAD) placement, sildenafil reduces PAP and PVR and facilitates weaning of parenteral pulmonary vasodilators while only minimally decreasing systemic blood pressure [172]. PDE5 inhibitors act synergistically with iNO [173–175] or iloprost [176]. Sildenafil also decreases rebound PH after iNO withdrawal [177]. In LVAD patients, sildenafil facilitates weaning from iNO and inotropes while providing additive reductions in PAP [178]. PDE5 inhibitors also decrease PVR, maintain systemic blood pressure, and improve myocardial perfusion after coronary artery bypass grafting [179, 180]. With a milrinone-like effect, sildenafil's inotropic actions are exerted at least in part through concomitant PDE3 inhibition [109]. Sildenafil effects occur after 15–30 min and peak after 30–60 min; half-life is 4 h. Like other PAH drugs, sildenafil may cause thrombocytopenia [181].

Interventional and Surgical Rescue Therapies

In patients with potentially reversible RVF in whom conventional support is failing or in transplant candidates, *BAS, VADs, or ECMO* may be used to temporarily stabilize the patient or to bridge them to surgery. Requirement for RVAD versus LVAD versus biventricular VAD depends on the etiology of acute RVF. LVADs or biventricular VADs are usually used for RVF secondary to LVF, with evidence of improved posttransplantation survival with LVAD placement [182, 183]. RVADs are used for isolated RVF, but data are limited [184]. If considering transplantation, early consultation for VAD placement is crucial to prevent further hemodynamic deterioration and development of multiorgan failure. Importantly, isolated RVADs may be insufficient or even deleterious in cases of increased afterload; extracorporeal membrane oxygenation (ECMO) may be more effective in unloading the RV [184]. ECMO is particularly beneficial if RVF is accompanied by severe hypoxemia. For RVF, venoarterial ECMO usually is the procedure of choice. A recent study demonstrated improved outcomes in awake, nonintubated patients as compared to mechanically ventilated ECMO patients awaiting lung transplantation, with improved survival at 6 months after transplant and shorter postoperative mechanical ventilation time [185].

> **Key Points**
> - The RV is embryologically, anatomically, physiologically, biochemically, and electrophysiologically different than the LV.
> - RVF is caused by alterations in RV preload, cardiac contractility/mechanics, and/or increased afterload.
> - Common causes are LV disease, valvular or congenital heart disease, pulmonary hypertension, and pulmonary embolism.
> - Key features of RVF are afterload sensitivity, ventricular interdependence, and RV ischemia.
> - Echocardiography and hemodynamic assessment, complemented by biomarkers and radiographic studies, are essential for diagnosis and risk stratification.

> - Treatment of RVF is directed toward the underlying etiology, complemented by general measures. RVF-directed therapies target alterations in preload, contractility/mechanics, and/or afterload; they are used (1) in addition to, (2) as a bridge to, or (3) as an alternate approach to primary treatments (the latter if no primary treatment is available or feasible).

Summary of Key Guidelines from Professional Societies

No RVF-specific guidelines exist. RV-directed approaches are discussed in an *AHA Statement on Massive and Submassive Pulmonary Embolism* [52] and a *Consensus Document on Pulmonary Hypertension* by the ACCF, AHA, ACCP, ATS, and PHA [49]. Recommendations in this chapter are derived from these documents.

References

1. Erzurum S, Rounds SI, Stevens T, et al. Strategic plan for lung vascular research: an NHLBI-ORDR workshop report. Am J Respir Crit Care Med. 2010;182(12):1554–62.
2. Voelkel NF, Quaife RA, Leinwand LA, et al. Right ventricular function and failure: report of a national heart, lung, and blood institute working group on cellular and molecular mechanisms of right heart failure. Circulation. 2006;114(17):1883–91.
3. Haddad F, Hunt SA, Rosenthal DN, Murphy DJ. Right ventricular function in cardiovascular disease, part I. Circulation. 2008;117:1436–48.
4. Greyson CR. Pathophysiology of right ventricular failure. Crit Care Med. 2008;36(1 Suppl):S57–65.
5. Garry DJ, Olson EN. A common progenitor at the heart of development. Cell. 2006;127(6):1101–4.
6. Buckingham M, Meilhac S, Zaffran S. Building the mammalian heart from two sources of myocardial cells. Nat Rev Genet. 2005;6(11):826–35.
7. Brown SB, Raina A, Katz D, Szerlip M, Wiegers SE, Forfia PR. Longitudinal shortening accounts for the majority of right ventricular contraction and improves after pulmonary vasodilator therapy in normal subjects and patients with pulmonary arterial hypertension. Chest. 2011;140(1):27–33.
8. Klima U, Guerrero JL, Vlahakes GJ. Contribution of the interventricular septum to maximal right ventricular function. Eur J Cardiothorac Surg. 1998;14(3):250–5.
9. MacNee W. Pathophysiology of cor pulmonale in chronic obstructive pulmonary disease. Part One. Am J Respir Crit Care Med. 1994;150(3):833–52.
10. Brooks WW, Bing OH, Blaustein AS, Allen PD. Comparison of contractile state and myosin isozymes of rat right and left ventricular myocardium. J Mol Cell Cardiol. 1987;19(5):433–40.
11. Rudolph AM. The changes in the circulation after birth. Their importance in congenital heart disease. Circulation. 1970;41(2):343–59.
12. Lowes BD, Minobe W, Abraham WT, et al. Changes in gene expression in the intact human heart. Downregulation of alpha-myosin

heavy chain in hypertrophied, failing ventricular myocardium. J Clin Invest. 1997;100(9):2315–24.

13. Wang GY, McCloskey DT, Turcato S, Swigart PM, Simpson PC, Baker AJ. Contrasting inotropic responses to alpha1-adrenergic receptor stimulation in left versus right ventricular myocardium. Am J Physiol Heart Circ Physiol. 2006;291(4):H2013–7.

14. Bristow MR, Minobe W, Rasmussen R, et al. Beta-adrenergic neuroeffector abnormalities in the failing human heart are produced by local rather than systemic mechanisms. J Clin Invest. 1992;89(3):803–15.

15. Denault AY, Chaput M, Couture P, Hebert Y, Haddad F, Tardif JC. Dynamic right ventricular outflow tract obstruction in cardiac surgery. J Thorac Cardiovasc Surg. 2006;132(1):43–9.

16. Lahm T, McCaslin CA, Wozniak TC, et al. Medical and surgical treatment of acute right ventricular failure. J Am Coll Cardiol. 2010;56(18):1435–46.

17. Haddad FDR, Murphy DJ, Hunt SA. Right ventricular function in cardiovascular disease, part II. Circulation. 2008;117:1717–31.

18. Vlahakes GJ, Turley K, Hoffman JI. The pathophysiology of failure in acute right ventricular hypertension: hemodynamic and biochemical correlations. Circulation. 1981;63(1):87–95.

19. Bogaard HJ, Natarajan R, Henderson SC, et al. Chronic pulmonary artery pressure elevation is insufficient to explain right heart failure. Circulation. 2009;120(20):1951–60.

20. Bogaard HJ, Abe K, Vonk Noordegraaf A, Voelkel NF. The right ventricle under pressure: cellular and molecular mechanisms of right-heart failure in pulmonary hypertension. Chest. 2009;135(3):794–804.

21. Haddad F, Ashley E, Michelakis ED. New insights for the diagnosis and management of right ventricular failure, from molecular imaging to targeted right ventricular therapy. Curr Opin Cardiol. 2010;25(2):131–40.

22. Pawlush DG, Musch TI, Moore RL. Ca2+-dependent heterometric and homeometric autoregulation in hypertrophied rat heart. Am J Physiol. 1989;256(4 Pt 2):H1139–47.

23. Nootens M, Kaufmann E, Rector T, et al. Neurohormonal activation in patients with right ventricular failure from pulmonary hypertension: relation to hemodynamic variables and endothelin levels. J Am Coll Cardiol. 1995;26(7):1581–5.

24. Le RJ, Fenstad ER, Maradit-Kremers H, et al. Syncope in adults with pulmonary arterial hypertension. J Am Coll Cardiol. 2011;58(8):863–7.

25. McGoon M, Gutterman D, Steen V, et al. Screening, early detection, and diagnosis of pulmonary arterial hypertension: ACCP evidence-based clinical practice guidelines. Chest. 2004;126(1 Suppl):14S–34.

26. Kelder JC, Cramer MJ, van Wijngaarden J, et al. The diagnostic value of physical examination and additional testing in primary care patients with suspected heart failure. Circulation. 2011;124(25):2865–73.

27. Piazza G, Goldhaber SZ. The acutely decompensated right ventricle: pathways for diagnosis and management. Chest. 2005;128(3):1836–52.

28. ZuWallack RL, Liss JP, Lahiri B. Acquired continuous murmur associated with acute pulmonary thromboembolism. Chest. 1976;70(4):557–9.

29. Hoeper MM, Mayer E, Simonneau G, Rubin LJ. Chronic thromboembolic pulmonary hypertension. Circulation. 2006;113(16):2011–20.

30. Fijalkowska A, Kurzyna M, Torbicki A, et al. Serum N-terminal brain natriuretic peptide as a prognostic parameter in patients with pulmonary hypertension. Chest. 2006;129(5):1313–21.

31. Klok FA, Mos IC, Huisman MV. Brain-type natriuretic peptide levels in the prediction of adverse outcome in patients with pulmonary embolism: a systematic review and meta-analysis. Am J Respir Crit Care Med. 2008;178(4):425–30.

32. Reesink HJ, Tulevski II, Marcus JT, et al. Brain natriuretic peptide as noninvasive marker of the severity of right ventricular dysfunction in chronic thromboembolic pulmonary hypertension. Ann Thorac Surg. 2007;84(2):537–43.

33. Benza RL, Miller DP, Gomberg-Maitland M, et al. Predicting survival in pulmonary arterial hypertension: insights from the Registry to Evaluate Early and Long-Term Pulmonary Arterial Hypertension Disease Management (REVEAL). Circulation. 2010;122(2):164–72.

34. Becattini C, Vedovati MC, Agnelli G. Prognostic value of troponins in acute pulmonary embolism: a meta-analysis. Circulation. 2007;116(4):427–33.

35. Nickel N, Kempf T, Tapken H, et al. Growth differentiation factor-15 in idiopathic pulmonary arterial hypertension. Am J Respir Crit Care Med. 2008;178(5):534–41.

36. Lankeit M, Kempf T, Dellas C, et al. Growth differentiation factor-15 for prognostic assessment of patients with acute pulmonary embolism. Am J Respir Crit Care Med. 2008;177(9):1018–25.

37. Forfia PR, Mathai SC, Fisher MR, et al. Hyponatremia predicts right heart failure and poor survival in pulmonary arterial hypertension. Am J Respir Crit Care Med. 2008;177(12):1364–9.

38. Sztrymf B, Souza R, Bertoletti L, et al. Prognostic factors of acute heart failure in patients with pulmonary arterial hypertension. Eur Respir J. 2010;35(6):1286–93.

39. Scherz N, Labarere J, Mean M, Ibrahim SA, Fine MJ, Aujesky D. Prognostic importance of hyponatremia in patients with acute pulmonary embolism. Am J Respir Crit Care Med. 2010;182(9):1178–83.

40. Haddad F, Peterson T, Fuh E, et al. Characteristics and outcome after hospitalization for acute right heart failure in patients with pulmonary arterial hypertension. Circ Heart Fail. 2011;4(6):692–9.

41. Quarck R, Nawrot T, Meyns B, Delcroix M. C-reactive protein: a new predictor of adverse outcome in pulmonary arterial hypertension. J Am Coll Cardiol. 2009;53(14):1211–8.

42. van der Meer RW, Pattynama PM, van Strijen MJ, et al. Right ventricular dysfunction and pulmonary obstruction index at helical CT: prediction of clinical outcome during 3-month follow-up in patients with acute pulmonary embolism. Radiology. 2005;235(3):798–803.

43. Forfia PR, Fisher MR, Mathai SC, et al. Tricuspid annular displacement predicts survival in pulmonary hypertension. Am J Respir Crit Care Med. 2006;174(9):1034–41.

44. Arkles JS, Opotowsky AR, Ojeda J, et al. Shape of the right ventricular Doppler envelope predicts hemodynamics and right heart function in pulmonary hypertension. Am J Respir Crit Care Med. 2011;183(2):268–76.

45. Chemla D, Castelain V, Herve P, Lecarpentier Y, Brimioulle S. Haemodynamic evaluation of pulmonary hypertension. Eur Respir J. 2002;20(5):1314–31.

46. Keogh AM, Mayer E, Benza RL, et al. Interventional and surgical modalities of treatment in pulmonary hypertension. J Am Coll Cardiol. 2009;54(1 Suppl):S67–77.

47. Humbert M, Sitbon O, Chaouat A, et al. Survival in patients with idiopathic, familial, and anorexigen-associated pulmonary arterial hypertension in the modern management era. Circulation. 2010;122(2):156–63.

48. Fitzpatrick 3rd JR, Frederick JR, Hsu VM, et al. Risk score derived from pre-operative data analysis predicts the need for biventricular mechanical circulatory support. J Heart Lung Transplant. 2008;27(12):1286–92.

49. McLaughlin VV, Archer SL, Badesch DB, et al. ACCF/AHA 2009 expert consensus document on pulmonary hypertension a report of the American College of Cardiology Foundation Task Force on Expert Consensus Documents and the American Heart Association developed in collaboration with the American College of Chest Physicians; American Thoracic Society, Inc.; and the Pulmonary Hypertension Association. J Am Coll Cardiol. 2009;53(17):1573–619.

50. Minai OA, Gudavalli R, Mummadi S, Liu X, McCarthy K, Dweik RA. Heart rate recovery predicts clinical worsening in patients with pulmonary arterial hypertension. Am J Respir Crit Care Med. 2012;185(4):400–8.

51. Nagaya N, Nishikimi T, Okano Y, et al. Plasma brain natriuretic peptide levels increase in proportion to the extent of right ventricular dysfunction in pulmonary hypertension. J Am Coll Cardiol. 1998;31(1):202–8.

52. Jaff MR, McMurtry MS, Archer SL, et al. Management of massive and submassive pulmonary embolism, iliofemoral deep vein thrombosis, and chronic thromboembolic pulmonary hypertension: a scientific statement from the American Heart Association. Circulation. 2011;123(16):1788–830.

53. Heresi GA, Tang WH, Aytekin M, Hammel J, Hazen SL, Dweik RA. Sensitive cardiac troponin I predicts poor outcomes in pulmonary arterial hypertension. Eur Respir J. 2012;39(4):939–44.

54. Torbicki A, Kurzyna M, Kuca P, et al. Detectable serum cardiac troponin T as a marker of poor prognosis among patients with chronic precapillary pulmonary hypertension. Circulation. 2003; 108(7):844–8.

55. Kempf T, Eden M, Strelau J, et al. The transforming growth factor-beta superfamily member growth-differentiation factor-15 protects the heart from ischemia/reperfusion injury. Circ Res. 2006;98(3):351–60.

56. Xu J, Kimball TR, Lorenz JN, et al. GDF15/MIC-1 functions as a protective and antihypertrophic factor released from the myocardium in association with SMAD protein activation. Circ Res. 2006;98(3):342–50.

57. Tunariu N, Gibbs SJ, Win Z, et al. Ventilation-perfusion scintigraphy is more sensitive than multidetector CTPA in detecting chronic thromboembolic pulmonary disease as a treatable cause of pulmonary hypertension. J Nucl Med. 2007;48(5):680–4.

58. Nagendran J, Michelakis E. MRI: one-stop shop for the comprehensive assessment of pulmonary arterial hypertension? Chest. 2007;132(1):2–5.

59. Vieillard-Baron A, Prin S, Chergui K, Dubourg O, Jardin F. Echo-Doppler demonstration of acute cor pulmonale at the bedside in the medical intensive care unit. Am J Respir Crit Care Med. 2002;166(10):1310–9.

60. Jardin F, Vieillard-Baron A. Monitoring of right-sided heart function. Curr Opin Crit Care. 2005;11(3):271–9.

61. Fisher MR, Forfia PR, Chamera E, et al. Accuracy of Doppler echocardiography in the hemodynamic assessment of pulmonary hypertension. Am J Respir Crit Care Med. 2009;179(7):615–21.

62. McConnell MV, Solomon SD, Rayan ME, Come PC, Goldhaber SZ, Lee RT. Regional right ventricular dysfunction detected by echocardiography in acute pulmonary embolism. Am J Cardiol. 1996;78(4):469–73.

63. Casazza F, Bongarzoni A, Capozi A, Agostoni O. Regional right ventricular dysfunction in acute pulmonary embolism and right ventricular infarction. Eur J Echocardiogr. 2005;6(1):11–4.

64. Platz E, Hassanein AH, Shah A, Goldhaber SZ, Solomon SD. Regional right ventricular strain pattern in patients with acute pulmonary embolism. Echocardiography. 2012;29(4):464–70.

65. Kaul S, Tei C, Hopkins JM, Shah PM. Assessment of right ventricular function using two-dimensional echocardiography. Am Heart J. 1984;107(3):526–31.

66. Rydman R, Soderberg M, Larsen F, Caidahl K, Alam M. Echocardiographic evaluation of right ventricular function in patients with acute pulmonary embolism: a study using tricuspid annular motion. Echocardiography. 2010;27(3):286–93.

67. Badano LP, Ginghina C, Easaw J, et al. Right ventricle in pulmonary arterial hypertension: haemodynamics, structural changes, imaging, and proposal of a study protocol aimed to assess remodelling and treatment effects. Eur J Echocardiogr. 2010;11(1):27–37.

68. Park JH, Park YS, Park SJ, et al. Midventricular peak systolic strain and Tei index of the right ventricle correlated with decreased right ventricular systolic function in patients with acute pulmonary thromboembolism. Int J Cardiol. 2008;125(3):319–24.

69. Dentali F, Bertolini A, Nicolini E, et al. Evaluation of right ventricular function in patients with a previous episode of pulmonary embolism using tissue Doppler imaging. Intern Emerg Med. 2011.

70. Hoeper MM, Barbera JA, Channick RN, et al. Diagnosis, assessment, and treatment of non-pulmonary arterial hypertension pulmonary hypertension. J Am Coll Cardiol. 2009;54(1 Suppl): S85–96.

71. Steele PM, Fuster V, Cohen M, Ritter DG, McGoon DC. Isolated atrial septal defect with pulmonary vascular obstructive disease – long-term follow-up and prediction of outcome after surgical correction. Circulation. 1987;76(5):1037–42.

72. La Vecchia L, Varotto L, Zanolla L, Spadaro GL, Fontanelli A. Right ventricular function predicts transplant-free survival in idiopathic dilated cardiomyopathy. J Cardiovasc Med (Hagerstown). 2006;7(9):706–10.

73. Badesch DB, Champion HC, Sanchez MA, et al. Diagnosis and assessment of pulmonary arterial hypertension. J Am Coll Cardiol. 2009;54(1 Suppl):S55–66.

74. Barst RJ, Gibbs JS, Ghofrani HA, et al. Updated evidence-based treatment algorithm in pulmonary arterial hypertension. J Am Coll Cardiol. 2009;54(1 Suppl):S78–84.

75. Halpern SD, Taichman DB. Misclassification of pulmonary hypertension due to reliance on pulmonary capillary wedge pressure rather than left ventricular end-diastolic pressure. Chest. 2009;136(1):37–43.

76. Tedford RJ, Hassoun PM, Mathai SC, et al. Pulmonary capillary wedge pressure augments right ventricular pulsatile loading. Circulation. 2012;125(2):289–97.

77. Champion HC, Michelakis ED, Hassoun PM. Comprehensive invasive and noninvasive approach to the right ventricle-pulmonary circulation unit: state of the art and clinical and research implications. Circulation. 2009;120(11):992–1007.

78. Marik PE, Cavallazzi R, Vasu T, Hirani A. Dynamic changes in arterial waveform derived variables and fluid responsiveness in mechanically ventilated patients: a systematic review of the literature. Crit Care Med. 2009;37(9):2642–7.

79. Lewis GD, Shah R, Shahzad K, et al. Sildenafil improves exercise capacity and quality of life in patients with systolic heart failure and secondary pulmonary hypertension. Circulation. 2007;116(14): 1555–62.

80. Ghio S, Gavazzi A, Campana C, et al. Independent and additive prognostic value of right ventricular systolic function and pulmonary artery pressure in patients with chronic heart failure. J Am Coll Cardiol. 2001;37(1):183–8.

81. Costard-Jackle A, Fowler MB. Influence of preoperative pulmonary artery pressure on mortality after heart transplantation: testing of potential reversibility of pulmonary hypertension with nitroprusside is useful in defining a high risk group. J Am Coll Cardiol. 1992;19(1):48–54.

82. Butler J, Chomsky DB, Wilson JR. Pulmonary hypertension and exercise intolerance in patients with heart failure. J Am Coll Cardiol. 1999;34(6):1802–6.

83. Mereles D, Ehlken N, Kreuscher S, et al. Exercise and respiratory training improve exercise capacity and quality of life in patients with severe chronic pulmonary hypertension. Circulation. 2006; 114(14):1482–9.

84. McLaughlin VV, Rich S. Pulmonary hypertension. Curr Probl Cardiol. 2004;29(10):575–634.

85. McLaughlin VV, Archer SL, Badesch DB, et al. ACCF/AHA 2009 expert consensus document on pulmonary hypertension: a report of the American College of Cardiology Foundation Task Force on Expert Consensus Documents and the American Heart Association: developed in collaboration with the American College of Chest Physicians, American Thoracic Society, Inc., and the Pulmonary Hypertension Association. Circulation. 2009;119(16):2250–94.

86. Handoko ML, de Man FS, Happe CM, et al. Opposite effects of training in rats with stable and progressive pulmonary hypertension. Circulation. 2009;120(1):42–9.

87. Badesch DB, Abman SH, Simonneau G, Rubin LJ, McLaughlin VV. Medical therapy for pulmonary arterial hypertension: updated ACCP evidence-based clinical practice guidelines. Chest. 2007;131(6):1917–28.

88. Bogaard HJ, Natarajan R, Mizuno S, et al. Adrenergic receptor blockade reverses right heart remodeling and dysfunction in pulmonary hypertensive rats. Am J Respir Crit Care Med. 2010; 182(5):652–60.

89. Reiter MJ, Reiffel JA. Importance of beta blockade in the therapy of serious ventricular arrhythmias. Am J Cardiol. 1998;82(4A):9I–19.

90. Packer M, Coats AJ, Fowler MB, et al. Effect of carvedilol on survival in severe chronic heart failure. N Engl J Med. 2001; 344(22):1651–8.

91. Drummond GA, Squire IB. The cardiac insufficiency bisoprolol study II. Lancet. 1999;353(9161):1361.

92. Hjalmarson A, Goldstein S, Fagerberg B, et al. Effects of controlled-release metoprolol on total mortality, hospitalizations, and well-being in patients with heart failure: the Metoprolol CR/XL Randomized Intervention Trial in congestive heart failure (MERIT-HF). MERIT-HF Study Group. JAMA. 2000;283(10): 1295–302.

93. Provencher S, Herve P, Jais X, et al. Deleterious effects of beta-blockers on exercise capacity and hemodynamics in patients with portopulmonary hypertension. Gastroenterology. 2006;130(1): 120–6.

94. Quaife RA, Christian PE, Gilbert EM, Datz FL, Volkman K, Bristow MR. Effects of carvedilol on right ventricular function in chronic heart failure. Am J Cardiol. 1998;81(2):247–50.

95. Massie B, Kramer BL, Topic N, Henderson SG. Hemodynamic and radionuclide effects of acute captopril therapy for heart failure: changes in left and right ventricular volumes and function at rest and during exercise. Circulation. 1982;65(7):1374–81.

96. Cargill RI, Lipworth BJ. Lisinopril attenuates acute hypoxic pulmonary vasoconstriction in humans. Chest. 1996;109(2):424–9.

97. Rich S, Seidlitz M, Dodin E, et al. The short-term effects of digoxin in patients with right ventricular dysfunction from pulmonary hypertension. Chest. 1998;114(3):787–92.

98. Zamanian RT, Haddad F, Doyle RL, Weinacker AB. Management strategies for patients with pulmonary hypertension in the intensive care unit. Crit Care Med. 2007;35(9):2037–50.

99. Barst RJ, Rubin LJ, Long WA, et al. A comparison of continuous intravenous epoprostenol (prostacyclin) with conventional therapy for primary pulmonary hypertension. The Primary Pulmonary Hypertension Study Group. N Engl J Med. 1996;334(5):296–302.

100. Badesch DB, Tapson VF, McGoon MD, et al. Continuous intravenous epoprostenol for pulmonary hypertension due to the scleroderma spectrum of disease. A randomized, controlled trial. Ann Intern Med. 2000;132(6):425–34.

101. Sitbon O, Humbert M, Nunes H, et al. Long-term intravenous epoprostenol infusion in primary pulmonary hypertension: prognostic factors and survival. J Am Coll Cardiol. 2002;40(4):780–8.

102. McLaughlin VV, Gaine SP, Barst RJ, et al. Efficacy and safety of treprostinil: an epoprostenol analog for primary pulmonary hypertension. J Cardiovasc Pharmacol. 2003;41(2):293–9.

103. Rubin LJ, Badesch DB, Barst RJ, et al. Bosentan therapy for pulmonary arterial hypertension. N Engl J Med. 2002;346(12):896–903.

104. Galie N, Badesch D, Oudiz R, et al. Ambrisentan therapy for pulmonary arterial hypertension. J Am Coll Cardiol. 2005;46(3):529–35.

105. Galie N, Ghofrani HA, Torbicki A, et al. Sildenafil citrate therapy for pulmonary arterial hypertension. N Engl J Med. 2005;353(20): 2148–57.

106. Galie N, Brundage BH, Ghofrani HA, et al. Tadalafil therapy for pulmonary arterial hypertension. Circulation. 2009;119(22): 2894–903.

107. Califf RM, Adams KF, McKenna WJ, et al. A randomized controlled trial of epoprostenol therapy for severe congestive heart failure: the Flolan International Randomized Survival Trial (FIRST). Am Heart J. 1997;134(1):44–54.

108. Teerlink JR. Reversal of left ventricular remodeling: role of the endothelin pathway. J Card Fail. 2002;8(6 Suppl):S494–9.

109. Nagendran J, Archer SL, Soliman D, et al. Phosphodiesterase type 5 is highly expressed in the hypertrophied human right ventricle, and acute inhibition of phosphodiesterase type 5 improves contractility. Circulation. 2007;116(3):238–48.

110. Yin J, Kukucka M, Hoffmann J, et al. Sildenafil preserves lung endothelial function and prevents pulmonary vascular remodeling in a rat model of diastolic heart failure. Circ Heart Fail. 2011;4(2):198–206.

111. Michelakis E, Tymchak W, Lien D, Webster L, Hashimoto K, Archer S. Oral sildenafil is an effective and specific pulmonary vasodilator in patients with pulmonary arterial hypertension: comparison with inhaled nitric oxide. Circulation. 2002;105(20):2398–403.

112. Guazzi M, Vicenzi M, Arena R, Guazzi MD. PDE5 inhibition with sildenafil improves left ventricular diastolic function, cardiac geometry, and clinical status in patients with stable systolic heart failure: results of a 1-year, prospective, randomized, placebo-controlled study. Circ Heart Fail. 2011;4(1):8–17.

113. Blum A. Treating heart failure with sildenafil. Congest Heart Fail. 2009;15(4):181–5.

114. Ghofrani HA, Wiedemann R, Rose F, et al. Sildenafil for treatment of lung fibrosis and pulmonary hypertension: a randomised controlled trial. Lancet. 2002;360(9337):895–900.

115. Zisman DA, Schwarz M, Anstrom KJ, Collard HR, Flaherty KR, Hunninghake GW. A controlled trial of sildenafil in advanced idiopathic pulmonary fibrosis. N Engl J Med. 2010;363(7):620–8.

116. Collard HR, Anstrom KJ, Schwarz MI, Zisman DA. Sildenafil improves walk distance in idiopathic pulmonary fibrosis. Chest. 2007;131(3):897–9.

117. Han MK, Bach D, Hagan P, Yow E, Flaherty K, Toews G, Anstrom K, Martinez F. Sildenafil preserves exercise capacity in patients with idiopathic pulmonary fibrosis and right-sided ventricular dysfunction. CHEST. 2013;143(6):1699–1708.

118. Blanco I, Gimeno E, Munoz PA, et al. Hemodynamic and gas exchange effects of sildenafil in patients with chronic obstructive pulmonary disease and pulmonary hypertension. Am J Respir Crit Care Med. 2010;181(3):270–8.

119. Barbera JA, Roger N, Roca J, Rovira I, Higenbottam TW, Rodriguez-Roisin R. Worsening of pulmonary gas exchange with nitric oxide inhalation in chronic obstructive pulmonary disease. Lancet. 1996;347(8999):436–40.

120. Zielinski J, Tobiasz M, Hawrylkiewicz I, Sliwinski P, Palasiewicz G. Effects of long-term oxygen therapy on pulmonary hemodynamics in COPD patients: a 6-year prospective study. Chest. 1998;113(1):65–70.

121. Stolz D, Rasch H, Linka A, et al. A randomised, controlled trial of bosentan in severe COPD. Eur Respir J. 2008;32(3):619–28.

122. Rothman A, Sklansky MS, Lucas VW, et al. Atrial septostomy as a bridge to lung transplantation in patients with severe pulmonary hypertension. Am J Cardiol. 1999;84(6):682–6.

123. Reichenberger F, Pepke-Zaba J, McNeil K, Parameshwar J, Shapiro LM. Atrial septostomy in the treatment of severe pulmonary arterial hypertension. Thorax. 2003;58(9):797–800.

124. Sandoval J, Gaspar J, Pulido T, et al. Graded balloon dilation atrial septostomy in severe primary pulmonary hypertension. A therapeutic alternative for patients nonresponsive to vasodilator treatment. J Am Coll Cardiol. 1998;32(2):297–304.

125. Olsson JK, Zamanian RT, Feinstein JA, Doyle RL. Surgical and interventional therapies for pulmonary arterial hypertension. Semin Respir Crit Care Med. 2005;26(4):417–28.

126. Hoetzenecker K, Ankersmit HJ, Bonderman D, et al. Atrial septal defect repair after a 10-month treatment with bosentan in a patient with severe pulmonary arterial hypertension: a case report. J Thorac Cardiovasc Surg. 2009;137(3):760–1.

127. Jamieson SW, Kapelanski DP, Sakakibara N, et al. Pulmonary endarterectomy: experience and lessons learned in 1,500 cases. Ann Thorac Surg. 2003;76(5):1457–62; discussion 1462–54.

128. Kurzyna M, Dabrowski M, Bielecki D, et al. Atrial septostomy in treatment of end-stage right heart failure in patients with pulmonary hypertension. Chest. 2007;131(4):977–83.

129. Mendeloff EN, Meyers BF, Sundt TM, et al. Lung transplantation for pulmonary vascular disease. Ann Thorac Surg. 2002;73(1): 209–17; discussion 217–9.

130. Gillebert TC, Sys SU, Brutsaert DL. Influence of loading patterns on peak length-tension relation and on relaxation in cardiac muscle. J Am Coll Cardiol. 1989;13(2):483–90.

131. Handoko ML, Lamberts RR, Redout EM, et al. Right ventricular pacing improves right heart function in experimental pulmonary arterial hypertension: a study in the isolated heart. Am J Physiol Heart Circ Physiol. 2009;297(5):H1752–9.

132. Kalogeropoulos AP, Georgiopoulou VV, Howell S, et al. Evaluation of right intraventricular dyssynchrony by two-dimensional strain echocardiography in patients with pulmonary arterial hypertension. J Am Soc Echocardiogr. 2008;21(9):1028–34.

133. Lopez-Candales A, Dohi K, Rajagopalan N, et al. Right ventricular dyssynchrony in patients with pulmonary hypertension is associated with disease severity and functional class. Cardiovasc Ultrasound. 2005;3:23.

134. Stojnic BB, Brecker SJ, Xiao HB, Helmy SM, Mbaissouroum M, Gibson DG. Left ventricular filling characteristics in pulmonary hypertension: a new mode of ventricular interaction. Br Heart J. 1992;68(1):16–20.

135. McAlister FA, Ezekowitz J, Hooton N, et al. Cardiac resynchronization therapy for patients with left ventricular systolic dysfunction: a systematic review. JAMA. 2007;297(22):2502–14.

136. Hardziyenka M, Surie S, de Groot JR, et al. Right ventricular pacing improves haemodynamics in right ventricular failure from pressure overload: an open observational proof-of-principle study in patients with chronic thromboembolic pulmonary hypertension. Europace. 2011;13(12):1753–9.

137. Hoeper MM, Granton J. Intensive care unit management of patients with severe pulmonary hypertension and right heart failure. Am J Respir Crit Care Med. 2011;184(10):1114–24.

138. Hebert PC, Wells G, Blajchman MA, et al. A multicenter, randomized, controlled clinical trial of transfusion requirements in critical care. Transfusion Requirements in Critical Care Investigators, Canadian Critical Care Trials Group. N Engl J Med. 1999;340(6): 409–17.

139. Rivers E, Nguyen B, Havstad S, et al. Early goal-directed therapy in the treatment of severe sepsis and septic shock. N Engl J Med. 2001;345(19):1368–77.

140. Groenveld HF, Januzzi JL, Damman K, et al. Anemia and mortality in heart failure patients a systematic review and meta-analysis. J Am Coll Cardiol. 2008;52(10):818–27.

141. Ventilation with lower tidal volumes as compared with traditional tidal volumes for acute lung injury and the acute respiratory distress syndrome. The Acute Respiratory Distress Syndrome Network. New Engl J Med. 2000;342(18):1301–8.

142. Vieillard-Baron A, Jardin F. Why protect the right ventricle in patients with acute respiratory distress syndrome? Curr Opin Crit Care. 2003;9(1):15–21.

143. Zamanian RT, Haddad F, Doyle RL, Weinacker AB. Management strategies for patients with pulmonary hypertension in the intensive care unit. Crit Care Med. 2007;35:2037–50.

144. Balanos GM, Talbot NP, Dorrington KL, Robbins PA. Human pulmonary vascular response to 4 h of hypercapnia and hypocapnia measured using Doppler echocardiography. J Appl Physiol. 2003; 94(4):1543–51.

145. Bindslev L, Jolin-Carlsson A, Santesson J, Gottlieb I. Hypoxic pulmonary vasoconstriction in man: effects of hyperventilation. Acta Anaesthesiol Scand. 1985;29(5):547–51.

146. Kerbaul F, Rondelet B, Motte S, et al. Effects of norepinephrine and dobutamine on pressure load-induced right ventricular failure. Crit Care Med. 2004;32(4):1035–40.

147. Vizza CD, Rocca GD, Roma AD, et al. Acute hemodynamic effects of inhaled nitric oxide, dobutamine and a combination of the two in patients with mild to moderate secondary pulmonary hypertension. Crit Care. 2001;5(6):355–61.

148. Chen EP, Bittner HB, Davis Jr RD, Van Trigt 3rd P. Milrinone improves pulmonary hemodynamics and right ventricular function in chronic pulmonary hypertension. Ann Thorac Surg. 1997;63(3):814–21.

149. Hentschel T, Yin N, Riad A, et al. Inhalation of the phosphodiesterase-3 inhibitor milrinone attenuates pulmonary hypertension in a rat model of congestive heart failure. Anesthesiology. 2007;106(1):124–31.

150. Solina A, Papp D, Ginsberg S, et al. A comparison of inhaled nitric oxide and milrinone for the treatment of pulmonary hypertension in adult cardiac surgery patients. J Cardiothorac Vasc Anesth. 2000;14(1):12–7.

151. Khazin V, Kaufman Y, Zabeeda D, et al. Milrinone and nitric oxide: combined effect on pulmonary artery pressures after cardiopulmonary bypass in children. J Cardiothorac Vasc Anesth. 2004;18(2):156–9.

152. De Backer D, Biston P, Devriendt J, et al. Comparison of dopamine and norepinephrine in the treatment of shock. N Engl J Med. 2010;362(9):779–89.

153. Kerbaul F, Rondelet B, Demester JP, et al. Effects of levosimendan versus dobutamine on pressure load-induced right ventricular failure. Crit Care Med. 2006;34(11):2814–9.

154. Missant C, Rex S, Segers P, Wouters PF. Levosimendan improves right ventriculovascular coupling in a porcine model of right ventricular dysfunction. Crit Care Med. 2007;35(3):707–15.

155. Angle MR, Molloy DW, Penner B, Jones D, Prewitt RM. The cardiopulmonary and renal hemodynamic effects of norepinephrine in canine pulmonary embolism. Chest. 1989;95(6):1333–7.

156. Rossaint R, Gerlach H, Schmidt-Ruhnke H, et al. Efficacy of inhaled nitric oxide in patients with severe ARDS. Chest. 1995;107(4):1107–15.

157. Kaisers U, Busch T, Deja M, Donaubauer B, Falke KJ. Selective pulmonary vasodilation in acute respiratory distress syndrome. Crit Care Med. 2003;31(4 Suppl):S337–42.

158. Meldrum DR, Shames BD, Meng X, et al. Nitric oxide downregulates lung macrophage inflammatory cytokine production. Ann Thorac Surg. 1998;66(2):313–7.

159. Bhorade S, Christenson J, O'Connor M, Lavoie A, Pohlman A, Hall JB. Response to inhaled nitric oxide in patients with acute right heart syndrome. Am J Respir Crit Care Med. 1999;159(2):571–9.

160. George I, Xydas S, Topkara VK, et al. Clinical indication for use and outcomes after inhaled nitric oxide therapy. Ann Thorac Surg. 2006;82(6):2161–9.

161. Ardehali A, Hughes K, Sadeghi A, et al. Inhaled nitric oxide for pulmonary hypertension after heart transplantation. Transplantation. 2001;72(4):638–41.

162. Fattouch K, Sbraga F, Bianco G, et al. Inhaled prostacyclin, nitric oxide, and nitroprusside in pulmonary hypertension after mitral valve replacement. J Card Surg. 2005;20(2):171–6.

163. Christenson J, Lavoie A, O'Connor M, Bhorade S, Pohlman A, Hall JB. The incidence and pathogenesis of cardiopulmonary deterioration after abrupt withdrawal of inhaled nitric oxide. Am J Respir Crit Care Med. 2000;161(5):1443–9.

164. Badesch DB, Abman SH, Ahearn GS, et al. Medical therapy for pulmonary arterial hypertension: ACCP evidence-based clinical practice guidelines. Chest. 2004;126(1 Suppl):35S–62.

165. Gomberg-Maitland M, Olschewski H. Prostacyclin therapies for the treatment of pulmonary arterial hypertension. Eur Respir J. 2008;31(4):891–901.

166. Khan TA, Schnickel G, Ross D, et al. A prospective, randomized, crossover pilot study of inhaled nitric oxide versus inhaled prostacyclin in heart transplant and lung transplant recipients. J Thorac Cardiovasc Surg. 2009;138(6):1417–24.

167. Rex S, Schaelte G, Metzelder S, et al. Inhaled iloprost to control pulmonary artery hypertension in patients undergoing mitral valve surgery: a prospective, randomized-controlled trial. Acta Anaesthesiol Scand. 2008;52(1):65–72.

168. De Wet CJ, Affleck DG, Jacobsohn E, et al. Inhaled prostacyclin is safe, effective, and affordable in patients with pulmonary hypertension, right heart dysfunction, and refractory hypoxemia after cardiothoracic surgery. J Thorac Cardiovasc Surg. 2004;127(4):1058–67.

169. Theodoraki K, Rellia P, Thanopoulos A, et al. Inhaled iloprost controls pulmonary hypertension after cardiopulmonary bypass. Can J Anaesth. 2002;49(9):963–7.

170. Winterhalter M, Simon A, Fischer S, et al. Comparison of inhaled iloprost and nitric oxide in patients with pulmonary hypertension during weaning from cardiopulmonary bypass in cardiac surgery: a prospective randomized trial. J Cardiothorac Vasc Anesth. 2008;22(3):406–13.

171. Voswinckel R, Reichenberger F, Enke B, et al. Acute effects of the combination of sildenafil and inhaled treprostinil on haemodynamics and gas exchange in pulmonary hypertension. Pulm Pharmacol Ther. 2008;21(5):824–32.

172. Trachte AL, Lobato EB, Urdaneta F, et al. Oral sildenafil reduces pulmonary hypertension after cardiac surgery. Ann Thorac Surg. 2005;79(1):194–7; discussion 194–7.

173. Lepore JJ, Maroo A, Pereira NL, et al. Effect of sildenafil on the acute pulmonary vasodilator response to inhaled nitric oxide in adults with primary pulmonary hypertension. Am J Cardiol. 2002;90(6):677–80.

174. Lepore JJ, Maroo A, Bigatello LM, et al. Hemodynamic effects of sildenafil in patients with congestive heart failure and pulmonary hypertension: combined administration with inhaled nitric oxide. Chest. 2005;127(5):1647–53.

175. Nagamine J, Hill LL, Pearl RG. Combined therapy with zaprinast and inhaled nitric oxide abolishes hypoxic pulmonary hypertension. Crit Care Med. 2000;28(7):2420–4.

176. Ghofrani HA, Wiedemann R, Rose F, et al. Combination therapy with oral sildenafil and inhaled iloprost for severe pulmonary hypertension. Ann Intern Med. 2002;136(7):515–22.

177. Atz AM, Wessel DL. Sildenafil ameliorates effects of inhaled nitric oxide withdrawal. Anesthesiology. 1999;91(1):307–10.

178. Klodell Jr CT, Morey TE, Lobato EB, et al. Effect of sildenafil on pulmonary artery pressure, systemic pressure, and nitric oxide utilization in patients with left ventricular assist devices. Ann Thorac Surg. 2007;83(1):68–71; discussion 71.

179. Fung E, Fiscus RR, Yim AP, Angelini GD, Arifi AA. The potential use of type-5 phosphodiesterase inhibitors in coronary artery bypass graft surgery. Chest. 2005;128(4):3065–73.

180. Urdaneta F, Lobato EB, Beaver T, et al. Treating pulmonary hypertension post cardiopulmonary bypass in pigs: milrinone vs. sildenafil analog. Perfusion. 2008;23(2):117–25.

181. Philip A, Ramchandani S, Dorrance K, Dorrance C. Sildenafil-induced thrombocytopenia. Ann Intern Med. 2008;149(6):437–9.

182. Liden H, Haraldsson A, Ricksten SE, Kjellman U, Wiklund L. Does pretransplant left ventricular assist device therapy improve results after heart transplantation in patients with elevated pulmonary vascular resistance? Eur J Cardiothorac Surg. 2009;35(6):1029–34; discussion 1034–5.

183. Zimpfer D, Zrunek P, Sandner S, et al. Post-transplant survival after lowering fixed pulmonary hypertension using left ventricular assist devices. Eur J Cardiothorac Surg. 2007;31(4):698–702.

184. Berman M, Tsui S, Vuylsteke A, Klein A, Jenkins DP. Life-threatening right ventricular failure in pulmonary hypertension: RVAD or ECMO? J Heart Lung Transplant. 2008;27(10):1188–9.

185. Fuehner T, Kuehn C, Hadem J, et al. Extracorporeal membrane oxygenation in awake patients as bridge to lung transplantation. Am J Respir Crit Care Med. 2012;185(7):763–8.

Thoracic Aortic Disease

23

Bulat A. Ziganshin and John A. Elefteriades

23

Abstract

The incidence of aortic pathology is increasing at an alarming rate, with no identified reasons for this trend. According to the Center for Disease Control and Prevention, aortic aneurysms are the 15th most common cause of death in individuals older than age 65 years. The majority of aortic diseases are silent and lack clear pathognomonic symptoms that would make their timely detection easier for the physician. Because of the silent nature of thoracic aortic aneurysm, devastating complications such as aortic dissection and rupture often prove a lethal first manifestation. Thoracic aortic aneurysm is largely a genetic disease with strong familial inheritance. Although a virulent disease, thoracic aortic aneurysm is an indolent process with the aortic growth rate of approximately 0.1 cm/year. This chapter discusses the current understanding of the pathophysiology of thoracic aortic diseases, the current diagnostic approaches, and up-to-date management strategies based on recent guidelines and published literature.

Keywords

Thoracic aortic aneurysm • Aortic dissection • Surgical treatment of thoracic aneurysm

"There is no disease more conducive to clinical humility than aneurysm of the aorta."
"The tragedies of life are largely arterial."

– Sir William Osler (1849–1919) [1]

B.A. Ziganshin, MD (✉)
Section of Cardiac Surgery, Department of Surgery,
Aortic Institute of Yale-New Haven Hospital,
Yale University School of Medicine, 333 Cedar Street,
New Haven, CT 06510, USA

Department of Surgical Diseases # 2,
Kazan State Medical University,
Butlerov Street, 49, Kazan 420012, Russia
e-mail: bulat.ziganshin@yale.edu

J.A. Elefteriades, MD
Section of Cardiac Surgery, Department of Surgery,
Aortic Institute of Yale-New Haven Hospital,
Yale University School of Medicine,
333 Cedar Street, New Haven,
CT 06510, USA
e-mail: john.elefteriades@yale.edu

Introduction

Diseases of the thoracic aorta are among the most challenging human illnesses that a physician can encounter. We call thoracic aortic disease "the Silent Killer" [2] because, in the absolute majority of the patients, thoracic aortic aneurysm does not cause symptoms; often, the first symptom is either death or a major complication that threatens to produce death, such as aortic rupture or dissection. Despite the insidious and virulent nature of thoracic aortic aneurysm, considerable progress has been made over the past two decades in understanding the natural history and behavior of thoracic aortic disease—thus reading "the enemy's playbook" [3].

The aorta itself is much more than just a passive vessel that carries blood. Significant evidence has been accumulated to prove that an aorta is rather an active organ with complex intrinsic biology and sophisticated mechanical properties. Pathophysiological mechanisms that compromise the function of this vitally important organ lead to aortic aneurysm formation, dissection, and rupture.

K. Stergiopoulos, D.L. Brown (eds.), *Evidence-Based Cardiology Consult*,
DOI 10.1007/978-1-4471-4441-0_23, © Springer-Verlag London 2014

According to the latest data from the Center for Disease Control and Prevention, approximately 13,000 people die annually in the United States of aortic aneurysms in various anatomic localizations, with almost 80 % of these deaths among people 65 years and older. This makes aortic aneurysms the 19th leading cause of death in all individuals and the 15th most common in individuals older than age 65 years [4]. It is noteworthy that aortic aneurysms cause more deaths than the human immunodeficiency virus. Even though these figures are impressive, they almost certainly represent underestimates of the true prevalence of aortic disease in the population because many aneurysm-related deaths (especially for the ascending aorta) are likely classified as "cardiac" and not tabulated in the aneurysm figures.

The estimated incidence of thoracic aortic aneurysm is approximately 10 per 100,000 patient-years. Women and men have a similar incidence, but the age at diagnosis is a decade later in women (1970s) than in men (1960s) [5]. It is worrisome that population-based studies have shown that the incidence of aortic disease is increasing rather dramatically. This has been demonstrated in geographic regions with stable self-contained populations with little out- or in-migration, like Olmsted County (Minnesota, USA) and Malmö (Sweden) [6, 7]. The reasons for such an increase in aortic disease incidence are yet to be understood.

Although cardiac surgeons manage advanced thoracic aortic disease, the diagnosis and medical care of patients with aortic pathology remains largely in the province of cardiologists (especially with regard to the ascending aorta). Therefore, it is crucial for cardiologists to be experienced in detecting and managing patients with thoracic aortic disease. This chapter will discuss the current understanding of the pathophysiology of thoracic aortic aneurysm and move on to diagnostic approaches and management strategies based on the most recent guidelines and published literature.

Pathophysiology

Anatomy of the Thoracic Aorta

In order to understand the mechanisms of thoracic aortic disease, it is essential to understand the normal anatomy of the aorta. Anatomically the thoracic aorta is divided into four parts:

- *Aortic root* – starts at the aortic valve annulus, includes the aortic valve cusps and the sinuses of Valsalva, which give rise to two coronary arteries, and ends at the sinotubular junction. Normally the aortic root is slightly wider in diameter than the ascending aorta.
- *Ascending aorta* – includes the tubular portion of the aorta, which extends upwards from the aortic root (the sinotubular junction) to the level of the origin of the

brachiocephalic trunk. No arteries branch from this part of the aorta.
- *Aortic arch* – the transverse aorta, which connects the ascending aorta to the descending aorta. It starts just above the ascending aorta and includes the origin of all head and neck vessels—the brachiocephalic trunk, the left carotid artery, and the left subclavian artery. The aortic arch extends to the isthmus between the origin of the left subclavian artery and the ligamentum arteriosum.
- *Descending aorta* – the longest part of the thoracic aorta, which extends from the level where the aortic arch ends to the level of the diaphragm. The descending aorta gives rise to numerous intercostal arteries and also provides branches that supply the spinal cord.

Just like any other large blood vessel in the human body, the aortic wall is composed of three main layers: *tunica intima*, *tunica media*, and the *tunica adventitia*. The aortic tunica media is largely composed of lamellae of elastic fibers and is interposed with collagen and a small number of smooth muscle cells. The media is the thickest layer of the aorta; the distensible elastic fibers serve to absorb the force of the pulse pressure. The adventitia is the thin outer layer, composed of indistensible collagen fibers which provide tensile strength to prevent deformation or rupture. Despite being so thin, the adventitia is highly respected by surgeons, who feel it is the "strength layer" of the aorta and is essential for secure suturing of aortic tissues. Lastly, the intima has no significant differences from other human blood vessels and is composed of a single layer of endothelial cells that are seated on the internal elastic lamina. As is well known, the endothelium has remarkably complex biological functions.

For clinical purposes, we commonly measure the aorta based on the anatomy discussed above (Fig. 23.1).

Types of Aortic Pathology

Four main types of aortic pathology have been identified that account for most thoracic aortic disease:

1. *Aortic aneurysm* is defined as an enlargement of the aorta greater than 1½ times its normal size [8]. Aneurysmal dilatation of the thoracic aorta may occur through a variety of mechanisms and will be discussed further in this chapter.
2. *Rupture of aortic aneurysm* is a self-explanatory term, which refers to an acute condition that should not, however, be confused with rupture of an acute aortic dissection or an acute aortic transection.
3. *Acute aortic dissection* refers to a very specific process of separation of layers of the aorta from each other with blood under pressure entering between the layers and propagating the separation to various extents. It is very

Fig. 23.1 Anatomic sites for measuring the size of the aorta

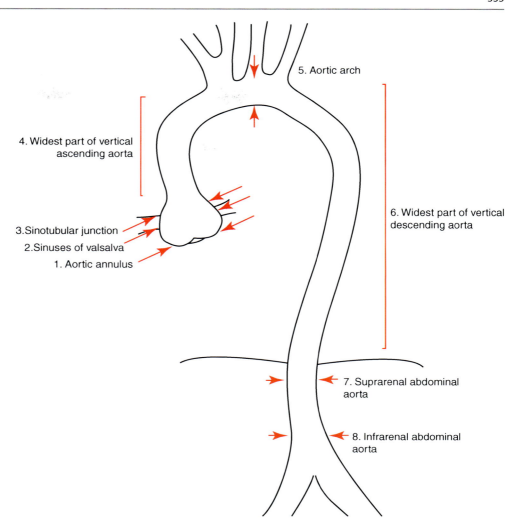

5. Aortic arch

4. Widest part of vertical ascending aorta

6. Widest part of vertical descending aorta

3. Sinotubular junction

2. Sinuses of valsalva

1. Aortic annulus

7. Suprarenal abdominal aorta

8. Infrarenal abdominal aorta

important to note here that in order for a dissection to occur, the aortic wall must nearly always be affected by structural disease of the media (Fig. 23.2).

4. *Acute aortic transection* is a traumatic phenomenon, with disruption of the wall of the aorta, without a propagating dissection. Contrary to aortic dissection, the aortic wall is intrinsically normal and resistant to the dissection process.

It is not uncommon for the three related but distinct entities—rupture of aortic aneurysm, aortic dissection, and acute aortic transection—to be confused in terminology. We have illustrated these different types of acute aortic pathology in Fig. 23.3.

Etiology and Pathogenesis of Thoracic Aortic Aneurysm Formation

Historically, the pathophysiology of aortic dilatation has been attributed to cystic medial degeneration of the aortic wall, which is characterized by disruption and loss of elastic fibers accompanied by increased deposition of proteoglycans. This is generally considered a noninflammatory mechanism of aneurysm formation; however recent studies (including one from our group) have challenged this concept by demonstrating the presence of inflammatory cell infiltration in aneurysmal aortic tissue [9, 10].

Current understanding of aortic wall function stresses the importance of maintaining a delicate homeostasis of vascular smooth muscle cells and extracellular matrix proteins in the medial layer of the aorta. This delicate balance preserves the mechanical and functional properties of the aorta and allows the aortic wall to sustain high pressures throughout life. However, when this balance is shifted toward excessive *degradation* of the extracellular matrix due to various molecular processes, which overrides its *synthesis*, the aortic wall becomes weaker and more vulnerable to mechanical stress, which leads to progressive aortic expansion and, ultimately, rupture [11, 12].

The activity of matrix metalloproteinases (MMPs)—a specific subset of proteolytic enzymes that degrade medial

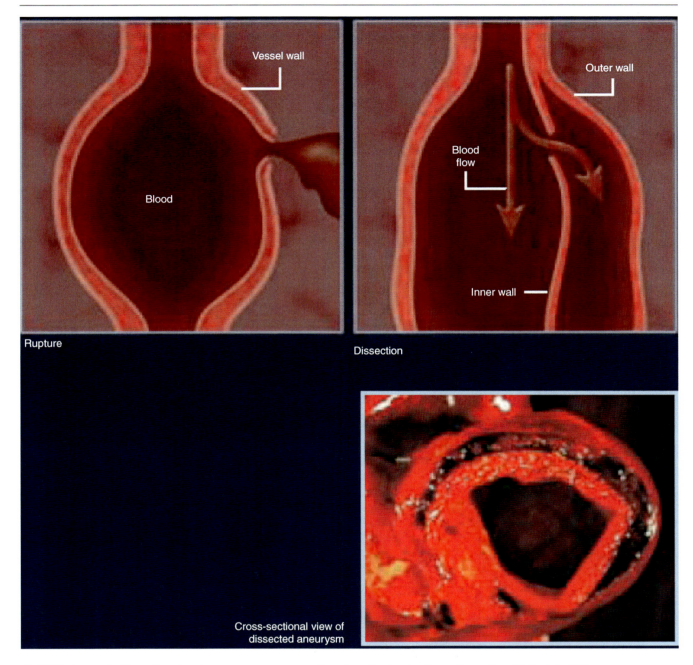

Fig. 23.2 Schematic illustration of aortic aneurysm rupture and dissection (Reprinted with permission from Elefteriades [2])

elastin, fibrillin, and collagen—has been established as a major pathophysiologic mechanism for aortic aneurysm formation. MMP involvement, particularly the MMP-2 and MMP-9 subtypes, has been demonstrated in patients with abdominal aortic aneurysm [13–16] and thoracic aortic aneurysm [11, 12, 17, 18].

Under normal conditions MMP tissue activity is regulated by the presence of tissue inhibitors of metalloproteinases (TIMPs). We have found a marked elevation of proteolytic enzymes (MMPs 1, 2, and 9) and a marked depression of the inhibitory enzymes (TIMPs) in ascending aortic aneurysms and dissections [11]. Thus, we concluded that in aneurysm patients, the balance between MMPs and TIMPs is shifted strongly toward increased proteolysis, which correlates with the observed degradation of the aortic wall. Our current belief is that aneurysm patients are genetically programmed to manifest excessive MMP activity, leading ultimately to degradation and thinning of the aortic wall [19]. This is shown in Fig. 23.4, in which the wall of a patient's aorta became so thin in a 6-cm aneurysm that a ruler placed behind can be seen

Fig. 23.3 Three commonly confused conditions: (**a**) acute aortic transection; (**b**) degenerative aneurysm of the descending aorta; (**c**) acute aortic dissection (Reproduced with permission from John A. Elefteriades, MD, the author)

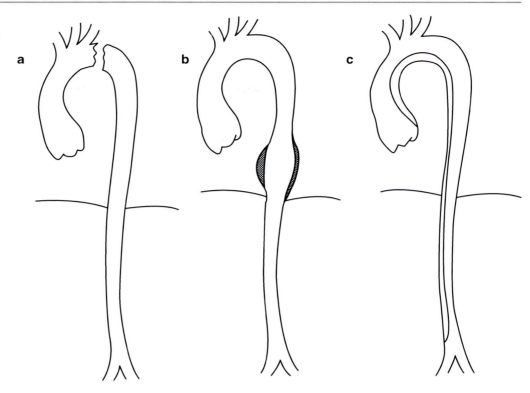

Fig. 23.4 Wall of the aorta became so thin in a 6-cm aneurysm that a ruler placed behind it can be seen through the tissue (Reprinted with permission from Elefteriades [19])

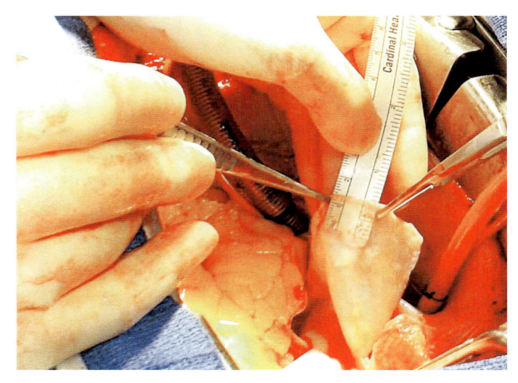

through the tissue. It is hard to imagine how such a thin structure was transmitting the cardiac output to all organs of the body without rupturing under arterial pressure. The recognition of this pathophysiologic mechanism of aneurysm development raises the potential for innovative drug therapy, such as matrix protease inhibitors, in order to produce a slowing or halting of the evolution of thoracic aneurysm disease.

The current confluence of inflammatory, proteolytic, and smooth muscle abnormalities in producing aortic aneurysms is schematized in Fig. 23.5.

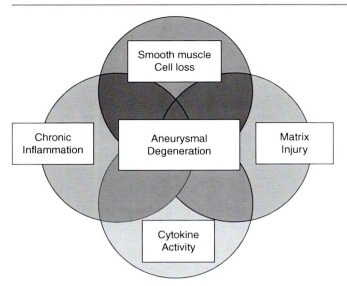

Fig. 23.5 Diagram illustrating multiple pathophysiological components that overlap and contribute to aortic aneurysm formation (Reprinted from Hackmann et al. [16])

Inflammation is now known to play an important role in aneurysm formation, and this is abundantly apparent in inflammatory conditions producing thoracic aortic aneurysm: giant cell arteritis, syphilitic aortitis, mycotic aneurysm (often caused by bacterial endocarditis), Takayasu's arteritis, rheumatoid arthritis, psoriatic arthritis, ankylosing spondylitis, reactive arthritis, Wegener's granulomatosis, and Reiter syndrome [20].

There has been a long-standing belief that aortic aneurysms may represent a late degenerative stage of atherosclerotic disease [21, 22], establishing atherosclerosis as one of the causative factors for aneurysm formation. This concept, however, has been heavily debated and seriously challenged in the literature over the years [23–25]. Although the role of atherosclerosis in aneurysm formation is still unclear [26], the current understanding is that atherosclerosis is seen significantly less frequently in the ascending aorta [25], as opposed to the descending aorta. When atherosclerosis is observed in the ascending aorta, it is usually superimposed on medial degenerative disease and hence not playing the role of a primary etiological factor [27]. At the same time atherosclerosis and risk factors such as hypertension, hypercholesterolemia, and smoking are known to play an important role in the development of descending thoracic and abdominal aneurysms (Fig. 23.6) [27].

Genetic Nature of Thoracic Aortic Aneurysm

The genetic nature of thoracic aortic aneurysms has been widely studied and currently accepted. The main genetic syndromes proven to be associated with development of thoracic aortic aneurysms and presentation with dissections

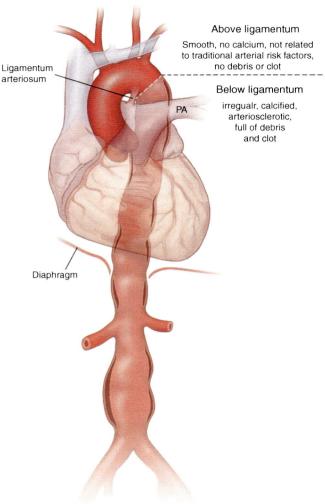

Fig. 23.6 Aortic aneurysm is really two diseases: ascending disease differs markedly from descending/abdominal disease. *PA* pulmonary artery (Reprinted with permission from Elefteriades and Farkas [28])

at smaller aortic diameters than usual include Marfan syndrome, Loeys-Dietz syndrome, Turner syndrome, and Ehlers-Danlos syndrome [20, 29] (Table 23.1).

Marfan syndrome is by far the most common genetic syndrome that causes aneurysms of the aortic root and cystic medial degeneration due to a mutation in the fibrillin-1 gene; however, Marfan accounts for only 5 % of thoracic aortic aneurysms and dissections [28] and is the "tip of the genetic iceberg." The other syndromes listed above are even less common. Currently there is growing evidence that a significant portion of the remaining 95 % of patients with thoracic aortic aneurysm also harbors genetic abnormalities responsible for aneurysm formation. We constructed approximately 500 family trees of patients with thoracic aortic aneurysm or dissection, which showed that 21 % of the probands have at least one family member with a known aneurysm somewhere in the arterial tree [30, 31]. The predominant

Table 23.1 Genetic syndromes associated with thoracic aortic aneurysm and dissection

Genetic syndrome	Common clinical features	Genetic defect	Diagnostic test	Comments of aortic disease
Marfan syndrome	Arachnodactyly, dolichostenomelia, kyphoscoliosis, dolichocephaly, and pectus deformities	FBN1 mutations[a]	Ghent diagnostic criteria	Surgical repair when the aorta reaches 5.0 cm unless there is a family history of AoD at <5.0 cm, a rapidly expanding aneurysm or presence of significant aortic valve regurgitation
	Joint laxity		DNA for sequencing	
	Recurrent or incisional hernias			
	Striae atrophicae			
	Ectopia lentis			
	Dural ectasia			
Loeys-Dietz syndrome	Bifid uvula or cleft palate	TGFBR2 or TGFBR1 mutations	DNA for sequencing	Surgical repair recommended at an aortic diameter of ≥4.2 cm by TEE (internal diameter) or 4.4 to ≥4.6 cm by CT and/or MRI (external diameter)
	Arterial tortuosity			
	Hypertelorism			
	Skeletal features similar to MFS			
	Craniosynostosis			
	Aneurysms and dissections of other arteries			
Ehlers-Danlos syndrome, vascular form	Thin, translucent skin	COL3A1 mutations	DNA for sequencing	Surgical repair is complicated by friable tissues
	Gastrointestinal rupture		Dermal fibroblasts for analysis of type III collagen	Noninvasive imaging recommended
	Rupture of the gravid uterus			
	Rupture of medium-sized to large arteries			
Turner syndrome	Short stature	45,X karyotype	Blood (cells) for karyotype analysis	AoD risk is increased in patients with bicuspid aortic valve, aortic coarctation, hypertension, or pregnancy
	Primary amenorrhea			
	Bicuspid aortic valve			
	Aortic coarctation			
	Webbed neck, low-set ears, low hairline, broad chest			

Reproduced with permission from Hiratzka et al. [29]

AoD indicates aortic dissection, *COL3A1* type III collagen, *CT* computed tomographic imaging, *FBN1* fibrillin-1, *MFS* Marfan syndrome, *MRI* magnetic resonance imaging, *TEE* transesophageal echocardiogram, *TGFBR1* transforming growth factor-beta receptor type I, and *TGFBR2* transforming growth factor-beta receptor type II

[a]The defective gene at a second locus for MFS is TGFBR2 but the clinical phenotype as MFS is debated

pattern of inheritance of familial thoracic aortic aneurysms is autosomal dominant, which means that a child needs to inherit the "aneurysm gene" from only one parent in order to be affected; however other inheritance patterns are also expressed. It is also evident that the actual inheritance rate is bound to be much higher than 21 %, since many family members may have a thoracic aortic aneurysm and not even be aware of that. Milewicz and colleagues found the exact same 21 % rate of family patterns [32].

Our studies also show that the location of the aneurysm in the proband has a strong impact on the site at which family members develop their aneurysms. Probands with an aneurysm of the ascending aorta have family members with predominantly ascending aortic aneurysms. On the contrary, probands with aneurysms of the descending thoracic aorta most commonly have family members with abdominal aortic aneurysms. This analysis fits a concept that aneurysm disease divides itself into two entities at the ligamentum arteriosum: above the ligament is one disease and below the ligament is another (see Fig. 23.6). Above the ligamentum, the disease is

nonarteriosclerotic in nature, while below the ligamentum, arteriosclerosis is abundant [28].

Significant progress has been achieved in identifying the genes and their mutations that are responsible for aortic aneurysms occurring in families. These mutations include thoracic aortic aneurysm and dissection 1 (which accounts for 20–30 % of familial cases), familial aortic aneurysm 1, transforming growth factor-beta receptor 2 (which accounts for 5 % of cases), smooth muscle α-actin (ACTA2), and myosin heavy chain 11 (Table 23.2) [33–38]. Milewicz and colleagues have done groundbreaking work in identifying these mutations. Our group has undertaken intensive efforts toward identifying the specific genetic aberrations that underlie familial inheritance in the hope of developing a widely sensitive genetic screening test for thoracic aortic aneurysm. We studied 30,000 ribonucleic acid (RNA) expression patterns in the blood of patients with thoracic aortic aneurysm and compared them with those of control patients. We found that a 41-single nucleotide polymorphism panel could discriminate quite well between patients with and without aneurysm via a simple blood test [39].

Table 23.2 Gene defects associated with familial thoracic aortic aneurysm and dissection

Defective gene leading to familial thoracic aortic aneurysms and dissection	Contribution to familial thoracic aortic aneurysms and dissection	Associated clinical features
TGFBR2 mutations	4 %	Thin, translucent skin
		Arterial or aortic tortuosity
		Aneurysm of arteries
MYH11 mutations	1 %	Patent ductus arteriosus
ACTA2 mutations	14 %	Livedo reticularis
		Iris flocculi
		Patent ductus arteriosus
		Bicuspid aortic valve

Reproduced with permission from Hiratzka et al. [29]

Abbreviations: *TGFBR2* transforming growth factor-beta receptor type II, *MYH11* myosin heavy chain 11, smooth muscle, *ACTA2* actin, alpha 2, smooth muscle aorta

Table 23.3 Comparison of epidemiology of Marfan disease (MFD) and bicuspid aortic valve, with special reference to number of cases of aortic dissection brought on by disease

Aortic manifestations of connective tissue disease		
	Incidence	Likelihood of aortic dissection
Marfan syndrome	0.01 % (1 in 10,000)	40 %
Bicuspid aortic valve	1–2 %	5 %

Reproduced with permission from Elefteriades and Rizzo [49]

Note: Bicuspid aortic valve causes 25 times more acute aortic dissections than Marfan syndrome. Dissection usually occurs long before onset of significant aortic stenosis

Bicuspid Aortic Valve

In terms of etiology, numerous studies recognize the role of a bicuspid aortic valve in aneurysm and dissection [40–48]. The structure of the thoracic aorta in patients born with a bicuspid aortic valve is different from the normal aorta, which establishes favorable conditions for these patients to develop aortic aneurysm and dissection. Aortic dissection in bicuspid aortic valve patients often occurs before the onset of aortic stenosis and its associated symptoms. Because bicuspid valve disease is so common (the most common congenital lesion of the human heart—1–2 % of the general population), it actually causes more dissections than the much more commonly appreciated Marfan syndrome (which occurs in only 1/10,000 human beings). The relevant arithmetic is shown in Table 23.3, which emphasizes the critical role of bicuspid valve in the generation of aortic dissection.

Anatomical Categorization of Thoracic Aortic Aneurysms

1. *Ascending aortic aneurysms* – are typically fusiform and may extend into the aortic arch. Ascending aortic aneurysms can be divided into three categories,

according to the pattern of involvement of the aortic root (Fig. 23.7):

   (a) Supracoronary type aneurysm. In this type, the aortic annulus is normal size, as is the short segment of aorta between the annulus and the coronary orifices.

   (b) Marfanoid type aneurysm (whether or not the patient has Marfan syndrome). This type is often termed *annuloaortic ectasia*, emphasizing that the aortic annulus and the most proximal portion of the aorta are dilated.

   (c) Tubular type aneurysm. This is a category midway between the other two types in configuration. The aortic annulus and proximal aorta are somewhat, but not markedly, dilated. The uniform caliber throughout the ascending aorta gives this category a tubular appearance.

2. *Descending aortic aneurysms*. In contrast to the ascending aorta, the majority of aneurysms of the descending thoracic aorta are associated with atherosclerosis. These may extend to the level of the abdominal aorta, are typically fusiform, and often begin just distal to the origin of the left subclavian artery.

3. *Thoracoabdominal aneurysms*. As suggested by the nomenclature, thoracoabdominal aortic aneurysms possess features of both thoracic and abdominal aortic aneurysms. Although they constitute only about 3 % of all aortic aneurysms, thoracoabdominal aneurysms are considered a separate class because of the diffuse and extensive aortic involvement and special considerations for surgical repair, which often require reimplantation of the visceral arteries.

Natural History of Thoracic Aortic Aneurysm

The natural history of thoracic aortic aneurysm is quite diverse, reflecting the broad spectrum of etiologies that cause this disease. At Yale we have conducted extensive studies to understand the natural history of thoracic aortic aneurysm development in order to be able to predict its behavior—in other words—to "read the enemy's playbook."

Fig. 23.7 Three common patterns of ascending aortic aneurysm disease: supracoronary, annuloaortic ectasia, and tubular (Reprinted with permission from Elefteriades [3])

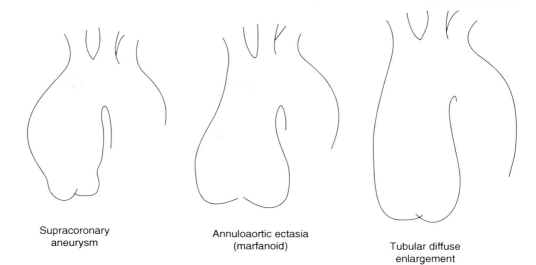

Supracoronary
aneurysm

Annuloaortic ectasia
(marfanoid)

Tubular diffuse
enlargement

Although thoracic aortic aneurysm is a virulent disease, the dilated aorta grows very slowly, in an indolent fashion. The rate of aortic growth is approximately 0.1 cm/year, whereas the descending aorta tends to grow somewhat faster than the ascending aorta (Fig. 23.8) [50]. Thus, an aneurysm takes decades of adult life to come to fruition. The only situation in which the thoracic aorta truly grows rapidly in a short time occurs when there has been an intercurrent aortic dissection.

Knowing the rate of aortic growth, the next question is—what is the appropriate size at which the diseased aorta needs to be replaced before a dissection or rupture occurs? Our analysis revealed abrupt "hinge points" in aneurysm size at which rupture or dissection becomes likely to occur. In the case of ascending aortic aneurysm, the hinge point is 6.0 cm, which is indicative of the fact that 31 % of the patients will have suffered rupture or dissection by the time their thoracic aneurysm reaches this size. For the descending aorta, the hinge point is slightly higher—7.0 cm, but by the time this size is reached, 43 % of the patients will have suffered a devastating complication [50–52]. These clinical "hinge points" are illustrated in Fig. 23.9. Based on these findings we were able to develop evidence-based criteria for surgical intervention for thoracic aortic aneurysm (which will be discussed later).

As our data became more robust, we were able to calculate the yearly rate of rupture or dissection for thoracic aortic aneurysms based on the size of the aorta (Table 23.4). These data allow the physician to form a reasonable estimate of the patient's risk of aortic dissection, rupture, or death for each future year of life if the aneurysmal aorta is not resected. It should be noted that the risk of adverse events is extremely high—14.1 %—for patients whose aneurysms have exceeded 6 cm in diameter [52].

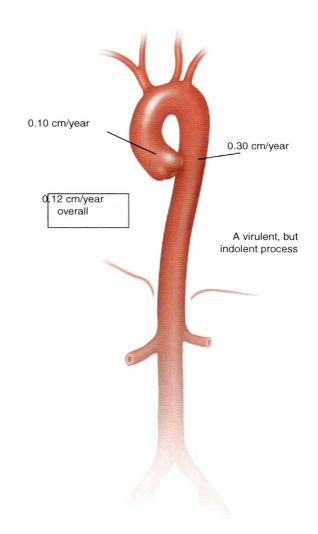

0.10 cm/year

0.30 cm/year

0.12 cm/year
overall

A virulent, but
indolent process

Fig. 23.8 Growth rates of the ascending and descending thoracic aorta—a virulent but indolent process (Reprinted with permission from Elefteriades and Farkas [28])

Fig. 23.9 The increase in risk of rupture or dissection as the aorta enlarges to specific dimensions. The hinge point is at 6 cm for the ascending aorta and 7 cm for the descending aorta (Reproduced from Coady et al. [50])

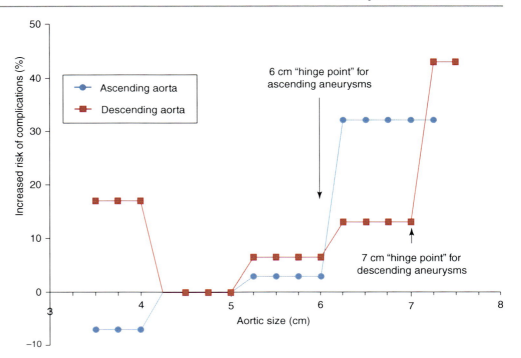

Table 23.4 Yearly rates of rupture, dissection, or death related to aortic size

	Aortic size			
Yearly risk (cm)	>3.5	>4	>5	>6
Rupture (%)	0.0	0.3	1.7	3.6
Dissection (%)	2.2	1.5	2.5	3.7
Death (%)	5.9	4.6	4.8	10.8
Any of the above (%)	7.2	5.3	6.5	14.1

Reproduced with permission from Elefteriades [52]

Aortic Dissection

Aortic dissection is known to be the most common cause of death related to the human aorta [53]. (Many cases masquerade as "heart attacks.") The typical aortic dissection process begins with a tear through the intima and inner media at one specific site. Blood under pressure rushes in between the separated layers, propagating further dissection longitudinally along the aorta. The split occurs within the tunica media: the intima and inner media are forced inward, while the outer media and adventitia are forced outward. This separation of layers creates two lumens, within which the blood flows—the true lumen and the false lumen. Dissection is an acute process that occurs in a chronically degenerated aorta. The danger of aortic dissection lies in its unique ability to compromise blood flow to any organ of the human body. We illustrate this in Fig. 23.10, which shows schematically how the pressurized false lumen occludes branch vessels causing acute organ ischemia with devastating outcomes [54].

Aortic dissections are commonly classified into Type A dissections, which involve the ascending aorta, and Type B dissections, which involve in the descending aorta. The two types are distinguished by the location of the inciting intimal tear. Tears usually occur in two very specific locations: (1) in the ascending aorta, 2–3 cm above the coronary arteries, and (2) in the descending aorta, 1–2 cm beyond the left subclavian artery. The first type of tear produces ascending dissection and the second produces descending dissection. It should be noted that ascending dissections usually go around the aortic arch and commonly further involve the descending and abdominal portions of the aorta as well [3].

The term *dissecting aneurysm of the aorta* causes much confusion with chronic "arteriosclerotic" aneurysms. It is best not to think of acute aortic dissection as an aneurysm in the first place. Until the point that the acute dissection occurs, the aorta may not be dramatically aneurysmal. After the dissection has occurred, although the aorta usually has widened acutely, it is the splitting of layers that has caused the widening; that splitting of layers constitutes the crucial pathophysiologic event. It is best to term this acute phenomenon an "acute aortic dissection" rather than an "aneurysm" of any type [54].

It is very important to understand what is the acute trigger for an aorta to dissect. A very common misconception is that the occurrence of dissection is random in a susceptible patient. Aortic dissection follows circadian and diurnal patterns, with a preponderance of instances in the winter months and in the early morning hours, when blood pressure is known to be highest. Our studies have shown that in the majority of patients, episodes of severe emotional upset or

Fig. 23.10 Schematic illustration of branch vessel occlusion by tense false lumen during typical aortic dissection (**a** and **b**) and its relief by reentry of blood into the true lumen (**c**) (Reprinted with permission from John A. Elefteriades, MD, the author)

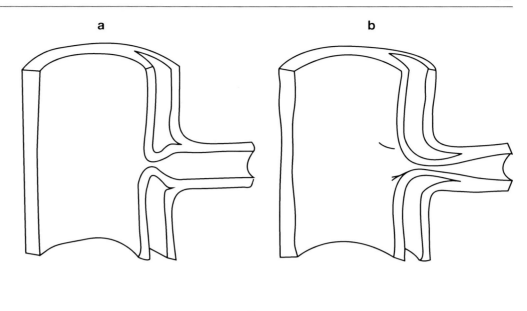

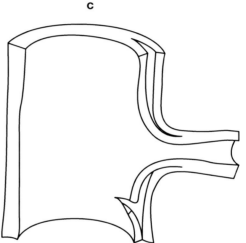

extreme physical exertion precede the dissection, suggesting their role as causative factors [55, 56].

Other variants of aortic dissection (besides typical dissection) include *intramural hematoma* and *penetrating aortic ulcer* (Fig. 23.11). An intramural hematoma has no dissection flap that separates the true and false lumen; it is usually located circumferentially around the aortic lumen, rather than obliquely oriented across the aortic lumen. Intramural hematomas may arise from small intimal tears that cannot be detected radiographically or from the rupture of the vasa vasorum (the small blood vessels that supply the aortic wall itself). However, this pathogenesis is unproven and a matter debate in the literature. A penetrating aortic ulcer is a localized penetration deep into the wall of the aorta, which disrupts the internal elastic lamina and erodes into the media. In some cases, this penetration may mimic or initiate aortic dissection, pseudoaneurysm formation, intramural hematoma, or rupture. Importantly, contrary to typical aortic dissection,

neither intramural hematomas nor penetrating ulcers occlude branch vessels.

Diagnosis

Clinical Presentation

We will discuss the clinical presentation of two of the most common thoracic aortic entities, which are very different in terms of presenting symptoms, namely, thoracic aortic aneurysm and thoracic aortic dissection:

Thoracic Aortic Aneurysm
The greatest challenge for physicians in detecting thoracic aortic aneurysm lies in the fact that in the absolute majority of affected individuals (90–95 %), the aneurysms are clinically silent and do not cause any symptoms. It is very

Fig. 23.11 Variant forms of aortic dissection: typical dissection, penetrating aortic ulcer, and intramural hematoma of the aorta (Reprinted with permission from Elefteriades [3])

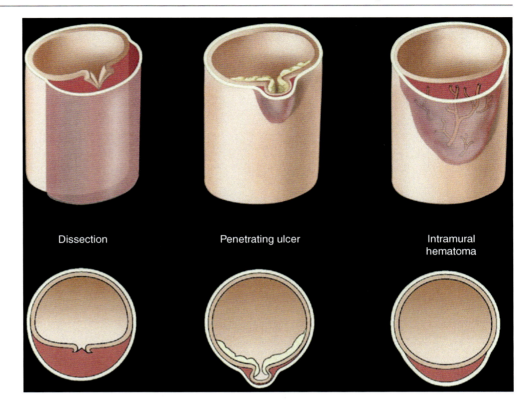

Dissection   Penetrating ulcer   Intramural hematoma

common for first symptom to be either death or a major complication that threatens to produce death—rupture or dissection. Thus, only a very small number of patients (5–10 %) are "fortunate" enough to experience some early symptoms of aneurysm formation, which permits early detection and adequate management.

Pain is the most common symptom that an aneurysm can produce. This symptom can be attributed to stretching of the aortic tissue or impingement on adjacent structures. Pain from the ascending aorta is typically felt retrosternally, while descending aortic aneurysm usually causes interscapular back pain. Pain in the lateral or posterior chest may be present when the growing aneurysm starts to compress surrounding structures or to erode into adjacent bones, such as the ribs or vertebral bodies. Aneurysm-related pain is often difficult to distinguish from other sources of pain. However, the patient can often discriminate deep visceral pain from pain of various superficial or musculoskeletal origins. Many people suffer from lower back pain, which is musculoskeletal in origin. However, back pain caused by an aneurysm is usually different from musculoskeletal back pain, because it is independent of position and type of activity. The *interscapular* location for pain from the descending aorta is, fortunately for diagnosis, rarely a musculoskeletal symptom.

If a rupture of an aortic aneurysm occurs acutely, it is very likely to produce symptoms, usually severe pain, followed by a loss of consciousness, or death due to internal hemorrhage. Rupture of the ascending aorta produces chest pain and shock from cardiac tamponade, while rupture of a descending or thoracoabdominal aortic aneurysm produces hypovolemic shock, with the associated pain felt in a distribution corresponding to the anatomic location of the process.

Thoracic aortic aneurysms can also produce other symptoms besides pain. For example, ascending aortic aneurysms can cause progressive heart failure due to severe aortic regurgitation, the underlying cause of which is the enlargement of the aortic root and loss of coaptation of valve leaflets that are pulled apart by the dilated root. In some cases, ascending aortic aneurysm can cause respiratory symptoms by distorting the trachea. Symptoms such as hoarseness or dysphagia can be attributed to aneurysms of the aortic arch or descending aorta which can damage the recurrent laryngeal nerve or cause direct impingement on the esophagus. Hemoptysis can be a very important and ominous symptom suggestive that a descending aortic aneurysm may have eroded directly into the lung parenchyma or bronchi. Similarly, if an erosion occurs into the esophagus, hematemesis would be the presenting symptom [3].

Thoracic Aortic Dissection

It is much more common for patients suffering an aortic dissection to present with symptoms. According to data from the International Registry of Aortic Dissection (IRAD), severe pain with an abrupt onset is the most common presenting symptom [57]. The pain is usually very intense and described as tearing, shearing, or stabbing in quality. This is very much consistent with the pathophysiology of aortic dissection, since an actual "tear" does occur within the aorta. Most patients would describe this pain as the worst pain they have ever experienced in their lives. The pain can migrate and change locations as the dissection propagates. For the Type A (ascending) dissections, sharp substernal pain is most characteristic with occasional radiation to the neck. For the Type B (descending) dissections, the pain is usually localized in the back, between the scapulae [58]. Dissection pain can be variable; for example, in 15 % of patients with aortic dissection, the pain is gradual in onset rather than abrupt, and in 10 % the pain is not severe [57, 59]. Also it is important to note that pain maybe completely absent in 10 % of the patients leading to a late presentation, months or years after the acute event [58].

Other symptoms of aortic dissection can include pleuritic pain, angina from true myocardial ischemia, abdominal pain, shortness of breath from aortic regurgitation, oliguria from renal ischemia, leg pain, neurologic deficit with transient cerebral ischemia or stroke, peripheral neurologic symptoms, and syncope. Such a variety of presenting symptoms and signs are so nonspecific that dissection may be overlooked initially in up to 40 % of cases. Therefore, deservingly, aortic dissection is referred to as "The Great Masquerader," since in many patients it does not present in the "classical fashion" but rather can mimic and present itself as a disease of any organ. After all, every organ receives its blood flow from the aorta and this source of flow can be disturbed by the dissection flap. Thus, whenever any combination of cardiac, neurologic, abdominal, or vascular abnormalities cannot be otherwise explained, one must consider aortic dissection as a possible unifying diagnosis; having a low threshold to obtain an appropriate diagnostic imaging study is essential [59, 60]. At the same time, it is not uncommon for the diagnosis not to be made until postmortem examination in a disturbingly large fraction of patients [61]. The mortality rate of untreated thoracic aortic dissection approaches an alarming 1–2 % per each hour during the first 48 h, 89 % at 14 days, and 90 % at 3 months [62]. All of this difficulty of diagnosis combined with the very high stakes of a missed dissection creates a malpractice "maelstrom" [60].

The most recent 2010 ACCF/AHA/AATS/ACR/ASA/SCA/SCAI/SIR/STS/SVM guidelines for the diagnosis and management of patients with thoracic aortic disease (further—ACCF/AHA guidelines) recommend that the clinician perform a focused physical examination for patients presenting with a history of acute cardiac and noncardiac symptoms associated with a significant likelihood of thoracic aortic disease, which should include a careful and complete search for arterial perfusion differentials in both upper and lower extremities, evidence of visceral ischemia, focal neurological deficits, a murmur of aortic regurgitation, vascular bruits, and findings compatible with possible cardiac tamponade (level of evidence: C) [29].

Table 23.5 Potential biomarkers for diagnosis and/or monitoring of aortic diseases

Indicators of ongoing thrombosis
D-dimer
Plasmin
Fibrinogen
Matrix metalloproteinases
Inflammatory markers
Cytokines
CD4+ CD28− T cells
C-reactive protein
Markers of collagen turnover
Elastin peptide
Others
Endothelin
Hepatocyte growth factor
Homocysteine
Genetic markers
Ribonucleic acid signature

Reproduced with permission from Elefteriades and Farkas [28]

Biomarkers for Thoracic Aortic Aneurysm

Due to the fact that thoracic aortic aneurysm is a predominantly silent disease, but at the same time virulent and potentially lethal, there is an urgent need for discovery of biomarkers of this disease which would permit detection of aneurysm in the general population, monitoring of its condition and progress, and prediction of complications. No such biomarker currently exists. Many potential biomarkers have been identified and are currently being studied for their clinical value and significance (Table 23.5) [28, 63]. However, the majority of these biomarkers are still far from routine clinical application.

The D-dimer is one potential biomarker that has been shown to be effective in clinical practice for detecting patients with acute aortic dissection. D-dimer is a degradation product of fibrin cross-linking in a clot. This test is sensitive for detecting ongoing intravascular thrombosis. D-dimer testing has been already implemented into clinical practice to rule out pulmonary embolism [64]. Recent studies have shown that in patients with acute aortic dissections, elevated levels of circulating D-dimer have been found [65–68]. D-dimer has a remarkable reported sensitivity of 99 % in early detection of acute aortic dissection [68]. Two meta-analyses have also shown the effectiveness of D-dimer assays in diagnosing aortic dissection [69, 70]. The level of D-dimer elevation reflects the extent of aortic dissection. At the same time it is of utmost importance to note that D-dimer is extremely nonspecific, being elevated in pulmonary embolism and coronary thrombosis—essentially in any state in which thrombosis and thrombolysis occur [28]. However, because D-dimer elevation occurs after the dissection, it is not useful as a predictor of the acute disease.

Table 23.6 Essential elements of aortic imaging reports

1. The location at which the aorta is abnormal

2. The maximum diameter of any dilatation, measured from the external wall of the aorta, perpendicular to the axis of flow, and the length of the aorta that is abnormal

3. For patients with presumed or documented genetic syndromes at risk for aortic root disease measurements of aortic valve, sinuses of Valsalva, sinotubular junction, and ascending aorta

4. The presence of internal filling defects consistent with thrombus or atheroma

5. The presence of IMH, PAU, and calcification

6. Extension of aortic abnormality into branch vessels, including dissection and aneurysm, and secondary evidence of end-organ injury (e.g., renal or bowel hypoperfusion)

7. Evidence of aortic rupture, including periaortic and mediastinal hematoma, pericardial and pleural fluid, and contrast extravasation from the aortic lumen

8. When a prior examination is available, direct image-to-image comparison to determine if there has been any increase in diameter

Reproduced with permission from Hiratzka et al. [29]
IMH indicates intramural hematoma and PAU indicates penetrating aortic ulcer

Because the efficacy and safety of using D-dimer as a screening test have not been tested in a large clinical trial, the ACCF/AHA guidelines do not yet recommend serum D-dimer screening for all patients being evaluated for aortic dissection [29].

Radiographic Imaging

In the present era, thoracic aortic aneurysms are most often identified as incidental findings on a computed tomographic scan (or echocardiogram, or magnetic resonance imaging study) that is usually done for a completely separate reason. Occasionally, a chest X-ray done routinely or for pulmonary symptoms suggests the presence of aortic aneurysm, which is later confirmed on computed tomographic (CT) imaging. Detection of aneurysms through these means provides an unparalleled opportunity to prevent aortic-related death via early detection [3].

The current ACCF/AHA guidelines recommend the use of four imaging techniques to determine the presence and progression of thoracic aortic disease—chest X-ray, echocardiography, computed tomographic imaging (CT), and magnetic resonance imaging (MR). Essential elements of aortic imaging studies are listed in Table 23.6:

1. *Chest X-ray* is a very useful screening test for thoracic aortic diseases. An experienced physician will be able to suspect and identify chronic aortic aneurysms on an X-ray. An ascending aneurysm bulges just to the right of the mid-mediastinal contour. A descending aortic aneurysm produces a widened paravertebral stripe. An arch aneurysm produces an enlarged aortic knob. For dissection, chest radiography will usually provide clues, most commonly, widening of the mediastinal shadow, pleural effusion, or inward displacement of aortic medial calcification. Although chest X-ray rarely conclusively establishes the diagnosis of aortic disease, it can suggest acute or chronic aortic pathology and lead to subsequent testing for more definitive diagnosis [3, 29, 71].

2. *Echocardiography* can be performed via two different approaches—transthoracic echocardiography (TTE) and transesophageal echocardiography (TEE). Echocardiography can detect the presence of aortic enlargement and associated cardiac pathology that suggests the underlying etiology of the aortic disease. A TTE can visualize the proximal several centimeters of the ascending aorta, to just above the sinotubular junction in a patient with good echocardiographic windows. A TEE is able to visualize the majority of the ascending and descending aorta, while being partially blinded to the aortic arch due to the interposed tracheal air column. Echocardiography also provides information about pericardial effusion/tamponade, valve function, and left ventricular function. A major limitation of both TTE and TEE is the frequent appearance of artifacts that mimic a dissection flap. It is therefore essential that the echocardiographer has the requisite experience to distinguish true dissection flaps from such artifacts. It is, however, important to note that echocardiography demonstrates good sensitivity and specificity for diagnosing aortic pathology [3, 28, 29, 71].

3. *Computed tomography* (*CT*). This imaging technique makes it possible to visualize the entire length of the aorta in the axial, sagittal, and coronal planes, with very high resolution of the images. This permits 3-dimensional reconstruction of the whole aorta in images that replicate anatomic specimens. CT also has the advantage of being highly time-efficient, thus permitting imaging in even the sickest patients. The primary diagnostic criterion for aortic dissection by contrast CT is the demonstration of two contrast-filled lumens separated by an intimal flap. These characteristics render CT a very convenient and reliable method for detection of aortic pathology, with both sensitivity and specificity of the method approaching 100 % [3, 28, 29, 71].

4. *Magnetic resonance* (*MR*) *imaging* has proven to be the most accurate diagnostic method for aortic disease, with sensitivity and specificity even exceeding those of CT. It is also very important to note that MR is completely non-invasive, has no associated ionizing radiation exposure, and can be performed without the use of potentially nephrotoxic contrast media. MR produces extremely high-resolution images that allow good differentiation between adjacent tissues. MR has been shown to be very good in detecting typical aortic dissection and its variants, intramural hematoma and penetrating ulcer. The procedure itself takes time to be performed and thus is not applicable in acute settings when a patient presents in

Table 23.7 A Summary of the major strengths and limitations of CT, TTE, TEE, and MRI

	Strengths	Limitations
TTE	Rapid/portable bedside use	Limited spatial resolution
	Can assess for AI, LV function, pericardial effusion, and/or tamponade	Anatomic window limited to aortic root and heart and cannot assess extent of dissection beyond aortic root
	May identify dissection of aortic root/proximal aorta	
TEE	Portable	Limited view of distal ascending aorta ("blind spot")
	Excellent spatial resolution	Cannot assess distal abdominal aorta
	Safe in hemodynamically unstable patient	Potential false-positive from reverberation artifact
	Fast diagnosis (complete study in <30 min)	
	May be used intraoperatively	
	Assessment of cardiac anatomy/function	
CT	Rapid exam	May miss small tears or entry site
	Offers excellent resolution of aorta, including aortic arch and branch vessels	Cannot assess cardiac or valvular function
	Shows extent of dissection into branch vessels	Moderate contrast exposure/risk nephrotoxicity
		Limited use in hemodynamically unstable patient
MRI	Highest accuracy, sensitivity, and specificity	Limited availability
	Can identify even very small aortic tears	Expensive
	Safer contrast media	Limited use in hemodynamically unstable patient
	Excellent depiction of arch and branch vessels	Incompatible with implanted metal devices or prostheses
		Rarely used as initial test (<2 %)

Modified and reproduced with permission from Raghupathy and Eagle [72]

Abbreviations: *CT* computed tomography, *MRI* magnetic resonance imaging, *TEE* transesophageal echocardiography, *TTE* transthoracic echocardiography

an unstable condition. The use of this technique is limited to patients without metallic implants (e.g., pacemakers) [3, 28, 29, 71].

The advantages and limitations of TTE, TEE, CT, and MR are listed in Table 23.7.

There is, however, a point of caution that we would like to raise among physicians evaluating diagnostic images of the thoracic aorta. Often the key decision on how to manage an aortic aneurysm depends on the size of the aorta. Most of the diagnostic techniques (echocardiography, CT, MR) permit us to measure the aortic diameter at various locations. However, each of the imaging techniques provides specific sources of error in the measurement of aortic size, which may be misleading and cause tactical errors in selecting the treatment strategy. For example, TTE can give us information regarding the size of the proximal part of the ascending aorta but may miss an aneurysm of the midportion or upper ascending aorta. On the other hand, reviewing axial CT images alone is also not a reliable method of evaluating the size of the aortic root and proximal part of the ascending aorta, since these portions of the aorta are rarely confined to the plane of the axial images (perpendicular to the longitudinal axis of the body); obliquity may suggest a misleadingly large size of the proximal aorta (Fig. 23.12). The same is true for axial CT images of the aortic arch and the peridiaphragmatic portion of the descending aorta, both of which produce an oblong rather than a circular contour and can lead to errors in assessing the maximal size of the oblong-shaped aorta. Thus, it is extremely important to understand the geometric complexity of the human aorta, take into account the limitations of the imaging modalities, and evaluate the size and shape of the aorta from all avail-

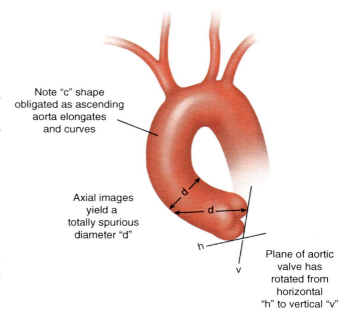

Note "c" shape obligated as ascending aorta elongates and curves

Axial images yield a totally spurious diameter "d"

Plane of aortic valve has rotated from horizontal "h" to vertical "v"

Fig. 23.12 Confounding of ascending aortic measurements due to elongation and "C" shape of ascending aorta. Image shows gross elongation of the ascending aorta, forcing the aorta into a C-shape and obligating the aortic valve to take a nearly vertical plane of orientation. On an axial computed tomographic image, this common anatomy would markedly confound measurement of proximal aortic diameter. Note the difference between a horizontal diameter (as in an axial image) and a diameter perpendicular to the long axis of the aorta (Reprinted with permission from Elefteriades and Farkas [28])

able planes and angles to be able to visualize a full 3-dimensional picture of the aorta [28]. We also caution physicians regarding the danger of comparing the current image of the aorta (either by echocardiography, CT, or MR) with only the last prior image of the aorta. As we have shown above, the aorta grows very slowly; hence it is of utmost importance to make comparisons with the *very first available image*, even if it means searching or sending for earlier studies [28, 73].

The ACCF/AHA guidelines recommend screening for aortic size of all the first-degree relatives of patients who have been found to have familial aortic aneurysm, genetic syndromes that cause aneurysm formation, or who are diagnosed with bicuspid aortic valve [28–30].

Management

The management of thoracic aortic diseases depends on the pathological process and the location of the disease within the aorta. For the simplicity of presentation and understanding, we will divide management into four main categories—medical and surgical treatment and treatment of acute and chronic aortic conditions.

Medical Treatment of Chronic Thoracic Aortic Aneurysm

The ACCF/AHA guidelines recommend implementation of stringent control of hypertension, lipid profile optimization, and smoking cessation, as well as optimization of other atherosclerosis-related risk factors in patients with small aneurysms not requiring surgery, as well as for patients who are not considered surgical or stent-graft candidates [29].

The goal of antihypertensive therapy in patients with chronic thoracic aortic diseases is blood pressure less than 140/90 mmHg, or even 130/80 mmHg for patients with diabetes or chronic renal disease. Blood pressure reduction aims at reducing the risk of stroke, myocardial infarction, heart failure, and cardiovascular death [29, 74–78]. Beta-blockers, angiotensin-converting enzyme inhibitors, or angiotensin receptor blockers are recommended for effective blood pressure control. For patients with thoracic aortic aneurysm, the guidelines recommend lowering the blood pressure to the maximal extent that can be tolerated by the patient without adverse effects [29]. The effectiveness of beta-blocking medications is still largely unproven and even controversial. The major concerns regarding beta-blockers lie in the evidence that they decrease the elasticity of the aortic wall, which is already compromised by aneurysm disease. However, while no proof of efficacy is yet available, the use of beta-blockers has become standard practice [3, 28].

The best available level of evidence (level A) for the effectiveness of a statin to achieve target low-density lipid cholesterol of less than 70 mg/dL (shown in studies for gen-

eral control of atherosclerosis) is also true for patients with atherosclerotic aneurysm [29, 79–81]. Thus, statin therapy should be recommended for patients with chronic aortic aneurysms which are suspicious for being atherosclerotic in origin. A study conducted by our group has also shown that statin use is associated with a lower mortality rate and a reduced rate of death, rupture, dissection, and need for surgical repair in patients with thoracic aortic aneurysms [82].

Many other options for medical treatment of aortic aneurysm have been proposed, which include the antibiotic doxycycline (a matrix metalloproteinase inhibitor), anti-inflammatory agents (COX-2 inhibitors), and immunosuppressants, among other agents. While none of these agents are of proven clinical benefit, several are undergoing clinical trials [16, 28, 83].

Medical therapy should be administered to patients only with small ascending and descending aortic aneurysms. Asymptomatic patients with degenerative thoracic aneurysm, chronic aortic dissection, intramural hematoma, penetrating aortic ulcer, mycotic aneurysm, or pseudoaneurysm, who are otherwise suitable candidates and for whom the ascending aorta or aortic sinus diameter is 5.5 cm or greater, should be strongly considered for surgical repair. Patients with Marfan syndrome (and other genetic syndromes) should undergo elective aortic replacement at smaller aortic root diameter (less than 5.0 cm). Also if a patient's ascending aorta grows at a rate faster than 0.5 cm/year, surgical treatment should be considered. A size criterion of 6.0 cm or greater of the descending aorta should be considered for surgical treatment. It should be noted that these size criteria apply to asymptomatic patients. Patients with symptoms suggestive of aortic origin should be evaluated for prompt surgical intervention regardless of the size of the aorta, unless life expectancy from comorbid conditions is limited or quality of life is substantially impaired [28, 29, 50, 84].

Medical Treatment of Acute Aortic Events (Dissection, Rupture)

Urgent surgical consultation should be obtained for all patients diagnosed with thoracic aortic dissection regardless of the anatomic location (ascending versus descending) as soon as the diagnosis is made or highly suspected [29]. Medical therapy as a sole means of treatment is only appropriate for patients with dissection of the descending aorta and nonsurgical candidates with ascending aortic dissection. However, regardless of whether the dissection is ascending or descending, or whether or not the patient will be taken emergently to the operating room, the currently accepted medical therapy must be instituted immediately to discourage rupture or extension of the dissection. For surgical candidates, medical therapy will be an interim measure.

The backbone of medical therapy in acute dissection is "anti-impulse therapy," which includes beta-blockade and afterload reduction. The pathophysiological rationale for such combination therapy is that aortic dissection propagates more vigorously when either blood pressure or force of cardiac contraction is excessive [85].

Nitroglycerin or nitroprusside is usually used for blood pressure control, because of their effectiveness, their rapid onset of action, and their quick cessation of action upon discontinuation. Angiotensin-converting enzyme inhibitors have also been used for this purpose [29]. The recommended systolic blood pressure range for patients with acute dissection is 90–100 mmHg, if the patient can tolerate such pressures without manifesting neurologic dysfunction or oliguria. However, in older patients it is not always possible to drop the systolic blood pressure below 120–130 mmHg. It is very important to remember that vasodilator therapy should not be initiated prior to rate control, so as to avoid associated reflex tachycardia that may increase aortic wall stress, leading to propagation or expansion of a thoracic aortic dissection [29].

It is also essential to decrease the force of cardiac contraction, because the drop in blood pressure by afterload reduction alone actually increases the sheer stress on the aortic wall. Decreasing the force of cardiac contraction is usually accomplished by administering a short-acting beta-blocking drug like esmolol. Another approach is administration of the alpha- and beta-adrenergic antagonist labetalol by intravenous infusion. Beta-blockers alter the morphology of the arterial pulse wave, which should be blunted by decreasing the force of cardiac contraction. The dp/dt, reflected in the upslope of the initial portion of the aortic pulse wave, must be decreased (Fig. 23.13) [85]. In patients with clear contraindications to beta-blockade, calcium channel-blocking agents such as verapamil should be utilized as an alternative for rate control and modification of the force of cardiac contraction [3, 29, 83].

Anti-impulse therapy is the appropriate initial response once the diagnosis of any type of acute aortic dissection or related process is entertained. Such therapy should be undertaken even while imaging studies are being performed to confirm the diagnosis of aortic dissection and to define the anatomic type, location, and extent of the process, as well as while definitive decisions regarding treatments strategies are being made.

Surgical Treatment of Chronic Thoracic Aortic Aneurysm

A variety of surgical techniques have been described over the years for different types and locations of thoracic aneurysms. Surgery of the ascending aorta, the aortic arch, and in some cases even of the descending aorta requires arresting the

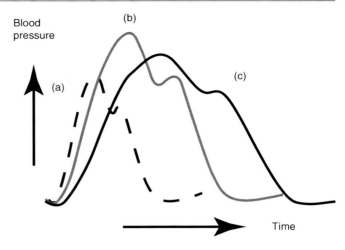

Fig. 23.13 Pharmacologic anti-impulse therapy. Diagram of aortic pressure curves under various conditions. The *continuous grey line* (**b**) represents the baseline state. Administration of a vasodilator agent such as nitroprusside is represented by the *dashed curve* (**a**). Beta-blockade administration is represented by the *continuous black line* (**c**) (Reprinted with permission from Sanz et al. [85])

heart for the duration of aortic reconstruction and instituting artificial blood circulation via the use of a cardiopulmonary bypass machine.

In patients without significant dilatation of the aortic root (see Fig. 23.7, supracoronary aneurysm), in elderly patients, and in young patients with concomitant aortic valve disease, separate aortic valve and ascending aortic replacement should be performed. However, in patients with Marfan and other genetic syndromes, who have a dilated aortic root (see Fig. 23.7, annuloaortic ectasia), the operation should include excision of the sinuses of Valsalva in combination with either a valve-sparing operation or if not feasible, complete root replacement with a valved graft conduit [29]. Although "valve-sparing" techniques, proposed by Yacoub and David and coworkers [86–89], have recently gained extreme popularity, further long-term follow-up is still needed to determine whether the efficacy of such operations will challenge the current "gold standard" for aortic root aneurysm—composite graft replacement [90]. Either technique requires meticulous reimplantation of coronary arteries into the newly implanted aortic graft.

Surgical techniques in approaching aneurysms of the aortic arch have evolved over time, and the fact that so many different techniques have been proposed suggests that there is no one surgical approach that will suit all patients and all surgeons. The greatest challenge in aortic arch surgery is the need to interrupt normal blood perfusion to the brain through the head vessels, while they are reimplanted into the new graft. Performing such an operation without adequate cerebral protection from ischemic injury is bound to cause severe postoperative neurological complications. There is still much

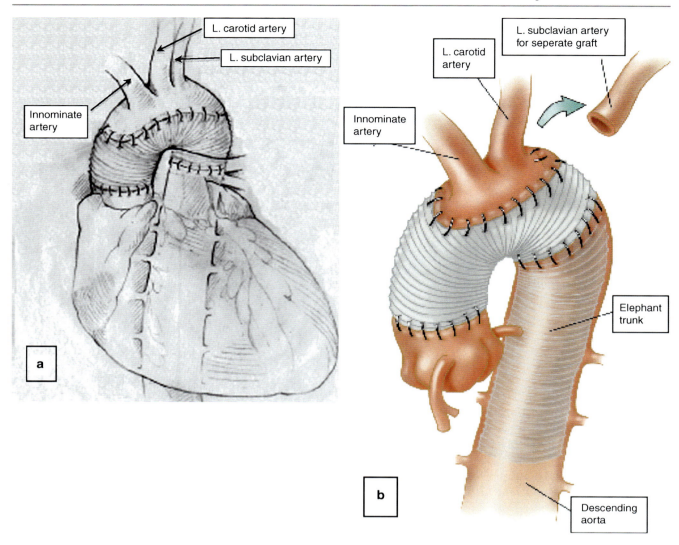

Fig. 23.14 (**a**) Traditional technique of aortic arch reconstruction. (**b**) Alternative technique that we prefer to the traditional one, as a 2-vessel smaller pedicle is quicker and easier to anastomose with the aortic graft than a 3-vessel pedicle (Reprinted with permission from Ziganshin and Elefteriades [91])

debate in the literature regarding the techniques of reimplanting the head vessels and the methods for cerebral protection during aortic arch surgery.

Depending on the location and extent of the aneurysm, complete or partial arch replacement can be performed [29, 91]. The head and neck vessels (namely, the innominate artery, the left carotid artery, and the left subclavian artery) are usually reimplanted into the prosthetic graft in one patch with a rim of the native aortic tissue (Fig. 23.14a). However, prefabricated branched grafts, which require an individual anastomosis to be performed for each of the great vessels, can also be used. At our institution we favor an alternative technique of aortic arch reconstruction, which involves reimplanting two of the great vessels—the innominate artery and the left carotid artery—into the prosthetic graft as a single

patch (see Fig. 23.14b), while the left subclavian artery is anastomosed to the aorta after termination of cardiopulmonary bypass. The advantage of this technique resides in the shorter time required to reimplant the head vessels and resume normal physiological blood flow to the brain [91, 92].

Cerebral protection techniques during aortic arch surgery have also been subject to rigorous debate, and institutional experience is currently recognized as a very important factor in selection of the best brain protection strategy. To date three main approaches to cerebral protection have been developed and widely used: deep hypothermic circulatory arrest, selective antegrade brain perfusion, and retrograde brain perfusion [91]. These techniques used alone or in combination are recommended for minimization of brain injury during surgical repairs of the ascending aorta and transverse aortic arch [29].

Table 23.8 Advantages and disadvantages of cerebral protection techniques

Technique	Advantage	Danger	Comment
DHCA	Safe for short periods of circulatory arrest Avoids cross-clamping an already diseased aorta	Questions of safety for long periods of circulatory arrest, increased incidence of permanent neurologic injury with >45 min of circulatory arrest, and conflicting data on transient effects with shorter (approximately 25 min) ischemia	Generally used in more straight forward cases Many of the survey's respondents commented on use of DHCA with SACP
RCP	Permits longer periods of circulatory arrest than with straight DHCA	Requires the handling of sclerotic vessels; may result in the release of emboli	Technique most often used Controversies regarding ideal site of cannulation for optimal perfusion
ACP	Flushes cerebral vasculature of toxic metabolic products and microemboli	Perfusion may be limited to the brain's surface	

Reproduced with permission from Ziganshin and Elefteriades [91]
Abbreviations: *DHCA* deep hypothermic circulatory arrest, *RCP* retrograde cerebral perfusion, *ACP* antegrade cerebral perfusion

However, none of the techniques has unequivocally demonstrated clear-cut superiority over the others. Of the three protective strategies, retrograde cerebral perfusion, which delivers blood to the brain through the venous system in a retrograde fashion, is becoming increasingly less popular among cardiothoracic surgeons because of published evidence, which suggests that very little oxygen is actually delivered to the brain tissue during venous perfusion [93, 94]. Antegrade cerebral perfusion maintains blood flow to the brain via selective cannulation of the arterial vessels; thus, perfusion is achieved in a physiologic antegrade fashion. During the last decade, this technique has become the most popular method of brain protection, and excellent results have been reported [95–97]. However, at our institution we favor deep hypothermic circulatory arrest (DHCA), which has been the preferred technique for aortic surgery for many years and whose results have withstood the test of time. DHCA requires cooling the patient to 18–19 °C followed by total termination of blood flow in the entire body for up to 40 min. This time frame allows an experienced surgical team to perform essentially any complex aortic arch reconstruction. We advocate DHCA because it is an extremely safe, simple, and effective technique that does not require any additional complex perfusion adjuncts [91, 98, 99]. Table 23.8 presents the advantages and disadvantages of the three techniques for this critically important type of aortic surgery [91].

Surgical treatment of aneurysms of the descending and thoracoabdominal aorta allows a choice of performing either an open surgical replacement of the descending aorta with a tube graft or an endovascular procedure that involves the use of a stent-graft. According to the ACCF/AHA guidelines for patients with chronic dissection, particularly if associated with a connective tissue disorder but without significant comorbid disease and a descending thoracic aortic diameter exceeding 5.5 cm, open repair is recommended. For patients with degenerative or traumatic aneurysms of the descending thoracic aorta exceeding 5.5 cm, saccular aneurysms, or postoperative pseudoaneurysms, endovascular stent-grafting should be strongly considered when feasible. For patients with thoracoabdominal aneurysms, in whom endovascular stent-graft options are limited and surgical morbidity is elevated, elective surgery is recommended if the aortic diameter exceeds 6.0 cm, or even earlier if a connective tissue disorder such as Marfan or Loeys-Dietz syndrome is present [29, 84].

One of the main issues in surgery of the descending thoracic aorta is protection of the lower body organs during the period of time that the aorta is cross-clamped and the anastomoses are being established. The spinal cord is the organ most vulnerable to ischemia. Arterial blood supply of the spinal cord is segmental, and viability of the spinal cord cells can be dependent on an artery (arteria magna or artery of Adamkiewicz) or arteries arising from the low intercostal or lumbar territory (T8 to L2)—which is temporarily or permanently excluded in the process of thoracoabdominal surgery. Intraoperative perfusion of the lower body by blood aspirated from the left atrium appears to be helpful in combating paraplegia. Other techniques believed to be protective include mild systemic hypothermia, cerebrospinal fluid drainage to decrease ambient pressure on the spinal cord, and intercostal artery reimplantation [3, 29, 100, 101]. These techniques have decreased the frequency of the dreaded complication of paraplegia, but paraplegia has not by any means been eliminated, following either open or endovascular procedures, especially for extensive or re-operative resection.

Surgical Treatment of Acute Dissections of the Thoracic Aorta

A differentiated approach is required when dealing with different types of dissections. The current guidelines give the following recommendations regarding thoracic aortic dissections:

Acute thoracic ascending (Type A) aortic dissections require emergent surgical repair because of the high risk of associated life-threatening complications such as rupture, aortic insufficiency, or myocardial infarction from coronary artery involvement [29]. Emergent surgical treatment of acute ascending dissections usually includes replacement of the ascending aorta, in some cases together with replacement of the aortic valve and the dissected aortic arch.

Acute descending (Type B) aortic dissections should be managed medically by "anti-impulse" therapy with beta-blockers and afterload-reducing medications (discussed previously) unless life-threatening complications develop, such as malperfusion syndrome, progression of dissection, enlarging aneurysm, inability to control blood pressure, or continued symptoms (pain). Data from our institution shows that about two-thirds of patients with Type B dissections have a completely uncomplicated course of the disease on anti-impulse medical therapy alone. In cases, in which a life-threatening complication does develop, surgical intervention strategy should be determined by the "complication-specific" approach to descending aortic dissection [102, 103]:

- In cases of realized aortic rupture, the only appropriate surgical treatment is direct surgical aortic replacement with a tube graft (or a stent-graft) to prevent exsanguination. Stent-grafting is a viable surgical alternative.
- When the complication is organ ischemia from branch vessel occlusion, we favor the fenestration procedure, which is a method for decompressing the false lumen of the dissected aorta [104, 105]. This permits outflow of blood from the false lumen, reduces the intraluminal pressure, and relieves branch vessel obstruction. Fenestration can now be done by an endovascular as well as a surgical approach.
- Lastly, if the complication is threatened (impending) rupture (manifested by continued pain or rapid aortic expansion), surgical aortic replacement of the aorta is indicated. This can also be performed by an endovascular approach.

After successful management of the initial acute dissection, patients are observed closely for the first month, with repeat aortic imaging. After that point, it is uncommon for the dissection to extend, cause symptoms, or rupture in the short to midterm. The patients are then followed as chronic aneurysm patients. Over years, some will develop enlargement of the dissected aorta (now chronically dissected and aneurysmal) requiring resection [3].

Endovascular Treatment of Descending Thoracic Aortic Dissections

Endovascular therapy of aortic disease (thoracic and abdominal) is gaining popularity in the current enthusiasm for less invasive procedures. Recently a randomized study was conducted in Europe to evaluate stent therapy for patients doing well beyond 2 weeks after uncomplicated type B aortic dissection. The hope was that "tacking down" the dissection flap would lead to later benefit. Alas, the trial showed severe early mortality and complications subsequent to stent therapy. There was no survival advantage over medical therapy alone [28, 106]. Currently there is no evidence to substantiate the superiority of endovascular stent therapy over medical management for acute aortic dissections.

In general, in the rapidly developing field of endovascular interventions for thoracic aortic disease, we believe that the enthusiasm for stent therapy must be balanced against the tremendous advances in open therapy for thoracic aortic aneurysm, which has set a very high standard of safety and effectiveness [28, 107, 108]. Durability continues to be a problem for endovascular therapies, contrasted with the durability of open techniques [109, 110]. We must avoid "irrational exuberance" for endovascular therapies, restraining application for aneurysms that pose a true threat to a patient's longevity according to the symptom and size criteria enumerated above.

The current ACCF/AHA guidelines for the diagnosis and management of patients with thoracic aortic disease do not recommend any type of endovascular therapy for acute aortic dissections [29].

Key Points
- Aortic aneurysms are the 19th leading cause of death in all individuals and the 15th most common in individuals older than age 65 years. The estimated incidence of thoracic aortic aneurysm is approximately 10 per 100,000 patient years and is increasing for unknown reasons.
- The pathophysiology of aortic dilatation is historically attributed to cystic medial degeneration of the aortic wall which is characterized by disruption and loss of elastic fibers and increased deposition of proteoglycans. We now know that a complex interplay of genetics, proteolysis, inflammation, and smooth muscle cell death leads to aneurysm development.
- Thoracic aortic aneurysm is largely a genetic disease with strong familial inheritance patterns that produce manifest aneurysm is 21 % of family members of aneurysm patients.
- Although a virulent disease, thoracic aortic aneurysm is an indolent process. The aneurysmal thoracic aorta grows at approximately 0.1 cm/year.
- Aortic dissection is the most common cause of death related to the human aorta. Many of these deaths are misdiagnosed as myocardial infarction.

- Aortic dissection has been called "The Great Masquerader" because it can produce symptoms related to virtually any organ.
- Echocardiography, computed tomography, and magnetic resonance imaging are all informative noninvasive methods for diagnosing and evaluating thoracic aortic aneurysm.
- In asymptomatic patients with chronic aortic aneurysm, surgical treatment should be performed for the ascending aorta larger than 5.5 cm and for the descending aorta larger than 6.0 cm. Earlier intervention for Marfan and familial cases should be considered.
- Acute ascending aortic dissection (Type A) must be treated with emergent open surgical approach.
- Uncomplicated descending aortic dissections (Type B) should be treated medically by "anti-impulse" therapy with beta-blockers and afterload-reducing medications.
- Endovascular treatment has not been proven to be beneficial for Type B dissections as compared to medical treatment and is not recommended as an alternative for treatment of acute aortic dissections.

References

1. Osler W, Bean RB, Bean WB. Aphorisms from his bedside teachings and writings. Springfield: Thomas; 1961.
2. Elefteriades JA. Beating a sudden killer. Sci Am. 2005;293(2): 64–71.
3. Elefteriades JA. Thoracic aortic aneurysm: reading the enemy's playbook. Curr Probl Cardiol. 2008;33(5):203–77.
4. National Center for Injury Prevention and Control. WISQARS leading causes of death reports, 1999–2007. http://webappa.cdc.gov/sasweb/ncipc/leadcaus10.html. Accessed 10 Apr 2012.
5. Clouse WD, Hallett Jr JW, Schaff HV, Gayari MM, Ilstrup DM, Melton 3rd LJ. Improved prognosis of thoracic aortic aneurysms: a population-based study. JAMA. 1998;280(22):1926–9.
6. Clouse WD, Hallett Jr JW, Schaff HV, et al. Acute aortic dissection: population-based incidence compared with degenerative aortic aneurysm rupture. Mayo Clin Proc. 2004;79(2):176–80.
7. Acosta S, Ogren M, Bengtsson H, Bergqvist D, Lindblad B, Zdanowski Z. Increasing incidence of ruptured abdominal aortic aneurysm: a population-based study. J Vasc Surg. 2006;44(2): 237–43.
8. Johnston KW, Rutherford RB, Tilson MD, Shah DM, Hollier L, Stanley JC. Suggested standards for reporting on arterial aneurysms. Subcommittee on Reporting Standards for Arterial Aneurysms, Ad Hoc Committee on Reporting Standards, Society for Vascular Surgery and North American chapter, International Society for Cardiovascular Surgery. J Vasc Surg. 1991;13(3): 452–8.
9. He R, Guo DC, Estrera AL, et al. Characterization of the inflammatory and apoptotic cells in the aortas of patients with ascending thoracic aortic aneurysms and dissections. J Thorac Cardiovasc Surg. 2006;131(3):671–8.
10. Tang PC, Coady MA, Lovoulos C, et al. Hyperplastic cellular remodeling of the media in ascending thoracic aortic aneurysms. Circulation. 2005;112(8):1098–105.
11. Koullias GJ, Ravichandran P, Korkolis DP, Rimm DL, Elefteriades JA. Increased tissue microarray matrix metalloproteinase expression favors proteolysis in thoracic aortic aneurysms and dissections. Ann Thorac Surg. 2004;78(6):2106–10.
12. Sinha I, Bethi S, Cronin P, et al. A biologic basis for asymmetric growth in descending thoracic aortic aneurysms: a role for matrix metalloproteinase 9 and 2. J Vasc Surg. 2006;43(2):342–8.
13. Thompson RW, Parks WC. Role of matrix metalloproteinases in abdominal aortic aneurysms. Ann N Y Acad Sci. 1996;800: 157–74.
14. McMillan WD, Pearce WH. Increased plasma levels of metalloproteinase-9 are associated with abdominal aortic aneurysms. J Vasc Surg. 1999;29(1):122–7; discussion 127–9.
15. Mao D, Lee JK, VanVickle SJ, Thompson RW. Expression of collagenase-3 (MMP-13) in human abdominal aortic aneurysms and vascular smooth muscle cells in culture. Biochem Biophys Res Commun. 1999;261(3):904–10.
16. Hackmann AE, Thompson RW, LeMaire SA. Long term suppressive therapy: clinical reality and future prospects. In: Elefteriades JA, editor. Acute aortic disease, vol. 61. New York: Informa Healthcare; 2007. p. 309–30.
17. LeMaire SA, Wang X, Wilks JA, et al. Matrix metalloproteinases in ascending aortic aneurysms: bicuspid versus trileaflet aortic valves. J Surg Res. 2005;123(1):40–8.
18. Ikonomidis JS, Jones JA, Barbour JR, et al. Expression of matrix metalloproteinases and endogenous inhibitors within ascending aortic aneurysms of patients with bicuspid or tricuspid aortic valves. J Thorac Cardiovasc Surg. 2007;133(4):1028–36.
19. Elefteriades JA. Thoracic aortic aneurysm: reading the enemy's playbook. Yale J Biol Med. 2008;81(4):175–86.
20. Ince H, Nienaber CA. Etiology, pathogenesis and management of thoracic aortic aneurysm. Nat Clin Pract Cardiovasc Med. 2007; 4(8):418–27.
21. Zarins CK, Glagov S, Vesselinovitch D, Wissler RW. Aneurysm formation in experimental atherosclerosis: relationship to plaque evolution. J Vasc Surg. 1990;12(3):246–56.
22. Reed D, Reed C, Stemmermann G, Hayashi T. Are aortic aneurysms caused by atherosclerosis? Circulation. 1992;85(1): 205–11.
23. Agmon Y, Khandheria BK, Meissner I, et al. Is aortic dilatation an atherosclerosis-related process? Clinical, laboratory, and transesophageal echocardiographic correlates of thoracic aortic dimensions in the population with implications for thoracic aortic aneurysm formation. J Am Coll Cardiol. 2003;42(6):1076–83.
24. Silence J, Collen D, Lijnen HR. Reduced atherosclerotic plaque but enhanced aneurysm formation in mice with inactivation of the tissue inhibitor of metalloproteinase-1 (TIMP-1) gene. Circ Res. 2002;90(8):897–903.
25. Achneck H, Modi B, Shaw C, et al. Ascending thoracic aneurysms are associated with decreased systemic atherosclerosis. Chest. 2005;128(3):1580–6.
26. Estrera AL, Miller CC, Azizzadeh A, Safi HJ. Thoracic aortic aneurysms. Acta Chir Belg. 2006;106(3):307–16.
27. Zarins CK, Xu C, Glagov S. Atherosclerotic enlargement of the human abdominal aorta. Atherosclerosis. 2001;155(1):157–64.
28. Elefteriades JA, Farkas EA. Thoracic aortic aneurysm clinically pertinent controversies and uncertainties. J Am Coll Cardiol. 2010;55(9):841–57.
29. Hiratzka LF, Bakris GL, Beckman JA, et al. ACCF/AHA/AATS/ACR/ASA/SCA/SCAI/SIR/STS/SVM guidelines for the diagnosis and management of patients with thoracic aortic disease. A report of the American College of Cardiology Foundation/American Heart Association Task Force on practice guidelines,

American Association for Thoracic Surgery, American College of Radiology, American Stroke Association, Society of Cardiovascular Anesthesiologists, Society for Cardiovascular Angiography and Interventions, Society of Interventional Radiology, Society of Thoracic Surgeons, and Society for Vascular Medicine. J Am Coll Cardiol. 2010;55(14):e27–129.

30. Coady MA, Davies RR, Roberts M, et al. Familial patterns of thoracic aortic aneurysms. Arch Surg. 1999;134(4):361–7.

31. Albornoz G, Coady MA, Roberts M, et al. Familial thoracic aortic aneurysms and dissections – incidence, modes of inheritance, and phenotypic patterns. Ann Thorac Surg. 2006;82(4):1400–5.

32. Biddinger A, Rocklin M, Coselli J, Milewicz DM. Familial thoracic aortic dilatations and dissections: a case control study. J Vasc Surg. 1997;25(3):506–11.

33. Milewicz DM, Michael K, Fisher N, Coselli JS, Markello T, Biddinger A. Fibrillin-1 (FBN1) mutations in patients with thoracic aortic aneurysms. Circulation. 1996;94(11):2708–11.

34. Putnam EA, Zhang H, Ramirez F, Milewicz DM. Fibrillin-2 (FBN2) mutations result in the Marfan-like disorder, congenital contractural arachnodactyly. Nat Genet. 1995;11(4):456–8.

35. Hasham SN, Willing MC, Guo DC, et al. Mapping a locus for familial thoracic aortic aneurysms and dissections (TAAD2) to 3p24-25. Circulation. 2003;107(25):3184–90.

36. Hasham SN, Lewin MR, Tran VT, et al. Nonsyndromic genetic predisposition to aortic dissection: a newly recognized, diagnosable, and preventable occurrence in families. Ann Emerg Med. 2004;43(1):79–82.

37. Guo DC, Pannu H, Tran-Fadulu V, et al. Mutations in smooth muscle alpha-actin (ACTA2) lead to thoracic aortic aneurysms and dissections. Nat Genet. 2007;39(12):1488–93.

38. Wang L, Guo DC, Cao J, et al. Mutations in myosin light chain kinase cause familial aortic dissections. Am J Hum Genet. 2010;87(5):701–7.

39. Wang Y, Barbacioru CC, Shiffman D, et al. Gene expression signature in peripheral blood detects thoracic aortic aneurysm. PLoS One. 2007;2(10):e1050.

40. Ward C. Clinical significance of the bicuspid aortic valve. Heart. 2000;83(1):81–5.

41. Russo CF, Mazzetti S, Garatti A, et al. Aortic complications after bicuspid aortic valve replacement: long-term results. Ann Thorac Surg. 2002;74(5):S1773–6; discussion S1792–9.

42. Borger MA, Preston M, Ivanov J, et al. Should the ascending aorta be replaced more frequently in patients with bicuspid aortic valve disease? J Thorac Cardiovasc Surg. 2004;128(5):677–83.

43. Fedak PW, David TE, Borger M, Verma S, Butany J, Weisel RD. Bicuspid aortic valve disease: recent insights in pathophysiology and treatment. Expert Rev Cardiovasc Ther. 2005;3(2):295–308.

44. Cecconi M, Nistri S, Quarti A, et al. Aortic dilatation in patients with bicuspid aortic valve. J Cardiovasc Med (Hagerstown). 2006;7(1):11–20.

45. Davies RR, Kaple RK, Mandapati D, et al. Natural history of ascending aortic aneurysms in the setting of an unreplaced bicuspid aortic valve. Ann Thorac Surg. 2007;83(4):1338–44.

46. Friedman T, Mani A, Elefteriades JA. Bicuspid aortic valve: clinical approach and scientific review of a common clinical entity. Expert Rev Cardiovasc Ther. 2008;6(2):235–48.

47. Michelena HI, Khanna AD, Mahoney D, et al. Incidence of aortic complications in patients with bicuspid aortic valves. JAMA. 2011;306(10):1104–12.

48. Nathan DP, Xu C, Plappert T, et al. Increased ascending aortic wall stress in patients with bicuspid aortic valves. Ann Thorac Surg. 2011;92(4):1384–9.

49. Elefteriades JA, Rizzo JA. Epidemiology: incidence, prevalence, and trends. In: Elefteriades JA, editor. Acute aortic disease, vol. 61. New York: Informa Healthcare; 2007. p. 89–97.

50. Coady MA, Rizzo JA, Hammond GL, et al. What is the appropriate size criterion for resection of thoracic aortic aneurysms? J Thorac Cardiovasc Surg. 1997;113(3):476–91.

51. Coady MA, Rizzo JA, Goldstein LJ, Elefteriades JA. Natural history, pathogenesis, and etiology of thoracic aortic aneurysms and dissections. Cardiol Clin. 1999;17(4):615–35.

52. Elefteriades JA. Natural history of thoracic aortic aneurysms: indications for surgery, and surgical versus nonsurgical risks. Ann Thorac Surg. 2002;74(5):S1877–80.

53. Anagnostopoulos CE. Acute aortic dissections. Baltimore: University Park Press; 1975.

54. Elefteriades JA, Geha AS, Cohen LS. House officer guide to ICU care: fundamentals of management of the heart and lungs. 2nd ed. New York: Raven; 1994.

55. Hatzaras IS, Bible JE, Koullias GJ, Tranquilli M, Singh M, Elefteriades JA. Role of exertion or emotion as inciting events for acute aortic dissection. Am J Cardiol. 2007;100(9):1470–2.

56. Elefteriades JA. Timing of acute aortic events: how does dissection pick a date, time and moment to occur? In: Elefteriades JA, editor. Acute aortic disease, vol. 61. New York: Informa Healthcare; 2007. p. 169–71.

57. Hagan PG, Nienaber CA, Isselbacher EM, et al. The international registry of acute aortic dissection (IRAD): new insights into an old disease. JAMA. 2000;283(7):897–903.

58. Thrumurthy SG, Karthikesalingam A, Patterson BO, Holt PJ, Thompson MM. The diagnosis and management of aortic dissection. BMJ. 2011;344:d8290.

59. Isselbacher EM. The symptoms and signs of acute aortic dissection: clinical diagnosis of "the great masquerader". In: Elefteriades JA, editor. Acute aortic disease, vol. 61. New York: Informa Healthcare; 2007. p. 29–38.

60. Elefteriades JA, Barrett PW, Kopf GS. Litigation in nontraumatic aortic diseases – a tempest in the malpractice maelstrom. Cardiology. 2008;109(4):263–72.

61. von Kodolitsch Y, Schwartz AG, Nienaber CA. Clinical prediction of acute aortic dissection. Arch Intern Med. 2000;160(19):2977–82.

62. Nienaber CA, Eagle KA. Aortic dissection: new frontiers in diagnosis and management: part I: from etiology to diagnostic strategies. Circulation. 2003;108(5):628–35.

63. Trimarchi S, Sangiorgi G, Sang X, et al. In search of blood tests for thoracic aortic diseases. Ann Thorac Surg. 2010;90(5):1735–42.

64. American College of Emergency Physicians Clinical Policies Committee, Clinical Policies Committee Subcommittee on Suspected Pulmonary Embolism. Clinical policy: critical issues in the evaluation and management of adult patients presenting with suspected pulmonary embolism. Ann Emerg Med. 2003;41(2):257–70.

65. Weber T, Hogler S, Auer J, et al. D-dimer in acute aortic dissection. Chest. 2003;123(5):1375–8.

66. Eggebrecht H, Naber CK, Bruch C, et al. Value of plasma fibrin D-dimers for detection of acute aortic dissection. J Am Coll Cardiol. 2004;44(4):804–9.

67. Akutsu K, Sato N, Yamamoto T, et al. A rapid bedside D-dimer assay (cardiac D-dimer) for screening of clinically suspected acute aortic dissection. Circ J. 2005;69(4):397–403.

68. Ohlmann P, Faure A, Morel O, et al. Diagnostic and prognostic value of circulating D-dimers in patients with acute aortic dissection. Crit Care Med. 2006;34(5):1358–64.

69. Marill KA. Serum D-dimer is a sensitive test for the detection of acute aortic dissection: a pooled meta-analysis. J Emerg Med. 2008;34(4):367–76.

70. Shimony A, Filion KB, Mottillo S, Dourian T, Eisenberg MJ. Meta-analysis of usefulness of D-dimer to diagnose acute aortic dissection. Am J Cardiol. 2011;107(8):1227–34.

71. Danias PG. Imaging of aneurysms and dissections: chest X-ray, echo, computed tomography, magnetic resonance imaging. In: Elefteriades JA, editor. Acute aortic disease, vol. 61. New York: Informa Healthcare; 2007. p. 39–61.

72. Raghupathy A, Eagle K. Putting it all together: symptoms, signs, and images. In: Elefteriades JA, editor. Acute aortic disease, vol. 61. New York: Informa Healthcare; 2007. p. 67–86.

73. Elefteriades JA, Rizzo JA, Coady MA. Thoracic aorta. Radiology. 1999;211(3):889.

74. Ogden LG, He J, Lydick E, Whelton PK. Long-term absolute benefit of lowering blood pressure in hypertensive patients according to the JNC VI risk stratification. Hypertension. 2000;35(2):539–43.

75. Neal B, MacMahon S, Chapman N. Blood Pressure Lowering Treatment Trialists' Collaboration. Effects of ACE inhibitors, calcium antagonists, and other blood-pressure-lowering drugs: results of prospectively designed overviews of randomised trials. Blood pressure lowering treatment trialists' collaboration. Lancet. 2000;356(9246):1955–64.

76. Hunt SA, Baker DW, Chin MH, et al. ACC/AHA guidelines for the evaluation and management of chronic heart failure in the adult: executive summary. A report of the American College of Cardiology/American Heart Association Task Force on practice guidelines (committee to revise the 1995 guidelines for the evaluation and management of heart failure). J Am Coll Cardiol. 2001;38(7):2101–13.

77. ALLHAT Officers and Coordinators for the ALLHAT Collaborative Research Group. The Antihypertensive and Lipid-Lowering Treatment to Prevent Heart Attack Trial. Major outcomes in high-risk hypertensive patients randomized to angiotensin-converting enzyme inhibitor or calcium channel blocker vs diuretic: the antihypertensive and lipid-lowering treatment to prevent heart attack trial (ALLHAT). JAMA. 2002;288(23):2981–97.

78. Lewington S, Clarke R, Qizilbash N, Peto R, Collins R. Prospective Studies Collaboration. Age-specific relevance of usual blood pressure to vascular mortality: a meta-analysis of individual data for one million adults in 61 prospective studies. Lancet. 2002; 360(9349):1903–13.

79. Kurzencwyg D, Filion KB, Pilote L, et al. Cardiac medical therapy among patients undergoing abdominal aortic aneurysm repair. Ann Vasc Surg. 2006;20(5):569–76.

80. Leurs LJ, Visser P, Laheij RJ, Buth J, Harris PL, Blankensteijn JD. Statin use is associated with reduced all-cause mortality after endovascular abdominal aortic aneurysm repair. Vascular. 2006;14(1):1–8.

81. Evans J, Powell JT, Schwalbe E, Loftus IM, Thompson MM. Simvastatin attenuates the activity of matrix metalloprotease-9 in aneurysmal aortic tissue. Eur J Vasc Endovasc Surg. 2007;34(3): 302–3.

82. Jovin IS, Duggal M, Ebisu K, et al. Comparison of the effect on long-term outcomes in patients with thoracic aortic aneurysms of taking versus not taking a statin drug. Am J Cardiol. 2012;109(7):1050–4.

83. Danyi P, Elefteriades JA, Jovin IS. Medical therapy of thoracic aortic aneurysms: are we there yet? Circulation. 2011;124(13): 1469–76.

84. Svensson LG, Kouchoukos NT, Miller DC, et al. Expert consensus document on the treatment of descending thoracic aortic disease using endovascular stent-grafts. Ann Thorac Surg. 2008;85 (1 Suppl):S1–41.

85. Sanz J, Einstein AJ, Fuster V. Acute aortic dissection: anti-impulse therapy. In: Elefteriades JA, editor. Acute aortic disease, vol. 61. New York: Informa Healthcare; 2007. p. 229–48.

86. Yacoub MH, Gehle P, Chandrasekaran V, Birks EJ, Child A, Radley-Smith R. Late results of a valve-preserving operation in patients with aneurysms of the ascending aorta and root. J Thorac Cardiovasc Surg. 1998;115(5):1080–90.

87. David TE, Ivanov J, Armstrong S, Feindel CM, Webb GD. Aortic valve-sparing operations in patients with aneurysms of the aortic root or ascending aorta. Ann Thorac Surg. 2002;74(5):S1758–61; discussion S1792–9.

88. de Oliveira NC, David TE, Ivanov J, et al. Results of surgery for aortic root aneurysm in patients with Marfan syndrome. J Thorac Cardiovasc Surg. 2003;125(4):789–96.

89. David TE, Maganti M, Armstrong S. Aortic root aneurysm: principles of repair and long-term follow-up. J Thorac Cardiovasc Surg. 2010;140(6 Suppl):S14–9; discussion S45–51.

90. Zafar MA, Farkas EA, Javier A, Anderson M, Gilani O, Elefteriades JA. Are thromboembolic and bleeding complications a drawback for composite aortic root replacement? Ann Thorac Surg. 2012;94(3):737–43.

91. Ziganshin B, Elefteriades JA. Does straight deep hypothermic circulatory arrest suffice for brain preservation in aortic surgery? Semin Thorac Cardiovasc Surg. 2010;22(4):291–301.

92. Stein LH, Elefteriades JA. Protecting the brain during aortic surgery: an enduring debate with unanswered questions. J Cardiothorac Vasc Anesth. 2010;24(2):316–21.

93. Ergin MA, Griepp EB, Lansman SL, Galla JD, Levy M, Griepp RB. Hypothermic circulatory arrest and other methods of cerebral protection during operations on the thoracic aorta. J Card Surg. 1994;9(5):525–37.

94. Reich DL, Uysal S, Ergin MA, Griepp RB. Retrograde cerebral perfusion as a method of neuroprotection during thoracic aortic surgery. Ann Thorac Surg. 2001;72(5):1774–82.

95. Di Eusanio M, Schepens MA, Morshuis WJ, Di Bartolomeo R, Pierangeli A, Dossche KM. Antegrade selective cerebral perfusion during operations on the thoracic aorta: factors influencing survival and neurologic outcome in 413 patients. J Thorac Cardiovasc Surg. 2002;124(6):1080–6.

96. Ogino H, Sasaki H, Minatoya K, et al. Evolving arch surgery using integrated antegrade selective cerebral perfusion: impact of axillary artery perfusion. J Thorac Cardiovasc Surg. 2008;136(3):641–8; discussion 948–9.

97. Sundt 3rd TM, Orszulak TA, Cook DJ, Schaff HV. Improving results of open arch replacement. Ann Thorac Surg. 2008;86(3):787–96; discussion 787–96.

98. Gega A, Rizzo JA, Johnson MH, Tranquilli M, Farkas EA, Elefteriades JA. Straight deep hypothermic arrest: experience in 394 patients supports its effectiveness as a sole means of brain preservation. Ann Thorac Surg. 2007;84(3):759–66; discussion 766–7.

99. Percy A, Widman S, Rizzo JA, Tranquilli M, Elefteriades JA. Deep hypothermic circulatory arrest in patients with high cognitive needs: full preservation of cognitive abilities. Ann Thorac Surg. 2009;87(1):117–23.

100. Hilgenberg AD. Spinal cord protection for thoracic aortic surgery. Cardiol Clin. 1999;17(4):807–13, x.

101. Elefteriades JA, Coady MA, Nikas DJ, Kopf GS, Gusberg RJ. "Cobrahead" graft for intercostal artery implantation during descending aortic replacement. Ann Thorac Surg. 2000;69(4):1282–4.

102. Elefteriades JA, Hartleroad J, Gusberg RJ, et al. Long-term experience with descending aortic dissection: the complication-specific approach. Ann Thorac Surg. 1992;53(1):11–20; discussion 20–1.

103. Elefteriades JA, Lovoulos CJ, Coady MA, Tellides G, Kopf GS, Rizzo JA. Management of descending aortic dissection. Ann Thorac Surg. 1999;67(6):2002–5; discussion 2014–19.

104. Elefteriades JA, Hammond GL, Gusberg RJ, Kopf GS, Baldwin JC. Fenestration revisited. A safe and effective procedure for descending aortic dissection. Arch Surg. 1990;125(6):786–90.

105. Pradhan S, Elefteriades JA, Sumpio BE. Utility of the aortic fenestration technique in the management of acute aortic dissections. Ann Thorac Cardiovasc Surg. 2007;13(5):296–300.

106. Nienaber CA, Rousseau H, Eggebrecht H, et al. Randomized comparison of strategies for type B aortic dissection: The INvestigation of STEnt grafts in aortic dissection (INSTEAD) trial. Circulation. 2009;120(25):2519–28.

107. Achneck HE, Rizzo JA, Tranquilli M, Elefteriades JA. Safety of thoracic aortic surgery in the present era. Ann Thorac Surg. 2007;84(4):1180–5.

108. Clagett GP. EVAR, TEVAR, FEVAR, too far? Perspect Vasc Surg Endovasc Ther. 2008;20(2):115–9.

109. EVAR trial participants. Endovascular aneurysm repair and outcome in patients unfit for open repair of abdominal aortic aneurysm (EVAR trial 2): randomised controlled trial. Lancet. 2005;365(9478):2187–92.

110. De Bruin JL, Baas AF, Buth J, et al. Long-term outcome of open or endovascular repair of abdominal aortic aneurysm. N Engl J Med. 2010;362(20):1881–9.

Cardiovascular Issues and Renal Disease

24

Firas Yazigi, Usman Hashmi, Henry Yuan, Karthiek Narala, and Peter A. McCullough

Abstract

The increasing prevalence of both chronic kidney disease (CKD) and cardiovascular disease requires a better understanding by physicians in practice. The regular emergence of newer data continues to support the unique and complex interaction between the kidney and the heart. CKD has been associated with increased risk of in-hospital death and major bleeding in patients with acute coronary syndromes (ACS). A higher level of risk stratification is required for these patients. Contrast-induced acute kidney injury requires a comprehensive management strategy in patients receiving percutaneous therapy for ACS. Patients with CKD are susceptible to cardiorenal syndromes which complicate bidirectional organ dysfunction and are particularly challenging to manage. Treatment and prevention methods continue to be adjusted to better incorporate the new improvements and recommendations in everyday clinical practice. In light of newer guidelines, nephrologists and cardiologists must work in tandem for better diagnosis and management. Imaging and laboratory diagnostic testing are now being utilized with better insight pertinent to each disease process. Medications and dosages must be adjusted with respect to the underlying physiology and pathophysiology of the two entities. Certain cardiovascular diseases (VHD, arrhythmias, PAD) are being looked at from a different angle, hoping for improvements in therapies. Further advances in the understanding of pathophysiological mechanisms at work in patients with CKD will continue to lead to new diagnostic and therapeutic targets in this high-risk population.

Keywords

Chronic kidney disease • Cardiovascular disease • Dialysis • Acute kidney injury • Renal transplant • Valvular heart disease • Cardiorenal syndrome • Peripheral arterial disease

F. Yazigi, MD (✉) • U. Hashmi, MD
Department of Cardiology, St. John Providence Health System,
22101 Moross Rd., 2nd Floor, VEP Cath Lab,
Detroit, MI 48236, USA
e-mail: firas.yazigi@stjohn.org; usman.hashmi@stjohn.org

H. Yuan, MD
Department of Nephrology, Johns Hopkins Hospital,
22101 Moross Rd., 2nd Floor, VEP Cath Lab,
Detroit, MI 48236, USA
e-mail: henry.yuan@stjohn.org

K. Narala, MD
Department of Internal Medicine, St. John Providence Health
System, 22101 Moross Rd., 2nd Floor, VEP Cath Lab,
Detroit, MI 48236, USA
e-mail: karthiek.narala@stjohn.org

P.A. McCullough, MD, MPH, FACC, FACP, FAHA
Department of Providence Park Clinical Research,
St. John Providence Health System,
47601 Grand River, B125, Novi, MI 48374, USA
e-mail: peteramccullough@gmail.com

K. Stergiopoulos, D.L. Brown (eds.), *Evidence-Based Cardiology Consult*,
DOI 10.1007/978-1-4471-4441-0_24, © Springer-Verlag London 2014

Introduction: Heart Disease and the Kidney

Chronic kidney disease (CKD) was estimated to affect more than 20 million Americans in 2010 [1]. Approximately half a million patients in the USA were established on dialysis treatment by the end of 2008 with a mortality rate approaching 151.7 deaths per 1,000 patient years, contributing to health costs exceeding 39.5 billion in public and private spending for the end-stage renal disease (ESRD) program [2]. Of all causes of deaths in the USA in 2006, 26 % – or more than 1 in every 4 – were caused by heart disease [3]. Higher cardiovascular and all-cause mortality increase exponentially as glomerular filtration rate (GFR) declines, with the largest increase seen when GFR drops below 60 ml/min/1.73 m^2 [4]. Besides sharing this high disease prevalence, the heart and kidney also share a very unique and interactive relationship that allows for the control of the body hemodynamic functions and maintenance of homeostasis. A complex regulatory network that includes the renin-angiotensin-aldosterone system, autonomic nervous system, and the natriuretic peptides connects these two organs to facilitate a precise physiologic response to different circumstances. Hypertension (HTN) and diabetes mellitus (DM) affect both the heart and the kidney, leading to combined CKD and cardiovascular disease (CVD). Approximately, 50 % of cases of ESRD are attributed to DM. In addition to the other traditional cardiac risk factors, patients with renal disease develop a constant proinflammatory and prothrombotic state [5]. Recent evidence proves CKD to be an independent risk factor for the development of coronary artery disease (CAD) and to be associated with a worse prognosis from CVD [6, 7]. This unique interaction has its own implications in terms of understanding the pathology, pathophysiology, and disease manifestation of CVD in CKD patients.

Acute Coronary Syndromes in Patients with CKD

Chronic kidney disease has been associated with increased risk of in-hospital death and major bleeding in patients with acute coronary syndromes (ACS). Additionally, patients with renal dysfunction often have more comorbidities and are less likely to receive guideline-based therapies [8]. Moreover, patients with advanced kidney disease are less likely to be included in trials studying ACS [9]. It has been demonstrated that patients with CKD presenting to the emergency department with chest pain have a 40 % cardiovascular event rate at 30 days [10].

A higher level of risk stratification is required for these patients, not only for the acute cardiac condition they present with but also for potential complications that can result from

therapy implemented in the form of medications and/or invasive testing.

Platelet dysfunction and potential dosing errors in the setting of anticoagulant use place these patients at higher risk of bleeding [11]. Coronary angiography carries the risk of contrast-induced acute kidney injury (CI-AKI), while percutaneous coronary intervention (PCI) in this population is associated with higher rates of complications including bleeding, thrombosis, and procedural failure [12].

While the latest 2007 American College of Cardiology/American Heart Association guidelines briefly describe patients with renal disease as a unique subset of patients who experience ACS, a more detailed overview can be found in the 2011 European Guidelines. A unifying theme in both guidelines is the importance of integrating renal function into treatment decisions (as many drugs for ACS are renally eliminated) and for risk stratification. Chronic kidney disease is classified into five distinct stages by The National Kidney Foundation and is best categorized according to GFR calculated by the MDRD equation. Commonly in clinical practice, creatinine clearance is used in place of GFR. Creatinine is the by-product of muscle metabolism. Thus, lower body weight (less muscle mass), advanced age, and women require special consideration when using it as a biomarker, as levels may not closely reflect actual kidney function.

This categorization of renal function allows for the appropriate selection of drugs and proper dose adjustments based on renal function. Drugs which may be contraindicated or require dose reduction based on impaired kidney function include low molecular weight heparin (LMWH), fondaparinux, bivalirudin, and glycoprotein IIb/IIIa inhibitors [13].

Presentation and Diagnosis of ACS in CKD Patients: Biomarkers

Patients with CKD may have elevated cardiac biomarkers such as troponins and creatinine kinase without the clinical suspicion for ACS. The mechanism for nonischemic, chronic troponin elevation in CKD is not fully understood and has been associated with chronic uremic skeletal myopathy [14], clinically unrecognized silent micro-infarctions, heart failure [15], and left ventricular hypertrophy (LVH) [16]. At this time, it has not been reliably demonstrated that troponin elevation is due to decreased renal clearance by the diseased kidney. For example, in a transplanted kidney with improved renal function, troponin elevation may still be seen [17].

Additionally, the clinician must recognize the potential for silent ischemia and atypical presentations of CAD in CKD patients [18]. In fact, one study found that only 17 % of patients with ESRD experienced angina [19]. Electrocardiogram (ECG) data can be difficult to interpret in the setting of LVH and the electrolyte and conduction disturbances common in these patients [20]. Data from large biomarker trials have excluded patients with renal failure even though there is clear data supporting increased risk and mortality with troponin elevation [21].

Troponin-T (TnT) elevation is seen in 53 % of patients with renal failure without clinical features of ACS [20], while troponin-I (TnI) is not as frequently elevated. This fact, along with the potentially more cardiac-specific nature of TnI, may suggest that TnI may be a more reliable biomarker for cardiac necrosis in patients with renal insufficiency [22]. In addition, TnI was found to decrease by 86 % after dialysis, whereas TnT levels increased [23].

The recommended biomarker-guided strategy at this time for diagnosing and managing myocardial injury in CKD/ESRD patients should be the serial measurement of troponins with attention to the trend in values. Also, TnI may have more reliability in patients with CKD when compared to cTnT.

Medical Therapy for ACS in CKD

In the absence of contraindications, patients with CKD should receive the same guideline-based therapies for ACS as other patients. Angiotensin converting enzyme (ACE) inhibitors and statins have been shown to reduce cardiovascular event risk in subgroups of patients with renal dysfunction. Aspirin, beta-blockers, ACE inhibitors, angiotensin receptor blockers, aldosterone receptor antagonists, and statins have demonstrated favorable outcomes in patients with renal dysfunction and should be utilized per guidelines.

The most commonly used thienopyridenes clopidogrel (Plavix), prasugrel (Effient), and ticagrelor do not require dose modification. Interestingly, patients with severe renal impairment (clearance 5–15 ml/min) and moderate renal impairment (clearance 30–60 ml/min) showed lower inhibition (25 %) of platelet aggregation when on clopidogrel [24]. The Study of Platelet Inhibition and Patient Outcomes (PLATO) trial population included those with CKD but excluded dialysis patients, showing more absolute benefit and a greater reduction of ischemic events with ticagrelor compared with clopidogrel in patients with advanced CKD [25].

Enoxaparin in patients with renal insufficiency (creatinine >2.5 mg/dl, creatinine clearance of <30 cc/min) requires dose adjustment. Dosing can be monitored with anti-factor Xa levels, and if the assay is unavailable, patients should be switched to unfractionated heparin. The Global Registry of Acute Coronary Events (GRACE) showed an increased risk of bleeding with unfractionated heparin (UFH) similar to that of LMWH in patients with renal dysfunction [26]. When

fondaparinux was compared with enoxaparin in patients with severe renal dysfunction, data from the Fifth Organization to Assess Strategies in Acute Ischemic Syndromes (OASIS-5) showed a lower risk of bleeding complications. Bivalirudin (Angiomax) is currently the only direct thrombin inhibitor approved for the treatment of ACS. Renal clearance of Angiomax was reduced approximately 20 % in patients with moderate to severe renal impairment and was decreased 80 % in dialysis patients. No reduction in bolus dose is needed for any level of renal dysfunction.

Clinical trials and guidelines continue to support glycoprotein IIb/IIIa inhibitors (GPI) in high-risk patients with ACS in whom PCI is planned (Class I, Level A) [27]. There are currently three available GPI in the USA. All three require a careful clinical assessment of bleeding risk prior to use in patients with renal failure. Abciximab (ReoPro) is the only GPI that does not require dose adjustment for renal function. Fifty percent of eptifibatide (Integrilin) is cleared renally in patients with renal failure; thus, a dose reduction of the infusion to 1 µg/kg/min is recommended in patients with CrCl <50 m/min, and the drug's use is contraindicated in patients with CrCl <30 ml/min. Tirofiban requires dose reduction, for a CrCl <30 ml/min. The infusion dose should be decreased by 50 % (Tables 24.1, 24.2, and 24.3).

Revascularization Therapy in CKD Patients with ACS

Percutaneous coronary revascularization leads to better long-term survival in patients with CKD presenting with ACS [41]. When readily available, PCI continues to be the treatment of choice despite presence of CKD for acute ST-segment elevation MI [42]. In a recent meta-analysis, benefit was seen in patients with CKD 3 and CKD 4 (though underrepresented) for an early invasive therapy for non-ST elevation MI and/or unstable angina, while CKD 5 patients were not included [43]. A Swedish study suggests harm with an early invasive strategy for CKD 5 patients [44].

Adequately powered randomized clinical trials comparing surgical revascularization versus PCI in patients with advanced renal disease are lacking. The ARTS-1 (Arterial Revascularization Therapies Study) found no significant difference in the endpoints of death, MI, or stroke when comparing PCI and coronary artery bypass graft surgery (CABG) in 290 patients with CrCl <60 ml/min, though markedly lower revascularization rates were seen in the CABG arm [45].

Chronic kidney disease patients have increased operative complication risks. Death after CABG is 9–12.2 % in CKD 5 patients and three to seven times higher in CKD4-5 patients versus non-CKD patients. A more recent study showed a 71 % decrease in risk of death in ESRD patients

Table 24.1 Oral agents used for chronic coronary disease and acute coronary syndrome

Class	Medication	Normal dose	CKD patient population	Notes
Antiplatelet	Aspirin	Acute MI 160–325 mg PO as soon as possible	All dialysis patients with CAD not allergic to aspirin should receive aspirin	Metabolism: liver, microsomal enzyme system
		MI prophylaxis 81–162 mg PO daily	Withholding aspirin before surgery is usually unnecessary	Renal clearance: 80–100 % 24–72 h
		PTCA 325 mg PO 2 h presurgery, then 160–325 mg PO maintenance	There are no data on use of aspirin in primary prevention of CVD in dialysis patients	Excretion: principally in urine (80–100 %), sweat, saliva, feces
		Unstable angina 75–162 mg PO daily		
Antiplatelet (ADP receptor antagonists)	Clopidogrel (Plavix)	Unstable angina, non-ST-segment elevation myocardial infarction 300–600 mg initial loading dose, follow by 75 mg PO daily in combination with aspirin ST-segment elevation myocardial infarction 75 mg PO daily in combination with aspirin 75–162 mg/day Recent MI 75 mg PO daily	No specific dosing adjustments in CKD patients	Metabolism: CYP3A4, CYP2C19 (predominantly), and others to generate active metabolite; also by esterase to an inactive metabolite Excretion: urine and feces
	Prasugrel (Effient)	Acute coronary syndrome Loading dose: 60 mg PO once Maintenance dose: 10 mg PO daily with aspirin 81–325 mg/day; bleeding risk may increase if weight <60 kg – consider 5 mg PO daily (efficacy/safety not established)	No specific dose adjustments Increased risk of bleeding, monitor closely	Metabolism: liver; CYP450 such as 2B6, 2C9/19 (minor), and 3A4 substrate; 2B6 (weak) inhibitor Excretion: urine (68 %) and feces (27 %)
ACE inhibitors			The dosing schedules may need to be individualized for each dialysis session in order to avoid intradialytic hypotension	
ARBs			As a first-line of treatment in the majority of patients, we propose the use of ACE inhibitors or ARBs. The latter also reduce LVH in hemodialysis patients, and may be more potent than ACE inhibitors [28, 29] Levels of ARBs do not change significantly during hemodialysis	
Beta-blockers			Hemodialysis reduces blood levels of atenolol, acebutolol, and nadolol; by contrast, levels of carvedilol and labetalol do not change significantly	
	Metoprolol (Lopressor)	Acute MI Metoprolol tartrate: 2.5–5 mg rapid IV q2–5 min, up to 15 mg over 10–15 min, then 15 min after last IV and receiving 15 mg IV	No specific dose adjustments	Dialyzable: yes Metabolism: hepatic CYP2D6
		Or 50 mg PO q6 h×48 h, then 50–100 mg PO BID	Recommend close monitoring for side effects	Metabolites: inactive
		Angina Metoprolol tartrate: initially 50 mg PO BID then titrated to 200 mg PO BID Metoprolol succinate (Toprol XL): 100 mg PO daily, no more than 400 mg/day	Consider avoiding extended release preparation in renal insufficiency	Excretion: urine 95 %

Table 24.1 (continued)

Class	Medication	Normal dose	CKD patient population	Notes
	Esmolol (Brevibloc)	1. Immediate control: for intraoperative treatment, give an 80 mg (approximately 1 mg/kg) bolus dose over 30 s followed by a 150 mcg/kg/min infusion, if needed. Max infusion rate: 300 mcg/kg/min	No specific dose adjustments	Metabolism: extensively metabolized by esterase in cytosol of red blood cells
		2. Gradual control: for postoperative treatment, give loading dosage infusion of 500 mcg/kg/min over 1 min followed by a 4-min infusion of 50 mcg/kg/min. If no effect within 5 min, repeat loading dose, and follow with infusion increased to 100 mcg/kg/min		Metabolites: major acid metabolite (ASL-8123), methanol (inactive) Excretion: urine <1–2 %
	Carvedilol	Hypertension and post-MI protection 6.25–25 mg PO BID Start at 6.25 mg PO BID, then increase q3–14 days to 12.5 mg PO BID, then 25 mg PO BID	No specific dose adjustments In a small study of dialysis patients with dilated cardiomyopathies, carvedilol was found to improve LV function and decrease hospitalization, cardiovascular deaths and total mortality [30]	
CCBs		In UA/NSTEMI patients where beta-blockers are contraindicated, a non-dihydropyridine calcium channel blocker should be given as initial therapy in the absence of clinically significant LV dysfunction or other contraindications (level of evidence: B) [31]	No specific dose adjustments The medical management of chronic CAD in dialysis patients should follow that of the general population and use of CCBs as indicated The hemodynamic and electrophysiological effects of CCBs are markedly different from each other, and these differences should be evaluated when selecting a suitable therapy	
HMG-CoA reductase inhibitors	Simvastatin	Cardiovascular event protection	With the Study of Heart and Renal Protection (SHARP), lipid lowering with statin + ezetimibe is beneficial in patients with kidney insufficiency [32]	Metabolism: liver, CYP450
		20 mg combined with 10 mg ezetimibe Max dose: 40 mg PO qPM	Severe impairment: consider starting dose at 5 mg qPM	Excretion: bile primarily, urine <2 %
	Atorvastatin	Cardiovascular event protection 10 mg PO daily	No specific dose adjustments Atorvastatin 10 mg in patients with kidney dysfunction revealed a significantly lower risk of the primary endpoint (nonfatal MI or cardiac death) in the atorvastatin group when compared with placebo	Metabolism: liver, CYP450 Excretion: bile primarily, urine <2 %
	Fluvastatin	Cardiovascular event protection 40 mg PO BID Extended release: 80 mg PO daily	No specific dose adjustments Caution for increased risk of rhabdomyolysis A multicenter, randomized, double-blind, placebo-controlled trial of 40–80 mg fluvastatin was conducted in kidney transplant recipients [33] Fluvastatin reduced low-density lipoprotein cholesterol concentrations by 32 %. The fluvastatin group experienced a third fewer cardiac death and nonfatal myocardial infarctions than the placebo group. Coronary intervention procedures and other secondary endpoints were not significantly different between the two groups	Excretion: feces 90 %, urine 5 %

(continued)

Table 24.1 (continued)

Class	Medication	Normal dose	CKD patient population	Notes
	Pravastatin	Cardiovascular event protection Start 40 mg PO daily, may adjust dose q4wk, 80 mg max	Start at 10 mg PO daily in patients with renal dysfunction A randomized trial of pravastatin versus placebo in with patients with previous MI and chronic renal insufficiency [34]. The incidence of coronary death or nonfatal MI was lower in patients receiving pravastatin, suggesting that pravastatin is effective for secondary prevention of cardiovascular events in persons with mild chronic kidney insufficiency	Excretion: feces 70 %, urine 20 %

Nitrates	Nitroglycerin	2 % ointment:
		Angina
		  0.5–2 in. applied in AM and 6 h later to truncal skin
		Heart failure
		  1.5 in., increase by 0.5–1 in. up to 4 in., q4 h
		Sublingual: 0.4 mg for relief of chest pain in ACS
		Sublingual: 0.3–0.6 mg SL q5min
		Maximum: 3 doses within 15 min
			No specific dose adjustments
			Care must be used to avoid hypotension in low volume states such as dialysis sessions
				Metabolism: mainly in the liver, extrahepatic sites such as vascular wall, red blood cells
				
				Excretion: urine

Antianginal	Ranolazine (Ranexa)	500–1,000 mg PO BID Max: 2,000 mg/day	No specific dose adjustments Prolongs QTc. Recommend close monitoring, particularly in those with renal insufficiency	Excretion: urine 73–75 %, feces 25 %

ACE angiotensin converting enzyme, *ACS* acute coronary syndromes, *ADP* adenosine diphosphate, *ARB* angiotensin receptor blocker, *CAD* coronary artery disease, *CCB* calcium channel blocker, *CKD* chronic kidney disease, *CVD* cardiovascular disease, *HMG-CoA* hydroxymethylglutaryl coenzyme A, *LV* left ventricle, *LVH* left ventricular hypertrophy, *MI* myocardial infarction, *PTCA* percutaneous transluminal coronary angioplasty, *UA/NSTEMI* unstable angina/non-ST-elevated myocardial infarction

Table 24.2 Intravenous antiplatelet agents for unstable angina/non-ST-elevated myocardial infarction and ST-elevated myocardial infarction

Class	Medication	Normal dose	CKD patient population	Notes
Glycoprotein IIb/IIIa inhibitors			When a glycoprotein IIb/IIIa antagonist is used, abciximab and tirofiban should be considered preferred agents, since no dosing changes are required for abciximab, and dialysis-specific dosing recommendations are available for tirofiban Increased bleeding but reduced in-hospital mortality in CKD patients with ACS treated with IIb/IIIa antagonists has also been shown [35]	

	Abciximab (ReoPro)	Adjunct to PCI
		  0.25 mg/kg IV bolus over at least 1 min, 10–60 min before start of PCI, then
		  0.125 mcg/kg/min (not to exceed 10 mcg/min) continuous IV infusion×12 h
		Unstable angina with PCI planned within 24 h
		  0.25 mg/kg IV bolus over at least 1 min, then
		  0.125 mcg/kg/min (not to exceed 10 mcg/min) IV infusion×18–24 h concluding 1 h post-PCI
			No specific dose adjustments
			Abciximab should also be considered as adjunctive therapy in ACS in dialysis patients
			In CKD, safety of abciximab was shown for creatinine >2.0 mg/dl [36]
			Although increased bleeding with abciximab in renal failure has been reported [37], other studies have shown no increase in bleeding for renal failure versus no renal failure for abciximab in PCI [38]
				Metabolism: others; CYP450, unknown
				
				Excretion: urine

Table 24.2 (continued)

Class	Medication	Normal dose	CKD patient population	Notes
	Eptifibatide (Integrilin)	ACS	Creatinine clearance <50 ml/min:	Metabolism: others; minimal; CYP450, unknown
		180 mcg/kg IV bolus, then	ACS: 180 mcg/kg IV, then continuous infusion 1 mcg/kg/min	Excretion: urine 50 %
		2 mcg/kg/min IV for up to 72 h	Hemodialysis: not defined	
		PCI	Hemodialysis: safety and use during hemodialysis not established	
		180 mcg/kg IV, then		
		Continuous infusion 2 mcg/kg/min with another 180 mcg/kg IV bolus 10 min after first bolus		
		Continue infusion for at least 12 h		
	Tirofiban (Aggrastat)	In patients undergoing PCI, tirofiban not recommended as an alternative to abciximab [39]	Creatinine clearance <30 ml/min	Excretion: urine 65 % (primarily unchanged), feces 25 % (primarily unchanged)
		ACS	Reduce dose to 50 % of normal rate	
		0.4 mcg/kg/min IV for 30 min, then		
		0.1 mcg/kg/min IV for 48–108 h		
		PCI		
		Continue 0.1 mcg/kg/min IV through procedure and for 12–24 h after		

ACS acute coronary syndromes, *CKD* chronic kidney disease, *PCI* percutaneous coronary intervention

Table 24.3 Anticoagulants for unstable angina/non-ST-elevated myocardial infarction and ST-elevated myocardial infarction

Class	Medication	Normal dose	CKD patient population	Notes
Indirect factor Xa inhibitors	Unfractionated heparin (UFH)	Recommended dosage and desired aPTT values per institutional protocol	Suggested starting dose heparin 50 IU/kg bolus, then 18 IU/kg/h. Monitor aPTT values and adjust accordingly per local protocol	Metabolism: liver (partial)
		PCI: 60–100 units/kg IV × 1		Metabolites: none
		Target ACT 250–350 s; in patients receiving glycoprotein IIb/IIIa inhibitor, give 50–70 units/kg IV × 1 to target ACT 200 s		Excretion: urine
		STEMI, adjunct treatment, streptokinase use:		
		Dose		
		<80 kg: 800 units/h		
		>80 kg: 1,000 units/h		
		Start: 5,000 units IV × 1		
		Adjust dose to target aPTT 50–75 s		
		NSTEMI		
		12–15 units/kg/h i.v.		
		Start: 60–70 units/kg i.v. × 1; max 5,000 units bolus, max rate 1,000 units/h		
		Adjust dose to target aPTT 50–75 s		
	Low molecular weight heparin	Unstable angina, non-Q-wave MI	STEMI: <75 years old, CrCl <30	Excretion: urine 40 %
		1 mg/kg SC BID		
		STEMI	30 mg IV bolus × 1 plus 1 mg/kg SC × 1, then 1 mg/kg SC qDay	
		<75 years old:		
	Enoxaparin (Lovenox)	30 mg IV bolus × 1 plus 1 mg/kg SC × 1, then 1 mg/kg SC q12h	STEMI: >75 years old, CrCl <30:	
		PCI patients: additional 0.3 mg/kg IV bolus if last s.c. given >8 h before balloon inflation		
		>75 years old:	1 mg/kg SC qDay	
		0.75 mg/kg SC q12 h (no IV bolus)		

(continued)

Table 24.3 (continued)

Class	Medication	Normal dose	CKD patient population	Notes
Direct factor Xa inhibitor	Fondaparinux (Arixtra)	UA/NSTEMI	CrCl 30–50 ml/min: use with caution	Excretion: urine (primarily unchanged)
		Conservative strategy	CrCl <30 ml/min: not indicated	
		2.5 mg SC daily		
		During PCI		
		Add UFH 50–60 units/kg IV bolus for prophylaxis of catheter thrombosis [40]		
Direct thrombin inhibitors	Bivalirudin (Angiomax)	Intended for use with aspirin 300–325 mg/day	CrCl 10–29: usual bolus dose, then initial infusion of 1 mg/kg/h IV up to 4h	Excretion: urine
		0.75 mg/kg IV bolus initially, followed by continuous infusion at rate of 1.75 mg/kg/h for duration of procedure	Hemodialysis: usual bolus dose, then initial infusion 0.25 mg/kg/h IV, up to 4h	Dialyzable: yes, with 25 % reduction in levels
		Perform ACT 5 min after bolus dose	Bivalirudin is a direct thrombin inhibitor specifically studied in dialysis patients with dosing recommendations and should be preferentially considered	
		May administer additional 0.3 mg/kg bolus if necessary		
		May continue infusion following PCI beyond 4 h (optional post-PCI, at discretion of treating healthcare provider) initiated at rate of 0.2 mg/kg/h for up to 20 h PRN		
	Dabigatran (Pradaxa)	Indicated for prevention of stroke and thromboembolism associated with nonvalvular atrial fibrillation	CrCl 15–30 ml/min: 75 mg PO BID	Excretion: urine 7 %, feces 86 %
		CrCl >30 ml/min	CrCl <15 ml/min or hemodialysis: not indicated	
		150 mg PO BID	For patients currently taking dabigatran, wait 12 h (CrCl ≥30 ml/min) or 24 h (CrCl <30 ml/min) after the last dose of dabigatran before initiating treatment with a parenteral anticoagulant	
			If possible, discontinue dabigatran 1–2 days (CrCl ≥50 ml/min) or 3–5 days (CrCl <50 ml/min) before invasive or surgical procedures because of the increased risk of bleeding	

ACT activated clotting time, *aPTT* activated partial thromboplastin time, *CKD* chronic kidney disease, *CrCl* creatinine clearance, *MI* myocardial infarction, *NSTEMI* non-ST-elevated myocardial infarction, *PCI* percutaneous coronary intervention, *STEMI* ST-elevated myocardial infarction, *UA* unstable angina, *UFH* unfractionated heparin

who received CABG over PCI [46]. Conflicting studies with incomplete data along with the existence of referral bias demonstrate that this area needs more dedicated research.

Adverse Outcomes of Invasive Procedures: Contrast-Induced Acute Kidney Injury

Contrast-induced acute kidney injury (CI-AKI), the third leading cause of hospital-associated renal failure, is diagnosed when there is a 25 % increase in serum creatinine from baseline or a 0.5 mg/dl increase in the absolute creatinine value within 48–72 h after the administration of intravenous contrast [47]. A newer definition of CI-AKI that can be used is the Acute Kidney Injury Criteria of a rise of ≥0.3 mg/dl at 48 h after exposure. Other causes of renal failure should be considered before establishing the diagnosis of CI-AKI including volume depletion (prerenal azotemia without AKI), interstitial nephritis, and systemic atheroembolism. Serum creatinine usually peaks in 2–5 days, followed by a gradual return to baseline over 14 days. The exact incidence of CI-AKI might be under reported, as post-catheterization patients are commonly discharged shortly after the procedure [47]. Pathophysiology is related to transient renal ischemia (~2 h), direct contrast toxicity (several days), and in some cases superimposed aortic microembolization of atheromatous debris to the kidney.

Though preexisting CKD is the most common risk factor for the development of CI-AKI, concomitant diabetes increases overall risk by two- to fourfold. Additional risk factors include age, hypertension, heart failure, metabolic syndrome, anemia, multiple myeloma, hypoalbuminemia, and prior renal transplant. The cardiologist must be cautious of potential substrates for hemodynamic instability such as hypovolemia, ejection fraction less than 40 %, hypotension, and intra-aortic balloon pump counterpulsation therapy. The volume of contrast, its composition, osmolality, ionicity, and viscosity are also contributing factors [47]. Patients with CKD undergoing cardiac catheterization experience more major adverse cardiovascular events (MACE), longer hospital stays, and higher costs [48]. Though there exists no definitive treatment once CI-AKI develops, a great deal of effort has been focused in preventing the syndrome from occurring.

Intravenous hydration remains the central tenant in prevention of CI-AKI. Post-procedure volume expansion is more important than pre-procedure hydration. Intravascular volume expansion, preferably with normal saline, promotes renal blood flow and counteracts the decreased renal perfusion that occurs for up to 20 h after contrast exposure. This also prevents medullary hypoxemia and preserves nitric oxide production that helps to enhance the elimination of contrast. Normal saline is superior to half normal saline in expanding intravascular. Increased delivery of sodium to the distal nephron prevents deleterious renin-angiotensin activation. The CIN Consensus Working Panel recommends the use of isotonic crystalloids (1–15 mml/kg/h) 3–12 h pre-procedure and continuously for 6–24 h post-procedure [49]. For hospitalized patients, volume expansion should begin 6 h pre-procedure and be continued for 6–14 h post-procedure. For outpatients, fluids can be initiated 3 h prior and continued for 12 h after procedure. Patients with compensated congestive heart failure should still be given volume but at a lower rate. Decompensated heart failure patients should undergo hemodynamic monitoring if possible with continuation of diuretics. Iodixanol is the contrast agent of choice for patients at risk for CI-AKI due to its nonionic, isosmolar properties and studies showing lower rates of CI-AKI [50, 51]. Contrast volume should be kept to 100 ml, with the risk of CI-AKI increasing by 12 % for each 100 ml of dye used beyond the initial 100 ml. Nephrotoxic agents such as NSAIDs, cyclosporine, and amphotericin should be discontinued 24 h before procedure in patients at risk. Metformin should also be discontinued and resumed 48 h later in the setting of normal renal function to avoid risk of lactic acidosis. There are no firm recommendations regarding the discontinuation of ACEs and ARBs at this time.

Other potential therapies continue to be investigated but cannot be recommended at this time. The almost ubiquitous utilization of *N*-acetylcysteine (NAC) was finally challenged in the ACT trial (Acetylcysteine for Prevention of Renal Outcomes in Patients Undergoing Coronary and Peripheral Vascular Angiography) in Brazil. In this large, randomized control trial of 2,308 patients, Berwanger et al. found no differences in incidence of CIN in the control and NAC group (12.7 % in each). Secondary outcomes such as need for dialysis and total mortality also did not differ. Additionally, the groups did not differ in the types of contrast dye utilized [32]. Guidelines will certainly be updated to reflect these findings in addition to promoting development of therapies with measurable benefit. Forced diuresis with mannitol and furosemide predisposes to dehydration and can worsen CI-AKI. A lower incidence of CI-AKI was found in patients treated with statins pre-procedure (4.37 % versus 5.93 %), but prospective trials are still required before recommendations can be made.

Cholesterol macroembolization syndrome should be suspected in patients with acute renal failure, hypereosinophilia, livedo reticularis, or blue toe syndrome, especially if the patient has had recent vascular procedures such as cardiac catheterization. Typically, presenting weeks or months after such procedures, it can be distinguished temporally from CI-AKI which occurs 24–48 h post-procedure. In a prospective study of 1,579 patients undergoing coronary angiography, clinical evidence of cholesterol emboli was present in 1 patient (0.06 %). Renal effects of the syndrome may range from spontaneous resolution to ESRD requiring dialysis.

Nephrogenic Systemic Fibrosis

The connection between gadolinium and renal failure leading to nephrogenic systemic fibrosis (NSF) was first described in a case series of 13 patients [52]. All patients with NSF have a history of renal failure with most on renal replacement therapy, whether it be hemodialysis or peritoneal dialysis or have a history of renal transplantation. Though an uncommon condition, it is clinically of importance as it may be linked to increased morbidity and mortality [53]. With reduced renal clearance, both gadolinium and gadodiamide have longer circulatory times and dissociate from the chelated state and allow presentation of unbound gadolinium to immune and satellite cells in connective tissue. The mechanism at play is not well understood, though hypotheses implicate a circulating fibrocyte which becomes activated by gadolinium exposure and begins to deposit excess collagen [54]. The disease itself results in a scleroderma-like condition with gadolinium deposition primarily occurring in the skin but can affect the tissues of any organs [55].

The risks and benefits of gadolinium in cardiac MRI should be carefully considered by the cardiologist. If the test is deemed of critical lifesaving importance, it should be discussed with the patient, with the risks of this disease entity described. Studies have shown that dialysis decreases the amount of gadolinium but has no effect on residual tissue deposits and thus does not prevent against NSF development [56]. The cardiologist should coordinate with the patient's nephrologist to initiate early dialysis, and even arrange the testing on the patient's dialysis day. There is no evidence at this time to initiate temporary dialysis in patients who are not already on dialysis.

Dyslipidemia in CKD

Though potentially treatable, dyslipidemias in CKD patients are not aggressively managed by clinicians due to questions about safety and unclear evidence demonstrating benefit in this patient group [57]. Complex lipid abnormalities, primarily low HDL-C and increased plasma triglycerides, result from the intricate dysregulation of lipoprotein metabolism in patients with CKD [58] and can be found in all stages of CKD. Reduced plasma levels of ApoA-I and ApoA-II as evidenced by reduced genetic expression of these apoproteins at HDL production sites in the liver result in low HDL-C levels [59]. In addition, chronic inflammation leading to reduced levels of albumin also contributes to lower HDL-C levels [58]. Increases in ApoC-III, a strong inhibitor of lipoprotein lipase whose purpose is to degrade triglyceride particles, can partly explain high triglyceride levels.

Key studies have highlighted lipid management in patients with mild to moderate CKD. The Heart Protection Study enrolled 20,000 subjects evaluating the benefits of 40 mg of daily simvastatin. In this group, 1,329 patients had CKD, their creatinine levels ranging from 1.3 to 2.3 mg/dl. An 11 % absolute risk reduction (ARR) for the outcomes of total morality and fatal and nonfatal vascular events was seen, in comparison to an ARR of 5.4 % for the entire study population [60]. A subgroup of 1,700 patients from the Cholesterol and Recurrent Events (CARE) study with creatinine clearance <75 ml/min experienced a 4 % ARR in death from CAD or symptomatic nonfatal MI when treated with 40 mg of pravastatin daily. In the ALERT (Assessment of Lescol in Renal Transplant) trial which was a randomized double-blind placebo-controlled trial of 2,102 renal transplant patients who had a mean serum creatinine of 1.6 mg/dl, a 17 % risk reduction in combined primary endpoints of cardiac death, nonfatal MI, or coronary intervention was observed in patients treated with fluvastatin [33]. When cardiac death and nonfatal MI were analyzed as the primary

endpoint, a 35 % risk reduction was seen [61]. In the VA-HIT (Veteran's Affairs High-Density Lipoprotein Intervention Trial) study of the 2,500 men enrolled, 1,000 had creatinine clearance <75 ml/min with a post hoc analysis showing a 27 % relative risk reduction and a 6.3 % ARR in fatal and nonfatal MI associated with gemfibrozil therapy [62].

Patients on hemodialysis (CKD 5) have a 10–30 times higher morbidity and mortality from CVD than the general population [63]. Observational data suggests benefit in treating dyslipidemia in dialysis patients. Statin users in the US Renal Data System Dialysis Morbidity and Mortality Study (3,700 patients on hemodialysis followed for 2 years) had a 32 % relative risk reduction in total mortality, while fibrate users had no reduction in cardiovascular or total mortality [64]. Statin users in the Dialysis Outcomes Practice Patterns Study had a 31 % relative risk reduction in total mortality compared to non-statin users [65]. The 4D (Die Deutsche Diabetes Dialyse Studie) trial studied statin use prospectively in a randomized controlled fashion in hemodialysis patients, finding, in contrast with observational data, an increased risk of fatal stroke. Criticism of this study was that patients had such severe atherosclerosis (on hemodialysis for 2 years, 50 % were smokers, 50 % had prior MI) that they were beyond benefit of statin therapy [66]. The randomized controlled SHARP trial (Study of Heart and Renal Protection) revealed combination therapy with simvastatin and ezetimibe in 9,270 patients with CKD and ESRD to decrease the risk of "major atherosclerotic events" by 17 %. Therapy resulted in a 25 % reduction in nonhemorrhagic stroke, a 27 % reduction in coronary revascularization, and a 21 % reduction in any revascularization [67]. Observational data of dialysis patients reveals a "reverse epidemiology" showing lower cholesterol levels to be associated with higher mortality rates [68]. This finding was derived from data from more than 12,000 hemodialysis patients and revealed that patients with a total cholesterol level less than 100 mg/dl had four times the risk of death when compared to patients with total cholesterols ranging from 200 to 250 mg/dl [69]. A 10-year prospective study of 1,167 Japanese patients on hemodialysis confirmed low cholesterol to be associated with higher all-cause mortality. The same study found low cholesterol to correlate with low albumin and higher CRP level, suggesting a link between low cholesterol, malnutrition, and inflammation [70].

Current National Kidney Foundation Kidney Disease Outcome Quality Initiative (K/DOQI) guidelines recommend a target LDL of below 100 in patients with CKD [71] with first-line therapy being statins at doses similar to those in clinical trials. Statins have a positive safety profile in CKD, dialysis, and renal transplant recipients [34]. There is insufficient evidence to conclude that statins through their pleiotropic effects actually prevent the decline of renal function. Atorvastatin has a <2 % renal excretion and does not require dose adjustment for GFR <30 ml/min/1.73 m^2 [72]. Fluvastatin also has minimal kidney excretion and does not utilize the CYP-3A4 metabolism pathway. In addition, its pharmacokinetics are unchanged in hemodialysis or peritoneal dialysis patients [73, 74].

Fibric acids, such as gemfibrozil, are most effective in the treatment of hypertriglyceridemia in these patients [75] although the overall benefit is unclear. The VA-HIT trial demonstrated a significantly lower risk of the primary endpoint of coronary death and nonfatal MI. However, there was no effect on total mortality, and therapy was linked with significant decline in renal function. Fibrates in combination with statins may pose an increased risk for rhabdomyolysis in patients with CKD. Gemfibrozil elevates plasma levels of all statins except fluvastatin [76]. The dose of gemfibrozil should be reduced to 600 mg/day for patients with GFR <60 ml/min/1.73 and avoided altogether in patients with GFR <15 ml/min/1.73 m^2 [77]. When treating mixed dyslipidemias, the National Lipid Association recommends avoiding the maximum dose of statin in combination with a fibrate [77]. Guidelines from the National Kidney Foundation (NKF) advise decreasing the dose of niacin by 50 % for GFR <15 mg/ml/1.73 m^2 [72]. Omega-3 fatty acids are safe in CKD patients and have limited drug interactions [31].

Perioperative Cardiac Evaluation of the Renal Transplant Recipient

Kidney transplant is the definitive treatment of choice for ESRD, potentially offering patients longer survival and better quality of life. As of 2009, more than 80,000 patients await kidney and kidney-pancreas transplant [78]. As already highlighted in this chapter, this population of patients carries a higher prevalence of CAD, and whether pre- or posttransplant, CVD continues to be the most common cause of death. In fact, posttransplant, 30 % of all overall deaths, with the highest rates occurring early after transplant, are attributed to CVD [79]. Nearly half of all deaths 30 days posttransplant are due to cardiac events [80]. Additionally, the posttransplant medication regimen of steroids and calcineurin inhibitors can worsen hypertension and dyslipidemia. The interaction of statins and calcineurin inhibitors may result in undertreatment of lipid abnormalities [81].

As part of the multidisciplinary transplant process, all patients should be evaluated for ischemic heart disease. At baseline, a history, physical examination, ECG, and chest x-ray should be ordered along with an assessment of functional status. Many questions and an overall lack of consensus exist on how to optimally approach cardiovascular risk assessment in patients where further advanced cardiac testing is needed. In fact, in a 1993 survey of US transplant centers and cardiac evaluation practices by Ramos et al., it was found that cardiac stress test screening was nearly standard practice, being obtained in 67 % of asymptomatic patients (age over 52), 86 % of diabetics, and 68 % of asymptomatic patients with multiple risk factors [82]. The ACC/AHA guidelines advise a cardiovascular evaluation based on patient symptoms and functional status. The American Society of Transplantation recommends stress testing for all "high-risk patients" defined as those with renal disease from diabetes, prior ischemia, or having two or more CAD risk factors (age ≥45 years in men and 55 in women, smoking, diabetes, hypertension, dyslipidemia, LVH). The evidence for acting on positive stress tests is less clear but would likely follow those of accepted guidelines for revascularization.

Noninvasive cardiac testing such as myocardial perfusion imaging with dipyridamole thallium/sestamibi scintigraphy (DSS) and dobutamine stress echocardiography (DSE) has been studied in patients with ESRD. De Lima et al. studied 125 renal transplant candidates with coronary angiography and noninvasive testing. They found DSS to have a sensitivity and specificity of 58 and 67 %, respectively, and DSE to have a sensitivity of only 44 %, with a better specificity of 87 %. The patients were followed for 4 years and only coronary angiography was able to reliably predict patients at risk. The authors concluded that noninvasive testing was probably inadequate in transplant patients who are already at high risk. Coronary angiography offers the ability to exclude significant CAD while carrying the risk of CI-AKI and atheroembolic disease (Fig. 24.1).

Congestive Heart Failure (CHF) and Cardiorenal Syndrome (CRS)

CHF and renal dysfunction often coexist, and primary dysfunction in one organ system often causes or exacerbates dysfunction in the other. Impaired cardiac output, for example, may result in decreased renal perfusion and progression of CKD. Conversely, progression of CKD may lead to sodium and water retention, hypertension, volume overload, and worsening cardiac dysfunction. The reciprocal nature of cardiac and renal disease can further be appreciated in the following observations: (1) impaired renal function in CHF correlates with cardiovascular morbidity and mortality [83], and (2) CKD patients have significant cardiovascular morbidity/mortality, most of them dying from such causes before reaching ESRD [84].

The term cardiorenal syndrome (CRS) has been applied to describe the bidirectional nature of cardiac and renal disease. A recent classification of CRS has been proposed which takes into account the time frame and pathophysiology of concomitant heart and renal dysfunctions. Under this classification, CRS is subdivided into subtypes according to the primary organ of dysfunction and the temporal sequence of events [85].

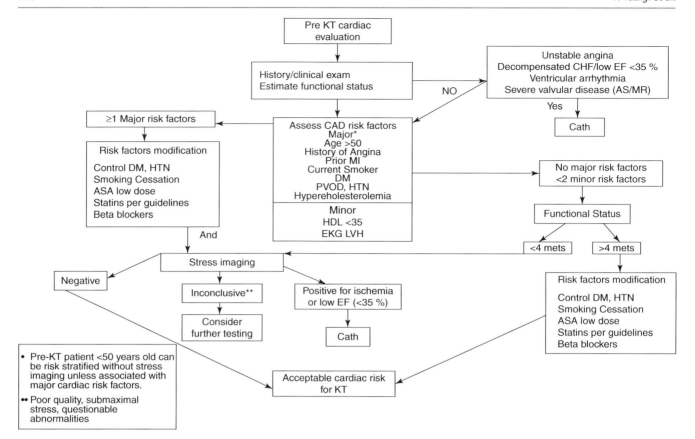

Fig. 24.1 Preoperative algorithm for renal transplantation. *KT* kidney transplant, *EF* ejection fraction, *HTN* hypertension, *MI* myocardial infarction (Adapted from [152])

Pathophysiology

Type 1 Acute Cardiorenal Syndrome: Acute Heart Failure Causing Renal Dysfunction/Injury. This subtype refers to an abrupt worsening of cardiac function leading to acute kidney injury (AKI). In decompensated HF, excessive activation of the renin-angiotensin-aldosterone system (RAAS) and the sympathetic nervous system (SNS) has been considered the hallmark of the disease process. These pathways are responsible for the excessive release of neurohormonal mediators such as angiotensin II, vasopressin, and norepinephrine resulting in increased sodium retention and vasoconstriction. This ultimately leads to increased cardiac preload and kidney congestion, which is thought to play a crucial role in renal dysfunction [85].

Type 2 Chronic Cardiorenal Syndrome: Chronic Heart Failure Causing Renal Dysfunction/Injury. This subtype refers to chronic abnormalities in cardiac function causing progressive chronic kidney disease. The proposed pathophysiology for renal dysfunction in this setting is similar to that of CRS type 1. The ESCAPE trial (Evaluation Study of Congestive Heart Failure and Pulmonary Artery Catheterization Effectiveness) clearly demonstrated a link between rising serum creatinine levels and right atrial pressures, suggesting that renal congestion may be more important than previously thought [86]. Additional factors which may contribute to the progressive renal deterioration relate to the pharmacological treatment for chronic CHF. These include excessive diuresis, early RAAS blockade, and drug-induced hypotension, which may contribute to worsening renal dysfunction [87].

Type 3 Acute Renocardiac Syndrome: Acute Renal Failure Causing Heart Dysfunction/Injury. This subtype consists of an abrupt worsening of renal function causing acute cardiac dysfunction. AKI can result in acute volume overload, electrolyte derangements, and accumulation of uremic toxins, which may lead to cardiac dysfunction [85].

Type 4 Chronic Renocardiac Syndrome: CKD Causing Heart Disease/Dysfunction/Injury. This subtype refers to disease of the heart that develops as a result of CKD. Cardiac disease in CKD patients is common, and cardiac-specific mortality rates are 10- to 20-fold higher compared to non-CKD populations. Progression of CKD usually leads to salt and water retention, hypertension, left ventricular hypertrophy/remodeling, and vascular calcification with accelerated atherosclerosis which ultimately result in the development of cardiac dysfunction [88].

Type 5 Cardiorenal Syndrome: Any Systemic Condition That Causes Simultaneous Renal and Cardiac Dysfunction/Injury. Also known as secondary CRS, both the heart and the kidney are simultaneously affected by a systemic illness, which can be either acute or chronic. An example of type 5 CRS is sepsis, a condition in which patients often develop concomitant renal and cardiac dysfunction [85].

Diagnostic Markers

Classic markers such as serum creatinine rise when renal injury is already established. More sensitive biomarkers for the early detection and prognostication of AKI are currently under investigation. These include the neutrophil gelatinase-associated lipocalin (NGAL), interleukin-18 (IL-18), cystatin C, and kidney injury molecule-1 (KIM-1). The usefulness of these biomarkers is still questioned, and adequately powered multicenter clinical trials are needed for further evaluation before they can be adopted into clinical practice [89].

B-type natriuretic peptide (BNP) is a marker of myocyte stress and is often used to diagnose and manage CHF. Its usefulness, however, is unclear as the serum concentrations are influenced by kidney function [90].

Treatment

A stepwise approach has been proposed for the treatment of CRS. This involves an initial evaluation in which adherence to medication regimen/salt restriction is optimized; arrhythmias, cardiac dyssynchrony, and anatomic abnormalities (ischemia, valvular disease, pericardial effusion) are recognized and treated; anemia is controlled (iron repletion, erythropoietin-stimulating agents); and key pharmacologic agents are optimized (diuretics, ACE inhibitors, ARBs, spironolactone, digoxin, afterload-reducing agents). In the presence of worsening renal function, ineffective diuresis, or persistent CHF, an effort to reevaluate for concurrent renal disease is indicated. Initiation of vasopressor/inotropic therapy or extracorporeal ultrafiltration should be considered in the setting of persistent hypotension, renal dysfunction, or CHF [91].

Extracorporeal Ultrafiltration

Peritoneal Dialysis (PD): Intermittent PD has been shown to be effective for fluid removal, improving NYHA class, bridging to cardiac transplantation, decreasing duration of hospitalization, and improving quality of life [92]. The safety of PD, however, has not been well established as there is evidence of increased peritoneal infection and PD-induced electrolyte derangements which may worsen cardiac rhythm control. In addition, the large peritoneal fluid volumes used can potentially affect respiration, which may already be compromised in CHF [91].

Conventional Hemodialysis or Hemofiltration: Intermittent hemodialysis for fluid removal in CHF has been shown to be effective and safe [93]. The major risk associated with this type of ultrafiltration (UF) is hemodynamic instability due to excessive fluid removal, which can potentially lead to hypovolemia, hypotension, and decreased renal function. The key to avoiding hemodynamic instability is to slow the UF rate which has led to longer and ultimately continuous treatment modalities [91]. In the recent UNLOAD trial (Ultrafiltration Versus Intravenous Diuretics for Patients Hospitalized for Acute Decompensated Heart Failure) in which CHF patients were randomized to early UF or IV diuretics, early UF was associated with a significantly greater rate of fluid loss than diuretic therapy with statistically similar rises in serum creatinine, BUN, sodium levels, heart failure scores, episodes of hypotension, and hospital length of stay. UF therapy proved to be safe, without increased mortality or hemorrhage compared with those undergoing standard care. Caution, however, should be undertaken to minimize the potential collateral effect of continuous renal replacement therapy (CRRT) on decreasing the therapeutic levels of medications used in treatment.

Valvular Heart Disease and Renal Dysfunction

Valvular heart disease (VHD) is commonly observed in patients with CKD and is related to the disturbances in serum levels of calcium and phosphorus due to secondary hyperparathyroidism. Other risk factors for VHD in renal patients include DM, hypertension, uremia, anemia, and infective endocarditis. The underlying pathology for valvular disease involves valvular and/or annular calcification as well as thickening of the valve apparatus, which can lead to either regurgitation or stenosis of the valve.

Mitral annular calcification (MAC) is frequently seen on echocardiography in patients with CKD/ESRD and is estimated to affect 10–50 % of these patients. Hyperphosphatemia plays a major role in MAC development in the renal failure population [94]. Aortic valve calcification (AVC) is usually seen later in the course of the kidney disease and is more often observed in patients who have been on dialysis for a few years [95, 96]. AVC, like MAC, is directly related to elevations in the calcium-phosphorus product in CKD patients. Valve sclerosis (thickening of the valve), which usually affects the aortic and mitral valves, is very common in CKD/ESRD patients. Although not directly related to progression to aortic stenosis (AS), aortic sclerosis has been shown to be associated with increased cardiovascular mortality [97].

The evaluation of suspected VHD in patients with CKD/ESRD is not different from that done in the general population. However, the evaluation process may be more challenging in renal patients due to the changes in volume status (which would affect physical examination and echocardiography findings) and other medical conditions frequently encountered in these patients [98]. Two-dimensional echocardiography is the recommended modality for evaluation and serial follow-up when indicated.

The incidence of AS in hemodialysis (HD) patients is estimated to be about 3.3 %/year according to one study [99]. The same study showed worse outcome of AS in HD patients compared with the general population, although clinical progression and symptoms of AS were not different between groups. The medical literature has limited data regarding the prevalence/incidence of mitral stenosis in renal failure patients [100].

Valvular regurgitation (including aortic, mitral, and tricuspid) is very common in HD/CKD patients and is thought to be of functional origin due to the increased volume status in these patients [101, 102]. Valvular regurgitation may be managed medically with control of volume and blood pressure in patients with functional valvular regurgitation.

Treatment options for VHD in renal patients are the same compared with the general population as indicated by the ACC/AHA guidelines. When surgery is recommended, the decision for selection of the valve (bioprosthetic versus mechanical) should be individualized based on risks and benefits. The risk of thromboembolism is high in the setting of calcified valves (MAC, AVC). Calcific embolism is not frequently recognized in renal patients but can be fatal and should be always considered in this population [103].

Pericardial Disease in Renal Failure

The morbidity and mortality of pericardial disease in patients with renal dysfunction has significantly decreased with advancements in renal replacement therapy (RRT). Pericardial disease in CKD/ESRD patients is classified into *uremic pericarditis* which usually develops before RRT or within 8 weeks of its initiation, *dialysis pericarditis* which occurs after being stabilized on dialysis for at least 8 weeks, and *chronic constrictive pericarditis* [104]. The reported incidence of pericarditis in patients with CKD/ESRD varies greatly with an average estimate of 8–20 % [105, 106]. The underlying etiology of pericarditis in renal dysfunction is believed to be related to retention of toxic metabolites [107, 108]. Immunologic injury and volume overload have been also suggested as a possible cause. Other types of pericarditis

(viral, bacterial) can also develop. The clinical features of pericarditis in renal failure patients are similar to those observed in nonuremic patients and classically involve pleuritic chest pain that worsens in the reclining position [109]. The typical diffuse ST elevation on ECG is not usually seen in uremic pericarditis [110]. Acute uremic pericarditis usually resolves rapidly once dialysis (hemodialysis or peritoneal) is initiated. Dialysis pericarditis is treated by intensifying the dialysis regimen [111]. Anti-inflammatory medications have limited effect when intensive dialysis has failed. In both, uremic and dialysis pericarditis, when a moderate to large pericardial effusion exists with evidence of hemodynamic compromise on clinical or echocardiographic evaluation, pericardial drainage should be performed preferably via a surgical pericardial window procedure [112, 113]. Asymptomatic patients with pericardial effusion should be monitored with serial transthoracic echocardiographic evaluation.

Arrhythmias and Renal Failure

The high prevalence of CAD along with electrolyte abnormalities, metabolic acidosis, and uremic milieu all combine to place the patient with CKD at high risk for cardiac arrhythmias [114]. Inflammation associated with renal dysfunction [115, 116] is believed to play a major role in the pathogenesis of atrial arrhythmias [117, 118].

Approximately one in four patients with ESRD dies suddenly with no clear cause [119]. More frequent implantable cardioverter defibrillator (ICD) therapy episodes occur in CKD/ESRD patients [119, 120]. Elevated defibrillation threshold and failure of ICD therapy have been frequently reported in CKD/ESRD patients [121]. An increased short-term mortality along with higher complication rates following ICD implant has been observed in ESRD patients [122]. Given these findings, the utility of ICDs for primary prevention in this subset of patients is currently under investigation.

One in five patients with CKD experiences atrial fibrillation, which is two to three times higher than the rate estimated in the general population [123]. In addition, CKD has been shown to be a strong predictor of new-onset AF in hypertensive patients [124]. The prevalence of AF is 13 % in patients on hemodialysis and 7 % in patients undergoing peritoneal dialysis in the US renal data system (USRDS) [125]. ESRD patients with known AF have an annual mortality rate of 5 % compared with only 2 % in those without it [12]. The presence of AF in CKD patients indicates an increased mortality risk. Whether AF is an independent risk factor for overall mortality in CKD or is a marker of risk has not been determined. The risk of stroke is markedly increased in CKD patients with AF compared to the general population [126]. According to one study, thromboembolic event rates were about 24 % per year in hemodialysis patients with AF compared to 5 % in those with normal sinus rhythm. The use of oral anticoagulation for stroke prevention in CKD patients with AF has not been widely studied [127]. Many of the safety studies and large clinical trials regarding anticoagulation have excluded CKD patients. In addition, patients with renal disease have both a prothrombotic state that leads to higher rates of thromboembolism and a coagulopathy resulting in an increased bleeding risk [128–130]. CHADS2 and HASBLED scores have not been validated in CKD patients, but they are considered a useful foundation in approaching this complex situation where the clinician has to perform individual risk stratification [131, 132]. Dabigatran is an oral direct thrombin inhibitor that has been approved by the Food and Drug Administration (FDA) for stroke prevention in nonvalvular AF. Exposure to dabigatran is increased by renal impairment and correlates with the severity of renal dysfunction. A decrease in the dose and/or an increase in the administration interval in these patients may be appropriate. In patients with ESRD, dabigatran can be partly removed from the plasma by hemodialysis [133]. The FDA approved dabigatran 150 mg twice daily in CKD stage 3 patients and a reduced dose of 75 mg twice daily in CKD stage 4 patients.

CKD patients who have arrhythmias should receive the same guideline-based therapy as others. The major differences in management are mainly related to medication dose adjustments based on renal function (Tables 24.1, 24.2, and 24.3).

Peripheral Arterial Disease in CKD

Chronic kidney disease has been recently determined to be an independent risk factor for atherosclerosis [134]. Peripheral arterial disease (PAD) is commonly encountered in patients with CKD. However, it has not been extensively studied in this group of patients [135].

Estimates of the prevalence of PAD in patients with ESRD range from 15 to 25 % depending on the geographic location and the diagnostic criteria [136, 137]. In patients with CKD, the incidence and prevalence of PAD are higher than in the general population. However, the lack of a unified definition of the disease has contributed to difficulties in obtaining accurate epidemiologic data [138, 139].

The traditional risk factors for PAD such as male gender, advanced age, coronary artery disease, diabetes mellitus, hypertension, smoking, and hyperlipidemia also hold true for patients with renal disease. The role of hyperphosphatemia, hyperparathyroidism, and vascular calcification in developing lower limb atherosclerosis in patients with renal dysfunction is not clear [140, 141].

The presentation of PAD as classified by 2005 ACC/AHA guidelines is as follows: asymptomatic (20–50 %), atypical leg pain (40–50 %), classic claudication (10–35 %), and critical limb ischemia (1–2 %) [142]. The symptoms of PAD in CKD patients are not different. However, compared to those who have normal kidney function, patients with CKD have higher mortality rates, and they are more likely to develop critical limb ischemia and higher rates of limb loss following revascularization. In patients with ESRD, symptoms of PAD may be exacerbated after inserting lower extremity hemodialysis access.

The diagnosis of PAD in patients with renal dysfunction can be made using the same noninvasive techniques used in the general population, including ABI (ankle-brachial index with diagnostic value of <0.9), TBI (toe-brachial index), segmental limb pressures, exercise treadmill testing, and ultrasonography. Clinicians must be aware of the limitation of ABI as a diagnostic tool due to the high prevalence of medial arterial calcification in this subgroup of patients which would falsely increase lower extremity pressure values [138]. Iodinated contrast arteriography remains the gold standard for diagnosis of PAD. Both magnetic resonance angiography (MRA) and computed tomography angiography (CTA) can serve as an alternative means of diagnosis [143]. The risks of CI-AKI and NSF must be considered and prevention measures should be employed.

Although it has not been studied specifically in this subset of patients, aggressive risk factor reduction is generally recommended as a secondary prevention strategy in CKD patients with PAD. This approach includes the use of statin therapy [144], antihypertensive medications, smoking cessation, and optimal control of blood glucose in diabetics. Exercise rehabilitation program is still the first-line therapy in PAD patients with intermittent claudication. This approach can be generalized to CKD patients since randomized studies in this population are lacking.

Although it has not been studied in the CKD population, antiplatelet therapy is recommended for renal disease patients with PAD based on large clinical trials (including CKD patients) that showed a reduction in cardiovascular events and death [145]. Aspirin is usually recommended over clopidogrel due to its low cost and proven efficacy [146]. Cilostazol, a phosphodiesterase inhibitor, is usually prescribed in patients with intermittent claudication, and it has been shown to be effective in multiple clinical trials, although it has not been studied exclusively in CKD population [147, 148]. Revascularization therapy is indicated in patients who fail medical treatment and have limiting persistent symptoms or for patients with critical limb ischemia, as recommended by the ACC/AHA guidelines. The comparative effectiveness of percutaneous versus surgical revascularization in CKD patients has not been studied. Both share a high mortality rate post-procedure in ESRD patients compared to the general population [149, 150]. Amputation is considered the last resort when revascularization measures fail. An increased risk of death has been reported in CKD patients with PAD after amputation [151].

Summary

Chronic kidney disease accelerates atherosclerosis and its complications including ACS. Contrast-induced acute kidney injury must be considered and managed in patients who are receiving PCI therapy for ACS. Multiple drugs need careful adjustment in this setting. Chronic CAD in CKD is responsive to lipid lowering therapies. Patients with CKD are susceptible to cardiorenal syndromes which lead to bidirectional organ dysfunction and are particularly difficult to manage. Both valvular heart disease and arrhythmias are more common in CKD but do not have special management implications in the presence of renal dysfunction. The understanding of pathophysiological mechanisms at work in patients with CKD in the future will likely lead to new diagnostic and therapeutic targets in this high-risk population.

Key Points
- CKD has been associated with increased risk of in-hospital death and major bleeding in patients with acute coronary syndromes (ACS).
- Contrast-induced acute kidney injury requires a comprehensive management strategy in patients receiving percutaneous therapy for ACS.
- Patients with CKD are susceptible to cardiorenal syndromes which complicate bidirectional organ dysfunction and are particularly challenging to manage.

References

1. Centers for Disease Control and Prevention (CDC). National chronic kidney disease fact sheet: general information and national estimates on chronic kidney disease in the United States, 2010. Atlanta: U.S. Department of Health and Human Services (HHS), CDC; 2010.
2. USRDS 2010 Annual Data Report. United States renal data system. Website: www.usrds.org/adr.htm. Accessed 8 Nov 2010. (The USRDS end-stage renal disease incident and prevalent quarterly update is available at: www.usrds.org/qtr/default.html).
3. Heron MP, Hoyert DL, Murphy SL, Xu JQ, Kochanek KD, Tejada-Vera B. Deaths: final data for 2006. Nat Vital Stat Rep;57(14). Hyattsville: National Center for Health Statistics; 2009:1–2.
4. Go AS, Chertow GM, Fan D, McCulloch CE, Hsu CY. Chronic kidney disease and the risks of death, cardiovascular events, and hospitalization. N Engl J Med. 2004;351:1296–305.
5. Shlipak MG, Fried LF, Cushman M, Manolio TA, Peterson D, Stehman-Breen C, Bleyer A, Newman A, Siscovick D, Psaty B. Cardiovascular mortality risk in chronic kidney disease: comparison of traditional and novel risk factors. JAMA. 2005;293: 1737–45.
6. Sarnak MJ, Levey AS, Schoolwerth AC, Coresh J, Culleton B, Hamm LL, McCullough PA, Kasiske BL, Kelepouris E, Klag MJ, Parfrey P, Pfeffer M, Raij L, Spinosa DJ, Wilson PW, American Heart Association Councils on Kidney in Cardiovascular Disease, High Blood Pressure Research, Clinical Cardiology, and Epidemiology and Prevention. Kidney disease as a risk factor for development of cardiovascular disease: a statement from the American Heart Association Councils on Kidney in Cardiovascular Disease, High Blood Pressure Research, Clinical Cardiology, and Epidemiology and Prevention. Circulation. 2003;108(17):2154.
7. Shlipak MG, Liu HH, Schiller NB, Whooley MA. Association between renal insufficiency and inducible ischemia in patients with coronary artery disease: the heart and soul study. J Am Soc Nephrol. 2003;14(12):3233.
8. Hanna EB, Chen AY, Roe MT, Wiviott SD, Fox CS, Saucedo JF. Characteristics and in-hospital outcomes of patients with non-ST-segment elevation myocardial infarction and chronic kidney disease undergoing percutaneous coronary intervention. JACC Cardiovasc Interv. 2011;4(9):1002–8.
9. De Servi S, Guastoni C, Mariani M, Poli A, D'Urbano M, Poletti F, Seveso G. Chronic renal failure in acute coronary syndromes. G Ital Cardiol (Rome). 2006;7(4 Suppl 1):30S–5.
10. McCullough PA, Nowak RM, Foreback C, Tokarski G, Tomlanovich MC, Khoury N, Weaver WD, Sandberg KR, McCord J. Emergency evaluation of chest pain in patients with advanced kidney disease. Arch Intern Med. 2002;162(21):2464–8.
11. Alexander KP, Chen AY, Roe MT, et al. Excess dosing of antiplatelet and antithrombin agents in the treatment of non-ST-segment elevation acute coronary syndromes. JAMA. 2005; 294:3108–16.
12. Coca SG, Krumholz HM, Garg AX, Parikh CR. Underrepresentation of renal disease in randomized controlled trials of cardiovascular disease. JAMA. 2006;296:1377–84.
13. Kirtane AJ, Piazza G, Murphy SA, Budiu D, Morrow DA, Cohen DJ, Peterson E, Lakkis N, Herrmann HC, Palabrica TM, Gibson CM. Correlates of bleeding events among moderate to high-risk patients undergoing percutaneous coronary intervention and treated with eptifibatide: observations from the PROTECT-TIMI-30 trial. J Am Coll Cardiol. 2006;47:2374–9.
14. Diesel W, Emms M, Knight BK, et al. Morphological features of the myopathy associated with chronic renal failure. Am J Kid Dis. 1993;22:677–84.
15. Antman EM, Grudzien C, Mitchell RN, Sacks DB. Detection of unsuspected myocardial necrosis by rapid bedside assay for cardiac troponin T. Am Heart J. 1997;133:596–8.
16. Diris JH, Hackeng CM, Kooman JP, et al. Impaired renal clearance explains elevated troponin T fragments in hemodialysis patients. Circulation. 2004;109:23.
17. Fredericks S, Chang R, Gregson H, et al. Circulating cardiac troponin T in patients before and after renal transplantation. Clin Chim Acta. 2001;310:199–203.
18. Aronow WS, Ahn C, Mercando AD, Epstein S. Prevalence of coronary artery disease, complex ventricular arrhythmias, and silent myocardial ischemia and incidence of new coronary artery events in older persons with chronic renal insufficiency and with normal renal function. Am J Cardiol. 2000;86:1142–3.
19. Zawada ET, Stinson JB, Done G. New perspectives on coronary artery disease in hemodialysis patients. South Med J. 1982;75:694–6.
20. Freda BJ, Tang WH, Van Lente F, Peacock WF, Francis GS. Cardiac troponins in renal insufficiency: review and clinical implications. J Am Coll Cardiol. 2002;40:2065–71.

21. Antman EM, Tanasijevic MJ, Thompson B, et al. Cardiac-specific troponin-I levels to predict the risk of mortality in patients with acute coronary syndromes. N Engl J Med. 1996;335:1342.

22. Martin GS, Becker BN, Schulman G. Cardiac troponin-I accurately predicts myocardial injury in renal failure. Nephrol Dial Transplant. 1998;13:1709–12.

23. Wayand D, Baum H, Schatzle G, Scharf J, Neumeier D. Cardiac troponin T and I in end-stage renal failure. Clin Chem. 2000;46:1345–50.

24. Sanofi U.S. Medication Guide Revised Dec 2011 Distributed by: Bristol-Myers Squibb/Sanofi Pharmaceuticals Partnership Bridgewater. Available http://products.sanofi.us/plavix/plavix.html#section-11.5.

25. Becker RC, Bassand JP, Budaj A, Wojdyla DM, James SK, Cornel JH, et al. Bleeding complications with the P2Y12 receptor antagonists clopidogrel and ticagrelor in the PLATelet inhibition and patient outcomes (PLATO) trial. Eur Heart J. 2011;32(23): 2933–44.

26. Collet JP, Montalescot G, Agnelli G, Van de Werf F, Gurfinkel EP, Lopez-Sendon J, Laufenberg CV, Klutman M, Gowda N, Gulba D. Non-ST-segment elevation acute coronary syndrome in patients with renal dysfunction: benefit of low-molecular-weight heparin alone or with glycoprotein IIb/IIIa inhibitors on outcomes. The Global Registry of Acute Coronary Events. Eur Heart J. 2005;26:2285–93.

27. Braunwald E, Antman EM, Beasley JW, et al. ACC/AHA guideline update for the management of patients with unstable angina and non-ST segment elevation myocardial infarction – 2002 summary article: a report of the American College of Cardiology/American Heart Association Task Force on Practice Guidelines (Committee on the Management of Patients with Unstable Angina). Circulation. 2002;106:1893–900.

28. Paoletti E, Cassottana P, Bellino D, et al. Left ventricular geometry and adverse cardiovascular events in chronic hemodialysis patients on prolonged therapy with ACE inhibitors. Am J Kidney Dis. 2002;40(4):728–36.

29. Shibasaki Y, Masaki H, Nishiue T, et al. Angiotensin II type 1 receptor antagonist, losartan, causes regression of left ventricular hypertrophy in end-stage renal disease. Nephron. 2002;90(3): 256–61.

30. Cice G, Ferrara L, D'Andrea A, et al. Carvedilol increases two-year survival in dialysis patients with dilated cardiomyopathy: a prospective, placebo-controlled trial. J Am Coll Cardiol. 2003;41: 1438–44.

31. Bays H. Clinical overview of Omacor: a concentrated formulation of omega-3 polyunsaturated fatty acids. Am J Cardiol. 2006;98:71i–6.

32. Investigators ACT. Acetylcysteine for prevention of renal outcomes in patients undergoing coronary and peripheral vascular angiography: main results from the Randomized Acetylcysteine for Contrast-Induced Nephropathy Trial (ACT). Circulation. 2011;124: 1250–9.

33. Holdaas H, Fellstrom B, Jardine AG, et al. Effect of fluvastatin on cardiac outcomes in renal transplant recipients: a multicentre, randomised, placebo-controlled trial. Lancet. 2003;361:2024–31.

34. Tonelli M, Moyé L, Sacks FM, Kiberd B, Curhan G. Cholesterol and Recurrent Events (CARE) Trial Investigators. Pravastatin for secondary prevention of cardiovascular events in persons with mild chronic renal insufficiency. Ann Intern Med. 2003;138(2):98–104.

35. Freeman RV, Mehta RH, Al Badr W, et al. Influence of concurrent renal dysfunction on outcomes of patients with acute coronary syndromes and implications of the use of glycoprotein IIb/IIIa inhibitors. J Am Coll Cardiol. 2003;41(5):718–24.

36. Jeremias A, Bhatt DL, Chew DP, et al. Safety of abciximab during percutaneous coronary intervention in patients with chronic renal insufficiency. Am J Cardiol. 2002;89(10):1209–11.

37. Frilling B, Zahn R, Fraiture B, et al. Comparison of efficacy and complication rates after percutaneous coronary interventions in patients with and with renal insufficiency treated with abciximab. Am J Cardiol. 2002;89(4):450–2.

38. Best PJ, Lennon R, Gersh BJ, et al. Safety of abciximab in patients with chronic renal insufficiency who are undergoing percutaneous coronary interventions. Am Heart J. 2003;146(2):345–50.

39. Harrington RA, Becker RC, Cannon CP, et al. Antithrombotic therapy for non-ST segment elevation acute coronary syndromes: American College of Chest Physicians evidence-based clinical practice guidelines (8th edition). Chest. 2008;133:670S–707.

40. Mehta SR, Granger CB, Eikelboom JW, et al. Efficacy and safety of fondaparinux versus enoxaparin in patients with acute coronary syndromes undergoing percutaneous coronary intervention: results from the OASIS-5 trial. J Am Coll Cardiol. 2007;50(18):1742–51.

41. Keeley EC, Kadakia R, Soman S, Borzak S, McCullough PA. Analysis of long-term survival after revascularization in patients with chronic kidney disease presenting with acute coronary syndromes. Am J Cardiol. 2003;92(5):509–14.

42. Chan MY, Becker RC, Sim LL, et al. Reperfusion strategy and mortality in ST-elevation myocardial infarction among patients with and without impaired renal function. Ann Acad Med Singapore. 2010;39:179–84.

43. Charytan DM, Wallentin L, Lagerqvist B, et al. Early angiography in patients with chronic kidney disease: a collaborative systematic review. Clin J Am Soc Nephrol. 2009;4:1032–43.

44. Szummer K, Lundman P, Jacobson SH, et al. Influence of renal function on the effects of early revascularization in non-ST-elevation myocardial infarction: data from the Swedish Web-System for Enhancement and Development of Evidence-Based Care in Heart Disease Evaluated According to Recommended Therapies (SWEDEHEART). Circulation. 2009;120:851–8.

45. Ix JH, Mercado N, Shlipak MG, et al. Association of chronic kidney disease with clinical outcomes after coronary revascularization: the Arterial Revascularization Therapies Study (ARTS). Am Heart J. 2005;149:512–9.

46. Szczech LA, Reddan DN, Owen WF, et al. Differential survival after coronary revascularization procedures among patients with renal insufficiency. Kidney Int. 2001;60:292–9.

47. Contrast-Induced Nephropathy Renu Bansal, Chief Editor: Vecihi Batuman. E-Medicine (www.emedicine.com) Updated 29 July 2011. Available at: http://emedicine.medscape.com/article/246751-overview.

48. Ilkhanoff L, Carver J. Contrast-induced nephropathy and cardiac catheterization: evidence in support of using the iso-osmolar contrast agent. 2005. Available at: http://www.invasivecardiology.com/article/3990.

49. Friedewald VE, Goldfarb S, Laskey WK, et al. The editor's round-table: contrast-induced nephropathy. Am J Cardiol. 2007;100(3): 544–51.

50. Aspelin P, Aubry P, Fransson SG, Strasser R, Willenbrock R, Berg KJ. Nephrotoxicity in high-risk patients study of iso-osmolar and low-osmolar non-ionic contrast media study investigators. N Engl J Med. 2003;348(6):491–9.

51. Davidson CJ, Laskey WK, Hermiller JB, Harrison JK, Matthai Jr W, Vlietstra RE, et al. Randomized trial of contrast media utilization in high-risk PTCA: the COURT trial. Circulation. 2000; 101(18):2172–7.

52. Marckmann P, Skov L, Rossen K, et al. Nephrogenic systemic fibrosis: suspected causative role of gadodiamide used for contrast-enhanced magnetic resonance imaging. J Am Soc Nephrol. 2006; 17(9):2359–62.

53. Todd DJ, Kagan A, Chibnik LB, Kay J. Cutaneous changes of nephrogenic systemic fibrosis: predictor of early mortality and association with gadolinium exposure. Arthritis Rheum. 2007;56(10): 3433–41.

54. Cowper SE, Kuo PH, Bucala R. Nephrogenic systemic fibrosis and gadolinium exposure: association and lessons for idiopathic fibrosing disorders. Arthritis Rheum. 2007;56(10):3173–5.

55. Gibson SE, Farver CF, Prayson RA. Multiorgan involvement in nephrogenic fibrosing dermopathy: an autopsy case and review of the literature. Arch Pathol Lab Med. 2006;130(2):209–12.

56. Broome DR, Cottrell AC, Kanal E. Response to "will dialysis prevent the development of nephrogenic systemic fibrosis after gadolinium-based contrast administration?". AJR Am J Roentgenol. 2007;189:W234–5.

57. Vaziri ND. Dyslipidemia of chronic renal failure: the nature, mechanisms, and potential consequences. Am J Physiol Renal Physiol. 2005;290:F262–72.

58. Vaziri ND, Moradi H. Mechanisms of dyslipidemia of chronic renal failure. Hemodial Int. 2006;10:1–7.

59. Vaziri ND, Deng G, Liang K. Hepatic HDL receptor, SR-B1 and Apo A-I expression in chronic renal failure. Nephrol Dial Transplant. 1999;14:1462–6.

60. Harper CR, Jacobson TA. Managing dyslipidemia in chronic kidney disease. J Am Coll Cardiol. 2008;51(25):2375–84. ISSN:0735-1097/08jacc.2008.03.02.

61. Jardine AG, Holdaas H, Fellstrom B, et al. Fluvastatin prevents cardiac death and myocardial infarction in renal transplant recipients: post-hoc subgroup analyses of the ALERT study. Am J Transplant. 2004;4:988–95.

62. Tonelli M, Collins D, Robins S, Bloomfield H, Curhan GC. Veterans' Affairs High-Density Lipoprotein Intervention Trial Investigators. Gemfibrozil for secondary prevention of cardiovascular events in mild to moderate chronic renal insufficiency. Kidney Int. 2004;66:1123–30.

63. Parfrey PS, Foley RN, Harnett JD, Kent GM, Murray D, Barre PE. Outcome and risk factors of ischemic heart disease in chronic uremia. Kidney Int. 1996;49:1428–34.

64. Seliger SL, Weiss NS, Gillen DL, et al. HMG-CoA reductase inhibitors are associated with reduced mortality in ESRD patients. Kidney Int. 2002;61:297–304.

65. Andreucci VE, Fissell RB, Bragg-Gresham JL, et al. Dialysis outcomes and Practice Patterns Study (DOPPS) data on medications in hemodialysis patients. Am J Kidney Dis. 2004;44:61–7.

66. Wanner C, Krane V, Marz W, et al. Atorvastatin in patients with type 2 diabetes mellitus undergoing hemodialysis. N Engl J Med. 2005;353:238–48.

67. Baigent C, Landray MJ, Reith C, behalf of the SHARP Investigators. The effects of lowering LDL cholesterol with simvastatin plus ezetimibe in patients with chronic kidney disease (Study of Heart and Renal Protection): a randomized placebo-controlled trial. Lancet. 2011;377(9784):2181–92.

68. Kasiske BL. Hyperlipidemia in patients with chronic renal disease. Am J Kidney Dis. 1998;32(5 Suppl 3):S142–56.

69. Lowrie EG, Lew NL. Death risk in hemodialysis patients: the predictive value of commonly measured variables and an evaluation of death rate differences between facilities. Am J Kidney Dis. 1990;15:458–82.

70. Iseki K, Yamazato M, Tozawa M, Takishita S. Hypocholesterolemia is a significant predictor of death in a cohort of chronic hemodialysis patients. Kidney Int. 2002;61:1887–93.

71. Bolton K, Coresh J, Culleton B et al. KDOQI Clinical Practice Guidelines for Chronic Kidney Disease: Evaluation, Classification, and Stratification. National Kidney Foundation. Available at: www.kidney.org/professionals/kdoqi/guidelines.cfm.

72. Kidney Disease Outcomes Quality Initiative (K/DOQI) Group. K/DOQI clinical practice guidelines for managing dyslipidemia in chronic kidney disease. Am J Kidney Dis. 2003;41 Suppl 3:S1–237.

73. Corsini A, Holdass H. Fluvastatin in the treatment of dyslipidemia associated with chronic kidney failure and renal transplantation. Ren Fail. 2005;27:259–73.

74. Blum CB. Comparison of properties of four inhibitors of 3-hydroxy-3-methylglutaryl-coenzyme a reductase. Am J Cardiol. 1994;73:3D.

75. Nishizawa Y, Shoji T, Nishitani H, et al. Hypertriglyceridemia and lowered apolipoprotein C-II/C-III ratio in uremia: effect of a fibric acid, clinofibrate. Kidney Int. 1993;44:1352.

76. Jacobson TA, Zimmerman FH. Fibrates in combination with statins in the management of dyslipidemia. J Clin Hypertens. 2006;8:35–41.

77. Davidson MH, Armani A, McKenney JM, Jacobson TA. Safety considerations with fibrate therapy. Am J Cardiol. 2007;99:3C–18.

78. Health Resources and Services Administration, U.S. Department of Health & Human Services. Organ Procurement and Transplant Network Database. Available at: http://optn.transplant.hrsa.gov/. Accessed 21 Jan 2009.

79. U.S. Renal Data System: USRDS. 2008 annual data report. Bethesda: National Institutes of Health, National Institute of Diabetes and Digestive and Kidney Diseases; 2008. Atlas of ESRD, transplantation, Figure 7.31. Available at: http://www.usrds.org/2008/view/esrd_07.as.

80. Ojo AO, Hanson JA, Wolfe RA, Leichtman AB, Agodoa LY, Port FK. Long-term survival in renal transplant recipients with graft function. Kidney Int. 2000;57:307–13.

81. Fishbane S. Cardiovascular risk evaluation before kidney transplantation. Am Soc Nephrol. 2005;16:843–5.

82. Ramos EL, Kasiske BL, Alexander SR, Danovitch GM, Harmon WE, Kahana L, Kiresuk TJ, Neylan JF. The evaluation of candidates for renal transplantation: the current practice of U.S. transplant centers. Transplantation. 1994;57:490–7.

83. Ryckelynck JP, et al. Peritoneal UF and treatment-resistant heart failure. Nephrol Dial Transplant. 1998;13:56–9.

84. United States Renal Data System Atlas of Chronic Kidney Disease & End-Stage Renal Disease in the United States 2007 Annual Data Report volume ii. Available at: http://www.usrds.org/2007/ref_07.pdf.

85. Ronco C, Haapio M, House AA, et al. Cardiorenal syndrome. J Am Coll Cardiol. 2008;52:1527.

86. Nohria A, Hasselblad V, Stebbins A, et al. Cardiorenal interactions-insights from the ESCAPE trial. J Am Coll Cardiol. 2007;51:1268–74.

87. Greenberg A, et al. Primer on kidney diseases. 5th ed. Philadelphia: Saunders/Elsevier; 2009.

88. Goel S, et al. Classification and pathophysiology of cardiorenal syndrome. ASN Kidney News. 2010; p. 9.

89. Yazigi F, et al. Which marker should we use to assess acute renal injury? http://biomarkers.cardiosource.org/Hot-Topics/2011/04/Which-marker-should-we-use-to-assess-acute-renal-injury.aspx.

90. Herzog C, et al. Cardiovascular disease in chronic kidney disease. A clinical update from Kidney Disease: Improving Global Outcomes (KDIGO). Kidney Int. 2011;80:572–86.

91. Floege J, et al. Comprehensive clinical nephrology. Philadelphia: Saunders/Elsevier; 2010. p. 853–7. Chapter 71.

92. Gotloib L, et al. Peritoneal dialysis in refractory end-stage congestive heart failure: a challenge facing a no-win situation. Nephrol Dial Transplant. 2005;20 Suppl 7:vii32–6.

93. Costanzo MR, et al. Early ultrafiltration versus intravenous diuretics for patients hospitalized for acute decompensated heart failure. J Am Coll Cardiol. 2007;49:675–83.

94. Forman MB, Virmani R, Robertson RM, Stone WJ. Mitral annular calcification in chronic renal failure. Chest. 1984;85(3):367.

95. London GM, Pannier B, Marchais SJ, Guerin AP. Calcification of the aortic valve in the dialyzed patient. J Am Soc Nephrol. 2000;11(4):778.

96. Straumann E, Meyer B, Misteli M, Blumberg A, Jenzer HR. Aortic and mitral valve disease in patients with end stage renal failure on long-term haemodialysis. Br Heart J. 1992;67(3):236.

97. Cosmi JE, Kort S, Tunick PA, Rosenzweig BP, Freedberg RS, Katz ES, Applebaum RM, Kronzon I. The risk of the development of aortic stenosis in patients with "benign" aortic valve thickening. Arch Intern Med. 2002;162(20):2345.

98. K/DOQI Workgroup. K/DOQI clinical practice guidelines for cardiovascular disease in dialysis patients. Am J Kidney Dis. 2005;45(4 Suppl 3):S1.

99. Ureña P, Malergue MC, Goldfarb B, Prieur P, Guédon-Rapoud C, Pétrover M. Evolutive aortic stenosis in hemodialysis patients: analysis of risk factors. Nephrologie. 1999;20(4):217.

100. D'Cruz IA, Madu EC. Progression to calcific mitral stenosis in end-stage renal disease. Am J Kidney Dis. 1995;26(6):956.

101. Lavie CJ, Hebert K, Cassidy M. Prevalence and severity of Doppler-detected valvular regurgitation and estimation of right-sided cardiac pressures in patients with normal two-dimensional echocardiograms. Chest. 1993;103(1):226.

102. Stinebaugh J, Lavie CJ, Milani RV, Cassidy MM, Figueroa JE. Doppler echocardiographic assessment of valvular heart disease in patients requiring hemodialysis for end-stage renal disease. South Med J. 1995;88(1):65.

103. Li Y, Muench A, McGregor DH, Wiegmann TB. Cerebral, myocardial and cutaneous ischemic necrosis associated with calcific emboli from aortic and mitral valve calcification in a patient with end-stage renal disease. Clin Nephrol. 2002;57(6):468.

104. Renfrew R, Buselmeier TJ, Kjellstrand CM. Pericarditis and renal failure. Annu Rev Med. 1980;31:345–60.

105. Rutsky EA, Rostand SG. Treatment of uremic pericarditis and pericardial effusion. Am J Kidney Dis. 1987;10:2–8.

106. Compty CM, Cohen SL, Shapiro FL. Pericarditis in chronic uremia and its sequels. Ann Intern Med. 1971;75:173–83.

107. Barach AL. Pericarditis in chronic nephritis. Am J Med Sci. 1922;163:44–59.

108. Marini PV, Hull AR. Uremic pericarditis: a review of incidence and management. Kidney Int. 1975;2:163–6.

109. Alpert MA, Ravenscraft MD. Pericardial involvement in end-stage renal disease. Am J Med Sci. 2003;325(4):228.

110. Gunukula SR, Spodick DH. Pericardial disease in renal patients. Semin Nephrol. 2001;21(1):52.

111. Tseng JR, Lee MJ, Yen KC, Weng CH, Liang CC, Wang IK, Chang CT, Lin-Tan DT, Lin JL, Yen TH. Course and outcome of dialysis pericarditis in diabetic patients treated with maintenance hemodialysis. Kidney Blood Press Res. 2009;32(1):17.

112. Ifudu O, Int J. Daily dialysis in hemodialysis patients with pericardial effusion: where are the data? Artif Organs. 1999;22(7):469.

113. Spodick DH. Acute cardiac tamponade. N Engl J Med. 2003;349(7):684.

114. Soman SS, Sandberg KR, Borzak S, et al. The independent association of renal dysfunction and arrhythmias in critically ill patients. Chest. 2002;122:669.

115. Panichi V, Migliori M, De Pietro S, Taccola D, Bianchi AM, Norpoth M, Metelli MR, Giovannini L, Tetta C, Palla R. C reactive protein in patients with chronic renal diseases. Ren Fail. 2001;23:551–62.

116. Shlipak MG, Fried LF, Crump C, Bleyer AJ, Manolio TA, Tracy RP, Furberg CD, Psaty BM. Elevations of inflammatory and procoagulant biomarkers in elderly persons with renal insufficiency. Circulation. 2003;107:87–92.

117. Aviles RJ, Martin DO, Apperson-Hansen C, Houghtaling PL, Rautaharju P, Kronmal RA, Tracy RP, Van Wagoner DR, Psaty BM, Lauer MS, Chung MK. Inflammation as a risk factor for atrial fibrillation. Circulation. 2003;108:3006–10.

118. Chung MK, Martin DO, Sprecher D, Wazni O, Kanderian A, Carnes CA, Bauer JA, Tchou PJ, Niebauer MJ, Natale A, Van Wagoner DR. C-reactive protein elevation in patients with atrial arrhythmias: inflammatory mechanisms and persistence of atrial fibrillation. Circulation. 2001;104:2886–91.

119. Green D, Roberts PR. Ventricular arrhythmias and sudden death in patients with chronic kidney disease. J Ren Care. 2010;36 Suppl 1:54–60.

120. Korantzopoulos P, Liu T, Li L, Goudevenos JA, Li G. Implantable cardioverter defibrillator therapy in chronic kidney disease: a meta-analysis. Europace. 2009;11(11):1469–75. Epub 2009 Oct 6.

121. Wase A, Basit A, Nazir R, et al. Impact of chronic kidney disease upon survival among implantable cardioverter-defibrillator recipients. J Interv Card Electrophysiol. 2004;11:199.

122. Dasgupta A, Montalvo J, Medendorp S, et al. Increased complication rates of cardiac rhythm management devices in ESRD patients. Am J Kidney Dis. 2007;49:656–63.

123. Soliman EZ, Prineas RJ, Go AS, Xie D, Lash JP, Rahman M, Ojo A, Teal VL, Jensvold NG, Robinson NL, Dries DL, Bazzano L, Mohler ER, Wright JT, Feldman HI. Chronic Renal Insufficiency Cohort (CRIC) Study Group. Chronic kidney disease and prevalent atrial fibrillation: the Chronic Renal Insufficiency Cohort (CRIC). Am Heart J. 2010;159(6):1102–7.

124. Horio T, Iwashima Y, Kamide K, Tokudome T, Yoshihara F, Nakamura S, Kawano Y. Chronic kidney disease as an independent risk factor for new-onset atrial fibrillation in hypertensive patients. J Hypertens. 2010;28(8):1738–44.

125. US Renal Data System. USRDS 2005 annual data report: atlas of end-stage renal disease in the United States. Bethesda: National Institutes of Health, National Institute of Diabetes and Digestive and Kidney Diseases; 2005.

126. Nakayama M, Metoki H, Terawaki H, Ohkubo T, Kikuya M, Sato T, Nakayama K, Asayama K, Inoue R, Hashimoto J, Totsune K, Hoshi H, Ito S, Imai Y. Kidney dysfunction as a risk factor for first symptomatic stroke events in a general Japanese population-the Ohasama study. Nephrol Dial Transplant. 2007; 22:1910–5.

127. Abbott KC, Trespalacios FC, Taylor AJ, Agodoa LY. Atrial fibrillation in chronic dialysis patients in the United States: risk factors for hospitalization and mortality. BMC Nephrol. 2003;4:1–10.

128. Boccardo P, Remuzzi G, Galbusera M. Platelet dysfunction in renal failure. Semin Thromb Hemost. 2004;30:579–89.

129. Tveit DP, Hypolite IO, Hshieh P, Cruess D, Agodoa LY, Welch PG, Abbott KC. Chronic dialysis patients have high risk for pulmonary embolism. Am J Kidney Dis. 2002;39:1011–7.

130. Iseki K, Kinjo K, Kimura Y, Osawa A, Fukiyama K. Evidence for high risk of cerebral haemorrhage in chronic dialysis patients. Kidney Int. 1993;44:1086–90.

131. Gage BF, Waterman AD, Shannon W, Boechler M, Rich MW, Radford MJ. Validation of clinical classification schemes for predicting stroke: results from the National Registry of Atrial Fibrillation. JAMA. 2001;285:2864–70.

132. Dahri K, Loewen P. The risk of bleeding with warfarin: a systematic review and performance analysis of clinical prediction rules. Thromb Haemost. 2007;98:980–7.

133. Stangier J, Rathgen K, Stähle H, Mazur D. Influence of renal impairment on the pharmacokinetics and pharmacodynamics of oral dabigatran etexilate: an open-label, parallel-group, single-centre study. Clin Pharmacokinet. 2010;49(4):259–68. doi:10.2165/11318170-000000000-00000.

134. Garg AX, Clark WF, Haynes RB, House AA. Moderate renal insufficiency and the risk of cardiovascular mortality: results from the NHANES I. Kidney Int. 2002;61(4):1486.

135. O'Hare A, Johansen K. Lower-extremity peripheral arterial disease among patients with end-stage renal disease. J Am Soc Nephrol. 2001;12(12):2838.

136. O'Hare AM, Hsu CY, Bacchetti P, Johansen KL. Peripheral vascular disease risk factors among patients undergoing hemodialysis. J Am Soc Nephrol. 2002;13(2):497.

137. Rajagopalan S, Dellegrottaglie S, Furniss AL, Gillespie BW, Satayathum S, Lameire N, Saito A, Akiba T, Jadoul M, Ginsberg N, Keen M, Port FK, Mukherjee D, Saran R. Peripheral arterial disease in patients with end-stage renal disease: observations from

the Dialysis Outcomes and Practice Patterns Study (DOPPS). Circulation. 2006;114(18):1914.

138. Leskinen Y, Salenius JP, Lehtimäki T, Huhtala H, Saha H. The prevalence of peripheral arterial disease and medial arterial calcification in patients with chronic renal failure: requirements for diagnostics. Am J Kidney Dis. 2002;40(3):472.

139. Fowkes FG, Housley E, Cawood EH, Macintyre CC, Ruckley CV, Prescott RJ. Edinburgh Artery Study: prevalence of asymptomatic and symptomatic peripheral arterial disease in the general population. Int J Epidemiol. 1991;20(2):384.

140. Boaz M, Weinstein T, Matas Z, Green, Smetana S. Peripheral vascular disease and serum phosphorus in hemodialysis: a nested case-control study. Clin Nephrol. 2005;63(2):98.

141. Chan CT, Mardirossian S, Faratro R, Richardson RM. Improvement in lower-extremity peripheral arterial disease by nocturnal hemodialysis. Am J Kidney Dis. 2003;41(1):225.

142. White JW, White RA, Rosenfield KA, Sacks D, Stanley JC, Taylor LM Jr, Halperin CJL, Hiratzka LF, Murphy WRC, Olin JW, Puschett JB, Hirsch AT, Haskal ZJ, Hertzer NR, Bakal CW, Creager MA, Jonathan. ACC/AHA 2005 practice guidelines for the management of patients with peripheral arterial disease (lower extremity, renal, mesenteric, and abdominal aortic). Circulation. 2006; 113(11):e463.

143. Koelemay MJ, Lijmer JG, Stoker J, Legemate DA, Bossuyt P. Magnetic resonance angiography for the evaluation of lower extremity arterial disease: a meta-analysis. JAMA. 2001; 285(10):1338.

144. Feringa HH, Karagiannis SE, Chonchol M, Vidakovic R, Noordzij PG, Elhendy A, van Domburg RT, Welten G, Schouten O, Bax JJ, Berl T, Poldermans D. Lower progression rate of end-stage renal disease in patients with peripheral arterial disease using statins or angiotensin-converting enzyme inhibitors. J Am Soc Nephrol. 2007;18(6):1872.

145. Clagett GP, Sobel M, Jackson MR, Lip GY, Tangelder M, Verhaeghe R. Antithrombotic therapy in peripheral arterial occlusive disease: the Seventh ACCP Conference on Antithrombotic and Thrombolytic Therapy. Chest. 2004;126 (3 Suppl):609S.

146. CAPRIE Steering Committee. A randomised, blinded, trial of clopidogrel versus aspirin in patients at risk of ischaemic events (CAPRIE). CAPRIE Steering Committee. Lancet. 1996; 348(9038):1329.

147. Beebe HG, Dawson DL, Cutler BS, Herd JA, Strandness Jr DE, Bortey EB, Forbes WP. A new pharmacological treatment for intermittent claudication: results of a randomized, multicenter trial. Arch Intern Med. 1999;159(17):2041.

148. Money SR, Herd JA, Isaacsohn JL, Davidson M, Cutler B, Heckman J, Forbes WP. Effect of cilostazol on walking distances in patients with intermittent claudication caused by peripheral vascular disease. J Vasc Surg. 1998;27(2):267.

149. Harrington EB, Harrington ME, Schanzer H, Haimov M. End-stage renal disease – is infrainguinal limb revascularization justified? J Vasc Surg. 1990;12(6):691.

150. O'Hare AM, Sidawy AN, Feinglass J, Merine KM, Daley J, Khuri S, Henderson WG, Johansen KL. Influence of renal insufficiency on limb loss and mortality after initial lower extremity surgical revascularization. J Vasc Surg. 2004; 39(4):709.

151. O'Hare AM, Feinglass J, Reiber GE, Rodriguez RA, Daley J, Khuri S, Henderson WG, Johansen KL. Postoperative mortality after nontraumatic lower extremity amputation in patients with renal insufficiency. J Am Soc Nephrol. 2004;15(2):427.

152. Karthikeyan V, Ananthasubramaniam K. Coronary risk assessment and management options in chronic kidney disease patients prior to kidney transplantation. Curr Cardiol Rev. 2009;5(3): 177–86.

Cardiac Tumors and Masses

25

Justina C. Wu

Abstract

Cardiac masses may present themselves upon investigation of cardiovascular symptoms, systemic manifestations, or incidentally upon screening. The differential diagnosis, workup, and subsequent management are heavily dependent upon the presenting clinical setting and the individual patient. In the broadest terms, a mass may be a benign or malignant tumor, a degenerative or infectious process, a normal but prominent structure, or even merely an imaging artifact that has been misinterpreted.

Armed with a basic knowledge of the most common entities and the demographic in which they typically present, together with an awareness of the pathways in which cancer or masses can involve the heart, one may then choose the most appropriate cardiac imaging modality and workup to diagnose and treat the patient.

In this chapter, the most common masses affecting the heart are presented with updated strategies for further refining the differential diagnosis. Initial treatment strategies and recommendations based on the available literature are presented.

Keywords

Cardiac tumors • Cardiac masses • Cancer • Echocardiography • MRI

Introduction

There are few accurate figures on the overall prevalence of cardiac masses discovered incidentally as compared to those that are discovered during evaluation of cardiac or cancer-related symptoms. Among primary tumors of the heart, it is estimated that up to 90 % or more are detected incidentally. However, it is highly likely that with the increasing use of thoracic imaging overall, as well as a growing population being screened and treated for heart disease or cancer, the overall detection rate of cardiac masses in general is increasing, particularly in developed nations.

Cardiac tumors are so rare (ranging from 1 to 2 % in general autopsy series, but up to 4–8 % in cancer patient autopsies) that routine screening is not performed, even in demographics known to be at a higher risk of cancer involving the heart (Fig. 25.1) [1–5]. Rather, it is far more common to unexpectedly encounter a cardiac mass upon imaging or surgery of the heart for an unrelated reason, or upon ancillary testing of a patient undergoing treatment for a noncardiac malignancy. More rarely, symptoms from a cardiac tumor may point towards the heart as a source, as in the case of systemic embolization or pericardial involvement. Only the larger masses will actually cause obstruction of cardiac inflow or outflow. Often, a pattern of concomitant cardiovascular, neurologic and/or pulmonic, and systemic sequelae offers clues to the presence of a cardiac tumor.

J.C. Wu, MD, PhD, FACC
Department of Medicine, Harvard Medical School,
Brigham and Women's Hospital, 75 Francis St.,
Boston, MA 02115, USA
e-mail: jcwu@partners.org

The online version of this chapter (doi:10.1007/978-1-4471-4441-0_25) contains supplementary material, which is available to authorized users.

This chapter will discuss (1) clinical manifestations of tumors and their pathologic effects on the heart, (2) common tumor locations, (3) epidemiology and oncologic types, (4) imaging modalities for parsing the differential diagnosis, (5) treatment algorithms, and (6) entities that may mimic or present as masses (pseudo-neoplasms).

Clinical Manifestations and Pathophysiology

Cardiac tumors may cause symptoms by a variety of mechanisms, primarily dependent upon the location of the mass and, to a lesser extent, by the type of tumor. Large masses may cause obstruction to cardiac chamber inflow (i.e., superior vena cava obstruction) or outflow. A classic example is that of a large left atrial myxoma intermittently obstructing the mitral valve (Fig. 25.2 and Videos 25.1a, 25.1b). Inflow obstruction of either side of the heart may cause syncope, and outflow obstruction may lead to symptoms of congestive heart failure. Embolic sequelae are also a common manifestation of even smaller tumors: left-sided tumors may be suspected when there are emboli thrown to key vascular beds in the CNS, limbs, kidneys, and spleen or even to the coronary arteries. Right-sided tumors may cause pulmonary emboli or paradoxical emboli (if an intracardiac shunt such as a patent foramen ovale is present). A pattern of embolic

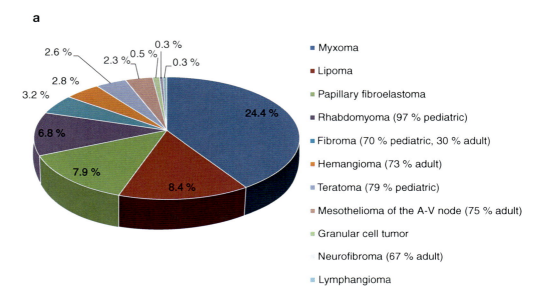

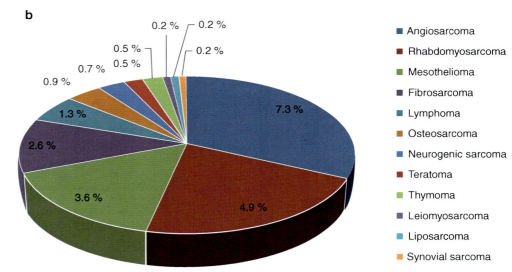

Fig. 25.1 (a–c) Frequency distribution of cardiac tumors. (a) Primary benign tumors of the heart. (b) Primary malignant tumors of the heart. (c) Secondary tumors metastatic to the heart (a and b, Adapted from McAllister et al. [2]). (1) Percentages are the percent of total primary tumors, n=533 (408 benign and 125 malignant). (2) Pericardial and bronchogenic cysts, with represent 16.7 % (n=89) of all primary cardiac masses in this autopsy series, are excluded from the above analysis. (3) Pediatric was defined as patients ≤15 years old. (c, Adapted from Butany et al. [1]). N=255, study population was ≥14 years old)

Fig. 25.1 (continued)

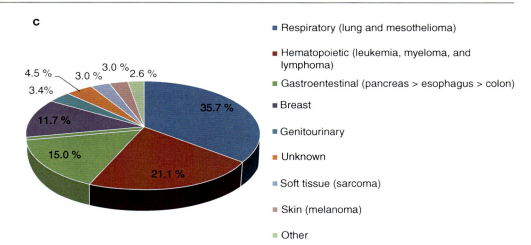

- ■ Respiratory (lung and mesothelioma)
- ■ Hematopoietic (leukemia, myeloma, and lymphoma)
- ■ Gastroentestinal (pancreas > esophagus > colon)
- ■ Breast
- ■ Genitourinary
- ■ Unknown
- ■ Soft tissue (sarcoma)
- ■ Skin (melanoma)
- ■ Other

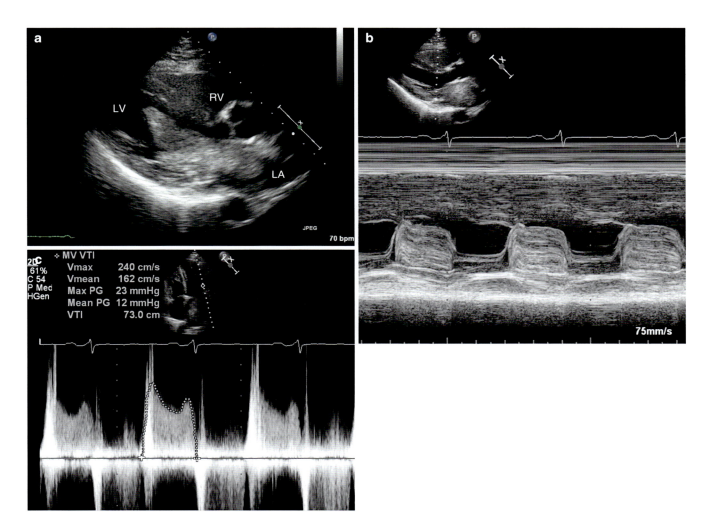

Fig. 25.2 Left atrial myxoma (**a**) viewed in parasternal echo window. This large (8×5 cm) mass was attached to the interatrial septum and prolapsed through the mitral valve into the left ventricle. (**b**) M-mode across the mitral leaflets, showing the tumor mass prolapsing between the two mitral leaflets in diastole. (**c**) Spectral Doppler of mitral flow. The tumor causes mitral stenosis (peak and mean gradients of 23 and 12 mmHg) and significant mitral regurgitation (Videos 25.1a and 25.1b) Apical four-chamber (1a) and parasternal short-axis (1b) views show tethering of the myxoma to the interatrial septum and prolapse through the mitral valve into the left ventricle. This was associated with the characteristic tumor "plop" on auscultation

"showering" causing organ infarcts in multiple territories should always cause one to suspect a cardiac source and is a strong indication for echocardiography [6]. Valvular regurgitation can be another mechanism leading to heart failure due to a mass tethering or interfering with leaflet closure, causing valvular incompetence and volume overload. Tumors that directly invade the heart may cause symptoms by creating arrhythmias (paroxysmal tachyarrhythmias or heart block if the AV conducting system is invaded), areas of impaired contractility, restrictive disease, and congestive heart failure. More commonly, however, either direct invasion or metastatic (hematogenous or lymphangitic) seeding of the pericardium leads to pericardial effusion which may manifest as dyspnea and hypotension due to cardiac tamponade or constriction.

Certain types of cancers, such as myxomas, are notorious for producing systemic or constitutional symptoms, such as fever, malaise, fatigue, rash, arthralgias, and weight loss, perhaps via humoral pathways. There are only rare tumor markers for cardiac tumors, dependent upon the primary type of cancer (e.g., interleukin-6 levels may be elevated in myxomas); however, laboratory testing may generally reveal an unexplained anemia and elevated erythrocyte sedimentation rate. There is no known hereditary or causative etiology for primary cardiac neoplasms, and only very rare disease associations (e.g., Carney complex in association with atrial myxomas and rhabdomyoma occurrence in patients with tuberous sclerosis) are known [7].

Tumors that are thought to be more likely to embolize are those associated with the aortic valve or left atrium [8], those that appear more mobile, or those with friable elements [9, 10]. In the case of cardiac myxoma, emboli have been found to be more frequently associated with those that are small or have a villous appearance. Papillary fibroelastomas that are larger (>1 cm) and more mobile are more frequently associated with embolic sequelae including coronary, CNS, retinal artery, and pulmonary emboli. Interestingly, in these studies, there is an inverse correlation with valvular regurgitation, possibly because the smaller, hemodynamically insignificant tumors are allowed to remain within the patients for longer periods of time, increasing the cumulative risk of embolization. Advanced malignancies that have metastasized to the heart obviously confer their own secondary risks with regard to hypercoagulability and marantic endocarditis, both of which are additional factors contributing to recurrent thromboembolization.

Common Tumor Locations

The location of the tumor is often the best clue as to type of tumor, with the overall tumor appearance playing only a secondary role in identification (see Table 25.1 for summary) [11]. When considering the source of the tumor, one should always consider the patient's age and comorbidities, as well as examine the cardiovascular structures adjacent to the tumor for clues. The most common tumor presenting in the left atrium is the cardiac myxoma, a primary benign cancer which typically is attached to the interatrial septum and can grow large enough to obstruct the left atrium, causing mitral stenosis and a renowned tumor "plop" on auscultation [12]. However, other tumors such as bronchogenic carcinomas may invade the left atrium via the pulmonary veins. In patients with rheumatic disease or atrial fibrillation, a thrombus should also definitely be considered in the differential. Right atrial tumors frequently are found to be myxomas as well, but invasion of this chamber by nephroblastoma, hepatic or adrenal tumors, or extension from inferior vena cava thrombi should also be considered. Lung and thyroid cancers have been known to invade the right atrium by extension down the superior vena cava. Of the malignant cardiac tumors, angiosarcomas have been reported more frequently in the right heart. Fragmentation of right atrial tumors may lead to pulmonary emboli or paradoxical emboli through a patent foramen ovale, and tricuspid valve obstruction or regurgitation can cause symptoms of right heart failure.

Ventricular tumors are rare. Unlike atrial masses which tend to be intracavitary, ventricular masses are usually intramural. Rhabdomyomas are the most common pediatric cardiac tumors, occurring in the left ventricle in 80 % of cases, with 15 % of cases arising in the right ventricle. Fibromas are the second most common pediatric cardiac tumor, although adult cases have been reported. They tend to arise in the interventricular septum or left ventricular free wall, approximately five times more frequently than in the right ventricle [13].

Of the primary cardiac tumors arising from valvular tissue, papillary fibroelastomas are the most common type in adults. Most (<80 %) are found on left-sided (aortic or mitral) valves, although any valve may be affected, and 9 % present as multiple lesions. They usually cause symptoms via embolization of the tumor itself or associated thrombus. However, a significant proportion (30 % in some series) are incidentally discovered upon echocardiography, cardiac surgery, or at autopsy [9, 14].

Pericardial involvement in cancers may arise from direct invasion of tumor from adjacent lung or mediastinum (e.g., mesothelioma or lymphoma) or more diffuse involvement and effusive/constrictive changes. The most frequent causes of malignant pericardial disease are lung, lymphoma/leukemia, and breast cancer due to their relatively high prevalence [1–4, 15]. Of all malignancies, melanoma has the highest predilection to metastasize to the pericardium, but only 2 % of patients become symptomatic despite postmortem findings showing cardiac involvement in 38–50 % of cases [16].

Table 25.1 Site-specific differential diagnoses for cardiac tumors

	Oncologic	Also consider nonneoplastic masses	Normal or variant structures
Left atrium	Myxoma	Thrombus	Pulmonary vein ridge
	Bronchogenic carcinoma	Endocardial blood cyst	Lipomatous hypertrophy of the interatrial septum
	Sarcoma (involving wall/pericardium)		Interatrial septal aneurysm
	Hemangioma		External compression (hernia, thoracic aorta, bezoar)
	Paraganglioma		Atrial suture anastomosis post-heart transplant
			Inverted LA appendage (postoperative)
			Appendage pectinate muscles
			Echocardiographic artifact
Right atrium	Myxoma	Thrombus (deep venous or in situ) or fibrin cast (if prior indwelling catheter/wire)	Eustachian valve
	Nephroblastoma, renal cell cancer	Vegetation (on pacer/AICD wires)	Chiari network
	Hepatocellular carcinoma	Lipomatous hypertrophy of the interatrial septum	Crista terminalis
	Sarcoma (angiosarcoma)		Pectus excavatum
	Paraganglioma		
	Adrenal tumors		
Left ventricle	Rhabdomyoma (often multiple)	Thrombus	Calcified or multilobed papillary muscles
	Fibroma	Apical hypertrophic cardiomyopathy	Redundant mitral chordae
	Hamartoma		Trabeculations
	Purkinje cell tumors		
Right ventricle	Rhabdomyoma	Thrombus	Redundant tricuspid chordae
	Fibroma		Moderator band
Valves	Papillary fibroelastoma	Lambl's excrescence	Nodules of Arantius
	Myxoma	Caseous mitral annular calcification	Myxomatous/degenerative changes
	Hamartoma	Vegetation	Pannus, loose suture, bioglue or pledgets around prosthetic valves
	Lipomatous tumor	Marantic endocarditis	
		Abscess	
		Blood cyst	
		Rheumatoid nodule	
Pericardium	Malignant involvement from: lung, breast, lymphoma/leukemia, gastrointestinal tract, melanoma	Pericardial or bronchogenic cyst	Epicardial or mediastinal fat
	Mesothelioma	Rheumatoid nodule	Pectus excavatum
	Primary		Atelectatic lung or fibrin in pleural/peritoneal spaces
	Spindle cell tumor, fibrous tumors, lipoma, liposarcoma, teratoma		Vascular pseudoaneurysm
	Paraganglioma		

Common Tumor Types

Primary

Primary cardiac tumors are very rare, with an incidence ranging around 0.2 %, whereas tumors metastatic to the heart are over 20–40 times more frequent [1–5, 7]. These tumors are usually of mesothelial or epithelial origin [17]. *Myxomas* represent over 50 % of primary cardiac tumors in adults, followed by lipomas and papillary fibroelastomas

(see Fig. 25.2). Cardiac myxomas are believed to arise from mesenchymal (endocardial) cells and typically arise in the left atrium, often from the interatrial septum near the fossa ovalis with a stalk-like pedicle as an attachment point. Histologically, the tumor consists of abundant mucopolysaccharide matrix containing polygonal stellate cells without mitotic figures and vascular channels. Grossly and by cardiac imaging, myxomas frequently appear as a gelatinous, compact ovoid mass attached to the interatrial septum by a stalk, but the shape and surface characteristics may vary (Fig. 25.2

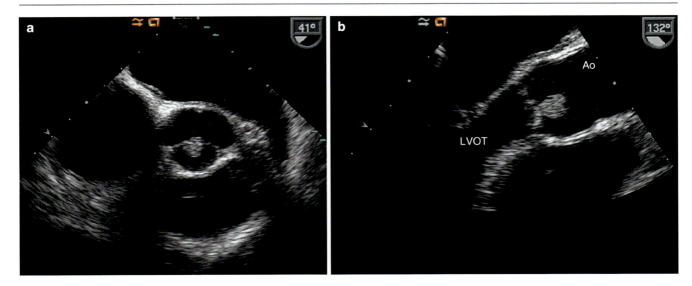

Fig. 25.3 Papillary fibroelastoma, seen on (**a**) TEE short-axis and (**b**) long-axis views, with Video 25.2 This 48-year-old female presented with palpitations. Stress echocardiography incidentally revealed a 1.1 cm mobile mass on the aortic aspect of the right coronary cusp. Although otherwise asymptomatic, resection was advised due to embolic risk. She underwent a minimally invasive surgery in which the tumor and its thin stalk were resected, with no further valve repair required

and Videos 25.1a, 25.1b). Attachments to the mitral valve have been described in a small percentage of cases. Smaller tumors tend to be more papillary or villous and friable and appear to be more inclined to embolize. The larger tumors may have a smoother, polyploid appearance and grow large enough to virtually fill the left atrial chamber and exert an obstructive effect on mitral inflow. Most myxoma cases arise sporadically in patients between 30 and 60 years of age, with a female predominance in most series. In approximately 7 % of cases, familial syndromes (Carney syndrome) associated with myxoma exist, in which skin myxomas, pigmented cutaneous lentigines, blue nevi, and endocrine or testicular tumors are concomitantly found, with an autosomal dominant pattern of inheritance. Myxomas in this latter group tend to occur earlier (<40 years), may be multicentric, and are more prone to recurrence [11, 12, 18].

Papillary fibroelastomas and lipomas are the next most common benign cardiac tumors in this population. Papillary fibroelastomas are the most common valvular cardiac tumor. Pathologists usually classify fibroelastomas as an advanced or more florid form of Lambl's excrescences, which are degenerative changes of the valves. Typically, the aortic valve (followed by the mitral valve in frequency) is involved, and the lesion consists of a hyalinized central mucopolysaccharide core lined by endocardial-type spindle cells. There is no clear distinction between a Lambl's excrescence and a papillary fibroelastoma as they appear to represent ends of a continuum, with growth over months to decades observed in expectantly followed cases [9]. On discovery, most are small (<0.2–1.0 cm); the larger entities have been alternatively

termed "giant Lambl's" excrescences. They have a tendency to appear on either side of the aortic valve or on the atrial side of mitral valves. Less frequently, they have also been known to arise on mitral chordae or papillary muscles. Occurrence on right-sided valves has been reported infrequently. Grossly the classic papillary fibroelastoma has innumerable filamentous avascular papillary fronds arising from the central stalk, giving the appearance of a "sea anemone" when resuspended in fluid. On echocardiography, they appear round, oval, or irregular in shape and appear homogenous in texture (Fig. 25.3 and Video 25.2). Nearly half have a short stalk, which confers more mobility. They are found most frequently in the elderly as solitary lesions (<10 % occur as a multiple). Shedding of the threadlike elements and/or associated clot accounts for the frequent presentation by embolization (transient ischemic attack or stroke, angina or sudden death) [9, 11, 14].

Lipomas (Fig. 25.4) are encapsulated collections of benign fat cells which often occur in subepicardial or subendocardial locations and may grow into the pericardial space. Although benign, usually discovered incidentally and easily distinguished by MRI imaging characteristics, these tumors tend to increase progressively and can cause mass effect, heart block, or tachyarrhythmias (Video 25.3). Pathologically lipomas can be difficult to distinguish from lipomatous hypertrophy of the interatrial septum, which is a normal finding particularly in elderly or obese patients (see later section on pseudotumors). However, lipomatous hypertrophy is due to an expansion of normal fat which stays confined to the interatrial septum and spares the fossa ovalis, producing a

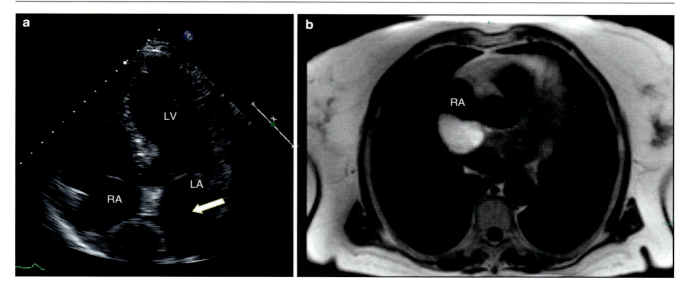

Fig. 25.4 Lipoma. This 82-year-old female had a history of lung cancer metastatic to the liver and bone. After experiencing syncope, she was found to have a cardiac mass (*arrow*) on echocardiography (**a**). The main differential diagnoses were lipomatous hypertrophy of the interatrial septum, lipoma, myxoma, or lung metastasis. (**b**) On cardiac MRI (T1-weighted short-axis images at the base of the heart), a well-circumscribed homogeneous mass was located posterior to the SVC and right atrium. It appeared hyperintense on both T1- and T2-weighted images, hypointense after fat suppression, and did not enhance during or after first-pass perfusion. Collectively the findings were consistent with lipoma. However, the patient subsequently developed complications (Video 25.3) from lung cancer including partial superior vena cava (SVC) syndrome and pericardial tamponade, requiring pericardiocentesis and, ultimately, a pericardial window for palliation (Courtesy of Swathy Kolli, MD, Brigham and Women's Hospital)

characteristic dumbbell-shaped mass. Although lipomatous hypertrophy may reach impressive thickness (1–2 cm), if the location is typical and there are no associated atrial arrhythmias or caval obstruction, no treatment is indicated [19].

Pericardial cysts are benign fluid-filled tumors of the parietal pericardium thought to be a congenital abnormality [20]. They may be solitary or multilocular and some have been documented to grow to massive (>20 cm) size [21]. They account for approximately 20 % of the benign primary cardiac masses (overall incidence 1:10,000) [2, 21] and commonly occur near the cardiophrenic borders (right more frequently than left) causing apparent cardiomegaly on chest X-ray and an encapsulated echolucent area on echocardiography [22]. Of known cases, 75 % are asymptomatic. However, if large they may cause atypical chest pain, breathlessness, atrial fibrillation, persistent cough, or compressive problems such as right ventricular outflow tract obstruction. Rare cases of cardiac tamponade due to intrapericardial rupture and hemorrhage have been reported [23].

Rhabdomyomas are the most common primary cardiac neoplasm in children and are usually found during the first year of life [24]. They tend to be found as solid intramyocardial lesions, containing striated myocyte fibers, and 90 % occur as multiple tumors. Although larger tumors have been known to cause arrhythmias, left ventricular outflow tract obstruction, and heart failure, most patients are asymptomatic. Half of the cases are associated with tuberous sclerosis.

Most regress spontaneously and, overall, these tumors are rare in young adults [2].

Fibroma is the second most common pediatric cardiac neoplasm [2–4]. They arise in the ventricular myocardial layer, are five times more common in the left ventricle, and are solid tumors consisting of fibroblasts. Tumors can become quite large and develop calcific foci. Unlike `rhabdomyomas, fibromas do not spontaneously regress and may grow to a size that obliterates the heart chamber, interferes with valvular function, or causes arrhythmia, necessitating surgical resection [25].

Very rare primary tumors arising within the heart are listed in Table 25.1 and Fig. 25.1a and include hemangiomas, hamartomas (Purkinje cell tumors), teratomas, and pericardial mesotheliomas. Some may have malignant potential or be otherwise life-threatening via paracrine or hemodynamic mechanisms.

Benign vs. Malignant

As discussed above, 75 % of primary cardiac tumors are benign, with myxomas clearly predominating in adults and rhabdomyomas being most frequent in the pediatric population. Of the 25 % of primary cardiac tumors that are malignant, 75 % are *sarcomas* (Fig. 25.1b) [1–4, 7]. There is no identified genetic linkage or predisposition to such neoplasms. In adults, *angiosarcoma* is the most common sarcoma. Angiosarcomas tend to arise in the right heart, particularly the right atrium, have a multilobulated form, and may completely obliterate the chamber and invade the vena cava and tricuspid apparatus. *Rhabdomyosarcoma* is the second most common malignant neoplasm of the adult heart, can arise in any cardiac chamber, and is multifocal in up to 60 % of cases. All share the common characteristics of rapid invasive growth and metastasis with frequent extension to the pericardium. The prognosis is dismal even with surgical excision and attempts at radio- and chemotherapy.

Secondary (Metastatic: With Pericardial Involvement)

In large autopsy series of cancer patients, 4–12 % have metastatic involvement of the heart. This number appears to be increasing due to increasing diagnostic tools, aggressive treatment of malignancies, and more thorough autopsies. Thus, secondary tumors outnumber primary cardiac tumors by 20–40 to 1 [1–5, 7]. In principle, any malignant tumor may metastasize to the heart. The most common primary neoplasm is bronchogenic carcinoma, followed by lymphomas and leukemia, breast cancer, and gastrointestinal (esophageal, pancreatic, or colon) cancer (see Fig. 25.1c). This almost certainly reflects the high prevalence of these neoplasms as well as the proximity of the primary source to the heart, since the actual rate of metastasis for most individual cancers is relatively low. The exception to this is malignant melanoma, which has a highest predilection (up to 50 % of cases) for cardiac metastasis. However, because of the relatively low prevalence of this cancer, it accounts for only 1 % of cases of cardiac metastasis [26]. Melanoma is followed next by leukemia and lymphoma (up to 33 % of patients die with cardiac infiltrates) and rare malignancies such as germ cell neoplasms and malignant thymoma in terms of predilection to metastasize to the heart. Despite finding involvement post-mortem, only a minority of melanoma (or other cancer) patients will actually manifest cardiac symptoms.

The most common site of involvement with metastatic disease is the pericardium followed by invasion of myocardium. Heart valves are rarely affected [4]. It is common for the cardiac metastases to be small and multiple, or alternatively they can cause diffuse thickening of the pericardium. However, bulky large solitary tumor lesions may also occur. Secondary tumors may invade the heart by direct extension, but transvenous migration and lymphatic or hematogenous routes also represent potential pathways to the heart (Fig. 25.5 and Video 25.4). The localization of the metastases tends to determine the patient's symptomatology rather than the histologic type.

Diagnostic Modalities

The cornerstone of detection and diagnosis of cardiac tumors has historically been *echocardiography*, due to its ease and widespread availability. Echocardiography has the advantages of being nonradioactive, easily portable, performed real time, and is able to not only visualize structural abnormalities but also discern any hemodynamic and valvular effects. The resolution of echocardiography is approximately 2 mm and even less for 5 MHz transesophageal probes, enabling very small masses (e.g., Lambl's excrescences) to be detected.

On echocardiography, however, tissue characterization is limited and tumors tend to be distinguished more by location rather than appearance. Nonetheless, important clues may be gleaned from the appearance of the tumor (size, solid vs. cystic, shape, degree of independent mobility, and friability), its attachments, and extent of myocardial, endocardial, or pericardial invasion. Properties such as calcification and cystic degeneration are viewed as echobright and echolucent areas on echocardiography, respectively (Fig. 25.6a, Video 25.5). Owing to the acoustic nature of the medium, echo artifacts may also arise and must be distinguished from true masses and normal structures before any invasive procedures are advised (see section on pseudotumors below). Obstruction to caval or valvular inflow is displayed as increases in peak spectral Doppler velocities and turbulence will manifest as a mosaic pattern on color Doppler imaging. Mitral stenosis and regurgitation caused by a left atrial myxoma prolapsing across the mitral valve is a classic example (see Fig. 25.2 and Videos 25.1a, 25.1b). The echocardiographic appearance of this entity is so pathognomic that usually no further workup is required before surgical resection. Similarly, papillary fibroelastomas occur so characteristically on the valves and so typically appear as filamentous or amorphous structures which shimmer, undulate, and prolapse that further assessment is usually not required (Fig. 25.3 and Video 25.2).

Echocardiography also offers a convenient way to monitor for recurrence, growth, or adverse sequelae posttreatment. This is particularly true in cases of pericardial involvement, when effusive or constrictive physiology and iatrogenic complications from pericardiocentesis may ensue. Transesophageal echocardiography (TEE) is recommended for better identification and delineation of tumor involvement particularly with regard to atrial and valvular involvement or when transthoracic imaging is technically difficult. One notable exception to this is when the results of a TEE would *not* change management, even when the source of embolus is known to be cardiac [6]. Most cardiac valves, pulmonary veins, and the proximal superior vena cava can be examined with greater clarity and resolution by TEE.

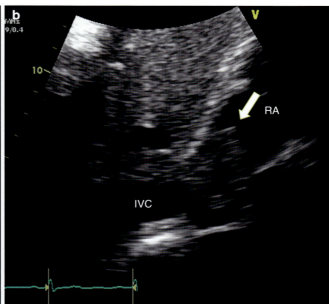

Fig. 25.5 Thrombus and renal cell cancer. (**a**) Apical four-chamber echocardiographic view of a mobile mass (*arrow*) in the right atrium which is not anchored to the interatrial septum and is seen in right atrial inflow views (Video 25.4). (**b**) Subcostal views reveal the mass (*arrow*) invading the right atrium from the inferior vena cava (*IVC*). Patient underwent right radical nephrectomy, caval resection, and extraction of renal cell carcinoma infiltrating the renal vein and extending into the IVC and right atrium via a combined subdiaphragmatic and atriotomy approach. The majority of the mass visualized in the right atrium was actually found to be tumor-associated thrombus

Beyond two-dimensional imaging, advanced echo techniques can prove particularly useful in specific scenarios. Three-dimensional (3D) echocardiography is useful for assessing the overall size, location, and attachments of intracavitary masses in real time. Doppler tissue imaging can reveal evidence of diastolic dysfunction due to infiltrative myocardial processes and monitor response to therapy [27]. Intravenous echocardiography contrast, which consists of sonicated microbubbles that pass freely through the pulmonary circulation, is useful for defining the borders of endocardium and masses in technically difficult cases. A more sophisticated use of echo contrast is to determine whether a tumor is neovascularized and, hence, more likely to be malignant as opposed to stromal [28]. While continuously infusing intravenous echo contrast, a "flash" of ultrasound waves with high mechanical index is used to destroy all microbubbles in the field, and the mass is then observed for reperfusion with the contrast. Vascular entities are more likely to be true tumors, whereas lack of perfusion by echo contrast is more indicative of a benign lesion, a normal finding, or thrombus. An example of the utility of intravenous echo contrast is shown in Video 25.6a.

A major advantage of echocardiography over the radiologic imaging modalities is the ability of echocardiography to visualize very small, fine, highly mobile structures which would not be adequately detected or displayed on the images of computed tomography (CT) and magnetic resonance imaging (MRI) which have slower acquisition times and frame rates. The resolution of transthoracic echocardiography is close to 2 mm and that of TEE is higher. Thus, papillary fibroelastomas, small mobile thrombi, and valvular lesions are far more likely to be detected and evaluated via ultrasound.

If a mass is detected on echocardiography without enough information to determine the probable etiology, it is appropriate to move on to other imaging modalities such as cardiac CT or MRI. In certain situations, all three modalities or even invasive procedures may be required to reliably make a definitive diagnosis [29].

Cardiac MRI is an excellent modality for evaluating cardiac masses because of its high resolution, ability to "cut" the heart in any imaging plane, and wider field of view enabling evaluation of adjacent extracardiac structures

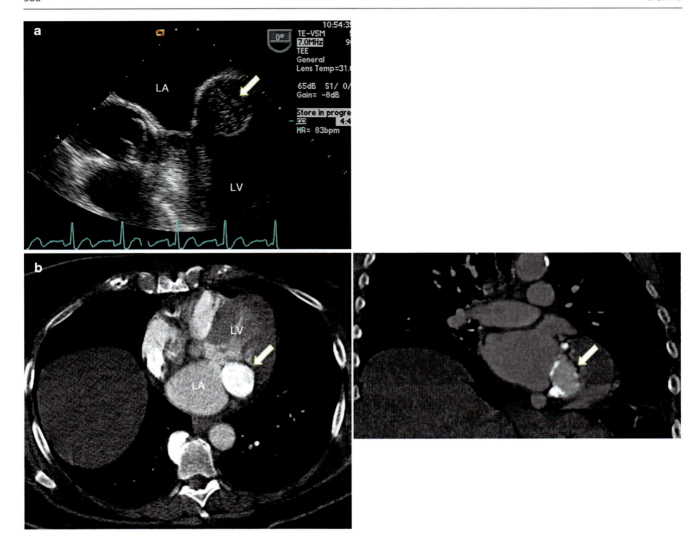

Fig. 25.6 Caseous mitral annular calcification. (**a** and Video 25.5) TEE apical five-chamber view zoomed in on a spherical 3.5 cm heterogeneously echogenic mass (*arrow*) which appears within the mitral annulus and protrudes into the left ventricular cavity in an 80-year-old female presenting with fever and retinal artery occlusion. Note the acoustic shadowing (black ray cast by calcification on the atrial surface of the mass, which prevents the ultrasound beams from passing through and obscures a narrow wedge of the left ventricle). (**b**) CT scan (*left panel*=short axis and *right panel*=coronal view) confirms dense calcification, which is typical of caseous calcification of the mitral annulus. Despite this, due to concern that the mass (*arrow*) might represent abscess or myxoma, it was surgically removed with reconstruction of the left ventricular wall and mitral valve replacement. Cultures were negative, and by pathology, only fibrous connective tissue with calcific degeneration and scant chronic inflammation was found (Courtesy of Frank J. Rybicki, MD and John D. Groarke, MD, Brigham and Women's Hospital)

(Video 25.6b). Of all the imaging modalities, MRI is able to display a greater range of soft tissue contrast. The higher intracellular and interstitial water content of malignant tissue and the increased vascularity are key features that distinguish malignant tumors on MRI. Detailed anatomic imaging is accomplished with standard spin-echo (T1-weighted) images. A higher degree of tissue characterization is achieved by T2-weighted imaging and T1 spin-echo techniques. Perfusion may be assessed with gadolinium enhancement. Myxomas will often appear heterogeneous in signal intensity on T1- and T2-weighted images and enhance with gadolinium contrast material (unlike thrombus). Lipomas have very homogenous high signal intensity on T1-weighted images (Fig. 25.4b) which will suppress on fat-saturated images. They do not enhance with gadolinium. Angiosarcomas are usually isointense relative to myocardium on T1-weighted images and hyperintense on T2-weighted images with a heterogeneous pattern of enhancement. Metastases from melanoma are usually hyperintense on T1-weighted imaging due to melanin content and enhance with gadolinium. MRI descriptions of the rarer cardiac tumors vary, and while there are few if any pathognomic features of any given histologic type, the signal characteristics, invasiveness, and vascularity or lack thereof can give strong clues as to origin [29].

Disadvantages of cardiac MRI include the need for electrocardiographic (ECG) gating which renders images in those with very irregular heart rates difficult, the possibility of dangerous or difficult imaging in those with implanted devices or claustrophobia, and the inability to demonstrate calcium in lesions. Gadolinium is contraindicated in patients with significant renal dysfunction. Patients with dyspnea or orthopnea may be unable to hold their breath in the supine position required.

Ultrafast electron beam or multidetector cardiac CT (ECG gated) is often helpful as an adjunct modality in patients in whom MRI is not an option, especially when the presence of calcium may help differentiate etiologies. It is particularly useful for confirming pericardial cysts and for distinguishing caseous mitral annular calcification from other masses (Fig. 25.6b). It may also distinguish fibromas, which tend to develop calcific foci, from rhabdomyomas. Neovascularization of malignant tumors may also be detected by CT angiography. The latest improvements in CT acquisition now allow for high-resolution thin slice 3D reconstruction, perfusion imaging, and cine images (3D plus time) which can convey cardiac function and tumor motion [30]. The disadvantages of CT include the use of ionizing radiation. Overall tissue resolution of cardiac CT is intermediate between echocardiography and MRI.

Although positron emission tomography (PET) scanning with ^{18}F-FDG has clear utility in diagnosing and staging noncardiac tumors, it currently has only a limited role in cardiac tumor imaging due to its low resolution and lack of specificity. However, whole-body scans with low-dose CT may be useful in differentiating benign from malignant tumors, in particular by excluding extracardiac metastases and, hence, can assist in preoperative assessment [31].

Treatment

Despite all the available advanced imaging tools, identification of a cardiac mass may still be challenging. The pseudomasses discussed in the next section are often more prevalent than true neoplasms. Suboptimal imaging, inaccessible location, or an elderly or debilitated patient may render a strategy of watchful waiting more prudent than pursuit of a tissue diagnosis, particularly when one cannot determine if a small mass is a true neoplasm, a thrombus, or an artifact. In some cases, a histologic diagnosis can be obtained invasively from discrete right-sided masses using transvenous access and echo-guided biopsy with a bioptome in order to direct definitive therapy. Pericardial effusions may be drained for cytologic analysis and symptomatic relief.

Once obtained, however, definitive diagnosis often simplifies the management: atrial myxomas should be promptly resected due to the risk of embolization and sudden death [10, 12, 13]. An autologous or bovine pericardial patch is used to reconstruct the interatrial septum or atrial free wall. The 20-year survival rate is approximately 85 %. Because there is a recurrence rate of approximately 5 %, serial follow-up with echocardiography is recommended. If Carney syndrome is diagnosed, all first-degree relatives should be screened.

Review of the literature with regard to papillary fibroelastomas has led to the following conclusions: larger papillary fibroelastomas, particularly those >1 cm and those with more mobility (i.e., possessing a stalk), appear more likely to cause embolic cardiac or neurologic events. However, embolization may be entirely unheralded. Thus, while it is relatively urgent that symptomatic patients undergo surgical excision, even asymptomatic patients should be considered if the lesion is left sided, large, and mobile (if the relative surgical risks are low) [9, 32]. Ideally the tumors may be resected while sparing overall valve integrity, avoiding the disadvantages of valve replacement. Very small asymptomatic papillary fibroelastomas in higher-risk patients may be monitored expectantly over time with echocardiography.

Experience has shown that lipomas grow slowly, and if the patient is asymptomatic, they may be merely observed over time. Rhabdomyomas in children tend to regress. Of the other benign primary cardiac tumors, the presence of associated symptoms such as obstruction to cardiac inflow or outflow, arrhythmias, or heart failure usually mandates operative resection and reconstruction of the involved cardiovascular structure. In virtually all cases of benign tumor resection, overall long-term outcomes are good with no significant recurrence rate [13].

For pericardial cysts, options include empiric observation. Percutaneous aspiration (with injection of a sclerosing agent such as alcohol) or video-assisted thoracotomy for resection is recommended only for cysts thought to be too symptomatic or high risk to follow [20].

In contrast, although primary solid malignant tumors of the heart are often resected requiring complex reconstruction of the heart, the results are disappointing [15]. If the tumor can be removed with clean margins and no metastases are detectable at diagnosis, the median survival increases from 5 to 6 months to over a year [33]. On the other hand, the presence of metastases implies that any surgical resection will likely only be palliative in nature. Overall prognosis correlates strongly with the histologic grade of malignancy [34]. Because of the rarity of these tumors, there is no standardized therapy: adjuvant chemotherapy (typically doxorubicin and ifosfamide) and radiation treatment of metastases may be offered, but the benefits are not yet clear. Because of their extracardiac location, pulmonary artery sarcomas appear more amenable to radiation therapy. Even with radical excision of cardiac sarcomas, local recurrence, infiltration, and metastases frequently recur; median survivals in most series range from 9 to 16 months. Alternative surgeries have been developed to try to improve this grim prognosis, including cardiac transplantation and autotransplantation (cardiac explantation, resection of the tumor with heart reconstruction ex vivo, and reimplantation). The series are small with mixed results but promising disease-free intervals in some cases [35]. Needless to say, referral to tertiary centers with specialized expertise is recommended.

Treatment of secondary malignancies involving the heart depends on symptomatology, the extent of cardiac involvement, and the nature of the underlying neoplasm. If there is significant pericardial effusion with signs of impending tamponade, pericardiocentesis is indicated. Analysis of the cytology of the fluid can give diagnostic and prognostic information. For instance, a significant percentage of both primary cardiac lymphoma (which most often occurs in Hodgkin's disease and immunocompromised or HIV-infected patients) and secondary lymphoma can regress markedly in response to systemic chemotherapy [36]. Even in advanced cases of disseminated carcinomas, a surgical or percutaneously created pericardial window can provide at least palliative relief for a meaningful period. Intracavitary metastatic heart tumors are rarer, but in patients who have already undergone extensive systemic therapy of the primary neoplasm, one might consider resection mainly to improve quality of life.

Pseudo-neoplasms

With the abundance of cardiac imaging being performed by various modalities, it is inevitable that normal or slight variants of normal structures, degenerative or acquired lesions, and noncancerous masses will be detected. The onus is upon the cardiologist or radiologist to distinguish between the following entities (summarized in Table 25.2) and a true neoplasm.

Masses such as thrombi and vegetations have obvious clinical implications. On echocardiography, thrombi appear relatively homogenous in echodensity and gel-like or deformable, although older thrombi may have more echobright regions and a compact immobile or laminated appearance. Clues that a mass is a thrombus include residing in areas of stasis such as the tip of the left atrial appendage or in a dyskinetic area of the ventricle (i.e., mural thrombi), "wisps" of spontaneous echo contrast (coagulating blood) associated with the surface, and associated cardiac conditions such as mitral stenosis, poor contractility, or atrial fibrillation. Rope-like or very elongated mobile masses in the right heart may actually represent thromboemboli from the deep venous system (Fig. 25.5b) and indicate that the inferior vena cava and pulmonary

Table 25.2 Pseudo-neoplasms of the heart

Nonneoplastic pathologies	Thrombus or fibrin
	Vegetation
	Pannus
	Fibrin casts of prior indwelling catheters or wires
Normal or variants	Focal upper septal hypertrophy
	Lipomatous hypertrophy of the interatrial septum
	Eustachian valve
	Chiari network
	False tendon
	Muscle bands, moderator band
	Multiheaded papillary muscles
	Redundant mitral or tricuspid chordae
	Left atrial chords
	Atrial appendage pectinate muscles
	Interatrial septal aneurysm
	Subaortic membrane
	Left atrial wall infoldings
	Crista terminalis
Degenerative	Lambl's excrescence
	Myxomatous mitral valve
	Focal valvular calcification
	Caseous mitral annular calcification
	Pseudoaneurysm
Extracardiac	Epicardial fat
	Esophageal hernias indenting the left atrial posterior wall
	Ectatic aorta or aortic aneurysms indenting the left atrium
	Vertebrae
	Thymus (in infants)
Echo (acoustic) artifacts	Pulmonary vein/atrial wall reflections (so-called Coumadin ridges)
	Reverberation or mirror artifact
Radiologic artifacts	Swirling from inhomogeneous i.v. contrast distribution

arteries should be inspected. Immobile thrombi or those in patients receiving anticoagulation frequently regress or remain stable [37].

Vegetations tend to have very irregular shapes and vary tremendously in size but have a predilection for forming on the upstream side of valves or at areas of flow turbulence. Valves with degenerative changes, prosthetic valves, and indwelling catheters or pacemaker/defibrillator leads are well-recognized niduses for infection. Thick, immobile, heaped-up irregular masses affixed to the annuli of older prosthetic valves may represent pannus (fibrovascular granulation tissue) which may interfere with both valve opening and closure. For both thrombi and vegetations, the larger and/or highly mobile masses that threaten the pulmonary or systemic and cerebral circulation with embolization or cause severe valvular dysfunction may compel emergent surgical resection.

It is not uncommon for a normal or normal variant of a structure to be mistaken for a potential neoplasm on echocardiography, since the transducer plane can only capture a two-dimensional slice of the heart. The most common error is mistaking lipomatous hypertrophy, upper septal hypertrophy, a redundant mitral chord or prominent/multilobed papillary muscle, interatrial septal aneurysm, or pericardial fat for a mass [11]. Unusually prominent degenerative changes such as valvular calcification or external compression of chambers of the heart by adjacent structures (e.g., from an esophageal hernia indenting the posterior wall of the left atrium) can all give the appearance of a large mass when viewed in one plane. Knowledge of the typical location of these abnormalities, use of echo contrast, and careful angling of the transducer plane to track the boundaries and attachments of these entities can reveal their nature. If still unclear, cardiac CT or MRI with contrast may be called upon for tissue characterization and examination of the adjacent extracardiac structures. Individual expertise in the interpretation of the initial imaging modality as well as judicious use of multimodality imaging should reduce the risk of imaging-specific artifacts.

Key Points

- Cardiac masses may present themselves upon investigation of cardiovascular symptoms, systemic manifestations, or incidentally upon screening.
- Among primary tumors of the heart, it is estimated that up to 90 % or more are detected incidentally.
- Cardiac tumors are so rare (ranging from 1 to 2 % in general autopsy series, but up to 4–8 % in cancer patient autopsies) that routine screening is not performed, even in demographics known to be at a higher risk of cancer involving the heart.
- Cardiac tumors may cause symptoms by a variety of mechanisms, primarily dependent upon the location of the mass and, to a lesser extent, by the type of tumor. Large masses may cause obstruction to cardiac chamber inflow (i.e., superior vena cava obstruction) or outflow.
- Tumors that are thought to be more likely to embolize are those associated with the aortic valve or left atrium, those that appear more mobile, or those with friable elements.
- The most common tumor presenting in the left atrium is the cardiac myxoma, a primary benign cancer which typically is attached to the interatrial septum and can grow large enough to obstruct the left atrium, causing mitral stenosis and a renowned tumor "plop" on auscultation.
- Ventricular tumors are rare.

- Primary cardiac tumors are very rare, with an incidence ranging around 0.2 %, whereas tumors metastatic to the heart are over 20–40 times more frequent.
- 75 % of primary cardiac tumors are benign, with myxomas clearly predominating in adults and rhabdomyomas being most frequent in the pediatric population.

References

1. Butany J, Leong SW, Carmichael K, Komeda M. A 30-year analysis of cardiac neoplasms at autopsy. Can J Cardiol. 2005; 21(8):675–80.
2. McAllister Jr HA, Fenoglio Jr JJ. Tumors of the cardiovascular system. In: Atlas of tumor pathology, Fascicle 15, vol. 2. Washington, DC: Armed Forces Institute of Pathology; 1978.
3. Burke A, Virmani R. Tumors of the heart and great vessels. In: Atlas of tumor pathology, Fascicle 16, vol. 3. Washington, DC: Armed Forces Institute of Pathology; 1996.
4. Lam KY, Dickens P, Chanc AC. Tumors of the heart. A 20-year experience with a review of 12,485 consecutive autopsies. Arch Pathol Lab Med. 1993;117:1027–31.
5. Silvestri F, Bussani R, Pavletic N, Mannone T. Metastases of the heart and pericardium. G Ital Cardiol. 1997;27:1252.
6. Douglas PS, Garcia MJ, Haines DE, et al. ACCF/ASE/AHA/ ASNC/HFSA/HRS/SCAI/SCCM/SCCT/SCMR 2011 appropriate use criteria for echocardiography. J Am Coll Cardiol. 2011;57: 1126–66.
7. Chahinian AP, Gutstein DE, Fuster V. Tumors of the heart and great vessels. In: Bast Jr RC, Kufe DW, Pollock RE, et al., editors. Holland-Frei cancer medicine. 5th ed. Hamilton: BC Decker; 2000. Chapter 91.
8. Elbardissi AW, Dearani JA, Daly RC, et al. Embolic potential of cardiac tumors and outcome after resection: a case-control study. Stroke. 2009;40:156–62.
9. Sun JP, Asher C, Yang XS, Cheng G, Scalia GM, Massed AG, et al. Clinical and echocardiographic characteristics of papillary fibroelastomas: a retrospective and prospective study in 162 patients. Circulation. 2001;103:2687–701.
10. Oliveira R, Branco L, Galrinho A, et al. Cardiac myxoma: a 13-year experience in echocardiographic diagnosis. Rev Port Cardiol. 2010;29:1087–100.
11. Peters PJ, Reinhardt S. The echocardiographic evaluation of intracardiac masses: a review. J Am Soc Echocardiogr. 2006;19: 230–40.
12. Reynen K. Cardiac myxomas. N Engl J Med. 1995;333: 1610–7.
13. ElBardissi AW, Dearani JA, Daly RC, et al. Analysis of benign ventricular tumors: long-term outcome after resection. J Thorac Cardiovasc Surg. 2008;135:1061–8.
14. Gowda RM, Khan IA, Nair CK, et al. Cardiac papillary fibroelastoma: a comprehensive analysis of 725 cases. Am Heart J. 2003;146: 404–10.
15. Abraham KP, Reddy V, Gattuso P. Neoplasms metastatic to the heart: review of 3314 consecutive autopsies. Am J Cardiovasc Pathol. 2009;3:195–8.
16. Gibs P, Cebon JS, Calafiore P, Robinson WQ. Cardiac metastases from malignant melanoma. Cancer. 1999;85:78–84.

17. Butany J, Nair V, Naseemuddin A, et al. Cardiac tumours: diagnosis and management. Lancet Oncol. 2005;6:219–28.
18. Carney JA. Differences between nonfamilial and familial cardiac myxoma. Am J Surg Pathol. 1985;9:53–5.
19. Zeebregts CJ, Hensens AG, Timmermans J, Pruszczynski MS, Lacquet LK. Lipomatous hypertrophy of the interatrial septum: indication for surgery? Eur J Cardiothorac Surg. 1997;11:785–7.
20. Maisch B, et al. The task force on the diagnosis and management of pericardial diseases of the European Society of Cardiology. Guidelines on the diagnosis and management of pericardial diseases executive summary. Eur Heart J. 2004;25:587–610.
21. Satur CMR, Hsin MKY, Dussek JE. Giant pericardial cysts. Ann Thorac Surg. 1996;61:208–10.
22. Patel J, Park C, Michaels J, Rosen S, Kort S. Pericardial cyst: case reports and a literature review. Echocardiography. 2004;21:269–72.
23. Shiraishi I, Yamagishi M, Kawakita A, Yamamoto Y, Hamaoka K. Acute cardiac tamponade caused by massive hemorrhage from pericardial cyst. Circulation. 2000;101:E196–7.
24. Beghetti M, Gow RM, Haney I, et al. Pediatric primary benign cardiac tumors: a 15-year review. Am Heart J. 1997;134:1107–14.
25. Parmley LF, Salley RK, Williams JP, Head 3rd GB. The clinical spectrum of cardiac fibroma with diagnostic and surgical considerations: noninvasive imaging enhances management. Ann Thorac Surg. 1988;45:455–65.
26. Roberts WC. Primary and secondary neoplasms of the heart. Am J Cardiol. 1997;80:671–82.
27. Gaspar A, Salome N, Nabais S, et al. Echocardiographic assessment of a cardiac lymphoma: beyond two-dimensional imaging. Eur J Cardiovasc Imaging. 2009;10:975–8.
28. Kirkpatrick JN, Wong T, Bednarz JE, et al. Differential diagnosis of cardiac masses using contrast echocardiographic perfusion imaging. J Am Coll Cardiol. 2004;43:1412–9.
29. Buckley O, Madan R, Kwong R, Rybicki FJ, Hunsaker A. Cardiac masses, part 2: key imaging features for diagnosis and surgical planning. Am J Roentgenol. 2011;197:W842–51.
30. Stanford W. Advances in cardiovascular CT imaging: CT clinical imaging. Int J Cardiovasc Imaging. 2005;21:29–37.
31. Rahbar K, Seifarth H, Schafers M, et al. Differentiation of malignant and benign cardiac tumors using 18F-FDG PET/CT. J Nucl Med. 2012;53:856–63.
32. Ngaage DL, Mullany CJ, Daly RC, et al. Surgical treatment of cardiac papillary fibroelastoma: a single center experience with eighty-eight patients. Ann Thorac Surg. 2005;80:1712–8.
33. Simpson L, Kumar SK, Okuno SH, et al. Malignant primary cardiac tumors: review of a single institution experience. Cancer. 2008;112:2440–6.
34. Donsbeck AV, et al. Primary cardiac sarcomas: an immunohistochemical and grading study with long-term follow-up of 24 cases. Histopathology. 1999;34:295–304.
35. Reardon MJ, Walkes J-C, Benjamin R. Therapy insight: malignant primary cardiac tumors. Nat Clin Pract Cardiovasc Med. 2006;3:548–53.
36. Ikeda H, Nakamura S, Nishimaki H, et al. Primary lymphoma of the heart: case report and literature review. Pathol Int. 2004;54:187–95.
37. Van Dantzig J, Delemarre BJ, Bot H, Visser CA. Left ventricular thrombus in acute myocardial infarction. Eur Heart J. 1996;17:1640–5.

Cardiovascular Complications of Chemotherapy: Anthracycline Cardiotoxicity

Raymond R. Russell III

Abstract

The anthracycline chemotherapeutic agents (doxorubicin, idarubicin, epirubicin) continue to play an important role in the treatment of certain malignancies. Their efficacy in treating cancer is related to the cumulative dose. Unfortunately, the risk of developing cardiotoxicity from these agents is also related to the cumulative dose. In this review, the incidence of anthracycline-mediated cardiotoxicity, the cellular mechanisms responsible for the cardiotoxicity, methods to detect cardiotoxicity, and strategies to treat and, more importantly, prevent the cardiotoxicity are discussed. Through close communication between the consulting cardiologist and the oncologist, a treatment plan can be developed that maximizes the tumoricidal activity of anthracyclines while minimizing the risk of cardiotoxicity.

Keywords

Anthracycline • Doxorubicin • Cardiotoxicity • Reactive oxygen species

Introduction

While great advances in molecularly targeted chemotherapeutic agents have led to significant improvements in survival for cancer patients, anthracycline agents, such as doxorubicin (Adriamycin), daunorubicin, and idarubicin, remain important therapeutic agents for the treatment of breast cancer, leukemias, and lymphomas. The efficacy of anthracyclines is related to the cumulative dose administered. However, the cumulative dose of anthracyclines is also responsible for the primary limiting toxicity, namely, cardiotoxicity. Shortly after the introduction of doxorubicin, the first major anthracycline to chemotherapy, it was recognized that treatment with this agent was associated with the development of congestive heart failure [1, 2]. Subsequent studies demonstrated that 2.2 % of patients receiving anthracyclines

developed heart failure [3, 4] and that there was a significant increase in the incidence of clinical heart failure (dyspnea on exertion, orthopnea, rales, or peripheral edema) at a cumulative dose of approximately 450 mg/m² [4]. Subsequent studies in patients with breast or lung cancer demonstrated objective evidence of left ventricular dysfunction, based on changes in the left ventricular ejection fraction (LVEF), at a cumulative dose of 300 mg/m² [5]. Patients who receive large bolus doses of doxorubicin are at greater risk for developing cardiotoxicity, while those who receive smaller, fractionated doses have a lower likelihood of developing cardiotoxicity [4].

In addition to frequency and size of individual doses, patients >65 years of age; those with preexisting left ventricular dysfunction or coronary artery disease, hypertension, and liver dysfunction; and those treated with other cardiotoxic therapies (radiation therapy, trastuzumab, cyclophosphamide) are also at greater risk for developing cardiotoxicity (Table 26.1). Furthermore, women are at greater risk than men for developing anthracycline-mediated cardiotoxicity after surviving childhood cancers [6]. Recent work has attempted to develop a scoring system, based on baseline factors, including age, weight, and performance status, in

R.R. Russell III, MD, PhD
Division of Cardiovascular Medicine,
Department of Internal Medicine,
Yale School of Medicine, 333 Cedar Street,
DCB 323, New Haven, CT 06520, USA
e-mail: raymond.russell@yale.edu

K. Stergiopoulos, D.L. Brown (eds.), *Evidence-Based Cardiology Consult*,
DOI 10.1007/978-1-4471-4441-0_26, © Springer-Verlag London 2014

Table 26.1 Risk factors for anthracycline-induced cardiotoxicity

Cumulative anthracycline dose
Age >65 years
Hypertension
Concomitant use of radiation therapy
Use of other cardiotoxic agents (e.g., cyclophosphamide, trastuzumab)
Liver dysfunction

addition to cumulative dose of anthracycline, that can predict the risk of cardiotoxicity in women receiving anthracyclines for breast cancer [7].

With increased experience with anthracyclines, the risk of cardiotoxicity has been more precisely defined. A retrospective analysis of three large multicenter trials of treatment of breast cancer and lymphoma demonstrated a significant increase in the incidence of left ventricular dysfunction at a cumulative dose of 250–300 mg/m^2 [5]. Approximately 12 % of breast cancer patients receiving 270 mg/m^2 of doxorubicin will have an ejection fraction <50 % after therapy [8]. In addition, it has been recognized that left ventricular dysfunction can occur many years after anthracycline treatment has been completed. This has been a particular problem for survivors of childhood malignancies, who may develop evidence of cardiotoxicity more than 10 years after cure from their cancer [9–11]. Up to 65 % of patients with a history of a childhood malignancy treated with doxorubicin have echocardiographic evidence of left ventricular contractile abnormalities [12]. In the Childhood Cancer Survivor Study, treatment with <250 mg/m^2 of anthracycline increased the risk of developing congestive heart failure 2.4-fold, and treatment with ≥250 mg/m^2 of doxorubicin increased the risk to 5.2-fold compared to individuals who did not receive anthracyclines [11].

As discussed in detail later in this review, the development of congestive heart failure and decreases in LVEF represent the most profound manifestation of anthracycline-mediated cardiotoxicity. However, more subtle forms of cardiac dysfunction and structural changes may occur with anthracycline-based chemotherapy, at much lower cumulative doses than those associated with systolic dysfunction. Although, histologic changes in the cardiomyocyte may occur at doses of 240 mg/m^2 [13, 14], these changes do not always correlate with the development of left ventricular systolic dysfunction.

Pathophysiology

The tumoricidal effects of the anthracyclines are based on disruption of DNA replication in rapidly dividing cancer cells through binding to topoisomerase II. However, the cardiotoxic effects of anthracyclines are not mediated through these mechanisms as there is little active replication of cardiac myocytes. It is believed that the primary mechanism

responsible for anthracycline-mediated cardiotoxicity is related to the generation of free radicals. Specifically, the metabolism of doxorubicin is initiated by the oxidation of doxorubicin to doxorubicinol, a free radical containing an unpaired electron, through the action of NADH dehydrogenase [15]. This unpaired electron is transferred to oxygen, generating superoxide radical [16]. In addition to the generation of superoxide radical through doxorubicin oxidation, doxorubicin can form reactive oxygen species through interaction with non-heme iron via the Fenton reaction [17, 18]. The production of reactive oxygen species results in activation of p38 MAP kinase [19, 20] which activates caspases 3 and 9, resulting in cardiomyocyte apoptosis [21–23].

Anthracycline-mediated cardiotoxicity can exist in two forms: acute or chronic cardiotoxicity. Acute cardiotoxicity generally occurs within 1 week of receiving anthracycline chemotherapy and is thought to be due to an inflammatory response [24–26]. It is associated with evidence of acute myocyte necrosis as evidenced by an increase in serum biomarker concentrations and a decrease in the LVEF. In addition, there has been a case report describing a patient who developed takotsubo cardiomyopathy following acute treatment with doxorubicin [27]. Fortunately, in contrast to the chronic cardiotoxicity caused by anthracyclines, the acute form generally resolves with normalization of left ventricular function.

Chronic anthracycline-mediated cardiotoxicity develops between 1 and 20 years after exposure to anthracycline agents [9]. As noted above, the incidence of left ventricular dysfunction increases with the cumulative dose of anthracycline. Because the final mechanism responsible for myocyte loss and left ventricular dysfunction in chronic anthracycline-mediated cardiotoxicity is apoptosis [28–30], there is usually no increase in the serum concentration of creatine kinase or troponin. Most importantly, the chronic form of anthracycline-mediated cardiotoxicity is usually irreversible.

Diagnosis

Assessment of Left Ventricular Function

The detection of anthracycline-mediated cardiotoxicity based on clinical history can be challenging given the fact that symptoms of fatigue, dyspnea, and peripheral edema can be caused by chemotherapy in the absence of left ventricular dysfunction due to factors such as anemia, aggressive hydration, and decreased nutritional intake. Therefore, careful attention to signs of congestive heart failure in the physical exam is essential. The current cornerstone for the diagnosis of anthracycline-mediated cardiotoxicity is serial assessment of LVEF. The most common methods for assessing LVEF in patients receiving chemotherapy are echocardiography and equilibrium radionuclide angiography (ERNA).

The two methods have their relative merits and limitations that must be weighed for individual patients. Two-dimensional echocardiography offers the benefits of providing structural information about the heart in addition to the assessment of LVEF with the added benefit of the absence of radiation exposure. In contrast, ERNA is inherently quantitative, since it is a count-based method to measure left ventricular volumes. However, unlike echocardiography, ERNA does not provide information on valvular function or cardiac morphology. In addition, ERNA requires labeling of red blood cells with technetium-99^m and is associated with a whole body exposure of approximately 2 mSv [31]. In studies that directly compare 2-dimensional echocardiography and ERNA, the latter modality appears to be more sensitive to detecting subtle changes in left ventricular function [32, 33]. Because of the additional structural and functional information afforded by echocardiography as well as the lack of radiation exposure, it is reasonable to utilize this modality as the preferred method to assess LVEF if ejection fraction is measured quantitatively using methods such as the Simpson's 2D method. Furthermore, 3-dimensional echocardiography may provide measurements of LVEF that are comparable to those determined by ERNA [34]. If the endocardial borders cannot be clearly visualized, echo contrast can be used to improve delineation of the left ventricular cavity. However, if the left ventricular cavity still cannot be adequately visualized, LVEF can be evaluated by ERNA. The most important factor is to use the same method, either echocardiography or ERNA, for all assessments to minimize variability.

Cardiotoxicity is generally defined by a decrease in LVEF below the lower limit of normal or an absolute decrease in LVEF of >10 %, even if the ejection fraction remains normal. Based on these criteria, recommendations have been established concerning the frequency of monitoring the LVEF and discontinuing anthracycline chemotherapy (Table 26.2). However, the risk of cardiotoxicity must be balanced by the likelihood of efficacy of anthracycline therapy in making the final decision concerning discontinuation of the anthracycline. It is for that reason that it is essential that an open dialogue is maintained between the cardiologist and oncologist.

Additional data obtained from echocardiography or ERNA may be useful in detecting cardiotoxicity earlier than the gross, late changes manifested by a decrease in LVEF, although these other measures have not been verified in large patient populations. Longitudinal strain, as assessed by echocardiography, decreases within 1 week of treatment with anthracyclines in patients with breast cancer [36]. Furthermore, decreases in longitudinal strain 3 months after receiving anthracyclines predict a subsequent decrease in LVEF [36]. Strain rate imaging has also demonstrated early subclinical changes in contractile function. Specifically, it has been demonstrated that echocardiographically derived strain rate is decreased in children 2 h after receiving anthracyclines [37]. As with strain

Table 26.2 Guidelines for monitoring of left ventricular function and discontinuation of anthracycline therapy

Patients with a normal baseline LVEF (≥50 %)

Repeat the study after 250–300 mg/m^2

Repeat the study after 400 mg/m^2 in patients with risk factors for cardiotoxicity[a] or after 450 mg/m^2 in patients with no risk factors

Repeat the study prior to each subsequent dose of anthracycline above 450 mg/m^2

If there is an absolute decrease in LVEF >10 % or to a value below 50 %, then discontinue therapy

Patients with an abnormal baseline LVEF (<50 %)

In patients with an LVEF >30 % but <50 %, repeat the study prior to each dose of anthracycline

Anthracycline therapy should not be initiated in patients with a baseline LVEF ≤30 %

If there is an absolute decrease in LVEF >10 % and/or an LVEF of ≤30 %, then discontinue therapy

Adapted from Schwartz et al. [35]

[a]Risk factors include age >65 years, hypertension, exposure to other cardiotoxic agents, and liver dysfunction

imaging, this decrease in longitudinal strain may persist for years after treatment with anthracyclines [38].

Similarly, ERNA evaluation of diastolic function, as measured by the peak filling rate (PFR), has demonstrated a decrease in PFR prior to a decrease in LVEF in patients receiving anthracyclines [39]. In addition, changes in the synchrony of left ventricular contraction as assessed by phase analysis have been identified in patients treated with anthracyclines [40], although no studies have been performed to determine if early changes in left ventricular synchrony predict subsequent decreases in the LVEF.

It is important to recognize, especially in older patients, that left ventricular dysfunction may be due to other causes. Therefore, in patients with risk factors for coronary artery disease or symptoms suggestive of myocardial ischemia, a workup for coronary artery disease should be considered. This is especially true in patients who develop left ventricular dysfunction at relatively low doses of anthracycline (<250 mg/m^2).

Endomyocardial Biopsy

Chronic anthracycline-mediated cardiotoxicity is associated with characteristic histopathologic changes [41, 42], including cytoplasmic vacuolization, mitochondrial swelling, myofibril dropout, and distention of the sarcoplasmic reticulum, which can be differentiated from changes that are seen with other causes of cardiomyopathy, such as viral myocarditis or giant cell myocarditis. As a result, endomyocardial biopsy has been given a class IIa (level of evidence: C) indication for use in diagnosing anthracycline-mediated cardiotoxicity by the American College of Cardiology (ACC) and the American Heart Association (AHA) [43]. As a matter of practicality, however, endomyocardial biopsy is rarely used to confirm a diagnosis of anthracycline-mediated cardiotoxicity, because the patient's presenting history generally does not support other diagnoses that would require endomyocardial biopsy to confirm.

Novel Methods to Identify Anthracycline-Mediated Cardiotoxicity

As noted above, a decrease in LVEF is a rather crude and late marker of anthracycline-mediated cardiotoxicity, and more sensitive methods to detect cardiomyocyte damage are needed to (1) identify heart muscle damage earlier than changes in LVEF and (2) identify patients at risk for cardiotoxicity prior to the initiation of anthracycline chemotherapy. Recent studies have demonstrated that individuals with an increase in the serum troponin I above the upper limit of normal 12–72 h after high-dose anthracycline infusion (200 mg/m^2 of epirubicin) were more likely to have a significant, persistent decrease in LVEF 7 months after receiving chemotherapy [44, 45], although the LVEF was still within the normal range. Subsequent studies have demonstrated that a persistent increase in troponin I 1 month after anthracycline treatment was associated with a greater decline in LVEF than if the troponin was elevated only around the time of treatment [46]. Furthermore, patients with an elevated troponin I at both the early and late time point had a greater combined cardiac event rate (sudden death, cardiac death, acute pulmonary edema, heart failure, asymptomatic left ventricular dysfunction, arrhythmias, and conduction disturbances) than patients with only an early increase in the biomarker. While this biomarker holds promise in identifying those patients at risk for the development of anthracycline-mediated cardiotoxicity, its value in patients receiving lower doses of anthracyclines has not been established. In children receiving lower doses of doxorubicin (median dose: 25 mg/m^2), there was no increase in the serum troponin T, although troponin I was not evaluated [47].

Personalized Identification of Risk of Anthracycline-Mediated Cardiotoxicity

With the greater ease and availability of genotyping, there is cause to believe that individualized assessment of risk of anthracycline-mediated cardiotoxicity may be achieved through the identification of genetic polymorphisms associated with this complication. In a study of the genetic determinants of anthracycline cytotoxicity, genome-wide linkage analysis studies of 24 individual human cell lines identified 30 genes associated with cytotoxicity. These genes were associated with signaling pathways, axon guidance pathways, and anchoring pathways. While the strength of this study was based on the unbiased genome-wide approach

to identifying genetic polymorphisms, the study focused on general cellular cytotoxicity, not cardiotoxicity [48]. In contrast, studies specifically directed at identifying genetic polymorphisms responsible for anthracycline-mediated cardiotoxicity have focused on candidate genes rather than using an unbiased approach. In a study of 1,697 patients with non-Hodgkin's lymphoma, the genes encoding NADP(H) oxidase and multidrug resistance protein 1 were identified as modulating the risk of developing anthracycline-mediated cardiotoxicity [49]. However, another study in patients with a variety of childhood cancers did not find an association between NADP(H) oxidase polymporphisms and the development of anthracycline-mediated cardiotoxicity, but there was a trend toward an association between polymorphisms in the carbonyl reductase 3 gene and cardiotoxicity [50]. While these studies suggest that genetic markers of cardiotoxicity may be present, unbiased genome-wide association study or exomic sequencing holds the promise for identifying a larger spectrum of candidate genes that might determine the susceptibility to anthracycline-mediated cardiotoxicity.

Management

Treatment of Established Cardiotoxicity

There are currently no therapies specific for the treatment of anthracycline-mediated cardiotoxicity. Rather, treatment follows the general AHA/ACC guidelines for the treatment of congestive heart failure [51] and focuses on aggressive treatment with ACE inhibitors, beta blockers, loop diuretics, and aldosterone-blocking agents. In patients with established anthracycline-mediated cardiotoxicity with an LVEF <45 %, the addition of enalapril (as well as carvedilol in some patients) normalized left ventricular function in 42 % of patients over a 36-month period [52]. Other studies also support a beneficial role for ACE inhibitors in patients with anthracycline-mediated cardiotoxicity [53]. However, the beneficial effects of ACE inhibition may not be permanent. In a retrospective study of survivors of childhood cancer with anthracycline-mediated cardiotoxicity, treatment with enalapril stabilized and even improved left ventricular fractional shortening for up to 6 years [54]. Unfortunately, there was a progressive deterioration in left ventricular function thereafter.

Beta blockers have been used in a limited number of patients to treat anthracycline-mediated cardiotoxicity. Case reports have illustrated improvement in LVEF in patients with anthracycline-mediated cardiotoxicity treated with either metoprolol or carvedilol [55–57]. In a retrospective, case–control study comparing patients with idiopathic cardiomyopathy to patients with anthracycline-mediated cardiotoxicity, treatment with beta blocker increased LVEF from 28 to 41 % in patients with anthracycline-mediated cardiotoxicity [58]. In one study comparing the effects of ACE inhibitors alone to ACE inhibitors plus beta blockers in patients with anthracycline-induced cardiotoxicity, therapy with the combination of the two agents was associated with greater improvement in LVEF [59].

The use of ACE inhibitors and/or beta blockers to treat individuals with anthracycline-mediated cardiotoxicity is based on small, retrospective studies or case reports bolstered by the more robust studies that have been performed for the general treatment of heart failure. Randomized, prospective trials will be required to evaluate the efficacy of these classes of drugs in the specific treatment of anthracycline-mediated cardiotoxicity.

The use of more advanced heart failure therapies, including implantable cardiac defibrillators, cardiac resynchronization therapy, ventricular assist devices, and cardiac transplantation, requires very careful consideration and multidisciplinary discussions involving the cardiologist, oncologist, and the patient and his/her family. These therapies must be individualized and the decision to implement them is based not only on cardiac factors but also on the oncologic status of the patient.

Prevention of Cardiotoxicity

The current established methods to prevent the development of anthracycline-mediated cardiotoxicity are based on two concepts: minimizing the exposure of doxorubicin to the cardiomyocytes and decreasing the generation of reactive oxygen species. With respect to the first concept, the early studies of anthracycline-mediated cardiotoxicity demonstrated that patients that received smaller, divided doses of anthracycline had a lower incidence of cardiotoxicity compared to those who received a larger, single dose of anthracycline [4]. This has led to many of the chemotherapeutic protocols currently in use.

Liposomal encapsulation of doxorubicin has also been used to decrease the cardiotoxicity associated with use of the drug. This occurs by preferentially increasing the accumulation of doxorubicin in tumors while also decreasing the clearance of the drug. A pegylated form of doxorubicin is available in the United States as a liposomal preparation (Doxil), although at the time of this review, there was a shortage of the drug. In studies of patients receiving >500 mg/m^2 of doxorubicin, use of Doxil was associated with a lower incidence of cardiotoxicity based on changes in LVEF and endomyocardial biopsy findings compared to the use of free doxorubicin [60]. Subsequent studies in patients with metastatic breast cancer who had received relatively lower doses of doxorubicin also demonstrated lower rates of cardiotoxicity with use of Doxil [61]. However, while the pegylated liposomal formulation of doxorubicin decreases its cardiotoxic effects, it can also decrease the tumoricidal effects of the drug [62]. A non-pegylated liposomal preparation of doxorubicin, Myocet, is available for use in Europe and Canada, but has not been approved by the Food and Drug Administration for use in the United States.

The second strategy to prevent anthracycline-mediated cardiotoxicity involves measures aimed at decreasing the production of reactive oxygen species. Multiple preclinical studies using cells in culture as well as nontransgenic and transgenic animal models have demonstrated that decreasing the production of reactive oxygen species will result in decreased cardiotoxicity of anthracyclines. However, the results of clinical trials of antioxidant therapy have not established a clear benefit of these therapies [63–65].

In contrast to therapies based on removing reactive oxygen species, one therapy based on preventing the production of reactive oxygen species has been shown to be cardioprotective in patients receiving anthracyclines. Dexrazoxane is a derivative of ethylenediaminetetraacetic acid (EDTA) that chelates intracellular iron, including iron complexed with doxorubicin, thereby decreasing the production of reactive oxygen species. Two multicenter trials of patients with breast cancer evaluated the cardioprotective value of dexrazoxane, with therapy initiated either at the beginning of anthracycline therapy or after a cumulative dose of 300 mg/m^2 had been achieved. With either strategy, the incidence of a significant decrease in LVEF was reduced with use of dexrazoxane [66, 67]; however, some data suggest that the cardiotoxic effect of doxorubicin is decreased with dexrazoxane therapy initiated at the beginning of anthracycline therapy [67, 68]. Based on this data, the use of dexrazoxane as a cardioprotective agent is recommended by the American Society of Clinical Oncology for patients treated with anthracyclines who have already received a cumulative dose of >300 mg/m^2 [69].

In addition to these proven strategies, other cardioprotective therapies have been proposed for patients receiving anthracyclines. In patients who have an increase in serum troponin I during anthracycline therapy, treatment with enalapril has been shown to prevent subsequent decreases in LVEF [70]. Similarly, treatment with carvedilol in patients who have received high cumulative doses of doxorubicin (>500 mg/m^2) decreases the likelihood of developing left ventricular dysfunction [71]. It must be kept in mind that these studies have included only a small number of patients and that larger, multicenter trials are necessary to determine the efficacy of such potentially cardioprotective treatment. Nevertheless it is not unreasonable to consider initiating these generally well-tolerated medications in patients with risk factors for anthracycline-mediated cardiotoxicity.

Conclusion

With the continued use of anthracycline-based cancer chemotherapy, risks of permanent left ventricular dysfunction and congestive heart failure remain a challenging clinical problem. Current methods to detect anthracycline-mediated cardiotoxicity remain relatively crude and only identify the problem after it has caused significant damage. As a result, the consulting cardiologist must pay close attention to patients receiving anthracyclines and consider the use of cardioprotective agents, including ACE inhibitors and beta blockers, early in the treatment of the patient. Optimization of the patient's therapy requires integration of the cardiologist into the team treating the patient's cancer.

Key Points

- Cardiotoxicity occurs as a cumulative-dose-dependent complication of anthracycline chemotherapy and can manifest up to 20 years after treatment is completed.
- Risk factors for developing anthracycline-mediated cardiotoxicity include age over 65 years, existing heart disease or left ventricular dysfunction, use of other cardiotoxic therapies, and liver dysfunction.
- Serial assessment of LVEF is essential for monitoring for anthracycline-mediated cardiotoxicity. While either transthoracic echocardiography or ERNA may be used to monitor LVEF, echocardiography offers additional structural and functional information.
- Decreases in LVEF of at least 10 % or below the lower limit of normal should be considered to reflect significant anthracycline-mediated cardiotoxicity, although it is important to consider other causes of cardiomyopathy, especially treatable causes, such as myocardial ischemia.
- Established anthracycline-mediated cardiotoxicity should be treated with standard heart failure therapy, including ACE inhibitors, beta blockers, and diuretics.
- There is evidence to suggest that cardioprotective therapy should be given to patients at risk for developing anthracycline-mediated cardiotoxicity. Both ACE inhibitors and the beta blocker, carvedilol, have been shown to provide cardioprotective effects in patients receiving anthracyclines.
- Decisions concerning the comprehensive care of patients receiving anthracyclines who either have developed cardiotoxicity or are at risk for anthracycline-mediated cardiotoxicity should be made collaboratively by the consulting cardiologist and the treating oncologist.

References

1. Tan C, et al. Daunomycin, an antitumor antibiotic, in the treatment of neoplastic disease. Clinical evaluation with special reference to childhood leukemia. Cancer. 1967;20(3):333–53.
2. Di Marco A, Cassinelli G, Arcamone F. The discovery of daunorubicin. Cancer Treat Rep. 1981;65 Suppl 4:3–8.
3. Lefrak EA, et al. A clinicopathologic analysis of adriamycin cardiotoxicity. Cancer. 1973;32(2):302–14.
4. Von Hoff DD, et al. Risk factors for doxorubicin-induced congestive heart failure. Ann Intern Med. 1979;91(5):710–7.
5. Swain SM, Whaley FS, Ewer MS. Congestive heart failure in patients treated with doxorubicin. Cancer. 2003;97(11):2869–79.
6. Lipshultz SE, et al. Female sex and drug dose as risk factors for late cardiotoxic effects of doxorubicin therapy for childhood cancer. N Engl J Med. 1995;332(26):1738–43.
7. Dranitsaris G, et al. The development of a predictive model to estimate cardiotoxic risk for patients with metastatic breast cancer receiving anthracyclines. Breast Cancer Res Treat. 2008;107(3):443–50.
8. Abu-Khalaf MM, et al. Long-term assessment of cardiac function after dose-dense and -intense sequential doxorubicin (A), paclitaxel (T), and cyclophosphamide (C) as adjuvant therapy for high risk breast cancer. Breast Cancer Res Treat. 2007;104(3):341–9.
9. Lipshultz SE, et al. Chronic progressive cardiac dysfunction years after doxorubicin therapy for childhood acute lymphoblastic leukemia. J Clin Oncol. 2005;23(12):2629–36.
10. Kremer LC, et al. Anthracycline-induced clinical heart failure in a cohort of 607 children: long-term follow-up study. J Clin Oncol. 2001;19(1):191–6.
11. Mulrooney DA, et al. Cardiac outcomes in a cohort of adult survivors of childhood and adolescent cancer: retrospective analysis of the Childhood Cancer Survivor Study cohort. BMJ. 2009;339:b4606.
12. Grenier MA, Lipshultz SE. Epidemiology of anthracycline cardiotoxicity in children and adults. Semin Oncol. 1998;25(4 Suppl 10):72–85.
13. Billingham ME, et al. Anthracycline cardiomyopathy monitored by morphologic changes. Cancer Treat Rep. 1978;62(6):865–72.
14. Bristow MR, et al. Doxorubicin cardiomyopathy: evaluation by phonocardiography, endomyocardial biopsy, and cardiac catheterization. Ann Intern Med. 1978;88(2):168–75.
15. Davies KJ, Doroshow JH. Redox cycling of anthracyclines by cardiac mitochondria. I. Anthracycline radical formation by NADH dehydrogenase. J Biol Chem. 1986;261(7):3060–7.
16. Doroshow JH, Davies KJ. Redox cycling of anthracyclines by cardiac mitochondria. II. Formation of superoxide anion, hydrogen peroxide, and hydroxyl radical. J Biol Chem. 1986;261(7):3068–74.
17. Kotamraju S, et al. Transferrin receptor-dependent iron uptake is responsible for doxorubicin-mediated apoptosis in endothelial cells: role of oxidant-induced iron signaling in apoptosis. J Biol Chem. 2002;277(19):17179–87.
18. Minotti G, et al. Doxorubicin cardiotoxicity and the control of iron metabolism: quinone-dependent and independent mechanisms. Methods Enzymol. 2004;378:340–61.
19. Kang YJ, et al. Suppression by metallothionein of doxorubicin-induced cardiomyocyte apoptosis through inhibition of p38 mitogen-activated protein kinases. J Biol Chem. 2000;275(18):13690–8.
20. Grethe S, et al. p38 MAPK downregulates phosphorylation of Bad in doxorubicin-induced endothelial apoptosis. Biochem Biophys Res Commun. 2006;347(3):781–90.
21. Chua CC, et al. Multiple actions of pifithrin-alpha on doxorubicin-induced apoptosis in rat myoblastic H9c2 cells. Am J Physiol Heart Circ Physiol. 2006;290(6):H2606–13.
22. Wu W, et al. Expression of constitutively active phosphatidylinositol 3-kinase inhibits activation of caspase 3 and apoptosis of cardiac muscle cells. J Biol Chem. 2000;275(51):40113–9.
23. Wang L, et al. Regulation of cardiomyocyte apoptotic signaling by insulin-like growth factor I. Circ Res. 1998;83(5):516–22.
24. Bristow MR, et al. Early anthracycline cardiotoxicity. Am J Med. 1978;65(5):823–32.
25. Buzdar AU, et al. Early and delayed clinical cardiotoxicity of doxorubicin. Cancer. 1985;55(12):2761–5.
26. Hayek ER, Speakman E, Rehmus E. Acute doxorubicin cardiotoxicity. N Engl J Med. 2005;352(23):2456–7.
27. Fernandez SF, Basra M, Canty JM. Takotsubo cardiomyopathy following initial chemotherapy presenting with syncope and cardiogenic shock – a case report and literature review. J Clin Exp Cardiol. 2001;2:124.

28. Dowd NP, et al. Inhibition of cyclooxygenase-2 aggravates doxorubicin-mediated cardiac injury in vivo. J Clin Invest. 2001;108(4):585–90.

29. Kotamraju S, et al. Oxidant-induced iron signaling in doxorubicin-mediated apoptosis. Methods Enzymol. 2004;378:362–82.

30. Kotamraju S, et al. Doxorubicin-induced apoptosis in endothelial cells and cardiomyocytes is ameliorated by nitrone spin traps and ebselen. Role of reactive oxygen and nitrogen species. J Biol Chem. 2000;275(43):33585–92.

31. Einstein AJ, et al. Radiation dose to patients from cardiac diagnostic imaging. Circulation. 2007;116(11):1290–305.

32. Corapcioglu F, et al. Evaluation of anthracycline-induced early left ventricular dysfunction in children with cancer: a comparative study with echocardiography and multigated radionuclide angiography. Pediatr Hematol Oncol. 2006;23(1):71–80.

33. Fatima N, et al. Assessing adriamycin-induced early cardiotoxicity by estimating left ventricular ejection fraction using technetium-99m multiple-gated acquisition scan and echocardiography. Nucl Med Commun. 2011;32(5):381–5.

34. Walker J, et al. Role of three-dimensional echocardiography in breast cancer: comparison with two-dimensional echocardiography, multiple-gated acquisition scans, and cardiac magnetic resonance imaging. J Clin Oncol. 2010;28(21):3429–36.

35. Schwartz RG, et al. Congestive heart failure and left ventricular dysfunction complicating doxorubicin therapy: seven-year experience using serial radionuclide angiocardiography. Am J Med. 1987;82(6):1109–18.

36. Stoodley PW, et al. Two-dimensional myocardial strain imaging detects changes in left ventricular systolic function immediately after anthracycline chemotherapy. Eur J Echocardiogr. 2011;12(12):945–52.

37. Ganame J, et al. Acute cardiac functional and morphological changes after Anthracycline infusions in children. Am J Cardiol. 2007;99(7):974–7.

38. Ganame J, et al. Myocardial dysfunction late after low-dose anthracycline treatment in asymptomatic pediatric patients. J Am Soc Echocardiogr. 2007;20(12):1351–8.

39. Cottin Y, et al. Impairment of diastolic function during short-term anthracycline chemotherapy. Br Heart J. 1995;73(1):61–4.

40. Alcan KE, et al. Early detection of anthracycline-induced cardiotoxicity by stress radionuclide cineangiography in conjunction with Fourier amplitude and phase analysis. Clin Nucl Med. 1985;10(3):160–6.

41. Mason JW, et al. Invasive and noninvasive methods of assessing adriamycin cardiotoxic effects in man: superiority of histopathologic assessment using endomyocardial biopsy. Cancer Treat Rep. 1978;62(6):857–64.

42. Singal PK, Iliskovic N. Doxorubicin-induced cardiomyopathy. N Engl J Med. 1998;339(13):900–5.

43. Cooper LT, et al. The role of endomyocardial biopsy in the management of cardiovascular disease: a scientific statement from the American Heart Association, the American College of Cardiology, and the European Society of Cardiology. Circulation. 2007;116(19):2216–33.

44. Cardinale D, et al. Left ventricular dysfunction predicted by early troponin I release after high-dose chemotherapy. J Am Coll Cardiol. 2000;36(2):517–22.

45. Cardinale D, et al. Myocardial injury revealed by plasma troponin I in breast cancer treated with high-dose chemotherapy. Ann Oncol. 2002;13(5):710–5.

46. Cardinale D, et al. Prognostic value of troponin I in cardiac risk stratification of cancer patients undergoing high-dose chemotherapy. Circulation. 2004;109(22):2749–54.

47. Clark SJ, et al. Cardiac troponin T following anthracycline chemotherapy in children and adolescents. J Chemother. 2007;19(3):332–4.

48. Duan S, et al. Mapping genes that contribute to daunorubicin-induced cytotoxicity. Cancer Res. 2007;67(11):5425–33.

49. Wojnowski L, et al. NAD(P)H oxidase and multidrug resistance protein genetic polymorphisms are associated with doxorubicin-induced cardiotoxicity. Circulation. 2005;112(24):3754–62.

50. Blanco JG, et al. Genetic polymorphisms in the carbonyl reductase 3 gene CBR3 and the NAD(P)H:quinone oxidoreductase 1 gene NQO1 in patients who developed anthracycline-related congestive heart failure after childhood cancer. Cancer. 2008;112(12):2789–95.

51. Jessup M, et al. 2009 Focused update: ACCF/AHA guidelines for the diagnosis and management of heart failure in adults: a report of the American College of Cardiology Foundation/American Heart Association Task Force on Practice Guidelines: developed in collaboration with the International Society for Heart and Lung Transplantation. Circulation. 2009;119(14):1977–2016.

52. Cardinale D, et al. Anthracycline-induced cardiomyopathy: clinical relevance and response to pharmacologic therapy. J Am Coll Cardiol. 2010;55(3):213–20.

53. Jensen BV, Skovsgaard T, Nielsen SL. Functional monitoring of anthracycline cardiotoxicity: a prospective, blinded, long-term observational study of outcome in 120 patients. Ann Oncol. 2002;13(5):699–709.

54. Lipshultz SE, et al. Long-term enalapril therapy for left ventricular dysfunction in doxorubicin-treated survivors of childhood cancer. J Clin Oncol. 2002;20(23):4517–22.

55. Fazio S, et al. Doxorubicin-induced cardiomyopathy treated with carvedilol. Clin Cardiol. 1998;21(10):777–9.

56. Mukai Y, et al. Five cases of anthracycline-induced cardiomyopathy effectively treated with carvedilol. Intern Med. 2004;43(11):1087–8.

57. Shaddy RE, et al. Efficacy and safety of metoprolol in the treatment of doxorubicin-induced cardiomyopathy in pediatric patients. Am Heart J. 1995;129(1):197–9.

58. Noori A, et al. Beta-blockade in adriamycin-induced cardiomyopathy. J Card Fail. 2000;6(2):115–9.

59. Tallaj JA, et al. Response of doxorubicin-induced cardiomyopathy to the current management strategy of heart failure. J Heart Lung Transplant. 2005;24(12):2196–201.

60. Safra T, et al. Pegylated liposomal doxorubicin (doxil): reduced clinical cardiotoxicity in patients reaching or exceeding cumulative doses of 500 mg/m². Ann Oncol. 2000;11(8):1029–33.

61. O'Brien ME, et al. Reduced cardiotoxicity and comparable efficacy in a phase III trial of pegylated liposomal doxorubicin HCl (CAELYX/Doxil) versus conventional doxorubicin for first-line treatment of metastatic breast cancer. Ann Oncol. 2004;15(3):440–9.

62. Halm U, et al. A phase II study of pegylated liposomal doxorubicin for treatment of advanced hepatocellular carcinoma. Ann Oncol. 2000;11(1):113–4.

63. Berthiaume JM, et al. Dietary vitamin E decreases doxorubicin-induced oxidative stress without preventing mitochondrial dysfunction. Cardiovasc Toxicol. 2005;5(3):257–67.

64. Bjelogrlic SK, et al. Activity of d, l-alpha-tocopherol (vitamin E) against cardiotoxicity induced by doxorubicin and doxorubicin with cyclophosphamide in mice. Basic Clin Pharmacol Toxicol. 2005;97(5):311–9.

65. Ladas EJ, et al. Antioxidants and cancer therapy: a systematic review. J Clin Oncol. 2004;22(3):517–28.

66. Swain SM, et al. Delayed administration of dexrazoxane provides cardioprotection for patients with advanced breast cancer treated with doxorubicin-containing therapy. J Clin Oncol. 1997;15(4):1333–40.

67. Swain SM, et al. Cardioprotection with dexrazoxane for doxorubicin-containing therapy in advanced breast cancer. J Clin Oncol. 1997;15(4):1318–32.

68. Trachtenberg BH, et al. Anthracycline-associated cardiotoxicity in survivors of childhood cancer. Pediatr Cardiol. 2011;32(3):342–53.

69. Hensley ML, et al. American Society of Clinical Oncology 2008 clinical practice guideline update: use of chemotherapy and radiation therapy protectants. J Clin Oncol. 2009;27(1):127–45.

70. Cardinale D, et al. Prevention of high-dose chemotherapy-induced cardiotoxicity in high-risk patients by angiotensin-converting enzyme inhibition. Circulation. 2006;114(23):2474–81.

71. Kalay N, et al. Protective effects of carvedilol against anthracycline-induced cardiomyopathy. J Am Coll Cardiol. 2006;48(11):2258–62.

Cardiotoxicity of Molecularly Targeted Chemotherapeutic Agents

Kerry Strong Russell

Abstract

The explosion of knowledge regarding the molecular underpinnings of cancer has led to rapid and significant improvements in oncologic therapy. However, little has been done to carefully define the impacts of these new treatments on cardiovascular health and disease. Many newer agents, by virtue of overlapping targets in tumors and normal cardiovascular tissues, have significant short- and long-term effects on cardiovascular structure and function. In this chapter, we will review (1) the wide variety of targeted therapies currently in use and their known, and potential, cardiovascular side effects; (2) the currently limited clinical trial data regarding prevention, diagnosis, and treatment of such side effects; and (3) the establishment and future of cardio-oncology as a novel field of research and clinical care.

Keywords

Molecularly targeted drugs • Chemotherapy • Cardiotoxicity • Cardiomyopathy • Trastuzumab • Tyrosine kinase inhibitors • Proteosome inhibitors • Angiogenesis inhibitors

Abbreviations

Abl	Abl kinase fused with Bcr in CML
Afib	Atrial fibrillation
AHA/ACC	American Heart Association/American College of Cardiology
AV	Atrioventricular
CAD	Coronary artery disease
CHB	Complete heart block
CHF	Congestive heart failure
EGFR	Epidermal growth factor receptor
ERNA	Equilibrium radionuclide angiography
HDAC	Histone deacetylase
Kit	c-Kit (CD117) kinase receptor for stem cell factor
LV	Left ventricle
LVEF	Left ventricular ejection fraction
mAb	Monoclonal antibody
MI	Myocardial infarction
mTOR	Mammalian target of rapamycin
PDGFR	Platelet-derived growth factor receptor
RAR	Retinoic acid receptor
SVT	Supraventricular tachycardia
TKI	Tyrosine kinase inhibitor
VEGF	Vascular endothelial growth factor
VEGFR	VEGF receptor

K.S. Russell, MD, PhD, FACC, FAHA
Internal Medicine, Department of Cardiovascular Medicine,
Yale University School of Medicine, Dana 321,
333 Cedar Street, New Haven, CT 06520-8017, USA
e-mail: kerry.russell@yale.edu

Introduction

With great power comes great responsibility – Voltaire

This ancient statement finds new applicability in the modern era of molecularly targeted chemotherapeutic agents. While the explosion of knowledge regarding the molecular underpinnings of cancer has led to rapid and significant improvements in therapy, little has been done to carefully define the impacts of these new treatments on cardiovascular health and disease. In this chapter, we will review (1) the wide variety of targeted

K. Stergiopoulos, D.L. Brown (eds.), *Evidence-Based Cardiology Consult*,
DOI 10.1007/978-1-4471-4441-0_27, © Springer-Verlag London 2014

therapies currently in use and their known, and potential, cardiovascular side effects; (2) the currently limited clinical trial data regarding prevention, diagnosis, and treatment of such side effects; and (3) the establishment and future of cardio-oncology as a novel field of research and clinical care.

What Are "Molecularly Targeted Chemotherapeutic Agents" and Why Are They Being Used?

The term "molecularly targeted" refers to a large group of relatively new chemotherapeutic drugs specifically designed to alter cellular signaling pathways crucial for oncogenesis and metastasis. These drugs can act either directly, altering signaling in cancer cells to interrupt their survival or proliferation (e.g., tyrosine kinase inhibitors) or promote their differentiation (e.g., retinoids), or indirectly, to interrupt tumor support systems (e.g., angiogenesis inhibitors). The strategy of selectively targeting crucial pathways or processes required for tumor cell survival and growth has revolutionized the treatment of a variety of hematologic and solid malignancies, dramatically improving length and quality of life for many patients. However, when the targeted pathways are also crucial for cardiovascular cell survival or function, interruption of these can lead to cardiovascular damage that can be reversible or irreversible. Years of prior experience with nontargeted cardiotoxic chemotherapeutic agents whose effects are largely irreversible (e.g., anthracyclines, reviewed in a Chap. 26) have led investigators to classify chemotherapeutic cardiotoxicity as Type I, that which is irreversible, and Type II, that which is largely reversible [1]. Though originally this classification system was based on the pathological findings of significant myocyte necrosis (as seen in Type I injury) versus very minimal or no myocyte necrosis (Type II injury), more recent data has blurred the reductionist boundary between these two classifications of cardiotoxicity, limiting the usefulness of this terminology [2]. As we will discuss below, the relative paucity of data regarding the pathological and pathophysiologic cardiovascular effects of most of the newer molecularly targeted chemotherapies limits our ability to currently predict long-term effects of these drugs, and most of the "reversibility" that classifies drugs in the Type II category is based on limited short-term follow-up.

What Types of Molecules and Pathways Are Being Targeted?

The types of molecular pathways currently being targeted are briefly summarized in Table 27.1 (also, see [3]). Critical signaling pathways for cancer cell growth including receptor and non-receptor signaling kinases have been targeted for treatment of breast, renal cell, lung, and other cancers. Drugs that inhibit some of these pathways are sometimes referred to as tyrosine kinase inhibitors (TKI). One of the most successful drugs in this class is trastuzumab (Herceptin), which has significantly improved prognosis in patients with erbB2/Her2-positive breast cancer [4, 31]. This is also one of the first of the molecularly targeted chemotherapeutic agents to show significant cardiotoxicity. Newer drugs, including mTOR and multi-kinase inhibitors, will require significantly broader and longer use before their full cardiotoxicity profile will be revealed. This will be discussed below.

Why Is Targeting These Pathways Toxic in the Cardiovascular System?

Many of the fundamentally important cellular signaling pathways used by cancer cells to survive and proliferate are also crucial for normal cardiovascular cell function and survival. Multiple cell types in the cardiovascular system, including cardiac myocytes, vascular endothelial and smooth muscle cells, and cells of the cardiac conduction system, are susceptible to interruption of these pathways. In addition, some of these molecularly targeted drugs can affect systemic processes (via both cardiovascular and non-cardiovascular targets) leading to adverse cardiovascular consequences including thromboembolism, hypertension, and dyslipidemia. These additional effects may have important short- and long-term consequences in patients with concomitant baseline cardiovascular risk factors or underlying cardiovascular disease.

Why Is Knowledge About the Cardiovascular Effects of These Drugs so Limited?

When faced with caring for patients undergoing potentially life-saving treatment with these new agents, one can quickly become frustrated by the paucity of good clinical trials data regarding the type, frequency, and outcomes of their cardiac side effects. Even worse, there is a near absence of data regarding identification of patients at risk, prevention, and treatment of cardiovascular complications from these therapies. There are a variety of reasons for the current state of knowledge. First, many of these agents are relatively new; therefore, large and long-term trial data are not available. Second, like most novel chemotherapeutic agents, many molecularly targeted agents have initially been trialed in patients with advanced cancer, who may have multiple comorbidities and whose long-term prognosis is poor. Thus, information on short-term effects may be modulated by concurrent additional cardiac risks and that on long-term effects is mostly lacking. Finally, cardiotoxicity monitoring in many older clinical trials was often superficial and cardiologists were rarely involved in this process. Luckily, largely in response to the significant and unexpected cardiotoxicity of the first generation of molecularly targeted agents (specifically trastuzumab), most clinical trials now involve

Table 27.1 Targeted drugs and cardiovascular side effects

Drug[a]	Target	Reported cardiovascular side effect[b]				Ref.[c]
		LV effects	Arrhythmia	Hypertension	Thromboembolism	
Tyrosine kinase pathway inhibitors						
Trastuzumab	ErbB2 (Her2/neu)	↓ LVEF, CHF	↑ QTc			[3–7]
Lapatinib						
Pertuzumab						
Gefetinib	ErbB1 (EGFR)				✓	[8]
Erlotinib						
Cetuximab						
Panitumumab						
Bevacizumab	VEGF	MI, CHF		✓	✓	[9, 10]
Multi-kinase pathway inhibitors						
Sorafenib	VEGFR, PDGFR,	↓ LVEF, CHF, MI	↑ QTc, AFib	✓	✓	[11–13]
Pazopanib	c-Kit, others					
Sunitinib						
Imatinib	Abl, c-Kit, PDGFR,	MI, CHF	↑ QTc, AFib,	✓	✓	[14]
Dasatinib	others		others			
Nilotinib						
mTOR inhibitors						
Temsirolimus	mTOR	CHF		✓	✓	[15]
Everolimus						
Hormone signaling pathway and hormone synthesis inhibitors						
Tamoxifen	Estrogen receptor	MI, CHF			✓	[16–20]
Toremifene						
Fulvestrant						
Bicalutamide	Androgen receptor	MI, CHF		✓		[21]
Anastrozole	Block hormone	MI		✓	✓	[22, 23]
Exemestane	synthesis					
Letrozole						
Other cellular pathway modulators						
Vorinostat	HDAC inhibitors	MI	↑ QTc, Afib		✓	[24]
Romidepsin						
Bexarotene	Retinoid (RAR)	↓ LVEF, CHF	✓	✓	✓	[25, 26]
Aliretinoin	agonists					
Tretinoin						
Bortezomib	Proteosome inhibitors	↓ LVEF, CHF, MI	↑ QTc, CHB			[27–30]

[a]For simplicity, generic names are used. Additional drugs are listed at http://www.cancer.gov/cancertopics/factsheet/Therapy
[b]Side effect may not have been reported for all drugs shown, but is listed if reported for any drug in category
[c]Information extracted from data package inserts and other information from manufacturers (available at the FDA website: http://www.fda.gov/) unless otherwise noted. Thus, many reported side effects may be based on small numbers with limited data regarding frequency in larger populations

better cardiotoxicity monitoring and include some level of cardiac specialty oversight. However, specific clinical trials aimed at risk assessment, prevention, and treatment are still scant.

Pathophysiology

The mechanistic reasons for cardiotoxicity of targeted agents can sometimes be predicted based on known roles for their targeted signaling pathways in the human cardiovascular system. However, this approach often incompletely identifies full risk and additional clinical data is essential.

Differences Between Human and Preclinical Models Limit Predictive Power of These Models for Clinical Side Effects

Predicting clinical cardiovascular toxicity based on preclinical models has failed to identify every potential adverse outcome for a number of reasons. An appreciation for these limitations is important because in order to fully understand the potential toxicity of each new agent, careful observation for early cardiovascular toxicity must be undertaken in the clinical setting. In some cases, drugs tailored to bind to human targets may not bind well to these same targets in non-human cells, limiting prediction of toxicity in these models. This is the case with trastuzumab, where this humanized monoclonal antibody binds poorly to non-human erbB receptors. Thus, cardiac toxicity was not predicted in pre-clinical models. Likewise, other targeted drugs may have altered binding or potency in humans versus other animals or in cell culture models. Susceptibility to induction of cell death may be significantly higher in normal cardiovascular cells compared to tumor cells, many of which express high levels of multidrug resistance genes. Finally, some cellular survival pathways being targeted in cancer cells may have overlapping or redundant mechanisms in non-human cells that are not present or function differently in humans.

Predicting Cardiotoxicity Based on Cell Targets

As described above, many of the cellular pathways and processes targeted by these new chemotherapeutic agents are important in non-cancer cells, including those of the cardiovascular system. In some cases, the cell-specific effects in the cardiovascular system have been studied. In others, adverse cardiovascular events have been described but the specific mechanism for these effects is not known.

Drugs That Target Cardiac Myocytes

Several of the kinases being targeted by these new chemotherapeutic agents play important roles in cardiac myocyte protection and survival. Thus, interruption of these crucial pathways may culminate in irreversible myocyte cell death. In addition, some of these therapies may also affect ion channel function and metabolic pathways in cardiac myocytes, leading to myocyte dysfunction. The finding that trastuzumab can (either alone or in synergy with anthracyclines) cause cardiomyopathy may not be surprising when one considers that cardiac myocytes also contain erbB2 receptors, the kinase targeted by trastuzumab in breast and other cancers [32]. This was not understood at the time trastuzumab first underwent clinical trials. Furthermore, signaling via erbB receptors has been shown to promote myocyte resistance to injury and survival, further supporting the concept that myocytes are a primary target in trastuzumab-induced cardiac dysfunction [32–35]. However, more recent data also suggests that vasculature may be an important target for anti-erbB-directed toxicity, highlighting the idea that more than one cell type may be affected [36].

A number of drugs targeting the phosphoinositide 3-kinase (PI3K)/AKT/mammalian target of rapamycin (mTOR)/S6-p70-kinase system are either in use or in development. This pathway also plays a crucial role in cardiomyocyte hypertrophy and survival [37]. Though the mTOR inhibitors currently in use appear to have limited cardiovascular side effects, additional targeting or combined targeting of these pathways may be anticipated to have cardiovascular side effects.

Proteosome inhibitors may have mixed effects, as in some models proteasome inhibition is detrimental to cardiomyocyte survival, whereas in others it is beneficial [38, 39]. Cases of fulminant congestive heart failure have been reported with some of these inhibitors; thus, investigation of potential cardiac toxicity will need to be done for each new drug [27].

Drugs That Target Vasculature

Because many tumors require extensive vasculature, targeted drugs that prevent angiogenesis or disrupt tumor vasculature have been attractive cancer therapeutics. The vascular-targeted (or antiangiogenic) therapeutics currently in use have many cardiovascular side effects, due to both direct effects on normal vasculature and additional systemic effects. One of the more important vascular/systemic side effects of these drugs is significant hypertension (discussed below) [40]. In addition, some of these drugs also target receptors on cardiac myocytes that are important for myocyte survival and have been found to be associated with increased risk of cardiomyopathy [11]. In animal models, targeting of these receptors synergized with hypertension to produce increased cardiac myocyte cell death (apoptosis), suggesting a potentially irreversible mode of action [41].

Diagnosis

In the era of nontargeted chemotherapeutics, the main offenders with regard to cardiotoxicity were anthracycline-based drugs. Since the most serious cardiovascular side effect of these drugs is cardiomyocyte death with subsequent declines in ventricular (LV) systolic function, detection of cardiotoxicity has predominantly been diagnosed by modalities aimed at quantitating this parameter (equilibrium radionuclide angiography (ERNA) or echocardiography). With so many newer targeted therapies whose cardiovascular effects are less well defined, cardiologists and oncologists are faced with the necessity to broadly monitor multiple cardiovascular parameters. In many cases, we have limited or poor tools for detecting early cardiovascular toxicity due to these drugs. Below, we will focus on the described manifestations of cardiovascular toxicity, with the caveat that in the clinical setting, diagnosis of cardiotoxicity is essentially based on exclusion of more common types of cardiovascular disease as causal agents.

Cardiomyopathy

Because many of the new targeted therapies interrupt signaling pathways crucial for cellular survival in cardiovascular cells as well as cancer, it does not seem surprising that damage from these agents may ultimately lead to cardiac dysfunction. Fortunately fulminant heart failure is rare with most of these new agents. However, it is important to understand that the long-term consequence of milder forms of cardiomyopathy is currently unclear, as most agents have been in use for only short periods of time. Subclinical declines in LV ejection fraction (LVEF) or the development of diastolic dysfunction that may be seen soon after treatment may progress over time or render the cardiovascular system more susceptible to subsequent injury from more common forms of heart disease. Few guidelines have been established regarding the appropriate form and timing of monitoring for changes in ventricular systolic and diastolic function in patients undergoing therapy with most of the newer targeted agents.

Trastuzumab is one of the few agents with recommended monitoring because it was one of the first targeted therapies clearly demonstrated to contribute to cardiomyopathy. Based on findings that trastuzumab can increase the risk of cardiomyopathy by four- to sixfold, it is recommended that cardiac monitoring be performed before treatment, every 3 months during treatment, at the end of treatment, and every 6 months after treatment for 2 years. Currently, the only specific parameter that is being monitored is LVEF, and measurement of this may be performed by radionuclide imaging (ERNA) or echocardiography. It is recommended that trastuzumab be withheld if (1) there is a ≥16 % absolute decrease in LVEF from baseline value or (2) there is a ≥10 % absolute decrease in LVEF from baseline to a value that is below the institutional lower limit of normal. In case of such changes in LVEF, it is recommended that trastuzumab be held for at least 4 weeks, followed by repeat evaluation of LVEF. If LVEF returns to a normal value that is ≤15 % lower than the baseline LVEF, trastuzumab may be restarted. If LVEF remains decreased for >8 weeks or trastuzumab is held on three occasions due to declines in LVEF, it should be permanently discontinued [42].

Other biomarkers of trastuzumab-induced cardiomyopathy include serum troponins [43] and myocardial strain assessed by echocardiography [44, 45]. Future studies aimed at determining whether early intervention in patients demonstrating elevations in serum troponin or decreases in myocardial strain will alter future risk of cardiomyopathy are necessary before routine clinical use of these parameters can be implemented. As implied by these guidelines, trastuzumab-induced declines in LVEF may or may not be reversible. Overall data suggests that >60 % of patients who have declines in LVEF will recover some function, on average by 6 months after cessation of treatment [46]. However, it is important to note that most large clinical trials of trastuzumab have not included longer-term (>12 months) follow-up of cardiac function, so it is unknown whether patients exposed to this drug will develop cardiomyopathy years after exposure, particularly as they are subject to additional cardiovascular disease processes that are more common with advanced age [2].

VEGF-targeted therapies such as bevacizumab and sunitinib have been found to be associated with an increased risk of heart failure [47–49]. The relative risk of these therapies is difficult to assess since many patients included in these analyses had prior cardiotoxic chemotherapy and may also have had additional underlying cardiac risk factors. For many other targeted therapies, only incidental data (often in the form of case reports) is available and few predictions can be made regarding the long-term effects on cardiac function for many of these drugs based on current information (see Table 27.1).

Underlying risk factors, including prior or concomitant treatment with other chemotherapies (especially anthracyclines), hypertension, coronary artery disease, or age >60 years, have been shown to place patients at increased risk for cardiomyopathy from trastuzumab [50, 51] and other signaling kinase inhibitors [11, 52]. It seems prudent, therefore, to assess for and minimize traditional cardiac risk factors where possible, though solid clinical trial data to support this notion does not yet exist.

Ischemia

Many of the targeted therapies aimed at tumor vasculature also have effects on normal vasculature in the heart and other organs [53, 54]. Patients with underlying cardiovascular disease may be particularly susceptible to such agents. Myocardial ischemia can occur in the setting of acute or chronic treatment with vascular-targeted therapies. Some case reports suggest that vasospasm, perhaps in vascular territories with underlying noncritical atheromatous disease, is a significant mechanism for promoting myocardial ischemia due to these agents, though no specific therapies based on this observation have been tested [55, 56].

Use of antihormone-targeted therapies, tamoxifen, aromatase inhibitors, and androgen antagonists, has been associated with a small increase in cardiac events, some of which are ischemic [57–59]. However, no well-controlled trials that allow calculation of relative risk in the setting of additional coronary risk factors currently exist. Because of potential adverse effects on lipid profiles in the setting of such therapies, additional monitoring in patients with prior dyslipidemia or additional cardiac risk factors seems warranted [60]. Additional factors such as hypertension or thromboembolism may be associated with targeted agents and promote myocardial ischemia.

Hypertension

Many of the vascular-targeted kinase inhibitors are associated with significant increases in systemic blood pressure [9]. Some of these agents are even associated with severe hypertension, including hypertensive crisis [10]. The presence of hypertension in the setting of targeted agents has been shown to exacerbate associated cardiomyopathy [11]. Though the development of hypertension during therapy with these agents is generally a biomarker for chemotherapeutic response, treatment of associated hypertension is likely to be crucial to reduce cardiovascular events in these patients [61, 62]. Hypertension may also exacerbate cardiomyopathy associated with other types of targeted therapies, e.g., trastuzumab [63]; thus, close attention to blood pressure during these therapies is also important for prevention and management of this complication.

Thromboembolism

Both the antihormone-targeted and vascular-targeted therapies can increase the risk of thromboembolic events [40, 64]. These can be both venous and arterial and can contribute to stroke or myocardial ischemia. Some studies suggest that polymorphisms in coagulation factors may play an important role in risk for thromboembolism in response to such therapies [65]. However, additional investigation is needed before routine use of such genetic or other testing can be used to determine which patients are at risk and how to manage this preventively.

Arrhythmias

Many targeted agents are associated with changes in electrical properties of the myocardium, either by direct channel modulation or by other less well-defined mechanisms. Vascular-targeted kinase inhibitors and histone deacetylase (HDAC) inhibitors can be associated with significant prolongation of the QT interval, including rare induction of ventricular arrhythmias [66–68]. QT prolongation, atrial arrhythmias, and complete heart block have also been seen with proteasome inhibition [28]. Based on these findings, it is recommended that all patients undergoing such therapies undergo baseline ECG assessment. Particular attention should be paid to patients receiving additional agents (e.g., antibiotics, antiemetics) that can additionally prolong QT. Many patients undergoing cancer therapy are particularly prone to electrolyte abnormalities that may also increase the pro-arrhythmic effects of these drugs. These electrolyte abnormalities should be carefully monitored and corrected to reduce such risk.

Management

Currently, there is no specific clinical trial data on prevention or management of the cardiovascular complications of targeted therapies. Decisions regarding use or cessation of these agents need to be made by a team approach with cardiologists and oncologists weighing the relative cardiac risk and oncologic benefit for any given therapy. Given the paucity of trial data, this assessment can be quite challenging. All recommendations must be considered level of evidence IIB at the current time. When managing patients undergoing potentially cardiovascular toxic chemotherapy, the following steps are recommended:

1. Pretreatment assessment should be performed in all patients undergoing potentially cardiovascular toxic therapy with targeted agents. This assessment should include a full traditional cardiovascular risk profile, because underlying risk may render the patient more susceptible to these therapies and this risk may potentially be modifiable. Family history should include coronary disease and stroke history as well as cardiomyopathy screening. Lipid profiles, electrolytes, serum glucose and renal function, blood pressure, careful cardiovascular review of systems, and baseline ECG should all be assessed to understand the overall cardiovascular risk of each patient. Recall that these agents can have significant effects on all these parameters, and understanding the pretreatment values can help discern whether abnormalities after treatment are due to the treatment itself or underlying nontreatment-related abnormalities. Because many of the agents are associated with cardiomyopathy, baseline assessment of LV function is generally routinely recommended. Though ERNA has traditionally been used due to its excellent quantitative characteristics for LVEF, improvements in echocardiographic imaging have made this modality equally effective in most patients. In addition, echocardiography has the benefit of increased sensitivity for additional anatomic and hemodynamic assessment compared to ERNA [69]. Echocardiography also has the advantage of not requiring additional radiation exposure. Generally, we prefer to use echocardiography, supplemented by ERNA where LVEF cannot be accurately assessed due to technical factors or is borderline (i.e., at or just below the lower limit of normal).

2. During treatment, assessment is based on the relative baseline risk of the patient, the targeted agent being used, and careful review of systems at the time of each administration of chemotherapy or follow-up visit. Of all these new agents, only trastuzumab has clearly defined time points for follow-up assessment of cardiac toxicity and this is only for follow-up of LVEF (see above). However, patients with baseline abnormalities (e.g., hypertension or borderline LVEF) should receive additional screening and follow-up throughout their therapy. Certainly, all patients receiving vascular-targeted therapies should have blood pressure assessment before each round of chemotherapy, and hypertension should be aggressively managed using current American Heart Association/American College of Cardiology (AHA/ACC) guidelines. Patients with decreases in LV systolic function or borderline LVEF may benefit from treatment with angiotensin-converting enzyme (ACE) inhibitors [63]. Management of congestive heart failure should also be done following current guidelines until additional data is available. ECG monitoring in patients receiving agents with known effects on QT interval is also important, particularly in those with borderline or prolonged baseline QT or other conduction abnormalities.

3. After treatment, follow-up depends on the baseline and during treatment cardiovascular findings. Again, only trastuzumab has clearly defined follow-up goals (up to 2 years monitoring of LVEF). Because most of these drugs have been in use for short PERIODS of time, long-term effects on cardiovascular function are largely unknown. We advocate that patients receiving any drug with known risk of cardiomyopathy should undergo posttreatment assessment of LVEF. The timing and frequency of this is the subject of much debate. Recommendations are being prepared by several imaging societies currently, though these will be based on consensus and large clinical trials are still necessary for best practice to be defined in this field.

Future of Cardio-oncology

Optimal design and use of targeted therapies will continue to require input from both cardiologists and oncologists to avoid cardiovascular toxicity. The finding of cardiovascular abnormalities (including hypertension, dyslipidemia, ECG abnormalities, or LV dysfunction) before, during, or after cancer therapy should be handled using standard treatment guidelines for prevention and treatment. Additional understanding of the mechanisms of cardiovascular toxicity may eventually lead to more specific modes of prevention and treatment or to design of targeted therapies that will affect tumor cells and vasculature preferentially over normal cardiovascular tissues.

Key Points

- Many targeted chemotherapeutic agents have the potential for adverse cardiovascular effects.
- Current diagnosis and management of cardiovascular toxicity from targeted agents is complicated by lack of sufficient data.
- Attributing any given cardiovascular disease to these agents is a diagnosis of exclusion and baseline assessment of cardiovascular risk is key for this diagnostic process.
- The consultant cardiologist must participate in a well-balanced dialogue with the patient and oncology team regarding use of these agents in patients with underlying cardiovascular disease or with new cardiovascular disease.
- Until better information is available, cardiovascular side effects should be treated according to standard AHA/ACC treatment guidelines for the specific finding (e.g., heart failure, hypertension).

References

1. Ewer MS, Lippman SM. Type II chemotherapy-related cardiac dysfunction: time to recognize a new entity. J Clin Oncol. 2005;23: 2900–2.
2. Telli ML, Hunt SA, Carlson RW, Guardino AE. Trastuzumab-related cardiotoxicity: calling into question the concept of reversibility. J Clin Oncol. 2007;25:3525–33.
3. Hedhli N, Russell K. Cardiotoxicity of molecularly targeted agents. Curr Cardiol Rev. 2011;7:221–33.
4. Piccart-Gebhart MJ, Procter M, Leyland-Jones B, Goldhirsch A, Untch M, Smith I, Gianni L, Baselga J, Bell R, Jackisch C, Cameron D, Dowsett M, Barrios CH, Steger G, Huang CS, Andersson M, Inbar M, Lichinitser M, Lang I, Nitz U, Iwata H, Thomssen C, Lohrisch C, Suter TM, Ruschoff J, Suto T, Greatorex V, Ward C, Straehle C, McFadden E, Dolci MS, Gelber RD. Trastuzumab after adjuvant chemotherapy in HER2-positive breast cancer. N Engl J Med. 2005;353:1659–72.
5. Tan-Chiu E, Yothers G, Romond E, Geyer Jr CE, Ewer M, Keefe D, Shannon RP, Swain SM, Brown A, Fehrenbacher L, Vogel VG, Seay TE, Rastogi P, Mamounas EP, Wolmark N, Bryant J. Assessment of cardiac dysfunction in a randomized trial comparing doxorubicin and cyclophosphamide followed by paclitaxel, with or without trastuzumab as adjuvant therapy in node-positive, human epidermal growth factor receptor 2-overexpressing breast cancer: NSABP B-31. J Clin Oncol. 2005;23:7811–9.
6. Hedhli N, Russell KS. Cytostatic drugs, neuregulin activation of erbB receptors, and angiogenesis. Curr Hypertens Rep. 2010;12:411–7.
7. Lenihan D, Suter T, Brammer M, Neate C, Ross G, Baselga J. Pooled analysis of cardiac safety in patients with cancer treated with pertuzumab. Ann Oncol. 2012;23:791–800.
8. Chaudhary P, Gajra A. Cardiovascular effects of EGFR (epidermal growth factor receptor) monoclonal antibodies. Cardiovasc Hematol Agents Med Chem. 2010;8:156–63.
9. Robinson ES, Khankin EV, Karumanchi SA, Humphreys BD. Hypertension induced by vascular endothelial growth factor signaling pathway inhibition: mechanisms and potential use as a biomarker. Semin Nephrol. 2010;30:591–601.
10. Ranpura V, Pulipati B, Chu D, Zhu X, Wu S. Increased risk of high-grade hypertension with bevacizumab in cancer patients: a meta-analysis. Am J Hypertens. 2010;23:460–8.
11. Khakoo AY, Kassiotis CM, Tannir N, Plana JC, Halushka M, Bickford C, Trent 2nd J, Champion JC, Durand JB, Lenihan DJ. Heart failure associated with sunitinib malate: a multitargeted receptor tyrosine kinase inhibitor. Cancer. 2008;112:2500–8.
12. Girardi F, Franceschi E, Brandes AA. Cardiovascular safety of VEGF-targeting therapies: current evidence and handling strategies. Oncologist. 2010;15:683–94.
13. Polcher M, Eckhardt M, Coch C, Wolfgarten M, Kubler K, Hartmann G, Kuhn W, Rudlowski C. Sorafenib in combination with carboplatin and paclitaxel as neoadjuvant chemotherapy in patients with advanced ovarian cancer. Cancer Chemother Pharmacol. 2010;66:203–7.
14. Atallah E. Nilotinib cardiac toxicity: should we still be concerned? Leuk Res. 2011;35:577–8.
15. Corporation NP AFINITOR – everolimus tablet drug label. 2009. http://dailymed.nlm.nih.gov/dailymed/archives/fdaDrugInfo.cfm?archiveid=14355.
16. Reis SE, Costantino JP, Wickerham DL, Tan-Chiu E, Wang J, Kavanah M. Cardiovascular effects of tamoxifen in women with and without heart disease: breast cancer prevention trial. National Surgical Adjuvant Breast and Bowel Project Breast Cancer Prevention Trial Investigators. J Natl Cancer Inst. 2001;93:16–21.
17. Bradbury BD, Lash TL, Kaye JA, Jick SS. Tamoxifen-treated breast carcinoma patients and the risk of acute myocardial infarction and newly-diagnosed angina. Cancer. 2005;103:1114–21.

18. Pyrhonen S, Valavaara R, Modig H, Pawlicki M, Pienkowski T, Gundersen S, Bauer J, Westman G, Lundgren S, Blanco G, Mella O, Nilsson I, Hietanen T, Hindy I, Vuorinen J, Hajba A. Comparison of toremifene and tamoxifen in post-menopausal patients with advanced breast cancer: a randomized double-blind, the 'nordic' phase III study. Br J Cancer. 1997;76:270–7.

19. Tominaga T, Kimijima I, Kimura M, Takatsuka Y, Takashima S, Nomura Y, Kasumi F, Yamaguchi A, Masuda N, Noguchi S, Eshima N. Effects of toremifene and tamoxifen on lipid profiles in post-menopausal patients with early breast cancer: interim results from a Japanese phase III trial. Jpn J Clin Oncol. 2010;40:627–33.

20. Smith MR, Malkowicz SB, Chu F, Forrest J, Sieber P, Barnette KG, Rodriquez D, Steiner MS. Toremifene improves lipid profiles in men receiving androgen-deprivation therapy for prostate cancer: interim analysis of a multicenter phase III study. J Clin Oncol. 2008;26:1824–9.

21. Martin-Merino E, Johansson S, Morris T, Garcia Rodriguez LA. Androgen deprivation therapy and the risk of coronary heart disease and heart failure in patients with prostate cancer: a nested case–control study in UK primary care. Drug Saf. 2011;34:1061–77.

22. Forbes JF, Cuzick J, Buzdar A, Howell A, Tobias JS, Baum M. Effect of anastrozole and tamoxifen as adjuvant treatment for early-stage breast cancer: 100-month analysis of the ATAC trial. Lancet Oncol. 2008;9:45–53.

23. Keating GM. Letrozole: a review of its use in the treatment of post-menopausal women with hormone-responsive early breast cancer. Drugs. 2009;69:1681–705.

24. Zhang L, Lebwohl D, Masson E, Laird G, Cooper MR, Prince HM. Clinically relevant QTc prolongation is not associated with current dose schedules of LBH589 (panobinostat). J Clin Oncol. 2008;26: 332–3; discussion 333–4.

25. De Botton S, Dombret H, Sanz M, Miguel JS, Caillot D, Zittoun R, Gardembas M, Stamatoulas A, Conde E, Guerci A, Gardin C, Geiser K, Makhoul DC, Reman O, de la Serna J, Lefrere F, Chomienne C, Chastang C, Degos L, Fenaux P. Incidence, clinical features, and outcome of all trans-retinoic acid syndrome in 413 cases of newly diagnosed acute promyelocytic leukemia. The European APL Group. Blood. 1998;92:2712–8.

26. Mahadeo KM, Dhall G, Ettinger LJ, Kurer CC. Exacerbation of anthracycline-induced early chronic cardiomyopathy with ATRA: role of B-type natriuretic peptide as an indicator of cardiac dysfunction. J Pediatr Hematol Oncol. 2010;32:134–6.

27. Jerkins J, Suciua A, Mazimbaa S, Calvo A. Bortezomib-induced severe congestive heart failure. Cardiol Res. 2010;1:20–3.

28. Dasanu CA. Complete heart block secondary to bortezomib use in multiple myeloma. J Oncol Pharm Pract. 2011;17:282–4.

29. Voortman J, Giaccone G. Severe reversible cardiac failure after bortezomib treatment combined with chemotherapy in a non-small cell lung cancer patient: a case report. BMC Cancer. 2006;6:129.

30. Takamatsu H, Yamashita T, Kotani T, Sawazaki A, Okumura H, Nakao S. Ischemic heart disease associated with bortezomib treatment combined with dexamethasone in a patient with multiple myeloma. Int J Hematol. 2010;91:903–6.

31. Romond EH, Perez EA, Bryant J, Suman VJ, Geyer Jr CE, Davidson NE, Tan-Chiu E, Martino S, Paik S, Kaufman PA, Swain SM, Pisansky TM, Fehrenbacher L, Kutteh LA, Vogel VG, Visscher DW, Yothers G, Jenkins RB, Brown AM, Dakhil SR, Mamounas EP, Lingle WL, Klein PM, Ingle JN, Wolmark N. Trastuzumab plus adjuvant chemotherapy for operable HER2-positive breast cancer. N Engl J Med. 2005;353:1673–84.

32. Zhao YY, Sawyer DR, Baliga RR, Opel DJ, Han X, Marchionni MA, Kelly RA. Neuregulins promote survival and growth of cardiac myocytes. Persistence of ErbB2 and ErbB4 expression in neonatal and adult ventricular myocytes. J Biol Chem. 1998;273:10261–9.

33. Fukazawa R, Miller TA, Kuramochi Y, Frantz S, Kim YD, Marchionni MA, Kelly RA, Sawyer DB. Neuregulin-1 protects ventricular myocytes from anthracycline-induced apoptosis via erbB4-dependent activation of PI3-kinase/Akt. J Mol Cell Cardiol. 2003;35:1473–9.

34. Pentassuglia L, Graf M, Lane H, Kuramochi Y, Cote G, Timolati F, Sawyer DB, Zuppinger C, Suter TM. Inhibition of ErbB2 by receptor tyrosine kinase inhibitors causes myofibrillar structural damage without cell death in adult rat cardiomyocytes. Exp Cell Res. 2009;315:1302–12.

35. Hedhli N, Huang Q, Kalinowski A, Palmeri M, Hu X, Russell RR, Russell KS. Endothelium-derived neuregulin protects the heart against ischemic injury. Circulation. 2011;123:2254–62.

36. Hedhli N, Dobrucki LW, Kalinowski A, Zhuang ZW, Wu X, Russell 3rd RR, Sinusas AJ, Russell KS. Endothelial-derived neuregulin is an important mediator of ischaemia-induced angiogenesis and arteriogenesis. Cardiovasc Res. 2012;93:516–24.

37. Aoyagi T, Matsui T. Phosphoinositide-3 kinase signaling in cardiac hypertrophy and heart failure. Curr Pharm Des. 2011;17:1818–24.

38. Zolk O, Schenke C, Sarikas A. The ubiquitin-proteasome system: focus on the heart. Cardiovasc Res. 2006;70:410–21.

39. Sohns W, van Veen TA, van der Heyden MA. Regulatory roles of the ubiquitin-proteasome system in cardiomyocyte apoptosis. Curr Mol Med. 2010;10:1–13.

40. Vaklavas C, Lenihan D, Kurzrock R, Tsimberidou AM. Anti-vascular endothelial growth factor therapies and cardiovascular toxicity: what are the important clinical markers to target? Oncologist. 2010;15:130–41.

41. Chintalgattu V, Ai D, Langley RR, Zhang J, Bankson JA, Shih TL, Reddy AK, Coombes KR, Daher IN, Pati S, Patel SS, Pocius JS, Taffet GE, Buja LM, Entman ML, Khakoo AY. Cardiomyocyte PDGFR-beta signaling is an essential component of the mouse cardiac response to load-induced stress. J Clin Invest. 2010;120:472–84.

42. FDA. 2010. U.S. BL 103792 supplement: Trastuzumab–Genentech, Inc. 4 of 32/Regional (First-Line AGC): Herceptin Final Labeling (sBLA 103792 5250 In Approval Letter).doc.

43. Cardinale D, Colombo A, Torrisi R, Sandri MT, Civelli M, Salvatici M, Lamantia G, Colombo N, Cortinovis S, Dessanai MA, Nole F, Veglia F, Cipolla CM. Trastuzumab-induced cardiotoxicity: clinical and prognostic implications of troponin I evaluation. J Clin Oncol. 2010;28:3910–6.

44. Stoodley PW, Richards DA, Hui R, Boyd A, Harnett PR, Meikle SR, Clarke J, Thomas L. Two-dimensional myocardial strain imaging detects changes in left ventricular systolic function immediately after anthracycline chemotherapy. Eur J Echocardiogr. 2011;12:945–52.

45. Sawaya H, Sebag IA, Plana JC, Januzzi JL, Ky B, Cohen V, Gosavi S, Carver JR, Wiegers SE, Martin RP, Picard MH, Gersztten RE, Halpern EF, Passeri J, Kuter I, Scherrer-Crosbie M. Early detection and prediction of cardiotoxicity in chemotherapy-treated patients. Am J Cardiol. 2011;107:1375–80.

46. Suter TM, Procter M, van Veldhuisen DJ, Muscholl M, Bergh J, Carlomagno C, Perren T, Passalacqua R, Bighin C, Klijn JG, Ageev FT, Hitre E, Groetz J, Iwata H, Knap M, Gnant M, Muehlbauer S, Spence A, Gelber RD, Piccart-Gebhart MJ. Trastuzumab-associated cardiac adverse effects in the herceptin adjuvant trial. J Clin Oncol. 2007;25:3859–65.

47. Choueiri TK, Mayer EL, Je Y, Rosenberg JE, Nguyen PL, Azzi GR, Bellmunt J, Burstein HJ, Schutz FA. Congestive heart failure risk in patients with breast cancer treated with bevacizumab. J Clin Oncol. 2011;29:632–8.

48. Chu TF, Rupnick MA, Kerkela R, Dallabrida SM, Zurakowski D, Nguyen L, Woulfe K, Pravda E, Cassiola F, Desai J, George S, Morgan JA, Harris DM, Ismail NS, Chen JH, Schoen FJ, Van den Abbeele AD, Demetri GD, Force T, Chen MH. Cardiotoxicity associated with tyrosine kinase inhibitor sunitinib. Lancet. 2007;370:2011–9.

49. Richards CJ, Je Y, Schutz FA, Heng DY, Dallabrida SM, Moslehi JJ, Choueiri TK. Incidence and risk of congestive heart failure in patients with renal and nonrenal cell carcinoma treated with sunitinib. J Clin Oncol. 2011;29:3450–6.

50. Seidman A, Hudis C, Pierri MK, Shak S, Paton V, Ashby M, Murphy M, Stewart SJ, Keefe D. Cardiac dysfunction in the trastuzumab clinical trials experience. J Clin Oncol. 2002;20:1215–21.

51. Jones AL, Barlow M, Barrett-Lee PJ, Canney PA, Gilmour IM, Robb SD, Plummer CJ, Wardley AM, Verrill MW. Management of cardiac health in trastuzumab-treated patients with breast cancer: updated United Kingdom National Cancer Research Institute recommendations for monitoring. Br J Cancer. 2009;100:684–92.

52. Trent JC, Patel SS, Zhang J, Araujo DM, Plana JC, Lenihan DJ, Fan D, Patel SR, Benjamin RS, Khakoo AY. Rare incidence of congestive heart failure in gastrointestinal stromal tumor and other sarcoma patients receiving imatinib mesylate. Cancer. 2010;116:184–92.

53. Kamba T, McDonald DM. Mechanisms of adverse effects of anti-VEGF therapy for cancer. Br J Cancer. 2007;96:1788–95.

54. Orphanos GS, Ioannidis GN, Ardavanis AG. Cardiotoxicity induced by tyrosine kinase inhibitors. Acta Oncol. 2009;48:964–70.

55. Arima Y, Oshima S, Noda K, Fukushima H, Taniguchi I, Nakamura S, Shono M, Ogawa H. Sorafenib-induced acute myocardial infarction due to coronary artery spasm. J Cardiol. 2009;54:512–5.

56. Naib T, Steingart RM, Chen CL. Sorafenib-associated multivessel coronary artery vasospasm. Herz. 2011;36:348–51.

57. Efstathiou JA, Bae K, Shipley WU, Hanks GE, Pilepich MV, Sandler HM, Smith MR. Cardiovascular mortality after androgen deprivation therapy for locally advanced prostate cancer: RTOG 85–31. J Clin Oncol. 2009;27:92–9.

58. Keating NL, O'Malley AJ, Freedland SJ, Smith MR. Diabetes and cardiovascular disease during androgen deprivation therapy: observational study of veterans with prostate cancer. J Natl Cancer Inst. 2010;102:39–46.

59. Mouridsen H, Keshaviah A, Coates AS, Rabaglio M, Castiglione-Gertsch M, Sun Z, Thurlimann B, Mauriac L, Forbes JF, Paridaens R, Gelber RD, Colleoni M, Smith I, Price KN, Goldhirsch A. Cardiovascular adverse events during adjuvant endocrine therapy for early breast cancer using letrozole or tamoxifen: safety analysis of BIG 1–98 trial. J Clin Oncol. 2007;25:5715–22.

60. Pritchard KI, Abramson BL. Cardiovascular health and aromatase inhibitors. Drugs. 2006;66:1727–40.

61. Jain RK, Duda DG, Willett CG, Sahani DV, Zhu AX, Loeffler JS, Batchelor TT, Sorensen AG. Biomarkers of response and resistance to antiangiogenic therapy. Nat Rev Clin Oncol. 2009;6:327–38.

62. Zhu X, Stergiopoulos K, Wu S. Risk of hypertension and renal dysfunction with an angiogenesis inhibitor sunitinib: systematic review and meta-analysis. Acta Oncol. 2009;48:9–17.

63. Oliva S, Cioffi G, Frattini S, Simoncini EL, Faggiano P, Boccardi L, Pulignano G, Fioretti AM, Giotta F, Lestuzzi C, Maurea N, Sabatini S, Tarantini L. Administration of angiotensin-converting enzyme inhibitors and beta-blockers during adjuvant trastuzumab chemotherapy for nonmetastatic breast cancer: marker of risk or cardioprotection in the real world? Oncologist. 2012;17:917–24.

64. Choueiri TK, Schutz FA, Je Y, Rosenberg JE, Bellmunt J. Risk of arterial thromboembolic events with sunitinib and sorafenib: a systematic review and meta-analysis of clinical trials. J Clin Oncol. 2010;28:2280–5.

65. Garber JE, Halabi S, Tolaney SM, Kaplan E, Archer L, Atkins JN, Edge S, Shapiro CL, Dressler L, Paskett ED, Kimmick G, Orcutt J, Scalzo A, Winer E, Levine E, Shahab N, Berliner N. Factor V Leiden mutation and thromboembolism risk in women receiving adjuvant tamoxifen for breast cancer. J Natl Cancer Inst. 2010;102:942–9.

66. Bagnes C, Panchuk PN, Recondo G. Antineoplastic chemotherapy induced QTc prolongation. Curr Drug Saf. 2010;5:93–6.

67. Bello CL, Mulay M, Huang X, Patyna S, Dinolfo M, Levine S, Van Vugt A, Toh M, Baum C, Rosen L. Electrocardiographic characterization of the QTc interval in patients with advanced solid tumors: pharmacokinetic- pharmacodynamic evaluation of sunitinib. Clin Cancer Res. 2009;15:7045–52.

68. Shah MH, Binkley P, Chan K, Xiao J, Arbogast D, Collamore M, Farra Y, Young D, Grever M. Cardiotoxicity of histone deacetylase inhibitor depsipeptide in patients with metastatic neuroendocrine tumors. Clin Cancer Res. 2006;12:3997–4003.

69. Karanth NV, Roy A, Joseph M, de Pasquale C, Karapetis C, Koczwara B. Utility of prechemotherapy echocardiographical assessment of cardiac abnormalities. Support Care Cancer. 2011;19:2021–6.

Evidence-Based Cardiovascular Management of Patients Receiving Radiotherapy to the Heart

28

B. Frazier Taylor, Suzanne B. Evans,
and Kenneth B. Roberts

Abstract

Historic and modern oncologic therapy techniques have the potential to adversely affect cardiovascular function. Depending on the disease, cancer therapy often requires radiotherapy (RT) to the chest, cardiotoxic chemotherapy, or both. A history of (or ongoing) RT to the heart may complicate the cardiovascular management of a patient. Radiotherapy is often thought to be selectively toxic to rapidly dividing cell populations, suggesting that tissues such as the heart and vessels would be relatively resistant. However, long-term outcome studies and more recent advances in imaging have given us a better understanding of the risks for both early and late cardiovascular complications of RT. While modern RT planning and treatment have reduced the dose to the heart, the risk to the cardiovascular system still remains. This review will attempt to give the reader comprehensive, up-to-date knowledge of the risks of RT to the heart, advances in treatment, advances in imaging for detecting adverse changes to the heart and the additive effects of chemotherapy, and other comorbidities on the effects of RT. Detailed recommendations are given for both the primary care physician as well as the cardiovascular team when managing patients who have received or are receiving RT to the heart.

Keywords

Radiotherapy • Dosimetry • Heart toxicity • Long-term complications • Acute complications • Cardiovascular imaging • Congestive heart failure (CHF) • Pericarditis • Coronary artery disease (CAD)

Introduction

Radiation therapy (RT) is an integral part of modern cancer care. Over 50 % of cancer patients will benefit from the use of therapeutic radiation at some point in their disease course.

B.F. Taylor, MD, PhD (✉)
Department of Therapeutic Radiology,
Yale New Haven Hospital, Yale School of Medicine,
208040, New Haven, CT 06520-8040, USA
e-mail: ben.taylor@yale.edu

S.B. Evans, MD, MPH • K.B. Roberts, MD
Department of Therapeutic Radiology,
Yale School of Medicine, Yale University School of Medicine,
208040, New Haven, CT 06520-8040, USA
e-mail: suzanne.evans@yale.edu; kenneth.roberts@yale.edu

Nonetheless, RT has been associated with toxicity and, arguably, the heart is one of the best known examples.

The two diseases in which the detrimental effects of radiation are best understood are breast cancer and Hodgkin's lymphoma. The excellent survival rates of these two conditions allow for long follow-up of patients with assessment of late toxicities.

It is helpful to understand that although the literature is full of reports of cardiotoxicity following breast cancer treatment and Hodgkin's lymphoma treatment, prior treatments bear little resemblance to the method by which modern RT is delivered. Hodgkin's disease treatment, for example, has shifted from relatively high-dose (40 Gy) total or subtotal nodal radiation (encompassing the mediastinal, supraclavicular, axillary, para-aortic, and sometimes pelvic and inguinofemoral nodes) to a combination of systemic chemotherapy paired with 20–30 Gy to an involved field of the initially diseased nodes. This reduction in both dose and volume undoubtedly minimizes the toxicity of treatment. A pediatric Hodgkin's lymphoma series has shown a reduction in late cardiac morbidity with reductions in mediastinal radiation doses; specifically cohorts receiving 36, 30, 25, 20, and 0 Gy had associated cardiac disease incidence rates at 25 years of follow-up of 21 %, 10, 6, 5, and 3 %, respectively [1]. Likewise, with breast cancer, treatment has shifted from the internal mammary nodal chain (located typically 3 cm lateral to the midline) with an *en face* "through-and-through" photon field in a "hockey stick" configuration [2] to 50 Gy delivered with orthovoltage to significantly more judicious use of internal mammary nodal treatment with megavoltage irradiation. Patients treated from this earlier era have been found to have a 10 % increase in mortality [3], largely driven by premature cardiac death. Examination of the treatment methods used previously reveals mean doses to the heart as high as 23 Gy [4], compared to the more modest mean heart doses of 3 Gy today [5].

The significance of the move to megavoltage radiation is that dose inhomogeneity was greatly improved. In Hodgkin's disease or treatment of seminoma in which the mediastinum was included, the use of orthovoltage radiation was particularly problematic. This lower energy radiation was not very penetrating and there were significant "hot spots" to the more superficial structures (like the anteriorly located coronary arteries) as a consequence of getting the prescription dose to the nodal targets surrounding the tracheobronchial tree. With modern techniques, there is a much more even dose delivery throughout the target area and the sensitive anteriorly located coronary arteries are more likely to be relatively spared.

Additionally, radiation delivered pre-1991 did not use computed tomography (CT) simulation. Simulation is the process by which radiation oncologists "map out" the radiation using CT data. This allows for more precise targeting as well as detailed analysis of the dose given to nearby organs from a given radiation plan. Prior to the early 1990s, all planning was done by fluoroscopy, taking a single measurement at the midpoint in the treated volume of the patient and prescribing the radiation on that basis. This did not always take into account varied patient thicknesses and contours which change the distribution of radiation. As a consequence, this often allowed for treatment "hot spots" in critical normal tissues like the heart due to inherent dose heterogeneity ; this can be better modulated in the modern era using 3-dimensional (3D) treatment planning and newer abilities that account for respiratory motion (4D planning).

Pathophysiology

The goal of oncologic RT is to aid in the cure or definitively cure localized malignancy. It is also used commonly for palliation of local disease. These goals are achieved by using ionizing radiation to induce cancer cell death via necrosis, mitotic catastrophe, apoptosis, or autophagy or by inhibiting a cell's ability to divide though induction of senescence. The largest contributing biochemical reaction responsible for induction of all of the aforementioned phenomena is DNA damage, specifically lethal DNA double-strand breaks (DSBs). Ionizing radiation causes DNA damage by both direct ionization but more commonly by indirect ionization through free radical formation by activation of water. While it is generally accepted that radiation is selective for rapidly dividing cells such as tumor cells or rapidly repopulating cells such as hematopoietic cells, there are potential side effects in any tissue treated with radiotherapy and cardiovascular tissue is no exception. Adverse effects are most commonly seen in the pericardium, but the myocardium can also be impacted resulting in congestive heart failure (CHF) due to restrictive cardiomyopathy and obstructive coronary artery disease (CAD) due to damage to the vascular endothelium. In addition, adverse effects can be seen in the microvasculature, conduction system, and valves. Patients with radiation-induced heart disease include survivors of Hodgkin's disease, non-Hodgkin's lymphoma, esophageal carcinoma, thymoma, lung cancer, breast cancer, and seminoma (given the historical practice of treating the mediastinum with radiation) [6].

The time to normal tissue injury and side effects depends on tissue kinetics of cell differentiation, loss, and repopulation. Acute injury is seen usually during the course of treatment (6–8 weeks) in tissues with rapid cell turnover such as the bone marrow, skin, and oropharyngeal, esophageal, and gastrointestinal mucosa. Subacute injury can occur 2 months to 1 year after the start of radiation such as with lung pneumonitis and is thought to occur during the "remodeling phase." Finally, late injury occurs in cells that are lost from the tissue at a slow rate, such as blood vessel endothelium, oligodendroglia or Schwann cells in neural tissue, tubule cells in the kidney, fibroblasts in skin and connective tissue, and osteoblasts and chondroblasts in bones. Timing and pathologic findings of late effects varies between tissues. In addition, infiltrating cells that secrete cytokines and growth factors [7] may also contribute to the pathogenesis of radiation effects unrelated to cell depletion such as in radiation gliosis [8] or fibrosis. Although rare, cardiovascular side effects can occur acutely as with acute pericarditis during irradiation but are more commonly seen as late, chronic health issues. Some clinical studies show no evidence of clinical cardiovascular risk of RT in adult patients with

Hodgkin's disease after more than 6 years following chemotherapy and RT [9] and in patients with early-stage left-sided breast cancer, after as long as 10 years of follow-up [10]. However, late radiation effects associated with atherosclerosis and heart disease can take decades to occur after irradiation [11–14]. In early-stage breast cancer, a difference in death due to cardiovascular disease and specifically ischemic heart disease was established between patients receiving high-dose-volume RT to the heart and non-irradiated controls after 4–5 years. Cumulative incidence curves continued to diverge up to 12 years later [15]. As patients live longer following cancer therapy, this becomes a more common and difficult problem to manage.

Pathology

In addition to the increased incidence of clinical cardiovascular symptoms secondary to RT, the effects of RT can be seen, measured, and quantified in the cardiovascular system. The first visible proof of radiation-related cardiovascular injury came from cardiac tissue analysis from surgical specimens and autopsy data. Pathologically evident abnormalities were limited to late time points after radiation. When the myocardium is involved, diffuse interstitial fibrosis occurs. In a pathology review of 27 specimens, 14/20 (70 %) had radiation-related disease in the pericardium (6 with effusions, 3 with constriction, and 2 with both). Twelve of 17 patients (71 %) showed radiation injury involving a total of 25 valves (9 mitral, 8 aortic, 5 tricuspid, and 3 pulmonary), 8 of which were clinically significant. Ten of 16 (63 %) exhibited radiation-related fibrosis of the myocardium, which was moderate to severe only in the 7 patients receiving more than 30 Gy. Two of 13 coronary arteries in relatively young men (26 and 44 years) with Hodgkin's disease [16] had "unequivocal radiation-induced obstructions."

Mechanisms

One possible mechanism of cardiovascular injury is damage to endothelial cells and subsequent induction of inflammatory responses. It has been hypothesized that the induction of late coronary effects is due to endothelial cell damage with reports of severe alterations in myocardial capillaries including irregularities of the endothelial cell membranes, cytoplasmic swelling, thrombosis, and wall rupture [17]. Quantitative analysis shows that the ratio of capillaries to myocytes may be reduced by as much as 50 % compared to untreated controls. Such a reduction in capillaries leads to ischemia and subsequent myocardial fibrosis [17]. Thus, radiation treatment produced a predictable and identifiable

sequence of events that is identifiable histologically in the myocardial microvasculature [18]. These findings are supported clinically as breast cancer patients receiving high doses to large volumes exhibit increased mortality from ischemic heart disease, but not from myocardial infarction, which implies radiation-induced microvascular damage to the heart rather than large vessel disease for this particular type of exposure between 4 and 12 years following treatment [15]. Other studies argue that fractionated and very low radiotherapy doses may cause endothelial damage by killing radiosensitive cell populations such as monocytes that may be required for maintaining the intima [19]. Irradiation and doxorubicin together dramatically show independent and additive organ effects as seen on light microscopy suggesting clinically additive but distinct mechanisms of injury [18]. Further studies are warranted, but it appears that radiotherapy has the potential to damage both microvascular and macrovascular structures resulting in clinically apparent abnormalities in virtually any area or function of the heart. There is a dose-volume dependence and the time from exposure to clinically apparent abnormality may vary greatly between specific heart tissues.

Diagnosis

Due to the clinically silent early effects of RT on cardiac tissue, the majority of data evaluating the effects and pathophysiology of radiation-induced cardiovascular change was previously based on long-term late effects such as clinical presentation with symptoms, intervention, and postmortem analysis. In addition to pathologic studies, long-term imaging studies have been able to demonstrate the pathophysiologic effects of RT. In 31 patients 20–28 years after radiotherapy, cardiac MRI found pathologic changes in 70 % of patients consisting of reduced left ventricular function (ejection fraction (EF) <55 %) in 23 %, hemodynamically significant valvular dysfunction in 42 %, late myocardial enhancement in 29 %, and perfusion deficits in 68 % [20]. Cardiac computed tomography (CT) with coronary artery calcium scoring is another method that has been reported as useful [21]. This method followed by CT angiography of the coronary arteries detected RT-related CAD from patients (age 35–60) with Hodgkin's lymphoma treated between ages 11 and 27 to a mediastinal dose range of 34–45 Gy. Calcium scores, a measurement of plaque and calcium deposition in the coronary arteries, were significantly greater when compared to other patients of similar ages [22]. In breast cancer patients undergoing RT, calcium scores may also prove to be a useful harbinger of clinically significant CAD [23]. But to add complexity to this concept, one study has suggested that calcium scores may be intrinsically higher in breast cancer patients relative to the general population even before any RT is delivered [24].

The most commonly used method for monitoring patients at risk of RT-induced cardiac side effects has been transthoracic echocardiography. Early attempts using echocardiography for post-RT surveillance initially revealed that women without heart disease showed a decrease in left ventricular (LV) function, but this change was transient and not associated with symptoms, normalizing within 6 months. After 6 months, a pericardial effusion was seen in one-third of patients [25]. New echocardiographic techniques, such as myocardial strain rate imaging (SRI), have the potential to detect early, silent, and preclinical RT-induced changes [26]. An example of this method was used in breast cancer patients receiving RT to the breast or chest wall. Standard echocardiography and SRI were used before RT, immediately after RT, and 2 months after RT. A reduction in strain was observed immediately after and 2 months post-RT in left-sided patients but not in right-sided patients [27]. Another recent study using conventional and tissue Doppler echocardiography before and 4–6 weeks after RT showed immediate detrimental effects of radiotherapy. After RT there was a decrease in early transmitral diastolic velocity (E), E/A ratio (indicating diastolic dysfunction), EF, early diastolic myocardial velocity (E_m), and E_m/A_m (A_m = late atrial diastolic myocardial velocity). There was also an increase in E-wave deceleration time, isovolumic relaxation time, isovolumic contraction time, and ejection time in patients treated for lung or breast cancer with mean heart dose of 13.1 Gy [28].

Myocardial perfusion imaging (MPI) and cardiac cine magnetic resonance imaging (MRI) are two additional methods for detecting early RT-induced changes. With a median interval of 12.3 months between RT and MPI, 7 of 18 lung cancer patients (39 %) with centrally located tumors receiving radiotherapy or concurrent chemoradiotherapy (CRT) demonstrated an MPI defect versus only 1 of 15 patients (7 %) in a control group [29]. Similarly in breast cancer patients receiving tangential RT, there were increased perfusion defects at 6 months with no additional change at 12 or 18 months [30]. On the contrary, another MPI study demonstrated new perfusion defects detected at 6, 12, 18, and 24 months following RT with incidences of 27, 29, 38, and 42 %, respectively. Although the loss of patients to follow-up over time somewhat influences these percentages, this data suggests a progressive increase in perfusion defects over time. These perfusion defects correlated with wall-motion abnormalities [31]. Finally, a recent study using cardiac cine MRI before, during, and after CRT for esophageal cancer demonstrated that CRT impairs left ventricular function at an early treatment stage (at 40 Gy during treatment and 0–12 days posttreatment).

In addition to imaging modalities, serum biomarkers for early signs of cardiac toxicity have been shown for predict

cardiac function decline from cancer therapy. For example, longitudinal strain reduction from baseline at 3 months and detectable high-sensitivity cardiac troponin I at 3 months were independent predictors of the development of cardiotoxicity at 6 months [32]. Elevation of troponin I, a marker of acute myocardial damage, after high-dose chemotherapy (usually containing an anthracycline, trastuzumab, or both) is sensitive and reliable at predicting the development of future LVEF depression [33–36]. The use of troponin I for the use as a biomarker for RT-induced heart toxicity in early left-sided breast cancer has been negative in two studies [37, 38], while another showed both brain natriuretic peptide (BNP) and troponin I were elevated due to radiotherapy although absolute levels were low [39]. Patients with left-sided breast cancer also show higher values of serum N-terminal pro-B-type natriuretic peptide (NT-proBNP) after RT when compared with non-RT-treated matched patients, and higher serum levels correlated high doses to small volumes of heart and ventricle [38]. In addition, novel biomarkers cardiotoxicity are emerging and the use of a multi-biomarker approach may allow for better identification for cardiac risk in patients treated with anticancer therapy [40].

Patient Variability, Anatomy, and Radiation Fields

Anatomy, location of radiotherapy portal, and dose distribution play a crucial role in the clinical presentation of cardiovascular complications. The age of the patient is also very important with the highest concern being with children. Patient anatomy plays a most important role in treatment variability and heart dose [41]. Radiation-induced heart complications also appear to be related to total dose (>30 Gy), radiated tissue volume, and fraction size (dose administered per treatment) [42]. Dose-volume analysis suggests that the larger the irradiated cardiac volume, the lower the total dose that can cause cardiac damage, although there are clearly small but critical volumes (such as irradiation of the left anterior descending coronary artery) that can cause clinically significant disease. In lung cancer patients treated with RT and concurrent CRT, central tumors have a higher likelihood of cardiovascular side effects [29]. In breast cancer, left-sided breast cancer patients treated in older generations clearly have increased risks of cardiovascular complications. A retrospective study of ~35,000 women in Denmark and Sweden demonstrated an increased mean heart dose in left-sided breast cancer patients than right-sided patients (6.7 Gy vs. 2.7 Gy) correlating with increased risk for acute myocardial infarction (Hazard Ratio (HR) 1.22), angina (HR 1.25), acute pericarditis (HR 2.16), and aortic valvular disease (HR 1.7) for left-sided disease

[43]. When stratified into high- and low-volume heart dose groups, the risk of death due to cardiovascular disease and specifically ischemic heart disease was increased relative to non-irradiated surgical controls in the high volume dose group [15]. Thus, the increased complication rate and death

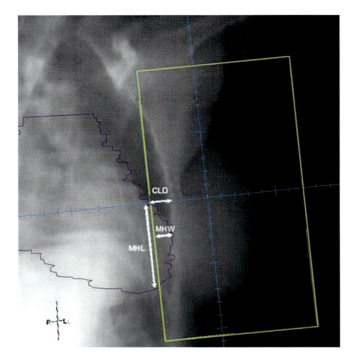

Fig. 28.1 Typical "beams eye view" of a breast tangent portal film, showing the radiotherapy treatment field. *MHW* maximum heart width, *CLD* central lung distance, *MHL* maximum heart length (From Correa et al. [44], with permission)

hazard is presumably due to increased heart dose. However, with sophisticated 3D treatment planning systems, we can now anticipate that in the subset of left-sided patients who would be at increased risk, and for those patients with little to no heart in the treatment field, cardiovascular complications should be minimal. Diagnostic abnormalities are higher in left-sided breast cancer patients with a larger median central lung distance (CLD). CLD is the measurement in the radiation portal beams eye view from chest wall to the radiation field edge in the lung (Fig. 28.1). Patients with RT-induced congestive heart failure (CHF) also have a larger median CLD [44]. Central lung distance is a surrogate for the amount of heart irradiated and was a commonly used method in the 2D era. Now that 3D dosimetry is widely available, more detailed patient-specific heart dosimetry is the preferred method for maximizing the safety of a radiotherapy plan.

When analyzing treatment planning, tangential fields for left-sided breast cancer results in a higher mean heart dose compared to right-sided breast cancer since the primary radiation fields include the anterior portion of the heart and a segment of the LAD [41]. Obstructive coronary artery disease is not only generally increased in left-sided patients but specifically in the middle and distal LAD and distal diagonal arteries, correlating with the radiated volumes (Fig. 28.2a, b) [45]. Adding the internal mammary nodal chain down to the fifth intercostal space as a target for RT also significantly increases heart dose [41]. This may deliver higher radiation doses to the proximal right coronary artery (RCA), particularly in right-sided breast cancers in which the IM nodes are being specifically targeted (Fig. 28.2c, d).

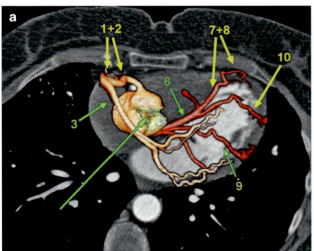

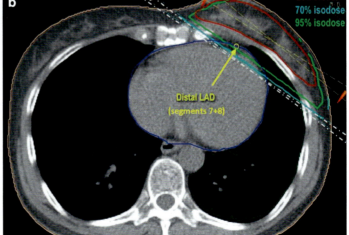

Fig. 28.2 (**a**) Coronary artery angiogram superimposed on computed tomography (CT) illustrating coronary arteries. Numerals *1–3* represent segments of the right coronary artery (RCA), *6–10* represent segments of the left anterior descending artery (LAD), and *5* represents left main coronary artery (LMCA), and left circumflex artery (LCX) segments not shown. Artery segments at increased risk (*1, 2, 7, 8* and *10*) are highlighted in *yellow*. (**b**) Dose distribution of a left-sided tangential breast field (From Nilsson et al. [45], with permission). Dose distribution in a right (**c**) and left (**d**) side internal mammary node (IMN) field (From Taylor et al. [41], with permission)

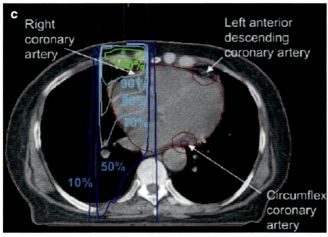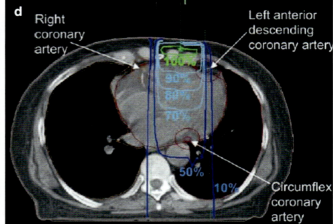

Fig. 28.2 (continued)

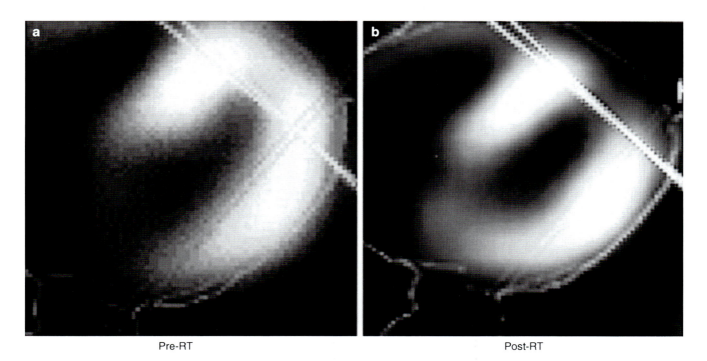

Pre-RT   Post-RT

Fig. 28.3 (**a**) Myocardial perfusion study demonstrating normal perfusion before RT and (**b**) perfusion deficit post-RT corresponding with radiation field (**b**) (From Marks et al. [31], with permission)

Imaging studies have also verified the specific location of RT-induced damage, linking the dosimetric studies on heart dose to clinical outcome and pathologic change. As described above, a reduction in myocardial strain was observed immediately after and 2 months post-RT in left-sided breast cancer patients, but there was a specific reduction in strain and strain rate after RT in the apical left ventricular (LV) segments of these patients, but not in mid or basal segments. Strain deficits were related to RT dose, as segments exposed to >3 Gy showed decrease in strain, but not in segments receiving <3 Gy [27]. Similarly, in left-sided breast cancer patients receiving tangential RT, there were increased perfusion (MPI) defects at 6 months specifically in the LAD distribution compared to pretreatment baseline. There were no increases in perfusion defects in the left circumflex (LCX) or RCA distributions. In multivariate analysis, the SPECT perfusion changes in the LAD distribution at 6 months were independently associated with the percent of LV irradiated [30]. Another MPI study noted new perfusion defects occurring in only 10–20 % of patients with less than 5 % of the LV included in the RT fields but as high as 50–60 % of patients with greater than 5 % of the LV treated (Fig. 28.3a, b) [31].

Chemotherapy and Comorbidities

Patients receiving radiotherapy often receive chemotherapeutic regimens before, after, and even during radiotherapy. Of all chemotherapeutic drugs, anthracyclines are the most recognized as being cardiotoxic. Anthracyclines such as doxorubicin often play a key role in the treatment of both Hodgkin's lymphoma and breast cancer. Unfortunately, this population of patients commonly receives radiation dose to the heart. Early pathologic studies showed that radiotherapy and doxorubicin separately caused increased fibrosis with capillary/arterial narrowing (sparing myocytes), and dramatic effects including vacuolization of cardiac myocytes (sparing vasculature), respectively. Combining the therapies resulted in abnormalities to both vasculature and myocytes [18, 46], but no additive histological effect on either. However, in a variety of animal models combining radiation and chemotherapy using different fractionation schedules, an additive effect was found when measuring the clinical manifestations and severity of myocardial lesions [47]. Clinical data, however, suggest that combined mediastinal radiotherapy and doxorubicin may be supra-additive in their respective risks of cardiac toxicity, particularly for congestive heart failure and valvular heart disease [48]. By itself, doxorubicin toxicity is exponentially dose dependent and increases dramatically when cumulative doses exceed 500 mg/m^2 in adults [49]. Toxicity may be decreased by continuous intravenous infusion [50]. Patient age is also a factor in both radiotherapy and anthracycline toxicity with pediatric patients being significantly more susceptible to cardiotoxicity [48, 51–53].

In addition to doxorubicin, many other chemotherapeutic agents may increase risk of acute and chronic cardiovascular disease. Of note is trastuzumab (Herceptin), which improves disease-free survival in Her2-positive breast cancer. While the additional incidence is not as large in magnitude as doxorubicin, adjuvant trastuzumab treatment is cardiotoxic, especially when given concomitantly with paclitaxel after doxorubicin and cyclophosphamide [54, 55]. Additionally, while tamoxifen is felt to be cardioprotective due to its favorable effect on the lipid profile, aromatase inhibitors do not have this favorable effect. As such, cardiovascular events are modestly higher on patients on aromatase inhibitors, although this is controversial [56]. Other therapeutic drugs associated with cardiotoxicity are reviewed elsewhere, and although milder and/or rare with regard to toxicity and incidence, their risks are not negligible [57, 58]. Such therapies include platinum agents, alkylating agents, taxanes, vinca alkaloids, biological agents (IL-2 and TNFα), hormonal therapy, monoclonal antibodies, targeted small molecules, and various other therapies such as all-trans-retinoic acid (ATRA) and arsenic trioxide (ATO).

While RT to the heart increases the risk of various forms of cardiovascular disease, independent comorbidities may have an additive effect on cardiovascular risk. For example, the risk of any heart disease in women receiving RT is higher for women diagnosed with ischemic heart disease prior to breast cancer diagnosis compared to all other women [43]. In SPECT perfusion changes in left-sided breast cancer patients receiving RT are independently associated with hormonal therapy ($p = 0.005$) and pre-RT hypercholesterolemia ($p = 0.006$), in addition to percent irradiated LV [30]. Thus, it should be assumed that radiation's effect on the cardiovascular system is enhanced by the common cardiac risk factors such as obesity, smoking, family history, diabetes mellitus, hyperlipidemia, hypertension, hormone therapy, and other cardiotoxic treatments such as trastuzumab and doxorubicin.

Management

Guidelines for accepted heart dose tolerance levels have been described. The minimum tolerance dose defined as a severe complication rate of 5 % at 5 years (TD 5/5) is 60, 45, and 40 Gy, where the volume of total heart treated is 1/3, 2/3, and 3/3, respectively. The maximum tolerance dose defined as severe complication rate of 50 % at 5 years (TD 50/5) is 70, 55, and 50 Gy treating 1/3, 2/3, and 3/3 of the heart volume, respectively [59]. When the whole heart and pericardium are irradiated, older experience from managing Hodgkin's lymphoma suggests an increasing risk for constrictive pericarditis above doses of 30 Gy. Doses of 15 Gy or lower have a negligible risk [60, 61]. The QUANTEC (Quantitative Analyses of Normal Tissue Effects in the Clinic) initiative recommends a heart volume of <10 % getting 25 Gy or more of in breast cancer patients [62].

With regard to Hodgkin's disease, doses >40 Gy to the mediastinum are associated with significantly increased risk of stroke, chronic heart failure, and myocardial infarction [63]. As noted, lower radiation doses (30, 25, 20, or 0 Gy vs. 36 Gy) result in significantly decreased risk of cardiac disease. Fortunately, more modern Hodgkin's combined modality therapy using lower radiation doses have been proven to be equally effective and we can expect reduction of late effects due to dose reduction [1]. In addition, subcarinal shield blocking at doses of 20–30 Gy can decrease the incidence of pericardial disease to 2.5 % [60]. Due to potentially large fields and the necessity for targeting the mediastinum, the benefits of 3D treatment planning may be more limited in Hodgkin's disease. Now that Hodgkin's lymphoma treatment includes low-dose involved-field radiotherapy (limiting radiotherapy only to the involved nodal area, not the next echelon), a movement towards further reducing the volume of mediastinal radiotherapy in what is termed "involved node radiotherapy" is expected to further decrease normal tissue and heart exposures [64, 65].

Since patient anatomy contributes the greatest variability to heart dose [41], 3D treatment planning is especially useful

Fig. 28.4 Dosimetry of a
left-sided breast tangential field
where heart dose was improved
from prone positioning due to
individual cardiac anatomy

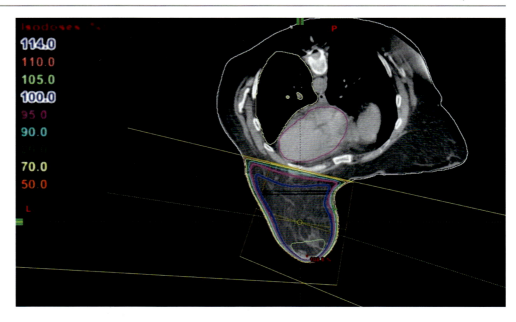

in breast cancer treatment. Death from RT-induced ischemic heart disease has substantially decreased over time suggesting that improvements in radiotherapy technique have resulted in reductions in toxicity. For example, each succeeding year after 1979, the hazard of ischemic heart disease death in left-sided breast cancer patients declined by 6 % compared to right-sided patients [66].

In addition to 3D treatment planning, patient position can improve normal tissue doses to lung and heart. For example, in breast cancer, prone treatment can decrease heart and lung dose in left-sided patients, in some cases completely excluding the heart from the field (Fig. 28.4). Prone positioning combined with advanced treatment planning such as intensity modulated radiotherapy (IMRT) has also been shown to improve heart and lung dose [67]. The prone position allows for breast tissue to fall away from the chest wall by gravity such that the radiation beams to cover the whole breast do not need to be deep to the chest wall (see Fig. 28.4). IMRT using multifield techniques, even in the supine position, may be used to minimize heart dose [68, 69]. Dynamic treatment techniques such as breath holding at deep inspiration can also greatly reduce heart dose. This technique is simple and can significantly reduce the cardiac volume included within the radiation portals by 40 % compared to end-tidal volume breath hold. Forced expiratory breath hold increases cardiac dose by 21 % [70].

Patients with heart disease induced by RT and chemoRT should be treated with angiotensin-converting enzyme inhibitors (ACEIs) or angiotensin receptor blockers (ARBs), beta blockers (BB), loop diuretics, and ICDs when indicated, similar to patients with non-RT-induced heart disease. In addition, other comorbidities for heart disease should be addressed in patients receiving RT to the heart. Interestingly,

proper cardiac treatment may be lacking in some patients receiving cardiotoxic therapy. In one study, 40 % of patients who received anthracycline and/or trastuzumab had decreased LVEF (<55 %) and of these, 40 % received ACEI or ARB therapy, 51 % received BB therapy, and 54 % of had cardiology consultation. Patients with asymptomatic decreased LVEF, 31 % received ACEI or ARB therapy, 35 % received BB therapy, and 42 % had cardiology consultation. Of those with symptomatic decreased LVEF, 100 % received BB therapy, 89 % received cardiology consultation, but only 67 % received ACEI or ARB therapy. Thus, cancer survivors in general are often not receiving treatment consistent with treatment guidelines [71].

In addition to early detection of patients at increased cardiac risk, discussed in the diagnosis section above, upfront presymptomatic medical therapy or cardioprotective agents concurrent with ongoing treatment may eventually play a role in preventing RT- and chemoRT-induced heart toxicity. For example, anthracycline cardiotoxicity may induce progressive deterioration of cardiac function continuing years after treatment. Patients who received an ACEI for more than 3 months have a remarkably potent and long-lasting recovery, while other non-treated patients did not spontaneously regain cardiac function [72]. In patients treated with high-dose cardiotoxic chemotherapy, early treatment with enalapril, an angiotensin-converting enzyme inhibitor (ACEI), prevented development of late cardiotoxicity in both non-randomized studies [36] and randomized studies where treatment was given only to high-risk patients with increased troponin I values [73]. Cardiotoxicity was defined as >10 % unit decrease in LVEF, where a 43 % incidence of cardiotoxicity was seen in the control group compared to 0 % incidence with enalapril ($p < 0.001$) [73]. Dexrazoxane, an iron chelator, prevents heart damage from anthracyclines with no effect on response rate or survival between the dexrazoxane and control groups. It is thought that if the risk of cardiac damage is expected to be high, it might be justified to use dexrazoxane in patients with cancer treated with anthracyclines. However, there is a theoretical risk of adverse effects with regard to efficacy of cancer therapy [74]. While neither ACEIs nor dexrazoxane has been used to correct or protect from RT-induced damage alone, it is not unreasonable to hypothesize a similar benefit for RT-induced heart toxicity pending adequate testing in the future.

Patients with Pacemakers and Implantable Cardioverter Defibrillators (ICDs)

It is very common to see and treat patients with implanted pacemakers and ICDs in the radiotherapy clinic. These implantable electronic devices typically have tolerances of 2–5 Gy depending on the manufacturer. Since the 1970s more sophisticated implantable devices have been manufactured, but the use of more radiosensitive metal-oxide semiconductors has decreased radiation tolerance. Tolerance also depends on type of radiotherapy, dose rate, and volume of device treated. Dose to device should always be calculated and devices should be removed or displaced out of the field if necessary [75, 76]. Removal should ideally be performed prior to formal radiotherapy planning to prevent treatment delay. In addition to potential dysfunction due to radiation damage, electric and magnetic fields generated by linear accelerators (LINACs) are another potential method of causing interference [76, 77].

In general, treatment of patients with pacemakers and ICDs is very safe. As long as the device is out of the direct radiation field and within factory described tolerance, multiple studies have shown that these patients can be treated safely without any documented device dysfunction suggesting scatter dose and electromagnetic fields are negligible [77, 78]. However, one prospective study showed that while treatment is safe, one patient with prostate cancer receiving IMRT had posttreatment device malfunction suggesting a small but potential risk even when the device is well out of the RT field [79]. Finally, it is unknown how radiotherapy affects the leads or site of lead implant in the heart. Despite the fact that complications and device malfunction are rare as long as appropriate precautions are taken, the device should be checked before, during (time interval is not standard and should be discussed with cardiology team), and after treatment as a precaution in pacer-dependent patients. In severe cardiac disease where patients are dependent on ICDs for continued survival, heart rate and blood pressure should be taken before and after each treatment with video-assisted EKG cardiac monitoring during treatment if necessary.

Key Points

- Cardiology consultation and follow-up for patients receiving thoracic RT are necessary. In patients with preexisting cardiac disease, close coordination prior to therapy is warranted with possible clearance needed from cardiologist prior to RT and chemoRT similar to presurgery evaluation.
- Serial cardiologic evaluation and possibly biomarker testing should be considered for all patients receiving thoracic RT [6].
- Early, presymptomatic treatment with ACEIs or ARBs can be considered in patients determined to be at high risk for RT-induced cardiac disease. Administration of concurrent cardioprotective agents, such as dexrazoxane, during treatment may be considered in high-risk patients pending additional evidence.
- Physicians should look for signs and symptoms of heart disease as well as instruct patients about specific signs of disease. Signs of disease include anginal pain, dyspnea, and diaphoresis for CAD; chest pain, dyspnea, cyanosis, peripheral edema, muffled heart sounds, venous distension, and pulsus paradoxus for pericarditis; dyspnea on exertion, peripheral edema, tachypnea, rales, hepatomegaly, syncope, and palpitations for cardiomyopathy with congestive heart failure (CHF); weakness, cough, dyspnea, new murmur, and pulsating liver for valvular disease; and palpitations and dyspnea for arrhythmias.
- Pericarditis
  - When constrictive pericarditis is secondary to irradiation or recurrent malignancy, open biopsy of the pericardium is advised.
  - Effusions are often asymptomatic, but if tamponade develops, pericardiocentesis is necessary.
- If chronic effusive-constrictive pericarditis develops, patients may require pericardiectomy.
- Medical therapy for heart disease such as CHF, arrhythmia, and CAD should be similar to patients without a history of RT to the chest.
  - Associated symptoms such as ascites and peripheral edema can be controlled with diuretics
- The treating radiation oncologist should counsel patients at the time of informed consent that thoracic radiation can contribute to cardiac risk. Patients should be made aware that while this risk factor cannot be modified after the radiation is given, modifying other preventable lifestyle risk factors is advisable. Primary care physicians should reinforce lifestyle changes to reduce cardiovascular

risk and consider aggressive blood pressure and glycemic control as well as aggressive lipid lowering.

- Surgical intervention for cardiovascular disease should be similar to patients without a history to RT with some caveats:
  - Coronary artery bypass graft surgery is a frequently used method of revascularization when percutaneous coronary intervention is not possible. With the young population of patients with cardiovascular disease secondary to RT, it has been proposed that arterial conduits would be superior to vein grafts. Unfortunately the internal thoracic arteries needed for a conduit can lie within the radiation field and may themselves be damaged or contain atherosclerosis. While coronary artery bypass and thoracic surgery is feasible in patients after chest irradiation, they may be at increased risk of surgical complications.
- Patients with pacemakers and ICDs can be treated safely, but a working relationship between radiation oncology and cardiology should be established early.
  - Device should be moved out of direct radiation field, prior to treatment planning if possible.
  - Device should be contoured and dose to device should always be calculated.
  - Device should be checked before, during, and after radiotherapy treatment.
- Despite the risk of cardiovascular disease clearly demonstrated historically, radiation remains a highly effective antineoplastic treatment. It should not be omitted from the care of patients solely based solely on concerns for cardiovascular risk.

References

1. Schellong G, Riepenhausen M, Bruch C, Kotthoff S, Vogt J, Bolling T, et al. Late valvular and other cardiac diseases after different doses of mediastinal radiotherapy for Hodgkin disease in children and adolescents: report from the longitudinal GPOH follow-up project of the German-Austrian DAL-HD studies. Pediatr Blood Cancer. 2010;55(6):1145–52.
2. Harris JR, Hellman S. Put the hockey stick on ice. Int J Radiat Oncol Biol Phys. 1988;15(2):497–9.
3. Cuzick J, Stewart H, Peto R, Baum M, Fisher B, Host H, et al. Overview of randomized trials of postoperative adjuvant radiotherapy in breast-cancer. Cancer Treat Rep. 1987;71(1):15–29.
4. Taylor CW, Nisbet A, McGale P, Goldman U, Darby SC, Hall P, et al. Cardiac doses from Swedish breast cancer radiotherapy since the 1950s. Radiother Oncol. 2009;90(1):127–35.
5. Evans SB, Sioshansi S, Moran MS, Hiatt J, Price LL, Wazer DE. Prevalence of poor cardiac anatomy in carcinoma of the breast treated with whole-breast radiotherapy: reconciling modern cardiac dosimetry with cardiac mortality data. Am J Clin Oncol. 2012; 35(6):587–92.
6. Vallebona A. Cardiac damage following therapeutic chest irradiation. Importance, evaluation and treatment. Minerva Cardioangiol. 2000;48(3):79–87.
7. Chiang CS, Hong JH, Stalder A, Sun JR, Withers HR, McBride WH. Delayed molecular responses to brain irradiation. Int J Radiat Biol. 1997;72(1):45–53.
8. Chiang CS, McBride WH, Withers HR. Radiation-induced astrocytic and microglial responses in mouse brain. Radiother Oncol. 1993;29(1):60–8.
9. Salloum E, Tanoue LT, Wackers FJ, Zelterman D, Hu GL, Cooper DL. Assessment of cardiac and pulmonary function in adult patients with Hodgkin's disease treated with ABVD or MOPP/ABVD plus adjuvant low-dose mediastinal irradiation. Cancer Invest. 1999;17(3):171–80.
10. Vallis KA, Pintilie M, Chong N, Holowaty E, Douglas PS, Kirkbride P, et al. Assessment of coronary heart disease morbidity and mortality after radiation therapy for early breast cancer. J Clin Oncol. 2002;20(4):1036–42.
11. Roychoudhuri R, Robinson D, Putcha V, Cuzick J, Darby S, Moller H. Increased cardiovascular mortality more than fifteen years after radiotherapy for breast cancer: a population-based study. BMC Cancer. 2007;7:9.
12. Orzan F, Brusca A, Conte MR, Presbitero P, Figliomeni MC. Severe coronary artery disease after radiation therapy of the chest and mediastinum: clinical presentation and treatment. Br Heart J. 1993;69(6):496–500.
13. Renner SM, Massel D, Moon BC. Mediastinal irradiation: a risk factor for atherosclerosis of the internal thoracic arteries. Can J Cardiol. 1999;15(5):597–600.
14. Clarke M, Collins R, Darby S, Davies C, Elphinstone P, Evans E, et al. Effects of radiotherapy and of differences in the extent of surgery for early breast cancer on local recurrence and 15-year survival: an overview of the randomised trials. Lancet. 2005;366(9503):2087–106.
15. Gyenes G, Rutqvist LE, Liedberg A, Fornander T. Long-term cardiac morbidity and mortality in a randomized trial of pre- and postoperative radiation therapy versus surgery alone in primary breast cancer. Radiother Oncol. 1998;48(2):185–90.
16. Veinot JP, Edwards WD. Pathology of radiation-induced heart disease: a surgical and autopsy study of 27 cases. Hum Pathol. 1996;27(8):766–73.
17. Fajardo LF, Stewart JR. Pathogenesis of radiation-induced myocardial fibrosis. Lab Invest. 1973;29(2):244–57.
18. Fajardo LF, Stewart JR. Experimental radiation-induced heart disease. I. Light microscopic studies. Am J Pathol. 1970;59(2):299–316.
19. Little MP, Tawn EJ, Tzoulaki I, Wakeford R, Hildebrandt G, Paris F, et al. Review and meta-analysis of epidemiological associations between low/moderate doses of ionizing radiation and circulatory disease risks, and their possible mechanisms. Radiat Environ Biophys. 2010;49(2):139–53.
20. Machann W, Beer M, Breunig M, Stork S, Angermann C, Seufert I, et al. Cardiac magnetic resonance imaging findings in 20-year survivors of mediastinal radiotherapy for Hodgkin's disease. Int J Radiat Oncol Biol Phys. 2011;79(4):1117–23.
21. Pletcher MJ, Tice JA, Pignone M. Use of coronary calcification scores to predict coronary heart disease. JAMA. 2004;291(15):1831–2.
22. Rademaker J, Schoder H, Ariaratnam NS, Strauss HW, Yahalom J, Steingart R, et al. Coronary artery disease after radiation therapy for Hodgkin's lymphoma: coronary CT angiography findings and calcium scores in nine asymptomatic patients. AJR Am J Roentgenol. 2008;191(1):32–7.

23. Leeuwen-Segarceanu EM, Bos WJ, Dorresteijn LD, Rensing BJ, der Heyden JA, Vogels OJ, et al. Screening Hodgkin lymphoma survivors for radiotherapy induced cardiovascular disease. Cancer Treat Rev. 2011;37(5):391–403.

24. Mast ME, Heijenbrok MW, Petoukhova AL, Scholten AN, Schreur JH, Struikmans H. Preradiotherapy calcium scores of the coronary arteries in a cohort of women with early-stage breast cancer: a comparison with a cohort of healthy women. Int J Radiat Oncol Biol Phys. 2012;83(3):853–8.

25. Ikaheimo MJ, Niemela KO, Linnaluoto MM, Jakobsson MJ, Takkunen JT, Taskinen PJ. Early cardiac changes related to radiation therapy. Am J Cardiol. 1985;56(15):943–6.

26. Stoodley PW, Richards DA, Meikle SR, Clarke J, Hui R, Thomas L. The potential role of echocardiographic strain imaging for evaluating cardiotoxicity due to cancer therapy. Heart Lung Circ. 2011; 20(1):3–9.

27. Erven K, Jurcut R, Weltens C, Giusca S, Ector J, Wildiers H, et al. Acute radiation effects on cardiac function detected by strain rate imaging in breast cancer patients. Int J Radiat Oncol Biol Phys. 2011;79(5):1444–51.

28. Dogan SM, Bilici HM, Bakkal H, Aydin M, Karabag T, Sayin MR, et al. The effect of radiotherapy on cardiac function. Coron Artery Dis. 2012;23:146–54.

29. Gayed IW, Liu HH, Wei X, Liao Z, Yusuf SW, Chang JY, et al. Patterns of cardiac perfusion abnormalities after chemoradiotherapy in patients with lung cancer. J Thorac Oncol. 2009;4(2):179–84.

30. Lind PA, Pagnanelli R, Marks LB, Borges-Neto S, Hu C, Zhou SM, et al. Myocardial perfusion changes in patients irradiated for left-sided breast cancer and correlation with coronary artery distribution. Int J Radiat Oncol Biol Phys. 2003;55(4):914–20.

31. Marks LB, Yu X, Prosnitz RG, Zhou SM, Hardenbergh PH, Blazing M, et al. The incidence and functional consequences of RT-associated cardiac perfusion defects. Int J Radiat Oncol Biol Phys. 2005;63(1):214–23.

32. Sawaya H, Sebag IA, Plana JC, Januzzi JL, Ky B, Cohen V, et al. Early detection and prediction of cardiotoxicity in chemotherapy-treated patients. Am J Cardiol. 2011;107(9):1375–80.

33. Cardinale D, Sandri MT, Colombo A, Colombo N, Boeri M, Lamantia G, et al. Prognostic value of troponin I in cardiac risk stratification of cancer patients undergoing high-dose chemotherapy. Circulation. 2004;109(22):2749–54.

34. Cardinale D, Sandri MT, Martinoni A, Borghini E, Civelli M, Lamantia G, et al. Myocardial injury revealed by plasma troponin I in breast cancer treated with high-dose chemotherapy. Ann Oncol. 2002;13(5):710–5.

35. Cardinale D, Sandri MT, Martinoni A, Tricca A, Civelli M, Lamantia G, et al. Left ventricular dysfunction predicted by early troponin I release after high-dose chemotherapy. J Am Coll Cardiol. 2000;36(2):517–22.

36. Cardinale D, Salvatici M, Sandri MT. Role of biomarkers in cardioncology. Clin Chem Lab Med. 2011;49(12):1937–48.

37. Hughes-Davies L, Sacks D, Rescigno J, Howard S, Harris J. Serum cardiac troponin T levels during treatment of early-stage breast cancer. J Clin Oncol. 1995;13(10):2582–4.

38. D'Errico MP, Grimaldi L, Petruzzelli MF, Gianicolo EA, Tramacere F, Monetti A, et al. N-terminal pro-B-type natriuretic peptide plasma levels as a potential biomarker for cardiac damage after radiotherapy in patients with left-sided breast cancer. Int J Radiat Oncol Biol Phys. 2012;82(2):e239–46.

39. Nellessen U, Zingel M, Hecker H, Bahnsen J, Borschke D. Effects of radiation therapy on myocardial cell integrity and pump function: which role for cardiac biomarkers? Chemotherapy. 2010;56(2):147–52.

40. Cardinale D, Cipolla CM. Assessment of cardiotoxicity with cardiac biomarkers in cancer patients. Herz. 2011;36(4):325–32.

41. Taylor CW, Nisbet A, McGale P, Darby SC. Cardiac exposures in breast cancer radiotherapy: 1950s-1990s. Int J Radiat Oncol Biol Phys. 2007;69(5):1484–95.

42. Giraud P, Cosset JM. Radiation toxicity to the heart: physiopathology and clinical data. Bull Cancer. 2004;91 Suppl 3:147–53.

43. McGale P, Darby SC, Hall P, Adolfsson J, Bengtsson NO, Bennet AM, et al. Incidence of heart disease in 35,000 women treated with radiotherapy for breast cancer in Denmark and Sweden. Radiother Oncol. 2011;100(2):167–75.

44. Correa CR, Das IJ, Litt HI, Ferrari V, Hwang WT, Solin LJ, et al. Association between tangential beam treatment parameters and cardiac abnormalities after definitive radiation treatment for left-sided breast cancer. Int J Radiat Oncol Biol Phys. 2008;72(2):508–16.

45. Nilsson G, Holmberg L, Garmo H, Duvernoy O, Sjogren I, Lagerqvist B, et al. Distribution of coronary artery stenosis after radiation for breast cancer. J Clin Oncol. 2012;30(4):380–6.

46. Fajardo LF, Eltringham JR, Steward JR. Combined cardiotoxicity of adriamycin and x-radiation. Lab Invest. 1976;34(1):86–96.

47. Eltringham JR, Fajardo LF, Stewart JR. Adriamycin cardiomyopathy: enhanced cardiac damage in rabbits with combined drug and cardiac irradiation. Radiology. 1975;115(2):471–2.

48. Aleman BM, van den Belt-Dusebout AW, de Bruin ML, 't Veer MB, Baaijens MH, de Boer JP, et al. Late cardiotoxicity after treatment for Hodgkin lymphoma. Blood. 2007;109(5):1878–86.

49. Swain SM, Whaley FS, Ewer MS. Congestive heart failure in patients treated with doxorubicin: a retrospective analysis of three trials. Cancer. 2003;97(11):2869–79.

50. Hortobagyi GN, Frye D, Buzdar AU, Ewer MS, Fraschini G, Hug V, et al. Decreased cardiac toxicity of doxorubicin administered by continuous intravenous infusion in combination chemotherapy for metastatic breast carcinoma. Cancer. 1989;63(1):37–45.

51. Hancock SL, Tucker MA, Hoppe RT. Factors affecting late mortality from heart disease after treatment of Hodgkin's disease. JAMA. 1993;270(16):1949–55.

52. Galper SL, Yu JB, Mauch PM, Strasser JF, Silver B, Lacasce A, et al. Clinically significant cardiac disease in patients with Hodgkin lymphoma treated with mediastinal irradiation. Blood. 2011;117(2):412–8.

53. van Dalen EC, Caron HN, Kremer LC. Prevention of anthracycline-induced cardiotoxicity in children: the evidence. Eur J Cancer. 2007;43(7):1134–40.

54. Tan-Chiu E, Yothers G, Romond E, Geyer Jr CE, Ewer M, Keefe D, et al. Assessment of cardiac dysfunction in a randomized trial comparing doxorubicin and cyclophosphamide followed by paclitaxel, with or without trastuzumab as adjuvant therapy in node-positive, human epidermal growth factor receptor 2-overexpressing breast cancer: NSABP B-31. J Clin Oncol. 2005;23(31):7811–9.

55. Slamon D, Eiermann W, Robert N, Pienkowski T, Martin M, Press M, et al. Adjuvant trastuzumab in HER2-positive breast cancer. N Engl J Med. 2011;365(14):1273–83.

56. Gandhi S, Verma S. Aromatase inhibitors and cardiac toxicity: getting to the heart of the matter. Breast Cancer Res Treat. 2007;106(1):1–9.

57. Bird BR, Swain SM. Cardiac toxicity in breast cancer survivors: review of potential cardiac problems. Clin Cancer Res. 2008;14(1):14–24.

58. Yeh ET, Tong AT, Lenihan DJ, Yusuf SW, Swafford J, Champion C, et al. Cardiovascular complications of cancer therapy: diagnosis, pathogenesis, and management. Circulation. 2004;109(25):3122–31.

59. Emami B, Lyman J, Brown A, Coia L, Goitein M, Munzenrider JE, et al. Tolerance of normal tissue to therapeutic irradiation. Int J Radiat Oncol Biol Phys. 1991;21(1):109–22.

60. Stewart JR, Fajardo LF, Gillette SM, Constine LS. Radiation injury to the heart. Int J Radiat Oncol Biol Phys. 1995;31(5):1205–11.

61. Carmel RJ, Kaplan HS. Mantle irradiation in Hodgkin's disease. An analysis of technique, tumor eradication, and complications. Cancer. 1976;37(6):2813–25.

62. Gagliardi G, Constine LS, Moiseenko V, Correa C, Pierce LJ, Allen AM, et al. Radiation dose-volume effects in the heart. Int J Radiat Oncol Biol Phys. 2010;76(3):S77–85.

63. Moser EC, Noordijk EM, van Leeuwen FE, le Cessie S, Baars JW, Thomas J, et al. Long-term risk of cardiovascular disease after treatment for aggressive non-Hodgkin lymphoma. Blood. 2006; 107(7):2912–9.

64. Girinsky T, Ghalibafian M. Radiotherapy of Hodgkin lymphoma: indications, new fields, and techniques. Semin Radiat Oncol. 2007;17(3):206–22.

65. Campbell BA, Voss N, Pickles T, Morris J, Gascoyne RD, Savage KJ, et al. Involved-nodal radiation therapy as a component of combination therapy for limited-stage Hodgkin's lymphoma: a question of field size. J Clin Oncol. 2008;26(32):5170–4.

66. Giordano SH, Kuo YF, Freeman JL, Buchholz TA, Hortobagyi GN, Goodwin JS. Risk of cardiac death after adjuvant radiotherapy for breast cancer. J Natl Cancer Inst. 2005;97(6):419–24.

67. Formenti SC, Gidea-Addeo D, Goldberg JD, Roses DF, Guth A, Rosenstein BS, et al. Phase I-II trial of prone accelerated intensity modulated radiation therapy to the breast to optimally spare normal tissue. J Clin Oncol. 2007;25(16):2236–42.

68. Smith W, Menon G, Wolfe N, Ploquin N, Trotter T, Pudney D. IMRT for the breast: a comparison of tangential planning techniques. Phys Med Biol. 2010;55(4):1231–41.

69. Cho BC, Hurkmans CW, Damen EM, Zijp LJ, Mijnheer BJ. Intensity modulated versus non-intensity modulated radiotherapy in the treatment of the left breast and upper internal mammary lymph node chain: a comparative planning study. Radiother Oncol. 2002;62(2):127–36.

70. Chen MH, Chuang ML, Bornstein BA, Gelman R, Harris JR, Manning WJ. Impact of respiratory maneuvers on cardiac volume within left-breast radiation portals. Circulation. 1997;96(10): 3269–72.

71. Yoon GJ, Telli ML, Kao DP, Matsuda KY, Carlson RW, Witteles RM. Left ventricular dysfunction in patients receiving cardiotoxic cancer therapies are clinicians responding optimally? J Am Coll Cardiol. 2010;56(20):1644–50.

72. Jensen BV, Skovsgaard T, Nielsen SL. Functional monitoring of anthracycline cardiotoxicity: a prospective, blinded, long-term observational study of outcome in 120 patients. Ann Oncol. 2002; 13(5):699–709.

73. Cardinale D, Colombo A, Sandri MT, Lamantia G, Colombo N, Civelli M, et al. Prevention of high-dose chemotherapy-induced cardiotoxicity in high-risk patients by angiotensin-converting enzyme inhibition. Circulation. 2006;114(23):2474–81.

74. van Dalen EC, Caron HN, Dickinson HO, Kremer LC. Cardioprotective interventions for cancer patients receiving anthracyclines. Cochrane Database Syst Rev. 2011;(6):CD003917.

75. Lambert P, Da Costa A, Marcy PY, Kreps S, Angellier G, Marcie S, et al. Pacemaker, implanted cardiac defibrillator and irradiation: management proposal in 2010 depending on the type of cardiac stimulator and prognosis and location of cancer. Cancer Radiother. 2011;15(3):238–49.

76. Hudson F, Coulshed D, D'Souza E, Baker C. Effect of radiation therapy on the latest generation of pacemakers and implantable cardioverter defibrillators: a systematic review. J Med Imaging Radiat Oncol. 2010;54(1):53–61.

77. Wadasadawala T, Pandey A, Agarwal JP, Jalali R, Laskar SG, Chowdhary S, et al. Radiation therapy with implanted cardiac pacemaker devices: a clinical and dosimetric analysis of patients and proposed precautions. Clin Oncol (R Coll Radiol). 2011;23(2):79–85.

78. Ferrara T, Baiotto B, Malinverni G, Caria N, Garibaldi E, Barboni G, et al. Irradiation of pacemakers and cardio-defibrillators in patients submitted to radiotherapy: a clinical experience. Tumori. 2010; 96(1):76–83.

79. Soejima T, Yoden E, NIshimura Y, Ono S, Yoshida A, Fukuda H, et al. Radiation therapy in patients with implanted cardiac pacemakers and implantable cardioverter defibrillators: a prospective survey in Japan. J Radiat Res. 2011;52(4):516–21.

Part IV

Cardiac Diseases in Patients with Concurrent Pregnancy

Normal Cardiovascular Adaptation to Pregnancy

29

Jérôme Cornette and Jolien W. Roos-Hesselink

Abstract

Normal pregnancy is characterized by profound hemodynamic changes. These begin early in pregnancy and include a fall in vascular resistance which induces an increase in blood volume and stroke volume. Heart rate and cardiac output also rise. Arterial blood pressure is reduced. The adaptation is most prominent in the first half of pregnancy. To cope with these hemodynamic challenges, the left ventricle hypertrophies, thereby preserving systolic and diastolic function. Peripheral arterial resistance is decreased and compliance and distensibility are increased. Venous capacitance is greatly enhanced.

Uteroplacental blood flow augments with gestation to meet the increased needs of a growing fetus. Maternal cerebral blood flow is reduced. The influence of these major macrovascular changes on microvascular perfusion remains to be elucidated. During labor and delivery, cardiac output further rises. Postpartum, most hemodynamic parameters are rapidly reversed within weeks. Structural changes normalize within several months.

Keywords

Pregnancy • Hemodynamic • Heart • Cardiac output • Ultrasound • Microcirculation

Introduction

Normal pregnancy is a unique physiological state. It imposes a profound challenge to the cardiovascular system in a relatively short period of time. These changes are necessary to meet the increased demands of a rapidly growing feto-placental unit. Fortunately, most young women have sufficient cardiovascular reserve. However, failure to achieve these adaptations is associated with maternal and fetal complications like hypertensive disorders and fetal growth restriction [1–6]. In women with preexisting heart disease, the work and volume load can cause deterioration in cardiac function [7–9].

J. Cornette, MD (✉)
Department of Obstetrics and Gynaecology, Erasmus MC,
Dr. Molewaterplein 60, Rotterdam 3015, The Netherlands
e-mail: j.cornette@erasmusmc.nl

J.W. Roos-Hesselink, MD, PhD
Department of Cardiology, Thoraxcenter, Erasmus MC,
Postbus 2040, Rotterdam 3062HK, The Netherlands
e-mail: j.roos@erasmusmc.nl

The cardiovascular system can be viewed as a closed circuit. The heart is the central core organ directing flow between the venous and arterial systems. Exchange of oxygen, carbon dioxide, and nutrients, the final goal of the circulation, takes place on a microcirculatory level in the capillaries. While central hemodynamics have been mostly studied due to the prominence and accessibility of the heart and large artery systems, knowledge about the venous compartment, local organ perfusion systems, and the microcirculation are equally essential for a complete understanding of the normal physiology of pregnancy. In this chapter we will discuss normal adaptation to pregnancy of the various components of the cardiovascular system.

Methods of Cardiovascular Monitoring

Hemodynamic monitoring is of clinical importance in the management of women with cardiovascular disease or severe hemodynamic complications like preeclampsia [10–13].

K. Stergiopoulos, D.L. Brown (eds.), *Evidence-Based Cardiology Consult*,
DOI 10.1007/978-1-4471-4441-0_29, © Springer-Verlag London 2014

Secondly, it can be of scientific interest in both healthy pregnant women and various other pregnancy complications [14, 15]. The ideal tool would be noninvasive, cheap, reliable, and easy to use at the bedside and offer a broad range of information. While different methods exist, experience and validation during pregnancy remain questionable for most of them [16, 17].

The pulmonary artery catheter (PAC) was often used in the 1980s and 1990s for the management of severe preeclampsia [10–13, 18–26]. As it measures both cardiac output and filling pressures, it contributed to the pathophysiological knowledge of the condition [10, 12, 23, 26]. Its invasive nature along with controversy about clinical benefit has abated the enthusiasm for this method such that it is now rarely used in pregnant women [27, 28]. However, it remains the gold standard for hemodynamic monitoring. Ideally, alternative methods should be validated in pregnancy against PAC [16].

Experience with pulse contour analysis in pregnancy (PiCCO®, LIDCO™ plus, FloTrac™/Vigileo™) is limited [14, 29, 30].

Thoracic bioimpedance has mainly been used for longitudinal hemodynamic cardiac output measurements in research settings [31–35]. While the method is simple, safe, and easy to use, there are some serious concerns about its accuracy, reliability, and validation [16, 36]. Thoracic bioreactance has been developed to overcome the limitations of impedance cardiography. It is based on changes in frequency rather than amplitude and therefore less susceptible to interference. Bioreactance holds promise but has not been validated and is rarely used in pregnancy [16, 17, 37]. Esophageal Doppler output measurements in pregnancy have shown poor agreements with thermodilution, and the method is not well tolerated by all women [38].

Transthoracic echocardiography has become a preferential method for the hemodynamic assessment of both ill and healthy pregnant women [39]. Its noninvasive nature allows bedside measurements, including structural and functional information. Most advanced obstetric ultrasound devices can be equipped with supplemental cardiac modules. As such, the method is accessible and can relatively easily be learned by caregivers with prior ultrasound experience. The Doppler method for cardiac output measurements has been validated in pregnancy against both thermodilution and Fick's method [40–46]. Additionally, ultrasound permits the investigation of peripheral arterial systems by the assessment of resistance and pulsatility indexes.

Finally cardiac MRI can be used in pregnancy [47]. Although expensive, it offers accurate structural and hemodynamic information and can be of great benefit in women with structural heart disease with suboptimal ultrasound image resolution [48]. While experience in pregnancy is limited, the technique is considered safe after the first trimester. Gadolinium contrast is best avoided [49].

Central Hemodynamics

Initiating Mechanisms

Cardiovascular adaptation starts very early in pregnancy. A primary fall in systemic and renal vascular tone induces an increase in the renal blood flow and glomerular filtration resulting in plasma volume expansion [50–54]. This is accompanied by a further reduction in systemic vascular resistance (SVR) and arterial pressure as well as an increase in stroke volume (SV) and cardiac output (CO) [39, 51, 55–60].

A substantial part of the adaptation occurs before the placenta becomes functional at around 8–12 weeks. In fact, similar changes as in early pregnancy have been observed in the luteal phase of the menstrual cycle [61]. It means that adaptation to pregnancy starts soon after ovulation and is probably triggered by substances produced by the corpus luteum. The exact mechanisms that initiate and sustain the primary fall in vascular resistance and subsequent hemodynamic adaptations remain to be elucidated. Reduced responsiveness to vasopressors such as angiotensin 2, thromboxane, and norepinephrine and increased sensitivity and production of vasodilators like prostacyclin and nitric oxide have been well described [62–65]. There are some indications that relaxin, a hormone structurally related to insulin, might be a key factor in initiating and sustaining the changes in pregnancy [63]. It is produced by the corpus luteum and, later, by the placenta and decidua and acts as a potent vasodilator through various nitric oxide pathways.

As mentioned before, the primary trigger is a fall in arterial and venous tone [50, 52, 66]. This leads to a rise in CO, a decrease in SVR, and reduction in mean arterial pressure [39, 50, 60, 67]. These changes are most prominent during the first trimester and reach a maximum in the second trimester when, remarkably, the nutritive requirements of the feto-placental unit still remain relatively small (Fig. 29.1).

Blood Volume

The expansion of blood volume is triggered by the state of vascular underfilling and the increased renal perfusion [50, 52–54, 68]. It rises gradually until 28–34 weeks and then plateaus until delivery [51]. The increase in plasma volume is more important as compared to the increase in red cell volume leading to a physiologic hemodilution [58, 69]. The total blood volume increases 50 % above nonpregnant values. Along with the drop in SVR, it allows high-flow low-resistance perfusion in order to meet the increased oxygen demands of the feto-placental unit and several maternal organs including the kidneys, skin, and heart [70]. Secondly, it forms a protective reserve for maternal blood loss around parturition.

Fig. 29.1 Hemodynamic changes in pregnancy, during labor, and postpartum. *CO* cardiac output, *SVR* systemic vascular resistance, *MAP* mean arterial pressure, *pp* postpartum

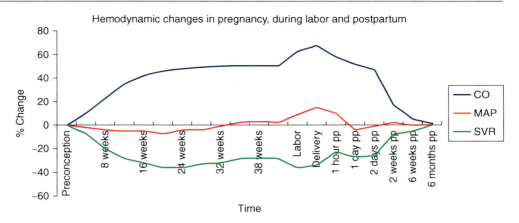

Vascular Resistance

Vascular resistance initially drops in the first and second trimester by 30–50 %, reaching its nadir by the end of the second trimester [39, 58–60, 67]. It then remains stable until the end of the third trimester to slightly rise again towards term. Plasma renin is increased and atrial natriuretic peptide (ANP) levels are reduced, indicating that volume expansion is proportional and in reaction to the vasodilatation and increased vascular capacitance [66, 68].

Cardiac Output, Stroke Volume, and Heart Rate

The increase in CO of 30–50 % mirrors the reduction in SVR. It is initiated by a rise in heart rate (HR) and subsequently accompanied by an increase in SV as soon as plasma volume expansion occurs [39, 50–53, 67]. After a rapid climb in the first half of pregnancy, it reaches a plateau in the second trimester after which it remains constant until the end of pregnancy [35, 39, 56, 60, 67, 71–73]. Towards term there is a slight reduction in SV which is probably compensated by an elevation in HR [39, 60, 67, 71, 72]. Some studies indicate a slight reduction in CO towards term due to this fall in SV [56, 74, 75]. This discrepancy probably reflects the large interpersonal variation between subjects and the limitations of the methods used to determine CO [39, 73]. The factors contributing to an elevation in SV during pregnancy are the increasing preload due to a rising blood volume and a reduction in afterload due to the decline in SVR.

More important than the slight variations between studies is the effect of maternal position on CO. As from 20 weeks gestation, supine position directly reduces maternal CO through aortocaval compression by the gravid uterus, thereby reducing preload and increasing afterload [47, 76]. Therefore, output should be measured in a left lateral position from as soon as 20 weeks gestation. Also in case of fetal or maternal distress, left lateral tilt is critical in enhancing output in the second half of pregnancy [77].

Blood Pressure

Both systolic and diastolic pressure fall early in gestation as a result of the reduction in SVR, reaching a nadir in the second trimester of 5–10 mmHg below values prior to pregnancy [67, 78–80]. In the third trimester, blood pressure gradually returns towards nonpregnant values.

Systemic Pressures

Central venous pressure remains within the normal nonpregnant range. The increased right ventricular preload, associated with volume expansion, is compensated for by afterload reduction through a decrease in pulmonary vascular resistance [18, 21, 52]. Left ventricular filling pressures (invasively reflected by pulmonary capillary wedge pressure) and pulmonary artery pressures, whether measured invasively or noninvasively, remain within normal nonpregnant ranges [21, 67].

Cardiac Adaptation

Left Ventricular Systolic Function and Mass

Assessment of left ventricular systolic function during pregnancy is mostly performed by ultrasound. It is complicated by the inherent limitations of the ultrasound technique as well as by the major fluctuation in loading conditions during pregnancy. As such, most standard indices are relatively indirect and only partly reflect different aspects of ventricular function. A good and complete denominator of global systolic function independent of loading conditions is still lacking. Newer techniques like tissue Doppler, strain analysis and speckle tracking are promising, as they offer additional information on left ventricular function.

Ejection fraction (EF) and fractional shortening (FS) are the most classic indices of left ventricular systolic function. They primarily reflect the function of the circumferential fibers of the myocardium. Both EF and FS probably slightly increase early in pregnancy, then remain constant until 30 weeks and subsequently slightly decrease towards term [25, 39, 56, 60, 67, 81]. The increase early in pregnancy suggests increased myocardial contractility. Still, there is discrepancy between several studies concerning the changes in EF and FS [72, 82]. It is probably due to the fact that the left ventricular volumes, used to calculate these parameters, are most often derived from the Teichholz formula, which is based on geometrical assumptions that are probably not met during pregnancy. While the Simpson methods of discs summation as well as 3D echocardiography are probably more accurate, they can be hampered by decreased echogenicity due to the cardiac axis displacement as well as engorgement of breast tissue during pregnancy.

Assessment of myocardial contractility using the less load-dependent ventricular end-systolic stress (ESS) and mean velocity of circumferential fiber thickening (Vcfc) relationship also offers conflicting results, although it seems that myocardial contractility is at least continuously preserved during pregnancy [67, 81, 83–85].

Analysis of left ventricular long axis function offers information on subendocardial longitudinally arranged fibers which are more prone to reflect subtle myocardial impairment. Apical M-mode measurements through the mitral annulus show an increase in left ventricular long axis displacement with gestation until 23 weeks with a subsequent decrease reaching values below preconceptional readings towards term [56]. Long axis shortening decreases significantly with gestation [71, 86]. Tissue Doppler of the mitral annulus, which is less load dependent, does not show any changes in S' velocity during pregnancy[71]. These findings also suggest that contractility and systolic function are preserved throughout pregnancy and might even be slightly enhanced in the first half of pregnancy.

The recent introduction of strain, strain rate analysis, as well as speckle tracking permits investigation of myocardial deformation and left ventricular twist (torsion) and untwist. A higher deformation rate in the first trimester suggests a state of increased contractility in response to the hemodynamic changes of early pregnancy [72]. In the third trimester, a small but significant reduction in longitudinal deformation and deformation rate is observed, without changes in circumferential and radial strain [72]. This reduction in longitudinal strain occurs despite an increase in global ventricular performance, reflected by left ventricular stroke work, suggesting that strain and strain rate are also influenced by loading conditions and chamber geometry. As such, they cannot be used as a surrogate for global myocardial function, but they are more sensitive than other conventional parameters in reflecting subtle changes in ventricular function.

Speckle tracking analysis shows that pregnancy is accompanied by an increase in left ventricular twist and twist velocity due to increased apical rotation without changes in untwist and untwist velocity [87, 88].

Structurally, pregnancy is characterized by a proportional increase of both chamber size and wall dimensions. This leads to an eccentric hypertrophy which is characteristic of volume loading conditions [5, 72]. Left atrial and ventricular diameters augment with increasing gestational age, reaching peaks at around 34 weeks [52, 57, 60, 67, 72, 89]. By term, left ventricular mass exceeds nonpregnant values by 50 % [57, 60, 67, 72]. This physiologic and reversible hypertrophy is similar to the one observed in endurance athletes. It is a compensatory mechanism, reducing wall stress by increasing wall thickness. As such, the necessary stroke volume can be achieved despite increases in both preload and afterload and reduced diastolic filling time [57].

In conclusion myocardial performance is increased during pregnancy. However, this is not uniformly reflected in all different markers of systolic function. This is probably related to the complex interaction between changes in left ventricular geometry, loading conditions, and limitations of the investigational methods. Globally one can conclude that myocardial function is preserved or slightly increased in normal healthy pregnancy, and the changes in left ventricular morphology and structure can be regarded as a physiological adaptation to the changes in loading conditions in order to preserve myocardial function.

Diastolic Function

As with left ventricular systolic function, the assessment of diastolic function is greatly influenced by the alterations in loading conditions during pregnancy. Pulsed wave Doppler analysis of the mitral valve shows an initial increase in E-wave (E) and A-wave (A) velocities as compared to pre-pregnancy values [57]. While early filling slightly diminishes with gestational age, the atrial contribution to ventricular filling increases leading to an increased A and decreased E/A ratio towards term [71, 90]. Doppler of the pulmonary venous flow shows a transient peak in systolic forward flow velocity in the second trimester, a gradual slight decrease in pulmonary venous diastolic velocity, and increase in pulmonary venous reversed flow at atrial contraction along with gestation [90]. With increasing myocardial hypertrophy, ventricular compliance and hence E-wave velocity diminishes, which partly explains this pattern of impaired relaxation. Nevertheless, the observed changes in pulsed wave Doppler of the mitral annulus mostly remain a reflection of changing loading conditions during pregnancy.

Load-independent tissue Doppler of the mitral annulus better demonstrate changes in diastolic function during pregnancy. There are no significant changes in either septal or lateral peak E' and A' velocities during normal gestation

[71, 86]. However, E/E′ ratio reaches the upper end of normality with a broadening of the range in the late third trimester, possibly reflecting a marginal increase in left ventricular filling pressure [71]. A slight increase in A′ with subsequent decrease in E′/A′ ratio is consistent with enhanced left atrial contraction [71]. The Tei index, which is a global measure for both left ventricular systolic and diastolic function, is characterized by a broader range during pregnancy compared to nonpregnant controls [71]. The absence of changes in untwist parameters using speckle tracking echocardiography further suggests normal diastolic function during pregnancy despite the volume overload [88].

In conclusion normal pregnancy is associated with normal diastolic function. Analysis of diastolic function best includes load-independent methods like tissue Doppler or speckle tracking in order to differentiate changing loading conditions from real diastolic dysfunction.

Labor and Delivery

During labor and delivery, maternal hemodynamics are influenced by several factors like anxiety, analgesia, uterine contractions, Valsalva maneuver, blood loss, and maternal position. An increase in SV and CO is observed from the beginning of the first stage of labor which further augments as dilation progresses [91–93]. During each contraction, 300–500 ml of blood from the uterine sinusoids is forced again in the systemic circulation thereby increasing preload [94]. Maternal discomfort and exertion can further increase the HR thereby augmenting CO 50 % above pre-labor values. Arterial pressure also increases during each contraction by about 15–20 mmHg (see Fig. 29.1). The changes can be more prominent in recumbent as compared to left lateral position due to caval compression as well as to occlusion of the distal aorta during contraction with redistribution of the stroke volume in the upper half of the body [58, 95]. It is evident that the abrupt onset and magnitude of these changes can pose a serious challenge to patients with cardiovascular disease.

Epidural analgesia also influences the hemodynamic changes during labor. Pain and anxiety are often reduced and both the fluid challenge and reactive vasodilatation can also influence loading conditions [96]. In controlled circumstances, the severe hemodynamic changes due to labor are often attenuated by epidural anesthesia.

Postpartum

The gradual hemodynamic adaptation to pregnancy is rapidly reversed after delivery.

Immediately postpartum, CO and SV are still elevated compared to pre-labor values [58, 91–93]. The massive auto-transfusion from the uterine blood volume and relief of caval obstruction compensate for postpartum blood loss [97]. Both SV and CO remain elevated for the first 24 h after which they gradually decline. The reduction is most prominent within the first 2 weeks postpartum but can continue until 6 months postpartum before reaching prepregnancy values [78, 97–99] (see Fig. 29.1).

Heart rate falls rapidly after delivery. Mean arterial pressure initially drops immediately postpartum but returns to pre-labor levels on the second day postpartum. It then gradually declines over the following 2 weeks [97]. Left atrial dimensions normalize within the first 2 weeks, reflecting the rapid normalization of blood volume in the puerperium [100].

While most cardiac adaptations progressively return to normal values within 6 months after delivery, some minor structural changes can remain longer or even become permanent [39, 55, 67, 78, 101, 102]. In subsequent pregnancies, hemodynamic adaptation is often more prompt and pronounced. The latter suggests that pregnancy induces some form of cardiovascular imprinting which is protective in further pregnancies and possibly later life.

Peripheral Systems

Arterial System

Changes in the systemic arterial circulation in normal pregnancy are characterized by a decreased peripheral resistance and increased arterial compliance and distensibility [103, 104]. The latter is mainly achieved by a reduction in smooth muscle tone, although there are some indications that some degree of structural vessel wall remodeling during pregnancy could also play a role.

Aortic valve cross-sectional area slightly increases between the first and third trimester [67, 83, 103]. Therefore, left ventricular outflow tract diameter should always be determined simultaneously with the velocity time integral, when assessing stroke volume by ultrasound at different gestational ages.

Global arterial compliance increases in the first trimester and remains elevated thereafter. The magnitude of peripheral wave reflection at the aorta is reduced [104, 105]. Noninvasive assessment of arterial stiffness by applanation tonometry, using pulse wave analysis and velocity, showed a transient decrease in augmentation index, with a nadir by the end of the second trimester. The reduction in central aortic blood pressure is more pronounced than the decline in peripheral blood pressure [105, 106].

Venous Hemodynamics

While the scientific interest in venous (patho) physiology is certainly less than their arterial and cardiac counterparts, the venous compartment nevertheless is important as it serves as a large volume reservoir storing approximately two thirds of total blood volume. In a state of extensive vascular expansion, it becomes even more prominent as it greatly contributes to the regulation of cardiac output. The splanchnic veins in particular serve as a major storage pool where much of the unstressed blood volume can remain and be mobilized when necessary [107]. In pregnancy, venous distensibility and capacitance are greatly increased. They return to prepregnancy values within 3 months postpartum [107–109]. Investigation of the venous hemodynamics can be performed noninvasively using Doppler ultrasound which also has a role in pathophysiological research of complicated hemodynamic syndromes such as preeclampsia [110].

Regional Blood Flows

Uterine Blood Flow

With increasing demands of nutrition and oxygen from the rapidly growing products of conception, several adaptations take place in the uterine circulation. From early gestation, uterine artery diameter progressively increases, while pulsatility and resistance indices decrease [31, 111–117]. Uterine blood flow increases from 50 ml/min in the first trimester to 500–750 ml/min at term [114, 116, 117]. The increase in uterine blood flow is not only in absolute terms but also in proportion to the total cardiac output [118].

The trophoblast invasion with arterial remodeling of spiral arteries allows appropriate uteroplacental exchange but also contributes to the reduction of arterial resistance [116].

Renal Blood Flow

It is very clear that renal hemodynamics play a major role in normal adaptation to pregnancy [54, 115]. Renal blood flow increases during pregnancy. While the results are less conclusive, renal artery resistance index probably rises during pregnancy, reaching a peak by the end of the second trimester and then slowly returning to normal values postpartum.

Cerebral Blood Flow

The cerebral circulation can be analyzed by noninvasive transcranial Doppler and MRI. Both Doppler technique and MRI technique show a decrease in middle cerebral artery velocity as well as a 20 % reduction in total cerebral blood flow at term [119–121].

The Microcirculation

The microcirculation is the site of exchange of oxygen and nutrients [122]. The importance of microcirculatory dysfunction, independent from macrocirculatory changes, is emerging in several pathological conditions such as sepsis and shock [123–125]. Research on microvascular parameters has mainly been hampered by technical difficulties. The gold standard, intravital microscopy, remains difficult outside the laboratory setting. Capillaroscopy, plethysmography, and laser Doppler have been used in pregnancy but are each hampered by several limitations [126–130]. More recent technical innovations like Orthogonal Polarization Spectral (OPS) imaging and Sidestream Dark Field (SDF) imaging are promising [131, 132]. They allow a combination of microvascular vessel density and flow velocity measurements at the bedside.

Thus far, microvascular research in pregnancy remains limited and mostly focused on pathological conditions like preeclampsia. Information on normal pregnancy is scarce and is mainly derived from healthy pregnant control groups. As such, it offers little information regarding the longitudinal adaptation to normal pregnancy. Anim-Nyame et al. showed a reduction in isovolumetric venous pressure as compared to nonpregnant controls [126]. Hassan et al. showed increased skin capillary density in pregnancy, reaching a peak by the end of the second trimester with subsequent gradual reduction to nonpregnant values 6 weeks postpartum [127].

Key Points

- Normal pregnancy is characterized by profound hemodynamic changes.
- A marked decline in systemic vascular resistance occurs early in pregnancy.
- Cardiac output rises dramatically, especially in the first half of pregnancy.
- To cope with these hemodynamic challenges, the left ventricle hypertrophies, thereby preserving systolic and diastolic function.
- During labor and delivery, cardiac output further rises. Postpartum, most hemodynamic parameters are rapidly reversed within weeks.
- Structural changes normalize within several months.

References

1. Bamfo JE, Kametas NA, Chambers JB, Nicolaides KH. Maternal cardiac function in normotensive and pre-eclamptic intrauterine growth restriction. Ultrasound Obstet Gynecol. 2008; 32:682–6.

2. Bosio PM, McKenna PJ, Conroy R, O'Herlihy C. Maternal central hemodynamics in hypertensive disorders of pregnancy. Obstet Gynecol. 1999;94:978–84.
3. De Paco C, Kametas N, Rencoret G, Strobl I, Nicolaides KH. Maternal cardiac output between 11 and 13 weeks of gestation in the prediction of preeclampsia and small for gestational age. Obstet Gynecol. 2008;111:292–300.
4. Duvekot JJ, Cheriex EC, Pieters FA, Menheere PP, Schouten HJ, Peeters LL. Maternal volume homeostasis in early pregnancy in relation to fetal growth restriction. Obstet Gynecol. 1995; 85:361–7.
5. Melchiorre K, Thilaganathan B. Maternal cardiac function in preeclampsia. Curr Opin Obstet Gynecol. 2011;23:440–7.
6. Vasapollo B, Valensise H, Novelli GP, Altomare F, Galante A, Arduini D. Abnormal maternal cardiac function precedes the clinical manifestation of fetal growth restriction. Ultrasound Obstet Gynecol. 2004;24:23–9.
7. Abbas AE, Lester SJ, Connolly H. Pregnancy and the cardiovascular system. Int J Cardiol. 2005;98:179–89.
8. Roos-Hesselink JW, Duvekot JJ, Thorne SA. Pregnancy in high risk cardiac conditions. Heart. 2009;95:680–6.
9. Siu SC, Colman JM, Sorensen S, Smallhorn JF, Farine D, Amankwah KS, et al. Adverse neonatal and cardiac outcomes are more common in pregnant women with cardiac disease. Circulation. 2002;105:2179–84.
10. Bolte AC, Dekker GA, van Eyck J, van Schijndel RS, van Geijn HP. Lack of agreement between central venous pressure and pulmonary capillary wedge pressure in preeclampsia. Hypertens Pregnancy. 2000;19:261–71.
11. Clark SL, Greenspoon JS, Aldahl D, Phelan JP. Severe preeclampsia with persistent oliguria: management of hemodynamic subsets. Am J Obstet Gynecol. 1986;154:490–4.
12. Cotton DB, Gonik B, Dorman K, Harrist R. Cardiovascular alterations in severe pregnancy-induced hypertension: relationship of central venous pressure to pulmonary capillary wedge pressure. Am J Obstet Gynecol. 1985;151:762–4.
13. Visser W, Wallenburg HC. Maternal and perinatal outcome of temporizing management in 254 consecutive patients with severe preeclampsia remote from term. Eur J Obstet Gynecol Reprod Biol. 1995;63:147–54.
14. Carlin A, Alfirevic Z. Physiological changes of pregnancy and monitoring. Best Pract Res Clin Obstet Gynaecol. 2008;22:801–23.
15. Cornette J, Duvekot J, Roos-Hesselink J, Hop W, Steegers E. Maternal and fetal haemodynamic effects of nifedipine in normotensive pregnant women. BJOG. 2010. doi:10.1111/j.1471-0528.2010.02794.x.
16. Lee AJ, Cohn JH, Ranasinghe JS. Cardiac output assessed by invasive and minimally invasive techniques. Anesthesiol Res Pract. 2011;2011:475151.
17. Mohammed I, Phillips C. Techniques for determining cardiac output in the intensive care unit. Crit Care Clin. 2010;26:355–64, table of contents.
18. Invasive hemodynamic monitoring in obstetrics and gynecology. ACOG technical bulletin number 175 – December 1992. Int J Gynaecol Obstet. 1993;42:199–205.
19. Wallenburg HC. Invasive hemodynamic monitoring in pregnancy. Eur J Obstet Gynecol Reprod Biol. 1991;42(Suppl):S45–51.
20. Clark SL, Cotton DB. Clinical indications for pulmonary artery catheterization in the patient with severe preeclampsia. Am J Obstet Gynecol. 1988;158:453–8.
21. Clark SL, Cotton DB, Lee W, Bishop C, Hill T, Southwick J, et al. Central hemodynamic assessment of normal term pregnancy. Am J Obstet Gynecol. 1989;161:1439–42.
22. Clark SL, Horenstein JM, Phelan JP, Montag TW, Paul RH. Experience with the pulmonary artery catheter in obstetrics and gynecology. Am J Obstet Gynecol. 1985;152:374–8.
23. Cotton DB, Lee W, Huhta JC, Dorman KF. Hemodynamic profile of severe pregnancy-induced hypertension. Am J Obstet Gynecol. 1988;158:523–9.
24. Gilbert WM, Towner DR, Field NT, Anthony J. The safety and utility of pulmonary artery catheterization in severe preeclampsia and eclampsia. Am J Obstet Gynecol. 2000;182:1397–403.
25. Mabie WC, DiSessa TG, Crocker LG, Sibai BM, Arheart KL. A longitudinal study of cardiac output in normal human pregnancy. Am J Obstet Gynecol. 1994;170:849–56.
26. Mabie WC, Ratts TE, Sibai BM. The central hemodynamics of severe preeclampsia. Am J Obstet Gynecol. 1989;161:1443–8.
27. Shure D. Pulmonary-artery catheters – peace at last? N Engl J Med. 2006;354:2273–4.
28. Vernon C, Phillips CR. Pulmonary artery catheters in acute heart failure: end of an era? Crit Care. 2009;13:1003.
29. Armstrong S, Fernando R, Columb M. Minimally- and non-invasive assessment of maternal cardiac output: go with the flow! Int J Obstet Anesth. 2011;20:330–40.
30. Bliacheriene F, Carmona MJ, Barretti Cde F, Haddad CM, Mouchalwat ES, Bortolotto MR, et al. Use of a minimally invasive uncalibrated cardiac output monitor in patients undergoing cesarean section under spinal anesthesia: report of four cases. Rev Bras Anestesiol. 2011;61:610–8, 334–8.
31. Heethaar RM, van Oppen AC, Ottenhoff FA, Brouwer FA, Bruinse HW. Thoracic electrical bioimpedance: suitable for monitoring stroke volume during pregnancy? Eur J Obstet Gynecol Reprod Biol. 1995;58:183–90.
32. Masaki DI, Greenspoon JS, Ouzounian JG. Measurement of cardiac output in pregnancy by thoracic electrical bioimpedance and thermodilution. A preliminary report. Am J Obstet Gynecol. 1989;161:680–4.
33. San-Frutos L, Engels V, Zapardiel I, Perez-Medina T, Almagro-Martinez J, Fernandez R, et al. Hemodynamic changes during pregnancy and postpartum: a prospective study using thoracic electrical bioimpedance. J Matern Fetal Neonatal Med. 2011;24:1333–40.
34. Scardo JA, Ellings J, Vermillion ST, Chauhan SP. Validation of bioimpedance estimates of cardiac output in preeclampsia. Am J Obstet Gynecol. 2000;183:911–3.
35. van Oppen AC, van der Tweel I, Alsbach GP, Heethaar RM, Bruinse HW. A longitudinal study of maternal hemodynamics during normal pregnancy. Obstet Gynecol. 1996;88:40–6.
36. Easterling TR, Benedetti TJ, Carlson KL, Watts DH. Measurement of cardiac output in pregnancy by thermodilution and impedance techniques. Br J Obstet Gynaecol. 1989;96:67–9.
37. Keren H, Burkhoff D, Squara P. Evaluation of a noninvasive continuous cardiac output monitoring system based on thoracic bioreactance. Am J Physiol Heart Circ Physiol. 2007;293:H583–9.
38. Penny JA, Anthony J, Shennan AH, De Swiet M, Singer M. A comparison of hemodynamic data derived by pulmonary artery flotation catheter and the esophageal Doppler monitor in preeclampsia. Am J Obstet Gynecol. 2000;183:658–61.
39. Duvekot JJ, Peeters LL. Maternal cardiovascular hemodynamic adaptation to pregnancy. Obstet Gynecol Surv. 1994;49:S1–14.
40. Belfort MA, Mares A, Saade G, Wen T, Rokey R. Two-dimensional echocardiography and Doppler ultrasound in managing obstetric patients. Obstet Gynecol. 1997;90:326–30.
41. Easterling TR, Carlson KL, Schmucker BC, Brateng DA, Benedetti TJ. Measurement of cardiac output in pregnancy by Doppler technique. Am J Perinatol. 1990;7:220–2.
42. Easterling TR, Watts DH, Schmucker BC, Benedetti TJ. Measurement of cardiac output during pregnancy: validation of Doppler technique and clinical observations in preeclampsia. Obstet Gynecol. 1987;69:845–50.
43. Lee W, Rokey R, Cotton DB. Noninvasive maternal stroke volume and cardiac output determinations by pulsed Doppler echocardiography. Am J Obstet Gynecol. 1988;158:505–10.

44. Robson SC, Boys RJ, Hunter S. Doppler echocardiographic estimation of cardiac output: analysis of temporal variability. Eur Heart J. 1988;9:313–8.

45. Robson SC, Dunlop W, Moore M, Hunter S. Combined Doppler and echocardiographic measurement of cardiac output: theory and application in pregnancy. Br J Obstet Gynaecol. 1987;94:1014–27.

46. Robson SC, Murray A, Peart I, Heads A, Hunter S. Reproducibility of cardiac output measurement by cross sectional and Doppler echocardiography. Br Heart J. 1988;59:680–4.

47. Rossi A, Cornette J, Johnson MR, Karamermer Y, Springeling T, Opic P, et al. Quantitative cardiovascular magnetic resonance in pregnant women: cross-sectional analysis of physiological parameters throughout pregnancy and the impact of the supine position. J Cardiovasc Magn Reson. 2011;13:31.

48. Kilner PJ, Geva T, Kaemmerer H, Trindade PT, Schwitter J, Webb GD. Recommendations for cardiovascular magnetic resonance in adults with congenital heart disease from the respective working groups of the European Society of Cardiology. Eur Heart J. 2010;31:794–805.

49. Chen MM, Coakley FV, Kaimal A, Laros Jr RK. Guidelines for computed tomography and magnetic resonance imaging use during pregnancy and lactation. Obstet Gynecol. 2008;112:333–40.

50. Chapman AB, Abraham WT, Zamudio S, Coffin C, Merouani A, Young D, et al. Temporal relationships between hormonal and hemodynamic changes in early human pregnancy. Kidney Int. 1998;54:2056–63.

51. Clapp 3rd JF, Seaward BL, Sleamaker RH, Hiser J. Maternal physiologic adaptations to early human pregnancy. Am J Obstet Gynecol. 1988;159:1456–60.

52. Duvekot JJ, Cheriex EC, Pieters FA, Menheere PP, Peeters LH. Early pregnancy changes in hemodynamics and volume homeostasis are consecutive adjustments triggered by a primary fall in systemic vascular tone. Am J Obstet Gynecol. 1993;169:1382–92.

53. Capeless EL, Clapp JF. Cardiovascular changes in early phase of pregnancy. Am J Obstet Gynecol. 1989;161:1449–53.

54. Duvekot JJ, Peeters LL. Renal hemodynamics and volume homeostasis in pregnancy. Obstet Gynecol Surv. 1994;49:830–9.

55. Hunter S, Robson SC. Adaptation of the maternal heart in pregnancy. Br Heart J. 1992;68:540–3.

56. Kametas NA, McAuliffe F, Cook B, Nicolaides KH, Chambers J. Maternal left ventricular transverse and long-axis systolic function during pregnancy. Ultrasound Obstet Gynecol. 2001;18:467–74.

57. Kametas NA, McAuliffe F, Hancock J, Chambers J, Nicolaides KH. Maternal left ventricular mass and diastolic function during pregnancy. Ultrasound Obstet Gynecol. 2001;18:460–6.

58. Metcalfe J, Ueland K. Maternal cardiovascular adjustments to pregnancy. Prog Cardiovasc Dis. 1974;16:363–74.

59. Ogueh O, Brookes C, Johnson MR. A longitudinal study of the maternal cardiovascular adaptation to spontaneous and assisted conception pregnancies. Hypertens Pregnancy. 2009;28:273–89.

60. Desai DK, Moodley J, Naidoo DP. Echocardiographic assessment of cardiovascular hemodynamics in normal pregnancy. Obstet Gynecol. 2004;104:20–9.

61. Chapman AB, Zamudio S, Woodmansee W, Merouani A, Osorio F, Johnson A, et al. Systemic and renal hemodynamic changes in the luteal phase of the menstrual cycle mimic early pregnancy. Am J Physiol. 1997;273:F777–82.

62. Carbillon L, Uzan M, Uzan S. Pregnancy, vascular tone, and maternal hemodynamics: a crucial adaptation. Obstet Gynecol Surv. 2000;55:574–81.

63. Conrad KP. Maternal vasodilation in pregnancy: the emerging role of relaxin. Am J Physiol Regul Integr Comp Physiol. 2011;301:R267–75.

64. Gant NF, Chand S, Whalley PJ, MacDonald PC. The nature of pressor responsiveness to angiotensin II in human pregnancy. Obstet Gynecol. 1974;43:854.

65. Nisell H, Hjemdahl P, Linde B. Cardiovascular responses to circulating catecholamines in normal pregnancy and in pregnancy-induced hypertension. Clin Physiol. 1985;5:479–93.

66. Schrier RW, Briner VA. Peripheral arterial vasodilation hypothesis of sodium and water retention in pregnancy: implications for pathogenesis of preeclampsia-eclampsia. Obstet Gynecol. 1991;77:632–9.

67. Robson SC, Hunter S, Boys RJ, Dunlop W. Serial study of factors influencing changes in cardiac output during human pregnancy. Am J Physiol. 1989;256:H1060–5.

68. Schrier RW. Pathogenesis of sodium and water retention in high-output and low-output cardiac failure, nephrotic syndrome, cirrhosis, and pregnancy (2). N Engl J Med. 1988;319:1127–34.

69. Pritchard JA. Changes in the blood volume during pregnancy and delivery. Anesthesiology. 1965;26:393–9.

70. Koller O. The clinical significance of hemodilution during pregnancy. Obstet Gynecol Surv. 1982;37:649–52.

71. Bamfo JE, Kametas NA, Nicolaides KH, Chambers JB. Maternal left ventricular diastolic and systolic long-axis function during normal pregnancy. Eur J Echocardiogr. 2007;8:360–8.

72. Savu O, Jurcut R, Giusca S, van Mieghem T, Gussi I, Popescu BA, et al. Morphological and functional adaptation of the maternal heart during pregnancy. Circ Cardiovasc Imaging. 2012;5:289–97.

73. van Oppen AC, Stigter RH, Bruinse HW. Cardiac output in normal pregnancy: a critical review. Obstet Gynecol. 1996;87:310–8.

74. Easterling TR, Benedetti TJ, Schmucker BC, Millard SP. Maternal hemodynamics in normal and preeclamptic pregnancies: a longitudinal study. Obstet Gynecol. 1990;76:1061–9.

75. McLennan FM, Haites NE, Rawles JM. Stroke and minute distance in pregnancy: a longitudinal study using Doppler ultrasound. Br J Obstet Gynaecol. 1987;94:499–506.

76. Kinsella SM, Lohmann G. Supine hypotensive syndrome. Obstet Gynecol. 1994;83:774–88.

77. Jeejeebhoy FM, Zelop CM, Windrim R, Carvalho JC, Dorian P, Morrison LJ. Management of cardiac arrest in pregnancy: a systematic review. Resuscitation. 2011;82:801–9.

78. Clapp 3rd JF, Capeless E. Cardiovascular function before, during, and after the first and subsequent pregnancies. Am J Cardiol. 1997;80:1469–73.

79. Grindheim G, Estensen ME, Langesaeter E, Rosseland LA, Toska K. Changes in blood pressure during healthy pregnancy: a longitudinal cohort study. J Hypertens. 2012;30:342–50.

80. Ochsenbein-Kolble N, Roos M, Gasser T, Huch R, Huch A, Zimmermann R. Cross sectional study of automated blood pressure measurements throughout pregnancy. BJOG. 2004;111:319–25.

81. Mone SM, Sanders SP, Colan SD. Control mechanisms for physiological hypertrophy of pregnancy. Circulation. 1996;94:667–72.

82. Gilson GJ, Samaan S, Crawford MH, Qualls CR, Curet LB. Changes in hemodynamics, ventricular remodeling, and ventricular contractility during normal pregnancy: a longitudinal study. Obstet Gynecol. 1997;89:957–62.

83. Katz R, Karliner JS, Resnik R. Effects of a natural volume overload state (pregnancy) on left ventricular performance in normal human subjects. Circulation. 1978;58:434–41.

84. Simmons LA, Gillin AG, Jeremy RW. Structural and functional changes in left ventricle during normotensive and preeclamptic pregnancy. Am J Physiol Heart Circ Physiol. 2002;283:H1627–33.

85. Colan SD, Borow KM, Neumann A. Left ventricular end-systolic wall stress-velocity of fiber shortening relation: a load-independent index of myocardial contractility. J Am Coll Cardiol. 1984;4:715–24.

86. Bamfo JE, Kametas NA, Nicolaides KH, Chambers JB. Reference ranges for tissue Doppler measures of maternal systolic and diastolic left ventricular function. Ultrasound Obstet Gynecol. 2007;29:414–20.

87. Tzemos N, Silversides CK, Carasso S, Rakowski H, Siu SC. Effect of pregnancy on left ventricular motion (twist) in women with aortic stenosis. Am J Cardiol. 2008;101:870–3.

88. Yoon AJ, Song J, Megalla S, Nazari R, Akinlaja O, Pollack S, et al. Left ventricular torsional mechanics in uncomplicated pregnancy. Clin Cardiol. 2011;34:543–8.

89. Yosefy C, Shenhav S, Feldman V, Sagi Y, Katz A, Anteby E. Left atrial function during pregnancy: a three-dimensional echocardiographic study. Echocardiography. 2012;29:1096–101.

90. Mesa A, Jessurun C, Hernandez A, Adam K, Brown D, Vaughn WK, et al. Left ventricular diastolic function in normal human pregnancy. Circulation. 1999;99:511–7.

91. Robson SC, Dunlop W, Boys RJ, Hunter S. Cardiac output during labour. Br Med J (Clin Res Ed). 1987;295:1169–72.

92. Kjeldsen J. Hemodynamic investigations during labour and delivery. Acta Obstet Gynecol Scand Suppl. 1979;89:1–252.

93. Ueland K, Hansen JM. Maternal cardiovascular dynamics. 3. Labor and delivery under local and caudal analgesia. Am J Obstet Gynecol. 1969;103:8–18.

94. Lee W, Rokey R, Miller J, Cotton DB. Maternal hemodynamic effects of uterine contractions by M-mode and pulsed-Doppler echocardiography. Am J Obstet Gynecol. 1989;161:974–7.

95. Danilenko-Dixon DR, Tefft L, Cohen RA, Haydon B, Carpenter MW. Positional effects on maternal cardiac output during labor with epidural analgesia. Am J Obstet Gynecol. 1996;175:867–72.

96. Patton DE, Lee W, Miller J, Jones M. Maternal, uteroplacental, and fetoplacental hemodynamic and Doppler velocimetric changes during epidural anesthesia in normal labor. Obstet Gynecol. 1991;77:17–9.

97. Robson SC, Boys RJ, Hunter S, Dunlop W. Maternal hemodynamics after normal delivery and delivery complicated by postpartum hemorrhage. Obstet Gynecol. 1989;74:234–9.

98. Robson SC, Dunlop W, Hunter S. Haemodynamic changes during the early puerperium. Br Med J (Clin Res Ed). 1987;294:1065.

99. Robson SC, Hunter S, Moore M, Dunlop W. Haemodynamic changes during the puerperium: a Doppler and M-mode echocardiographic study. Br J Obstet Gynaecol. 1987;94:1028–39.

100. Robson SC, Hunter S, Dunlop W. Left atrial dimension during early puerperium. Lancet. 1987;2:111–2.

101. Capeless EL, Clapp JF. When do cardiovascular parameters return to their preconception values? Am J Obstet Gynecol. 1991;165:883–6.

102. Turan OM, De Paco C, Kametas N, Khaw A, Nicolaides KH. Effect of parity on maternal cardiac function during the first trimester of pregnancy. Ultrasound Obstet Gynecol. 2008;32:849–54.

103. Hart MV, Morton MJ, Hosenpud JD, Metcalfe J. Aortic function during normal human pregnancy. Am J Obstet Gynecol. 1986;154:887–91.

104. Poppas A, Shroff SG, Korcarz CE, Hibbard JU, Berger DS, Lindheimer MD, et al. Serial assessment of the cardiovascular system in normal pregnancy. Role of arterial compliance and pulsatile arterial load. Circulation. 1997;95:2407–15.

105. Macedo ML, Luminoso D, Savvidou MD, McEniery CM, Nicolaides KH. Maternal wave reflections and arterial stiffness in normal pregnancy as assessed by applanation tonometry. Hypertension. 2008;51:1047–51.

106. Wykretowicz M, Krauze T, Guzik P, Piskorski J, Markwitz W, Wykretowicz A, et al. Arterial stiffness, central hemodynamics and wave reflection in normal pregnancy and control nonpregnant women. Eur J Obstet Gynecol Reprod Biol. 2011;159:49–52.

107. Gyselaers W, Mullens W, Tomsin K, Mesens T, Peeters L. Role of dysfunctional maternal venous hemodynamics in the pathophysiology of pre-eclampsia: a review. Ultrasound Obstet Gynecol. 2011;38:123–9.

108. Sakai K, Imaizumi T, Maeda H, Nagata H, Tsukimori K, Takeshita A, et al. Venous distensibility during pregnancy. Comparisons between normal pregnancy and preeclampsia. Hypertension. 1994;24:461–6.

109. Skudder Jr PA, Farrington DT, Weld E, Putman C. Venous dysfunction of late pregnancy persists after delivery. J Cardiovasc Surg (Torino). 1990;31:748–52.

110. Gyselaers W. Hemodynamics of the maternal venous compartment: a new area to explore in obstetric ultrasound imaging. Ultrasound Obstet Gynecol. 2008;32:716–7.

111. Deurloo KL, Bolte AC, Twisk JW, van Vugt JM. Longitudinal Doppler measurements of spiral artery blood flow in relation to uterine artery blood flow. J Ultrasound Med. 2009;28:1623–8.

112. Flo K, Wilsgaard T, Acharya G. A new non-invasive method for measuring uterine vascular resistance and its relationship to uterine artery Doppler indices: a longitudinal study. Ultrasound Obstet Gynecol. 2011;37:538–42.

113. Gomez O, Figueras F, Martinez JM, del Rio M, Palacio M, Eixarch E, et al. Sequential changes in uterine artery blood flow pattern between the first and second trimesters of gestation in relation to pregnancy outcome. Ultrasound Obstet Gynecol. 2006;28:802–8.

114. Konje JC, Kaufmann P, Bell SC, Taylor DJ. A longitudinal study of quantitative uterine blood flow with the use of color power angiography in appropriate for gestational age pregnancies. Am J Obstet Gynecol. 2001;185:608–13.

115. Ogueh O, Clough A, Hancock M, Johnson MR. A longitudinal study of the control of renal and uterine hemodynamic changes of pregnancy. Hypertens Pregnancy. 2011;30:243–59.

116. Bernstein IM, Ziegler WF, Leavitt T, Badger GJ. Uterine artery hemodynamic adaptations through the menstrual cycle into early pregnancy. Obstet Gynecol. 2002;99:620–4.

117. Flo K, Wilsgaard T, Vartun A, Acharya G. A longitudinal study of the relationship between maternal cardiac output measured by impedance cardiography and uterine artery blood flow in the second half of pregnancy. BJOG. 2010;117:837–44.

118. Thaler I, Manor D, Itskovitz J, Rottem S, Levit N, Timor-Tritsch I, et al. Changes in uterine blood flow during human pregnancy. Am J Obstet Gynecol. 1990;162:121–5.

119. Belfort MA, Tooke-Miller C, Allen Jr JC, Saade GR, Dildy GA, Grunewald C, et al. Changes in flow velocity, resistance indices, and cerebral perfusion pressure in the maternal middle cerebral artery distribution during normal pregnancy. Acta Obstet Gynecol Scand. 2001;80:104–12.

120. Lindqvist PG, Marsal K, Pirhonen JP. Maternal cerebral Doppler velocimetry before, during, and after a normal pregnancy: a longitudinal study. Acta Obstet Gynecol Scand. 2006;85:1299–303.

121. Zeeman GG, Hatab M, Twickler DM. Maternal cerebral blood flow changes in pregnancy. Am J Obstet Gynecol. 2003;189:968–72.

122. De Backer D, Ospina-Tascon G, Salgado D, Favory R, Creteur J, Vincent JL. Monitoring the microcirculation in the critically ill patient: current methods and future approaches. Intensive Care Med. 2010;36:1813–25.

123. De Backer D, Ortiz JA, Salgado D. Coupling microcirculation to systemic hemodynamics. Curr Opin Crit Care. 2010;16:250–4.

124. Trzeciak S, Dellinger RP, Parrillo JE, Guglielmi M, Bajaj J, Abate NL, et al. Early microcirculatory perfusion derangements in patients with severe sepsis and septic shock: relationship to hemodynamics, oxygen transport, and survival. Ann Emerg Med. 2007;49:88–98, e1–2.

125. Verdant C, De Backer D. How monitoring of the microcirculation may help us at the bedside. Curr Opin Crit Care. 2005;11:240–4.

126. Anim-Nyame N, Gamble J, Sooranna SR, Johnson MR, Sullivan MH, Steer PJ. Evidence of impaired microvascular function in pre-eclampsia: a non-invasive study. Clin Sci (Lond). 2003;104:405–12.

127. Hasan KM, Manyonda IT, Ng FS, Singer DR, Antonios TF. Skin capillary density changes in normal pregnancy and pre-eclampsia. J Hypertens. 2002;20:2439–43.
128. Houben AJ, de Leeuw PW, Peeters LL. Configuration of the microcirculation in pre-eclampsia: possible role of the venular system. J Hypertens. 2007;25:1665–70.
129. Rosen L, Ostergren J, Fagrell B, Stranden E. Mechanisms for edema formation in normal pregnancy and preeclampsia evaluated by skin capillary dynamics. Int J Microcirc Clin Exp. 1990;9:257–66.

130. Vollebregt KC, Boer K, Mathura KR, de Graaff JC, Ubbink DT, Ince C. Impaired vascular function in women with pre-eclampsia observed with orthogonal polarisation spectral imaging. BJOG. 2001;108:1148–53.
131. Bezemer R, Khalilzada M, Ince C. Recent advancements in microcirculatory image acquisition and analysis. Yearbook Intensive Care Emerg Med. 2008;2008:677–90.
132. De Backer D, Hollenberg S, Boerma C, Goedhart P, Buchele G, Ospina-Tascon G, et al. How to evaluate the microcirculation: report of a round table conference. Crit Care. 2007;11:R101.

Hypertension and Pregnancy

30

Letitia Acquah and Vesna D. Garovic

Abstract

Hypertension is the most common medical disorder encountered during pregnancy, affecting up to 10 % of all pregnancies. Hypertensive disorders are one of the major causes of pregnancy-related maternal deaths in the United States. Hypertension in pregnancy includes a spectrum of conditions, including preeclampsia-eclampsia, preeclampsia superimposed on chronic hypertension, chronic hypertension, and gestational hypertension. Unlike other hypertensive pregnancy disorders, preeclampsia is a multisystem disease, its distinctive feature being either sudden onset or worsening of preexisting proteinuria. Despite significant advances in our understanding of preeclampsia, the etiology of this condition remains elusive, resulting in a failure to develop specific screening, preventive, and treatment strategies. Delivery remains the mainstay of therapy for severe forms and anticipated life-threatening complications. The most important reason for the initiation of antihypertensive treatment in these patients is to prevent maternal cerebrovascular and cardiac complications. The optimal timing and choice of therapy for hypertensive pregnancy disorders involves carefully weighing the risk-versus-benefit ratio for each individual patient, with an overall goal of improving maternal and fetal outcomes. Finally, over the past decades, it has become increasingly clear that women with a history of preeclamptic compared to normotensive pregnancies are at increased risk for cardiovascular disease later in life. In this chapter, we summarize the mechanisms thought to be involved in hypertensive pregnancy disorders, review the current treatment guidelines, and outline some newer perspectives on management, including postpartum monitoring and treatment of conventional cardiovascular risk factors in the affected women.

Keywords

Hypertension in pregnancy • Gestational hypertension • Preeclampsia • Cardiovascular disease in women • Pregnancy outcomes

L. Acquah, MD, MSc, FACP
Divisions of General and Obstetric Medicine,
Department of Medicine,
Mayo Clinic, 200 First Street, SW,
Gonda 17 South, Rochester, MN 55905, USA
e-mail: acquah.letitia@mayo.edu

V.D. Garovic, MD (✉)
Division of Nephrology and Hypertension,
Mayo Clinic, 200 First Street, SW,
Rochester, MN 55905, USA
e-mail: garovic.vesna@mayo.edu

Introduction

Hypertension affects 10 % of pregnancies and covers a spectrum of hypertensive pregnancy disorders, including preeclampsia, eclampsia, and chronic and gestational hypertension (Table 30.1, Fig. 30.1) [1]. Approximately one-half of all hypertensive pregnancy disorders are due to preeclampsia, a hypertensive disorder which is unique to pregnancy and further characterized by proteinuria. Preeclampsia and related conditions, namely, eclampsia, its

K. Stergiopoulos, D.L. Brown (eds.), *Evidence-Based Cardiology Consult*,
DOI 10.1007/978-1-4471-4441-0_30, © Springer-Verlag London 2014

Table 30.1 Classification and definitions of hypertensive pregnancy disorders

Chronic hypertension	BP ≥140/±90 mmHg before pregnancy or before the 20th week of gestation
Preeclampsia-eclampsia	A pregnancy-specific disorder that is a multisystem disease characterized by hypertension ≥140/±90 mmHg, on at least two occasions at least 6 h apart, and proteinuria ≥300 mg in a 24 h urine collection; after 20 weeks gestation
	The convulsive form of preeclampsia is eclampsia and affects 0.1 % of all pregnancies
Preeclampsia superimposed on chronic hypertension	Up to 30 % of women with chronic hypertension develop preeclampsia, as heralded by the occurrence of de novo proteinuria in the third trimester. In women with chronic hypertension and preexisting proteinuria (i.e., before 20 weeks of gestation), the diagnosis of superimposed preeclampsia is likely with any of the following findings: sudden increase in proteinuria, sudden worsening of previously well-controlled blood pressure, new onset of thrombocytopenia, or elevated liver function tests
Gestational hypertension	New onset of hypertension ≥140/±90 mmHg, on at least two occasions at least 6 h apart, after 20 weeks gestation, in the absence of proteinuria (≤300 mg in a 24 h urine collection). If blood pressure returns to normal by 12 weeks postpartum, the diagnosis of transient hypertension of pregnancy can be assigned. If elevated blood pressure persists, the diagnosis of chronic hypertension is made

Fig. 30.1 Hypertensive pregnancy disorders. *The diagnosis of eclampsia, a convulsive form of preeclampsia, is based on new-onset seizures, in the absence of a previous history of a seizure disorder. *GW* gestational weeks, *HTN* hypertension. Reprinted with permission from Garovic [44]

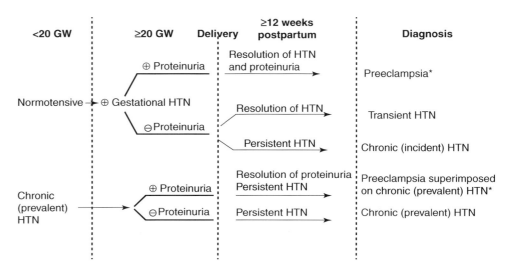

convulsive form, and HELLP syndrome (an acronym for *h*emolysis, *e*levated *l*iver enzymes, and *l*ow *p*latelet count), remain leading causes of fetal and maternal morbidity and mortality. Maternal complications occur as a consequence of hypertensive end-organ damage of the central nervous system (stroke), kidneys (acute renal failure), and heart (acute cardiac decompensation). In a study examining all maternal deaths after the 20th week of pregnancy, preeclampsia and eclampsia were responsible for 790 of 4,024 deaths between 1979 and 1992 [2]. The overall preeclampsia-eclampsia case-fatality rate was 6.4 cases per 10,000 cases at delivery. The burden is even higher in developing countries.

Over the last 50 years, much progress has been made in improving the treatment of preeclampsia with respect to blood pressure control and prevention of eclamptic seizures. However, the etiology of this condition remains elusive, resulting in a failure to develop specific screening, preventive, and treatment strategies. Delivery remains the mainstay of therapy for severe forms and anticipated life-threatening complications. As severe forms of preeclampsia commonly develop before 34 weeks of gestation, labor induction under these circumstances typically results in a preterm delivery and low birth weight with related neonatal complications.

Hypertensive pregnancy disorders may have an impact on public health well beyond the affected pregnancies [3]. Epidemiological studies have demonstrated consistently an association between an increased risk for cardiovascular disease in adulthood and a low birth weight, which, in children born to preeclamptic mothers, may occur as a consequence of either prematurity or intrauterine growth retardation. In addition, women with a history of hypertensive compared to normotensive pregnancies are at increased risk for cardiovascular disease later in life [4]. Therefore, improved screening, prevention, and treatment of hypertensive pregnancy disorders may not only optimize immediate pregnancy outcomes, but may have long-term impact on women and their children years after the affected pregnancies.

There are many factors to consider when contemplating the treatment of hypertension during pregnancy. These encompass maternal factors, including duration and severity of hypertension and presence of end-organ damage, as well as fetal factors, such as the safety of blood pressure medications and the potential for compromised uteroplacental and fetal circulation due to overzealous blood pressure control. The following discussion will address the pathophysiology of the various hypertensive pregnancy disorders, related diagnostic criteria, and treatment options.

Cardiovascular Adaptation to Normal Pregnancy

The normal physiological changes occurring in pregnancy facilitate adequate blood perfusion of the developing vascular bed and fetal circulation that are required for normal fetal development and growth [5].

During pregnancy, cardiac output is increased by about 50 %. At least half of the increase is accomplished within the first 8 weeks of pregnancy. The augmented cardiac output is attained through an increase in vascular volume (preload), a decrease in systemic vascular resistance (afterload), and an increase in chronotropy. The left ventricular ejection fraction remains unchanged throughout pregnancy.

The combination of increased preload and heart rate and decreased afterload has dramatic effects on systemic blood pressure. In general, blood pressure drops during the first and second trimesters, resulting in a reduction of about 10 mmHg in diastolic pressure by the end of the second trimester. Blood pressure typically increases during the third trimester and approximates prepregnancy values by the time of delivery.

Preload also can be affected by the size and position of the fetus. Supine positioning causes compression of the maternal inferior vena cava and a subsequent decrease in preload. The heart rate increases in an attempt to maintain cardiac output, but the net result of supine positioning may be decreased blood pressure and possibly decreased placental blood flow. For this reason, it is important for women to lie in the left lateral position rather than supine.

Renal changes include increased blood flow and a corresponding increase in glomerular filtration rate (GFR). Renal blood flow increases by about 75 % over prepregnancy values, and this leads to at least a 40 % increase in GFR. The serum creatinine concentration is appropriately decreased, to about 0.5 mg/dL. In fact, gravid women with a creatinine that would be considered "normal" in the nonpregnant state may have underlying renal insufficiency. Due to the increased blood flow, renal size increases by about 1–2 cm.

These changes in cardiovascular and renal physiology may not occur in women with preexisting cardiac and renal diseases or, alternatively, may unmask or worsen preexisting conditions, such as hypertension, in susceptible individuals.

Pathophysiology of Preeclampsia

There is accumulating evidence suggesting that endothelial dysfunction plays a central role in the pathogenesis of preeclampsia [6]. In addition, the fact that hypertension rapidly resolves upon the removal of products of conception has lead to several theories implicating structural and/or functional changes in the developing placenta as factors causing preeclampsia. In normal pregnancy, the invasive activity of cytotrophoblast leads to important changes in the spiral arteries (~100–150 in total), causing them to lose muscle and elastic tissue and undergo transformation into flaccid, large capacitance uteroplacental arteries [7]. These changes occur both in more superficial, decidual portions, and in deeper, myometrial segments during normal pregnancy [8–10]. The net result of these changes, frequently referred to as "physiological change" or "spiral artery remodeling," is an increased blood supply that meets the increased metabolic demands of the developing fetus and placenta. In preeclampsia, the placental spiral arteries fail to lose their musculoelastic layers ultimately leading to decreased placental perfusion [10, 11]. Placental hypoxia is viewed frequently as an early event that may cause placental production of soluble factors leading to endothelial dysfunction [12]. However, multiple research efforts have failed to identify one or more molecules of placental origin that can cause a reproducible effect on systemic endothelial function.

Recent reports have demonstrated that women with preeclampsia have elevated levels of the soluble receptor for vascular endothelial growth factor (VEGF) of placental origin [13]. This soluble receptor, also known as sFlt-1 (from fms-like tyrosine kinase receptor-1), may bind and neutralize VEGF and the closely related placental growth factor (PlGF), leading to decreases in free VEGF and PlGF levels, which are required for active fetal and placental angiogenesis during pregnancy [14]. Thus, elevated sFlt-1 levels may be the missing link between placental ischemia on one side and endothelial dysfunction, mediated by sFlt-1 neutralization of VEGF and PlGF, on the other. However, urine and serum measurements of circulating angiogenic proteins have not provided reliable screening tools for preeclampsia with the currently available techniques [15]. In addition, their roles as possible therapeutic targets remain to be determined. We have recently shown that proteinuria in preeclampsia is not merely a function of endothelial dysfunction, but likely a consequence of both disruption of the glomerular filtration barrier [16] and loss of glomerular epithelial cells, i.e., podocytes [17]. The clinical applicability of these findings remains to be determined.

Hypertensive Disorders of Pregnancy: Diagnostic Classifications

In 2000, the National High Blood Pressure Education Program (NHBPEP) working group on high blood pressure in pregnancy defined hypertension as a blood pressure ≥140 mmHg systolic and/or ≥90 mmHg diastolic on 2 occasions at least 6 h apart [1]. Blood pressures ≥160 mmHg systolic and/or ≥110 mmHg diastolic signify severe hypertension.

The hypertensive disorders of pregnancy are classified on the basis of clinical and laboratory abnormalities. Clinical criteria include signs such as hypertension, and symptoms such as headache or abdominal pain. Common laboratory tests used in the assessment of hypertension during pregnancy include urinalysis, hemoglobin, hematocrit, platelet count, serum uric acid, serum albumin, and kidney and liver function tests.

Pregnancy and Blood Pressure Measurement

The diagnosis of hypertension during pregnancy requires accurate measurements of both the systolic and diastolic pressures [1]. Ideally, this requires manual blood pressure measurements. Many automated machines have not been tested for use during pregnancy and, therefore, may provide unreliable readings. Obtaining a manual blood pressure is the best approach, using Korotkoff phase V (disappearance) rather than Korotkoff phase IV (muffling of sounds) to determine the diastolic pressure. In the clinical setting, blood pressure should be measured in the sitting position. In recumbent hospitalized patients, care must be taken to measure the blood pressure in the left lateral decubitus position to abrogate the blood pressure change caused by the compression of the inferior vena cava by the gravid uterus. In all cases, the arm in which the blood pressure is being measured should be maintained at the level of the heart to avoid spuriously low readings from elevation of the arm. Hypertension is diagnosed at a systolic pressure ≥140 mmHg and/or a diastolic pressure ≥90 mmHg.

Preeclampsia (previously termed pregnancy-induced hypertension and toxemia of pregnancy) is a pregnancy-specific disorder clinically characterized by hypertension and proteinuria that occurs after 20 weeks of gestation. Proteinuria is diagnosed in patients with ≥300 mg of protein in a 24-h urine specimen. When a 24-h specimen cannot be obtained, or if a diagnosis is urgently required, a dipstick result of 1+ or greater or a protein-to-creatinine ratio of 0.3 g/24 h will suffice. The 24-h urine collection, however, remains the gold standard and should be completed if possible.

Preeclampsia traditionally has been considered a disease of first pregnancy. However, women with a history of preeclampsia are at increased risk during subsequent pregnancies.

Table 30.2 Risk factors for preeclampsia

Diabetes mellitus
Renal disease
History of preeclampsia with previous pregnancies
Extremes of maternal age
Multiparity
Multiple gestations
Family history of preeclampsia
Chronic hypertension (either essential or secondary)
Thrombophilias
Trophoblastic disease (i.e., hydatidiform mole)
Autoimmune and connective tissue diseases

Several other risk factors are well recognized, which may aid in the early recognition of patients at risk (Table 30.2). For high-risk patients, the following laboratory values should be obtained early in pregnancy: hemoglobin, hematocrit, platelet count, serum uric acid, and creatinine level. In addition, patients should have a urinalysis, which, if confirming the presence of 1+ protein, should be followed by a 24-h urine protein measurement. Patients who develop hypertension in the second half of pregnancy should be tested biweekly, with additional testing to include serum transaminase levels, lactate dehydrogenase levels, and peripheral blood smear and serum albumin levels to monitor for hepatic dysfunction, hemolysis, and capillary leak, respectively. The role of early testing and serial measurements is to facilitate an early diagnosis of preeclampsia and to assess disease severity and progression.

Preeclampsia may develop de novo in previously healthy pregnant women or may occur in women with preexisting conditions, such as renal disease or chronic hypertension, i.e., superimposed preeclampsia. In women with chronic hypertension, but no proteinuria at baseline, preeclampsia is heralded by the development of proteinuria after 20 weeks gestation. Some women may have proteinuria at baseline, which can significantly complicate the diagnosis. In general, the development of severe hypertension (≥160 mmHg systolic and/or ≥110 mmHg diastolic) or any of the signs or symptoms of severe preeclampsia (Table 30.3) signifies the development of superimposed preeclampsia; up to 30 % of pregnancies in women with chronic hypertension may be affected.

Several different strategies have been evaluated for prevention of preeclampsia, including a low-salt diet [18], low-dose aspirin [19], antioxidants [20], and calcium [21] and magnesium supplements [22]. With the exception of calcium supplementation for calcium-deficient women and low-dose aspirin for women at high risk (i.e., those with a history of chronic hypertension and preeclampsia in a previous pregnancy), these approaches have failed to demonstrate reproducible benefits.

Table 30.3 Diagnostic criteria for severe preeclampsia

Criteria	Remarks
Severe hypertension	Blood pressure ≥160 systolic and/or ≥110 diastolic
Severe proteinuria	Protein ≥5 g in 24 h, or ≥3+ by dipstick
Renal impairment	Serum creatinine >1.2 mg/dL
Oliguria	Urine output <500 mL in 24 h
Microangiopathic hemolytic anemia[a]	Schistocytes on blood smear
Hepatic involvement[a]	Right upper quadrant pain (may herald hepatic rupture)
	Nausea, vomiting
	Elevated liver function test results (at least twice the upper limits of normal)
Thrombocytopenia[a]	Platelet count <100×10⁹/L
Neurological signs and symptoms[b]	Altered mental status, headache, visual changes, cerebrovascular events
Cardiovascular compromise	Pulmonary edema or cyanosis
Fetal complications	Fetal growth restriction
	Intrauterine fetal distress

[a]Presence of these findings should prompt consideration of HELLP syndrome
[b]May represent impending eclampsia

Chronic hypertension in pregnant women is diagnosed based on the presence of hypertension before the 20th week of gestation. The diagnosis may be difficult in young women with little or no medical history. Physiological changes during pregnancy lead to a fall in blood pressure during the first and second trimesters. In a woman with undiagnosed hypertension prior to pregnancy, this may lead to normal readings early in pregnancy. During the third trimester, the return to prepregnancy hypertensive values may lead to a false diagnosis of new-onset hypertension. While most patients with chronic hypertension fare well during pregnancy, those who develop superimposed preeclampsia are at a particularly high risk for cerebral hemorrhage and placental abruption.

Gestational hypertension is characterized by new-onset hypertension after the 20th week of gestation, in the absence of proteinuria. Women who develop gestational hypertension after 30 weeks gestation have a 10 % risk of progressing to preeclampsia; this risk is increased to 30 % in women who present before 30 weeks gestation. Women who do not develop proteinuria are diagnosed with either transient hypertension (normalization of blood pressure by 12 weeks postpartum) or chronic hypertension (elevated blood pressure and need for blood pressure treatments persisting after pregnancy and delivery).

During the first 5 postpartum days, blood pressures in normotensive women tend to be higher compared to pregnancy values, likely due to fluid shifts from the interstitial space and resultant transient rise in intravascular volume.

While hypertension in most of these women resolves by 2–4 weeks postpartum, some of these women may remain hypertensive and require antihypertensive treatment. A subset of these patients may progress to preeclampsia/eclampsia that, due to the onset after delivery, may represent a diagnostic challenge leading to delayed treatment.

HELLP syndrome is believed to be a deceptive form of preeclampsia, which presents with a distinctive and ominous triad of microangiopathic hemolytic anemia, hepatocellular injury, and consumption of platelets [23]. Right upper quadrant and epigastric pain may occur as a consequence of a hepatic hematoma and resultant stretching of Glisson's capsule. It may herald hepatic rupture, which is associated with high maternal and fetal mortality rates. Urgent delivery remains the mainstay of treatment for patients with HELLP syndrome. Retrospective analyses of HELLP syndrome patients, in whom urgent delivery was not undertaken, have documented an extremely high perinatal infant mortality of 70 % [24].

Eclampsia refers to the development of seizures in a woman with preeclampsia or gestational hypertension. While the classic presentation is the development of seizures in a woman with severe preeclampsia, up to 20 % of cases occur in women with no evidence of proteinuria and many cases occur in patients with mild hypertension. The mainstay of treatment is intravenous magnesium sulfate, which has been shown to be more effective than either phenytoin or diazepam for seizure prophylaxis in women with severe preeclampsia and for prevention of recurrent seizures in those with eclampsia [25].

Management

Preconception Counseling

Women with a history of hypertension should be evaluated before pregnancy for target organ damage, such as left ventricular hypertrophy, hypertensive nephropathy, and retinopathy, which will help establish blood pressure treatment goals. Patients with clinical clues suggestive of secondary hypertension (e.g., hard-to-control hypertension requiring more than three antihypertensive agents and/or indicative laboratory and clinical findings) should undergo a workup for secondary hypertension (primary hyperaldosteronism, pheochromocytoma, and renal artery stenosis). Therefore, prepregnancy counseling of women with chronic hypertension may require expertise outside the realm of obstetrics. Some forms of secondary hypertension, and particularly pheochromocytoma and renovascular hypertension, may further increase the risk for adverse pregnancy outcomes beyond that of essential hypertension; thus, surgery (for pheochromocytoma) or revascularization (for renal artery stenosis) should be considered before pregnancy. In this population of young women of childbearing age, these interventions may result in the cure of hypertension. Prepregnancy evaluation further should address changes in medications to those that have acceptable safety profiles in pregnancy and counseling regarding pregnancy risks. It is estimated that as many as 25 % of women with chronic hypertension may develop superimposed preeclampsia. These women are at a particularly high risk for cerebral hemorrhage and placental abruption. It remains unclear as to whether early treatment of chronic hypertension in pregnancy prevents preeclampsia [26]. In the absence of randomized prospective trials adequately powered to address this important clinical question, practicing physicians should treat chronically hypertensive women according to currently accepted national guidelines, which are presented and discussed below.

Initiation of Therapy and Treatment Goals

The rationale for treatment of mild-to-moderate hypertension in pregnancy (defined as a diastolic blood pressure 90–100 mmHg), along with therapeutic blood pressure goals, is the subject of an ongoing debate. Central to these disagreements is the lack of well-designed and adequately powered studies demonstrating reductions in obstetric complications with antihypertensive treatment for this degree of hypertension. Coupled with the concerns that fetal risks may be increased – due to both intrauterine exposure to medications with potential adverse effects and abrupt blood pressure lowering leading to a decrease in uteroplacental blood flow and fetal hemodynamic compromise – this is commonly used as an argument to discontinue antihypertensive drugs during pregnancy in women with hypertension predating their pregnancies. In addition, it is frequently assumed that hypertension of 4–5 months duration in a young woman (without other cardiovascular risk factors) does not affect her immediate and long-term cardiovascular health. The arguments against this approach come from evidence suggesting that mild chronic hypertension may lead to increased maternal and fetal risks [27] and that treatment of chronic hypertension may prevent progression to severe hypertension [26]. These unanswered questions underscore the need for prospective, randomized, and likely multicenter trials that will be adequately powered to compare the effects of different blood pressure targets on maternal and fetal outcomes. Based on the current guidelines, for purposes of treatment, hypertension during pregnancy may be divided into two general categories. The first includes the acute hypertensive syndromes of preeclampsia/eclampsia/HELLP syndrome. The second general category is chronic hypertension. According to the Working Group report of the NHBPEP, first-line oral and intravenous treatment is methyldopa and hydralazine, respectively [1].

Hypertension in Preeclamptic Patients

The acute hypertensive syndromes of preeclampsia/eclampsia/HELLP syndrome carry a high risk for maternal and fetal morbidity and mortality. The most important reason for the initiation of antihypertensive treatment in these patients is to prevent maternal cerebrovascular and cardiac complications. While hypertension in these settings can be treated medically, the definitive treatment remains delivery.

Most experts agree that therapy should be initiated for blood pressures of $\geq 160/110$ mmHg in order to decrease the incidence of maternal cardiac and cerebral events. It is common clinical practice to initiate treatment as the diastolic blood pressure approaches 100 mmHg [28]. The medications most commonly used for the urgent control of hypertension include intravenous hydralazine and labetalol. Oral agents may be considered if delivery is not expected within the next 48 h. Medications that may be used, along with their safety profiles, are summarized in Table 30.4. The NHBPEP guidelines suggest that preconception medications be continued in women with chronic hypertension who become pregnant, with the exception of angiotensin-converting enzyme inhibitors (ACEI) and angiotensin II receptor blockers (ARBs), as both have been associated with adverse fetal effects [29]. Commonly, antihypertensive medications other than methyldopa and hydralazine are being used more often in pregnancy (Table 30.4), particularly in patients for whom blood pressure control either cannot be achieved with these agents or because of intolerable side effects. Beta-blockers, with the exception of atenolol, and calcium channel blockers (CCBs) are acceptable medications that can be continued in patients with prepregnancy hypertension. The use of diuretic therapy during pregnancy has been controversial, primarily due to theoretical concerns. In the 1970s, physicians were advised that diuretics may actually be contraindicated because of the potential deleterious effects on placental blood flow. This recommendation was based on a study that has not been replicated [30]. Subsequent studies have indicated that diuretics are not associated with adverse perinatal effects [31]. The 2000 NHBPEP Working Group Report recognized that the major concern for the use of diuretics in pregnancy is primarily theoretical, as supporting evidence for their deleterious effects is lacking.

Control of blood pressure does not cure preeclampsia or prevent progression of preeclampsia; eclamptic seizures can occur when the blood pressure is only mildly elevated. Therefore, in addition to antihypertensive therapy, preeclamptic patients should receive seizure prophylaxis with intravenous magnesium sulfate that should be continued during labor and delivery and for at least 24 h after delivery. As magnesium is renally excreted, the rate of continuous infusion, but not the loading dose, should be adjusted, i.e.,

Table 30.4 Therapeutic options for treatment of hypertension in pregnancy

		Benefits	Risks
Central agents			
Preferred	Methyldopa	Proven safety and efficacy	Neuro-depressant side effects
Alternative	Clonidine	Efficacy similar to methyldopa	Unproven safety
Beta-blockers			
Preferred	Labetalol	Safety and efficacy similar to methyldopa. May be used for hypertensive urgency	Fetal bradycardia, neonatal hypoglycemia, decreased uteroplacental flow
Contraindicated	Atenolol	N/A	Intrauterine growth retardation
Calcium channel blockers			
Preferred	Nifedipine	Lowers blood pressure without affecting umbilical artery flow	Fetal distress, profound hypotension with magnesium
Alternative	Verapamil	Similar efficacy to other oral agents	Untested safety profile, risk of interaction with magnesium
Direct vasodilators			
Preferred	Hydralazine	Most efficacious oral agent	Maternal neuropathy, drug-induced lupus, neonatal thrombocytopenia and lupus
Alternative	Nitroprusside	Effective in severe hypertension	Cyanide and thiocyanate toxicity
Diuretics			
Preferred	Thiazide	Useful in chronic hypertension, renal failure, congestive heart failure	Volume contraction, electrolyte abnormalities
Contraindicated	Spironolactone	N/A	Possible fetal antiandrogen effects

decreased in women with renal failure. Serum magnesium levels should also be checked more frequently (every 1–2 h) in these women compared to women with normal renal function (every 4–6 h). Non-pharmacological treatment should include bed rest, which has been demonstrated to promote diuresis, lower blood pressure, and reduce premature labor. Salt restriction is not routinely recommended for women with preeclampsia who frequently are volume contracted; it may be advisable for women with histories of chronic hypertension who followed a low-sodium diet before pregnancy.

Chronic Hypertension in Pregnancy

For women with chronic hypertension, medications prescribed before pregnancy can be continued during pregnancy, except ACEI, ARBs, and atenolol. For pregnant patients with chronic hypertension, but on no treatment, therapy is usually instituted for a systolic pressure ≥150 mmHg and/or diastolic blood pressure ≥100 mmHg. Treatment thresholds are higher for pregnant than for non-pregnant patients due to the lack of studies to support the benefit of treatment for mild diastolic hypertension (90–99 mmHg) and concerns with respect to fetal safety, as treatment-induced blood pressure drops may be associated with impaired fetal growth [32]. An exception is made in women with evidence of end-organ damage: in the presence of renal disease, proteinuria, left ventricular hypertrophy, and retinopathy, antihypertensive therapy is initiated for a diastolic blood pressure ≥90 mmHg.

Perspectives

Similar to the general population, hypertension is the most common medical disorder encountered during pregnancy and remains one of the major causes of pregnancy-related maternal deaths in the United States [33]. However, treatment recommendations for hypertension in pregnancy, unlike those for the general population, have not evolved. For example, the elevations in systolic blood pressure in preeclamptic patients, at which pharmacotherapy is indicated, have not been established. Also, the prevailing view that pregnant women with hypertension are at low risk for cardiovascular complications within the short duration of pregnancy may be true for young, otherwise healthy women, but not those with advanced age at first pregnancy (a trend commonly described in developed countries), who may have subclinical evidence of vascular damage. New evidence that has emerged with respect to the pathophysiology of preeclampsia and the possible benefits of early treatment of hypertension in the general population may affect future guidelines for the management of hypertension in pregnancy.

A study of 29 women with severe preeclampsia who developed strokes indicated that the systolic blood pressure was 155 mmHg or more in all women before the stroke. In contrast, the diastolic blood pressure was 105 mmHg or more in only 20 % of the affected women [34]. The authors suggested a paradigm shift and recommended the initiation of antihypertensive therapy when the systolic blood pressure reaches or exceeds 155–160 mmHg. In addition, posterior reversible encephalopathy syndrome (PRES), a clinically recognizable entity of neurological signs and symptoms, coupled with the neuroimaging findings of vasogenic edema in the posterior circulation, seems to occur at lower peak systolic blood pressure readings in pregnant [35, 36] compared to nonpregnant patients with hypertensive encephalopathy [35, 37]. One possible explanation is that the threshold at which an elevation in blood pressure may lead to brain edema may be decreased in pregnancy [38]. Finally, recent studies in nonpregnant populations have shown that treatment of hypertension of even short duration may decrease subsequent cardiovascular risks, i.e., result in better outcomes with earlier and more effective treatment [39, 40]. However, extrapolating these findings to hypertensive pregnant patients is difficult, mainly due to the significant differences in their overall cardiovascular risks, but underscores the need for future research focusing on immediate and long-term cardiovascular outcomes, as functions of blood pressure control, over the course of pregnancy.

Timing of Delivery

The decision to proceed with delivery can be made only after a careful assessment of risks to the fetus and mother. Consideration should be given to postponing delivery in pregnancies affected by preeclampsia before 32 weeks gestation, as the fetus is still immature and may suffer profound consequences due to incomplete respiratory development. This approach is only reasonable in cases where the maternal risk is relatively low, such as in mild hypertension without evidence of hepatic or cerebral involvement. Outpatient management can be considered for mild preeclampsia: an asymptomatic patient with treatment-responsive hypertension in the absence of marked proteinuria (<1 g/24 h) undergoing regular monitoring for evidence of progression to more severe disease.

Induction of labor should be entertained in circumstances of adequate fetal development or progression to severe forms of hypertensive disease, irrespective of fetal maturity. For women requiring delivery prior to 34 weeks gestation, corticosteroid therapy should be initiated in order to accelerate fetal lung development. In the case of severe hypertension, a trial of antihypertensive therapy may be undertaken. If an adequate response is not observed in 24–48 h, the high risk of maternal cerebral or cardiac events should prompt consideration of delivery. Other indications for urgent delivery include HELLP syndrome, progressive renal failure, premonitory signs of eclampsia, or fetal distress.

Future Complications

Traditionally, the cardiovascular complications of hypertensive pregnancy disorders were believed to be confined to pregnancy, and elimination of the placenta was felt to be akin to cure. In recent years, however, observational studies have consistently demonstrated that women with a history of hypertensive pregnancies are more likely to develop hypertension, ischemic heart disease, or stroke later in life [41]. The highest risk was reported for women with severe forms of preeclampsia who delivered prematurely. The likely mechanism for this association is that these two conditions share several common risk factors, such as renal disease and diabetes mellitus, which may lead to hypertensive pregnancy disorders and cardiovascular disease at different times in a woman's life. Alternatively, hypertensive pregnancy disorders may result in metabolic and vascular changes that might increase the overall cardiovascular risk later in life [42]. Either way, a history of hypertensive pregnancy disorders may aid in identifying women at risk for future cardiovascular disease. Primary prevention in these women should focus on lifestyle modifications (exercise, weight loss, and smoking cessation), early detection of cardiovascular disease risk factors, and treatment according to evidence-based national guidelines [43].

> **Key Points**
> - The etiology and pathogenesis of preeclampsia remain elusive.
> - No reliable early marker for preeclampsia currently exists.
> - The risk for superimposed preeclampsia is ≥25 % in women with a history of chronic hypertension.
> - The only definitive treatment for preeclampsia and eclampsia is delivery.
> - The goal of hypertension treatment is to prevent maternal cardiovascular complications, as treatment of hypertension does not prevent preeclampsia.
> - Severe maternal complications include stroke, acute renal failure, and acute cardiac decompensation; adverse fetal outcomes include prematurity, intrauterine growth retardation, and intrauterine demise.
> - Affected women may be at a greater risk for cardiovascular disease later in life. As such, they should receive advice regarding established preventive lifestyle measures, and their modifiable risk factors should be treated according to current guidelines.

Summary of the Key Guidelines

The National High Blood Pressure Education Program (NHBPEP) Working Group on High Blood Pressure in Pregnancy [1]

1. Classification of the hypertensive pregnancy disorders
   - Chronic hypertension
   - Preeclampsia-eclampsia

- Preeclampsia superimposed on chronic hypertension
- Gestational hypertension
2. Diagnostic criteria
   - Hypertension: blood pressure ≥140 mmHg systolic and/or ≥90 mmHg diastolic on 2 occasions at least 6 h apart
   - Proteinuria (which, together with hypertension, represent the diagnostic criteria for preeclampsia): ≥300 mg of protein in a 24-h urine specimen. When a 24-h specimen cannot be obtained, or if a diagnosis is urgently required, a dipstick result of 1+ or greater or a protein-to-creatinine ratio of 0.3 g/24 h
3. Treatment goals
   - Diastolic blood pressure <105 mmHg for acute hypertension associated with preeclampsia
   - Blood pressure <150/100 mmHg in pregnant patients with chronic hypertension
4. Preferred agents
   - Methyldopa for oral use
   - Hydralazine for intravenous use

Effectiveness-Based Guidelines for the Prevention of Cardiovascular Disease in Women: 2011 Update: A Guideline from the American Heart Association [43]

1. Preeclampsia may be an early indicator of cardiovascular risk.
2. A careful and detailed history of pregnancy complications should be obtained from women later in their lives.
3. Postpartum referral to a primary care physician or cardiologist, such that risk factors can be monitored and controlled years after pregnancy; their conventional risk factors should be treated according to current evidence-based guidelines.

References

1. Anonymous. Report of the National High Blood Pressure Education Program Working Group on high blood pressure in pregnancy. Am J Obstet Gynecol. 2000;183:S1–22 [comment].
2. MacKay AP, Berg CJ, Atrash HK. Pregnancy-related mortality from preeclampsia and eclampsia. Obstet Gynecol. 2001;97:533–8.
3. Garovic VD, Hayman SR. Hypertension in pregnancy: an emerging risk factor for cardiovascular disease. Nat Clin Pract Nephrol. 2007;3:613–22.
4. Garovic VD, Bailey KR, Boerwinkle E, Hunt SC, Weder AB, Curb JD, Mosley TH, Wiste JW, Turner ST. Hypertension in pregnancy as a risk factor for cardiovascular disease later in life. J Hypertens. 2010;28:826–33.
5. McLaughlin M, Roberts JM. Hemodynamic changes. In: Lindheimer MD, Roberts JM, Cunningham FG, editors. Chesley's hypertensive disorders in pregnancy. Stamford: Appleton & Lange; 1999. p. 69–102.
6. Roberts JM. Endothelial dysfunction in preeclampsia. Semin Reprod Endocrinol. 1998;16:5–15.
7. Ramsey EM. The story of the spiral arteries. J Reprod Med. 1981; 26:393–9.
8. Pijnenborg R, Anthony J, Davey DA, Rees A, Tiltman A, Vercruysse L, van Assche A. Placental bed spiral arteries in the hypertensive disorders of pregnancy. Br J Obstet Gynaecol. 1991;98:648–55.
9. Brosens JJ, Pijnenborg R, Brosens IA. The myometrial junctional zone spiral arteries in normal and abnormal pregnancies: a review of the literature. Am J Obstet Gynecol. 2002;187:1416–23.
10. Khong TY, De Wolf F, Robertson WB, Brosens I. Inadequate maternal vascular response to placentation in pregnancies complicated by pre-eclampsia and by small-for-gestational age infants. Br J Obstet Gynaecol. 1986;93:1049–59.
11. Meekins JW, Pijnenborg R, Hanssens M, McFadyen IR, van Asshe A. A study of placental bed spiral arteries and trophoblast invasion in normal and severe pre-eclamptic pregnancies. Br J Obstet Gynaecol. 1994;101:669–74.
12. Genbacev O, Zhou Y, Ludlow JW, Fisher SJ. Regulation of human placental development by oxygen tension. Science. 1997;277: 1669–72.
13. Levine RJ, Maynard SE, Qian C, Lim KH, England LJ, Yu KF, Schisterman EF, Thadhani R, Sachs BP, Epstein FH, Sibai BM, Sukhatme VP, Karumanchi SA. Circulating angiogenic factors and the risk of preeclampsia. N Engl J Med. 2004;350:672–83 [see comment].
14. Maynard SE, Min JY, Merchan J, Lim KH, Li J, Mondal S, Libermann TA, Morgan JP, Sellke FW, Stillman IE, Epstein FH, Sukhatme VP, Karumanchi SA. Excess placental soluble fms-like tyrosine kinase 1 (sFlt1) may contribute to endothelial dysfunction, hypertension, and proteinuria in preeclampsia. J Clin Invest. 2003; 111:649–58 [see comment].
15. Widmer M, Villar J, Benigni A, Conde-Agudelo A, Karumanchi SA, Lindheimer M. Mapping the theories of preeclampsia and the role of angiogenic factors: a systematic review. Obstet Gynecol. 2007;109:168–80.
16. Garovic VD, Wagner SJ, Petrovic LM, Gray CE, Hall P, Sugimoto H, Kalluri R, Grande JP. Glomerular expression of nephrin and synaptopodin, but not podocin, is decreased in kidney sections from women with preeclampsia. Nephrol Dial Transplant. 2007;22: 1136–43.
17. Garovic VD, Wagner SJ, Turner ST, Rosenthal DW, Watson WJ, Brost BC, Rose CH, Gavrilova L, Craigo P, Bailey KR, Achenbach J, Schiffer M, Grande JP. Urinary podocyte excretion as a marker for preeclampsia. Am J Obstet Gynecol. 2007;196:320.e321–7 [see comment].
18. Steegers EA, Eskes TK, Jongsma HW, Hein PR. Dietary sodium restriction during pregnancy; a historical review. Eur J Obstet Gynecol Reprod Biol. 1991;40:83–90.
19. Caritis S, Sibai B, Hauth J, Lindheimer MD, Klebanoff M, Thom E, VanDorsten P, Landon M, Paul R, Miodovnik M, Meis P, Thurnau G. Low-dose aspirin to prevent preeclampsia in women at high risk. National institute of child health and human development network of maternal-fetal medicine units. N Engl J Med. 1998;338:701–5.
20. Roberts JM, Myatt L, Spong CY, Thom EA, Hauth JC, Leveno KJ, Pearson GD, Wapner RJ, Varner MW, Thorp Jr JM, Mercer BM, Peaceman AM, Ramin SM, Carpenter MW, Samuels P, Sciscione A, Harper M, Smith WJ, Saade G, Sorokin Y, Anderson GB. Vitamins C and E to prevent complications of pregnancy-associated hypertension. N Engl J Med. 2010;362:1282–91.
21. Levine RJ, Hauth JC, Curet LB, Sibai BM, Catalano PM, Morris CD, DerSimonian R, Esterlitz JR, Raymond EG, Bild DE, Clemens JD, Cutler JA. Trial of calcium to prevent preeclampsia. N Engl J Med. 1997;337:69–76.
22. Spatling L, Spatling G. Magnesium supplementation in pregnancy. A double-blind study. Br J Obstet Gynaecol. 1988;95:120–5.

23. Weinstein L. Syndrome of hemolysis, elevated liver enzymes, and low platelet count: a severe consequence of hypertension in pregnancy. Am J Obstet Gynecol. 1982;142:159–67.

24. Wagner SJ, Craici IM, Hogan MC, Bailey KR, Garovic VD. The effect of early diagnosis and treatment on maternal and fetal outcomes in patients with HELLP syndrome. Biochem Med. 2007;17:60–70.

25. Duley L, Gulmezoglu AM, Henderson-Smart DJ, Chou D. Magnesium sulphate and other anticonvulsants for women with pre-eclampsia. Cochrane Database Syst Rev. 2010;CD000025.

26. Abalos E, Duley L, Steyn DW, Henderson-Smart DJ. Antihypertensive drug therapy for mild to moderate hypertension during pregnancy. Cochrane Database Syst Rev. 2007;CD002252

27. Ferrer RL, Sibai BM, Mulrow CD, Chiquette E, Stevens KR, Cornell J. Management of mild chronic hypertension during pregnancy: a review. Obstet Gynecol. 2000;96:849–60.

28. August P. Preeclampsia: new thoughts on an ancient problem. J Clin Hypertens. 2000;2:115–23.

29. Cooper WO, Hernandez-Diaz S, Arbogast PG, Dudley JA, Dyer S, Gideon PS, Hall K, Ray WA. Major congenital malformations after first-trimester exposure to ace inhibitors. N Engl J Med. 2006;354:2443–51.

30. Gant NF, Madden JD, Siteri PK, MacDonald PC. The metabolic clearance rate of dehydroisoandrosterone sulfate. III. The effect of thiazide diuretics in normal and future pre-eclamptic pregnancies. Am J Obstet Gynecol. 1975;123:159–63.

31. Collins R, Yusuf S, Peto R. Overview of randomised trials of diuretics in pregnancy. Br Med J. 1985;290:17–23.

32. von Dadelszen P, Ornstein MP, Bull SB, Logan AG, Koren G, Magee LA. Fall in mean arterial pressure and fetal growth restriction in pregnancy hypertension: a meta-analysis. Lancet. 2000;355:87–92.

33. Berg CJ, Callaghan WM, Syverson C, Henderson Z. Pregnancy-related mortality in the united states, 1998–2005. Obstet Gynecol. 2010;116:1302–9.

34. Martin Jr JN, Thigpen BD, Moore RC, Rose CH, Cushman J, May W. Stroke and severe preeclampsia and eclampsia: a paradigm shift focusing on systolic blood pressure. Obstet Gynecol. 2005;105:246–54.

35. Hinchey J, Chaves C, Appignani B, Breen J, Pao L, Wang A, Pessin MS, Lamy C, Mas JL, Caplan LR. A reversible posterior leukoencephalopathy syndrome. N Engl J Med. 1996;334:494–500.

36. Wagner SJ, Acquah L, Lindell E, Craici I, Wingo M, Rose C, White W, August P, Garovic V. Posterior reversible encephalopathy syndrome (PRES) and eclampsia: pressing the case for more aggressive blood pressure control. Mayo Clin Proc. 2011;86(9):851–6.

37. Fugate JE, Claassen DO, Cloft HJ, Kallmes DF, Kozak OS, Rabinstein AA. Posterior reversible encephalopathy syndrome: associated clinical and radiologic findings. Mayo Clin Proc. 2010;85:427–32.

38. Cipolla MJ. Cerebrovascular function in pregnancy and eclampsia. Hypertension. 2007;50:14–24.

39. Gradman AH, Basile JN, Carter BL, Bakris GL. Combination therapy in hypertension. J Am Soc Hypertens. 2010;4:42–50.

40. Weber MA, Julius S, Kjeldsen SE, Brunner HR, Ekman S, Hansson L, Hua T, Laragh JH, McInnes GT, Mitchell L, Plat F, Schork MA, Smith B, Zanchetti A. Blood pressure dependent and independent effects of antihypertensive treatment on clinical events in the value trial. Lancet. 2004;363:2049–51.

41. Bellamy L, Casas JP, Hingorani AD, Williams DJ. Pre-eclampsia and risk of cardiovascular disease and cancer in later life: systematic review and meta-analysis. BMJ. 2007;335:974 [see comment].

42. Zeeman GG, Fleckenstein JL, Twickler DM, Cunningham FG. Cerebral infarction in eclampsia. Am J Obstet Gynecol. 2004;190:714–20.

43. Mosca L, Benjamin EJ, Berra K, Bezanson JL, Dolor RJ, Lloyd-Jones DM, Newby LK, Piña IL, Roger VL, Shaw LJ, Zhao D, Beckie TM, Bushnell C, D'Armiento J, Kris-Etherton PM, Fang J, Ganiats TG, Gomes AS, Gracia CR, Haan CK, Jackson EA, Judelson DR, Kelepouris E, Lavie CJ, Moore A, Nussmeier NA, Ofili E, Oparil S, Ouyang P, Pinn VW, Sherif K, Smith SC, Sopko G, Chandra-Strobos N, Urbina EM, Vaccarino V, Wenger NK. Effectiveness-based guidelines for the prevention of cardiovascular disease in women – 2011 update. Circulation. 2011;123:1243–62.

44. Garovic VD. The role of angiogenic factors in the prediction and diagnosis of preeclampsia superimposed on chronic hypertension. Hypertension. 2012;59(3):555–7.

Cardiomyopathies, Heart Failure, and Pregnancy

31

Kathleen Stergiopoulos

Abstract

Women with cardiomyopathy are at risk for complications during and after pregnancy if they are unable to adapt to the hemodynamic changes of pregnancy. The hemodynamic challenges of pregnancy, labor, and delivery pose unique risks to this group of patients which can result in clinical decompensation with overt heart failure, arrhythmias, and even maternal death. A multidisciplinary approach and a controlled delivery are crucial to adequate management of patients with underlying heart disease. Preconception planning, proper counseling, and accurate risk assessment are essential and should be offered to women of childbearing age. In this chapter, the risk assessment of pregnancy in women with cardiomyopathy will be reviewed. In addition, the management of pregnant women with cardiomyopathies and heart failure will be discussed including consideration of issues at the time of labor and delivery.

Keywords

Cardiomyopathy • Pregnancy • Dilated cardiomyopathy • Heart failure • Hypertrophic cardiomyopathy • Noncompaction cardiomyopathy • BNP

Introduction

The hemodynamic changes that occur during pregnancy challenge the adaptability of the cardiovascular system in patients with preexisting heart disease. The greater metabolic and hemodynamic needs of pregnancy are accompanied by changes in blood volume, peripheral vascular resistance, and cardiac output. In women with underlying cardiomyopathy, however, the demands of pregnancy, labor, and delivery pose additional stressors that can lead to clinical decompensation, arrhythmias, and maternal death [1]. Although heart disease is present in only 0.2–4 % of all pregnant women in the industrialized world [2], data from the

K. Stergiopoulos, MD, PhD, FASE, FACC, FAHA
Division of Cardiology, Department of Medicine,
Stony Brook University School of Medicine,
Nichols Road, Health Sciences Center, T16-080,
Stony Brook, NY 11530-8167, USA
e-mail: kathleen.stergiopoulos@stonybrookmedicine.edu

United Kingdom suggests that a cardiac etiology is the most common cause of death among pregnant women in the developed world [3, 4]. Data from the Centers for Disease Control suggests that pregnancy-related mortality increased in the United States from 1998 to 2005 and the proportion of deaths related to cardiovascular disease has also increased [5, 6]. In a study that examined the characteristics of delivery and postpartum hospitalizations from 1995 to 2006 in the United States, about 1.4 % of delivery hospitalizations were complicated by chronic heart disease; an increase was found for specific congenital heart disease conditions, cardiac arrhythmias, cardiomyopathy, and congestive heart failure [7]. Moreover, the rate of postpartum hospitalizations in patients with chronic heart disease has tripled. Severe complications associated with delivery were more common in 2004–2006 than they were from 1995 to 1997 in patients with chronic heart disease. Registry data on pregnancy in women with heart disease have demonstrated a maternal mortality of 1 %, which may seem low but is 100 times higher than in healthy pregnant patients [8].

K. Stergiopoulos, D.L. Brown (eds.), *Evidence-Based Cardiology Consult*,
DOI 10.1007/978-1-4471-4441-0_31, © Springer-Verlag London 2014

Outcomes of pregnant women with preexisting dilated cardiomyopathy have been recently examined [9]. Heart failure, which typically occurred late in the pregnancy or postpartum, was the most common complication. Moreover, registry data has demonstrated that maternal mortality for pregnant women with heart disease was highest in the patients with cardiomyopathy [8]. In this chapter, cardiomyopathies that affect women of childbearing age and prepregnancy risk assessment will be reviewed. In addition, evaluation of cardiomyopathy during pregnancy, labor, and delivery will be addressed. Peripartum cardiomyopathy will not be discussed in detail, as this subject is as addressed in Chap. 33 [10–15].

Cardiomyopathy in Women of Childbearing Age

A diverse set of potential etiologies of cardiomyopathy exist for women of childbearing age. Table 31.1 outlines these etiologies, in no particular order or degree of incidence. Future studies are required to determine the incidence in developing and industrialized countries. Initial findings of the European Registry on Pregnancy and Heart disease (ROPAC) documented a 7 % prevalence of cardiomyopathy of 1,321 pregnant women with heart disease between 2007 and 2011 [8]. The most common etiologies described were dilated

Table 31.1 Etiologies of cardiomyopathy that affect women of childbearing age

Idiopathic dilated cardiomyopathy
Myocarditis
Viral cardiomyopathy
Chagas' disease
Lyme disease
Human immunodeficiency virus (HIV) infection
Ischemic heart disease
Infiltrative disease (restrictive cardiomyopathy)
Hypertrophic cardiomyopathy
Peripartum cardiomyopathy
Hypertensive disorders
Chemotherapy related (doxorubicin, trastuzumab)
Connective tissue disease (systemic lupus erythematosus)
Substance abuse (alcohol, cocaine)
Other
Stress-induced (takotsubo) cardiomyopathy
Noncompaction cardiomyopathy
Tachycardia-mediated cardiomyopathy
Endocrine related (thyroid dysfunction, acromegaly, pheochromocytoma)
Inherited/familial cardiomyopathy
Arrhythmogenic right ventricular dysplasia
Obstructive sleep apnea

Adapted with permission from Stergiopoulos et al. [16]

cardiomyopathy, peripartum cardiomyopathy, hypertrophic cardiomyopathy, and "other," which may include chemotherapy-related cardiomyopathy, among others. The differential diagnosis of heart failure in pregnancy is broad and includes valvular etiologies (aortic stenosis, aortic regurgitation, mitral stenosis, and mitral regurgitation), previously undiagnosed congenital heart disease, hypertensive heart disease, pregnancy associated myocardial infarction, and eclampsia or preeclampsia.

Preconception Evaluation, Risk Assessment, and Counseling

Preconception Evaluation

Women with known or suspected cardiomyopathy require a complete preconception evaluation and counseling in order to stratify the maternal and fetal risks of pregnancy. Preconception risk assessment and counseling are now considered class I recommendations by the European Society of Cardiology (ESC) for the management of pregnant women with cardiac disease as well as by American College of Cardiology/American Heart Association (ACC/AHA) guidelines for adults with congenital heart disease [17, 18]. A detailed history and physical exam, assessment of exercise capacity with New York Heart Association (NYHA) functional class, and a 12-lead electrocardiogram are essential (Table 31.2). Echocardiography is indicated in women with a history of known or suspected cardiomyopathy, valvular or congenital heart disease that may result in systemic ventricular dysfunction, significant dyspnea, or any symptoms or signs of heart failure [16]. Moreover, the echocardiogram can determine the etiology of the cardiomyopathy if not previously known and quantify the degree of pulmonary

Table 31.2 Preconception evaluation

Thorough history of cardiac symptoms and physical exam
12-lead electrocardiogram
Baseline exercise tolerance and NYHA functional class (exercise testing if needed)
Baseline echocardiogram
Assessment of ventricular function (right and left)
Assessment of pulmonary artery pressure
Presence and degree of valvular dysfunction
Assessment of stability of cardiac hemodynamics over time
Effective contraception until pregnancy desired
Adjustment of medications to prevent adverse fetal events
Genetics referral for patients with heritable cardiac lesion
Risk assessment of pregnancy, labor, and delivery
Discussion regarding breast feeding and need for medical therapy

Adapted with permission from Stergiopoulos et al. [16]
NYHA New York Heart Association Class

Table 31.3 Risk stratification for pregnant patients with cardiac disease

Risk assessment for adverse maternal and fetal outcomes based on CARPREG data

Any prior cardiac event or arrhythmia (heart failure, transient ischemic attack, stroke before pregnancy)

Baseline NYHA functional class >II or cyanosis

Systemic ventricular dysfunction (ejection fraction <40 %)

Left heart obstruction

    Mitral valve area <2 cm^2

    Aortic valve area <1.5 cm^2

    Peak LV outflow tract gradient >30 mmHg by echocardiography

Adapted from Siu et al. [23]

CARPREG risk score: For each predictor of adverse event, a point is assigned. Risk estimation of cardiovascular maternal complications is as follows:

0 point: 5 %

1 point: 27 %

>1 point: 75 %

NYHA New York Heart Association, *LV* left ventricular

Table 31.4 General principles of modified World Health Organization (WHO) classification of maternal cardiovascular risk

Risk class	Risk of pregnancy by medical condition
I	No detectable increased risk of maternal mortality and no/mild increase in morbidity
II	Small increased risk of maternal mortality or moderate increase in morbidity
III	Significantly increased risk of maternal mortality or severe morbidity. Expert counseling required. If pregnancy is decided upon, the intensive care specialist's cardiac and obstetric monitoring is needed throughout pregnancy, childbirth, and the postpartum period
IV	Extremely high risk of maternal mortality or severe comorbidity; pregnancy contraindicated. If pregnancy occurs termination should be discussed. If pregnancy continues, care as for class III

Adapted with permission from Regitz-Zagrosek et al. [17]

hypertension, valvular dysfunction, and left ventricular or systemic ventricular systolic function [19]. Poor functional status has been previously associated with maternal or fetal complications [20]. Functional capacity may be an important predictor of the ability to tolerate a pregnancy, regardless of the underlying lesion. In a recent study examining pregnancy outcomes in women with congenital heart disease, an abnormal chronotropic response to exercise correlated with adverse pregnancy outcomes [21]. Prior to conception, adjustment of medications to prevent adverse fetal events and toxicity should be addressed. Some women may require a genetics referral if a heritable cardiac lesion is known or suspected.

Estimation of Maternal Pregnancy Risk

In order to estimate the risk of pregnancy in a woman with preexisting heart disease, several approaches are now available. In general, the risk of complications increases with increasing disease complexity [22]. Risk estimation can be carried out using risk scores derived from studies involving diverse groups of women with various forms of heart disease. Siu and colleagues [23] developed a commonly used risk score (CARPREG; Table 31.3) to identify predictors of the development of unfavorable cardiac events in pregnant women with heart disease. This risk assessment may be used to allow for the establishment of a plan of management for the antepartum, peripartum, and postpartum periods. The risk score has been validated in several studies, although overestimation has been described [24]. Among pregnant women with known cardiac disease, poor prognostic factors include any of the following: prior cardiac events, prior arrhythmias, a NYHA functional class >II, peripheral

cyanosis, significant valvular or outflow tract obstruction, and systemic ventricular dysfunction with left ventricular ejection fraction (LVEF) <40 % [23, 25, 26]. When one or more of these features are combined, the risk is more than additive [23, 25, 26]. Women at elevated risk for adverse events should be managed by a multidisciplinary team at a tertiary care center equipped with the expertise to handle high-risk pregnancies – now considered a class I recommendation by the European Society of Cardiology (ESC) [27]. As part of a complete risk assessment, plans for monitoring at the time of labor and delivery and postpartum, type of delivery, anesthetic concerns, and need for antibiotic prophylaxis should be addressed.

The Task Force on the Management of Cardiovascular Diseases during pregnancy from the ESC recommends that maternal risk assessment be carried out according to a modified World Health Organization (WHO) risk classification [17, 28]. The WHO risk assessment integrates all known maternal cardiovascular risk factors including comorbid conditions and underlying heart disease. The application of previous risk assessment models has been limited by the inclusion of mainly congenital patients. The basic principles are shown in Table 31.4. In patients who are categorized as WHO class I, pregnancy risk for adverse events is very low and cardiology follow-up during pregnancy can be limited to 1–2 visits. In those patients who are WHO II, pregnancy risk is considered low or moderate, and follow-up every trimester at a minimum is indicated. For women who are WHO III, there is a high risk of complications and frequent (often monthly or twice monthly) visits are required. In conditions in which pregnancy is WHO IV, pregnancy is contraindicated. Notably, women at particularly high risk include those with pulmonary hypertension of any cause (Eisenmenger's syndrome), Marfan syndrome with aortopathy (aortic root >45 mm) [29], a history of peripartum cardiomyopathy with any residual impairment of left ventricular function, and severe left ventricular dysfunction (LVEF <30 %, NYHA III–IV) [15]. In these situations, patients are counseled against pregnancy altogether. In patients who become pregnant, termination should be offered. If termination is determined to be an unacceptable option for the patient, the pregnancy is considered high risk and is treated as WHO III.

Preconception Counseling

Along with preconception risk assessment, preconception counseling is essential [17, 30]. A study of women with congenital heart disease found that more than one third of women could not recall if they were ever counseled by a health-care provider or if they were ever informed of an increased risk for maternal complications [31]. Moreover, a similar proportion could not recall whether they were told of an increased risk of congenital heart disease in their offspring. Strict prenatal care and early risk stratification are fundamental measures to improve the prognosis of pregnancy in women with heart disease.

Contraceptive Choices in Women with Cardiomyopathies

Choice of contraception requires consideration of pregnancy risk, available contraception options as well as their risks and benefits, failure rates, understanding the consequences of unplanned pregnancy, and the preferences of the woman. Cardiologists are responsible for educating women about safe contraceptive options as they relate to their cardiac condition, a position recently endorsed by professional societies [28]. Furthermore, it is now a class I recommendation from the ESC guidelines that prepregnancy and postconception risk assessments and counseling are performed in all women with known or suspected congenital or acquired heart or aortic disease [14]. There is considerable room for improvement in this area. In a survey of women with congenital heart disease, it was noted that only half of the women surveyed had recalled receiving specific information about contraception from a nurse or physician [26] and many women do not use adequate methods of birth control [30].

Contraceptive options include (1) combined hormonal contraceptives (COCs; estrogen/progestin formulations), (2) progestin-only formulations, (3) intrauterine devices, (4) barrier methods, and (5) sterilization/permanent forms of contraception [31, 32]. The most comprehensive guidance comes from a British working group that developed guidelines for the use of COCs in women with heart disease using the WHO format [31, 33–35], which has recently been modified by the Centers for Disease Control [36]. Both estrogen and progestins have adverse cardiac effects. However, the most clinically important are those of estrogens which can cause thromboembolic events and hypertension. In women with severe systemic ventricular dysfunction, maternal complication rates of pregnancy are high and pregnancy is contraindicated. Due to the potential for thromboembolic complications, combined hormonal contraceptives in the form of pills, transdermal patches, or vaginal rings are not recommended. Monthly injectable formulations that contain medroxyprogesterone acetate are no longer appropriate for patients with heart failure because of the tendency for fluid retention [36]. Barrier methods and the levonorgestrel-releasing intrauterine devices are the safest and most effective options that can be used in women with cardiomyopathy and reduced systemic ventricular function, cyanotic heart disease, and advanced pulmonary hypertension [36]. A detailed discussion regarding family planning is indicated so that patients can better understand the risks of pregnancy and contraception.

Diagnosis of Heart Failure in Pregnancy

The clinical diagnosis of heart failure can be complicated in a pregnant woman. Symptoms such as dyspnea, fluid retention, palpitations, and fatigue are common in normal pregnancy. However, complaints of marked dyspnea on exertion, paroxysmal nocturnal dyspnea, orthopnea, and recumbent cough are most often pathologic. The physical examination findings of a normal pregnancy can often mimic disease. A thorough physical and echocardiographic evaluation can often clarify the differences between physiologic and pathologic changes. Serial physical examinations, as well as echocardiographic evaluations during pregnancy, perhaps as often as once a trimester, can aid in determining changes in clinical status and assist in the early diagnosis of heart failure. Physical examination findings such as the evaluation of jugular veins should be performed in the left lateral decubitus position so that the gravid uterus and fetus do not compress the inferior vena cava, inhibiting venous return. Mildly elevated jugular venous pressure is not pathologic in a pregnant woman. The presence of an S3 gallop in a patient with cardiomyopathy is nearly always pathologic, while an S3 can be noted in normal pregnant patients without any history of cardiac disease. An S4 gallop in any pregnant woman is always pathologic and should warrant further evaluation. Lower extremity edema, when more than mild, is often pathologic, especially when severe or progressive. However, lower extremity edema is common and can have multiple etiologies in the pregnant woman (i.e., deep vein thrombosis, nephrotic syndrome, heart failure). Pulmonary crackles are always pathologic in pregnancy.

Brain Natriuretic Peptide in Pregnancy

Increases in volume load during pregnancy are thought to be a central factor ultimately responsible for most cardiovascular clinical events. In the nonpregnant state, B-type natriuretic peptide (BNP) increases in response to this type of volume load and predicts adverse outcomes in a variety of cardiac conditions [32]. While clinical and echocardiographic predictors have been described [23], risk stratification of pregnant women with cardiomyopathy remains incomplete. BNP can be useful in the adjudication of suspected clinical events in pregnant women with heart disease [33]. BNP levels are elevated in many women with heart disease during pregnancy, compared with normal pregnant controls. Importantly, normal BNP values in women with heart disease predict a low probability of adverse events. While there is no definite cutoff value in pregnancy, BNP values of <100 pg/ml have a very high negative predictive value for adverse events. Notably, this data was derived from a study that included 20 % of women with cardiomyopathy and left ventricular dysfunction, suggesting that BNP measurement can be useful in this population. BNP was highest in this group of patients, in both those with and without clinical

events, suggesting that the volume load of pregnancy may be at least in part responsible for clinical deterioration. Future studies are required in larger numbers of women with heart disease and pregnancy. Nevertheless, BNP offers an attractive option for the potential early identification of deterioration in status, before acute events occur. This is particularly important in pregnant women with cardiomyopathy, as decompensation can be abrupt and adverse events harm both the mother and fetus.

Outcomes in Women with Cardiomyopathy in Pregnancy

Dilated Cardiomyopathy

Dilated cardiomyopathy (DCM) is defined as dilation of the left ventricle with impairment of systolic function (Fig. 31.1). Many causes of DCM have been identified, some of which are listed on Table 31.1. However, in up to 50 % of cases, the etiology is not identified [34] and is termed idiopathic. Genetic causes are exceedingly rare, with an estimated prevalence of 1:2,500 [35]. Pregnancy in women with dilated

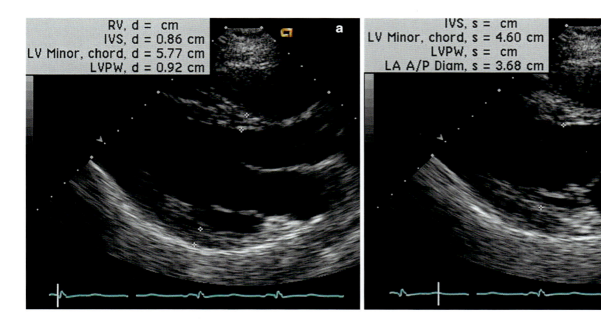

Fig. 31.1 A pregnant woman with familial dilated cardiomyopathy. A 25-year-old woman with a history of familial dilated cardiomyopathy with moderately reduced left ventricular systolic function prior to pregnancy. She had an implantable cardioverter defibrillator (ICD) placed for primary prevention of sudden cardiac death prior to pregnancy. She was hospitalized at 26 weeks gestation for congestive heart failure and appropriate ICD firing for ventricular tachycardia and was managed with in-hospital bed rest and medically with carvedilol, sotalol, and intermittent intravenous furosemide. She developed worsening heart failure and worsening left ventricular systolic dysfunction (LVEF

declined from 35 to 25 %) at 30–32 weeks gestation. Her heart failure was refractory and she was delivered at 33 weeks by urgent Cesarean section with epidural anesthesia and sedation and central and arterial lines for closer monitoring of her hemodynamics. Her postpartum course was unremarkable without further heart failure or arrhythmia. Panel **a** Parasternal long axis view (end-diastolic dimension) demonstrating mild left ventricular dilation and tethering of the mitral leaflets. Panel **b** Parasternal long axis view (end-systolic dimension). Panel **c** M-mode of the left ventricle demonstrating poor contractility, consistent with severe left ventricular systolic dysfunction

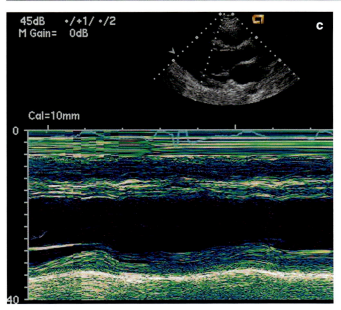

Fig. 31.1 (continued)

Late Effects of Pregnancy on the Cardiomyopathic Heart

Pregnancy appears to alter the natural history of the disease over the short term, perhaps partly related to the hemodynamic load of pregnancy, labor, and delivery, as well as the discontinuation of many crucial medications for the management of heart failure due to patient preference or contraindications. In women with moderate or severe left ventricular dysfunction, the 16-month event-free survival was worse in pregnant women compared with nonpregnant controls with a similar degree of baseline left ventricular impairment [9] (Fig. 31.2). Some authors propose increased oxidative stress causing additional damage to the left ventricle as a potential mechanism for worsening heart failure and event-free survival [38]. Future research is required to elucidate mechanisms of worsening left ventricular function during and after pregnancy.

cardiomyopathy has been associated with poor maternal outcomes. As such, pregnancy in women with a cardiomyopathy and LVEF <30 % are classified as WHO IV and is, therefore, contraindicated. Potential complications include arrhythmias, thromboembolism, heart failure, worsening left ventricular systolic function, and sudden cardiac death. Women with documented idiopathic or doxorubicin-induced cardiomyopathy with mild–severe left ventricular systolic dysfunction were examined as part of a larger prospective cohort study [9]. Nearly 40 % of pregnancies were complicated by at least 1 maternal cardiac event, defined as pulmonary edema, sustained arrhythmia, stroke, angina, myocardial infarction, cardiac arrest, or cardiac death. There were no cardiac deaths in this study up to 6 months postpartum. The most common adverse events were arrhythmias and heart failure. Predictors of adverse events were moderate or severe left ventricular dysfunction and/or NYHA functional class III or IV [9]. In a study of pregnant women with either dilated cardiomyopathy or peripartum cardiomyopathy from India, maternal mortality was nearly 16 % [36]. The mean ejection fraction was 32 % and approximately half were NYHA class IV [9]. Other investigators have described worsening of NYHA class during pregnancy and worsening fractional shortening and left ventricular end-diastolic dimension [37]. Both maternal and fetal death rates are higher in developing countries than developed countries in women with heart disease [8]. In the European Registry on Pregnancy and Heart disease, the highest maternal mortality was found in patients with cardiomyopathy [8] who also had the highest rate of heart failure and ventricular arrhythmias.

Left Ventricular Noncompaction Cardiomyopathy

Left ventricular noncompaction cardiomyopathy, also known as noncompaction cardiomyopathy (NCCM), is a cardiomyopathy characterized by a distinctive hypertrabeculated morphological appearance of the myocardium (Fig. 31.3). It appears to be a familial disease in up to 60 % of patients, demonstrating an autosomal dominant inheritance pattern but with considerable genetic heterogeneity [35]. The exact prevalence of NCCM is unclear but it may not be as rare as previously thought due to increasing recognition and diagnosis. Several affected genes have been described, with beta-myosin heavy chain (*MHY7*) being the most common, followed by myosin binding protein C (*MYBPC3*) and cardiac troponin T (*TNNT2*). Noncompaction of the left ventricular myocardium is felt to be due to intrauterine arrest of endocardial compaction, a process by which the loose interwoven meshwork of myocardial fibers of the developing embryonic myocardium fails to condense and deep intertrabecular recesses remain, causing a spongy appearance [39]. The diagnosis of NCCM can be made using echocardiography or cardiac magnetic resonance imaging; noncompacted areas are usually in the apical, inferior, and lateral walls of the left ventricle. Echocardiographic contrast aids in the diagnosis [40], but little data exist to support its use or safety in pregnancy. Magnetic resonance imaging is considered safe, especially after the first trimester. However, the risks of gadolinium use in pregnancy are not known; its use is not advisable in pregnancy at any time [41]. Prognosis in nonpregnant patients with noncompaction cardiomyopathy depends on the presence of symptoms. Asymptomatic patients have a

Fig. 31.2 Comparison of cardiac outcome in pregnant versus nonpregnant women with significant left ventricular dysfunction. Sixteen-month survival free from adverse events in pregnant women (*dashed line*) compared with nonpregnant women (*solid line*). Time zero is defined as (1) the first antenatal visit for pregnant women and (2) the index visit to the heart failure clinic for nonpregnant women (With permission from Grewal et al. [9])

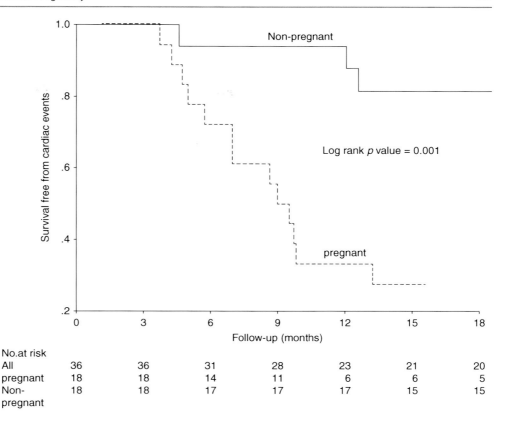

No.at risk							
	0	3	6	9	12	15	18
All	36	36	31	28	23	21	20
pregnant	18	18	14	11	6	6	5
Non-pregnant	18	18	17	17	17	15	15

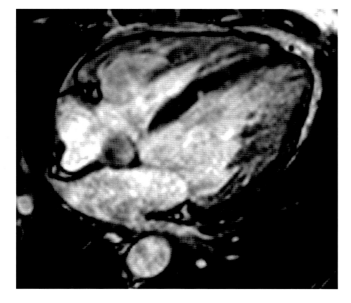

Fig. 31.3 Noncompaction cardiomyopathy. Four-chamber-view magnetic resonance imaging of a patient with noncompaction cardiomyopathy (Reproduced with permission from Stergiopoulos et al. [16])

good prognosis with few cardiovascular events [42], while patients presenting with heart failure (NYHA III or IV), sustained ventricular arrhythmias, stroke, embolic event, or an enlarged left atrium have an unfavorable prognosis [43]. Interestingly, left ventricular dimension and left ventricular systolic dysfunction are less strongly associated with outcome [42].

Experience with noncompaction cardiomyopathy and pregnancy is limited. Risk assessment would likely be similar to other cardiomyopathies during pregnancy. NCCM in itself has an increased thrombogenic risk with systemic embolism described in 4 % of symptomatic nonpregnant patients [42]. Moreover, pregnancy may be assumed to enhance this risk by inducing hypercoagulability. However, routine therapy with antiplatelet agents or anticoagulants cannot be routinely recommended in this group during pregnancy. Notably, underlying NCCM may be present in asymptomatic antepartum patents who cannot tolerate the hemodynamic stress of pregnancy resulting in clinical decompensation. Such a presentation may be confused with peripartum cardiomyopathy [44–47]. The importance of correctly diagnosing this type of cardiomyopathy relates to the classification of NCCM as a genetic disorder. First-degree relatives should be offered genetic screening and echocardiography to identify the disease in the asymptomatic phase [48].

Hypertrophic Cardiomyopathy

Hypertrophic cardiomyopathy (HCM) is the most common genetic cardiac disorder with an estimated prevalence of

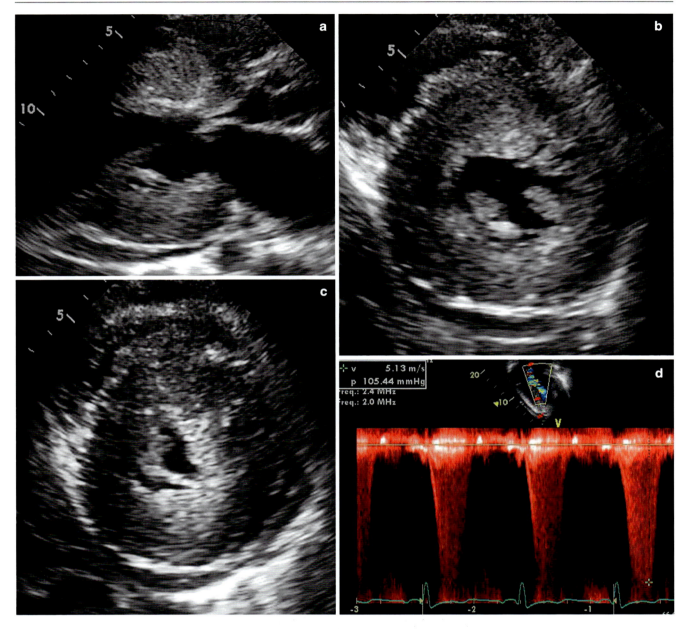

Fig. 31.4 Hypertrophic cardiomyopathy. Panel **a** Two-dimensional echocardiogram (parasternal long axis view) from a patient with hypertrophic cardiomyopathy who survived sudden cardiac death. The interventricular septum measures 3.1 cm. The common finding of a small posterior pericardial effusion is noted. Panels **b**, **c** End-diastolic (**b**) and systolic (**c**) short axis images demonstrating near obliteration of the left ventricular cavity at end systole. Panel **d** Continuous wave Doppler analysis of the left ventricular outflow tract (LVOT) obstruction (due to severe systolic anterior motion of the mitral valve, not shown) demonstrating severe LVOT obstruction (Figure reproduced with permission from Vainrib and Stergiopoulos [49])

1:500. Familial occurrence is as high as 90 %, mainly with autosomal dominant inheritance. Abnormalities in more than ten known genes are described, but mutations of the beta-myosin heavy chain and myosin binding protein C are the most commonly affected genes [35]. HCM is characterized by pathologic hypertrophy of the left ventricle, resulting in obstructive (Fig. 31.4) or nonobstructive forms. The clinical course and the risks during pregnancy are highly variable, ranging from asymptomatic to severe forms of heart failure, arrhythmias, and sudden cardiac death. Most women who experience no or mild symptoms prior to pregnancy are likely to be at low risk for complications [50–52]. However, the small subset of patients with significant symptoms prior to pregnancy are at increased risk of developing complications during pregnancy. Moreover, the higher the left ventricular outflow tract (LVOT) gradient is prior to pregnancy or in the first trimester, the greater the likelihood of cardiac events during pregnancy. Sudden death is a recognized complication of HCM during pregnancy, but the incidence is unclear [51]. Identifying patients at risk for sudden death is an important aspect of counseling and management, as is the treatment of arrhythmias and heart failure. Heart failure can be the first presentation during pregnancy or postpartum. Maternal morbidity is related to NYHA functional class before pregnancy and clinical deterioration is more common in patients with outflow tract obstruction. Special consideration must be given to the potential for decreased venous return at the time of labor and delivery, either due to acute blood loss or the Valsalva maneuver during delivery, which can create or exacerbate outflow tract obstruction. Beta-blockers are considered the mainstay of therapy in pregnancy, especially at the time of labor and delivery [17]. Vaginal delivery is uneventful in the majority of asymptomatic patients, despite possible hemodynamic complications during labor and delivery.

Subsequent Pregnancy in Women with a History of Peripartum Cardiomyopathy

Women with a history of peripartum cardiomyopathy may seek another pregnancy, as many women may be in the midst of family building when this occurs. There is sparse data available for counseling women in this regard. Elkayam et al. [53] noted in a study involving a small number of women that LVEF increased after the initial pregnancy but decreased again in the subsequent pregnancy. In addition, about half of the women in whom the ejection fraction did not normalize and who became pregnant had complications including heart failure, worsening ejection fraction, and death. Ejection fraction at the time of initial diagnosis impacts the outcome of subsequent pregnancy [54]. Based on limited evidence, women in whom the ejection fraction has not normalized and in whom the initial ejection fraction was less than 25 % should be counseled against subsequent pregnancy [14, 17]. Therefore, women with a history of peripartum cardiomyopathy and any residual impairment of left ventricular systolic function are considered WHO class IV (pregnancy is contraindicated). Women who are not candidates for another pregnancy require counseling regarding contraception or sterilization.

Pregnancy in the Heart Transplant Patient

Although this practice is evolving, pregnancy after cardiac transplantation has been generally discouraged by most centers. The potential risks to the prospective mother and concerns regarding maternal longevity and the teratogenic effects of immunosuppressant medications have been cited as the primary reasons [55]. Cardiac transplant recipients are asked to avoid pregnancy within the first year of transplantation as this is the period of highest risk for rejection after transplantation. Patients considered potentially suitable for pregnancy after transplantation are those with no rejection within 1 year, adequate and stable graft function, no acute infections, and maintenance of stable immunosuppressant medications. An important point regarding the physiology of the post-transplant heart is that the heart is denervated, with a loss of vagal tone, leading to higher-than-normal resting heart rates (typically 80–100 beats per minute or higher). Importantly, pregnancy causes a physiologic increase in the heart rate and the denervated heart may be more sensitive to circulating catecholamines and volume changes. In addition, the increased blood volume may cause hemodilution and affect serum drug levels. It appears that acute rejection is not increased in pregnant transplant recipients [56]. Infection remains a constant concern, the risk of which may be increased in pregnancy. Hypertension and preeclampsia are common and are major factors associated with the increased prevalence of preterm delivery and fetal growth restriction in transplant patients [57]. Teratogenic effects of immunosuppressant medications require discussion with the mother prior to pregnancy. However, the risks of rejection due to discontinuation of antirejection medications far outweigh the teratogenic risks. Often, medications require adjustment to the lowest effective dose. If rejection complicates a pregnancy, systolic and/or diastolic heart failure may become an issue. Antibiotic prophylaxis is required for transplant recipients with a transplant valvulopathy at the time of delivery according to guidelines [58]. Vaginal delivery is considered safe in this population.

Neonatal Outcomes

There is limited information available on neonatal outcomes of pregnant women with heart disease. In patients who are at high risk for maternal events, their fetuses are also at high risk for events. Thus, maternal and neonatal events are highly correlated. Neonatal complications occur in 20–28 % of patients with diverse cardiac conditions with a neonatal mortality of 1–4 % [25]. Maternal predictors of neonatal events in women with heart disease include baseline NYHA functional class II or greater, left heart obstruction, smoking during pregnancy, mechanical valve prosthesis, multiple gestation, and the use of oral anticoagulants during pregnancy [25]. The most common neonatal complications are premature birth and small for gestational age. Less commonly observed complications are respiratory distress syndrome, intraventricular hemorrhage, and death [24, 25]. Specifically in women with dilated cardiomyopathy, a fetal adverse event rate of 20 % is described with small for gestational age and preterm delivery being the most common [9]. There were no neonatal deaths in this study.

Management of Heart Failure in Pregnancy, Labor, and Delivery

Medical Therapy of Heart Failure in Pregnancy

The goals of therapy in a pregnant woman with heart failure are similar to those of a nonpregnant woman. These include relief of symptoms, control of hemodynamics, and treatment and/or reversal of precipitating factors such as anemia, infection, thyroid disorder, and arrhythmias. In addition, the continuation of medications that prolong survival should occur whenever possible. However, medications that are contraindicated throughout pregnancy (angiotensin-converting enzyme inhibitors or angiotensin receptor blockers) should not be used in pregnancy and should be discontinued prior to conception (Table 31.5).

Arrhythmias Associated with Cardiomyopathy

Arrhythmias are common in patients in the setting of preexisting structural heart disease. Supraventricular and ventricular arrhythmias requiring treatment develop in up to 15 % of patients with congenital heart disease during preg-

Table 31.5 Medical management of chronic heart failure in pregnancy

Drug/class	Purpose	Comment
Diuretics		
Furosemide	Generally reserved for treatment of pulmonary edema	Can result in uteroplacental hypoperfusion
	Use of lowest possible dose	Contraindicated in settings in which uteroplacental hypoperfusion is already reduced (IUGR, preeclampsia)
		FDA class C[a]
Digoxin	Not considered first-line therapy for heart failure in nonpregnant patients	Generally considered safe
	No improvement in mortality	Useful in treatment of persistent symptoms despite standard therapy
	Considered useful in pregnancy given limitations of medical armamentarium	FDA class C
Vasodilators		
Hydralazine	Commonly used oral antihypertensive agent in pregnancy	Demonstrated efficacy in hypertension
	Can be substituted for ACE inhibitor during pregnancy	Risk of hypotension
		Pregnancy already reduces SVR
		Avoid large or precipitous decreases in blood pressure
		FDA class C
ACE inhibitors/ARB	Proven benefit in treatment of chronic heart failure in nonpregnant patients	Contraindicated throughout pregnancy due to teratogenic effects. Associated with oligohydramnios, neonatal death secondary to renal failure, renal agenesis
		FDA class C for first trimester; D for second and third trimesters
Amlodipine	Alternative to ACE inhibitor in pregnancy	Can be used with hydralazine if needed
		FDA class C
Nitrates	May be used to treat decompensated heart failure	FDA class C
Beta-blockers		
Carvedilol, labetalol, metoprolol, propranolol	Essential component to chronic heart failure therapy	Generally safe and effective in pregnancy
	Agents that are beta-1 selective are preferable	Can cause IUGR
	Beta-blockers should be continued throughout pregnancy	Infants born to mothers on beta-blockers should be observed for at least 72 h after birth
		FDA class C
Aldosterone antagonists		
Spironolactone, eplerenone	Prolongs survival in selected heart failure patients	No data to support safety in pregnancy
	Not routinely used in pregnancy	FDA class D
Warfarin	Risk/benefit ratio needs to be discussed with the patient for treatment and prophylactic anticoagulation in severe left ventricular dysfunction	First trimester teratogenesis
		Dosing is complicated in pregnancy
		FDA class X

Adapted with permission from Stergiopoulos et al. [16]
ACE inhibitor, angiotensin-converting enzyme inhibitor, *ARB* angiotensin receptor blocker, *IUGR* intrauterine growth retardation, *SVR* systemic vascular resistance
[a]Food and Drug Administration (FDA) class: A (controlled studies show no risk), B (no evidence of human risk in controlled studies), C (risk cannot be ruled out), D (positive evidence of risk), X (contraindicated in pregnancy)

Table 31.6 Management of arrhythmias during pregnancy

Table 31.6 Management of arrhythmias during pregnancy

Management of supraventricular tachycardia (SVT)

For acute conversion of SVT, vagal maneuvers followed by adenosine (class I)

Immediate electrical cardioversion is recommended for any tachyarrhythmia with hemodynamic instability (class I)

For long-term management of SVT, digoxin or metoprolol/propranolol (class I)

Atenolol should not be used for any arrhythmia (class III)[a]

Management of ventricular tachycardia (VT)

For the long-term management of congenital long QT syndrome, beta-blocking agents are recommended during pregnancy and postpartum (class I)

For the long-term management of idiopathic sustained VT, oral metoprolol, propranolol, or verapamil is recommended (class I)

Immediate electrical cardioversion of VT is recommended for sustained, unstable, and stable VT (class I)

Adapted with permission from Regitz-Zagrosek et al. [17]

Classes I–III refer to European Society of Cardiology (ESC) classes of recommendation based on level of evidence and the strength of recommendation (REF)

[a]Atenolol is considered Food and Drug Administration (FDA) class D, due to hypospadias (first trimester), low birth weight, bradycardia, and hypoglycemia in the fetus (second and third trimester)

nancy [22]. In a study cohort of mainly women with structural heart disease, the recurrence rates of arrhythmias during pregnancy or the early postpartum period were elevated to 44 % in women with sinus rhythm at baseline [59]. Rhythm disturbances included recurrence of supraventricular tachycardia, atrial fibrillation or flutter, and ventricular tachycardia. Adverse fetal events were noted more commonly in women who developed antepartum arrhythmias compared to those that did not. Episodes of sustained tachyarrhythmia may not be well tolerated and can cause fetal and placental hypoperfusion. Table 31.6 summarizes the management of arrhythmias during pregnancy.

Atrial Flutter and Atrial Fibrillation

Atrial flutter and atrial fibrillation are considered uncommon in pregnancy unless structural heart disease or hyperthyroidism is present. A rapid ventricular response can result in hypotension and hemodynamic instability which can cause fetal and placental hypoperfusion. Therefore, in patients with hemodynamic instability, prompt electrical cardioversion is usually required to prevent further detrimental hemodynamic consequences to the fetus and mother.

In hemodynamically stable patients with structurally normal hearts, pharmacologic termination of atrial flutter or atrial fibrillation can be considered. In such cases, intravenous ibutilide or flecainide have been shown to be effective in pregnancy in a limited case series [60]. Amiodarone is not recommended as a frontline agent due to its toxic effects on the fetus. Rate control with atrioventricular nodal blocking agents such as digoxin, beta-blocking agents, and non-dihydropyridine calcium channel blockers

(verapamil, diltiazem) can be considered. Beta-blockers are recommended as the first-line agent, with calcium blockers as second-line agents (see Table 31.6) [17].

Indications for anticoagulation in the setting of cardioversion and for chronic thromboembolic prophylaxis follow the same recommendations for nonpregnant patients [61]. A decision regarding long-term anticoagulation in pregnancy would be assessed using established criteria, with either the CHADS2 or CHA_2DS_2VASc scores. Patients with a risk score of ≥ 2 are at elevated risk for thromboembolic events and full-dose anticoagulation with warfarin or low molecular weight heparin can be considered. The choice of anticoagulant is based on the stage of the pregnancy [62]. Subcutaneous low molecular weight heparin is used in the first trimester and the last month of pregnancy and must be dose-adjusted for body weight which often changes as pregnancy advances. Warfarin can be used for the second trimester without teratogenic effects on the fetus, but bleeding risks remain.

Labor and Delivery

A multidisciplinary approach is critical for the optimal management of patients at the time of labor and delivery [16]. Consultation among the patient's obstetrician, obstetrical anesthesiologist, and cardiologist is required by the onset of the third trimester with a clear understanding from the patient regarding the delivery plan. The decision regarding the timing and mode of delivery is made based on the hemodynamic status of the patient and obstetrical considerations [16]. Early delivery is not required in all patients with cardiomyopathies or heart failure; the decision is based on failure of the patient to respond to medical therapy and the overall hemodynamic status of the patient. Virtually all pregnant women with cardiac disease should expect an attempt at vaginal delivery, now considered a class I recommendation by the ESC guidelines on the management of pregnant women with heart disease [17], unless obstetric contraindications exist. A vaginal delivery often poses less hemodynamic risk, as Cesarean delivery is accompanied by approximately twice as much blood loss. Recommendations for the peripartum obstetric management of women with heart disease have traditionally included vaginal delivery unless the patient is unstable or obstetric indications exist, early induction of labor, shortening of the second stage of labor during vaginal delivery, and a low threshold for elective Cesarean section. However, a recent single center study using logistic regression and propensity matching compared women with heart disease to those without and demonstrated that women with heart disease were more likely to undergo induction of labor at term for logistic reasons rather than for the indication of maternal heart disease [63]. Assisted vaginal deliveries were more common, but the rates of Cesarean sections were the

Table 31.7 Management during labor and delivery and postpartum concerns

Multidisciplinary approach required
Use of vaginal delivery with excellent anesthesia, possibly with assisted second stage of labor
Left lateral decubitus position
Cesarean section – according to obstetric indications
Medical therapy – optimization of loading conditions
Anesthetic choices for labor and delivery in the setting of heart failure
General anesthesia
Volatile agents (sevoflurane, isoflurance, desflurane) can decrease SVR
Reserved for emergency situations
Rapid sequence induction can lead to cardiovascular instability
Mortality is highest at the time of induction and intubation
Regional anesthesia
Includes spinal, epidural, or combined spinal-epidural
Technique of choice in patients with heart failure and pregnancy for delivery
Offers afterload reduction and blunts hemodynamic response of labor and delivery
Low concentration of bupivacaine and lipophilic opiates allow for hemodynamic stability
Sedation
Can accompany regional techniques if needed
Agents such as propofol, midazolam, and fentanyl have been used without fetal issues
Aspiration risk exists
Postpartum concerns
Medical therapy to optimize loading conditions (treatment of pulmonary edema)
Hemodynamic and telemetry monitoring for 12–24 h
Consider options for contraception or sterilization

Adapted with permission from Stergiopoulos et al. [16]
SVR systemic vascular resistance

Table 31.8 Summary of guideline recommendations

Recommendations	Class (level)[a]
Prepregnancy risk assessment and counseling are indicated in all women with known or suspected congenital or acquired cardiovascular and aortic disease	I (C)
Vaginal delivery is recommended as first choice in most patients	I (C)
Women with dilated cardiomyopathy should be informed about the risk of deterioration of the condition during pregnancy and thereafter	I (C)
Women with heart failure during pregnancy should be treated according to current guidelines for nonpregnant patients, except for those medications that are contraindicated	I (B)
Beta-blockers can be considered for all patients with hypertrophic cardiomyopathy	II (C)
Subsequent pregnancy is not recommended if LVEF does not normalize in women with a history of peripartum cardiomyopathy	III (C)

Adapted from Regitz-Zagrosek et al. [17]
LVEF left ventricular ejection fraction
[a]Class of recommendation and level of evidence

same in both groups. Invasive cardiac monitoring was rarely used. Adverse maternal cardiac events were rare (2 % of pregnancies). A less aggressive approach may be used in the future, but more data are required. In contrast, in the European Registry on Pregnancy and Heart disease (ROPAC), 41 % of patients underwent Cesarean section, compared with 23 % of the general population studied [8]. Assisted vaginal delivery was performed commonly in 32 % of the vaginal deliveries. In a study of dilated cardiomyopathy patients, most deliveries were vaginal (81 %), and the most frequently used form of anesthesia was epidural in 86 % of patients [9]. Indications for Cesarean delivery were unrelated to preexisting cardiac disease in any one of these patients. Anesthetic considerations in pregnant women with chronic or new onset heart failure require a specialized approach and, when possible, should be planned in the antepartum period. These are reviewed in Tables 31.7 and 31.8.

> **Key Points**
> - Women with cardiomyopathy are at risk for complications during and after pregnancy if they are unable to adapt to the hemodynamic changes of pregnancy.
> - A diverse set of potential etiologies of cardiomyopathy exist for women of childbearing age.
> - Pregnancy risk can be estimated.
> - Pregnancy in women with a cardiomyopathy and left ventricular ejection fraction of <30 % is classified as World Health Organization class IV and is therefore contraindicated.
> - Potential complications include arrhythmias, thromboembolism, heart failure, worsening left ventricular systolic function, and cardiac death.
> - Most women with hypertrophic cardiomyopathy tolerate pregnancy well, except symptomatic patients prior to pregnancy and those with a high left ventricular outflow tract gradient.
> - Women with a history of peripartum cardiomyopathy and any residual impairment of left ventricular systolic function are considered WHO class IV.
> - A multidisciplinary approach is critical to the optimal management of patients at the time of labor and delivery.

References

1. Silversides CK, Colman JM. Physiologic changes in pregnancy. In: Oakley C, Warnes CA, editors. Heart disease in pregnancy. Malden: Blackwell Publishing; 2007. p. 173–85.
2. Weiss BM, von Segesser LK, Alon E, Seifert B, Turina MI. Outcome of cardiovascular surgery and pregnancy: a systematic review of the period 1984–1996. Am J Obstet Gynecol. 1998;179(6 Pt 1):1643–53.
3. 7th report of the confidential enquiries into maternal deaths in the UK. London: Royal College of Obstetrics and Gynecology; 2007.
4. Roos-Hesselink JW, Duvekot JJ, Thorne SA. Pregnancy in high risk cardiac conditions. Heart. 2009;95(8):680–6.
5. Berg CJ, Callaghan WM, Syverson C, Henderson Z. Pregnancy-related mortality in the United States, 1998 to 2005. Obstet Gynecol. 2010;116(6):1302–9.
6. Main EK. Maternal mortality: new strategies for measurement and prevention. Curr Opin Obstet Gynecol. 2010;22(6):511–6.
7. Kuklina E, Callaghan W. Chronic heart disease and severe obstetric morbidity among hospitalisations for pregnancy in the USA: 1995–2006. BJOG. 2011;118(3):345–52.
8. Roos-Hesselink JW, Ruys TP, Stein JI, et al. Outcome of pregnancy in patients with structural or ischaemic heart disease: results of a registry of the European Society of Cardiology. Eur Heart J. 2013; 34:657–65.
9. Grewal J, Siu SC, Ross H, Mason J, Balint O, Sermer M, Colman J, Silversides C. Pregnancy outcomes in women with dilated cardiomyopathy. J Am Coll Cardiol. 2010;55:45–52.
10. Sliwa K, Fett J, Elkayam U. Peripartum cardiomyopathy. Lancet. 2006;368(9536):687–93.
11. Gleicher N, Elkayam U. Peripartum cardiomyopathy, an autoimmune manifestation of allograft rejection? Autoimmun Rev. 2009; 8(5):384–7.
12. Elkayam U. Pregnancy and cardiovascular disease. In: Zipes DP, Libby P, Bonow RO, Braunwald U, editors. Braunwald's heart disease. 7th ed. Philadelphia: Elsevier; 1965.
13. Hilfiker-Kleiner D, Sliwa K, Drexler H. Peripartum cardiomyopathy: recent insights in its pathophysiology. Trends Cardiovasc Med. 2008;18(5):173–9.
14. Sliwa K, Hilfiker-Kleiner D, Petrie MC, et al. Current state of knowledge on aetiology, diagnosis, management, and therapy of peripartum cardiomyopathy: a position statement from the Heart Failure Association of the European Society of Cardiology Working Group on peripartum cardiomyopathy. Eur J Heart Fail. 2010;12(8):767–78.
15. Elkayam U. Clinical characteristics of peripartum cardiomyopathy in the United States: diagnosis, prognosis, and management. J Am Coll Cardiol. 2011;58(7):659–70.
16. Stergiopoulos K, Shiang E, Bench T. Pregnancy in patients with pre-existing cardiomyopathies. J Am Coll Cardiol. 2011;58(4): 337–50.
17. Regitz-Zagrosek V, Blomstrom Lundqvist C, Borghi C, et al. ESC guidelines on the management of cardiovascular diseases during pregnancy: the Task Force on the Management of Cardiovascular Diseases during Pregnancy of the European Society of Cardiology (ESC). Eur Heart J. 2011;32:3147–97.
18. Warnes CA, Williams RG, Bashore TM, et al. ACC/AHA 2008 guidelines for the management of adults with congenital heart disease: a report of the American College of Cardiology/American Heart Association Task Force on Practice Guidelines (writing committee to develop guidelines on the management of adults with congenital heart disease). Developed in Collaboration with the American Society of Echocardiography, Heart Rhythm Society, International Society for Adult Congenital Heart Disease, Society for Cardiovascular Angiography and Interventions, and Society of Thoracic Surgeons. J Am Coll Cardiol. 2008;52(23):e1–121.
19. Lang RM, Bierig M, Devereux RB, et al. Recommendations for chamber quantification: a report from the American Society of Echocardiography's Guidelines and Standards Committee and the Chamber Quantification Writing Group, developed in conjunction with the European Association of Echocardiography, a branch of the European Society of Cardiology. J Am Soc Echocardiogr. 2005;18(12):1440–63.
20. Shime J, Mocarski EJ, Hastings D, Webb GD, McLaughlin PR. Congenital heart disease in pregnancy: short- and long-term implications. Am J Obstet Gynecol. 1987;156(2):313–22.
21. Lui GK, Silversides CK, Khairy P, et al. Heart rate response during exercise and pregnancy outcome in women with congenital heart disease. Circulation. 2011;123(3):242–8.
22. Drenthen W, Pieper PG, Roos-Hesselink JW, et al. Outcome of pregnancy in women with congenital heart disease: a literature review. J Am Coll Cardiol. 2007;49(24):2303–11.
23. Siu SC, Sermer M, Colman JM, et al. Prospective multicenter study of pregnancy outcomes in women with heart disease. Circulation. 2001;104(5):515–21.
24. Drenthen W, Boersma E, Balci A, et al. Predictors of pregnancy complications in women with congenital heart disease. Eur Heart J. 2010;31(17):2124–32.
25. Siu SC, Colman JM, Sorensen S, et al. Adverse neonatal and cardiac outcomes are more common in pregnant women with cardiac disease. Circulation. 2002;105(18):2179–84.
26. Siu SC, Sermer M, Harrison DA, et al. Risk and predictors for pregnancy-related complications in women with heart disease. Circulation. 1997;96(9):2789–94.
27. Howlett JG, McKelvie RS, Costigan J, et al. The 2010 Canadian Cardiovascular Society guidelines for the diagnosis and management of heart failure update: heart failure in ethnic minority populations, heart failure and pregnancy, disease management, and quality improvement/assurance programs. Can J Cardiol. 2010;26(4):185–202.
28. Thorne S, MacGregor A, Nelson-Piercy C. Risks of contraception and pregnancy in heart disease. Heart. 2006;92(10):1520–5.
29. Elkayam U, Ostrzega E, Shotan A, Mehra A. Cardiovascular problems in pregnant women with the Marfan syndrome. Ann Intern Med. 1995;123(2):117–22.
30. Vasu S, Stergiopoulos K. Valvular heart disease in pregnancy. Hellenic J Cardiol. 2009;50(6):498–510.
31. Kovacs AH, Harrison JL, Colman JM, Sermer M, Siu SC, Silversides CK. Pregnancy and contraception in congenital heart disease: what women are not told. J Am Coll Cardiol. 2008;52(7): 577–8.
32. Berger R, Huelsman M, Strecker K, et al. B-type natriuretic peptide predicts sudden death in patients with chronic heart failure. Circulation. 2002;105(20):2392–7.
33. Tanous D, Siu SC, Mason J, et al. B-type natriuretic peptide in pregnant women with heart disease. J Am Coll Cardiol. 2010; 56(15):1247–53.
34. Felker GM, Thompson RE, Hare JM, et al. Underlying causes and long-term survival in patients with initially unexplained cardiomyopathy. N Engl J Med. 2000;342(15):1077–84.
35. Krul SP, van der Smagt JJ, van den Berg MP, Sollie KM, Pieper PG, van Spaendonck-Zwarts KY. Systematic review of pregnancy in women with inherited cardiomyopathies. Eur J Heart Fail. 2011;13(6):584–94.
36. Suri V, Aggarwal N, Kalpdev A, Chopra S, Sikka P, Vijayvergia R. Pregnancy with dilated and peripartum cardiomyopathy: maternal and fetal outcome. Arch Gynecol Obstet. 2013;287:195–9.

37. Katsuragi S, Omoto A, Kamiya C, et al. Risk factors for maternal outcome in pregnancy complicated with dilated cardiomyopathy. J Perinatol. 2012;32(3):170–5.

38. van den Berg MP, van Spaendonck-Zwarts KY, van Veldhuisen DJ. Dilated cardiomyopathy complicates pregnancy outcome: but how? J Am Coll Cardiol. 2010;55(20):2291; author reply 2291–2.

39. Kitao K, Ohara N, Funakoshi T, et al. Noncompaction of the left ventricular myocardium diagnosed in pregnant woman and neonate. J Perinat Med. 2004;32(6):527–31.

40. Jayan P, Shankarappa RK, Ananthakrishna R, Nanjappa MC. Isolated left ventricular noncompaction mimicking ventricular mass. Echocardiography. 2011;28(7):E137–9.

41. Kanal E, Barkovich AJ, Bell C, et al. ACR guidance document for safe MR practices: 2007. AJR Am J Roentgenol. 2007;188(6):1447–74.

42. Greutmann M, Mah ML, Silversides CK, et al. Predictors of adverse outcome in adolescents and adults with isolated left ventricular noncompaction. Am J Cardiol. 2012;109(2):276–81.

43. Lofiego C, Biagini E, Pasquale F, et al. Wide spectrum of presentation and variable outcomes of isolated left ventricular noncompaction. Heart. 2007;93(1):65–71.

44. Patel C, Shirali G, Pereira N. Left ventricular noncompaction mimicking peripartum cardiomyopathy. J Am Soc Echocardiogr. 2007;20(8):1009.e9–12.

45. Rehfeldt KH, Pulido JN, Mauermann WJ, Click RL. Left ventricular hypertrabeculation/noncompaction in a patient with peripartum cardiomyopathy. Int J Cardiol. 2010;139(2):e18–20.

46. Williams RI, Masani ND, Buchalter MB, Fraser AG. Abnormal myocardial strain rate in noncompaction of the left ventricle. J Am Soc Echocardiogr. 2003;16(3):293–6.

47. Bahl A, Swamy A, Sharma Y, Kumar N. Isolated noncompaction of left ventricle presenting as peripartum cardiomyopathy. Int J Cardiol. 2006;109(3):422–3.

48. Agmon Y, Connolly HM, Olson LJ, Khandheria BK, Seward JB. Noncompaction of the ventricular myocardium. J Am Soc Echocardiogr. 1999;12(10):859–63.

49. Vainrib A, Stergiopoulos K. Hypertrophic cardiomyopathy and pregnancy. Minerva Ginecol. 2012;64(5):399–407.

50. Thaman R, Varnava A, Hamid MS, et al. Pregnancy related complications in women with hypertrophic cardiomyopathy. Heart. 2003;89(7):752–6.

51. Autore C, Conte MR, Piccininno M, et al. Risk associated with pregnancy in hypertrophic cardiomyopathy. J Am Coll Cardiol. 2002;40(10):1864–9.

52. Alegria J, Nishimura RA. Hypertrophic cardiomyopathy and pregnancy. In: Oakley C, Warnes CA, editors. Heart disease in pregnancy. Malden: Blackwell Publishing; 2007. p. 173–85.

53. Elkayam U, Tummala PP, Rao K, et al. Maternal and fetal outcomes of subsequent pregnancies in women with peripartum cardiomyopathy. N Engl J Med. 2001;344(21):1567–71.

54. Habli M, O'Brien T, Nowack E, Khoury S, Barton JR, Sibai B. Peripartum cardiomyopathy: prognostic factors for long-term maternal outcome. Am J Obstet Gynecol. 2008;199(4):415.e1–5.

55. Ross LF. Ethical considerations related to pregnancy in transplant recipients. N Engl J Med. 2006;354(12):1313–6.

56. Armenti VT, Radomski JS, Moritz MJ, et al. Report from the National Transplantation Pregnancy Registry (NTPR): outcomes of pregnancy after transplantation. Clin Transpl. 2004:103–14.

57. Scott JR, Wagoner LE, Olsen SL, Taylor DO, Renlund DG. Pregnancy in heart transplant recipients: management and outcome. Obstet Gynecol. 1993;82(3):324–7.

58. Wilson W, Taubert KA, Gewitz M, et al. Prevention of infective endocarditis: guidelines from the American Heart Association: a guideline from the American Heart Association Rheumatic Fever, Endocarditis, and Kawasaki Disease Committee, Council on Cardiovascular Disease in the Young, and the Council on Clinical Cardiology, Council on Cardiovascular Surgery and Anesthesia, and the Quality of Care and Outcomes Research Interdisciplinary Working Group. Circulation. 2007;116(15):1736–54.

59. Silversides CK, Harris L, Haberer K, Sermer M, Colman JM, Siu SC. Recurrence rates of arrhythmias during pregnancy in women with previous tachyarrhythmia and impact on fetal and neonatal outcomes. Am J Cardiol. 2006;97(8):1206–12.

60. Kockova R, Kocka V, Kiernan T, Fahy GJ. Ibutilide-induced cardioversion of atrial fibrillation during pregnancy. J Cardiovasc Electrophysiol. 2007;18(5):545–7.

61. Fuster V, Ryden LE, Cannom DS, et al. ACC/AHA/ESC 2006 guidelines for the management of patients with atrial fibrillation – executive summary: a report of the American College of Cardiology/American Heart Association Task Force on Practice Guidelines and the European Society of Cardiology Committee for Practice Guidelines (writing committee to revise the 2001 guidelines for the management of patients with atrial fibrillation). J Am Coll Cardiol. 2006;48(4):854–906.

62. Elkayam U, Singh H, Irani A, Akhter MW. Anticoagulation in pregnant women with prosthetic heart valves. J Cardiovasc Pharmacol Ther. 2004;9(2):107–15.

63. Robertson JE, Silversides CK, Mah ML, et al. A contemporary approach to the obstetric management of women with heart disease. J Obstet Gynaecol Can. 2012;34(9):812–9.

Valvular Heart Disease and Pregnancy

32

Eric V. Krieger and Karen K. Stout

Abstract

The population of women with valvular disease who are of childbearing age continues to increase. Many will want to become pregnant or may present already pregnant, and in some cases, underlying valve disease will complicate pregnancy, increasing the risk for adverse outcomes for the mother and fetus. This chapter discusses the hemodynamic changes of pregnancy and the implications for patients with valve disease. Focus is on the physiology and outcomes of pregnancy with specific valve lesions. There is a discussion of particular issues that may be relevant in these patients, such as anticoagulation for mechanical valves and cardiac surgery during pregnancy. Issues to be addressed during labor and delivery are described. Ideally, women with valvular disease will present prior to pregnancy, allowing for preconceptual counseling. Thus, strategies to assess risk include currently available risk scores that can aid in counseling, regardless of specific valve abnormality.

Keywords

Pregnancy • Valvular disease • Aortic stenosis • Mitral stenosis • Mitral regurgitation • Aortic regurgitation • Tetralogy of Fallot • Mechanical valves • Pregnancy risk score

Introduction

Many women with valvular heart disease are of childbearing age and will want to become pregnant or will present for care already pregnant. In some cases, underlying valve disease will substantially complicate pregnancy and increase the risk for adverse outcomes for the mother and fetus. This chapter will discuss the hemodynamic changes of pregnancy, the outcomes of pregnancy with specific valve lesions, and the role of preconceptual counseling.

Hemodynamics of Pregnancy

The hemodynamic changes during pregnancy may worsen the hemodynamics of underlying valvular disease resulting in adverse outcomes for the mother and fetus. It is important to understand the hemodynamic changes of both pregnancy and delivery when counseling and managing women with valvular heart disease. As the changes during pregnancy are quite different than those during delivery, some patients may do well during pregnancy but have significant cardiovascular symptoms during delivery or in the first 24–48 h postpartum.

During pregnancy, cardiac output steadily increases by up to 50 % of baseline values. The increase in cardiac output is achieved by an increase in heart rate of up to 20 % and an increase in blood volume of up to 50 % that results in increased preload [1]. The increase in blood volume does not have a similar increase in red cell mass; therefore, there is a relative anemia of pregnancy that may further drive the increased cardiac output. The relative anemia is blunted by iron supplementation. The placenta is a low-resistance

E.V. Krieger, MD (✉) • K.K. Stout, MD
Division of Cardiology, Department of Medicine and Pediatrics, University of Washington/University of Washington Medical Center and Seattle Children's Hospital, 1959 NE Pacific, Box 356422, Seattle, WA 98195, USA
e-mail: ekrieger@u.washington.edu; stoutk@u.washington.edu

K. Stergiopoulos, D.L. Brown (eds.), *Evidence-Based Cardiology Consult*,
DOI 10.1007/978-1-4471-4441-0_32, © Springer-Verlag London 2014

vascular bed which contributes to decreasing systemic vascular resistance (SVR) through the course of pregnancy. The systemic blood pressure may be somewhat lower or may stay the same, depending on the relative balance of low SVR and increased cardiac output. Pulmonary artery pressures generally remain unchanged during pregnancy and delivery unless a disease process is present that causes increased pulmonary vascular resistance and pulmonary pressures. Systemic venous return may be impaired in later pregnancy by the gravid uterus which can compress the inferior vena cava when the patient is supine. Therefore, for significantly preload-dependent valve lesions, the left lateral decubitus position may be better tolerated.

During delivery, anxiety and pain contribute to marked increases in heart rate and blood pressure [2]. Uterine contractions result in an increase in venous return during the contraction which diminishes between contractions. Once the placenta is delivered, the SVR rises abruptly and there is an immediate return of up to 500 ml of blood back into the maternal circulation. The combination may raise left ventricular end-diastolic pressures and precipitate pulmonary edema. Over the first 2 weeks after delivery, extravascular volume is redistributed to the circulation which may result in additional volume.

In addition to the hemodynamic changes during pregnancy and delivery, there are changes to connective tissues necessary to facilitate delivery through an otherwise rigid pelvis. The impact of changing levels of matrix metalloproteinases and fibrinogen necessary for pelvic relaxation is systemic and can affect the aorta and other large arteries. Thus, for patients at risk for aortic dissection or rupture, pregnancy and the puerperium pose a particularly high-risk time due to hemodynamic and connective tissue changes [3, 4].

The hemodynamic changes of pregnancy are variably tolerated by women with valvular disease, depending on the nature and severity of the valve dysfunction. In general, patients with regurgitant lesions tolerate pregnancy well due to the decreased SVR. However, delivery itself, with the abrupt increases in vascular resistance and blood pressure, may be poorly tolerated in those with substantial regurgitation, especially if there is left ventricular (LV) dysfunction.

Alternatively, patients with stenotic lesions may tolerate pregnancy poorly due to the rise in cardiac output, blood volume, heart rate, and the relative anemia. The decrease in SVR and blood pressure may not be readily overcome in the face of severe LV obstructive lesions, particularly aortic stenosis. Delivery may be difficult because of the further increase in heart rate and blood pressure. Mixed lesions can be particularly difficult to predict; patients with significant mixed stenosis and regurgitation may tolerate pregnancy more poorly than similar degrees of isolated stenosis or regurgitation.

Physical Exam

On exam, systolic murmurs are heard in 80 % of pregnant women. These are generally flow murmurs, grades 1–2, and heard along the sternal borders. They may represent increased blood flow through the pulmonary artery and aorta, but are not reflective of pathologic changes. However, as in nonpregnant patients, any murmur that is loud (grade 3/6 or greater), any diastolic murmur, or any murmur with radiation patterns typical of significant valve dysfunction (carotids, apex, back) warrants further evaluation [5]. Lower extremity edema is common, but should not be severe in a normal pregnancy. Attention should be paid to the jugular venous pressure (JVP) and lung exam, as evidence of elevated JVP or pulmonary crackles are not typical of normal pregnancy.

Specific Valve Lesions

Aortic Stenosis

Most women of childbearing age with aortic stenosis have congenital aortic stenosis. Like other stenotic lesions, aortic valve gradients predictably rise during pregnancy due to increased transvalvular flow associated with the increased cardiac output and plasma volume seen during pregnancy. Cardiac output and stroke volume reach a peak by approximately 20 weeks of gestation and then plateau [6]. Although peak and mean gradients increase during pregnancy, valve area remains stable when calculated according to the continuity equation [7, 8]. Furthermore, women with aortic stenosis may have LV hypertrophy and reduced compliance [9] which can manifest as heart failure when intravascular volume and preload increase.

Maternal Risk

Although severe aortic stenosis is considered to be a high-risk lesion in pregnancy, mild-to-moderate aortic stenosis is well tolerated during pregnancy [8, 10]. However, because early series reported high maternal mortality in pregnant women with aortic stenosis [11], current guidelines recommend that women with severe or symptomatic aortic stenosis be advised to avoid pregnancy until the aortic stenosis is treated [12].

Women with more severe aortic stenosis are more likely to have adverse cardiovascular events during pregnancy [10, 13]. Women with mild or moderate stenosis (valve area >1.0 cm^2 and peak gradient <64 mmHg) rarely have life-threatening maternal cardiovascular complications during pregnancy [8]. However, approximately 10–15 % of women with severe aortic stenosis develop cardiac complications during pregnancy. The most common events are heart failure requiring diuretics (~7 %) or maternal arrhythmia (~3 %) [14]. Death remains very rare in modern series [8, 15, 16]. Nonetheless, when compared to other forms of congenital heart disease, congenital aortic stenosis remains a high-risk lesion, and many women will increase one New York Heart Association (NYHA) class during the course of pregnancy [16, 17]. Women who are symptomatic prior to pregnancy remain at very high risk and should be counseled against pregnancy until the obstruction is relieved.

There is some data to suggest that pregnancy may accelerate the need for aortic valve intervention late postpartum when compared with similar women who do not become pregnant [18]. However, as pregnancy is not known to affect aortic valve area or left ventricular function [8, 19], these data should be interpreted cautiously until they are confirmed.

Patients with bicuspid aortic valve have an intrinsic aortopathy which predisposes to dilation and dissection. Bicuspid aortic valve has been associated with dissections in pregnancy, and the risk appears to be greatest in women with an ascending aortic diameter >4 cm prior to pregnancy, with an average diameter at the time of dissection of 5.3 cm [20, 21]. However, given the high prevalence of bicuspid aortic valve in the general population and the rarity of dissection, the risk of dissection in women without substantial aortic dilation may not be as high as previously suspected and may, in part, be driven by selective reporting [21, 22]. Pregnancy in women with a bicuspid aortic valve and aortic diameters below or near 4 cm is probably not a major risk for dissection.

Fetal and Neonatal Risk

Severe aortic stenosis is a risk factor for adverse fetal and neonatal outcomes [10, 17]. Approximately 10–15 % of such pregnancies are associated with adverse fetal events, mostly premature delivery, small for gestational age, or respiratory distress syndrome [8, 14]. Not all authors have found an association between isolated aortic stenosis and adverse fetal and neonatal outcomes, however [16].

Some families with bicuspid aortic valve have an autosomal dominant pattern of inheritance with variable penetrance [23, 24] so recurrence in offspring is frequent.

Evaluation and Treatment

Echocardiography should be performed preconception, whenever possible [12]. B-type natriuretic peptide (BNP) can be helpful in managing aortic stenosis [25–27]. BNP levels behave similarly in pregnant and nonpregnant women [28]. Serial echocardiography will reliably demonstrate an increased transvalvular gradient during pregnancy. The development of LV systolic dysfunction or pulmonary hypertension is a cause for concern.

If symptoms develop during pregnancy, bed rest and diuretics are the mainstays of therapy. Inpatient diuresis and hemodynamic monitoring may be required. Balloon aortic valvuloplasty and aortic valve replacements have been performed in pregnant women with severe symptomatic aortic stenosis but present considerable fetal risk and are discussed in more detail elsewhere in this chapter [29–31].

Aortic Regurgitation

In women of childbearing age, aortic regurgitation is usually a result unicommissural or bicommissural aortic valve, prior intervention for aortic stenosis, prior endocarditis, or aortic root dilation from an intrinsic aortopathy.

Maternal Risk

Asymptomatic aortic regurgitation is generally well tolerated in pregnancy [16]. Chronic aortic regurgitation is characterized by high preload and high afterload. During pregnancy, preload increases but afterload falls [32] and diastole shortens due to tachycardia. This combination of decreased afterload and tachycardia could theoretically decrease aortic regurgitation [33] although this has not been rigorously demonstrated.

Patients with severe aortic regurgitation and depressed LV systolic function are more likely to develop heart failure or worsening of ejection fraction during surgery [34]. These patients meet established guideline criteria for aortic valve replacement [12] which should be performed prior to pregnancy. Patients with aortic regurgitation secondary to significant root dilation are at risk of dissection during pregnancy, particularly if the aortic diameter is >4 cm.

Fetal Risk

It does not appear that stable, asymptomatic aortic regurgitation with preserved LV systolic function increases obstetric or neonatal complications, although the number of women studied is relatively small [16].

Evaluation and Treatment

Bed rest and diuretic therapy should be used for symptomatic patients. Systemic vasodilators have been used with variable success in chronic aortic regurgitation in nonpregnant women. Notably, angiotensin-converting enzymes (ACE) inhibitors are contraindicated due to teratogenicity. Nifedipine has been used safely in pregnancy for other indications but has not been studied in the setting of aortic regurgitation in pregnancy [35].

Mitral Stenosis

Mitral stenosis in pregnancy is usually rheumatic in origin and is often diagnosed when a previously healthy woman develops heart failure in pregnancy.

Maternal Risk

Moderate or severe mitral stenosis is poorly tolerated during pregnancy and typically presents in the second trimester. The mitral valve gradient increases due to increased intravascular volume and increased cardiac output. Tachycardia preferentially shortens diastole which increases the transvalvular flow rate and further worsens the gradient across the mitral valve. High mitral valve gradients obligate left atrial hypertension, precipitate pulmonary edema, and may cause atrial fibrillation which can further increase heart rate and worsen pulmonary venous congestion and pulmonary edema.

The majority of women with moderate or severe mitral stenosis have a functional decline during pregnancy [10, 36]. Approximately 50 % of women with significant mitral stenosis will increase more than one NYHA functional class, a significantly worse outcome than is seen in other forms of valve disease. Approximately 75 % of women with significant mitral stenosis will be hospitalized during pregnancy, and most will require cardiac medications, mostly diuretics and beta-blockers. Women with a history of symptomatic mitral stenosis or associated pulmonary hypertension are at increased risk [10]. Maternal mortality is very rare.

Fetal Risk

Adverse fetal or neonatal risks complicate approximately 30 % of pregnancies in women with mitral stenosis. Adverse outcomes are more likely with more severe valve disease. Prematurity, small for gestational age, low birth weight, and respiratory distress syndrome are the most common complications [10, 36].

Evaluation and Treatment

An electrocardiogram should be performed to evaluate for atrial fibrillation and determine the possible need for anticoagulation during pregnancy. Echocardiography remains the gold standard for evaluation of mitral stenosis. The echocardiogram should determine the mitral valve morphology including the degree of leaflet thickening, presence and symmetry of commissural fusion, degree of valve calcification, and involvement of subvalvular shortening and thickening. Mitral regurgitation should also be graded and rheumatic involvement of other valves should be evaluated. The presence of associated pulmonary hypertension is important to determine as patients with pulmonary hypertension have worse outcomes [10].

It is reasonable to obtain an echocardiogram each trimester or if the patient develops a significant change in symptoms.

During pregnancy the mitral valve gradient increases, as described above. However, the mitral valve area as determined by the pressure-half-time method or by planimetry should remain stable through pregnancy [36].

Brain-type natriuretic peptide (BNP) levels correspond with the severity of mitral stenosis [37, 38] and can be useful to trend during pregnancy, particularly if signs and symptoms remain ambiguous. Healthy women without heart disease have stable and low levels of BNP throughout pregnancy [39]. If BNP remains low, this is reassuring. Conversely an elevated BNP in this population is associated with worse outcomes [40].

The mainstay of therapy is restricted activity, diuretics, and beta-blockers. Beta-blockers slow the heart rate and decrease mitral valve gradient. Diuretics provide relief of pulmonary congestion. The metabolism of metoprolol is often upregulated during pregnancy requiring higher doses. Thus, the dose should be titrated to clinical effect [41]. If atrial fibrillation develops, digoxin can be useful for additional rate control, and anticoagulation should be strongly considered.

Severe symptomatic mitral stenosis refractory to conservative medical therapy may require intervention during pregnancy. Patients with suitable valve morphology may be considered for balloon mitral valvuloplasty. Optimal timing is between 14 and 22 weeks in order to avoid radiation exposure during organogenesis. Balloon mitral valvuloplasty has been performed extensively during pregnancy with good maternal and fetal outcomes. Maternal mortality is <1 % and fetal demise is rare [42]. Radiation dose should be minimized but is generally considered safe if kept under 5 rads. If >10 rads of exposure takes place, consideration should be given to termination due to high rates of teratogenicity, central nervous system abnormalities, or increased risk of childhood leukemias [43]. Transesophageal echocardiography can be used to minimize fluoroscopy time [44]. Acutely, left atrial pressure acutely decreases on average by 13 mmHg, valve area increases, and pulmonary pressures normalize in most patients [42, 45]. If the patient is not a candidate for balloon mitral valvuloplasty, surgical commissurotomy or mitral valve replacement can be considered. As discussed elsewhere, the risk of fetal demise remains high (>10 %) when cardiopulmonary bypass is used in pregnancy [31, 44, 46].

Women with mitral stenosis are at high risk for pulmonary edema in the peripartum and immediate postpartum period. Pain and stress associated with labor precipitate tachycardia. Beta-blockers and adequate analgesia and anesthesia can mitigate this. Often an arterial catheter is placed for hemodynamic monitoring, particularly if intravenous beta-blockers are used. Pulmonary artery catheters have been used in severe pulmonary edema in order to guide therapy but are less frequently used in the contemporary era. At the time of delivery, afterload and intravascular volume abruptly rise which can lead to acute pulmonary edema. Aggressive diuresis (>200 cc/h) in the immediate postpartum period is often required, and regular clinical evaluations for the first 48 h postpartum are required to monitor for decompensation.

Mitral Regurgitation

The most common etiologies of mitral regurgitation in pregnancy are prior endocarditis, myxomatous degeneration, rheumatic disease, and mitral valve prolapse.

Maternal Risk

Mild and moderate mitral regurgitation are usually well tolerated during pregnancy because the decrease of SVR in pregnancy decreases the severity of the mitral regurgitation. Severe mitral regurgitation can lead to pulmonary congestion, particularly in the second and third trimesters [16, 34]. Supraventricular arrhythmias can also precipitate deterioration, usually in the second and third trimesters. Women with atrial arrhythmias, reduced LV systolic function, and prior symptomatic heart failure are at highest risk.

Fetal Risk

Fetal risk is elevated in women with symptoms of heart failure, arrhythmias, or decreased LV systolic function. In well-compensated patients, fetal risk does not appear markedly elevated [16].

Evaluation and Treatment

Prepregnancy echocardiography should be used to grade the severity of regurgitation, evaluate for associated pulmonary hypertension, and exclude LV systolic dysfunction. Patients with pulmonary hypertension or reduced LV ejection fraction should be referred for valve surgery prior to pregnancy [12]. During pregnancy, the severity of mitral regurgitation does not change markedly and LV function generally remains stable [34]. Diuretics and activity restriction are the mainstays of therapy for mitral regurgitation during pregnancy.

Pulmonic Regurgitation

Pulmonic regurgitation in pregnancy is usually secondary to prior palliation for pulmonic stenosis or tetralogy of Fallot. In these instances, pulmonary regurgitation is usually severe and present since infancy; right ventricular dilation is common.

Maternal Risk

Pregnancy is well tolerated in most women with pulmonary regurgitation. In the largest series of women undergoing pregnancy with pulmonary regurgitation, there were no

deaths. Supraventricular tachycardia was the most frequent complication, affecting 2–6 % of women, but may be less common in women who are treated with adequate doses of diuretics [47]. Women with more severe pulmonary regurgitation seem to be at greatest risk for the development of right heart failure [13, 17, 47–49], and right heart failure is more common in those with preexisting right ventricular systolic dysfunction [13]. However, symptomatic right heart failure is usually effectively treated with diuretics and long-term sequelae are uncommon. Residual anatomic defects associated with the original congenital heart lesion, such as peripheral pulmonary artery stenosis or LV systolic dysfunction, also increase the risk of adverse maternal outcomes [47].

Fetal Risk

Fetal risk is not well defined in this population but appears to be low. Depending on the underlying congenital heart defect, there may be considerable (>5 %) risk of inheritance. A 22q11.2 microdeletion (DiGeorge syndrome) is found in approximately 6 % of patients with tetralogy of Fallot and may be difficult to diagnose clinically [50, 51]. Inheritance is 50 %. Fluorescence in situ hybridization (FISH) testing for 22q11.2 microdeletion is clinically available and should be discussed with women with tetralogy of Fallot as part of their preconception counseling.

Evaluation and Treatment

Because adverse maternal outcomes are closely linked to associated anatomic defects such as LV systolic dysfunction, peripheral pulmonary stenosis, and pulmonary hypertension, the preconception echocardiogram should look for these findings and, when possible, be performed at a center with expertise in congenital heart disease [52]. Volume status should be monitored at each clinic visit, and diuretics should be used to treat signs of right heart failure. During normal pregnancy intravascular volume increases, and a right ventricular heave, elevated JVP, and lower extremity edema are common which can lead to the erroneous diagnosis of right heart failure in the compensated patient [43]. BNP can help guide therapy when physical findings are ambiguous [38, 39, 53].

Pulmonic Stenosis

Pulmonic stenosis in pregnant women is congenital or postoperative.

Maternal Risk

In one large series of 60 women with pulmonary stenosis undergoing pregnancy, approximately 40 % had been previously repaired and had residual pulmonic stenosis. There were no adverse maternal events [17]. This excellent outcome was confirmed in subsequent series [16, 47]. However, one large study demonstrated a 15 % incidence of hypertension-related disorders of pregnancy (pregnancy-induced hypertension, preeclampsia, eclampsia) which is higher than the 8 % seen in the general population. Thromboembolic complications were also higher than expected (~2 %) [54]. These findings are limited by study design and require further validation.

Fetal Risk

As in other valvular abnormalities, fetal risk is elevated in women with heart failure, arrhythmias, or associated pulmonary hypertension. In the absence of these findings, fetal outcomes are usually good [17, 34]. The risk of miscarriage or preterm delivery may be as high as 19 and 16 %, respectively, slightly higher than the general population [54]. The risk of congenital heart disease in the offspring of women with isolated pulmonic stenosis is approximately 3 % [54, 55].

Evaluation and Management

During echocardiography for pulmonic stenosis, it is important to distinguish right ventricular systolic pressure (calculated from the tricuspid regurgitation jet velocity) from pulmonary artery systolic pressure (calculated by subtracting maximum pulmonic valve gradient from the right ventricular systolic pressure). Pulmonic valve gradient (and consequently right ventricular systolic pressure) increases during pregnancy, but pulmonary pressures should remain normal. The rare women who develop right heart failure due to pulmonic stenosis should be treated with diuretics.

Risk Scores

Several models have been developed in order to predict maternal and neonatal risk (Fig. 32.1). These are discussed in detail in Chap. 34. A comparison of the most commonly used scoring systems is summarized on Table 32.1.

Prosthetic Valves

For women who have high-risk or symptomatic valve disease prior to pregnancy, elective valve replacement or repair, if possible, prior to conception is indicated. The selection of the appropriate valve type is challenging because biologic valves are safer in pregnancy for the mother and fetus but have limited life span which requires future reoperation [56, 57].

Biologic Valves in Pregnancy

The major advantage of biologic valves is their reduced thrombogenicity such that they do not require anticoagulation during pregnancy and are associated with fewer maternal, obstetric, and neonatal complications than mechanical valves.

However, biologic valve degeneration is accelerated in younger patients [57–60]. As many as 73 % of patients younger than 30 years of age have substantial valve deterioration within 10 years compared with only 17 % of patients older than 60 years of age [61]. This means that women with biologic valves placed in their 20s or 30s will require several valve replacements over their lifetime, and redo operations have substantially increased operative mortality [59]. Newer generation bioprosthetic valves are likely more durable than older bioprosthetic valves with one author reporting valve survival of >90 % at 12 years, even in younger patients [62], but robust confirmatory data is lacking [63].

Pericardial valves, autografts, and homgrafts may have superior durability in younger patients when compared to porcine bioprosthetic valves [57, 59, 64]. In young patients with aortic valve disease, a Ross procedure places a pulmonary autograft into the aortic position, and a homgraft is placed in the pulmonic position. However, patients who undergo the Ross procedure are predisposed to degeneration of the neo-pulmonic as well as the neo-aortic valves and can be predisposed to neo-aortic root dilation as well. There has been enormous variability in the long-term outcomes of patients who have undergone the Ross procedure, and results are highly dependent upon the surgeon and institution [65].

There is conflicting information as to whether pregnancy accelerates degeneration of biologic valves [66–69]. Several authors have found high rates of valve failure in young patients who have become pregnant, but this phenomenon may be in part due to the fact that these patients are younger which is an established risk factor for biologic valve deterioration. Furthermore, these studies are generally of earlier generation biologic valves which are believed to have reduced longevity compared with contemporary valves. However, several recent studies comparing young women with biologic valves who did and did not become pregnant did not find any evidence of accelerated valve deterioration in the 43 women who became pregnant [57, 69, 70].

One option favored by many institutions is to recommend a biologic valve during childbearing years which subsequently gets changed to a mechanical valve. While this strategy may necessitate an additional operation, that risk is partially offset by the lower rate of complications during pregnancy.

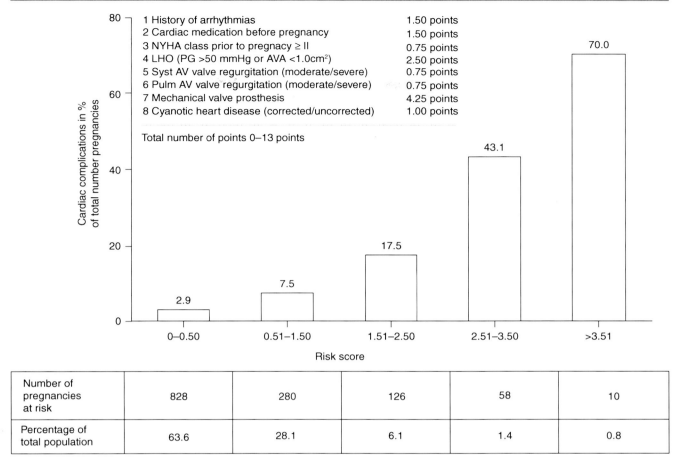

Fig. 32.1 The modified risk score for cardiac complications during completed (20 weeks of gestation) pregnancies in women with congenital heart disease (expressed as % of the total number of completed pregnancies). *AV* atrioventricular, *AVA* aortic valve area, *LHO* left heart obstruction, *NYHA* New York Heart Association, *PG* peak gradient, *Pulm* pulmonary, *Syst* systemic (Adapted with permission from Drenthen et al. [16])

Table 32.1 Comparison of risk factors for adverse maternal adverse outcomes

	ACC/AHA guidelines [12]	Siu et al. [17]	Drenthen et al. [16]	Khairy et al. [13]
Study group		599 pregnancies, 224 women with heart disease	1,302 pregnancies in women with congenital heart disease	90 pregnancies, 54 women with congenital heart disease
History		Prior cardiac event or arrhythmia	Prior arrhythmia cardiac medication prior to pregnancy	Prior history of heart failure, smoking history, weight
NYHA class	AR, MS, MR with class III–IV symptoms	NYHA >II or cyanosis	NYHA >2	NYHA ≥2
Valve lesion	AS with or without symptoms Mechanical prosthesis	Left heart obstruction	≥Moderate mitral regurgitation ≥Moderate tricuspid regurgitation Left heart obstruction (AVA <1 cm², pressure gradient >50 mmHg) Mechanical prosthesis	Severe pulmonic regurgitation
Ejection fraction	AV or MV disease with EF <40 %	Systemic ventricular dysfunction (EF <40 %)		Decreased subpulmonic ventricular EF

ACC/AHA American College of Cardiology/American Heart Association, *AR* aortic regurgitation, *MS* mitral stenosis, *MR* mitral regurgitation, *AS* aortic stenosis, *AV* aortic valve, *MV* mitral valve, *AVA* aortic valve area, *NYHA: NYHA* New York Heart Association, *EF* ejection fraction, *mmHg* millimeters of mercury

Mechanical Valves in Pregnancy

Pregnancy is a hypercoagulable state which increases the risk of mechanical valve thrombosis so effective uninterrupted anticoagulation is absolutely essential throughout [71–73]. Strategies for anticoagulation are discussed below.

Maternal Complications

The maternal complication rate is consistently found to be high in women with mechanical valves [71–76]. The thromboembolic rate during pregnancy ranges from 2.4 to 10.3 % depending on the type of valve and the strategy of anticoagulation used [71]. With ineffective anticoagulation the thromboembolic rate is as high as 60 % [74]. Even with effective anticoagulation, women with mechanical valves are at high risk during pregnancy and should be managed by an interdisciplinary team which includes a cardiologist, high-risk obstetrician, and an anticoagulation clinic with expertise in pregnancy.

Maternal mortality rate is ~2.9 % and is usually due to thromboembolic complications. Mortality is even higher in women with inadequate anticoagulation. The risk of major bleeding at the time of delivery is 2.5 %, but others have reported rates as high as 10 % [74, 77]. The presence of a mechanical valve increases maternal risk 75-fold [16].

Fetal Complications

The rate of fetal complications is closely linked to the strategy of anticoagulation used during pregnancy and is discussed in more detail below. In women with mechanical valves, the overall rate of spontaneous abortion is approximately 25 %, and the rate of congenital fetal anomalies is approximately 3.5 % and is substantially higher in women who take warfarin during the first trimester [74].

Anticoagulation for Mechanical Valves in Pregnancy

The most important consideration when selecting an anticoagulation regimen during pregnancy is to ensure therapeutic uninterrupted anticoagulation. There is no universally accepted anticoagulation strategy as maternal risk needs to be balanced against fetal risk. Each anticoagulation strategy has significant limitations and challenges. Therefore, the appropriate strategy needs to be individualized and thoroughly discussed with the patient. Women at the highest risk for thromboembolic complications (those with older generation mechanical atrioventricular valve, prior thromboembolic complication, multiple mechanical valves, or atrial fibrillation and a mechanical valve) may require more intensive anticoagulation which increases fetal risk and the risk of

Table 32.2 Recommended anticoagulant regimens in pregnant women with mechanical heart valves [78]

ACCP guidelines. The selection of any of the following regiments is acceptable
1. Adjusted-dose bid LMWH throughout pregnancy 　Doses adjusted to achieve the manufacturer's peak anti-Xa LMWH 4 h postinjection
2. Adjusted-dose UFH throughout pregnancy 　Administered subcutaneously every 12 h in doses adjusted to keep the mid-interval aPTT at least twice control or attain an anti-Xa heparin level of 0.35–0.70 U/ml
3. UFH or LMWH (as above) until the 13th week, with substitution by vitamin K antagonists until close to delivery when UFH or LMWH is resumed

Modified from Bates et al. [78]
ACCP American College of Chest Physicians, *LMWH* low molecular weight heparin, *UFH* unfractionated heparin, *aPTT* activated partial thromboplastin time

maternal hemorrhage. The most comprehensive guidelines for anticoagulation during pregnancy are provided by the American College of Chest Physicians in 2012, and treatment options are summarized in Table 32.2 [78].

- *Warfarin throughout pregnancy*: The use of warfarin throughout pregnancy is associated with the lowest rate of maternal thromboembolism but the highest rate of fetal malformation. For most women, the risk of fetal complications makes uninterrupted warfarin an unappealing choice. It may be a reasonable option for women at the highest risk of thromboembolic complication after careful discussion with the patient and obstetrician. Women should be transitioned to a shorter-acting agent (dose-adjusted low molecular weight heparin or dose-adjusted unfractionated heparin) at week 35 to avoid labor while on warfarin which increases maternal and fetal hemorrhagic complications. The rate of maternal thromboembolism is as low as 3.9 % in women treated with uninterrupted warfarin, a significantly lower rate than is seen in other strategies of anticoagulation during pregnancy [74, 79].For women at highest risk of thrombotic complication, low-dose aspirin can be added [78]. The overall risk of warfarin embryopathy (midfacial hypoplasia, skeletal anomalies, central nervous system abnormalities, and developmental delay) among women treated with warfarin during the first trimester ranges from 3.7 to 7.3 % in two large systematic reviews [74, 78, 80]. Some authors believe the rate is even higher [59]. Warfarin embryopathy appears to be restricted to women who take warfarin during the first trimester. The rate of warfarin embryopathy is dose related and is lower in women who require less than 5 mg/day [81]. The rate of spontaneous abortion is also higher in women who take warfarin during the first trimester. For many women and providers, the risk of teratogenicity is unacceptable and therefore an alternative regimen is selected.

- *Heparin (either unfractionated or low molecular weight) during the first trimester followed by warfarin*: Because warfarin embryopathy appears to be highest in the first trimester, the approach of using heparin during the first trimester followed by warfarin has been used. This option has lower thrombotic risk than using heparin throughout pregnancy [74] and lower fetal risk than uninterrupted warfarin. In order to minimize fetal risk, heparin should replace warfarin by week 6. Frequent pregnancy testing is reasonable in women taking warfarin so that the transition can be made in a timely fashion.
  - Dose-adjusted low molecular weight heparin (preferred) or dose-adjusted unfractionated heparin can be used in the first trimester. Because dosing can be unpredictable in pregnancy, dose adjustment is mandatory (see below).
  - Unfractionated heparin can be given as a continuous infusion or as twice daily subcutaneous dosing.
  - While warfarin embryopathy is not common if use is restricted to second and third trimester, minor neurodevelopmental problems may be slightly more common in children exposed to warfarin during the later trimesters [82].
  - After 12 weeks the patient is transitioned to warfarin until week 35.
- *Heparin throughout pregnancy:* Patients at lowest risk for thromboembolic complications (bileaflet tilting disk in the aortic position, no atrial fibrillation or prior thromboembolic complication) may consider a heparin throughout pregnancy. Neither unfractionated heparin nor low molecular weight heparin crosses the placenta, and teratogenicity is not increased [78]. The rate of maternal thromboembolic complication is highest in women on heparin throughout pregnancy (compared to women who take warfarin) and ranges from 8.6 to 15 % [74, 76, 83]. Careful dose adjustment likely reduces the risk of thromboembolic complications. The majority of cases of valve thrombosis in women taking low molecular weight heparin occur in those receiving a fixed, weight-based dose [83].
  - Fixed, weight-based dosing of either unfractionated heparin or low molecular weight heparin is associated with unacceptable levels of thrombosis and is contraindicated [83]. The therapeutic dose often fluctuates throughout pregnancy so regular monitoring is required [84].
  - Unfractionated heparin is associated with higher rates of heparin-induced thrombocytopenia and osteoporosis. Continuous infusion is also associated with catheter complications such as infection or endocarditis.
- Fondaparinux, parenteral direct thrombin inhibitors, oral direct thrombin inhibitors (dabigatran), and oral anti-Xa inhibitors (rivaroxaban, apixaban) should be avoided in pregnancy [78].
  - *Dose monitoring*See Table 32.2.

Valve Thrombosis in Pregnancy

Despite adequate anticoagulation, the risk of valve thrombosis is elevated in pregnancy. Valve thrombosis is potentially catastrophic and should be diagnosed quickly. Echocardiography, transesophageal echocardiography, and fluoroscopy can all be used to clarify the mechanism of valve thrombosis. Surgery has traditionally been the mainstay of therapy for mechanical valve thrombosis, but thrombolytics are used with increasing frequency and may have better outcomes in patients with severe symptoms or LV dysfunction, particularly if the thrombus is less than 1 cm by transesophageal echocardiography [85–87]. There are no prospective trials on the use of thrombolytic therapy in pregnancy. However, teratogenicity is not described and fetal loss is approximately 6 %. Major maternal hemorrhage is common if delivery is within 24 h of therapy [88].

For patients who are not candidates for thrombolytic therapy during pregnancy, emergent valve replacement is an option. As discussed below, cardiac surgery with cardiopulmonary bypass carries a high rate of fetal loss [88].

Cardiac Surgery During Pregnancy

For women who have symptoms refractory to medical therapy or acute valve dysfunction not amenable to thrombolytic therapy, cardiac surgery during pregnancy remains an option. Fetal loss rate is approximately 15–30 %. The maternal mortality rate is also high (7–13 %), reflecting the severity of illness in this population [31, 46, 89, 90]. Higher NYHA functional class and emergency surgery are associated with worse maternal and fetal outcomes [90]. The effects of cardiopulmonary bypass on placental circulation are not well defined. When feasible, surgery should be avoided during the first trimester to avoid teratogenicity. Coordination between the obstetrical team and cardiac team is critical. Continuous fetal heart monitoring should be performed throughout the perioperative period.

Labor and Delivery

Pregnant women with significant valvular disease should be delivered in centers with expertise in their management. The optimal care is delivered by a multidisciplinary team of obstetricians, cardiologists, and anesthesiologists who can anticipate the hemodynamic perturbations of labor and delivery, treat any that arise, and are prepared for acute deterioration in the maternal or fetal condition.

As a general rule, labor and delivery should be "short and pain-free" in women with significant valve disease. Vaginal delivery is preferred unless obstetric indications dictate a cesarean section. The only circumstance where guidelines recommend a cesarean delivery on the basis of maternal heart disease is for women with Marfan syndrome and aortic dilation. The general goal is to allow maternal pushing as long as tolerated, but be ready to assist the second stage of labor. Adequate treatment of pain and anxiety typically involves an epidural or local blocks, in addition to intravenous pain medication or anxiolytics as needed. Caution should be taken with those patients who may not tolerate the decrease in afterload associated with an epidural. Either an alternative approach should be considered or appropriate medical therapy to support blood pressure should be readily available. Anticoagulation may impact the ability to perform an epidural, particularly if enoxaparin is used on the day prior to delivery.

Some patients may benefit from invasive monitoring during pregnancy, such as an arterial line or pulmonary artery catheter. One experienced center reported a steady decline in their use of invasive monitoring as they gained more experience in the delivery of patients with significant heart disease [91].

Preconceptual Counseling

Ideally, all women with heart disease should receive preconceptual counseling regarding the risks of pregnancy, including maternal risk and any anticipated fetal issues, such as medication exposure or inheritance of congenital heart disease. As with the management of these patients, this counseling is best done by practitioners with expertise, especially in patients with significant valve disease. Comprehensive counseling can be provided by either the cardiologist or the obstetrician expected to care for the patient during pregnancy. However, it is ideal for the patient to meet with both the cardiologist and the obstetrician. In some cases, women with mild disease who will likely have a normal pregnancy and delivery are under the misconception that they are at increased risk. On the other end of the spectrum, some women with severe symptomatic valve disease may not understand the high-risk nature of pregnancy or the possible need for valve intervention prior to any anticipated pregnancy.

Preconceptual counseling should take into account the patient's functional status, heart disease history, exam, and echocardiographic findings. Some patients may benefit from additional testing, such as other imaging (magnetic resonance imaging or computed tomography) or exercise testing. Counseling should include not only an assessment of risk but discussion of what can be done to minimize the likelihood of complications during pregnancy, how labor and delivery will be managed, and what medications may be necessary. Many women will be under the assumption that a cesarean section is obligatory or that medications cannot be used during pregnancy, while others hope for "natural" or even at home deliveries; thus, establishing the patient's expectations and desires

Table 32.3 Key components of preconceptual counseling

Accurately identify all relevant lesion
Assess symptoms and physical exam
Assess functional status
Consider exercise testing
Address medications
Meet with maternal-fetal medicine specialist
Discuss recurrence risk
Fetal echocardiogram

is an important part of counseling. Since there is an increased risk of fetal congenital heart disease in women with congenital heart disease, counseling must include assessment of this risk. Fetal echocardiography is appropriate for all women with congenital heart disease and the role, and limitations of fetal echocardiography should be discussed as part of preconceptual counseling. In summary, counseling will be individualized, tailored to the patient's valve disease, severity of disease, presence of symptoms, need for medications, and desires surrounding pregnancy, labor and delivery, and the inheritance patterns of the maternal heart disease (Table 32.3). For those patients for whom pregnancy isn't advised, effective contraception must be addressed and provided. For women who meet criteria for valve intervention, either catheter based or surgical, these should be completed prior to pregnancy. However, if women are not otherwise in need of a valve procedure, it is not generally recommended to pursue intervention solely to make pregnancy "safer."

Key Points

- The hemodynamic changes of pregnancy are variably tolerated by women with valvular disease, depending on the nature and severity of the valve dysfunction.
- Severe aortic stenosis is considered to be a high-risk lesion in pregnancy.
- Mitral stenosis in pregnancy is usually rheumatic in origin and is often first diagnosed when a previously healthy woman develops heart failure in pregnancy.
- Moderate or severe mitral stenosis is poorly tolerated during pregnancy and typically presents in the second trimester. The mitral valve gradient increases due to increased intravascular volume, increased cardiac output, and tachycardia.
- The majority of women with moderate or severe mitral stenosis have a functional decline during pregnancy.
- Preconceptual counseling should take into account the patient's functional status, heart disease history, physical exam, and echocardiographic findings.
- For women who have high-risk or symptomatic valve disease prior to pregnancy, elective valve replacement prior to conception is indicated.

References

1. Easterling TR, Benedetti TJ, Schmucker BC, Millard SP. Maternal hemodynamics in normal and preeclamptic pregnancies: a longitudinal study. Obstet Gynecol. 1990;76:1061–9.

2. Robson SC, Dunlop W, Hunter S. Haemodynamic changes during the early puerperium. Br Med J (Clin Res Ed). 1987;294:1065.

3. Meijboom LJ, Drenthen W, Pieper PG, Groenink M, van der Post JA, Timmermans J, Voors AA, Roos-Hesselink JW, van Veldhuisen DJ, Mulder BJ. Obstetric complications in Marfan syndrome. Int J Cardiol. 2006;110(1):53–9.

4. Donnelly RT, Pinto NM, Kocolas I, Yetman AT. The immediate and long-term impact of pregnancy on aortic growth rate and mortality in women with Marfan syndrome. J Am Coll Cardiol. 2012;60: 224–9.

5. Mishra M, Chambers JB, Jackson G. Murmurs in pregnancy: an audit of echocardiography. BMJ. 1992;304:1413–4.

6. Hunter S, Robson SC. Adaptation of the maternal heart in pregnancy. Br Heart J. 1992;68:540–3.

7. Otto CM. The practice of clinical echocardiography. Philadelphia: Saunders/Elsevier; 2007.

8. Silversides CK, Colman JM, Sermer M, Farine D, Siu SC. Early and intermediate-term outcomes of pregnancy with congenital aortic stenosis. Am J Cardiol. 2003;91:1386–9.

9. Grossman W, McLaurin LP. Diastolic properties of the left ventricle. Ann Intern Med. 1976;84:316–26.

10. Hameed A, Karaalp IS, Tummala PP, Wani OR, Canetti M, Akhter MW, Goodwin I, Zapadinsky N, Elkayam U. The effect of valvular heart disease on maternal and fetal outcome of pregnancy. J Am Coll Cardiol. 2001;37:893–9.

11. Arias F, Pineda J. Aortic stenosis and pregnancy. J Reprod Med. 1978;20:229–32.

12. Bonow RO, Carabello BA, Chatterjee K, de Leon Jr AC, Faxon DP, Freed MD, Gaasch WH, Lytle BW, Nishimura RA, O'Gara PT, O'Rourke RA, Otto CM, Shah PM, Shanewise JS. 2008 focused update incorporated into the ACC/AHA 2006 guidelines for the management of patients with valvular heart disease: a report of the American College of Cardiology/American Heart Association Task Force on Practice Guidelines (writing committee to revise the 1998 guidelines for the management of patients with valvular heart disease). Endorsed by the Society of Cardiovascular Anesthesiologists, Society for Cardiovascular Angiography and Interventions, and Society of Thoracic Surgeons. J Am Coll Cardiol. 2008;52: e1–142.

13. Khairy P, Ouyang DW, Fernandes SM, Lee-Parritz A, Economy KE, Landzberg MJ. Pregnancy outcomes in women with congenital heart disease. Circulation. 2006;113:517–24.

14. Drenthen W, Pieper PG, Roos-Hesselink JW, van Lottum WA, Voors AA, Mulder BJ, van Dijk AP, Vliegen HW, Yap SC, Moons P, Ebels T, van Veldhuisen DJ. Outcome of pregnancy in women with congenital heart disease: a literature review. J Am Coll Cardiol. 2007;49:2303–11.

15. Yap SC, Drenthen W, Pieper PG, Moons P, Mulder BJ, Mostert B, Vliegen HW, van Dijk AP, Meijboom FJ, Steegers EA, Roos-Hesselink JW. Risk of complications during pregnancy in women with congenital aortic stenosis. Int J Cardiol. 2008;126:240–6.

16. Drenthen W, Boersma E, Balci A, Moons P, Roos-Hesselink JW, Mulder BJ, Vliegen HW, van Dijk AP, Voors AA, Yap SC, van Veldhuisen DJ, Pieper PG. Predictors of pregnancy complications in women with congenital heart disease. Eur Heart J. 2010;31:2124–32.

17. Siu SC, Sermer M, Colman JM, Alvarez AN, Mercier LA, Morton BC, Kells CM, Bergin ML, Kiess MC, Marcotte F, Taylor DA, Gordon EP, Spears JC, Tam JW, Amankwah KS, Smallhorn JF, Farine D, Sorensen S. Prospective multicenter study of pregnancy outcomes in women with heart disease. Circulation. 2001;104:515–21.

18. Tzemos N, Silversides CK, Colman JM, Therrien J, Webb GD, Mason J, Cocoara E, Sermer M, Siu SC. Late cardiac outcomes after pregnancy in women with congenital aortic stenosis. Am Heart J. 2009;157:474–80.

19. Tzemos N, Silversides CK, Carasso S, Rakowski H, Siu SC. Effect of pregnancy on left ventricular motion (twist) in women with aortic stenosis. Am J Cardiol. 2008;101:870–3.

20. Immer FF, Bansi AG, Immer-Bansi AS, McDougall J, Zehr KJ, Schaff HV, Carrel TP. Aortic dissection in pregnancy: analysis of risk factors and outcome. Ann Thorac Surg. 2003;76:309–14.

21. McKellar SH, MacDonald RJ, Michelena HI, Connolly HM, Sundt 3rd TM. Frequency of cardiovascular events in women with a congenitally bicuspid aortic valve in a single community and effect of pregnancy on events. Am J Cardiol. 2011;107:96–9.

22. Oskoui R, Lindsay Jr J. Aortic dissection in women <40years of age and the unimportance of pregnancy. Am J Cardiol. 1994;73:821–3.

23. Lewin MB, Otto CM. The bicuspid aortic valve: adverse outcomes from infancy to old age. Circulation. 2005;111:832–4.

24. Garg V. Molecular genetics of aortic valve disease. Curr Opin Cardiol. 2006;21:180–4.

25. Gerber IL, Stewart RA, Legget ME, West TM, French RL, Sutton TM, Yandle TG, French JK, Richards AM, White HD. Increased plasma natriuretic peptide levels reflect symptom onset in aortic stenosis. Circulation. 2003;107:1884–90.

26. Lim P, Monin JL, Monchi M, Garot J, Pasquet A, Hittinger L, Vanoverschelde JL, Carayon A, Gueret P. Predictors of outcome in patients with severe aortic stenosis and normal left ventricular function: role of B-type natriuretic peptide. Eur Heart J. 2004;25: 2048–53.

27. Patel S, Grayburn PA, High ST, Rosnes J, Choi JW. Usefulness of serial brain natriuretic peptide measurements for managing aortic valve stenosis in pregnancy. Proc (Bayl Univ Med Cent). 2009; 22:226–9.

28. Resnik JL, Hong C, Resnik R, Kazanegra R, Beede J, Bhalla V, Maisel A. Evaluation of B-type natriuretic peptide (BNP) levels in normal and preeclamptic women. Am J Obstet Gynecol. 2005;193: 450–4.

29. Lao TT, Adelman AG, Sermer M, Colman JM. Balloon valvuloplasty for congenital aortic stenosis in pregnancy. Br J Obstet Gynaecol. 1993;100:1141–2.

30. Myerson SG, Mitchell AR, Ormerod OJ, Banning AP. What is the role of balloon dilatation for severe aortic stenosis during pregnancy? J Heart Valve Dis. 2005;14:147–50.

31. John AS, Gurley F, Schaff HV, Warnes CA, Phillips SD, Arendt KW, Abel MD, Rose CH, Connolly HM. Cardiopulmonary bypass during pregnancy. Ann Thorac Surg. 2011;91:1191–6.

32. Edouard DA, Pannier BM, London GM, Cuche JL, Safar ME. Venous and arterial behavior during normal pregnancy. Am J Physiol. 1998;274:H1605–12.

33. Marcus FI, Ewy GA, O'Rourke RA, Walsh B, Bleich AC. The effect of pregnancy on the murmurs of mitral and aortic regurgitation. Circulation. 1970;41:795–805.

34. Lesniak-Sobelga A, Tracz W, KostKiewicz M, Podolec P, Pasowicz M. Clinical and echocardiographic assessment of pregnant women with valvular heart diseases – maternal and fetal outcome. Int J Cardiol. 2004;94:15–23.

35. Walters BNJ, Redman CWG. Treatment of severe pregnancy-associated hypertension with the calcium-antagonist nifedipine. Br J Obstet Gynaecol. 1984;91:330–6.

36. Silversides CK, Colman JM, Sermer M, Siu SC. Cardiac risk in pregnant women with rheumatic mitral stenosis. Am J Cardiol. 2003;91:1382–5.

37. Chadha DS, Karthikeyan G, Goel K, Malani SK, Seth S, Singh S, Dhall A, Bhargava B. N-terminal pro-BNP plasma levels before and after percutaneous transvenous mitral commissurotomy for mitral stenosis. Int J Cardiol. 2010;144:238–40.

38. Iltumur K, Karabulut A, Yokus B, Yavuzkir M, Taskesen T, Toprak N. N-terminal proBNP plasma levels correlate with severity of mitral stenosis. J Heart Valve Dis. 2005;14:735–41.

39. Hameed AB, Chan K, Ghamsary M, Elkayam U. Longitudinal changes in the b-type natriuretic peptide levels in normal pregnancy and postpartum. Clin Cardiol. 2009;32:E60–2.

40. Tanous D, Siu SC, Mason J, Greutmann M, Wald RM, Parker JD, Sermer M, Colman JM, Silversides CK. B-type natriuretic peptide in pregnant women with heart disease. J Am Coll Cardiol. 2010;56:1247–53.

41. Wadelius M, Darj E, Frenne G, Rane A. Induction of cyp2d6 in pregnancy. Clin Pharmacol Ther. 1997;62:400–7.

42. Esteves CA, Munoz JS, Braga S, Andrade J, Meneghelo Z, Gomes N, Maldonado M, Esteves V, Sepetiba R, Sousa JE, Palacios IF. Immediate and long-term follow-up of percutaneous balloon mitral valvuloplasty in pregnant patients with rheumatic mitral stenosis. Am J Cardiol. 2006;98:812–6.

43. Zipes DP, Braunwald E. Braunwald's heart disease : a textbook of cardiovascular medicine. Philadelphia: W.B. Saunders; 2005.

44. Hameed AB, Mehra A, Rahimtoola SH. The role of catheter balloon commissurotomy for severe mitral stenosis in pregnancy. Obstet Gynecol. 2009;114:1336–40.

45. Ben Farhat M, Gamra H, Betbout F, Maatouk F, Jarrar M, Addad F, Tiss M, Hammami S, Chahbani I, Thaalbi R. Percutaneous balloon mitral commissurotomy during pregnancy. Heart. 1997;77:564–7.

46. Avila WS, Gouveia AM, Pomerantzeff P, Bortolotto MR, Grinberg M, Stolf N, Zugaib M. Maternal-fetal outcome and prognosis of cardiac surgery during pregnancy. Arq Bras Cardiol. 2009;93:9–14.

47. Greutmann M, Von Klemperer K, Brooks R, Peebles D, O'Brien P, Walker F. Pregnancy outcome in women with congenital heart disease and residual haemodynamic lesions of the right ventricular outflow tract. Eur Heart J. 2010;31:1764–70.

48. Veldtman GR, Connolly HM, Grogan M, Ammash NM, Warnes CA. Outcomes of pregnancy in women with tetralogy of Fallot. J Am Coll Cardiol. 2004;44:174–80.

49. Meijer JM, Pieper PG, Drenthen W, Voors AA, Roos-Hesselink JW, van Dijk AP, Mulder BJ, Ebels T, van Veldhuisen DJ. Pregnancy, fertility, and recurrence risk in corrected tetralogy of Fallot. Heart. 2005;91:801–5.

50. Beauchesne LM, Warnes CA, Connolly HM, Ammash NM, Grogan M, Jalal SM, Michels VV. Prevalence and clinical manifestations of 22q11.2 microdeletion in adults with selected conotruncal anomalies. J Am Coll Cardiol. 2005;45:595–8.

51. Rauch R, Hofbeck M, Zweier C, Koch A, Zink S, Trautmann U, Hoyer J, Kaulitz R, Singer H, Rauch A. Comprehensive genotype-phenotype analysis in 230 patients with tetralogy of Fallot. J Med Genet. 2010;47:321–31.

52. Warnes CA, Williams RG, Bashore TM, Child JS, Connolly HM, Dearani JA, del Nido P, Fasules JW, Graham Jr TP, Hijazi ZM, Hunt SA, King ME, Landzberg MJ, Miner PD, Radford MJ, Walsh EP, Webb GD, Smith Jr SC, Jacobs AK, Adams CD, Anderson JL, Antman EM, Buller CE, Creager MA, Ettinger SM, Halperin JL, Krumholz HM, Kushner FG, Lytle BW, Nishimura RA, Page RL, Riegel B, Tarkington LG, Yancy CW. ACC/AHA 2008 guidelines for the management of adults with congenital heart disease: a report of the American College of Cardiology/American Heart Association Task Force on Practice Guidelines (writing committee to develop guidelines on the management of adults with congenital heart disease). Developed in collaboration with the American Society of Echocardiography, Heart Rhythm Society, International Society for Adult Congenital Heart Disease, Society for Cardiovascular Angiography and Interventions, and Society of Thoracic Surgeons. J Am Coll Cardiol. 2008;52:e143–263.

53. Oosterhof T, Tulevski II, Vliegen HW, Spijkerboer AM, Mulder BJ. Effects of volume and/or pressure overload secondary to congenital heart disease (tetralogy of Fallot or pulmonary stenosis) on right ventricular function using cardiovascular magnetic resonance and B-type natriuretic peptide levels. Am J Cardiol. 2006;97:1051–5.

54. Drenthen W, Pieper PG, Roos-Hesselink JW, Schmidt AC, Mulder BJ, van Dijk AP, Vliegen HW, Sollie KM, Voors AA, Ebels T, van Veldhuisen DJ. Non-cardiac complications during pregnancy in women with isolated congenital pulmonary valvar stenosis. Heart. 2006;92:1838–43.

55. Driscoll DJ, Michels VV, Gersony WM, Hayes CJ, Keane JF, Kidd L, Pieroni DR, Rings LJ, Wolfe RR, Weidman WH. Occurrence risk for congenital heart defects in relatives of patients with aortic stenosis, pulmonary stenosis, or ventricular septal defect. Circulation. 1993;87:I114–20.

56. Curtis SL, Marsden-Williams J, Sullivan C, Sellers SM, Trinder J, Scrutton M, Stuart AG. Current trends in the management of heart disease in pregnancy. Int J Cardiol. 2009;133:62–9.

57. North RA, Sadler L, Stewart AW, McCowan LM, Kerr AR, White HD. Long-term survival and valve-related complications in young women with cardiac valve replacements. Circulation. 1999;99:2669–76.

58. Yun KL, Craig Miller D, Moore KA, Scott Mitchell R, Oyer PE, Stinson EB, Robbins RC, Reitz BA, Shumway NE. Durability of the Hancock MO bioprosthesis compared with standard aortic valve bioprostheses. Ann Thorac Surg. 1995;60 Suppl 2:S221–8.

59. Elkayam U, Bitar F. Valvular heart disease and pregnancy: part II: prosthetic valves. J Am Coll Cardiol. 2005;46:403–10.

60. Jeejeebhoy FM. Prosthetic heart valves and management during pregnancy. Can Fam Physician. 2009;55:155–7.

61. Jamieson WR, Rosado LJ, Munro AI, Gerein AN, Burr LH, Miyagishima RT, Janusz MT, Tyers GF. Carpentier-Edwards standard porcine bioprosthesis: primary tissue failure (structural valve deterioration) by age groups. Ann Thorac Surg. 1988;46:155–62.

62. Bach DS, Metras J, Doty JR, Yun KL, Dumesnil JG, Kon ND. Freedom from structural valve deterioration among patients aged < or = 60 years undergoing freestyle stentless aortic valve replacement. J Heart Valve Dis. 2007;16:649–55; discussion 656.

63. El Oakley R, Kleine P, Bach DS. Choice of prosthetic heart valve in today's practice. Circulation. 2008;117:253–6.

64. Gao G, Wu Y, Grunkemeier GL, Furnary AP, Starr A. Durability of pericardial versus porcine aortic valves. J Am Coll Cardiol. 2004;44:384–8.

65. David TE. Ross procedure at the crossroads. Circulation. 2009;119:207–9.

66. Bortolotti U, Milano A, Mazzucco A, Valfre C, Russo R, Valente M, Schivazappa L, Thiene G, Gallucci V. Pregnancy in patients with a porcine valve bioprosthesis. Am J Cardiol. 1982;50:1051–4.

67. Badduke BR, Jamieson WR, Miyagishima RT, Munro AI, Gerein AN, MacNab J, Tyers GF. Pregnancy and childbearing in a population with biologic valvular prostheses. J Thorac Cardiovasc Surg. 1991;102:179–86.

68. Hanania G, Thomas D, Michel PL, Garbarz E, Age C, Millaire A, Acar J. Pregnancy and prosthetic heart valves: a French cooperative retrospective study of 155 cases. Eur Heart J. 1994;15:1651–8.

69. Cleuziou J, Horer J, Kaemmerer H, Teodorowicz A, Kasnar-Samprec J, Schreiber C, Lange R. Pregnancy does not accelerate biological valve degeneration. Int J Cardiol. 2010;145:418–21.

70. Avila WS, Rossi EG, Grinberg M, Ramires JA. Influence of pregnancy after bioprosthetic valve replacement in young women: a prospective five-year study. J Heart Valve Dis. 2002;11:864–9.

71. Abildgaard U, Sandset PM, Hammerstrom J, Gjestvang FT, Tveit A. Management of pregnant women with mechanical heart valve prosthesis: thromboprophylaxis with low molecular weight heparin. Thromb Res. 2009;124:262–7.

72. Vural KM, Ozatik MA, Uncu H, Emir M, Yurdagok O, Sener E, Tasdemir O. Pregnancy after mechanical mitral valve replacement. J Heart Valve Dis. 2003;12:370–6.

73. Salazar E, Izaguirre R, Verdejo J, Mutchinick O. Failure of adjusted doses of subcutaneous heparin to prevent thromboembolic phenomena in pregnant patients with mechanical cardiac valve prostheses. J Am Coll Cardiol. 1996;27:1698–703.

74. Chan WS, Anand S, Ginsberg JS. Anticoagulation of pregnant women with mechanical heart valves: a systematic review of the literature. Arch Intern Med. 2000;160:191–6.

75. Curtis SL, Trinder J, Stuart AG. Acute thrombosis of a prosthetic mitral valve in pregnancy in spite of adjusted-dose low-molecular-weight heparin and aspirin. J Heart Valve Dis. 2008;17:133–4.

76. McLintock C, McCowan LM, North RA. Maternal complications and pregnancy outcome in women with mechanical prosthetic heart valves treated with enoxaparin. BJOG. 2009;116:1585–92.

77. Sillesen M, Hjortdal V, Vejlstrup N, Sorensen K. Pregnancy with prosthetic heart valves – 30 years' nationwide experience in Denmark. Eur J Cardiothorac Surg. 2011;40:448–54.

78. Bates SM, Greer IA, Middeldorp S, Veenstra DL, Prabulos AM, Vandvik PO. VTE, thrombophilia, antithrombotic therapy, and pregnancy: antithrombotic therapy and prevention of thrombosis, 9th ed: American college of chest physicians evidence-based clinical practice guidelines. Chest. 2012;141:e691S–736.

79. Bian C, Wei Q, Liu X. Influence of heart-valve replacement of warfarin anticoagulant therapy on perinatal outcomes. Arch Gynecol Obstet. 2012;285(2):347–51.

80. Frewin R, Chisholm M. Anticoagulation of women with prosthetic heart valves during pregnancy. Br J Obstet Gynaecol. 1998;105:683–6.

81. Vitale N, De Feo M, De Santo LS, Pollice A, Tedesco N, Cotrufo M. Dose-dependent fetal complications of warfarin in pregnant women with mechanical heart valves. J Am Coll Cardiol. 1999;33:1637–41.

82. Farquharson RG, Quenby S, Greaves M. Antiphospholipid syndrome in pregnancy: a randomized, controlled trial of treatment. Obstet Gynecol. 2002;100:408–13.

83. Oran B, Lee-Parritz A, Ansell J. Low molecular weight heparin for the prophylaxis of thromboembolism in women with prosthetic mechanical heart valves during pregnancy. Thromb Haemost. 2004;92:747–51.

84. Barbour LA, Oja JL, Schultz LK. A prospective trial that demonstrates that dalteparin requirements increase in pregnancy to maintain therapeutic levels of anticoagulation. Am J Obstet Gynecol. 2004;191:1024–9.

85. Caceres-Loriga FM, Perez-Lopez H, Morlans-Hernandez K, Facundo-Sanchez H, Santos-Gracia J, Valiente-Mustelier J, Rodiles-Aldana F, Marrero-Mirayaga MA, Betancourt BY, Lopez-Saura P. Thrombolysis as first choice therapy in prosthetic heart valve thrombosis. A study of 68 patients. J Thromb Thrombolysis. 2006;21:185–90.

86. Lengyel M. Thrombolysis should be regarded as first-line therapy for prosthetic valve thrombosis in the absence of contraindications. J Am Coll Cardiol. 2005;45:325; author reply 326.

87. Tong AT, Roudaut R, Ozkan M, Sagie A, Shahid MS, Pontes Junior SC, Carreras F, Girard SE, Arnaout S, Stainback RF, Thadhani R, Zoghbi WA. Transesophageal echocardiography improves risk assessment of thrombolysis of prosthetic valve thrombosis: results of the international pro-tee registry. J Am Coll Cardiol. 2004;43:77–84.

88. Turrentine MA, Braems G, Ramirez MM. Use of thrombolytics for the treatment of thromboembolic disease during pregnancy. Obstet Gynecol Surv. 1995;50:534–41.

89. Weiss BM, von Segesser LK, Alon E, Seifert B, Turina MI. Outcome of cardiovascular surgery and pregnancy: a systematic review of the period 1984–1996. Am J Obstet Gynecol. 1998;179:1643–53.

90. Arnoni RT, Arnoni AS, Bonini RC, de Almeida AF, Neto CA, Dinkhuysen JJ, Issa M, Chaccur P, Paulista PP. Risk factors associated with cardiac surgery during pregnancy. Ann Thorac Surg. 2003;76:1605–8.

91. Robertson JE, Silversides CK, Mah ML, Kulikowski J, Maxwell C, Wald RM, Colman JM, Siu SC, Sermer M. A contemporary approach to the obstetric management of women with heart disease. J Obstet Gynaecol Can. 2012;34:812–9.

Peripartum Cardiomyopathy

Abdallah Georges Kfoury, Kismet D. Rasmusson,
Kimberly D. Brunisholz, T. Flint Porter,
and Benjamin D. Horne

Abstract

Peripartum cardiomyopathy (PPCM) is an uncommon but important form of left ventricular systolic dysfunction with global implications. Its pathophysiology is likely multifactorial and may include a genetic predisposition. Our understanding of PPCM has been challenged by the lack of prospective studies and large registries. The clinical presentation, diagnostic assessment, and treatment usually mirror those of other forms of dilated cardiomyopathy. However, pregnancy status and breastfeeding are important considerations. While acknowledging that a fair number of patients with PPCM will have recovery of cardiac function, advanced heart failure therapies should be considered in a timely manner to improve short- and long-term outcomes. Subsequent pregnancies are associated with increased risk for the mother and fetus and generally should be discouraged, even in the setting of normalized ventricular function. Further advances in the knowledge of PPCM will stem from an emerging prospective study and through creating large-scale national/international registries.

Keywords

Peripartum cardiomyopathy • Heart failure • Pregnancy

A.G. Kfoury, MD, FACC (✉)
Department of Cardiology, Intermountain Medical Center,
5121 South Cottonwood Street, LL1,
Salt Lake City, UT 84107, USA
e-mail: akfoury@imail.org

K.D. Rasmusson, MSN, FNP-BC
Heart Failure Program Development Lead,
Intermountain Medical Center, University of Utah College
of Nursing, The Heart Institute, Heart Failure and Transplant
Program, 5121 South Cottonwood Street, LL1,
Salt Lake City, UT 84017, USA
e-mail: kismet.rasmusson@imail.org

K.D. Brunisholz, MST, CRCC
Department of Cardiovascular Research, Intermountain Medical
Center, Intermountain Heart Institute, 5121 South Cottonwood
Street, Salt Lake City, UT 84157, USA
e-mail: kim.brunisholz@imail.org

T.F. Porter, MD, MPH
Division of Maternal-Fetal Medicine, Department of Obstetrics
and Gynecology, Intermountain Medical Center, University
of Utah, 5121 South Cottonwood Street, Suite #100,
Salt Lake City, UT 84107, USA
e-mail: flint.porter@imail.org

B.D. Horne, PhD, MPH
Division of Genetic Epidemiology, Intermountain Medical Center
and University of Utah, Intermountain Heart Institute,
5121 South Cottonwood Street,
Salt Lake City, UT 84157, USA
e-mail: benjamin.horne@imail.org

Introduction

Peripartum cardiomyopathy (PPCM) is an uncommon but increasingly recognized type of cardiomyopathy that affects otherwise healthy women during late pregnancy, delivery, or afterwards. Heart failure during pregnancy has been recognized since the late nineteenth century [1]. Although the medical literature first reported it as a clinical entity in 1937 [2], it was not until 1971 that the term "peripartum cardiomyopathy" was proposed by Demakis et al. to include the specific diagnostic criterion of onset between the last month of pregnancy and 5 months following

K. Stergiopoulos, D.L. Brown (eds.), *Evidence-Based Cardiology Consult*,
DOI 10.1007/978-1-4471-4441-0_33, © Springer-Verlag London 2014

Table 33.1 Comparison of PPCM definitions

2000 National Institutes of Health	2010 European Society of Cardiology
4 criteria:	
1. HF developed within the last month of pregnancy or within 5 months of delivery	1. An idiopathic cardiomyopathy presenting with HF
2. Absence of other identifiable etiology of HF	2. Presenting in the last month of pregnancy or in the months following delivery
3. No prior cardiac history	3. No other cause of HF is found
4. Evidence of left ventricular systolic dysfunction	4. Diagnosis of exclusion
	5. Left ventricular ejection fraction <45 %

The ESC definition is less strict on the diagnostic time frame and the level of left ventricular dysfunction
PPCM peripartum cardiomyopathy, *HF* heart failure

delivery [3]. Since that time, diagnostic criteria have evolved to include systolic dysfunction (i.e., left ventricular ejection fraction (LVEF) ≤45 %) and the absence of any other identifiable cause of heart failure. PPCM was formally defined in 2000 by the National Institutes of Health [4]. As our understanding of this uncommon condition has evolved, so has its definition [5]. Table 33.1 compares the working definitions of PPCM.

While the true incidence of PPCM is unknown, it is likely underreported, and large variations by chronological era and geographic region exist. Estimates of the incidence of PPCM are 1 case for every 2,000–4,000 live births, affecting roughly 1,000–2,000 women annually in the United States [6]. The rate is reportedly much higher in other countries, such as South Africa (1:1,000), Haiti (1:300), or Nigeria (1:100) [5]. PPCM has also been reported in Caucasians, Japanese, Chinese, Indians, and Korean women but much less commonly in Hispanic women. PPCM is not restricted to any particular childbearing age, but in 58 % of cases the age at presentation is greater than 30 years [7].

PPCM currently ranks as one of the leading causes of pregnancy-related morbidity and mortality [8, 9] with a high rate of relapse with subsequent pregnancies [10, 11]. Outcomes with PPCM are highly variable among patients with the potential in some for full recovery of LV function. Yet, a substantial proportion requires chronic medical therapy and possibly advanced cardiac interventions such as mechanical circulatory support or heart transplantation. While little is known about morbidity and mortality risks in offspring, one population-based cohort study reported that neonates born to women with PPCM were more likely to be premature, have low or very low birth weight, be small for gestational age, and have lower 5-min Apgar scores compared to those born to healthy mothers [12].

Numerous predisposing factors for PPCM have been identified, but few have been validated with large population-based studies and the definitive etiology remains unclear. Risk factors that have been proposed include tocolytic therapy, preeclampsia or toxemia, gestational hypertension, multiparity and multiple gestation, older age, and non-Caucasian ethnicity [4, 9, 13]. Although these risk factors have been associated with a higher incidence of PPCM, they cannot conclusively predict who will or will not develop PPCM.

Given that PPCM occurs around a life event that otherwise should be "normal" and joyful in healthy females, the diagnosis can impart substantial hardship on patients and their families. The emotional and psychological distress PPCM patients endure has not been studied, and it is likely that additional social and mental support is required. The extent of this assistance is usually proportional to the severity of illness and the patient's ability to proceed with usual activities of life without undue limiting symptoms.

Pathophysiology

Despite extensive research on the underlying etiology, to date no definitive causes have been identified and PPCM remains a diagnosis of exclusion. PPCM can be distinguished from other forms of cardiomyopathy mostly by its occurrence during or around pregnancy. Evidence suggests that multiple triggers may initiate the disease, although the pathologic process still remains uncertain.

Oxidative Stress and Excessive Prolactin Production

Recent studies point to a mechanistic cascade involving oxidative stress, the prolactin-cleaving protease cathepsin D, and the hormone prolactin to explain the pathophysiology of PPCM. During pregnancy and delivery, oxidative stress appears to trigger cathepsin D expression in cardiomyocytes, which cleaves the 23 kDa prolactin into a 16 kDa fragment. Expression of 16 kDa prolactin has been found in mice models (with a cardiac-specific deletion for signal transducer and activator of transcription-3) to cause vasoconstriction, apoptosis, inflammation, and dissociation of the capillary structures within the endothelial cells, which can potentially lead to damage to or impair metabolism and contractility of cardiomyocytes [14–16]. This theory is supported by small clinical reports of postpartum women with PPCM responding to treatment with the dopamine D2 receptor agonist, bromocriptine, which has been shown to reduce secretion of prolactin from the posterior pituitary gland [15, 17]. Whereas treatment with bromocriptine prevents the development of PPCM in mice models, forced myocardial expression of 16 kDa prolactin results in the cardiac phenotype of PPCM, providing additional evidence for this theory of the pathogenesis of PPCM [17].

Systemic Inflammation and Apoptosis

Myocardial disruption due to systemic inflammation and apoptosis may also play a role in the pathophysiology of PPCM. Serum markers of inflammatory processes including soluble death receptor sFas/Apo-1, C-reactive protein (CRP), interferon gamma (IFN-γ), tumor necrosis factor-alpha (TNF-α), and interleukin-1 and interleukin-6 (IL1 and IL6) have all been shown to be elevated in patients with PPCM [13, 18, 19]. Plasma levels of the apoptosis signaling surface receptor Fas/APO-1 not only correlate with the severity of LV dysfunction at diagnosis but are also an independent predictor of subsequent mortality [18]. An investigation into the effects of inhibition of TNF-α with pentoxifylline in patients with PPCM already receiving optimal medical therapy demonstrated clinical improvement in a small nonrandomized study of treated patients ($n = 30$) compared with controls ($n = 29$) [20]. CRP levels have been shown to be positively correlated with LV end-systolic and end-diastolic diameters and negatively with EF in 100 PPCM patients at presentation [18].

Viral Pathology

Viral infection in the mother leading to the development of myocarditis may be another possible mechanism for cardiac dysfunction in PPCM. The identification of viral infection, including cardiotropic enteroviruses in PPCM, has been reported. However, this data is far from conclusive [21]. The incidence of myocarditis on endomyocardial biopsies ranges widely (9–78 %) across studies with small cohorts of PPCM patients [22–25].

Abnormal Immune Response

An abnormal autoimmune response to fetal antigens released into the maternal blood has been suggested as a possible contributor to the development and progression of PPCM [26]. High titers of autoantibodies against selected cardiac tissue proteins have been shown to be present in a majority of women with the diagnosis of PPCM [27]. In a larger multicenter international study, Warraich et al. compared IgG profiles against cardiac myosin heavy chain in patients with PPCM, idiopathic dilated cardiomyopathy, and normal controls [28]. All IgG subclasses were elevated in PPCM compared to idiopathic dilated cardiomyopathy. Furthermore, the levels of these antibodies were correlated with clinical presentation and New York Heart Association (NYHA) functional class.

Other Possible Etiologies

Other proposed hypotheses to explain PPCM include abnormal hemodynamic response (i.e., increased cardiac demand during pregnancy, hypertension), nutritional deficits (i.e., deficiency of micronutrients such as selenium), or excess (i.e., salt) hormonal abnormalities, possible genetic links, and other environmental factors [4, 13]. Overall, it seems that a multifactorial mechanism may be at play, and further investigation is required to determine the extent to which these factors may be interlinked to produce the clinical phenotype of PPCM.

Familial, Heritable, and Genetic Associations with PPCM

The genetic predisposition to PPCM is poorly understood. In fact, both the 2006 American Heart Association (AHA) and the 2008 European Society of Cardiology (ESC) classification systems for cardiomyopathies state that PPCM does not have a genetic basis. The AHA classification tree labels PPCM as "acquired," [29], while the ESC system classifies PPCM as "nonfamilial" [30]. While the heritable influences on PPCM have not been studied in depth, limited evidence suggests that PPCM does occur within families [31–34].

The clustering of PPCM within similar populations and in families leads to the possibility of inherited sources of disease. The genetic causes for PPCM have only begun to be explored with some early evidence of a genetic association existing for a few proposed genetic loci. These include loci identified through the study of other similar conditions and a few genetic variants validated in research studies that specifically evaluated the genetics of PPCM.

Various cardiomyopathies have a genetic basis [35], and a few studies of PPCM have evaluated whether mutations discovered for other cardiomyopathies also lead to PPCM due to similar pathophysiology [36, 37]. In one [36] molecular genetic analysis of index cases in five dilated cardiomyopathy families, three PPCM patients showed no mutations in the cardiomyopathy genes LMNA, TNNT2, and MYH7, while one patient had a TNNC1 mutation (Gln50Arg). The second study reported that 45 PPCM cases were found in 42 families

Table 33.2 Signs, symptoms, and possible findings with diagnostic testing

Symptoms	Signs	Possible aberrations on diagnostic tests
Dyspnea	Jugular venous distention	*BNP*: elevation fivefold higher
Orthopnea	Tachypnea	*CRP and hsCRP*: may be mildly elevated
Paroxysmal nocturnal dyspnea	Hypoxia	*OxLDL and INF-γ*: significantly elevated
Cough	Tachycardia	*ECG*: ST-T wave abnormalities, sinus tachycardia, left bundle branch block, left ventricular hypertrophy, new onset atrial or ventricular arrhythmias, conduction abnormalities
Edema	Rales	*CXR*: cardiomegaly, pulmonary congestion, interstitial infiltrates, pleural effusion
Chest pain/pressure	Third heart sound/S3	*Echocardiogram*: left ventricular systolic dysfunction with or without dilation, right ventricular enlargement with reduced function, restrictive pattern, mitral and tricuspid valve regurgitation
Palpitations	Right ventricular heave	*Cardiac MRI*: fibrosis, thrombus
Abdominal pain/discomfort	Laterally displaced PMI	
Fatigue	Murmur of mitral or tricuspid valve regurgitation	
Activity intolerance	Edema	

PMI point of maximal impulse, *BNP* brain natriuretic peptide, *CRP* c-reactive protein, *hsCRP* high sensitivity CRP, *oxLDL* oxidized low-density lipoprotein, *IFN-γ* interferon gamma, *TNF* tumor necrosis factor, *ECG* electrocardiogram, *CXR* chest X-ray, *MRI* magnetic resonance imaging

with familial cardiomyopathy and that genetic testing of 14 of the PPCM cases showed mutations in six of the cases, including one mutation each in the cardiomyopathy genes *MYH7*, *SCN5A*, *TNNT2*, *PSEN2*, *MYBPC3*, and *MYH6* (no cardiomyopathy mutations were found in any of the 14 genes among 253 controls) [37].

In the only genome-wide association study of PPCM-associated variants to date, more than 500,000 single nucleotide polymorphisms were studied in 41 PPCM cases and 49 age-discordant (elderly) cardiovascular disease-free patients [38]. One polymorphism (rs258415) on chromosome 12 near the *PTHLH* gene was significantly associated with PPCM ($p=2.1 \times 10^{-8}$) after multiple-testing correction (requiring $p<9.0 \times 10^{-8}$). This association was validated when the 41 cases were compared to a second set of $n=654$ controls, when a separate set of 30 cases were compared to multiple sets of controls, and when 29 pregnancy-associated cardiomyopathy cases were evaluated [38].

Thus, despite current international consensus statements on cardiomyopathies, the etiology of PPCM is, at least in part, found in genetic factors. Genetic knowledge about PPCM should stimulate improvements in the detection and treatment of PPCM.

Presentation, Diagnosis, and Management

Because PPCM occurs in otherwise healthy females, the diagnosis is often missed or comes late when the clinical presentation of acute heart failure becomes more evident. Recognizing heart failure in a pregnant female is often challenged by differentiating between mild symptoms of a normal pregnancy due to plasma volume expansion versus those of the pathologic condition of PPCM [4]. When symptoms appear to be out of proportion to a normal pregnancy, PPCM should be suspected and definitive evaluation undertaken so that appropriate treatment may be initiated. There are no signs or symptoms specific to PPCM. Instead, patients typically present with congestive (shortness of breath, dyspnea on exertion, cough) or low-flow (fatigue, exercise intolerance) symptoms that are common to systolic heart failure from any cause. Signs on physical exam will vary depending on the patient's acuity and whether a single or both ventricles are involved. Signs and symptoms can be subtle and mild in a stable outpatient or severe and catastrophic in another with cardiogenic shock (Table 33.2). A scored, patient-administered test quantifying the degree of symptoms (orthopnea, dyspnea, cough, edema, excessive weight gain, palpitations) may be useful if PPCM is suspected [39]. A higher score represents a higher symptom burden that in turn necessitates confirmatory testing for PPCM. Early diagnosis of PPCM and initiation of treatment are crucial since delays in treatment often lead to poorer outcomes [8].

When PPCM is suspected, the following steps summarized in Table 33.2 aid in confirming the diagnosis (see algorithm on Fig. 33.1):

1. A careful history including determining the onset of symptoms related to pregnancy and to exclude prior cardiac disease or other contributing comorbidities
2. A thorough physical examination as is done in heart failure of other etiologies
3. Diagnostic testing that includes an assessment of LV function, chest X-ray, electrocardiogram, and laboratory testing

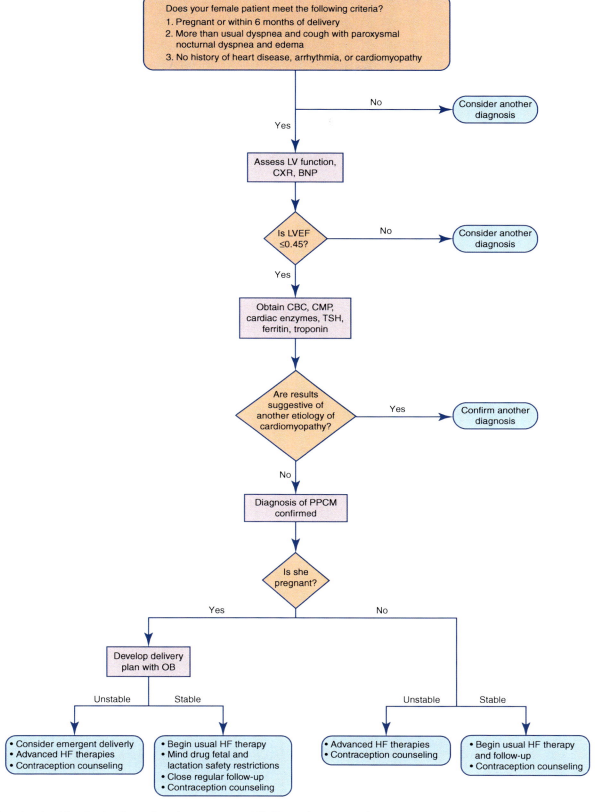

Fig. 33.1 An algorithm for the diagnosis and management of PPCM. *PPCM* peripartum cardiomyopathy, *LV* left ventricular, *CXR* chest X-ray, *BNP* B-type natriuretic peptide, *LVEF* left ventricular ejection fraction, *CBC* complete blood count, *CMP* comprehensive metabolic panel, *TSH* thyroid-stimulating hormone, *OB* obstetrics, *HF* heart failure

Table 33.3 Medication safety profile during pregnancy

FDA pregnancy category B	FDA pregnancy category C	FDA pregnancy category D	FDA pregnancy category X
Dobutamine	Amlodipine	Amiodarone	Warfarin
Enoxaparin	Bisoprolol	Candesartan	
Eplerenone	Bumetanide	Captopril (second, third trimester)	
Ethacrynic acid	Captopril (first trimester)	Enalapril (second, third trimester)	
Hydrocholorothiazide	Carvedilol	Irbesartan	
Sotalol	Digoxin	Lisinopril	
Torsemide	Diltiazem	Losartan (second, third trimester)	
	Dopamine	Telmisartan	
	Enalapril (first trimester)	Trandolapril (second, third trimester)	
	Furosemide	Valsartan	
	Hydralazine		
	Isosorbide mononitrate		
	Isosorbide dinitrate		
	Lisinopril (first trimester)		
	Losartan (first trimester)		
	Metoprolol succinate		
	Mexiletine		
	Milrinone		
	Nitroprusside		
	Spironolactone		
	Trandolapril (first trimester)		
	Verapamil		
	Unfractionated heparin		

FDA (Food and Drug Administration) Pregnancy Category: A, controlled studies show no risk to fetus; B, *either* animal studies show no risk *and* there are no controlled trials in humans *or* animals have shown risk *but* controlled trials in humans showed no risk; C, no evidence of risk in humans but animal studies show increased risk to fetus; D, positive evidence of risk in humans; X, contraindicated in humans. For reference: www.drugs.com/pregnancy

The differential diagnosis of PPCM includes other forms of cardiomyopathy, primary valvular heart disease, anemia, thyroid disorders, myocardial infarction, sepsis, severe preeclampsia, and amniotic fluid or pulmonary embolism [40, 41].

Diagnostic imaging is most easily performed with echocardiography. Cardiac magnetic resonance imaging (MRI) as an adjunctive imaging modality may be considered to assess and quantify the degree of LV dysfunction, to detect the presence of an intracardiac thrombus, and possibly to detect inflammatory changes during the acute phase of the disease [42], although controversy exists in terms of the ability of MRI to differentiate PPCM from other forms of cardiomyopathy [43]. The routine use of endomyocardial biopsy is not recommended [44]; however, it may be used to exclude autoimmune myocarditis when suspected [45]. Brain natriuretic peptides (BNP) or N-terminal pro-BNP (NT-pro-BNP) can be elevated in PPCM [19] and should be assessed to aid in the diagnosis. An elevated cardiac troponin T has been found to negatively correlate with LVEF at 6 months [46].

Treating PPCM for the most part will be similar to other cardiomyopathies with the exception of addressing pregnancy status and desire to breastfeed. A pregnant patient with PPCM will require counseling regarding the risk of continuing with the pregnancy, timing and mode of delivery,

and the safety of medications during pregnancy and lactation (Tables 33.3 and 33.4). Ultimately, management decisions will vary based on pregnancy status and the presence of hemodynamic instability (Fig. 33.2). When hemodynamic instability is evident in a pregnant female, rapid decision-making should include specialists in heart failure, intensive care medicine, and high-risk obstetrics/perinatology to provide multidisciplinary care [5]. Treatment should focus on providing symptomatic relief of congestion and restoring hemodynamic stability and may include diuretic therapy, oxygen in the presence of hypoxia, noninvasive positive pressure ventilation, and afterload reduction. Invasive hemodynamic monitoring, intravenous inotropes, vasopressors, and mechanical intubation should be considered if required to improve the hemodynamic profile.

Hemodynamic instability in a pregnant PPCM patient should prompt decisions about early delivery. Otherwise, careful symptom and hemodynamic monitoring of both mother and fetus should occur until delivery [5]. If possible, a vaginal delivery is preferred [47]. During pregnancy, diuretics should be used cautiously in order to avoid decreases in placental blood flow; nitrates and hydralazine should be used preferentially over the angiotensin-converting enzyme (ACE) inhibitor or angiotensin receptor blockers (ARBs); beta-1 selective beta-blockers are preferred.

Previously, breastfeeding had been encouraged, not only for the benefits to the infant but because breastfeeding women have been reported to have higher rates of recovery of LV

Table 33.4 Heart failure medication safety profile during lactation

Drugs and lactation (LactMed) database[a]		
Likely safe	Avoid if possible	No information
Benazepril[b]	Amiodarone	Amlodipine
Captopril[b]	Bumetanide	Bisoprolol
Digoxin, oral	Ethacrynic acid	Candesartan
Enalapril[b]	Furosemide	Carvedilol
Enoxaparin	Sotalol	Diltiazem
Hydrochlorothiazide	Torsemide	Eplerenone
Hydralazine		Irbesartan
Metoprolol		Lisinopril
Quinapril[b]		Losartan
Spironolactone		Mexiletine
Unfractionated heparin		Nitroglycerin
Verapamil		Ramipril
Warfarin		Sotalol
		Telmisartan
		Trandolapril
		Valsartan

[a]http://toxnet.nlm.nih.gov/cgi-bin/sis/search
[b]Ingested amounts of ACE inhibitors from a mother's milk are not expected to cause adverse effects; however, use caution in neonates and preterm infants to avoid hypotension. World Health Organization (WHO) and American Academy of Pediatrics (AAP) drugs and lactation ratings may differ from above

function [48]. However, this practice is presently controversial due to the potential role of prolactin in the development of PPCM [5].

Principles of chronic management of PPCM will mirror those of systolic heart failure of other etiologies [44]. The duration of ongoing therapy in the setting of normalized LV function is not clear. Recovery of LV function has been found to occur within 2–12 months [9, 49–51]. For this reason, it has been thought that ACE inhibitors (or ARBs) and beta-blockers should be continued at least for 1 year, if not indefinitely. There is not yet enough evidence to guide decisions to discontinue therapy. Limited reports have shown mixed results in outcomes after medical therapy was discontinued in the setting of normalized LV function [8, 51]. The response to therapy should be monitored with echocardiography to assess for recovery or the need for further heart failure therapies such as resynchronization therapy or an internal cardioverter defibrillator (ICD) for persistent LV dysfunction. Because recovery of LV function may be delayed, early interventions with an ICD or transplant should be avoided, if possible, to allow for the full extent of myocardial recovery [5, 48]. In the interim, wearable external defibrillators and mechanical assist devices as a bridge to recovery may be reasonable [5, 48, 49]. Patients with PPCM with persistently reduced LVEF should have close surveillance and aggressive treatment and ultimately be considered for advanced heart failure therapies [52]. Early consideration of mechanical

Is the patient hemodynamically unstable?			
		No	**Yes**
Is the patient currently pregnant?	**No**	• Heart failure specialist consult • Usual heart failure treatment (ACEi or ARB, BB, AA, digoxin) • Usual follow up to assess response to treatment • Address lactation preferences & medication safety profile • Consider anticoagulation • Discuss future pregnancy and family planning	• Heart failure specialist & critical care consult • Risk assessment/prognostication • Advanced heart failure therapies: mechanical circulatory support &/or cardiac transplantation • Consider anticoagulation-warfarin • Discuss future pregnancy and family planning
	Yes	• Heart failure specialist consult • High risk obstetric & perinatology consult • Delivery planning: mode and timing • Planned fetal monitoring • Heart failure treatment (diuretics, digoxin, nitrates, hydralazine) • Consider anticoagulation- LMWH • Avoid ACEi or ARB, AA, coumadin • Close clinical monitoring; monthly visit and echocardiogram	• Heart failure specialist & critical care consult • High risk obstetric & perinatology consult • Fetal monitoring • Risk assessment/prognostication • May use dobutamine, milrinone and nitroglycerine (nitroprusside- cautiously) • Advanced heart failure therapies: mechanical circulatory support &/or cardiac transplantation • Delivery planning: mode and timing vs. pregnancy termination • Consider anticoagulation

Fig. 33.2 PPCM management based on pregnancy status and hemodynamic stability. *ACEi* angiotensin-converting enzyme inhibitor, *ARB* angiotensin receptor blocker, *BB* beta-blocker, *AA* aldosterone antagonist, *LMWH* low molecular weight heparin

circulatory support should be made when cardiogenic shock is present. Mechanical circulatory support can be used as a bridge to recovery, since a significant portion of patients will have LV recovery by 6 months, or as a bridge to decision for cardiac transplantation [52].

Anticoagulation to treat or prevent thromboembolic events may be necessary given the hypercoagulable state observed during pregnancy and in the early postpartum months [53, 54]. Atrial fibrillation, pulmonary embolism, and deep vein thrombosis are clear indications for systemic anticoagulation that may occur in patients with PPCM. During pregnancy, low molecular weight heparin is safest, since it does not cross the placenta. Warfarin has been found to be teratogenic, particularly in the first trimester of pregnancy and therefore should not be used during that period [55]. Other treatments for PPCM with limited experience include bromocriptine, pentoxifylline, and immune globulin.

The extent of recovery of cardiac function following PPCM has important implications on outcomes and especially on determining the safety of future pregnancies. One of the largest database analyses in PPCM to date included 187 patients in the United States that showed ventricular function returned to normal in 61 % of patients; an initial LVEF >30 % was the only predictor of recovery [49]. This confirms other studies that suggest that a higher LVEF, without dilation, at the time of diagnosis confers a lower risk of recurrence or poor outcomes after a subsequent pregnancy [48, 49, 56]. Freedom from recurrence of PPCM cannot be guaranteed, as even groups with recovered ventricular function have had reductions in LVEF with a subsequent pregnancy [57]. In general, women with a history of PPCM should be discouraged from attempting another pregnancy, particularly those with residual cardiac dysfunction [58]. The risk of recurrent heart failure is high in subsequent pregnancy, especially in those who do not have complete recovery of LV function [59]. In the largest study to date, 20 % of women with a history of PPCM developed recurrent heart failure in a subsequent pregnancy [48]. No maternal deaths were reported in this study. In contrast, 40 % of women with persistent cardiac dysfunction after PPCM had recurrent heart failure in a subsequent pregnancy and the maternal mortality was 19 %.

Obstetric Considerations

Antenatal PPCM, by definition, is diagnosed during the last month of pregnancy (>36 weeks' gestation). Because the clinical course is variable and difficult to predict [60], most authorities recommend delivery at the time of diagnosis. The timing and mode of delivery depends largely on the fetal and maternal clinical status [48]. The obstetric management of patients with PPCM should be geared toward an expeditious delivery in order to minimize maternal and fetal risks. A team approach to intrapartum and postpartum care is imperative and should include input from the obstetrician and/or a maternal-fetal medicine specialist, the cardiologist, an intensivist, a neonatologist, and an anesthesiologist with special expertise in cardiac disease.

Vaginal delivery is preferred for women in stable condition and may attenuate the hemodynamic fluctuations that accompany parturition. However, a long induction of labor in a medically unstable patient increases the likelihood of maternal and fetal morbidity and mortality. Cesarean delivery is more rapid and allows easier coordination of care among experienced medical personnel. However, when compared to vaginal delivery, cesarean delivery is associated with more blood loss, increased postoperative pain, a slower recovery, and increased risk of complications such as infection, thromboembolism, and damage to surrounding pelvic organs [61].

Recommendations for family planning should be initiated soon after delivery. The number of contraceptive options available to women with a history of PPCM varies according to postpartum cardiac function. More permanent methods of contraception such as tubal ligation or vasectomy should be strongly considered [59]. Women with residual LV dysfunction should avoid the use of combination hormonal contraceptive devices because of the increased risk of thromboembolism associated with estrogen.

Outcomes

Much of what is known about outcomes for patients with PPCM has been limited to case reports and small observational series. Large global registries or prospective studies are lacking. Existing PPCM outcomes data vary considerably. Roughly half of patients with PPCM recover cardiac function on usual heart failure therapy within 6 months of diagnosis [8, 24, 51, 62]. This is a greater degree of recovery than non-peripartum women or men with new onset heart failure [63]. Recovery was as high as 78 % in one PPCM database created through internet participation [50]. The time to recovery ranges from 2 to 9 months [9, 51, 64] with continued recovery up to 1 year [51, 65]. Lower LVEF at baseline ($\leq$25 %), non-Caucasian race, and delayed diagnosis predicted major adverse events, with most occurring within the first year of diagnosis [8]. Conversely, a preliminary LVEF >30 % and LV end-diastolic dimension (LVEDD) <5.5–6.0 cm at the time of diagnosis was predictive of ventricular recovery [49]. Other predictors of LV recovery include low baseline levels of biomarkers [19, 46], diagnosis after delivery, presence of gestational hypertension/preeclampsia, and breastfeeding [50].

Factors associated with lack of recovery include a dilated heart (LVEDD >5.6 cm), presence of LV thrombus, and African-American race.

Internal cardioverter defibrillators are placed in 4–16 % of patients [8, 64]. Cardiac transplantation was considered in up to 23 % [56] and performed in 6–11 % of PPCM patients [8, 24, 51, 65, 66]. The use of mechanical support has been low at 2 % [8] or 3 % [47, 58]. A recent analysis of the United Network for Organ Sharing (UNOS) database revealed that the 485 cardiac transplant recipients who were transplanted for PPCM were younger than other recipients, had higher sensitization, and higher acuity and listing status [67]. Posttransplant, they had more rejection, poorer graft survival, and shorter graft half-life compared to all other recipients, males and other females [67]. Patients bridged with mechanical support experienced improved survival [68].

Mortality rates for PPCM in the United States range from 0 to 19 % [6, 51, 58, 67]. In the last decade, mortality in both Haiti and South Africa was 15 % [13, 69, 70], whereas in Turkey it was as high as 30 % [70].

Discontinuation of heart failure therapy in patients with PPCM is controversial. Some studies have documented no worsening of LV function after medical therapy was discontinued where as others have found deterioration in LV function with medication withdrawal [48, 50].

Key Points

- Peripartum cardiomyopathy (PPCM) is an uncommon but important form of systolic heart failure with global implications.
- Its pathophysiologic process is likely multifactorial and may include a genetic predisposition.
- Our understanding of PPCM has been challenged by the lack of prospective studies and large registries.
- The clinical presentation, diagnostic assessment, and treatment usually mirror that of other forms of cardiomyopathy.
- Subsequent pregnancies are risky and generally should be discouraged, even in the setting of normalized cardiac function.

References

1. Richie C. Clinical contributions to the pathology, diagnosis, and treatment of certain chronic disease of the heart. Edinb Med Surg J. 1849;2(333).
2. Hull E, Hafkesbring E. "Toxic" postpartal heart disease. New Orleans Med Surg J. 1937;89:550.
3. Demakis JG, Rahimtoola SH. Peripartum cardiomyopathy. Circulation. 1971;44(5):964–8.
4. Pearson GD, et al. Peripartum cardiomyopathy: national heart, lung, and blood institute and office of rare diseases (National Institutes of Health) workshop recommendations and review. JAMA. 2000;283(9):1183–8.
5. Sliwa K, et al. Current state of knowledge on aetiology, diagnosis, management, and therapy of peripartum cardiomyopathy: a position statement from the Heart Failure Association of the European Society of Cardiology Working Group on peripartum cardiomyopathy. Eur J Heart Fail. 2010;12(8):767–78.
6. Mielniczuk LM, et al. Frequency of peripartum cardiomyopathy. Am J Cardiol. 2006;97(12):1765–8.
7. Pyatt JR, Dubey G. Peripartum cardiomyopathy: current understanding, comprehensive management review and new developments. Postgrad Med J. 2011;87(1023):34–9.
8. Goland S, et al. Clinical profile and predictors of complications in peripartum cardiomyopathy. J Card Fail. 2009;15(8):645–50.
9. Elkayam U, et al. Pregnancy-associated cardiomyopathy: clinical characteristics and a comparison between early and late presentation. Circulation. 2005;111(16):2050–5.
10. Sliwa K, et al. Outcome of subsequent pregnancy in patients with documented peripartum cardiomyopathy. Am J Cardiol. 2004; 93(11):1441–3, A10.
11. Sliwa K, Tibazarwa K, Hilfiker-Kleiner D. Management of peripartum cardiomyopathy. Curr Heart Fail Rep. 2008;5(4):238–44.
12. Gunderson EP, et al. Epidemiology of peripartum cardiomyopathy: incidence, predictors, and outcomes. Obstet Gynecol. 2011;118(3): 583–91.
13. Sliwa K, Fett J, Elkayam U. Peripartum cardiomyopathy. Lancet. 2006;368(9536):687–93.
14. Corbacho AM, Martinez De La Escalera G, Clapp C. Roles of prolactin and related members of the prolactin/growth hormone/placental lactogen family in angiogenesis. J Endocrinol. 2002;173(2): 219–38.
15. Hilfiker-Kleiner D, et al. A cathepsin D-cleaved 16 kDa form of prolactin mediates postpartum cardiomyopathy. Cell. 2007;128(3): 589–600.
16. Hilfiker-Kleiner D, Sliwa K, Drexler H. Peripartum cardiomyopathy: recent insights in its pathophysiology. Trends Cardiovasc Med. 2008;18(5):173–9.
17. Hilfiker-Kleiner D, et al. Recovery from postpartum cardiomyopathy in 2 patients by blocking prolactin release with bromocriptine. J Am Coll Cardiol. 2007;50(24):2354–5.
18. Sliwa K, et al. Peripartum cardiomyopathy: inflammatory markers as predictors of outcome in 100 prospectively studied patients. Eur Heart J. 2006;27(4):441–6.
19. Forster O, et al. Reversal of IFN-gamma, oxLDL and prolactin serum levels correlate with clinical improvement in patients with peripartum cardiomyopathy. Eur J Heart Fail. 2008;10(9):861–8.
20. Sliwa K, et al. The addition of pentoxifylline to conventional therapy improves outcome in patients with peripartum cardiomyopathy. Eur J Heart Fail. 2002;4(3):305–9.
21. Fett JD. Viral infection as a possible trigger for the development of peripartum cardiomyopathy. Int J Gynaecol Obstet. 2007;97(2): 149–50.
22. Sanderson JE, Olsen EG, Gatei D. Peripartum heart disease: an endomyocardial biopsy study. Br Heart J. 1986;56(3):285–91.
23. Midei MG, et al. Peripartum myocarditis and cardiomyopathy. Circulation. 1990;81(3):922–8.
24. Felker GM, et al. Myocarditis and long-term survival in peripartum cardiomyopathy. Am Heart J. 2000;140(5):785–91.
25. Bultmann BD, et al. High prevalence of viral genomes and inflammation in peripartum cardiomyopathy. Am J Obstet Gynecol. 2005; 193(2):363–5.
26. Ansari AA, et al. Autoimmune mechanisms as the basis for human peripartum cardiomyopathy. Clin Rev Allergy Immunol. 2002; 23(3):301–24.

27. Lamparter S, Pankuweit S, Maisch B. Clinical and immunologic characteristics in peripartum cardiomyopathy. Int J Cardiol. 2007; 118(1):14–20.

28. Warraich RS, et al. Impact of pregnancy-related heart failure on humoral immunity: clinical relevance of G3-subclass immunoglobulins in peripartum cardiomyopathy. Am Heart J. 2005;150(2): 263–9.

29. Maron BJ, et al. Contemporary definitions and classification of the cardiomyopathies: an American Heart Association Scientific Statement from the Council on Clinical Cardiology, Heart Failure and Transplantation Committee; Quality of Care and Outcomes Research and Functional Genomics and Translational Biology Interdisciplinary Working Groups; and Council on Epidemiology and Prevention. Circulation. 2006;113(14):1807–16.

30. Elliott P, et al. Classification of the cardiomyopathies. Kardiol Pol. 2008;66(5):533–40; discussion 541–2.

31. Massad LS, et al. Familial peripartum cardiomyopathy after molar pregnancy. Obstet Gynecol. 1993;81(5 (Pt 2)):886–8.

32. Pierce JA, Price BO, Joyce JW. Familial occurrence of postpartal heart failure. Arch Intern Med. 1963;111:651–5.

33. Pearl W. Familial occurrence of peripartum cardiomyopathy. Am Heart J. 1995;129(2):421–2.

34. Fett JD, et al. Mother-daughter peripartum cardiomyopathy. Int J Cardiol. 2002;86(2–3):331–2.

35. Cowan J, et al. Genetic testing and genetic counseling in cardiovascular genetic medicine: overview and preliminary recommendations. Congest Heart Fail. 2008;14(2):97–105.

36. van Spaendonck-Zwarts KY, et al. Peripartum cardiomyopathy as a part of familial dilated cardiomyopathy. Circulation. 2010;121(20): 2169–75.

37. Morales A, et al. Rare variant mutations in pregnancy-associated or peripartum cardiomyopathy. Circulation. 2010;121(20):2176–82.

38. Horne BD, et al. Genome-wide significance and replication of the chromosome 12p11.22 locus near the PTHLH gene for peripartum cardiomyopathy. Circ Cardiovasc Genet. 2011;4(4):359–66.

39. Fett JD. Validation of a self-test for early diagnosis of heart failure in peripartum cardiomyopathy. Crit Pathw Cardiol. 2011;10(1): 44–5.

40. Ray P, Murphy GJ, Shutt LE. Recognition and management of maternal cardiac disease in pregnancy. Br J Anaesth. 2004;93(3): 428–39.

41. Abboud J, et al. Peripartum cardiomyopathy: a comprehensive review. Int J Cardiol. 2007;118(3):295–303.

42. Renz DM, et al. New insights into peripartum cardiomyopathy using cardiac magnetic resonance imaging. Rofo. 2011;183(9):834–41.

43. Mouquet F, et al. Characterisation of peripartum cardiomyopathy by cardiac magnetic resonance imaging. Eur Radiol. 2008;18(12): 2765–9.

44. Hunt SA, et al. 2009 focused update incorporated into the ACC/ AHA 2005 guidelines for the diagnosis and management of heart failure in adults: a report of the American College of Cardiology Foundation/American Heart Association Task Force on Practice Guidelines: developed in collaboration with the International Society for Heart and Lung Transplantation. Circulation. 2009; 119(14):e391–479.

45. Cooper LT, et al. The role of endomyocardial biopsy in the management of cardiovascular disease: a scientific statement from the American Heart Association, the American College of Cardiology, and the European Society of Cardiology. Circulation. 2007;116(19): 2216–33.

46. Hu CL, et al. Troponin T measurement can predict persistent left ventricular dysfunction in peripartum cardiomyopathy. Heart. 2007;93(4):488–90.

47. Velickovic IA, Leicht CH. Peripartum cardiomyopathy and cesarean section: report of two cases and literature review. Arch Gynecol Obstet. 2004;270(4):307–10.

48. Elkayam U. Clinical characteristics of peripartum cardiomyopathy in the United States: diagnosis, prognosis, and management. J Am Coll Cardiol. 2011;58(7):659–70.

49. Goland S, et al. Evaluation of the clinical relevance of baseline left ventricular ejection fraction as a predictor of recovery or persistence of severe dysfunction in women in the United States with peripartum cardiomyopathy. J Card Fail. 2011;17(5):426–30.

50. Safirstein JG, et al. Predictors of left ventricular recovery in a cohort of peripartum cardiomyopathy patients recruited via the internet. Int J Cardiol. 2012;154(1):27–31.

51. Amos AM, Jaber WA, Russell SD. Improved outcomes in peripartum cardiomyopathy with contemporary. Am Heart J. 2006;152(3): 509–13.

52. Francis GS, et al. ACCF/AHA/ACP/HFSA/ISHLT 2010 clinical competence statement on management of patients with advanced heart failure and cardiac transplant: a report of the ACCF/AHA/ ACP Task Force on Clinical Competence and Training. J Am Coll Cardiol. 2010;56(5):424–53.

53. Gynaecologists R.C.o.O.a. Reducing the risk of thromboembolism during pregnancy, birth, and the puerperium. Guideline no. 37. 2009;London: RCOG.

54. James AH, et al. Venous thromboembolism during pregnancy and the postpartum period: incidence, risk factors, and mortality. Am J Obstet Gynecol. 2006;194(5):1311–5.

55. Holzgreve W, Carey JC, Hall BD. Warfarin-induced fetal abnormalities. Lancet. 1976;2(7991):914–5.

56. Bozkurt B, et al. Intravenous immune globulin in the therapy of peripartum cardiomyopathy. J Am Coll Cardiol. 1999;34(1):177–80.

57. Fett JD. Personal commentary: monitoring subsequent pregnancy in recovered peripartum cardiomyopathy mothers. Crit Pathw Cardiol. 2009;8(4):172–4.

58. Elkayam U, et al. Maternal and fetal outcomes of subsequent pregnancies in women with peripartum cardiomyopathy. N Engl J Med. 2001;344(21):1567–71.

59. Karaye KM, Henein MY. Peripartum cardiomyopathy: a review article. Int J Cardiol. 2013;164(1):33–8.

60. Fett JD, Christie LG, Murphy JG. Brief communication: outcomes of subsequent pregnancy after peripartum cardiomyopathy: a case series from Haiti. Ann Intern Med. 2006;145(1):30–4.

61. Reimold SC, Rutherford JD. Peripartum cardiomyopathy. N Engl J Med. 2001;344(21):1629–30.

62. Elkayam U, Goland S. Bromocriptine for the treatment of peripartum cardiomyopathy. Circulation. 2010;121(13):1463–4.

63. Ecker JL, Frigoletto Jr FD. Cesarean delivery and the risk-benefit calculus. N Engl J Med. 2007;356(9):885–8.

64. Cooper LT, et al. Myocardial recovery in peripartum cardiomyopathy: prospective comparison with recent onset cardiomyopathy in men and nonperipartum women. J Card Fail. 2012;18(1):28–33.

65. Rasmusson K, et al. Long term outcomes in patients with peripartum cardiomyopathy and no recovery of left ventricular function. J Card Fail. 2010;16:S97.

66. Witlin AG, Mabie WC, Sibai BM. Peripartum cardiomyopathy: an ominous diagnosis. Am J Obstet Gynecol. 1997;176(1 Pt 1): 182–8.

67. Rasmusson K, et al. Peripartum cardiomyopathy: post-transplant outcomes from the united network for organ sharing database. J Heart Lung Transplant. 2012;31(2):180–6.

68. Rasmusson K, et al. Predictors of graft survival in heart transplant recipients with peripartum cardiomyopathy: insights from the United Network for Organ Sharing (UNOS) database. J Heart Lung Transplant. 2012;31(4S):S137.

69. Fett JD, et al. Five-year prospective study of the incidence and prognosis of peripartum cardiomyopathy at a single institution. Mayo Clin Proc. 2005;80(12):1602–6.

70. Brar SS, et al. Incidence, mortality, and racial differences in peripartum cardiomyopathy. Am J Cardiol. 2007;100(2):302–4.

Congenital Heart Disease: Pregnancy and Contraception

Rachael Hatton, Jack M. Colman, Matthew Sermer, Samuel C. Siu, and Candice K. Silversides

Abstract

Due to surgical advances, most children born with congenital heart disease (CHD) now survive to adulthood and, as a consequence, there is a growing population of young women with CHD of childbearing age. The superimposed hemodynamic stress of pregnancy in this population can contribute to complications for the women and their babies. Potential maternal cardiac complications include deterioration in ventricular function, heart failure, arrhythmias, thromboembolic events, and endocarditis. Therefore, risk assessment and management of pregnancy is an important aspect of their care. This chapter will review the physiologic changes associated with pregnancy, focusing on the interaction between these changes and the congenitally abnormal heart, considerations for preconception counseling and assessment of pregnancy risk in women with CHD, and management of common cardiovascular complications in this population.

Keywords

Congenital heart disease • Pregnancy • Pregnancy risk assessment • Contraceptive choices • Valvular heart disease • Anticoagulation

R. Hatton, BMed, FRACP
Division of Cardiology, University of Toronto,
Mount Sinai Hospital and University Health Network,
Toronto General Hospital, 200 Elizabeth Avenue,
Toronto, ON M5G 2C2, Canada
e-mail: rachael.hatton@uhn.ca

J.M. Colman, MD, FRCPC
Division of Cardiology, University of Toronto, Mount Sinai
Hospital and University Health Network, Mount Sinai Hospital,
600 University Avenue, Toronto,
ON M5G 1X5, Canada
e-mail: j.colman@utoronto.ca

M. Sermer, MD, FRCSC
Department of Obstetrics and Gynecology,
University of Toronto, Mount Sinai Hospital,
600 University Avenue, 19-316B,
Toronto, ON M5G 1X5, Canada
e-mail: msermer@mtsinai.on.ca

S.C. Siu, MD, SM
Division of Cardiology, Department of Medicine,
University of Western Ontario, Schulich School of Medicine
and Dentistry, 339 Windermere Road,
London, ON N6A 5A5, Canada
e-mail: samuel.siu@lhsc.on.ca

C.K. Silversides, MD, MS, FRCPC (✉)
Division of Cardiology,
University of Toronto, Mount Sinai Hospital
and University Health Network, OPG Building,
700 University Avenue, Toronto, ON M5T 1Z5, Canada
e-mail: candice.silversides@uhn.ca

Introduction

Due to surgical advances, most children born with congenital heart disease (CHD) now survive to adulthood [1–3] and, as a consequence, there is a growing population of young women with CHD of childbearing age. The superimposed hemodynamic stress of pregnancy in this population can contribute to complications for the women and their babies. Potential maternal cardiac complications include deterioration in ventricular function, heart failure, arrhythmias, thromboembolic events, and endocarditis. Therefore, risk assessment and management of pregnancy is an important aspect of their care.

This chapter will review the physiologic changes associated with pregnancy, focusing on the interaction between

K. Stergiopoulos, D.L. Brown (eds.), *Evidence-Based Cardiology Consult*,
DOI 10.1007/978-1-4471-4441-0_34, © Springer-Verlag London 2014

these changes and the congenitally abnormal heart, considerations for preconception counseling and assessment of pregnancy risk in women with CHD, and management of common cardiovascular complications in this population.

Pathophysiology

Plasma volume increases by an average of 40–50 % during pregnancy. A relatively greater increase in plasma volume compared to red cell volume results in a physiologic anemia of pregnancy [4, 5]. In early pregnancy, the cardiac output increases as a consequence of increased stroke volume and, later in pregnancy, an increase in heart rate contributes to a further increase in cardiac output. Although there is significant individual variation, cardiac output peaks at 25–50 % above non-gravid levels during the second trimester [6–11]. During labor, cardiac output increases beyond peak pregnancy levels, with additional increments during contractions when as much as 500 mL of blood may be returned to the circulation from the contracting uterus [12]. At full cervical dilatation, cardiac output is as much as 30 % above pre-labor output [5]. Regional anesthesia modulates these effects by causing peripheral vasodilation, while supine positioning can reduce venous return due to compression of the inferior vena cava.

Women with obstructive lesions such as mitral or aortic stenosis who are asymptomatic prior to pregnancy may become symptomatic for the first time as a result of the increased cardiac output. An inability to increase cardiac output due to a fixed obstruction to flow can elevate left-sided intracardiac pressure, thus predisposing to heart failure and arrhythmias [13]. Regurgitant lesions are generally better tolerated in pregnancy than stenotic lesions. However, for women with repaired tetralogy of Fallot with residual severe pulmonic regurgitation and dilated or dysfunctional right ventricles, the additional volume load can contribute to the development of arrhythmias and right heart failure [14, 15].

The mean arterial pressure falls in association with a decline in the diastolic blood pressure, reaching a nadir at approximately 20 weeks' gestation before returning to normal or supranormal levels by 38 weeks' gestation [5, 7]. Fluctuations in blood pressure during pregnancy, brought about by changes in vascular resistance and cardiac output, can lead to decompensation in some women with CHD. For example, in women with large intracardiac shunts associated with pulmonary hypertension or Eisenmenger syndrome, decreases in peripheral vascular resistance may facilitate increases in right-to-left shunting and result in cyanosis. Low oxygen saturations are associated with recurrent miscarriage, poor fetal growth, and intrauterine growth retardation [16].

Pregnancy is a prothrombotic state exposing women to a substantially higher risk of venous thrombotic events compared to nonpregnant women; this risk extends into the postpartum period [17, 18]. The propensity to thrombosis associated with pregnancy can be particularly dangerous for some women with CHD. Women with right-to-left shunt lesions are at risk of systemic thromboembolism [19]. Women with a univentricular circulation following a Fontan palliation are at risk for pulmonary thromboembolism during pregnancy. Women with mechanical valves are at risk for thromboembolic complications, including valve thrombosis and cardioembolic stroke. Valve thrombosis can be fatal; the risk is highly dependent on the type of anticoagulant used [20] and will be discussed in more detail below.

Diagnosis

Occasionally, the hemodynamic stress of pregnancy will lead to symptoms or accentuation of physical findings and the recognition of a new diagnosis of CHD. More commonly, however, women with CHD will be aware of their cardiac condition prior to pregnancy. A full history and examination should focus on delineating the underlying cardiac diagnosis as well as any palliative or corrective surgeries or interventions. Risk factors for adverse outcomes should be identified including signs and symptoms of heart failure, arrhythmias, chest pain or syncope, as well as an obstetric history capturing details pertaining to maternal, fetal, and neonatal outcomes during previous pregnancies. In familial conditions such as Marfan syndrome, other connective tissue disorders, or in women with syndromic clinical features, a detailed family history should be emphasized. A history of sudden or unexplained death in family members may point to a diagnosis of familial aortopathy, cardiomyopathy, or arrhythmia. Genetic testing of the patient (and family), preimplantation genetic diagnosis, or chorionic villus sampling may be considered in some instances. Fetal echocardiography can identify major CHD in the fetus [21, 22]. Postnatal pediatric cardiology assessments can be helpful to exclude minor CHD not detected by fetal echocardiographic screening [23].

Maternal functional status and baseline oxygen saturation should be documented as they are important determinants of outcome during pregnancy [16]. The medication history is important to identify drugs that are potentially toxic to the fetus, such as angiotensin-converting enzyme inhibitors (ACEI) and warfarin.

All pregnant women with CHD should have a standard 12-lead electrocardiogram and a transthoracic echocardiogram, both of which are safe during pregnancy. The hemodynamic changes of a normal pregnancy may produce small increases in the left- and right-sided chamber dimensions and transvalvular gradients on echocardiography [24]. A Holter ambulatory monitor should be considered to identify the mechanism of symptomatic arrhythmias. In women with CHD, an exercise stress test can be helpful for prepregnancy risk assessment; an abnormal chronotropic response to exercise has been associated with adverse pregnancy outcomes [25]. If an exercise stress test is felt to be necessary during pregnancy to guide management, a submaximal stress test to a peak heart rate of 80 % of predicted maximum can be performed safely [26]. Cardiac biomarkers such as B-type natriuretic peptide (BNP) may help to adjudicate the basis of symptoms during pregnancy that might be of cardiac origin [27].

Investigations requiring radiation exposure should be considered in situations where alternative diagnostic tests do not yield the necessary information. When clinically indicated, diagnostic tests, such as chest x-rays, should not be withheld. Radiation exposure of less than 0.5 mGy is not thought to be deleterious to the developing fetus. A chest x-ray exposes the fetus to approximately 0.002 mGy and computed tomography (CT) of the chest, approximately 0.2 mGy [28, 29]. If complete visualization of the thoracic aorta is necessary to clarify complex cardiac anatomy, a cardiac MRI does not expose the patient or fetus to radiation and is likely safe [30, 31]. Use of gadolinium as MRI contrast during pregnancy is not recommended because the long-term effects of gadolinium on the developing fetus are not known [26].

Management

General Approach to the Assessment of Pregnancy Risk

Although most women with CHD do well during pregnancy, they are at increased risk of adverse cardiac events during pregnancy and the early postpartum period compared to normal women [19]. Adverse cardiovascular events occur in approximately 10–20 % of pregnancies in women with congenital heart disease [19, 32, 33]. Arrhythmias and heart failure are the most common, although cardiac arrest, cerebrovascular events, endocarditis, and aortic dissections also occur [19, 32, 34, 35]. The probability of maternal cardiac complications varies according to the underlying cardiac lesion and overall cardiac status of the mother. Certain high-risk conditions need special consideration: pulmonary arterial hypertension [36], Marfan syndrome with dilated aortic root [37–39], significant ventricular dysfunction [35, 40], symptomatic left ventricular inflow or outflow tract obstruction [35, 41], and history of peripartum cardiomyopathy, especially if there is residual left ventricular systolic dysfunction after the index pregnancy [42, 43] (Table 34.1).

Not only does pregnancy pose short-term risks to the mother but it may also have long-term implications for women with CHD [38, 45, 46]. For instance, women with subaortic right ventricles are at risk of deterioration in ventricular function after pregnancy [45], women with Marfan

Table 34.1 Classification of maternal cardiac risk during pregnancy

Risk Class	Description	Examples
I	Uncomplicated, small, or mild	Pulmonary stenosis
		Ventricular septal defect
		Patent ductus arteriosus
		Mitral valve prolapse with no more than trivial regurgitation
	Successfully repaired simple lesions	Ostium secundum atrial septal defect
		Ventricular septal defect
		Patent ductus arteriosus
		Total anomalous pulmonary venous connection
II	If otherwise uncomplicated and well	Unoperated atrial septal defect
		Repaired tetralogy of Fallot
		Most arrhythmias
II–III	Depending on the patient	Mild left ventricular impairment
		Hypertrophic cardiomyopathy
		Native or tissue valvular disease not considered WHO IV
		Marfan syndrome without aortic dilatation
III	Subaortic right ventricle	Congenitally corrected transposition of the great arteries
		Simple transposition of the great arteries post-Mustard or Senning procedure
	Anticoagulation-dependent valve disease	Mechanical valve
	Other complex congenital heart disease	Post-Fontan operation
		Cyanotic heart disease
		Other complex congenital heart disease
IV	Subaortic ventricular pathology	NYHA III–IV
		Subaortic ventricular ejection fraction <30 %
		Severe left ventricular outflow tract obstruction
		Previous peripartum cardiomyopathy with any residual impairment of left ventricular systolic function
	Pulmonary vascular disease	Pulmonary arterial hypertension from any cause
	Aortopathy	Marfan syndrome with aorta dilated >40 mm

Adapted from Thorne et al. [44]. Used with permission
Risk classification (WHO [World Health Organization] definition of risk): I – Morbidity and mortality not appreciably higher than for the general population; II – Small increased risk of morbidity and mortality; III – Significant increase in the risk of morbidity and mortality, management in a high-risk pregnancy program is recommended; IV – Risk of morbidity and mortality is prohibitively high, termination should be recommended

Fig. 34.1 Adverse maternal cardiac events following pregnancy. (**a**) Late risk of adverse maternal cardiac events stratified according to the presence or absence of cardiac event in pregnancy. (**b**) Late risk of adverse maternal cardiac events stratified according to the CARPREG risk scores of 0, 1, or >1 (Adapted from Balint et al. [46]. Used with permission)

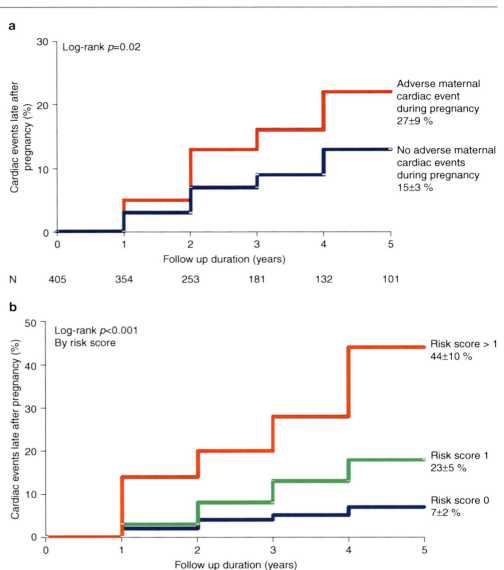

syndrome and a dilated aortic root are at risk of accelerated aortic dilation after pregnancy [38], and women with aortic stenosis are more likely to have valve interventions after pregnancy [47]. Women with CHD who experience adverse cardiovascular events during pregnancy are at increased risk of additional adverse cardiovascular events late after pregnancy [46] (Fig. 34.1a, b).

The goals of preconception assessment include optimization of the maternal cardiac condition, counseling addressing the risk of pregnancy and long-term consequences for both mother and child, and planning for medication adjustment in anticipation of or at the time of pregnancy, when necessary. When pregnancy is considered to be very high risk, appropriate advice regarding the efficacy and safety of various contraception options should be discussed. In this instance, other options that may be discussed include adoption or surrogacy.

Assessment of Maternal Cardiac Risk

Preconception assessment is an important component of pregnancy management. When estimating pregnancy risk, both global or general cardiac risk factors and lesion-specific risks need to be considered. Two common tools for global risk assessment are the Cardiac Disease in Pregnancy (CARPREG) score and the ZAHARA score [34, 35] (Table 34.2). The CARPREG score is based on a prospective multicenter Canadian study of pregnancy outcomes in 599 women with heart disease (Fig. 34.2). The CARPREG study identified four predictors of adverse pregnancy outcome. One point is allocated for presence of each of the 4 risk factors: prior cardiac event, baseline New York Heart Association (NYHA) functional class >2 or cyanosis, left heart obstruction, and systemic ventricular systolic function <40 %. Risk can then be estimated based on the total score.

Table 34.2 The CARPREG and ZAHARA risk scores

CARPREG risk predictors	Weighted risk
Prior cardiac event or arrhythmia	1
Baseline NYHA class > II or cyanosis	1
Left heart obstruction (MVA <2 cm², AVA <1.5 cm² or peak LVOT gradient >30 mmHg)	1
Reduced systemic ventricular systolic function (LVEF <40 %)	1
Maximum possible score	4

CARPREG score	Risk of cardiac event
0	5 %
1	27 %
>1	75 %

ZAHARA risk predictors	Weighted risk
History of arrhythmias	1.5
Baseline NYHA class >1	0.75
Left heart obstruction (PG >50 mmHg or AVA <1 cm²)	2.5
Cardiac medication prior to pregnancy	1.5
Systemic AV valve regurgitation (mod/severe)	0.75
Pulmonic AV valve regurgitation (mod/severe)	0.75
Mechanical valve prosthesis	4.25
Cyanotic heart disease (corrected/uncorrected)	1.0
Maximum possible Score	13

ZAHARA score	Risk of cardiac event
0–0.5	2.9 %
0.51–1.5	7.5 %
1.51–2.5	17.5 %
2.51–3.5	43.1 %
>3.51	70 %

Adapted from Siu et al. [35] and Drenthen et al. [34]
NYHA New York Heart Association, *MVA* mitral valve area, *AVA* aortic valve area, *LVOT* left ventricular outflow tract, *AV* atrioventricular, *LVEF* left ventricular ejection fraction, *PG* peak gradient

The CARPREG risk score has been validated by other groups [32]. The ZAHARA score was based on 1,302 completed pregnancies in women with CHD. The ZAHARA study identified 9 risk factors related to adverse maternal cardiac events and a weighted scoring system was devised based on those risk factors. Some women with high-pregnancy risk, such as those with Marfan syndrome with dilated aortas or those who have undergone Fontan operations, may not have been represented in the large cohort studies from which the global risk predictors were derived. Thus, their pregnancy risk is not captured by the global risk scoring systems. Therefore, in addition to the global risk scores, it is important to integrate risk information about a specific lesion when available A general approach to risk on a lesion-by-lesion basis, taking into account known lesion-specific risk information, has been proposed (Table 34.2).

Low-Risk Cardiac Lesions

Pregnancies in women with pulmonary stenosis, repaired total anomalous pulmonary venous return, and small or repaired atrial septal defect, ventricular septal defect, or patent ductus arteriosus are considered low risk for adverse cardiac events during pregnancy [48–50]. Women with unrepaired isolated atrial septal defect have low rates of cardiac complications but may be at risk for other complications such as preeclampsia or small for gestational age births.

Intermediate and High Risk Cardiac Lesions

Women with simple lesions with significant residua or sequelae are at intermediate risk. In addition, many CHD lesions fall into the intermediate-risk category such as congenitally corrected transposition of the great arteries and complete transposition of the great arteries following an atrial switch operation. When assessing pregnancy risk in women with these conditions, it is important to also consider general risk predictors such as subaortic ventricular function or functional capacity, as these factors can have a major impact on pregnancy risk. These women are at risk for developing heart failure and systemic ventricular dysfunction which may persist after pregnancy in some cases [45, 51]. In one series, subaortic right ventricular dysfunction progressed in 25 % of pregnancies and was irreversible in 75 % of the cases in which it had progressed during pregnancy [35]. Following a Fontan operation, women require careful risk evaluation prior to pregnancy. They are at risk for arrhythmia, heart failure, and thromboembolism [52, 53]. While women with Fontan operations can do well during pregnancy, for some women, such as those with failing Fontan circulation or impaired subaortic ventricular function, pregnancy can be associated with substantial risk. The late effects of pregnancy on the single ventricle are unknown. Miscarriage rates are high in this population (up to 50 %), and premature labor is common [52, 53]. Women with cyanotic heart disease are at risk for developing heart failure and arrhythmias even if they do not have pulmonary hypertension [16].

Specific High-Risk Cardiac Lesions

Marfan Syndrome
Due to the hemodynamic and perhaps hormonal changes of pregnancy, aortic dilation and dissection can occur during and shortly after pregnancy in women with Marfan syndrome and preexisting aortopathy. Progressive aortic dilatation occurs in some women and is a risk factor for dissection [38, 54]. Aortic

Fig. 34.2 Estimation of adverse cardiovascular outcomes according to the CARPREG risk score. Frequency of maternal primary cardiac events, as predicted by the risk index and observed in the derivation and validation groups (in which 1 point is allocated for each of four risk factors: prior cardiac event, baseline New York Heart Association (NYHA) functional class >2 or cyanosis, left heart obstruction, and systemic ventricular systolic function <40 %) (From Siu et al. [35]. Used with permission)

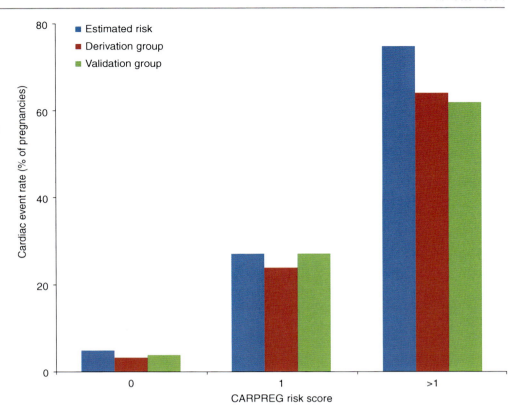

dissection occurs in approximately 3 % of pregnancies [55]. Risk can be stratified according to aortic dimensions and is highest in women with significant dilation (>44 mm) of the proximal aorta and in the peripartum period [54, 56, 57].

Eisenmenger Syndrome

Pregnancy risk in women with pulmonary arterial hypertension, including Eisenmenger syndrome, remains very high with mortality rates of approximately 30 % [26, 36, 58, 59]. Even with advanced therapies for pulmonary arterial hypertension such as prostacyclin analogues, pregnancy risk remains high [36]. Women, therefore, should be advised to use safe and efficacious contraception to avoid becoming pregnant [44, 60].

Mechanical Valves

Women requiring anticoagulation for mechanical valves during pregnancy face a high rate of early fetal loss, up to 25 % [20, 61]. The risk of valve thrombosis in pregnancy varies from 4 to 30 % depending on the regime of anticoagulation employed [20, 61, 62]. In addition to the type of anticoagulant used, the location and type of valve and the history of valve or other thrombosis impact the risk of valve thrombosis. Major bleeding is less common, occurring in 2.5 % of pregnancies, mostly in the peripartum period [20]. Fetal embryopathy occurs in 5–11 % of cases of women using warfarin throughout the first trimester;

there is some evidence that this risk is dose related [20, 63].

Aortic Stenosis

Women with mild and moderate aortic stenosis usually tolerate pregnancy well [13, 64]. However, heart failure has been reported in up to 16 % of women with severe aortic stenosis [13, 41, 64, 65]. Although rare, maternal deaths have been reported [41]. Most cases of congenital aortic stenosis in pregnant women are due to bicuspid aortic valve disease, and some of these women will have an associated aortopathy [66, 67]. Although women with bicuspid valve aortopathy are at risk of aortic dissection, the risk appears to be significantly lower than for women with Marfan syndrome [37]. Risk assessment should include an echocardiogram to assess the degree of aortic stenosis and an exercise stress test to assess functional capacity and ensure adequate blood pressure response to exercise [26].

Assessment of Fetal and Neonatal Risk

Women with CHD have an increased risk of fetal and neonatal complications in pregnancy [33] primarily related to a high prevalence of prematurity, low birth weight for gestational age, and transmission of heart diseases to offspring. Overall risk of adverse fetal and neonatal events is more than twice that of normal pregnancies, and it is further increased in women with obstetric risk factors (history of premature birth, incompetent cervix or cesarean section, intrauterine growth retardation, antepartum bleeding, uterine or placental abnormalities), with multiple gestation, who are smokers, and who require anticoagulation [33]. Adverse fetal outcomes are particularly common in patients with cyanotic heart disease. Women with oxygen saturations less than 85 % prior to pregnancy have been reported to have live birth rates of only 12 % [16] as well as a high incidence of premature birth and low birth weights for gestational age [16].

The transmission rate of CHD to offspring of women with CHD is approximately 3–5 % [32, 33, 68, 69]. However, women with conditions with autosomal dominant transmission, such as Marfan syndrome or 22q11 deletion syndrome, will transmit to 50 % of their fetuses. Genetic counseling prior to pregnancy is appropriate for all women with CHD and especially so when the transmission risk is high.

Assessment of Obstetric Risk

In common with all women, those with CHD are at risk of obstetric complications including pregnancy-induced hypertension, preeclampsia or eclampsia, premature rupture of the membranes, premature labor, and postpartum hemorrhage. However, because of limited cardiac reserve and other alterations of physiology, women with CHD may tolerate such obstetric complications less well and their onset may be the trigger for cardiac decompensation of various types. Hypertensive disorders of pregnancy are more common in women with transposition of the great arteries, aortic coarctation, aortic stenosis, pulmonic stenosis, and pulmonary atresia with ventricular septal defect [19]. Postpartum hemorrhage is more common in women with cyanotic heart disease [16].

Contraception Options

When considering contraception in women with CHD, it is important to consider the following: (1) the risk of pregnancy for the mother, (2) available forms of contraception and their risks and benefits, (3) failure rates and the consequences of an unplanned pregnancy, and (4) preferences of the woman [70]. Possible contraception options include barrier methods, combined oral contraceptives (estrogen/progestin), progestin-only methods, intrauterine devices, sterilization, and emergency contraception. The use of inappropriate contraception can expose the woman to adverse events; however, contraception is often not discussed or the discussion is not recalled [71–73]. In one study of women with CHD, 20 % were using a form of contraception contraindicated in their heart condition, while nearly 30 % of women considered high risk for pregnancy were using no contraception [73]. The number of women who had not been counseled about contraception or the risk of pregnancy approached 50 % [73].

Barrier methods such as male condoms have been shown to have high failure rates with unintended pregnancies occurring in as many as 20 % of cases [74]. Thus, although there are no contraindications to their use in patients with CHD, they are not recommended as a sole form of contraception on grounds of inadequate efficacy.

Combined hormonal contraceptives as oral tablets, transdermal patches, and vaginal rings contain estrogen and progestins. When used correctly, they can be very efficacious [74]. However, they have been associated with venous and arterial thrombosis [75–78] and are therefore not advisable in women with intracardiac shunts who are at risk for paradoxical emboli, women with a univentricular circulation [79, 80] or Eisenmenger syndrome [70] who are at risk pulmonary emboli, and women with mechanical valves who are at risk for valve thrombosis [20, 44, 60, 70].

Most progesterone-only pills have higher failure rates than combined hormonal contraceptives [74]. Intramuscular injections (Depo-Provera®), subdermal devices (Implanon®), and intrauterine devices (Mirena®) using progesterone are more efficacious than the oral pill formulation. Progesterone-only preparations have not been associated with venous or arterial thrombosis and thus are suitable for many women with cardiac disease (Table 34.3) [81]. Care must be taken when implanting intrauterine devices in women with a univentricular circulation as insertion may induce a vagal response and cause circulatory collapse.

Emergency contraceptive pills are safe for women with CHD but can interfere with warfarin metabolism and, thus, INR monitoring is recommended [70].

Women who have a prohibitively high-pregnancy risk may need to consider permanent forms of contraception. Female sterilization by minimally invasive procedures, such as laparoscopic tubal ligation, is relatively safe for many women with CHD. However, the insufflation of carbon dioxide into the abdominal cavity can raise intra-abdominal pressure to a degree that venous return to the heart can be impaired. In susceptible women, such as those with a Fontan circulation, this can produce circulatory collapse. The general anesthetic used for a laparoscopic procedure can also cause adverse hemodynamic changes in women with CHD. Thus, the risks need to be carefully considered and discussed with the patient. Laparoscopic tubal ligation in women with CHD should be performed by experienced operators with a cardiac anesthesiologist and in a center where appropriate cardiac support is available. The Essure® and Adiana® systems are alternative, less invasive approaches to sterilization [82]. The Essure system employs stainless steel coils inserted in the fallopian tubes [83, 84] and the Adiana system uses a silicone matrix to obstruct the fallopian tubes [83, 85, 86]. Women with CHD

Table 34.3 Risk of combined hormonal contraceptives in women with congenital heart disease

WHO class 1 Always usable	WHO class 2 Broadly usable	WHO class 3 Caution with use		WHO class 4 Do not use	
Minor valve lesions: Mitral valve prolapse with mild regurgitation Bicuspid aortic valves with normal function Mild pulmonic stenosis	Tissue prosthetic valve lacking WHO 3 or 4 features	Thrombotic risk, even on warfarin	Mechanical valves: bileaflet valves	Thrombotic risk, even on warfarin	Mechanical valves: Bjork-Shiley, Starr-Edwards, any tricuspid
Repaired coarctation with no hypertension or aneurysm	Uncomplicated mild native mitral or aortic valve disease		Previous thromboembolism		Pulmonary hypertension from any cause
Simple congenital lesions repaired in childhood and with no sequelae	Most arrhythmias other than atrial fibrillation or flutter		Atrial arrhythmia		Dilated cardiomyopathy LV dysfunction from any cause with EF <30 %
	Past cardiomyopathy fully recovered, including peripartum cardiomyopathy				Fontan circulation
	Uncomplicated Marfan syndrome				
	Congenital heart disease lacking any WHO 3 or 4 features: Small left to right shunts not reversible with physiological maneuvers	Risk of paradoxical embolism	Potential reversal of left to right shunt Unoperated ASD	Risk of paradoxical embolism	Cyanotic heart disease; pulmonary AVM

Adapted from Thorne et al. [44]. Used with permission
WHO World Health Organization, *ASD* atrial septal defect, *LV* left ventricle, *EF* ejection fraction, *AVM* arteriovenous malformation

may have a shortened life span such that the male partner may outlive his spouse and wish to father children with a new partner. This needs to be discussed if male sterilization is being considered [70].

Approach to Management During Pregnancy

All women with CHD should be reviewed at least once during pregnancy by a cardiologist with expertise in pregnancy and CHD [26]. For women with low-risk cardiac lesions, this assessment may simply serve to provide reassurance. Women with moderate- or high-risk congenital lesions (World Health Organization (WHO) classification II–IV, Table 34.1) will require more frequent follow-up during pregnancy and should be managed by physicians with expertise in pregnancy and heart disease. A multidisciplinary approach to care is recommended with input from cardiology, high-risk obstetrics (maternal-fetal medicine), and obstetric anesthesia [26]. The focus of care for women with intermediate- and high-risk lesions includes regular surveillance, management of complications, and working closely with high-risk obstetrics and obstetric anesthesia to determine the optimal strategy for labor and delivery. A management plan should be developed, recorded, and made easily available to all care providers.

A woman's cardiac status, functional reserve, and perceived ability to cope with the stress of labor and delivery will ultimately determine the approach to management of the puerperium. Almost all women with CHD can undergo a vaginal delivery. Cesarean delivery is rarely required for cardiac indications. Cesarean delivery should be considered in patients with aortic dilatation greater than 45 mm, aortic dissection, and acute severe decompensated heart failure and for women presenting in spontaneous preterm labor while on anticoagulation [26].

Induction of labor can be safely performed in women with CHD when necessary and has not been associated with higher rates of cesarean section than in normal controls [87]. Women should labor in the left lateral position to minimize compression of the inferior vena cava. A carefully titrated epidural anesthetic is recommended for most patients with CHD to mitigate the elevation of cardiac output associated with the pain of labor. Care must be taken to avoid systemic hypotension with regional anesthetics, particularly in patients with left heart obstructive lesions, Fontan circulation, or Eisenmenger syndrome [26]. During the second stage of labor, women with CHD and limited cardiac reserve or Fontan circulation should avoid the Valsalva maneuver by avoiding maternal expulsive efforts. The presenting part can descend unaided during contractions followed by an assisted delivery. Noninvasive cardiac monitoring with telemetry or oximetry may be useful for some women with CHD during labor and delivery, but invasive monitoring (pulmonary artery or arterial catheters) is rarely needed [88].

Immediate postpartum management centers on ensuring adequate hemostasis, as well as minimizing the risk of thromboembolic phenomena with elastic support stockings and early mobilization. Although most of the pregnancy changes in hemodynamics resolve soon after delivery, complete return to baseline does not occur until 6 months postpartum. Therefore, women should continue to be followed up after delivery for up to 6 months or until they have returned to baseline function.

Management of Maternal Cardiac Complications

Heart Failure

Heart failure complicating pregnancy has been reported in 5–17 % of pregnancies in women with CHD [19, 32, 33]. As with other complications in pregnancy, event rates are dependent on the underlying cardiac lesion. Rates are highest in women with systemic ventricular systolic dysfunction [45, 89], left-sided outflow tract lesions [41, 90], pulmonary atresia/VSD [46], or Eisenmenger syndrome [36, 59, 91].

Differentiating between symptoms of heart failure and symptoms of a normal pregnancy can be difficult. Measuring the BNP level in these instances can be helpful [27]. The peak hemodynamic changes of pregnancy occur during the last trimester and congestive heart failure is more likely to occur during this trimester [40]. There is also an increased risk at the time of labor and delivery secondary to increases in cardiac output and autotransfusion from the contracting uterus. Continuing use of and dosages of heart failure medications should be reconsidered prior to discharge from hospital, because dosing may differ in the nonpregnant state. Ongoing heart failure management may be required in the postpartum period.

The mainstays of heart failure therapy in the nonpregnant population include beta-blockers, angiotensin-converting enzyme (ACE) inhibitors, spironolactone, and diuretics. In pregnant women, ACE inhibitors are contraindicated due to their negative impact on fetal renal development, particularly in the second and third trimester [92].Although one study suggested an increased risk with first-trimester exposure to ACE inhibitors [93], subsequent studies have not supported this finding [94–96]. Spironolactone is not recommended because of its antiandrogenic effects. Hydralazine is an alternative afterload-reducing agent that can be used with relative safety at all stages of pregnancy. Beta-blockers (except atenolol) are often used during pregnancy after a discussion with the mother of the risks and benefits. Atenolol has been implicated to a greater extent than other beta-blockers in lower birth weight babies and is often avoided during pregnancy [97, 98]. Diuretics can be used for symptomatic relief but dehydration should be avoided.

Arrhythmias

Arrhythmias requiring treatment in pregnancy have been reported in 2–5 % of pregnancies in women with CHD, but the incidence is higher in women with transposition of the great arteries who have undergone an atrial switch procedure [19], Ebstein anomaly, or Fontan operation [53]. Mitral stenosis, whether congenital or rheumatic in origin, is associated with atrial arrhythmias, predominantly atrial fibrillation [41, 99]. Most arrhythmias during pregnancy are atrial in origin. Atrial arrhythmias are poorly tolerated in some subgroups of women with CHD. For instance, in women with a Fontan circulation, atrial arrhythmia can result in the rapid development of right atrial thrombus, pulmonary emboli, and heart failure. In women with impaired ventricular function, loss of atrial contribution to ventricular filling can reduce cardiac output, raising atrial pressure, and result in congestive cardiac failure. In these groups of women, aggressive treatment of atrial arrhythmias is often necessary. Ventricular arrhythmias are less common during pregnancy and, when identified, structural heart disease should be excluded and the arrhythmia should be treated, often in conjunction with a cardiac electrophysiologist.

Direct current cardioversion can be performed safely for the acute management of symptomatic arrhythmias associated with hemodynamic instability [26]. In the management of maternal atrial arrhythmias, the shock is synchronized to the mother's QRS signal, but not to the fetal QRS signal. Defibrillation pads/paddles should be positioned to minimize exposure of the uterus to the defibrillator discharge. Chemical cardioversion of supraventricular tachycardias can be safely attempted with adenosine after vagal maneuvers fail. Beta-blockers or digoxin are often used for the treatment of atrial arrhythmias [26]. Treatment of ventricular arrhythmias is more complicated and should be individualized. Amiodarone is only used during pregnancy in exceptional instances, because of potential adverse effects on the fetal thyroid. Electrophysiology studies and ablation procedures are reserved for refractory cases because they expose the fetus to ionizing radiation [26].

Marfan Syndrome and Aortic Dilation and Dissection

Women with Marfan syndrome and other aortopathies, such as Loeys-Dietz syndrome or vascular (formerly type IV) Ehlers-Danlos syndrome, are at risk for aortic complications during pregnancy. In women with Marfan syndrome and dilated aortic roots, avoidance of pregnancy until after aortic root replacement is recommended. Recommendations for the absolute aortic dimension requiring prepregnancy intervention vary among guidelines. The American Heart

Association/American College of Cardiology guidelines for the diagnosis and management of patients with thoracic aortic disease suggest that surgical intervention should occur if the aortic dimension is greater than 40 mm [100], whereas the European Society of Cardiology taskforce on the management of cardiovascular disease during pregnancy suggests intervention if the aortic dimension is greater than 45 mm [26]. The Canadian Cardiovascular Society consensus conference on the management of adults with congenital heart disease suggests intervention if the aortic dimension is greater than 44 mm [101]. During pregnancy, beta-blocker therapy is recommended for women with Marfan syndrome in the hope of limiting progressive dilation or dissection of the aorta. This recommendation is based upon limited data examining the use of beta-blockers in the nonpregnant Marfan population [26, 101–105]. There may be late effects of pregnancy on the dilated aorta in women with Marfan syndrome. One small study showed that women with an aortic diameter greater than 40 mm at the start of pregnancy had higher rates of aortic root dilation following pregnancy, when compared to nonpregnant controls [26]. Another study showed that a larger increase in aortic diameter during pregnancy and the absence of beta-blocker therapy were associated with a higher rate of long-term adverse outcomes [106].

Women with aortopathy should be followed every 6–8 weeks throughout pregnancy with serial echocardiographic assessment of the proximal thoracic aorta [26, 101, 102]. Aortic dissection should be immediately excluded in any pregnant woman with acute severe chest pain. In cases of acute aortic dissection during pregnancy, management is similar to that in the nonpregnant patient and is considered a medical emergency. Blood pressure control and surgical assessment are paramount. There is significant associated maternal and fetal morbidity and mortality, particularly in the setting of type A dissection [37].

Anticoagulation of Mechanical Valves

Warfarin, unfractionated heparin, and low molecular weight heparin (LMWH) are all associated with high rates of spontaneous abortion in early pregnancy (approximately 15–25 %), thought to be related, at least in part, to subplacental bleeding [20, 62]. Pregnancy is a prothrombotic state and is associated with significant maternal thromboembolic risk in women with mechanical heart valves. Valve thrombosis, when it occurs, is associated with maternal mortality in 40 % of cases and therefore effective anticoagulation is of utmost importance. Warfarin and other vitamin K antagonists are associated with lower rates of valve thrombosis when compared to heparin formulations. The risk of valve thrombosis is approximately 4 % with oral anticoagulants used throughout pregnancy, 9–10 % when unfractionated heparin is substituted in the first trimester and at term only (a vitamin K antagonist is used from the 13th to the 36th week of gestation), and up to 30 % when unfractionated heparin is used throughout pregnancy [20, 61, 62]. Rates of thromboembolic complications during pregnancy in women using low molecular weight heparins vary between 5 and 20 % [61, 62, 107, 108]. Warfarin has superior maternal safety but is associated with embryopathy following exposure during the 6th–12th weeks of gestation [109]. Warfarin embryopathy has been identified in as high as 11 % of pregnancies where warfarin was given throughout the first trimester [20]. However, some data suggest that when a dose of less than 5 mg of warfarin per day provides adequate anticoagulation, the risk of embryopathy with first-trimester use is lower [63, 110]. Heparin does not cross the placenta and is not teratogenic but is associated with higher rates of maternal thrombotic complications [20].

Guidelines for the management of anticoagulation in pregnant women with mechanical valves are available from the European Society of Cardiology task force on the management of cardiovascular disease during pregnancy [26], the American College of Cardiology/American Heart Association guidelines for the management of patients with valvular heart disease [111], and the American College of Chest Physicians evidence-based clinical practice guidelines on antithrombotic therapy and prevention of thrombosis [112]. Recommendations for anticoagulation management differ slightly among the three groups. The 2012 guidelines from the American College of Chest Physicians and the 2011 recommendations from the European Society of Cardiology are shown in Table 34.4.

When warfarin is used, close monitoring of the INR is required. With low molecular weight heparin, anti-factor Xa levels should be measured every 2–4 weeks during pregnancy and should be maintained at 0.8–1.2 U/mL 4–6 h after administration (peak level). Even at this level, pre-dose concentrations can be subtherapeutic [26]. Although thrombotic complications have occurred in patients on therapeutic doses of anticoagulants, patient non-compliance and subtherapeutic dosing are the best recognized risk factors for thromboembolic events in these women [62, 114].

Valve thrombosis should be suspected in patients presenting with progressive dyspnea, embolic events (TIA, stroke, ischemic chest pain), or cardiac collapse. Transesophageal echocardiography or other imaging should be performed immediately to exclude valve thrombosis. When valve thrombosis is identified urgent, surgical assessment is critical [115]. Fibrinolytics may be a feasible option for critical patients, although experience is limited. Risks include embolization and subplacental bleeding [26, 116, 117].

Major bleeding complicates 2.5 % of pregnancies requiring anticoagulation, mostly at the time of delivery [20]. Thus, the timing and mode of delivery must be carefully planned. Since warfarin therapy exposes the fetus to a risk of intracranial hemorrhage, a cesarean delivery is indicated unless maternal warfarin has been replaced with heparin at least 2 weeks prior to labor to reduce the risk of fetal intracranial hemorrhage [26].

Table 34.4 American college of chest physicians guidelines on the use of antithrombotic therapies in pregnant women with mechanical valves

Recommendation	Grade of recommendation
For women requiring long-term vitamin K antagonists who are attempting pregnancy and are candidates for LMWH substitution, frequent pregnancy tests are recommended with substitution of LMWH for vitamin K antagonists when pregnancy is achieved rather than switching to LMWH while attempting pregnancy	Grade 2C
Avoid the use of oral direct thrombin (e.g., dabigatran) and anti-Xa (e.g., rivaroxaban, apixaban) inhibitors	Grade 1C
For pregnant women with mechanical heart valves, one of the following anticoagulant regimens is recommended in preference to no anticoagulation: (a) Adjusted-dose bid LMWH throughout pregnancy. Doses be adjusted to achieve the manufacturer's peak anti-Xa LMWH 4 h postsubcutaneous injection or (b) Adjusted-dose UFH throughout pregnancy administered subcutaneously every 12 h in doses adjusted to keep the mid-interval aPTT at least twice control or attain an anti-Xa heparin level of 0.35–0.70 U/mL or (c) UFH or LMWH (as above) until the 13th week, with substitution by vitamin K antagonists until close to delivery when UFH or LMWH is resumed	Grade 1A
In women judged to be at very high risk of thromboembolism in whom concerns exist about the efficacy and safety of UFH or LMWH as dosed above (e.g., older generation prosthesis in the mitral position or history of thromboembolism), vitamin K antagonists throughout pregnancy with replacement by UFH or LMWH (as above) close to delivery are recommended, rather than one of the regimens above	Grade 2C

Adapted from Bates et al. [112, 113] Used with Permission
Grade 1A – Strong recommendation, high-quality evidence. Benefits clearly outweigh risks. Recommendation can apply to most patients
Grade 1B – Strong recommendation, moderate-quality evidence. Benefits clearly outweigh risks. Recommendations can apply to most patients
Grade 1C – Strong recommendation, low- or very low-quality evidence. Benefits clearly outweigh risks. Recommendations can apply to most patients
Grade 2A – Weak recommendation, high-quality evidence. Benefits closely balanced with risks. Best action may differ depending on patient circumstances
Grade 2B – Weak recommendation, moderate-quality evidence. Benefits closely balanced with risks. Best action may differ depending on patient circumstances
Grade 2C – Weak recommendation, low- or very low-quality evidence. Other alternatives may be equally reasonable
UFH unfractionated heparin, *LMWH* low molecular weight heparin

Eisenmenger Syndrome and Pulmonary Arterial Hypertension

The risk of pregnancy in women with pulmonary arterial hypertension (PAH), including PAH secondary to congenital heart disease such as Eisenmenger syndrome, remains prohibitively high [26, 36]. Women should be advised to use adequate and safe contraception so to avoid becoming pregnant [44, 60]. The endothelin-1 receptor antagonist bosentan can reduce the effectiveness of progesterone-only pills [44].

For women with Eisenmenger syndrome who become pregnant, notwithstanding the risk involved, multidisciplinary care is critical. This includes involvement of cardiologists with expertise in adult congenital heart disease, pulmonary hypertension physicians, maternal-fetal medicine specialists (high-risk obstetricians), and obstetric anesthetists. Advanced therapies for PAH (prostacyclin analogues, phosphodiesterase inhibitors) should be considered. Endothelin-1 receptor antagonists, such as bosentan, are teratogenic in animals and are not recommended in pregnancy [26]. Frequent follow-up is advisable throughout pregnancy with serial transthoracic echocardiography to monitor pulmonary pressures and right ventricular function. Some experts also follow serial serum BNP levels. In women with intracardiac right-to-left shunts, the peripheral vasodilation associated with pregnancy can increase the degree of shunting resulting in worsening cyanosis. Supplemental oxygen can be used but will likely not reverse the cyanosis. Restriction of physical activities is also

recommended. Up-titration of PAH therapy may be required as pregnancy progresses, particularly if symptoms are worsening despite diuretic therapy. Right heart failure can be managed with diuretics, such as furosemide, using caution to avoid hypovolemia. Patients with preexisting indications for

> **Key Points**
> - Pregnancy poses a hemodynamic burden that can result in complications in some women with congenital heart disease.
> - The stress of pregnancy may also have long-term implications on cardiac function, disease progression, and mortality.
> - All women with congenital heart disease who are contemplating pregnancy should be counseled regarding pregnancy risk and risks to long-term health.
> - Global risk assessment tools, such as the CARPREG and ZAHARA scores, can help to estimate the risk of cardiovascular complications during pregnancy. These estimates of risk should be supplemented with lesion-specific data if available.
> - In cases where the risk is unacceptably high, management should focus on the appropriate use of safe contraception, including permanent contraception.

- Women with pulmonary arterial hypertension, Marfan syndrome with dilated aortas, severe subaortic ventricular dysfunction, severe symptomatic left heart obstructive lesions, and prior peripartum cardiomyopathy with residual ventricular impairment remain at high risk of adverse outcomes including death and should be advised not to become pregnant.
- If a woman at intermediate or high risk of an adverse cardiac outcome during pregnancy chooses to proceed with pregnancy, regular clinical and echocardiographic follow-up during pregnancy and the early postpartum is advised.
- Common cardiovascular complications include heart failure and arrhythmias. Most complications can be managed with medical therapy.
- Labor and delivery should be planned in advance with input from cardiologists, maternal-fetal medicine specialists (high-risk obstetricians), and obstetric anesthetists. Plans should be documented and disseminated.
- Cesarean delivery is rarely indicated for cardiac reasons.
- The hemodynamic and other changes of pregnancy do not resolve immediately postpartum, and therefore, women remain at risk for postpartum complications.

anticoagulation should consider continuing that therapy throughout pregnancy.

Prematurity is common in women with Eisenmenger syndrome [36]. A planned vaginal or cesarean delivery is preferable to an emergency cesarean delivery, and the mode of delivery should be based on the expertise available at each center [26]. A regional anesthetic approach has been associated with less mortality than a general anesthetic in this population of women [36].

Maternal deaths often occur in the postpartum period and women should therefore not be discharged early but rather should be monitored in hospital for an extended period up to 1 week [58].

Guidelines

Recommendations pertaining to pregnancy risk assessment in women with congenital heart disease are available in the European Society of Cardiology task force on the management of cardiovascular diseases during pregnancy [26], the American Heart Association/American College of Cardiology guidelines for the management of adults with congenital heart disease [102], and the Canadian Cardiovascular Society consensus conference on the management of adults with congenital heart disease [101, 118, 119].

The most comprehensive recommendations pertaining to management of cardiovascular complications during pregnancy are in the European Society of Cardiology task force on the management of cardiovascular diseases during pregnancy [26]. Management recommendations for specific conditions can be found in other guidelines. The European Society of Cardiology task force on the management of cardiovascular disease during pregnancy [26], the American College of Cardiology/American Heart Association guidelines for the management of patients with valvular heart disease [111], and the American College of Chest Physicians Evidence-Based Clinical Practice Guidelines on Antithrombotic Therapy and Prevention of Thrombosis [112] provide recommendations for anticoagulation management in women with mechanical heart valves during pregnancy. Management recommendations for thoracic aortic aneurysms can be found in the American Heart Association/American College of Cardiology guidelines for the diagnosis and management of patients with thoracic aortic disease [100]. Recommendations for management of arrhythmias can be found in the joint American Heart Association/American College of Cardiology and European Society of Cardiology guidelines on the management of ventricular arrhythmias and the prevention of sudden cardiac death [120], the guidelines for the management of patients with supraventricular arrhythmias [121], and the guidelines for the management of patients with atrial fibrillation [122]. Recommendations on antibiotic prophylaxis at the time of labor and delivery can be found in the American Heart Association/American College of Cardiology guideline update on valvular heart disease: focused update on infective endocarditis [123].

References

1. Marelli AJ, Mackie AS, Ionescu-Ittu R, Rahme E, Pilote L. Congenital heart disease in the general population: changing prevalence and age distribution. Circulation. 2007;115:163–72.
2. Warnes CA, Liberthson R, Danielson GK, et al. Task force 1: the changing profile of congenital heart disease in adult life. J Am Coll Cardiol. 2001;37:1170–5.
3. Moons P, Bovijn L, Budts W, Belmans A, Gewillig M. Temporal trends in survival to adulthood among patients born with congenital heart disease from 1970 to 1992 in Belgium. Circulation. 2010;122:2264–72.
4. Pritchard JA. Changes in the blood volume during pregnancy and delivery. Anesthesiology. 1965;26:393–9.
5. Hunter S, Robson SC. Adaptation of the maternal heart in pregnancy. Br Heart J. 1992;68:540–3.
6. Easterling TR, Benedetti TJ, Schmucker BC, Millard SP. Maternal hemodynamics in normal and preeclamptic pregnancies: a longitudinal study. Obstet Gynecol. 1990;76:1061–9.
7. Gilson GJ, Mosher MD, Conrad KP. Systemic hemodynamics and oxygen transport during pregnancy in chronically instrumented, conscious rats. Am J Physiol. 1992;263:H1911–8.

8. Gilson GJ, Samaan S, Crawford MH, Qualls CR, Curet LB. Changes in hemodynamics, ventricular remodeling, and ventricular contractility during normal pregnancy: a longitudinal study. Obstet Gynecol. 1997;89:957–62.

9. Robson SC, Hunter S, Boys RJ, Dunlop W. Serial study of factors influencing changes in cardiac output during human pregnancy. Am J Physiol. 1989;256:H1060–5.

10. Karamermer Y, Roos-Hesselink JW. Pregnancy and adult congenital heart disease. Expert Rev Cardiovasc Ther. 2007;5:859–69.

11. Hennessy TG, MacDonald D, Hennessy MS, et al. Serial changes in cardiac output during normal pregnancy: a Doppler ultrasound study. Eur J Obstet Gynecol Reprod Biol. 1996;70:117–22.

12. Robson SC, Dunlop W, Boys RJ, Hunter S. Cardiac output during labour. Br Med J (Clin Res Ed). 1987;295:1169–72.

13. Yap SC, Drenthen W, Pieper PG, et al. Risk of complications during pregnancy in women with congenital aortic stenosis. Int J Cardiol. 2008;126:240–6.

14. Veldtman GR, Connolly HM, Grogan M, Ammash NM, Warnes CA. Outcomes of pregnancy in women with tetralogy of Fallot. J Am Coll Cardiol. 2004;44:174–80.

15. Greutmann M, Von Klemperer K, Brooks R, Peebles D, O'Brien P, Walker F. Pregnancy outcome in women with congenital heart disease and residual haemodynamic lesions of the right ventricular outflow tract. Eur Heart J. 2010;31:1764–70.

16. Presbitero P, Somerville J, Stone S, Aruta E, Spiegelhalter D, Rabajoli F. Pregnancy in cyanotic congenital heart disease. Outcome of mother and fetus. Circulation. 1994;89:2673–6.

17. Marik PE. Venous thromboembolism in pregnancy. Clin Chest Med. 2010;31:731–40.

18. Pabinger I, Grafenhofer H. Thrombosis during pregnancy: risk factors, diagnosis and treatment. Pathophysiol Haemost Thromb. 2002;32:322–4.

19. Drenthen W, Pieper PG, Roos-Hesselink JW, et al. Outcome of pregnancy in women with congenital heart disease: a literature review. J Am Coll Cardiol. 2007;49:2303–11.

20. Chan WS, Anand S, Ginsberg JS. Anticoagulation of pregnant women with mechanical heart valves: a systematic review of the literature. Arch Intern Med. 2000;160:191–6.

21. Allan LD, Crawford DC, Chita SK, Tynan MJ. Prenatal screening for congenital heart disease. Br Med J (Clin Res Ed). 1986;292:1717–9.

22. Wan AW, Jevremovic A, Selamet Tierney ES, et al. Comparison of impact of prenatal versus postnatal diagnosis of congenitally corrected transposition of the great arteries. Am J Cardiol. 2009;104:1276–9.

23. Thangaroopan M, Wald RM, Silversides CK, et al. Incremental diagnostic yield of pediatric cardiac assessment after fetal echocardiography in the offspring of women with congenital heart disease: a prospective study. Pediatrics. 2008;121:e660–5.

24. Campos O. Doppler echocardiography during pregnancy: physiological and abnormal findings. Echocardiography. 1996;13:135–46.

25. Lui GK, Silversides CK, Khairy P, et al. Heart rate response during exercise and pregnancy outcome in women with congenital heart disease. Circulation. 2011;123:242–8.

26. Regitz-Zagrosek V, Blomstrom Lundqvist C, Borghi C, et al. ESC Guidelines on the management of cardiovascular diseases during pregnancy: the Task Force on the Management of Cardiovascular Diseases during Pregnancy of the European Society of Cardiology (ESC). Eur Heart J. 2011;32:3147–97.

27. Tanous D, Siu SC, Mason J, et al. B-type natriuretic peptide in pregnant women with heart disease. J Am Coll Cardiol. 2010;56:1247–53.

28. Wang PI, Chong ST, Kielar AZ, et al. Imaging of pregnant and lactating patients: part 2, evidence-based review and recommendations. AJR Am J Roentgenol. 2012;198:785–92.

29. Ain DL, Narula J, Sengupta PP. Cardiovascular imaging and diagnostic procedures in pregnancy. Cardiol Clin. 2012;30:331–41.

30. Kok RD, de Vries MM, Heerschap A, van den Berg PP. Absence of harmful effects of magnetic resonance exposure at 1.5 T in utero during the third trimester of pregnancy: a follow-up study. Magn Reson Imaging. 2004;22:851–4.

31. Clements H, Duncan KR, Fielding K, Gowland PA, Johnson IR, Baker PN. Infants exposed to MRI in utero have a normal paediatric assessment at 9 months of age. Br J Radiol. 2000;73:190–4.

32. Khairy P, Ouyang DW, Fernandes SM, Lee-Parritz A, Economy KE, Landzberg MJ. Pregnancy outcomes in women with congenital heart disease. Circulation. 2006;113:517–24.

33. Siu SC, Colman JM, Sorensen S, et al. Adverse neonatal and cardiac outcomes are more common in pregnant women with cardiac disease. Circulation. 2002;105:2179–84.

34. Drenthen W, Boersma E, Balci A, et al. Predictors of pregnancy complications in women with congenital heart disease. Eur Heart J. 2010;31:2124–32.

35. Siu SC, Sermer M, Colman JM, et al. Prospective multicenter study of pregnancy outcomes in women with heart disease. Circulation. 2001;104:515–21.

36. Bedard E, Dimopoulos K, Gatzoulis MA. Has there been any progress made on pregnancy outcomes among women with pulmonary arterial hypertension? Eur Heart J. 2009;30:256–65.

37. Immer FF, Bansi AG, Immer-Bansi AS, et al. Aortic dissection in pregnancy: analysis of risk factors and outcome. Ann Thorac Surg. 2003;76:309–14.

38. Meijboom LJ, Vos FE, Timmermans J, Boers GH, Zwinderman AH, Mulder BJ. Pregnancy and aortic root growth in the Marfan syndrome: a prospective study. Eur Heart J. 2005;26:914–20.

39. McKellar SH, MacDonald RJ, Michelena HI, Connolly HM, Sundt 3rd TM. Frequency of cardiovascular events in women with a congenitally bicuspid aortic valve in a single community and effect of pregnancy on events. Am J Cardiol. 2011;107:96–9.

40. Grewal J, Siu SC, Ross HJ, et al. Pregnancy outcomes in women with dilated cardiomyopathy. J Am Coll Cardiol. 2009;55:45–52.

41. Hameed A, Karaalp IS, Tummala PP, et al. The effect of valvular heart disease on maternal and fetal outcome of pregnancy. J Am Coll Cardiol. 2001;37:893–9.

42. Goland S, Modi K, Bitar F, et al. Clinical profile and predictors of complications in peripartum cardiomyopathy. J Card Fail. 2009;15:645–50.

43. Sliwa K, Fett J, Elkayam U. Peripartum cardiomyopathy. Lancet. 2006;368:687–93.

44. Thorne S, MacGregor A, Nelson-Piercy C. Risks of contraception and pregnancy in heart disease. Heart. 2006;92:1520–5.

45. Guedes A, Mercier LA, Leduc L, Berube L, Marcotte F, Dore A. Impact of pregnancy on the systemic right ventricle after a Mustard operation for transposition of the great arteries. J Am Coll Cardiol. 2004;44:433–7.

46. Balint OH, Siu SC, Mason J, et al. Cardiac outcomes after pregnancy in women with congenital heart disease. Heart. 2010;96:1656–61.

47. Tzemos N, Silversides CK, Colman JM, et al. Late cardiac outcomes after pregnancy in women with congenital aortic stenosis. Am Heart J. 2009;157:474–80.

48. Yap SC, Drenthen W, Meijboom FJ, et al. Comparison of pregnancy outcomes in women with repaired versus unrepaired atrial septal defect. BJOG. 2009;116:1593–601.

49. Yap SC, Drenthen W, Pieper PG, et al. Pregnancy outcome in women with repaired versus unrepaired isolated ventricular septal defect. BJOG. 2010;117:683–9.

50. Zuber M, Gautschi N, Oechslin E, Widmer V, Kiowski W, Jenni R. Outcome of pregnancy in women with congenital shunt lesions. Heart. 1999;81:271–5.

51. Canobbio MM, Morris CD, Graham TP, Landzberg MJ. Pregnancy outcomes after atrial repair for transposition of the great arteries. Am J Cardiol. 2006;98:668–72.

52. Canobbio MM, Mair DD, van der Velde M, Koos BJ. Pregnancy outcomes after the Fontan repair. J Am Coll Cardiol. 1996;28:763–7.

53. Drenthen W, Pieper PG, Roos-Hesselink JW, et al. Pregnancy and delivery in women after Fontan palliation. Heart. 2006;92:1290–4.

54. Mulder BJ, Meijboom LJ. Pregnancy and Marfan syndrome: an ongoing discussion. J Am Coll Cardiol. 2012;60:230–1.

55. Goland S, Elkayam U. Cardiovascular problems in pregnant women with Marfan syndrome. Circulation. 2009;119:619–23.

56. Elkayam U, Ostrzega E, Shotan A, Mehra A. Cardiovascular problems in pregnant women with the Marfan syndrome. Ann Intern Med. 1995;123:117–22.

57. Rossiter JP, Repke JT, Morales AJ, Murphy EA, Pyeritz RE. A prospective longitudinal evaluation of pregnancy in the Marfan syndrome. Am J Obstet Gynecol. 1995;173:1599–606.

58. Kiely DG, Condliffe R, Webster V, et al. Improved survival in pregnancy and pulmonary hypertension using a multiprofessional approach. BJOG. 2010;117:565–74.

59. Weiss BM, Zemp L, Seifert B, Hess OM. Outcome of pulmonary vascular disease in pregnancy: a systematic overview from 1978 through 1996. J Am Coll Cardiol. 1998;31:1650–7.

60. Thorne S, Nelson-Piercy C, MacGregor A, et al. Pregnancy and contraception in heart disease and pulmonary arterial hypertension. J Fam Plann Reprod Health Care. 2006;32:75–81.

61. Yinon Y, Siu SC, Warshafsky C, et al. Use of low molecular weight heparin in pregnant women with mechanical heart valves. Am J Cardiol. 2009;104:1259–63.

62. McLintock C, McCowan LM, North RA. Maternal complications and pregnancy outcome in women with mechanical prosthetic heart valves treated with enoxaparin. BJOG. 2009;116:1585–92.

63. Vitale N, De Feo M, De Santo LS, Pollice A, Tedesco N, Cotrufo M. Dose-dependent fetal complications of warfarin in pregnant women with mechanical heart valves. J Am Coll Cardiol. 1999;33:1637–41.

64. Silversides CK, Colman JM, Sermer M, Farine D, Siu SC. Early and intermediate-term outcomes of pregnancy with congenital aortic stenosis. Am J Cardiol. 2003;91:1386–9.

65. Lao TT, Sermer M, MaGee L, Farine D, Colman JM. Congenital aortic stenosis and pregnancy – a reappraisal. Am J Obstet Gynecol. 1993;169:540–5.

66. Morgan-Hughes GJ, Roobottom CA, Owens PE, Marshall AJ. Dilatation of the aorta in pure, severe, bicuspid aortic valve stenosis. Am Heart J. 2004;147:736–40.

67. Siu SC, Silversides CK. Bicuspid aortic valve disease. J Am Coll Cardiol. 2010;55:2789–800.

68. Burchill L, Greenway S, Silversides CK, Mital S. Genetic counseling in the adult with congenital heart disease: what is the role? Curr Cardiol Rep. 2011;13:347–55.

69. Ouyang DW, Khairy P, Fernandes SM, Landzberg MJ, Economy KE. Obstetric outcomes in pregnant women with congenital heart disease. Int J Cardiol. 2010;144:195–9.

70. Silversides CK, Sermer M, Siu SC. Choosing the best contraceptive method for the adult with congenital heart disease. Curr Cardiol Rep. 2009;11:298–305.

71. Leonard H, O'Sullivan JJ, Hunter S. Family planning requirements in the adult congenital heart disease clinic. Heart. 1996;76:60–2.

72. Kovacs AH, Harrison JL, Colman JM, Sermer M, Siu SC, Silversides CK. Pregnancy and contraception in congenital heart disease: what women are not told. J Am Coll Cardiol. 2008;52:577–8.

73. Vigl M, Kaemmerer M, Seifert-Klauss V, et al. Contraception in women with congenital heart disease. Am J Cardiol. 2010;106:1317–21.

74. Trussell J. Contraceptive failure in the United States. Contraception. 2011;83:397–404.

75. Lidegaard O. Oral contraceptives, pregnancy and the risk of cerebral thromboembolism: the influence of diabetes, hypertension, migraine and previous thrombotic disease. Br J Obstet Gynaecol. 1995;102:153–9.

76. Poulter NR, Chang CL, Farley TMM, et al. Acute myocardial infarction and combined oral contraceptives: results of an international multicentre case-control study. WHO Collaborative Study of Cardiovascular Disease and Steroid Hormone Contraception. Lancet 1997;349:1202–9.

77. Poulter NR, Chang CL, Meirik O, et al. Venous thromboembolic disease and combined oral contraceptives: results of international multicentre case-control study. World Health Organization Collaborative Study of Cardiovascular Disease and Steroid Hormone Contraception. Lancet 1995;346:1575–82.

78. Lidegaard O, Lokkegaard E, Jensen A, Skovlund CW, Keiding N. Thrombotic stroke and myocardial infarction with hormonal contraception. N Engl J Med. 2012;366:2257–66.

79. Tsang W, Johansson B, Salehian O, et al. Intracardiac thrombus in adults with the Fontan circulation. Cardiol Young. 2007;17:646–51.

80. Varma C, Warr MR, Hendler AL, Paul NS, Webb GD, Therrien J. Prevalence of "silent" pulmonary emboli in adults after the Fontan operation. J Am Coll Cardiol. 2003;41:2252–8.

81. Vasilakis C, Jick H, del Mar Melero-Montes M. Risk of idiopathic venous thromboembolism in users of progestagens alone. Lancet. 1999;354:1610–1.

82. Palmer SN, Greenberg JA. Transcervical sterilization: a comparison of essure(r) permanent birth control system and adiana(r) permanent contraception system. Rev Obstet Gynecol. 2009;2:84–92.

83. Abbott J. Transcervical sterilization. Curr Opin Obstet Gynecol. 2007;19:325–30.

84. Wittmer MH, Famuyide AO, Creedon DJ, Hartman RP. Hysterosalpingography for assessing efficacy of Essure microinsert permanent birth control device. AJR Am J Roentgenol. 2006;187:955–8.

85. Anderson TL, Vancaillie TG. The Adiana System for permanent contraception: safety and efficacy at 3 years. J Minim Invasive Gynecol. 2011;18:612–6.

86. Vancaillie TG, Harrington DC, Anderson JM. Mechanism of action of the Adiana((R)) device: a histologic perspective. Contraception. 2011;84:299–301.

87. Oron G, Hirsch R, Ben-Haroush A, et al. Pregnancy outcome in women with heart disease undergoing induction of labour. BJOG. 2004;111:669–75.

88. Goldszmidt E, Macarthur A, Silversides C, Colman J, Sermer M, Siu S. Anesthetic management of a consecutive cohort of women with heart disease for labor and delivery. Int J Obstet Anesth. 2010;19:266–72.

89. Therrien J, Barnes I, Somerville J. Outcome of pregnancy in patients with congenitally corrected transposition of the great arteries. Am J Cardiol. 1999;84:820–4.

90. Elkayam U, Bitar F. Valvular heart disease and pregnancy part I: native valves. J Am Coll Cardiol. 2005;46:223–30.

91. Weiss BM, Hess OM. Pulmonary vascular disease and pregnancy: current controversies, management strategies, and perspectives. Eur Heart J. 2000;21:104–15.

92. Ratnapalan S, Koren G. Taking ACE inhibitors during pregnancy. Is it safe? Coll Fam Physicians Can. 2002;48:1047–9.

93. Cooper WO, Hernandez-Diaz S, Arbogast PG, et al. Major congenital malformations after first-trimester exposure to ACE inhibitors. N Engl J Med. 2006;354:2443–51.

94. Caton AR, Bell EM, Druschel CM, et al. Antihypertensive medication use during pregnancy and the risk of cardiovascular malformations. Hypertension. 2009;54:63–70.

95. Lennestal R, Otterblad Olausson P, Kallen B. Maternal use of antihypertensive drugs in early pregnancy and delivery outcome, notably the presence of congenital heart defects in the infants. Eur J Clin Pharmacol. 2009;65:615–25.

96. Li DK, Yang C, Andrade S, Tavares V, Ferber JR. Maternal exposure to angiotensin converting enzyme inhibitors in the first trimester and risk of malformations in offspring: a retrospective cohort study. BMJ. 2011;343:d5931.

97. Lip GY, Beevers M, Churchill D, Shaffer LM, Beevers DG. Effect of atenolol on birth weight. Am J Cardiol. 1997;79:1436–8.

98. Lydakis C, Lip GY, Beevers M, Beevers DG. Atenolol and fetal growth in pregnancies complicated by hypertension. Am J Hypertens. 1999;12:541–7.

99. Silversides CK, Colman JM, Sermer M, Siu SC. Cardiac risk in pregnant women with rheumatic mitral stenosis. Am J Cardiol. 2003;91:1382–5.

100. Hiratzka LF, Bakris GL, Beckman JA, et al. ACCF/AHA/AATS/ACR/ASA/SCA/SCAI/SIR/STS/SVM guidelines for the diagnosis and management of patients with thoracic aortic disease: a report of the American College of Cardiology Foundation/American Heart Association Task Force on Practice Guidelines, American Association for Thoracic Surgery, American College of Radiology, American Stroke Association, Society of Cardiovascular Anesthesiologists, Society for Cardiovascular Angiography and Interventions, Society of Interventional Radiology, Society of Thoracic Surgeons, and Society for Vascular Medicine. Circulation. 2010;121:e266–369.

101. Silversides CK, Kiess M, Beauchesne L, et al. Canadian Cardiovascular Society 2009 consensus conference on the management of adults with congenital heart disease: outflow tract obstruction, coarctation of the aorta, tetralogy of Fallot, Ebstein anomaly and Marfan's syndrome. Can J Cardiol. 2010;26:e80–97.

102. Warnes CA, Williams RG, Bashore TM, et al. ACC/AHA 2008 guidelines for the management of adults with congenital heart disease: a report of the American College of Cardiology/American Heart Association Task Force on Practice Guidelines (writing committee to develop guidelines on the management of adults with congenital heart disease). Developed in Collaboration with the American Society of Echocardiography, Heart Rhythm Society, International Society for Adult Congenital Heart Disease, Society for Cardiovascular Angiography and Interventions, and Society of Thoracic Surgeons. J Am Coll Cardiol. 2008;52:e143–263.

103. Salim MA, Alpert BS, Ward JC, Pyeritz RE. Effect of beta-adrenergic blockade on aortic root rate of dilation in the Marfan syndrome. Am J Cardiol. 1994;74:629–33.

104. Shores J, Berger KR, Murphy EA, Pyeritz RE. Progression of aortic dilatation and the benefit of long-term beta-adrenergic blockade in Marfan's syndrome. N Engl J Med. 1994;330:1335–41.

105. Ladouceur M, Fermanian C, Lupoglazoff JM, et al. Effect of beta-blockade on ascending aortic dilatation in children with the Marfan syndrome. Am J Cardiol. 2007;99:406–9.

106. Donnelly RT, Pinto NM, Kocolas I, Yetman AT. The immediate and long-term impact of pregnancy on aortic growth rate and mortality in women with Marfan syndrome. J Am Coll Cardiol. 2012;60:224–9.

107. Rowan JA, McCowan LM, Raudkivi PJ, North RA. Enoxaparin treatment in women with mechanical heart valves during pregnancy. Am J Obstet Gynecol. 2001;185:633–7.

108. Oran B, Lee-Parritz A, Ansell J. Low molecular weight heparin for the prophylaxis of thromboembolism in women with prosthetic mechanical heart valves during pregnancy. Thromb Haemost. 2004;92:747–51.

109. Iturbe-Alessio I, Fonseca MC, Mutchinik O, Santos MA, Zajarias A, Salazar E. Risks of anticoagulant therapy in pregnant women with artificial heart valves. N Engl J Med. 1986;315:1390–3.

110. Cotrufo M, De Feo M, De Santo LS, et al. Risk of warfarin during pregnancy with mechanical valve prostheses. Obstet Gynecol. 2002;99:35–40.

111. Bonow RO, Carabello BA, Chatterjee K, et al. 2008 Focused update incorporated into the ACC/AHA 2006 guidelines for the management of patients with valvular heart disease: a report of the American College of Cardiology/American Heart Association Task Force on Practice Guidelines (writing committee to revise the 1998 guidelines for the management of patients with valvular heart disease): endorsed by the Society of Cardiovascular Anesthesiologists, Society for Cardiovascular Angiography and Interventions, and Society of Thoracic Surgeons. Circulation. 2008;118:e523–661.

112. Bates SM, Greer IA, Middeldorp S, Veenstra DL, Prabulos AM, Vandvik PO. VTE, thrombophilia, antithrombotic therapy, and pregnancy: antithrombotic therapy and prevention of thrombosis, 9th ed: American college of chest physicians evidence-based clinical practice guidelines. Chest. 2012;141:e691S–736.

113. Guyatt GH, Norris SL, Schulman S, et al. Methodology for the development of antithrombotic therapy and prevention of thrombosis guidelines: Antithrombotic Therapy and Prevention of Thrombosis, 9th ed: American College of Chest Physicians Evidence-Based Clinical Practice Guidelines. Chest. 2012;141:53S–70.

114. Salazar E, Izaguirre R, Verdejo J, Mutchinick O. Failure of adjusted doses of subcutaneous heparin to prevent thromboembolic phenomena in pregnant patients with mechanical cardiac valve prostheses. J Am Coll Cardiol. 1996;27:1698–703.

115. Weiss BM, von Segesser LK, Alon E, Seifert B, Turina MI. Outcome of cardiovascular surgery and pregnancy: a systematic review of the period 1984–1996. Am J Obstet Gynecol. 1998;179:1643–53.

116. Turrentine MA, Braems G, Ramirez MM. Use of thrombolytics for the treatment of thromboembolic disease during pregnancy. Obstet Gynecol Surv. 1995;50:534–41.

117. Kurzrok S, Singh AK, Most AS, Williams DO. Thrombolytic therapy for prosthetic cardiac valve thrombosis. J Am Coll Cardiol. 1987;9:592–8.

118. Silversides CK, Salehian O, Oechslin E, et al. Canadian Cardiovascular Society 2009 consensus conference on the management of adults with congenital heart disease: complex congenital cardiac lesions. Can J Cardiol. 2010;26:e98–117.

119. Silversides CK, Dore A, Poirier N, et al. Canadian Cardiovascular Society 2009 consensus conference on the management of adults with congenital heart disease: shunt lesions. Can J Cardiol. 2010;26:e70–9.

120. Zipes DP, Camm AJ, Borggrefe M, et al. ACC/AHA/ESC 2006 guidelines for management of patients with ventricular arrhythmias and the prevention of sudden cardiac death: a report of the American College of Cardiology/American Heart Association Task Force and the European Society of Cardiology Committee for Practice Guidelines (writing committee to develop guidelines for management of patients with ventricular arrhythmias and the prevention of sudden cardiac death): developed in collaboration with the European Heart Rhythm Association and the Heart Rhythm Society. Circulation. 2006;114:e385–484.

121. Blomstrom-Lundqvist C, Scheinman MM, Aliot EM, et al. ACC/AHA/ESC guidelines for the management of patients with supraventricular arrhythmias – executive summary. A report of the American College of Cardiology/American Heart Association Task Force on Practice Guidelines and the European Society of Cardiology Committee for Practice Guidelines (writing committee to develop guidelines for the management of patients with supraventricular arrhythmias) developed in collaboration with NASPE-Heart Rhythm Society. J Am Coll Cardiol. 2003;42:1493–531.

122. Wann LS, Curtis AB, January CT, et al. ACCF/AHA/HRS focused update on the management of patients with atrial fibrillation (updating the 2006 guideline): a report of the American College of Cardiology Foundation/American Heart Association Task Force on Practice Guidelines. Circulation. 2011;123:104–23.

123. Nishimura RA, Carabello BA, Faxon DP, et al. ACC/AHA 2008 guideline update on valvular heart disease: focused update on infective endocarditis: a report of the American College of Cardiology/American Heart Association Task Force on Practice Guidelines: endorsed by the Society of Cardiovascular Anesthesiologists, Society for Cardiovascular Angiography and Interventions, and Society of Thoracic Surgeons. Circulation. 2008;118:887–96.

Part V

Management of Cardiovascular Disease in Patients Requiring Non-cardiac Surgery

Preoperative Cardiac Evaluation Before Noncardiac Surgery

35

Lee A. Fleisher

Abstract

Over the past 30 years, there has been a great deal of interest in defining the optimal preoperative cardiac evaluation before noncardiac surgery. From an evidence-based perspective, the studies transition from cohort studies involving risk assessment to cohort studies of interventions and finally to randomized controlled trials. Since 1996, there have been a series of evidence-based guidelines published from a diverse group of societies including the American Heart Association/American College of Cardiology Foundation, the American College of Physicians, and the European Society of Cardiology. While the specific details of the recommendations differ slightly, the overall approach is very similar. This chapter will review the evidence that underlies these guidelines and place it within the context of the optimal cardiology consultation.

Keywords

Preoperative evaluation • Noncardiac surgery • Risk assessment

Role of the Consultant

The role of the cardiac consultant is to identify the key questions and ensure that all the perioperative caregivers are considered when providing a response. The yield of a cardiology consultation, in terms of initiating new therapy or having a significant effect on patient management strategy prior to surgery, has been reported to vary from 10 % to more than 70 % [1]. A review of 146 medical consultations suggested that the majority of such consultations give little advice that impacts either perioperative management or outcome of the surgery [2].

Since these early reports, preoperative anesthetic clinics have become commonplace, and guidelines have been published beginning in 1996. As a result, more appropriate utilization of cardiology consultations has been observed recently [3].

Once the consultation has been requested, the consultant should review available patient data, obtain a history, and perform a physical examination that includes a comprehensive cardiovascular evaluation pertinent to the patient's problems and proposed surgery. It is critical for the consultant to determine the patient's cardiovascular status and whether the patient is in the optimal medical condition within the context of the surgical illness as well as to recommend any changes in medical therapy. Most importantly, the consultant should not use phrases such as "cleared for surgery" but rather provide recommendations for optimization of the patient's status and outcome.

Pathophysiology of Perioperative Cardiac Events

The presence of postoperative ischemia is strongly associated with myocardial infarction (MI) and cardiac death [4, 5].

L.A. Fleisher, MD
Department of Anesthesiology and Critical Care,
Perelman School of Medicine at the University of Pennsylvania,
3400 Spruce Street, Suite 680 Dulles,
Philadelphia, PA 19104, USA
e-mail: fleishel@uphs.upenn.edu

K. Stergiopoulos, D.L. Brown (eds.), *Evidence-Based Cardiology Consult*,
DOI 10.1007/978-1-4471-4441-0_35, © Springer-Verlag London 2014

However, the pathophysiology underlying postoperative ischemia is multifactorial, which influences the potential value of preoperative cardiac testing. Duvall studied 66 patients with perioperative myocardial infarction (MI) and demonstrated the distribution of demand, thrombotic, and nonobstructive MI to be 55, 26, and 19 %, respectively [6]. As a result, preoperative testing for significant coronary disease frequently fails to identify patients at risk of a postoperative cardiac event.

Clinical Assessment

Since the original manuscript by Goldman and colleagues in 1977 describing a Cardiac Risk Index, multiple investigators have validated various clinical risk indices for their ability to predict perioperative cardiac complications [7]. The most recent index was developed in a study of 4,315 patients aged 50 years or greater undergoing elective major noncardiac procedures in a tertiary care teaching hospital. The six independent predictors of complications included in a Revised Cardiac Risk Index (RCRI)were high-risk type of surgery, history of ischemic heart disease, history of congestive heart failure, history of cerebrovascular disease, preoperative treatment with insulin, and preoperative serum creatinine >2.0 mg/dl, with increasing cardiac complication rates noted with an increasing number of risk factors [8]. The RCRI has become the standard tool in the literature for assessing perioperative cardiac risk in a given individual and has been used to direct the decision to perform cardiovascular testing and implement perioperative management protocols. It has recently been validated for both short- and long-term cardiovascular outcomes [9]. It has also been shown to predict long-term quality of life [9]. Therefore, it can be used to help define both the short- and long-term risks of cardiovascular disease in the surgical patient.

A primary issue with all of these indices is that a simple estimate of risk does not help in refining perioperative management for an individual patient. Therefore, it is important that the consultant communicates the extent and stability of the patient's coronary artery disease rather than a simple statement of risk classification.

A thorough history should focus on cardiovascular risk factors and symptoms or signs of unstable cardiac disease states, such as myocardial ischemia with minimal exertion, active congestive heart failure, symptomatic valvular heart disease, and significant cardiac arrhythmias. The presence of unstable angina is associated with a 28 % incidence of perioperative MI [10]. Such patients would benefit from delaying elective surgery to address their coronary disease. For those patients with chronic stable angina, exercise tolerance appears to be a good method of assessing perioperative risk.

In virtually all studies, the presence of active congestive heart failure has been associated with increased perioperative cardiac morbidity [11]. In addition, multiple studies have demonstrated that reduced ejection fraction is associated with an increased incidence of perioperative cardiac events [12, 13]. Flu and colleagues performed echocardiography in vascular surgery patients and found that for open surgical procedures, asymptomatic systolic and diastolic left ventricular (LV) dysfunction were both associated with increased 30-day cardiovascular event rates (odds ratio (OR) 2.3, 95 % confidence interval [CI] 1.4–3.6 and 1.8, 95 % CI 1.1–2.9, respectively) and long-term cardiovascular mortality (hazard ratios 4.6, 95 % CI 2.4–8.5 and 3.0, 95 % CI 1.5–6.0, respectively) [14]. In patients undergoing endovascular surgery ($n = 356$), only symptomatic heart failure was associated with an increase in 30-day cardiovascular events and long-term cardiovascular mortality. These results suggest that stabilization of ventricular function and treatment of pulmonary congestion are prudent prior to elective surgery.

A recent MI has traditionally been an important predictor of perioperative risk. The more recent the MI, particularly within 3–6 months, the greater the perioperative risk. However, like the Goldman Cardiac Risk Index, medicine has changed and outcomes are improved. The classic Rao paper published in 1983 cited a reinfarction rate of nearly 30 % if noncardiac surgery occurred within 3 months of a prior infarction [15]. These reinfarctions had a very high mortality rate. With the advent of dedicated postoperative intensive care units, more vigilant monitoring, and early intervention, the postoperative reinfarction rate has decreased by almost an order of magnitude. The American Heart Association/American College of Cardiology Foundation (AHA/ACCF) guidelines advocate the use of ≤30 days as the acute period, with high risk continuing for 6–8 weeks [16]. After that time, a prior MI places the patient in the intermediate clinical risk category, and further risk stratification depends upon clinical symptoms.

For those patients without overt symptoms or history of coronary artery disease (CAD), the probability of CAD varies with the type and number of atherosclerotic risk factors present. Diabetes accelerates the progression of atherosclerosis, which can frequently be silent in nature, leading many clinicians to assume diabetes is a CAD equivalent and treating them as such. Diabetes is an independent risk factor for perioperative cardiac morbidity, and the preoperative treatment with insulin has been included in the RCRI. In attempting to determine the degree of the increased risk associated with diabetes, the treatment modality, length of the disease, and other associated end-organ dysfunction should be taken into account.

Hypertension has also been associated with an increased risk of myocardial ischemia and infarction. Those hypertensive patients with left ventricular hypertrophy and who are

Table 35.1 Active cardiac conditions for which the patient should undergo evaluation and treatment before noncardiac surgery

Condition	Examples
Unstable coronary syndromes	Unstable or severe angina (CCS class III or IV)
	Recent MI
Decompensated HF	NYHA functional class IV
	Worsening or new-onset HF
Significant arrhythmias	High-grade atrioventricular block
	Mobitz II atrioventricular block
	Third-degree atrioventricular heart block
	Symptomatic ventricular arrhythmias
	Supraventricular arrhythmias (including atrial fibrillation) with uncontrolled ventricular rate (HR >100 bpm at rest)
	Symptomatic bradycardia
	Newly recognized ventricular tachycardia
Severe valvular disease	Severe aortic stenosis (mean pressure gradient greater than 40 mmHg, aortic valve area less than 1.0 cm², or symptomatic)
	Symptomatic mitral stenosis (progressive dyspnea on exertion, exertional presyncope, or HF)

HR heart rate, *HF* heart failure, *MI* myocardial infarction, *CCS* Canadian Cardiovascular Society, *NYHA* New York Heart Association

undergoing noncardiac surgery are at a higher perioperative risk than normotensive patients [17]. There is a great deal of debate regarding a specific level of blood pressure that should trigger the delay or cancellation of a surgical procedure in a patient with poorly controlled or untreated hypertension. A sustained diastolic blood pressure >110 mmHg has traditionally triggered a delay in surgery although the data does not support such an assertion. In the absence of end-organ changes, such as renal insufficiency or left ventricular hypertrophy, it would seem appropriate to proceed with surgery. A randomized trial of treated hypertensive patients without known CAD who presented the morning of surgery with an elevated diastolic blood pressure was unable to demonstrate any difference in outcome between those who were actively treated and those in whom surgery was delayed [18]. In contrast, a patient with a markedly elevated blood pressure and the new onset of a headache should have surgery delayed for further evaluation and potential treatment. A list of active cardiac conditions for which nonemergent, noncardiac surgeries might be delayed are defined in Table 35.1.

Importance of the Type of Surgical Procedure

The type of surgical procedure influences the extent of the preoperative evaluation due to the potential range of perioperative hemodynamic and hemostatic changes among different operations (Table 35.2). There is little hard data to

Table 35.2 Cardiac risk stratification for noncardiac surgical procedures

Risk stratification	Procedure examples
Vascular (reported cardiac risk >5 %)	Aortic and other major vascular surgery
	Peripheral vascular surgery
Intermediate (reported cardiac risk 1–5 %)	Intraperitoneal and intrathoracic surgery
	Carotid endarterectomy
	Head and neck surgery
	Orthopedic surgery
	Prostate surgery
Low (reported cardiac risk <1 %)	Endoscopic procedures
	Superficial procedure
	Cataract surgery
	Breast surgery
	Ambulatory surgery

define the surgery-specific incidence of complications, and the rate may be very institution dependent. Eagle et al. published data on the incidence of perioperative MI and mortality by procedure for patients enrolled in the Coronary Artery Surgery Study (CASS) [19]. Higher-risk procedures for which coronary artery bypass grafting reduced the risk of noncardiac surgery compared to medical therapy included major vascular, abdominal, thoracic, and orthopedic surgery. Vascular surgery involves a unique group of patients in whom there is extensive evidence regarding preoperative testing and perioperative interventions. Endovascular stent placement is associated with lower perioperative risk, particularly the risk of death, but similar long-term mortality compared to open procedures [20]. Most importantly, the rate of mortality and cardiac morbidity varies greatly between hospitals, which is in part related to surgical volume [21]. Therefore, the surgical risk should be individualized by institution. Table 35.3 defines a general categorization of surgical procedures in the AHA/ACCF guidelines.

Importance of Exercise Tolerance

Exercise tolerance is one of the most important determinants of perioperative complications. If a patient can walk a mile without becoming short of breath, then the probability of extensive coronary artery disease is small. Alternatively, if patients develop dyspnea and chest pain with minimal exertion, then the probability of extensive coronary artery disease is high. Reilly and colleagues demonstrated that the likelihood of a serious complication was inversely related to the number of blocks that could be walked or flights of stairs that could be climbed [22]. Exercise tolerance can be assessed with formal treadmill testing or with a questionnaire that assesses activities of daily living (see Table 35.3).

Table 35.3 Estimated energy requirement for various activities

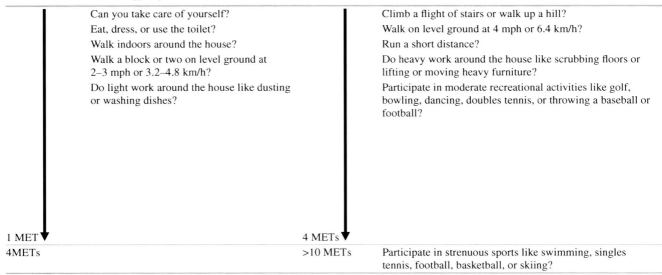

Can you take care of yourself?	Climb a flight of stairs or walk up a hill?
Eat, dress, or use the toilet?	Walk on level ground at 4 mph or 6.4 km/h?
Walk indoors around the house?	Run a short distance?
Walk a block or two on level ground at 2–3 mph or 3.2–4.8 km/h?	Do heavy work around the house like scrubbing floors or lifting or moving heavy furniture?
Do light work around the house like dusting or washing dishes?	Participate in moderate recreational activities like golf, bowling, dancing, doubles tennis, or throwing a baseball or football?
1 MET	4 METs
4METs	>10 METs

Participate in strenuous sports like swimming, singles tennis, football, basketball, or skiing?

Adapted from: Fleisher et al. [16] © 2007 American Heart Association, Inc.
MET metabolic equivalent

Approach to the Patient

Figure 35.1 presents in algorithmic form a framework for determining which patients are candidates for cardiac testing published in the 2007 guidelines. The guidelines are being updated and a new version will be published in 2014. Importantly, the value of adopting the algorithm depends upon local factors such as current perioperative risk and utilization of testing.

Step 1: The consultant should determine the urgency of non-cardiac surgery. In many instances, patient- or surgery-specific factors dictate an obvious strategy (e.g., emergent surgery) that may not allow for further cardiac assessment or treatment.

Step 2: Does the patient have one of the active cardiac conditions? In patients being considered for elective noncardiac surgery, the presence of unstable coronary disease, decompensated heart failure, severe arrhythmia, or valvular heart disease usually leads to cancellation or delay of surgery until the cardiac problem has been clarified and treated appropriately. Examples of unstable coronary syndromes include previous MI with evidence of residual ischemia by clinical symptoms or noninvasive study, unstable or severe angina, and new or poorly controlled ischemia-mediated heart failure. Depending on the results of the test or interventions and the risk of delaying surgery, it may be appropriate to proceed to the planned surgery with maximal medical therapy.

Step 3: Is the patient undergoing low-risk surgery? In these patients, since interventions based on cardiovascular testing in stable patients would rarely result in a change in management, it is appropriate to proceed with the planned surgical procedure.

Step 4: Does the patient have moderate functional capacity without symptoms? In highly functional asymptomatic patients, management will rarely be changed on the basis of results of any further cardiovascular testing, and it is therefore appropriate to proceed with the planned surgery. If the patient has poor functional capacity, is symptomatic, or has unknown functional capacity, then the presence of clinical risk factors will determine the need for further evaluation. If the patient has no clinical risk factors, then it is appropriate to proceed with the planned surgery, and no further change in management is indicated.

If the patient has 1 or 2 clinical risk factors, it is reasonable either to proceed with the planned surgery, with heart rate control, or to consider testing if it will change management. In patients with 3 or more clinical risk factors or if the patient is undergoing vascular surgery, recent studies suggest that testing should only be considered if it will change management. In nonvascular surgery in which perioperative morbidity related to the procedures ranges from 1 to 5 % (intermediate-risk surgery), there are insufficient data to determine the best strategy (proceeding with the planned surgery with tight heart rate control with beta-blockade or further cardiovascular testing if it will change management).

Choice of Diagnostic Test

There are multiple noninvasive diagnostic tests which have been proposed to evaluate the extent of CAD before noncardiac surgery. Although exercise electrocardiography has been the traditional method of evaluating individuals for the presence of CAD, patients with good exercise tolerance will

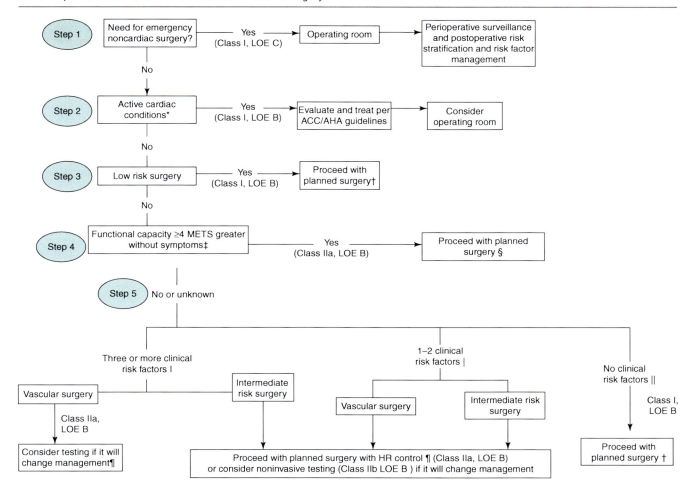

Fig. 35.1 Cardiac evaluation and care algorithm for noncardiac surgery based on active clinical conditions, known cardiovascular disease, or cardiac risk factors for patients 50 years of age or greater. The American Heart Association/American College of Cardiology Task Force on Perioperative Evaluation of Cardiac Patients for Noncardiac Surgery has proposed an algorithm regarding the need for further evaluation. This represents one of multiple algorithms proposed in the literature. It is based upon expert opinion and incorporates five steps. First, the clinician must evaluate the urgency of the surgery and the appropriateness of a formal preoperative assessment. Next, he or she must determine whether the patient has had a previous revascularization procedure or coronary evaluation. Those patients with unstable coronary syndromes should be identified, and appropriate treatment should be instituted. The decision to have further testing depends on the interaction of the clinical risk factors, surgery-specific risk, and functional capacity (Adapted with permission from Fleisher et al. [16]. © 2007 American Heart Association, Inc)

rarely benefit from further testing. Therefore, pharmacologic stress testing in patients unable to exercise or with poor functional capacity has become popular, particularly as a preoperative test in vascular surgery patients.

Several authors have shown that the presence of a redistribution defect on dipyridamole-thallium imaging in patients undergoing peripheral vascular surgery is predictive of postoperative cardiac events. In order to increase the predictive value of the test, several strategies have been suggested. Lung uptake, left ventricular cavity dilation, and redistribution defect size on nuclear imaging have all been shown to be predictive of subsequent morbidity [23]. The appearance of new or worsened regional wall motion abnormalities on stress echocardiography is considered a positive test. The advantage of this test is that it is a dynamic assess-

ment of ventricular function. Dobutamine echocardiography has been studied and was found to have among the best positive and negative predictive values. Poldermans et al. demonstrated that the groups at greatest risk were those who demonstrated regional wall motion abnormalities at low heart rates [24]. The presence of five or more segments with new regional wall motion abnormalities denotes a high-risk group who did not benefit from perioperative beta-blockade in one trial [25]. Beattie and colleagues demonstrated that stress echocardiography has better negative predicative characteristics than thallium imaging [26]. They found that moderate-to-large perfusion defects on either test predicted postoperative MI and death.

As noted above, the presence of reduced ejection fraction is associated with an increased incidence of cardiac morbidity and mortality. Therefore, the current ACCF/ AHA guidelines instruct that assessment of left ventricular (LV) function (1) is reasonable for patients with dyspnea of unknown origin (recommendation IIa, level of evidence: C) and (2) is reasonable for patients with current or prior heart failure with worsening dyspnea or other change in clinical status if not performed within 12 months (recommendation IIa, level of evidence: C), (3) reassessment of LV function in clinically stable patients with previously documented cardiomyopathy is not well established (recommendation IIb, level of evidence: C), and (4) routine perioperative evaluation of LV function in patients is not recommended (recommendation III, level of evidence: B) [16].

Interventions for Patients with Documented CAD

There is increasing evidence that coronary revascularization before noncardiac surgery does not reduce the incidence of perioperative cardiac morbidity. McFalls and colleagues reported the results of a multicenter randomized trial in the Veterans Administration Health System in which patients with documented CAD on coronary angiography excluding those with left main disease or severely depressed ejection fraction (<20 %) were randomized to coronary artery bypass grafting (CABG) (59 %) or percutaneous coronary interventions (PCI) (41 %) versus routine medical therapy [27]. At 2.7 years after randomization, mortality in the revascularization group was not significantly different (22 %) than the no-revascularization group (23 %). Within 30 days after the vascular operation, a postoperative MI, defined by elevated troponin levels, occurred in 12 % of the revascularization group and 14 % of the no-revascularization group ($P=0.37$). In a follow-up analysis, Ward and colleagues reported improved outcomes in the subset who underwent CABG compared to PCI [28]. Poldermans and colleagues randomized 770 patients having major vascular surgery and considered as having intermediate cardiac risk, defined as the presence of 1 or 2 cardiac risk factors, to either undergo further risk stratification with stress imaging or proceed directly to surgery [29]. All patients received preoperative bisoprolol with a targeted heart rate (HR) of 60–65 initiated before and continued after surgery. The 30-day incidence of cardiac death and nonfatal MI was similar in both groups (1.8 % in the no testing group versus 2.3 % in the tested group). The conclusion of the authors was that further risk stratification in this group of patients considered at intermediate risk based on clinical history alone was unnecessary as long as perioperative beta-blockers were used and that testing only delayed necessary vascular surgery. The Poldermans study is currently under investigation because of scientific misconduct and should not be used to make recommendations.

The current evidence does not support the use of percutaneous coronary intervention (PCI) to reduce perioperative ischemic events, since the incidence of perioperative complications does not appear to be reduced in those patients in whom PCI was performed less than 90 days prior to surgery [30]. In patients with a prior coronary stent, the new guidelines suggest continuing aspirin therapy in all patients with a coronary stent and discontinuing clopidogrel for as short a time interval as possible for patients with bare-metal stents placed within 30 days or drug-eluting stents placed within 1 year.

There is now a great deal of evidence to suggest that perioperative medical therapy can be optimized in those patients with CAD as a means of reducing perioperative cardiovascular complications. Multiple studies have demonstrated improved outcome in patients given perioperative beta-blockers, especially if heart rate is controlled, although there is recent concern regarding the quality of the studies from the Erasmus group and the should not be used to support recommendations [31, 32]. Newer studies have demonstrated that beta-blockers may not be effective if heart rate is not well controlled or in lower-risk patients [33–35]. The Perioperative Ischemic Evaluation Study (POISE) trial randomized 8,351 high-risk beta-blocker naive patients to high-dose metoprolol CR versus placebo [36]. There was a significant reduction in the primary outcome of cardiovascular events, associated with a 30 % reduction in MI rate, but a significantly increased rate of 30-day all-cause mortality and stroke. Patients at intermediate risk were randomized to statin therapy, beta-blocker therapy, both (started on average 30 days in advance), or double placebo. Beta-blocker therapy was associated with significantly decreased cardiovascular events, while statin therapy was not [37]. The current ACCF/AHA guidelines on perioperative beta-blockade indicate that perioperative beta-blockade is a class I indication and should be used in patients previously on beta-blockers. The new recommendations advocate that beta-blockers titrated to heart rate and blood pressure are probably recommended for patients undergoing vascular surgery who are at high cardiac risk due to CAD or the finding of cardiac ischemia on preoperative testing (class IIa). A recent meta-analysis is excluding the Poldermans study suggests that acute initiation of beta-blockers is associated with increased mortality [38]. Wallace et al. reported that perioperative beta-blockade administered according to the perioperative cardiac risk reduction protocol is associated with a reduction in 30-day and 1-year mortality [39]. Perioperative withdrawal of beta-blockers is associated with increased mortality.

Other pharmacologic agents have also been shown to improve perioperative cardiac outcome. Most recently, perioperative statins have been shown to improve cardiac outcome. Durazzo and colleagues published a randomized trial of 200 vascular surgery patients in which statins were started an average of 30 days prior to vascular surgery [40]. A significant reduction in cardiovascular complications was demonstrated using this protocol. Le Manach and colleagues demonstrated that statin withdrawal greater than 4 days was associated with a 2.9 odds ratio of increased risk of cardiac morbidity in vascular surgery [41]. The recent guidelines advocate continuing statin therapy in patients currently taking statins as a class I indication.

> **Key Points**
> - Active cardiac conditions should be treated prior to elective surgery.
> - A stepwise algorithm should be used to assess preoperative cardiac risk and whether additional testing is required.
> - Exercise tolerance is one of the most important determinants of perioperative risk and the need for invasive monitoring.
> - Medical therapy can be optimized in those patients with coronary artery disease as a means of reducing perioperative cardiovascular complications.

References

1. Park KW. Preoperative cardiology consultation. Anesthesiology. 2003;98(3):754–62 [Research Support, Non-U.S. Gov't Review].
2. Katz RI, Cimino L, Vitkun SA. Preoperative medical consultations: impact on perioperative management and surgical outcome. Can J Anaesth. 2005;52(7):697–702.
3. Tsen LC, Segal S, Pothier M, Hartley LH, Bader AM. The effect of alterations in a preoperative assessment clinic on reducing the number and improving the yield of cardiology consultations. Anesth Analg. 2002;95(6):1563–8, table of contents.
4. Fleisher LA, Nelson AH, Rosenbaum SH. Postoperative myocardial ischemia: etiology of cardiac morbidity or manifestation of underlying disease. J Clin Anesth. 1995;7:97–102.
5. Mangano DT, Browner WS, Hollenberg M, London MJ, Tubau JF, Tateo IM, et al. Association of perioperative myocardial ischemia with cardiac morbidity and mortality in men undergoing noncardiac surgery. N Engl J Med. 1990;323:1781–8.
6. Duvall WL, Sealove B, Pungoti C, Katz D, Moreno P, Kim M. Angiographic investigation of the pathophysiology of perioperative myocardial infarction. Catheter Cardiovasc Interv. 2012;80(5):768–76.
7. Goldman L, Caldera DL, Nussbaum SR, Southwick FS, Krogstad D, Murray B, et al. Multifactorial index of cardiac risk in noncardiac surgical procedures. N Engl J Med. 1977;297:845–50.
8. Lee TH, Marcantonio ER, Mangione CM, Thomas EJ, Polanczyk CA, Cook EF, et al. Derivation and prospective validation of a simple index for prediction of cardiac risk of major noncardiac surgery. Circulation. 1999;100(10):1043–9.
9. Hoeks SE, Scholte Op Reimer WJ, van Gestel YR, Smolderen KG, Verhagen H, van Domburg RT, et al. Preoperative cardiac risk index predicts long-term mortality and health status. Am J Med. 2009;122(6):559–65.
10. Shah KB, Kleinman BS, Rao T, Jacobs HK, Mestan K, Schaafsma M. Angina and other risk factors in patients with cardiac diseases undergoing noncardiac operations. Anesth Analg. 1990;70:240–7.
11. Hammill BG, Curtis LH, Bennett-Guerrero E, O'Connor CM, Jollis JG, Schulman KA, et al. Impact of heart failure on patients undergoing major noncardiac surgery. Anesthesiology. 2008;108(4):559–67.
12. Mantha S, Roizen MF, Barnard J, Thisted RA, Ellis JE, Foss J. Relative effectiveness of four preoperative tests for predicting adverse cardiac outcomes after vascular surgery: a meta-analysis. Anesth Analg. 1994;79(3):422–33.
13. McEnroe CS, O'Donnell TF, Yeager A, Konstam M, Mackey WC. Comparison of ejection fraction and Goldman risk factor analysis to dipyridamole-thallium imaging 201 studies in the evaluation of cardiac morbidity after aortic aneurysm surgery. J Vasc Surg. 1990;11:497–504.
14. Flu WJ, van Kuijk JP, Hoeks SE, Kuiper R, Schouten O, Goei D, et al. Prognostic implications of asymptomatic left ventricular dysfunction in patients undergoing vascular surgery. Anesthesiology. 2010;112(6):1316–24 [Comparative Study Research Support, Non-U.S. Gov't].
15. Rao TK, Jacobs KH, El-Etr AA. Reinfarction following anesthesia in patients with myocardial infarction. Anesthesiology. 1983;59:499–505.
16. Fleisher LA, Beckman JA, Brown KA, Calkins H, Chaikof EL, Fleischmann KE, et al. 2009 ACCF/AHA focused update on perioperative beta blockade incorporated into the ACC/AHA 2007 guidelines on perioperative cardiovascular evaluation and care for noncardiac surgery: a report of the American College of Cardiology Foundation/American Heart Association Task Force on Practice Guidelines. Circulation. 2009;120(21):e169–276.
17. Hollenberg M, Mangano DT, Browner WS, London MJ, Tubau JF, Tateo IM. Predictors of postoperative myocardial ischemia in patients undergoing noncardiac surgery. The Study of Perioperative Ischemia Research Group [see comments]. JAMA. 1992;268(2):205–9.
18. Weksler N, Klein M, Szendro G, Rozentsveig V, Schily M, Brill S, et al. The dilemma of immediate preoperative hypertension: to treat and operate, or to postpone surgery? J Clin Anesth. 2003;15(3):179–83.
19. Eagle KA, Rihal CS, Mickel MC, Holmes DR, Foster ED, Gersh BJ. Cardiac risk of noncardiac surgery: influence of coronary disease and type of surgery in 3368 operations. CASS Investigators and University of Michigan Heart Care Program. Coronary Artery Surgery Study. Circulation. 1997;96(6):1882–7.
20. Archan S, Roscher CR, Fairman RM, Fleisher LA. Revised Cardiac Risk Index (Lee) and perioperative cardiac events as predictors of long-term mortality in patients undergoing endovascular abdominal aortic aneurysm repair. J Cardiothorac Vasc Anesth. 2010;24(1):84–90.
21. Birkmeyer JD, Warshaw AL, Finlayson SR, Grove MR, Tosteson AN. Relationship between hospital volume and late survival after pancreaticoduodenectomy. Surgery. 1999;126(2):178–83 [Research Support, Non-U.S. Gov't].
22. Reilly DF, McNeely MJ, Doerner D, Greenberg DL, Staiger TO, Geist MJ, et al. Self-reported exercise tolerance and the risk of serious perioperative complications. Arch Intern Med. 1999;159(18):2185–92.
23. Fleisher LA, Rosenbaum SH, Nelson AH, Jain D, Wackers FJT, Zaret BL. Preoperative dipyridamole thallium imaging and Holter monitoring as a predictor of perioperative cardiac events and long term outcome. Anesthesiology. 1995;83:906–17.
24. Poldermans D, Arnese M, Fioretti PM, Salustri A, Boersma E, Thomson IR, et al. Improved cardiac risk stratification in major vascular surgery with dobutamine-atropine stress echocardiography. J Am Coll Cardiol. 1995;26(3):648–53.

25. Boersma E, Poldermans D, Bax JJ, Steyerberg EW, Thomson IR, Banga JD, et al. Predictors of cardiac events after major vascular surgery: role of clinical characteristics, dobutamine echocardiography, and beta-blocker therapy. JAMA. 2001;285(14):1865–73.

26. Beattie WS, Abdelnaem E, Wijeysundera DN, Buckley DN. A meta-analytic comparison of preoperative stress echocardiography and nuclear scintigraphy imaging. Anesth Analg. 2006;102(1): 8–16.

27. McFalls EO, Ward HB, Moritz TE, Goldman S, Krupski WC, Littooy F, et al. Coronary-artery revascularization before elective major vascular surgery. N Engl J Med. 2004;351(27): 2795–804.

28. Ward HB, Kelly RF, Thottapurathu L, Moritz TE, Larsen GC, Pierpont G, et al. Coronary artery bypass grafting is superior to percutaneous coronary intervention in prevention of perioperative myocardial infarctions during subsequent vascular surgery. Ann Thorac Surg. 2006;82(3):795–800; discussion –1.

29. Poldermans D, Bax JJ, Schouten O, Neskovic AN, Paelinck B, Rocci G, et al. Should major vascular surgery be delayed because of preoperative cardiac testing in intermediate-risk patients receiving beta-blocker therapy with tight heart rate control? J Am Coll Cardiol. 2006;48(5):964–9.

30. Posner KL, Van Norman GA, Chan V. Adverse cardiac outcomes after noncardiac surgery in patients with prior percutaneous transluminal coronary angioplasty. Anesth Analg. 1999;89(3): 553–60.

31. Mangano DT, Layug EL, Wallace A, Tateo I. Effect of atenolol on mortality and cardiovascular morbidity after noncardiac surgery. Multicenter Study of Perioperative Ischemia Research Group. N Engl J Med. 1996;335(23):1713–20.

32. Poldermans D, Boersma E, Bax JJ, Thomson IR, van de Ven LL, Blankensteijn JD, et al. The effect of bisoprolol on perioperative mortality and myocardial infarction in high-risk patients undergoing vascular surgery. Dutch Echocardiographic Cardiac Risk Evaluation Applying Stress Echocardiography Study Group [see comments]. N Engl J Med. 1999;341(24):1789–94.

33. Juul AB, Wetterslev J, Gluud C, Kofoed-Enevoldsen A, Jensen G, Callesen T, et al. Effect of perioperative beta blockade in patients with diabetes undergoing major non-cardiac surgery: randomised placebo controlled, blinded multicentre trial. BMJ. 2006;332(7556): 1482.

34. Lindenauer PK, Pekow P, Wang K, Mamidi DK, Gutierrez B, Benjamin EM. Perioperative beta-blocker therapy and mortality after major noncardiac surgery. N Engl J Med. 2005;353(4):349–61.

35. Yang H, Raymer K, Butler R, Parlow J, Roberts R. The effects of perioperative beta-blockade: results of the Metoprolol after Vascular Surgery (MaVS) study, a randomized controlled trial. Am Heart J. 2006;152(5):983–90.

36. Devereaux PJ, Yang H, Yusuf S, Guyatt G, Leslie K, Villar JC, et al. Effects of extended-release metoprolol succinate in patients undergoing non-cardiac surgery (POISE trial): a randomised controlled trial. Lancet. 2008;371(9627):1839–47.

37. Goei D, Flu WJ, Hoeks SE, Galal W, Dunkelgrun M, Boersma E, et al. The interrelationship between preoperative anemia and N-terminal pro-B-type natriuretic peptide: the effect on predicting postoperative cardiac outcome in vascular surgery patients. Anesth Analg. 2009;109(5):1403–8.

38. Bouri S, Shun-Shin MJ, Cole GD, Mayet J, Francis DP. Meta-analysis of secure randomised controlled trials of β-blockade to prevent perioperative death in non-cardiac surgery. Heart. 2013. [Epub ahead of print].

39. Wallace AW, Au S, Cason BA. Association of the pattern of use of perioperative beta-blockade and postoperative mortality. Anesthesiology. 2010;113(4):794–805.

40. Durazzo AE, Machado FS, Ikeoka DT, De Bernoche C, Monachini MC, Puech-Leao P, et al. Reduction in cardiovascular events after vascular surgery with atorvastatin: a randomized trial. J Vasc Surg. 2004;39(5):967–75; discussion 75–6.

41. Le Manach Y, Godet G, Coriat P, Martinon C, Bertrand M, Fleron MH, et al. The impact of postoperative discontinuation or continuation of chronic statin therapy on cardiac outcome after major vascular surgery. Anesth Analg. 2007;104(6):1326–33, table of contents.

Perioperative Myocardial Infarction

Santiago Garcia and Edward O. McFalls

Abstract

The proportion of elderly patients with significant cardiac comorbidities undergoing noncardiac operations is likely to increase in the future. A perioperative myocardial infarction is associated with high in-hospital mortality and poor long-term outcomes. The majority of these events are clinically and electrocardiographically silent requiring active surveillance with cardiac biomarkers (preferably troponins).

Most myocardial infarctions in the perioperative period result from a mismatch between oxygen supply and demand in patients with stable coronary artery disease. Most of the research in the field has been focused on risk stratification and prevention prior to the noncardiac operation with little emphasis in best treatment strategies after the event has occurred. Clinical trials are needed to define the role of adjunct pharmacology and cardiac imaging, including angiography, in this special population.

Keywords

Noncardiac surgery • Myocardial infarction • Prevention • Treatment

Introduction

The number of patients undergoing noncardiac surgery worldwide is growing, and annually 500,000–900,000 of these patients will experience perioperative cardiac death, nonfatal perioperative myocardial infarction (PMI), or cardiac arrest [1]. For several reasons, the magnitude of this problem will increase over the next several decades. First, patients with coronary artery disease (CAD) are living longer as a result of medical advances [2]. Second, there has been a trend toward more invasive therapies being administered to elderly patients [3]. Finally, surgical treatments have evolved and in many cases can now be performed through minimally invasive procedures [4]. All of these factors, coupled with a rapid demographic growth in emerging economies, suggest that the number of surgical procedures and subsequent cardiac complications are likely to increase severalfold in the future.

A PMI is associated with a high in-hospital mortality and poor long-term outcomes [5–7], particularly among high-risk patients undergoing vascular surgery [8]. Understandably, most research efforts have been aimed at identifying patients more likely to suffer perioperative cardiac events (Table 36.1) and finding strategies to mitigate this risk in the preoperative period [9–12]. Unfortunately, there is a paucity of high-quality, clinical trial data to help the clinician in the management of these often complex patients after the cardiac event has occurred. A firm grasp of the pathophysiology is necessary to develop successful treatment strategies.

S. Garcia, MD, FACC, FSCAI (✉) • E.O. McFalls, MD, PhD
Department of Cardiology, University of Minnesota/Minneapolis
VA Healthcare System, One Veterans Drive (111-C),
Minneapolis, MN 55417, USA
e-mail: garci205@umn.edu; mcfal001@umn.edu

K. Stergiopoulos, D.L. Brown (eds.), *Evidence-Based Cardiology Consult*,
DOI 10.1007/978-1-4471-4441-0_36, © Springer-Verlag London 2014

Table 36.1 Revised Cardiac Risk Index predicts risk of major cardiac complications at 30 days

	Derivation set ($n=2,893$)		Validation set ($n=1,422$)	
	Events	Rate, 95 % CI	Events	Rate, 95 % CI
0	5/1071	0.5 (0.2–1.1)	2/488	0.4 (0.5–1.5)
1	14/1106	1.3 (0.7–2.1)	5/567	0.9 (0.3–2.1)
2	18/506	3.6 (2.1–5.6)	17/258	6.6 (3.9–10.3)
≥3	19/210	9.1 (5.5–13.8)	12/109	11 (5.8–18.4)

The Revised Cardiac Risk Index (also known as Lee Index) is calculated by giving a score of 0, if absent, or 1, if present, to the following six variables: high-risk operation, history of cerebrovascular disease, history of coronary artery disease, history of congestive heart failure, creatinine >2 mg/dl, and insulin-dependent diabetes mellitus (From Lee et al. [9])

Patients with a calculated risk ≥5 % are considered high risk of having cardiac complications at 30 days

Pathophysiology

Unlike a spontaneous myocardial infarction, referred to as a Type I MI, the majority of postoperative, or Type 2, myocardial infarctions are thought to result from an imbalance between oxygen supply and demand [13] in the setting of severe established coronary artery disease (Fig. 36.1). The evidence to support this concept comes from clinical, angiographic, and pathological studies. Several studies using continuous electrocardiographic monitoring in high-risk vascular patients undergoing surgery have shown that tachycardia-related ST-segment depression is common in the postoperative period and is associated with increased in-hospital as well as long-term mortality [14, 15]. Peak troponin elevation, a surrogate marker for infarct size, cor-

Preoperative angiogram

Post operative angiogram

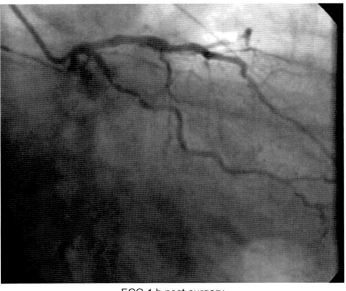
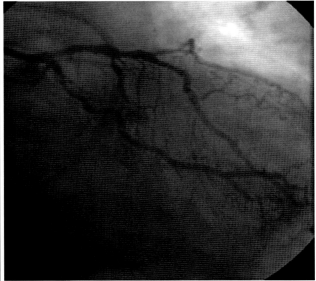

ECG 1 h post-surgery

ECG 48 h followig surgery

Fig. 36.1 This case illustrates the most common mechanism underlying postoperative myocardial infarction. This 73-year-old patient was part of the CARP trial and underwent randomization to medical therapy prior to open abdominal aortic aneurysm repair. He had 2-vessel coronary artery disease, which consisted of an occluded right coronary artery (not shown) and a severe (90 %) lesion in a large obtuse marginal branch. Forty-eight hours after the operation, his electrocardiogram

(*ECG*) showed supraventricular tachycardia with a heart rate of 125 beats per minute (bmp). Coronary angiography remained unchanged. However, in contrast to the ECG performed 1 h after the operation at a heart rate of 75 bmp, this ECG showed extensive ST depression in the anterolateral leads. His ECG returned to baseline with administration of diuretics and beta-blockers. Troponin I peaked at 6 µg/l

relates well with the duration of ST-segment depression [15]. Catecholamine levels rise during noncardiac surgery [16], and the magnitude of the rise is greater among patients with elevated troponin levels [17], which would suggest an association between catecholamines and myocardial necrosis probably mediated by fluctuations in heart rate and myocardial wall stress. In a landmark angiographic study, only 8 % of patients with peripheral arterial disease in need of major vascular surgery were found to have normal coronary arteries [18]. The prevalence of angiographic chronic total occlusions in patients with PMI or cardiac death is 81 % as opposed to only 29 % of matched control patients without PMI or cardiac death [19]. On average, patients with postoperative cardiac complications have 2 ±1.4 critical (>70 %) coronary stenoses in contrast to patients without postoperative complications who have less disease burden (0.7 ±1.2 stenoses). Two small autopsy studies have reported conflicting data on the incidence of coronary plaque rupture in patients with fatal PMI [20, 21]. Dawood et al. found plaque rupture in only 7 % of 42 autopsied patients [20]. In contrast, in a smaller study, Cohen et al. reported a higher incidence of plaque rupture (46 %) [21]. Differences between studies could be related to the timing of the autopsy relative to the occurrence of PMI.

Diagnosis

A joint European Society of Cardiology (ESC)/American College of Cardiology Foundation (ACCF)/American Heart Association (AHA)/World Heart Foundation (WHF) Task Force has redefined myocardial infarction as an event characterized by ischemic symptoms (i.e., chest pain or dyspnea), a typical rise and fall of cardiac biomarkers (preferably troponin) with at least one value above the 99th percentile of the upper reference limit, and electrocardiographic (ECG) changes consistent with myocardial ischemia or imaging evidence of new loss of viable myocardium (i.e., new perfusion defect) or wall motion abnormality [22].

Although this definition is useful for distinguishing spontaneous coronary events (Type I MI) from events that arise at the time of coronary revascularization (Type 4 and 5 MIs) [22], it does not take into account unique features of perioperative myocardial infarctions after noncardiac operations. For instance, the vast majority of coronary events that occur in the postoperative period are clinically silent as a result of sedation and analgesia. In a post hoc analysis of the PeriOperative ISchemia Evaluation (POISE) trial, 65.3 % of all patients with an MI did not have any ischemic symptoms [23]. Importantly, the 30-day mortality rate was similar for patients with an MI, regardless of the presence (9.7 %) or absence of ischemic symptoms (12.5 %). In support of this, our group has shown that the ECG is insensitive relative to cardiac troponin I to detect myocardial ischemia in the postoperative period (7 % vs. 50 %) [24]. Finally, after vascular surgery, the presence of ischemic ECG changes does not provide additional prognostic information regarding long-term mortality over and above that provided by a single peak troponin I measured within 48 h after vascular surgery (Fig. 36.2) [24]. Taken together, these observations emphasize the importance of widespread utilization of cardiac troponin in the perioperative period for the surveillance of myocardial infarction and risk stratification [25].

Management

Preventive Therapies

Therapies that have been proven to reduce PMI among patients undergoing noncardiac surgery include beta-blockers and statins.

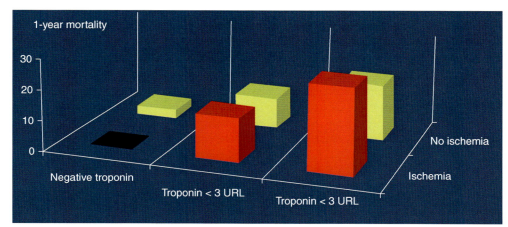

Fig. 36.2 One-year mortality among 468 patients undergoing vascular surgery relative to postoperative peak troponin I value and ischemic ECG changes. The addition of the ECG did not add prognostic information to the model with troponins alone (all p NS). Troponin values were classified as normal, low (+) ≥99th percentile but ≤3 times the URL, and high (+) ≥3 times the URL

Beta-Blockers

Mangano et al. [12] reported a 6 % absolute risk reduction in cardiac events at 6 months with atenolol among 200 male veterans undergoing noncardiac surgery. Poldermans et al. [26] reported a more dramatic 30 % absolute risk reduction with bisoprolol among 173 patients undergoing vascular surgery with evidence of myocardial ischemia on stress test. However, subsequent larger studies with metoprolol yielded negative results [27]. The landmark POISE trial, with over 8,300 patients enrolled, showed that although extended-release metoprolol 200 mg reduces PMI by 26 %, it is associated with a higher risk of death and stroke [28]. For every 1,000 patients treated with extended-release metoprolol, 15 nonfatal myocardial infarctions would be prevented, but 5 strokes and 8 deaths would be caused by it. Therefore, the POISE trial raised serious concerns about the safety of injudicious administration of high-dose beta-blockers in the perioperative period [29].

Statins

In the Dutch Echocardiographic Cardiac Risk Evaluation Applying Stress Echocardiography (DECREASE-III) study, high-dose fluvastatin reduced the composite of cardiovascular death and nonfatal myocardial infarction by 53 % among 457 patients undergoing vascular surgery [30]. In a smaller trial involving 100 vascular patients randomly assigned to 20 mg of atorvastatin or placebo, statins reduced cardiac events from 26 to 8 % at 6 months [10]. Statins may play a pivotal role in plaque stabilization by reducing circulating levels of inflammatory cytokines, increasing expression of nitric oxide synthase and reducing production of endothelin-1 and reactive oxygen species [31].

Coronary Revascularization

The Coronary Artery Prophylactic Revascularization trial (CARP) showed that a strategy of prophylactic revascularization was not superior to optimal medical therapy in preventing PMIs or improving long-term mortality among 510 veterans undergoing elective major vascular surgery [11]. Despite high utilization rates of statins and beta-blockers in the CARP trial, 16 % of patients suffered a PMI. Moreover, among patients with multiple risk factors and/or evidence of myocardial ischemia on nuclear imaging test, the incidence of PMI was 25 % [32]. Similarly to CARP, the DECREASE-V pilot study failed to show any benefit with prophylactic revascularization among 101 patients with multivessel CAD and abnormal stress test prior to vascular surgery (death or MI at 1 year 49 % vs. 44 %) [33]. These high event rates despite optimal medical therapy highlight the need for additional interventions for risk reduction among high-risk patients.

Therapeutic Interventions

Although robust data from randomized clinical trials is lacking, small studies have shown that interventions aimed at improving oxygen delivery and minimizing myocardial oxygen consumption are beneficial in this setting. The main goals of therapy are to prevent, or minimize, wide fluctuations in blood pressure and heart rate through beta-blockade, analgesia, and fluid administration with the intent to preserve optimal coronary perfusion pressure during diastole [13].

Martinez et al. randomized 80 patients with prolonged (≥20 min) ischemia after vascular surgery to beta-blockers, aspirin, nitrates, and optimization of oxygen supply-demand balance or control. At 6 months, patients treated for ischemia had lower mortality relative to control patients (8 % vs. 20 %). In the postoperative period, treated patients had lower median troponin values when compared to controls (3.3 ng/ml vs. 8.5 ng/ml) [34].

Anemia is an independent predictor of mortality after noncardiac surgery in the elderly [35]. Blood transfusion appears to improve survival in critically ill patients with CAD and hemoglobin <10 % [36]. However, this benefit is not seen among patients without CAD or among patients with a hematocrit >25 % with some studies reporting increased mortality and nosocomial infections associated with blood transfusions [37].

Cardiac Evaluation

Although there is no consensus with regard to the type (invasive angiography vs. imaging) and timing (in-hospital vs. 4–6 weeks after discharge) of cardiac evaluation after a PMI, registry data suggest that only a minority of patients with elevated biomarkers receive cardiac work-up after the event [38].

Given the high risk of bleeding immediately after noncardiac surgery, the use of emergency coronary angiography and stenting is usually reserved for patients with hemodynamic instability, ST elevation, or inability to control ischemic symptoms with medications. Among patients with coronary stents, it is important to consider stent thrombosis in the differential diagnosis if ischemic symptoms develop after noncardiac surgery, particularly if antiplatelet agents have been discontinued prior to the operation [39, 40]. These patients have a high mortality rate, and emergency coronary angiography with revascularization is appropriate.

Summary

As the number of surgical procedures continues to increase, the proportion of patients experiencing serious cardiac complications will likely follow this trend. Most of the efforts in the field have been focused on prevention and risk stratification prior to the operation with little emphasis put on best treatment strategies. Given that most of these events are clinically silent, surveillance of PMI with cardiac biomarkers is the first step toward recognizing this complication. Clinical trials focusing on patients with positive cardiac biomarkers are needed to define the role of additional therapies and cardiac imaging.

References

1. Devereaux PJ, Goldman L, Cook DJ, et al. Perioperative cardiac events in patients undergoing noncardiac surgery: a review of the magnitude of the problem, the pathophysiology of the events and methods to estimate and communicate risk. CMAJ. 2005;173(6): 627–34.
2. Ford ES, Ajani UA, Croft JB, et al. Explaining the decrease in U.S. deaths from coronary disease, 1980-2000. N Engl J Med. 2007; 356(23):2388–98.
3. Leon MB, Smith CR, Mack M, et al. Transcatheter aortic-valve implantation for aortic stenosis in patients who cannot undergo surgery. N Engl J Med. 2010;363(17):1597–607.
4. Nowygrod R, Egorova N, Greco G, et al. Trends, complications and mortality in peripheral vascular surgery. J Vasc Surg. 2006;43: 205–16.
5. Badner NH, Knil RL, Brown JE, et al. Myocardial infarction after noncardiac surgery. Anesthesiology. 1998;88:572–8.
6. Le Manach Y, Pereal A, Coriat P, et al. Early and delayed myocardial infarction after abdominal aortic surgery. Anesthesiology. 2005; 102:885–91.
7. Mangano DT, Browner WS, Hollenberg M, et al. Association of perioperative myocardial ischemia with cardiac mortality in men undergoing noncardiac surgery: the study of perioperative ischemia research group. N Engl J Med. 1990;323:1781–8.
8. McFalls E, Ward H, Moritz T, et al. Predictors and outcomes of a perioperative myocardial infarction following elective vascular surgery in patients with documented coronary artery disease: results of the coronary artery revascularization prophylaxis (CARP) trial. Eur Heart J. 2008;29:394–401.
9. Lee T, Marcantonio E, Mangione C, et al. Derivation and prospective validation of a simple index for prediction of cardiac risk of major noncardiac surgery. Circulation. 1999;100:1043–9.
10. Durazzo AE, Machado FS, Ikeoka DT, et al. Reduction in cardiovascular events after vascular surgery with atorvastatin: a randomized trial. J Vasc Surg. 2004;39(5):967–75; discussion 975–66.
11. McFalls E, Ward H, Moritz T, et al. Coronary-artery revascularization before elective major vascular surgery. N Engl J Med. 2004; 351:2795–804.
12. Mangano DT, Layug EL, Wallace A, Tateo I. Effect of atenolol on mortality and cardiovascular morbidity after noncardiac surgery. Multicenter Study of Perioperative Ischemia Research Group. N Engl J Med. 1996;335(23):1713–20.
13. Landesberg G, Beattie S, Mosseri M, Jaffe AS, Alpert JS. Perioperative myocardial infarction. Circulation. 2009;119: 2936–44.
14. Bottiger BW, Motsch J, Teschendorf P, et al. Postoperative 12-lead ECG predicts peri-operative myocardial ischaemia associated with myocardial cell damage. Anaesthesia. 2004;59:1083–90.
15. Landesberg G, Maseri M, Zahger D, et al. Myocardial infarction following vascular surgery: the role of prolonged, stress-induced. ST-depression-type ischemia. J Am Coll Cardiol. 2001;37: 1839–45.
16. Sametz W, Metzler H, Gries M, et al. Perioperative catecholamine changes in cardiac risk patients. Eur J Clin Invest. 1999;29:582–7.
17. Parker SD, Breslow MJ, Frank SM, et al. Catecholamine and cortisol responses to lower extremity revascularization: correlation with outcome variables. Crit Care Med. 1995;23:1954–61.
18. Hertzer N, Beven E, Young J, et al. Coronary artery disease in peripheral vascular patients: a classification of 1000 coronary angiograms and results of surgical management. Ann Surg. 1984; 199:223–33.
19. Ellis SG, Hertzer NR, Young JR, Brener S. Angiographic correlates of cardiac death and myocardial infarction complicating major nonthoracic vascular surgery. Am J Cardiol. 1996;77(12):1126–8.
20. Dawood MM, Gutpa DK, Southern J, et al. Pathology of fatal perioperative myocardial infarction: implications regarding pathophysiology and prevention. Int J Cardiol. 1996;57(1):37–44.
21. Cohen MC, Aretz TH. Histological analysis of coronary artery lesions in fatal postoperative myocardial infarction. Cardiovasc Pathol. 1999;8(3):133–9.
22. Thygesen K, Alpert J, Jaffe AS, et al. Third universal definition of myocardial infarction. Eur Heart J. 2012;33:2551–67.
23. Devereaux PJ, Xavier D, Pogue J, et al. Characteristics and short-term prognosis of perioperative myocardial infarction in patients undergoing noncardiac surgery: a cohort study. Ann Intern Med. 2011;154:523–8.
24. Garcia S, Marston N, Sandoval Y, et al. Prognostic value of 12-lead electrocardiogram and peak troponin I level after vascular surgery. J Vasc Surg. 2013;57(1):166–72.
25. Marston N, Brenes J, Garcia S, et al. Peak postoperative troponin levels outperform preoperative cardiac risk indices as predictors of long-term mortality after vascular surgery troponins and postoperative outcomes. J Crit Care. 2012;27:66–72.
26. Poldermans D, Boersma E, Bax JJ, et al. The effect of bisoprolol on perioperative mortality and myocardial infarction in high-risk patients undergoing vascular surgery. Dutch Echocardiographic Cardiac Risk Evaluation Applying Stress Echocardiography Study Group. N Engl J Med. 1999;341(24):1789–94.

27. Yang H, Raymer K, Butler R, Parlow J, Roberts R. The effects of perioperative beta-blockade: results of the Metoprolol after Vascular Surgery (MaVS) study, a randomized controlled trial. Am Heart J. 2006;152:983–90.

28. POISE STUDY GROUP, Devereaux P, Yang H, Yusuf S, et al. Effects of extended-release metoprolol succinate in patients undergoing non-cardiac surgery (POISE trial): a randomised controlled trial. Lancet. 2008;371:1839–47.

29. Mastracci TM, Aarts MA, Cassivi SD, Garcia S, McLean RF, McFalls EO, Members of the Evidence Based Reviews in Surgery Group. CAGS and ACS evidence based reviews in surgery. 34: effects of ß-blockers in patients undergoing noncardiac surgery. Can J Surg. 2010;53(5):342–4.

30. Schouten O, Boersma E, Hoeks SE, et al. Dutch Echocardiographic Cardiac Risk Evaluation Applying Stress Echocardiography Study Group (DECREASE). Fluvastatin and perioperative events in patients undergoing vascular surgery. N Engl J Med. 2009;361:980–9.

31. Liao JK, Laufs U. Pleiotropic effects of statins. Annu Rev Pharmacol Toxicol. 2005;45:89–118.

32. Garcia S, Moritz T, Goldman S, et al. Perioperative complications after vascular surgery are predicted by the revised cardiac risk index but are not reduced in high-risk subsets with preoperative revascularization. Circ Cardiovasc Qual Outcomes. 2009;2:73–7.

33. Poldermans D, Schouten O, Vidakovic R, et al. A clinical randomized trial to evaluate the safety of a noninvasive approach in high-risk patients undergoing major vascular surgery: the DECREASE-V Pilot Study. J Am Coll Cardiol. 2007;49(17):1763–9.

34. Martinez E, Kim L, Rosenfeld B, et al. Early detection and real-time intervention of postoperative myocardial ischemia: the STOPMI (Study for the Treatment of Perioperative Myocardial Ischemia) Study. Abstract presented at: Association of University Anesthesiologists; 16–18 May 2008; Durham.

35. Wu WC, Schifftner TL, Henderson WG, et al. Preoperative hematocrit levels and postoperative outcomes in older patients undergoing noncardiac surgery. JAMA. 2007;297(22):2481–8.

36. Deans KJ, Minneci PC, Suffredini AF, et al. Randomization in clinical trials of titrated therapies: unintended consequences of using fixed treatment protocols. Crit Care Med. 2007;35(6):1509–16.

37. Rao SV, Jollis JG, Harrington RA, et al. Relationship of blood transfusion and clinical outcomes in patients with acute coronary syndromes. JAMA. 2004;292(13):1555–62.

38. McFalls EO, Larsen G, Johnson GR, et al. Outcomes of hospitalized patients with non-acute coronary syndrome and elevated cardiac troponin level. Am J Med. 2011;124(7):630–5.

39. Brilakis ES, Banerjee S, Berger PB. Perioperative management of patients with coronary stents. J Am Coll Cardiol. 2007;49(22):2145–50.

40. Holmes Jr DR, Kereiakes DJ, Garg S, et al. Stent thrombosis. J Am Coll Cardiol. 2010;56(17):1357–65.

Management of Antiplatelet Agents in the Perioperative Setting

37

Ali O. Abualsaud and Mark J. Eisenberg

Abstract

Management of antiplatelet agents in the perioperative setting is a common clinical challenge. Although discontinuation of aspirin therapy in patients who are taking aspirin for primary or secondary prevention is common, premature cessation of antiplatelet therapy in a patient with a prior drug-eluting stent is the single most important predictor of stent thrombosis, which carries a high morbidity and mortality. Therefore, these patients should ideally continue their antiplatelet therapy throughout surgery. However, this approach to reducing the risk of stent thrombosis must be counterbalanced by the increased risk of surgical bleeding. Multiple factors require evaluation to appropriately balance the risk of stent thrombosis against the risk of surgical bleeding. These include the type and timing of surgery, type and location of coronary stents if present, extent of coronary artery disease, and patient-specific risk factors. In general, for patients with coronary stents, all elective surgeries should be delayed until dual antiplatelet therapy is no longer crucial. Most surgical procedures may be performed on aspirin with acceptable risk of bleeding.

Keywords

Antiplatelet agents • Perioperative • Stent thrombosis • Coronary stents • Surgical bleeding • Percutaneous coronary intervention

Management of antiplatelet agents in the perioperative setting is a challenging clinical dilemma. Antiplatelet agents are widely prescribed in primary and secondary prevention of various cardiovascular diseases such as coronary artery disease (CAD), peripheral arterial disease (PAD), and cerebrovascular disease. Antiplatelet therapy also plays a key role in the management of acute coronary syndromes (ACS).

A.O. Abualsaud, MBBS
Department of Cardiology,
McGill University Health Center/McGill Univesrity,
687 Pine Ave, West, Montreal, QC H3A 1A1, Canada
e-mail: ali.abualsaud@mail.mcgill.ca

M.J. Eisenberg, MD, MPH, FACC, FAHA (✉)
Divisions of Cardiology and Clinical Epidemiology,
Jewish General Hospital/McGill University, 3755 Cote-Ste-Catherine Rd/Room H-421, Montreal, QC H3T 1E2, Canada
e-mail: mark.eisenberg@mcgill.ca

However, their use becomes of paramount importance in patients who have undergone percutaneous coronary intervention (PCI) with stent insertion. In these patients, maintenance of dual antiplatelet therapy (DAPT) is essential for the prevention of stent thrombosis (ST), a catastrophic complication that carries a high morbidity and mortality.

It is estimated that 5 % of patients undergoing PCI will need surgery within 12 months after stent insertion, and 40 % of cases of ST occur in the perioperative setting, often when DAPT is held [1, 2]. Although antiplatelet agents are associated with an increased risk of surgical hemorrhage, the risk of preoperative cessation of antiplatelet drugs may outweigh the risk of surgical bleeding. Therefore, the routine practice of cessation of antiplatelet agents to avoid excess bleeding in patients undergoing surgical procedures should be avoided, and each patient must be managed on a case-by-case basis by balancing the risk of ST against the risk of bleeding.

K. Stergiopoulos, D.L. Brown (eds.), *Evidence-Based Cardiology Consult*,
DOI 10.1007/978-1-4471-4441-0_37, © Springer-Verlag London 2014

Fig. 37.1 Antiplatelet agents and their target receptors [3]. Abbreviations: *GP* glycoprotein, *PAR* protease-activated receptor, *ADP* adenosine diphosphate, *TXA$_2$* thromboxaneA$_2$. Reprinted by permission from Macmillan Publishers Ltd: Nature Reviews Cardiology 2011;8(10):547–559

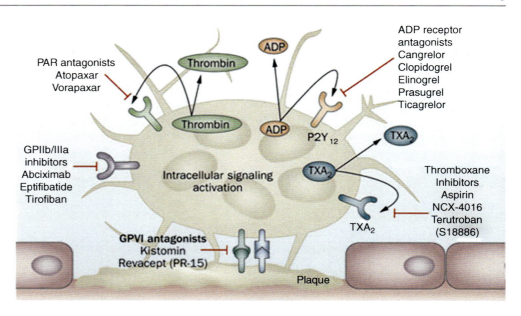

Table 37.1 Pharmacological properties of clinically used ADP-P2Y$_{12}$ inhibitors

Drug	Clopidogrel	Prasugrel	Ticagrelor
Class	Thienopyridine	Thienopyridine	Triazolopyrimidine
Reversibility	Irreversible	Irreversible	Reversible
Activation	Prodrug, limited by metabolization	Prodrug, not limited by metabolization	Active drug
Onset of action	2–4 h	30 min	30 min
Duration of action	3–10 days	5–10 days	3–4 days
Withdrawal before surgery	5 days	7 days	5 days

Adapted from Hamm et al. [18]

Antiplatelet Therapy in Coronary Artery Disease

Aspirin, an irreversible cyclooxygenase-1 (COX-1) inhibitor, and clopidogrel, an irreversible ADP-P2Y$_{12}$ receptor inhibitor, are the most widely prescribed antiplatelet therapies for CAD (Fig. 37.1) [3]. The addition of clopidogrel to aspirin as DAPT yields a synergistic effect, which is superior to aspirin alone in reducing cardiovascular death, myocardial infarction (MI), or stroke in patients with or at risk of CAD [4, 5]. Major bleeding is increased when both agents are used, but the benefit of DAPT outweighs the bleeding risk in patients with ACS [5].

Prasugrel and ticagrelor are novel ADP-P2Y$_{12}$ receptor inhibitors similar to clopidogrel, but with the properties of more rapid onset of action and more consistent platelet inhibition than clopidogrel (Fig. 37.1; Table 37.1). Both prasugrel and ticagrelor are superior to clopidogrel in the

reduction of cardiovascular death, MI, stroke, and ST in patients with ACS undergoing PCI. However, prasugrel is associated with an increased risk of major bleeding, including fatal bleeding, compared to clopidogrel [6, 7]. Unlike prasugrel, ticagrelor is a reversible platelet inhibitor and is not associated with a significant increase in the risk of major or fatal bleeding when compared to clopidogrel. Given its reversibility, ticagrelor may prove to be a suitable agent for perioperative use. However, restoration of platelet activity takes 3–4 days after discontinuation. Thus, similar to clopidogrel, ticagrelor should be discontinued at least 5 days prior to surgery.

Antiplatelet Therapy After Percutaneous Coronary Intervention

Percutaneous coronary intervention (PCI) is known to cause endothelial destruction and medial damage which heals by neointimal formation within 2–6 weeks after placement of a bare-metal stent (BMS) [8]. This healing process may be associated with intimal hyperplasia that leads to in-stent restenosis in approximately 16–32 % of cases after BMS [9, 10]. In order to reduce the rate of restenosis, drug-eluting stents (DES) were introduced in 2002. Despite their success in reducing the rate of in-stent restenosis to less than 10 %, the recognition of late and very late ST following DES placement raised many concerns regarding their safety [11]. When a DES is used, re-endothelialization and neointimal healing are delayed resulting in prolonged exposure of thrombogenic stent struts to blood facilitating platelet adherence, aggregation, and thrombus formation within the DES [8, 12]. Complete healing of a DES may take years during which time there is an ongoing risk of late and very late ST [13]. Available data suggest about a 0.6 % incremental risk of ST with DES compared to BMS [14].

According to the 2011 American College of Cardiology Foundation/American Heart Association/Society of Cardiovascular Angiography and Interventions (ACCF/AHA/SCAI) guidelines for PCI, aspirin should be continued indefinitely, and a $P2Y_{12}$ inhibitor should be given for at least 1 month and up to 12 months after PCI with a BMS and for at least 12 months after PCI with DES [15]. The 2011 updated guidelines for the management of UA/NSTEMI add that in patients with clinical features associated with an increased risk of ST, such as diabetes or renal insufficiency or procedural characteristics such as multiple stents or a treated bifurcation lesion, extension of DAPT beyond 12 months may be reasonable in patients with DES [16].

Stent Thrombosis

Stent thrombosis is a sudden and potentially catastrophic complication after PCI. It usually manifests as an acute MI, generally with ST-segment elevation, malignant arrhythmia, or death. Adding $P2Y_{12}$ inhibitors to aspirin is the standard of care after PCI with stent insertion as it reduces the rate of early stent thrombosis from 3.5 % with aspirin alone to 0.5 % with DAPT [17]. Although the optimal duration of DAPT is yet to be determined in patients with DES, available data suggest that long-term use of DAPT beyond 12 months may be reasonable for the prevention of very late stent thrombosis [16, 18].

Several risk factors for stent thrombosis with DES have been described (Table 37.2) [8, 19–23]. Early stent

Table 37.2 Risk factors for stent thrombosis in patients with drug-eluting stents (DES)

Acute coronary syndrome
Reduced left ventricular ejection fraction
Diabetes mellitus
Renal insufficiency
Hypercoagulable states (e.g., malignancy, surgery, diabetes)
Residual dissection
Incomplete stent apposition or under-expansion
Side branch occlusion
Left main coronary artery stent
Bifurcation
Long and narrow lesions
In-stent restenosis
Multivessel disease
Bypass graft
Stent surface
Hypersensitivity to polymer
Cessation of antiplatelets
Antiplatelet resistance

Adapted from references [8, 19, 21–23]

thrombosis and subacute stent thrombosis are thought to be related to procedure-related factors. In contrast, the single most important predictor of late and very late stent thrombosis is the premature cessation of DAPT [2, 19, 24, 25].

It is estimated that 5 % of patients with coronary stents will undergo a surgical procedure within the first year after PCI [1]. Furthermore, it has been reported that up to 40 % of cases of stent thrombosis with DES occur in the perioperative setting, commonly after the cessation of antiplatelet agents [2]. The increased rate of stent thrombosis in patients undergoing surgery early after PCI (<6 weeks with BMS and <12 months with DES) is likely related to the combination of a postoperative hypercoagulable state with decreased fibrinolysis, superimposed on the prothrombotic milieu of the delayed endothelialization of the stent [26]. In addition, cessation of antiplatelet agents likely triggers a rebound increase in platelet aggregation [27]. In patients with DES, discontinuation of DAPT has been associated with a 90-fold increase in ST and a mortality of 45 % [19]. A 9-fold increase in mortality has been demonstrated if thienopyridines are discontinued within the first 30 days of DES insertion [29]. ST has been shown to occur at a median of 7 days after cessation of DAPT. However, in patients maintained on aspirin with only thienopyridines discontinued, the median time to a coronary event was 122 days (Fig. 37.2) [31].

Fig. 37.2 Cumulative proportion of late stent thrombosis cases among patients who discontinued antiplatelet therapy [31]. (**a**) Within 1 year of discontinuing antiplatelet therapy. (**b**) Within 30 days of discontinuing antiplatelet therapy. Abbreviations: *ASA* acetylsalicylic acid

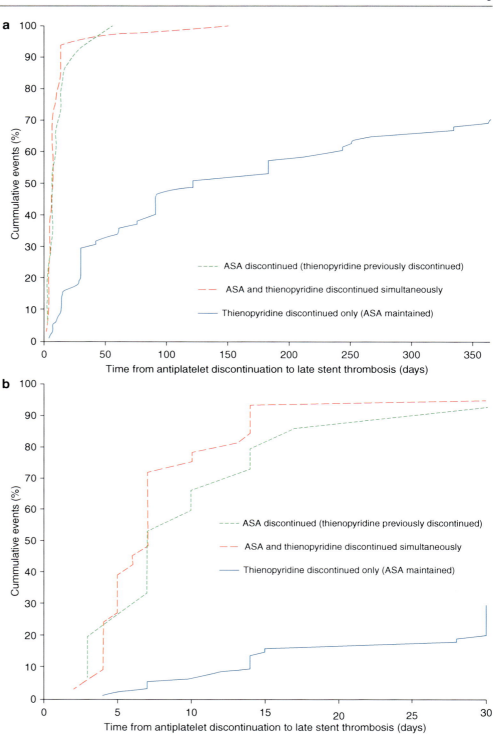

Perioperative Bleeding with Antiplatelet Therapy

Surgical Bleeding in Patients on Aspirin

A meta-analysis of 50,000 patients undergoing noncardiac surgery demonstrated that continuation of aspirin led to a 50 % increase in the risk of bleeding. However, this increased risk did not translate to a higher level of the severity of bleeding complications except in intracranial surgery and, possibly, transurethral resection of the prostate (TURP) [30]. Moreover, withdrawal of aspirin was associated with a higher incidence of cardiac, cerebral, and peripheral vascular events. In a randomized controlled trial of 220 patients undergoing surgery, maintenance of aspirin was associated with a 7.2 % reduction of acute MI, cardiac arrest, severe arrhythmia, or cardiovascular death within the first 30 postoperative days without an increase in bleeding complications [32].

In general the use of aspirin in dental surgery, anterior chamber ophthalmic surgery, dermatologic surgery, biopsies, and visceral surgery is not associated with an increased risk of bleeding complications or fatal bleeding [30]. Similarly, in patients undergoing gastrointestinal endoscopic procedures including biopsies and polypectomies, the use of aspirin alone has not been associated with an increased risk of bleeding [33]. In urologic surgery, initial reports suggested an increased risk of bleeding in patients undergoing TURP if aspirin was maintained [34]. However, more recent prospective and retrospective studies indicate that even though bleeding following TURP and transrectal prostate biopsy is increased, it is not associated with a need for blood transfusions, particularly if a laser was used [35, 36]. Studies evaluating bleeding in the setting of nephrectomy or radical prostatectomy are lacking. However, the use of robot-assisted radical prostatectomy and nephrectomy on aspirin is not associated with an increased risk of bleeding [37, 38]. In orthopedic surgery, the use of antiplatelet agents has not been associated with significant surgical morbidity or mortality except in orthopedic spinal surgery [30, 39]. In peripheral vascular surgery, aspirin use is associated with increased nonfatal bleeding but a decrease in perioperative mortality [40].

Surgical Bleeding in Patients on DAPT

The effect of DAPT on surgical bleeding has been most studied in cardiac surgery. Low-dose aspirin is associated with a low risk of excessive bleeding following coronary artery bypass surgery [41]. However, the addition of a thienopyridine to aspirin results in a significant increase in bleeding, blood product transfusion, ventilation requirements, length of hospital stay, and surgical re-exploration [42]. For this reason, the American College of Cardiology/American Heart Association/European Society of Cardiology (ACC/AHA/ESC) guidelines recommend that in patients undergoing coronary artery bypass surgery, $P2Y_{12}$ inhibitors should be withheld at least 5 days and up to 7 days prior to surgery unless the urgency of revascularization outweighs the risks of excess bleeding [18, 43].

Individual reports describe significant and even fatal postoperative hemorrhage with DAPT after vascular, orthopedic, and even endoscopic procedures [44–46]. However, larger studies demonstrate that, even though there is an increase in surgical bleeding and transfusion requirements, there is no change in mortality or surgical outcome [1, 28, 39, 47]. In transbronchial biopsy, the use of DAPT has been associated with significant bleeding in all cases. However, none of these bleeding events were fatal or required transfusions [45]. The use of clopidogrel is contraindicated in regional spinal or epidural anesthesia due to the risk of significant hematomas and spinal cord compression [48]. A prospective study evaluating

patients with coronary stents undergoing noncardiac surgery demonstrated a major adverse cardiac event (MACE) rate of 10.9 % and a bleeding complication rate of 9.5 % [49]. Complete cessation of antiplatelet agents was an independent predictor of MACE, whereas the use of antiplatelet agents was not a predictor of bleeding complications.

Collectively the data suggest that most surgical procedures can be performed at low risk on aspirin and potentially on DAPT and that the increased risk of perioperative hemorrhage is not necessarily associated with worsened morbidity, mortality, or surgical outcome. Therefore, the risk of stopping antiplatelet agents in patients with coronary stents might outweigh the risk of continuing them, particularly in high-risk patients.

Strategies for Perioperative Management of Antiplatelet Agents in Patients with Coronary Stents

Any decisions regarding the perioperative management of antiplatelet agents is based on a limited body of evidence. Management of these patients requires an individualized, multidisciplinary approach by the patient's cardiologist, surgeon, and anesthesiologist. The approach should take into consideration the type of surgery and its bleeding risk, the CAD burden and ischemic risk, the timing of surgery after an event or after PCI, if a DES was used or not, and the presence of concomitant risk factors of ST. Subsequently, the risk of surgical bleeding (Table 37.3) [39] should be weighed against the estimated risk of ST (Fig. 37.3).

Table 37.3 Hemorrhagic risk with noncardiac surgery

Surgical hemorrhagic risk	Type of surgery
Low	
Blood transfusion usually not required	Peripheral
	Plastic
	Biopsies
	Endoscopy
	Minor orthopedic
	Minor otolaryngologic
	Ophthalmic (anterior chamber)
	Dental
Intermediate	
Blood transfusion frequently required	Visceral
	Vascular
	Major orthopedic
	Major otolaryngologic
	Reconstructive
	Urology
High	
Possible bleeding in a closed space	Intracranial neurosurgery
	Spinal canal surgery
	Ophthalmic (posterior chamber)

Data adapted from Chassot et al. [39]

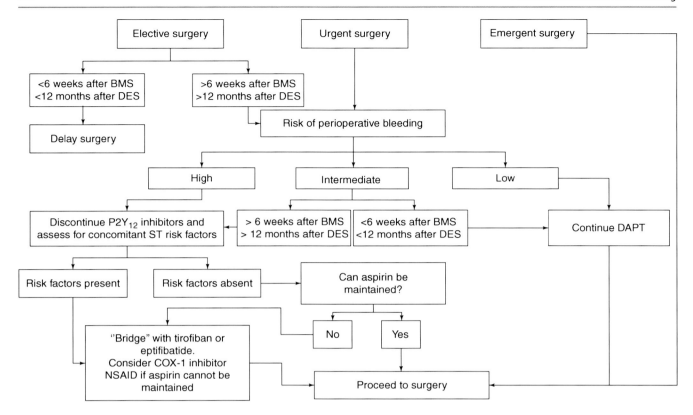

Fig. 37.3 Algorithm of perioperative management of patients with coronary stents [66]. Abbreviations: *COX* cyclooxygenase, *BMS* bare-metal stents, *DES* drug-eluting stent(s), *NSAID* nonsteroidal anti-inflammatory drug, *ST* stent thrombosis, *DAPT* dual antiplatelet therapy

Aspirin and P2Y$_{12}$ Inhibitor Throughout Surgery

American and European Cardiology Society guidelines recommend delaying all elective surgical procedures until the duration of DAPT is completed (Table 37.4) [18, 50–56]. Therefore, as a general approach, all elective procedures should be delayed at least 4–6 weeks after PCI with BMS and 12 months after PCI with DES. According to the 2009 ESC guidelines for preoperative cardiac risk assessment and perioperative cardiac management in noncardiac surgery, elective surgery should be delayed for a minimum of 6 weeks and optimally 3 months after a BMS [52]. However, if surgery cannot be delayed due to urgency, then maintenance of DAPT is of paramount importance as the risk of ST is significantly increased. The 2011 ESC guidelines on the management of non-ST elevation acute coronary syndrome (NSTEACS) state that most surgical procedures can be performed under DAPT or at least aspirin alone with acceptable rates of bleeding and that surgeons should be encouraged to operate under DAPT if bleeding risk is low or moderate [18]. This applies to most surgical procedures, except those in cases in which bleeding can occur in a closed space and could be catastrophic, such as intracranial, spinal, and posterior-chamber ophthalmic surgeries (see Table 37.3).

Discontinue P2Y$_{12}$ Inhibitor and Maintain Aspirin

The 2011 ESC guidelines for the management of NSTEACS state that interruption of DAPT for urgent surgical procedures 1 month after ACS while continuing aspirin in patients *without* a DES may be reasonable [18]. Similarly, in patients *with* a DES without concomitant risk factors of ST undergoing surgery more than 12 months after PCI, P2Y$_{12}$ inhibitors may be safely discontinued 5–7 days prior to surgery while maintaining aspirin. If risk factors of ST are present and the risk of perioperative bleeding is significantly high, then P2Y$_{12}$ inhibitors may be discontinued while aspirin is maintained, understanding that the patient is at increased risk of postoperative ST. Following surgery, P2Y$_{12}$ inhibitors should be started once the risk of bleeding is felt to be sufficiently low (ideally within the first 24 h) with a loading dose of either clopidogrel 300–600 mg,

Table 37.4 Summary of guidelines for perioperative management of antiplatelet agents in patients with coronary stents

Guidelines	BMS	DES	Bleeding risk necessitating AP cessation
2007 ACC/AHA guidelines on perioperative cardiovascular evaluation and care for noncardiac surgery [50]	Delay elective surgery for at least 4–6 weeks After 6 weeks proceed on aspirin	Delay elective surgery for at least 12 months After 12 months proceed on aspirin	Aspirin should be maintained if thienopyridines are discontinued and should be restarted as soon as possible Resuming DAPT perioperatively 12 m after PCI should be considered if risk factors of ST are present No evidence for use of warfarin, antithrombotics, or GP IIb/IIIa inhibitors
2007 ACC/AHA/SCAI/ACS/ADA Science advisory on prevention of premature discontinuation of DAPT in patients with coronary stents [51]	Delay elective procedures at least 1 month	Delay elective procedures at least 12 months	Aspirin should be maintained if thienopyridines are discontinued and should be restarted as soon as possible
2009 ESC guidelines for preoperative cardiac risk assessment and perioperative cardiac management in noncardiac surgery [52]	Delay elective surgery for at least 6 weeks and optimally for 3 months (Class I) After 3 months proceed on aspirin (Class I)	Delay elective surgery for at least 12 months After 12 months proceed on aspirin	Discontinue AP 5 days and optimally 10 days prior to surgery If surgery is urgent, transfusion of platelets or pro-hemostatic agents is recommended Resume AP within 24 h
2011 ESC guidelines for the management of ACS without persistent ST-segment elevation [18]	Interruption of DAPT after 1 month may be reasonable	If bleeding risk is low or moderate, surgeons should be encouraged to operate on DAPT	Discontinue clopidogrel or ticagrelor 5 days prior to surgery Discontinue prasugrel 7 days prior to surgery Bridging with GP IIb/IIIa inhibitors is not considered evidence-based yet
2011 Canadian Cardiovascular Society guidelines on the use of antiplatelet therapy [53]	Delay elective surgery for at least 6 weeks (Class I) If urgent surgery continue DAPT (Class I)	Delay elective surgery for at least 12 months (Class I) If urgent surgery continue DAPT (Class I)	Discontinue clopidogrel 7–10 days prior to surgery
2012 ACCP Perioperative management of antithrombotic therapy [55]	Delay elective surgery for 6 weeks If within 6 weeks continue DAPT	Delay elective surgery for 6 months (12 months in 2008 guidelines [54]) If within 6 months continue DAPT	Use of bridging with GP IIb/IIIa inhibitors is inadvisable due to lack of evidence
2010 Cardiac Society of Australia and New Zealand guidelines for the management of antiplatelet therapy in patients with coronary stents undergoing noncardiac surgery [63]	Delay elective surgery for at least 6 weeks and ideally for 3 months	Delay elective surgery for at least 12 months	Patient with high risk of ST requires monitored clinical setting in a facility with 24/7 PCI capacity Bridging with GP IIb/IIIa and heparin should be considered in high-risk patients
2006 Perioperative management of antiplatelet agents in patients with coronary stents: recommendations of a French Task Force [56]	Delay elective surgery for at least 4–6 weeks	Delay elective surgery for at least 6–12 months If within 6–12 months, continue DAPT	Discontinue DAPT 5–10 days before surgery Consider using another NSAID such as flurbiprofen (50 mg × 2, withdrawn 24 h before surgery) or LMWH (85–100 IU aXa per KG for 12 h)

Abbreviations: *BMS* bare-metal stent, *DES* drug-eluting stent, *DAPT* dual antiplatelet therapy, *ACC* American College of Cardiology, *AHA* American Heart Association, *ESC* European Society of Cardiology, *SCAI* Society of Cardiovascular Angiography and Interventions, *ACS* American College of Surgeons, *ADA* American Dental Association, *ACCP* American College of Chest Physicians, *PCI* percutaneous coronary intervention, *GP* glycoprotein, *NSAID* nonsteroidal anti-inflammatory drug, *AP* antiplatelet, *LMWH* low-molecular-weight heparin

prasugrel 60 mg, or ticagrelor 180 mg. Short-term discontinuation of thienopyridines has been shown to be relatively safe if aspirin is maintained; however, the risk of ST remains elevated [31].

"Bridging Therapy" with Glycoprotein IIb/IIIa Inhibitors

Glycoprotein (GP) IIb/IIIa inhibitors act by blocking fibrinogen-mediated cross-linking of platelets, thereby inhibiting platelet aggregation [57]. Abciximab causes a prolonged irreversible antagonism of GP IIb/IIIa leading to platelet aggregation inhibition that lasts for at least 48 h and up to 7 days and therefore should not be used perioperatively [58]. The synthetic peptides eptifibatide and tirofiban are competitive, reversible binders to GP IIb/IIIa receptors and dissociate rapidly. Their half-life is quite short, and platelet function is completely restored 2–4 h after stopping the infusion, making them potentially suitable for perioperative use [59].

Even though GP IIb/IIIa inhibitors have not been studied extensively in the perioperative setting, their successful use as a "bridge" when P2Y$_{12}$ inhibitors are stopped before surgery has been reported [60–62]. Two small series of patients, at high risk of both ST and surgical bleeding, demonstrated that bridging with eptifibatide was associated with a favorable postoperative outcome without increased perioperative hemorrhage [61, 62]. Perioperative bridging with tirofiban was evaluated in another prospective study of 30 patients undergoing high bleeding risk surgery within 1–12 months after PCI with DES. There were no MACE, and major bleeding was observed in two patients who did not require surgical re-exploration [60].

For patients with coronary stents who are at an increased risk of perioperative bleeding and a significant risk of ST (e.g., early after PCI) but who require surgery, bridging therapy with aspirin and a GP IIb/IIIa inhibitor could be considered, although limited data exist in support of this strategy. This entails stopping P2Y$_{12}$ inhibitors 5–7 days before surgery and admitting the patient to the hospital 2–4 days before surgery to begin tirofiban or eptifibatide which is discontinued 6 h before surgery. Importantly, the increased bleeding risk associated with GP IIb/IIIa inhibitor treatment also has to be considered.

Even though this strategy is not practical in most cases and is not considered evidence-based yet, it might be worthwhile in patients at extremely high risk of stent thrombosis. According to the 2010 Cardiac Society of Australia and New Zealand guidelines for the management of antiplatelet therapy in patients with coronary stents undergoing noncardiac surgery, bridging with GP IIb/IIIa inhibitors and heparin can be considered in high-risk patients [63].

Discontinue Aspirin and P2Y$_{12}$ Inhibitors and Consider Alternatives

If the risk of surgical bleeding is potentially catastrophic or fatal, such as in intracranial, spinal, and posterior-chamber ophthalmic surgeries, aspirin cessation might be necessary. In these cases aspirin and P2Y$_{12}$ inhibitors should be discontinued 5–7 days before surgery. Given the increased risk of ST with cessation of antiplatelet agents, intensive perioperative monitoring and early interventions are of paramount importance. Moreover, dual antiplatelet therapy should be reintroduced once the risk of hemorrhage is diminished.

Heparin has been considered as a substitute to aspirin or P2Y$_{12}$ inhibitors. However, heparin is an antithrombin agent, rather than an antiplatelet agent. The use of unfractionated heparin (UFH) and low-molecular-weight heparin (LMWH) has been proposed in the perioperative management of patients with coronary stents [64]. However, data on perioperative heparin use suggest increased mortality [1]. In addition, abrupt cessation of UFH may be associated with a rebound hypercoagulable state [65]. Finally, since ST is a platelet-mediated process, it is expected that antithrombin agents such as UFH and LMWH would not be ideal agents.

Management of Postoperative Stent Thrombosis

Given that ST most often presents as an STEMI, the most appropriate management is early reperfusion therapy. Since thrombolytic therapy is contraindicated postoperatively, due to the excessive bleeding risk, primary PCI is the treatment of choice for perioperative ST.

Conclusion

Management of antiplatelet agents in the perioperative setting remains a common clinical challenge. Premature cessation of antiplatelet therapy is the single most important predictor of ST, which carries a high morbidity and mortality, particularly in the perioperative setting. Therefore, patients ideally should continue their antiplatelet medications throughout surgery to reduce the risk of ST. However, this reduction is accompanied by an increased risk of surgical bleeding. All elective surgeries should be delayed until DAPT is no longer crucial. Most surgical procedures may be performed on aspirin with an acceptable risk of bleeding. However, if the bleeding risk is unacceptable on oral antiplatelets, then bridging with a GP IIb/IIIa inhibitor could be considered.

Key Points

- All patients with CAD should receive aspirin indefinitely, and a P2Y$_{12}$ inhibitor (clopidogrel, prasugrel, or ticagrelor) should be added and maintained for at least 1 month and up to 12 months after BMS insertion and for at least 12 months after DES insertion that may be extended beyond 12 months in patients with increased risk of ST.
- All elective surgical procedures should be delayed until the duration of DAPT is completed (at least 1 month after PCI with BMS and 12 months after PCI with DES).
- If surgery cannot be delayed due to urgency, then maintenance of DAPT is of paramount importance for the prevention of ST.
- Most surgical procedures can be performed under DAPT or at least aspirin alone with acceptable rates of bleeding.
- Interruption of DAPT for necessary surgical procedures 1 month after ACS in patients without a DES may be reasonable.
- In patients with DES without concomitant risk factors of ST undergoing surgery more than 12 months after PCI, P2Y$_{12}$ inhibitors may be safely discontinued 5–7 days prior to surgery while maintaining aspirin.

References

1. Vicenzi MN, et al. Coronary artery stenting and non-cardiac surgery – a prospective outcome study. Br J Anaesth. 2006;96(6):686–93.
2. Artang R, Dieter RS. Analysis of 36 reported cases of late thrombosis in drug-eluting stents placed in coronary arteries. Am J Cardiol. 2007;99(8):1039–43.
3. Yousuf O, Bhatt DL. The evolution of antiplatelet therapy in cardiovascular disease. Nat Rev Cardiol. 2011;8(10):547–59.
4. CAPRIE Steering Committee. A randomised, blinded, trial of clopidogrel versus aspirin in patients at risk of ischaemic events (CAPRIE). Lancet. 1996;348(9038):1329–39.
5. Mehta SR, Yusuf S. The clopidogrel in unstable angina to prevent recurrent events (CURE) trial programme; rationale, design and baseline characteristics including a meta-analysis of the effects of thienopyridines in vascular disease. Eur Heart J. 2000;21(24):2033–41.
6. Wiviott SD, et al. Prasugrel compared with high loading- and maintenance-dose clopidogrel in patients with planned percutaneous coronary intervention: the prasugrel in comparison to clopidogrel for inhibition of platelet activation and aggregation-thrombolysis in myocardial infarction 44 trial. Circulation. 2007;116(25):2923–32.
7. Wallentin L, et al. Ticagrelor versus clopidogrel in patients with acute coronary syndromes. N Engl J Med. 2009;361(11):1045–57.
8. Joner M, et al. Pathology of drug-eluting stents in humans: delayed healing and late thrombotic risk. J Am Coll Cardiol. 2006;48(1):193–202.
9. Fischman DL, et al. A randomized comparison of coronary-stent placement and balloon angioplasty in the treatment of coronary artery disease. Stent Restenosis Study Investigators. N Engl J Med. 1994;331(8):496–501.
10. Serruys PW, et al. A comparison of balloon-expandable-stent implantation with balloon angioplasty in patients with coronary artery disease. Benestent Study Group. N Engl J Med. 1994;331(8):489–95.
11. Holmes Jr DR, et al. Stent thrombosis. J Am Coll Cardiol. 2010;56(17):1357–65.
12. Kotani J, et al. Incomplete neointimal coverage of sirolimus-eluting stents: angioscopic findings. J Am Coll Cardiol. 2006;47(10):2108–11.
13. Awata M, et al. Serial angioscopic evidence of incomplete neointimal coverage after sirolimus-eluting stent implantation: comparison with bare-metal stents. Circulation. 2007;116(8):910–6.
14. Mauri L, et al. Stent thrombosis in randomized clinical trials of drug-eluting stents. N Engl J Med. 2007;356(10):1020–9.
15. Levine GN, et al. ACCF/AHA/SCAI Guideline for Percutaneous Coronary Intervention. A report of the American College of Cardiology Foundation/American Heart Association Task Force on Practice Guidelines and the Society for Cardiovascular Angiography and Interventions. J Am Coll Cardiol. 2011;58(24):e44–122.
16. Wright RS, et al. 2011 ACCF/AHA focused update incorporated into the ACC/AHA 2007 guidelines for the management of patients with unstable angina/non-ST-elevation myocardial infarction: a report of the American College of Cardiology Foundation/ American Heart Association Task Force on Practice Guidelines developed in collaboration with the American Academy of Family Physicians, Society for Cardiovascular Angiography and Interventions, and the Society of Thoracic Surgeons. J Am Coll Cardiol. 2011;57(19):e215–367.
17. Leon MB, et al. A clinical trial comparing three antithrombotic-drug regimens after coronary-artery stenting. Stent Anticoagulation Restenosis Study Investigators. N Engl J Med. 1998;339(23):1665–71.
18. Hamm CW, et al. ESC guidelines for the management of acute coronary syndromes in patients presenting without persistent ST-segment elevation: The Task Force for the management of acute coronary syndromes (ACS) in patients presenting without persistent ST-segment elevation of the European Society of Cardiology (ESC). Eur Heart J. 2011;32(23):2999–3054.
19. Iakovou I, et al. Incidence, predictors, and outcome of thrombosis after successful implantation of drug-eluting stents. JAMA. 2005;293(17):2126–30.
20. Colombo A, Corbett SJ. Drug-eluting stent thrombosis: increasingly recognized but too frequently overemphasized. J Am Coll Cardiol. 2006;48(1):203–5.
21. Park DW, et al. Frequency of and risk factors for stent thrombosis after drug-eluting stent implantation during long-term follow-up. Am J Cardiol. 2006;98(3):352–6.
22. Cutlip DE, et al. Stent thrombosis in the modern era: a pooled analysis of multicenter coronary stent clinical trials. Circulation. 2001;103(15):1967–71.
23. Kuchulakanti PK, et al. Correlates and long-term outcomes of angiographically proven stent thrombosis with sirolimus- and paclitaxel-eluting stents. Circulation. 2006;113(8):1108–13.
24. Auer J, et al. Risk of noncardiac surgery in the months following placement of a drug-eluting coronary stent. J Am Coll Cardiol. 2004;43(4):713; author reply 714–5.
25. Kaluza GL, et al. Catastrophic outcomes of noncardiac surgery soon after coronary stenting. J Am Coll Cardiol. 2000;35(5):1288–94.

26. Camenzind E, Steg PG, Wijns W. Stent thrombosis late after implantation of first-generation drug-eluting stents: a cause for concern. Circulation. 2007;115(11):1440–55; discussion 1455.

27. Ferrari E, et al. Coronary syndromes following aspirin withdrawal: a special risk for late stent thrombosis. J Am Coll Cardiol. 2005;45(3):456–9.

28. Sharma AK, et al. Major noncardiac surgery following coronary stenting: when is it safe to operate? Catheter Cardiovasc Interv. 2004;63(2):141–5.

29. Spertus JA, et al. Prevalence, predictors, and outcomes of premature discontinuation of thienopyridine therapy after drug-eluting stent placement: results from the PREMIER registry. Circulation. 2006;113(24):2803–9.

30. Burger W, et al. Low-dose aspirin for secondary cardiovascular prevention – cardiovascular risks after its perioperative withdrawal versus bleeding risks with its continuation – review and meta-analysis. J Intern Med. 2005;257(5):399–414.

31. Eisenberg MJ, et al. Safety of short-term discontinuation of antiplatelet therapy in patients with drug-eluting stents. Circulation. 2009;119(12):1634–42.

32. Oscarsson A, et al. To continue or discontinue aspirin in the perioperative period: a randomized, controlled clinical trial. Br J Anaesth. 2010;104(3):305–12.

33. Boustiere C, et al. Endoscopy and antiplatelet agents. European Society of Gastrointestinal Endoscopy (ESGE) Guideline. Endoscopy. 2011;43(5):445–61.

34. Watson CJ, et al. Identifiable factors in post-prostatectomy haemorrhage: the role of aspirin. Br J Urol. 1990;66(1):85–7.

35. Elzayat E, Habib E, Elhilali M. Holmium laser enucleation of the prostate in patients on anticoagulant therapy or with bleeding disorders. J Urol. 2006;175(4):1428–32.

36. Nielsen JD, et al. The effect of low-dose acetylsalicylic acid on bleeding after transurethral prostatectomy – a prospective, randomized, double-blind, placebo-controlled study. Scand J Urol Nephrol. 2000;34(3):194–8.

37. Patel VR, et al. Robot-assisted laparoscopic radical prostatectomy: perioperative outcomes of 1500 cases. J Endourol. 2008;22(10): 2299–305.

38. Parikh A, et al. Preoperative aspirin is safe in patients undergoing urologic robot-assisted surgery. J Endourol. 2012;26:852–6.

39. Chassot PG, Delabays A, Spahn DR. Perioperative antiplatelet therapy: the case for continuing therapy in patients at risk of myocardial infarction. Br J Anaesth. 2007;99(3):316–28.

40. Neilipovitz DT, Bryson GL, Nichol G. The effect of perioperative aspirin therapy in peripheral vascular surgery: a decision analysis. Anesth Analg. 2001;93(3):573–80.

41. Sun JC, et al. Should aspirin be discontinued before coronary artery bypass surgery? Circulation. 2005;112(7):e85–90.

42. Purkayastha S, et al. Does clopidogrel affect outcome after coronary artery bypass grafting? A meta-analysis. Heart. 2006;92(4):531–2.

43. Hillis LD, et al. ACCF/AHA guideline for coronary artery bypass graft surgery. A report of the American College of Cardiology Foundation/American Heart Association Task Force on Practice Guidelines. Developed in collaboration with the American Association for Thoracic Surgery, Society of Cardiovascular Anesthesiologists, and Society of Thoracic Surgeons. J Am Coll Cardiol. 2011;58(24):e123–210.

44. Chapman TW, et al. Haemorrhage associated with combined clopidogrel and aspirin therapy. Eur J Vasc Endovasc Surg. 2001; 22(5):478–9.

45. Ernst A, et al. Effect of routine clopidogrel use on bleeding complications after transbronchial biopsy in humans. Chest. 2006;129(3): 734–7.

46. Moore M, Power M. Perioperative hemorrhage and combined clopidogrel and aspirin therapy. Anesthesiology. 2004;101(3):792–4.

47. Wilson SH, et al. Clinical outcome of patients undergoing noncardiac surgery in the two months following coronary stenting. J Am Coll Cardiol. 2003;42(2):234–40.

48. Horlocker TT, et al. Regional anesthesia in the anticoagulated patient: defining the risks (the second ASRA consensus conference on neuraxial anesthesia and anticoagulation). Reg Anesth Pain Med. 2003;28(3):172–97.

49. Albaladejo P, et al. Non-cardiac surgery in patients with coronary stents: the RECO study. Heart. 2011;97(19):1566–72.

50. Fleisher LA, et al. ACC/AHA 2007 guidelines on perioperative cardiovascular evaluation and care for noncardiac surgery: a report of the American College of Cardiology/American Heart Association Task Force on Practice Guidelines (writing committee to revise the 2002 guidelines on perioperative cardiovascular evaluation for noncardiac surgery) developed in collaboration with the American Society of Echocardiography, American Society of Nuclear Cardiology, Heart Rhythm Society, Society of Cardiovascular Anesthesiologists, Society for Cardiovascular Angiography and Interventions, Society for Vascular Medicine and Biology, and Society for Vascular Surgery. J Am Coll Cardiol. 2007;50(17):e159–241.

51. Grines CL, et al. Prevention of premature discontinuation of dual antiplatelet therapy in patients with coronary artery stents: a science advisory from the American Heart Association, American College of Cardiology, Society for Cardiovascular Angiography and Interventions, American College of Surgeons, and American Dental Association, with representation from the American College of Physicians. J Am Coll Cardiol. 2007;49(6):734–9.

52. Poldermans D, et al. Guidelines for pre-operative cardiac risk assessment and perioperative cardiac management in non-cardiac surgery. Eur Heart J. 2009;30(22):2769–812.

53. Bell AD, et al. The use of antiplatelet therapy in the outpatient setting: Canadian Cardiovascular Society guidelines. Can J Cardiol. 2011;27(Suppl A):S1–59.

54. Douketis JD, et al. The perioperative management of antithrombotic therapy: American College of Chest Physicians Evidence-Based Clinical Practice Guidelines (8th Edition). Chest. 2008;133(6 Suppl):299S–339.

55. Douketis JD, et al. Perioperative management of antithrombotic therapy: antithrombotic therapy and prevention of thrombosis, 9th ed: American College of Chest Physicians Evidence-Based Clinical Practice Guidelines. Chest. 2012;141(2 Suppl):e326S–50.

56. Albaladejo P, et al. Perioperative management of antiplatelet agents in patients with coronary stents: recommendations of a French Task Force. Br J Anaesth. 2006;97(4):580–2.

57. Frishman WH, et al. Novel antiplatelet therapies for treatment of patients with ischemic heart disease: inhibitors of the platelet glycoprotein IIb/IIIa integrin receptor. Am Heart J. 1995;130(4):877–92.

58. Faulds D, Sorkin EM. Abciximab (c7E3 Fab). A review of its pharmacology and therapeutic potential in ischaemic heart disease. Drugs. 1994;48(4):583–98.

59. Kleiman NS. Pharmacokinetics and pharmacodynamics of glycoprotein IIb-IIIa inhibitors. Am Heart J. 1999;138(4 Pt 2):263–75.

60. Savonitto S, et al. Urgent surgery in patients with a recently implanted coronary drug-eluting stent: a phase II study of 'bridging' antiplatelet therapy with tirofiban during temporary withdrawal of clopidogrel. Br J Anaesth. 2010;104(3):285–91.

61. Bigalke B, et al. Perioperative antiplatelet therapy in patients at risk for coronary stent thrombosis undergoing noncardiac surgery. Clin Res Cardiol. 2009;98(5):335–9.

62. Chou S, et al. Bridging therapy in the perioperative management of patients with drug-eluting stents. Rev Cardiovasc Med. 2009;10(4):209–18.

63. Cardiac Society of Australia and New Zealand. Guidelines for the management of antiplatelet therapy in patients with coronary stents undergoing non-cardiac surgery. Heart Lung Circ. 2010;19(1): 2–10.

64. Broad L, et al. Successful management of patients with a drug-eluting coronary stent presenting for elective, non-cardiac surgery. Br J Anaesth. 2007;98(1):19–22.

65. Dent H, Lekic Z, Vicenzi M. Unfractionated heparin and coronary artery stenting. Br J Anaesth. 2006;97(4):582; author reply 582.

66. Abualsaud AO, Eisenberg MJ. Perioperative management of patients with drug-eluting stents. JACC Cardiovasc Interv. 2010;3(2):131–42.

Managing Anticoagulation in Patients with Mechanical Valves

38

Usman Baber, Nilusha Gukathasan, and Valentin Fuster

Abstract

As the burden of valvular heart disease increases worldwide, surgical valve replacement with mechanical prostheses continues to be an important treatment option for thousands of patients each year. All patients with mechanical heart valves require oral anticoagulation with vitamin K antagonists. The optimal dose and intensity of anticoagulation depends on patient- and valve-related risk factors. Clinical management is further complicated during pregnancy or surgery because antithrombotic therapy may need to be altered and decisions are often based on limited, observational data. Novel therapies that may overcome many of the inherent limitations associated with vitamin K antagonists are currently being developed and tested as alternative anticoagulants in different patient populations.

Keywords

Vitamin K antagonists • Mechanical heart valves • Valvular heart disease • Pregnancy • Perioperative management • Anticoagulation

Introduction

The worldwide burden of valvular heart disease continues to grow due to increases in life expectancy combined with the high incidence of rheumatic heart disease in developing nations [1]. The definitive treatment for many forms of valvular heart disease remains surgical substitution of a native valve with a biological or mechanical prosthesis. Not surprisingly, the rate of valve implantation worldwide is increasing by around 5–7 % per year due to this rising demand with approximately 250,000 valve replacements occurring annually. In addition, mechanical implants are favored over biological prostheses by a slim majority (55 % vs. 45 %) [2]. While the choice of valve is influenced by patient age, preferences, and risk factors for thromboembolism or bleeding, mechanical prostheses may be favored due to their longevity, durability, and structural integrity. Mechanical heart valves (MHV), however, are more thrombogenic than their biological counterparts, and mandatory lifelong anticoagulation is associated with substantial and potentially life-threatening bleeding complications. MHV prostheses may be categorized by the following designs: caged-ball, monoleaflet, and bileaflet [3, 4]. All valves have a regurgitant or washing jet to prevent thrombus formation and are comprised of three basic components: (1) occluder, (2) housing, and a (3) sewing ring. The occluder consists of one or more rigid moveable parts such as a ball, flat disc (tilting or free-floating), or two hinged leaflets (Fig. 38.1). The housing provides the

U. Baber, MD, MS • N. Gukathasan, MD
Department of Cardiology, Mount Sinai School of Medicine,
One Gustave L. Levy Place, New York, NY 10029, USA
e-mail: usman.baber@mountsinai.org;
nilusha.gukathasan@mountsinai.org

V. Fuster, MD, PhD (✉)
Zena and Michael A. Wiener Cardiovascular Institute
and the Marie-Josée and Henry R. Kravis Center
for Cardiovascular Health, One Gustave L. Levy Place,
New York, NY 10029, USA

Centro Nacional de Investigaciones Cardiovasculares
Carlos III (CNIC), Madrid, Spain

Department of Cardiology, Mount Sinai Medical Center,
New York, NY, USA
e-mail: valentin.fuster@mountsinai.org

K. Stergiopoulos, D.L. Brown (eds.), *Evidence-Based Cardiology Consult*,
DOI 10.1007/978-1-4471-4441-0_38, © Springer-Verlag London 2014

Caged ball valves		Single leaflet valves		Bileaflet valves	
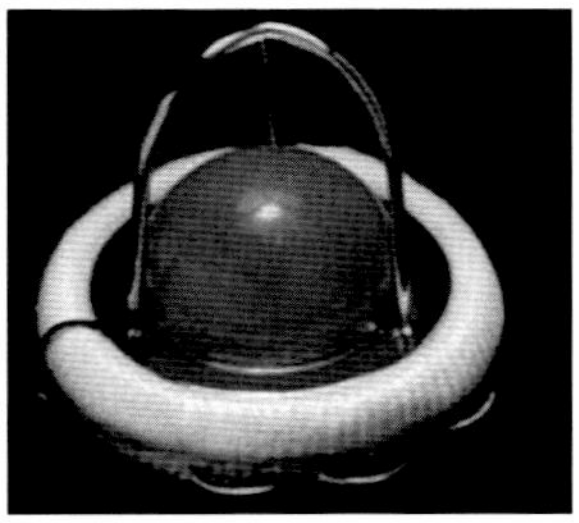		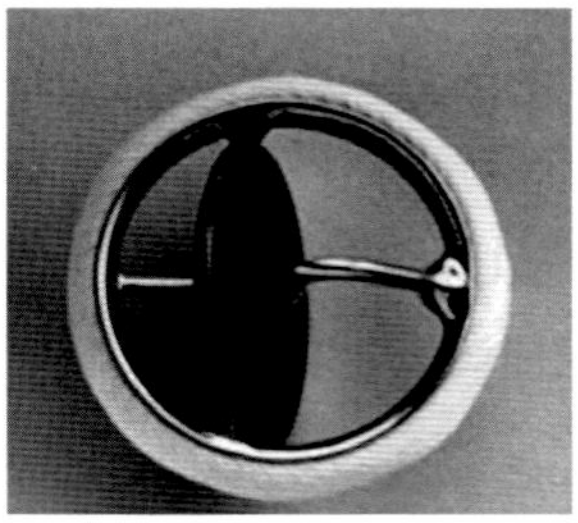		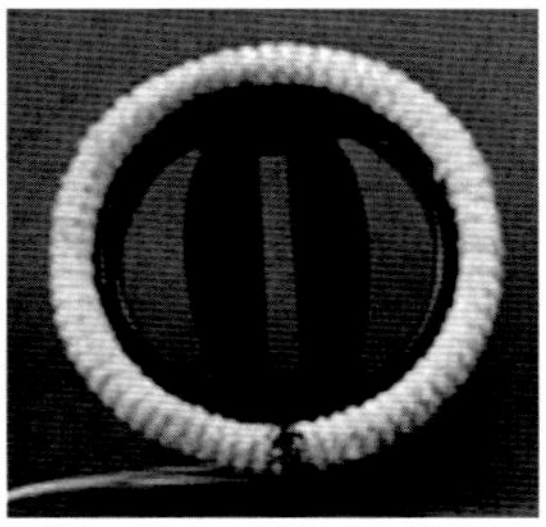	
Production years	Position/total implants	Production years	Position/total implants	Production years	Position/total implants
Starr–Edwards		**Bjork–shiley (Flat disc)**		**St. Jude Medical**	
1960–present	Aortic~80,000 Mitral~100,000	1969–1986	Aortic~157,000 Mitral~140,000	1977–present	Aortic~780,000 Mitral~520,000
Smeloff–Cutter		**Medtronic–hall**		**Carbomedics**	
1966–1988	Aortic } ~72,000 Mitral }	1977–present	Aortic~183,000 Mitral~122,000	1986–present	Aortic~307,000 Mitral~205,000
Magovern–Cromie		**Omni–Science**			
1962–1980	Aortic~ 7,300 Mitral < 200	1978–present	Aortic~ 72,000 Mitral < 26,000		
		Omni–Carbon			
		1984–present	Aortic~17,000 Mitral~13,000		

Fig. 38.1 Representative major mechanical heart valve structural designs, models, dates of production, and approximate number of implants (Adapter from Vongpatanasin et al. [4] and Gott et al. [3])

"seat" for the occluder and might include a cage-like structure or valve base and body. Pyrolytic carbon, a highly compatible and thromboresistant biomaterial that was first introduced in valve design in the mid-1970s, is now a major structural component of contemporary MHVs [5]. The basic valve design and structure of the six currently available mechanical prostheses in the United States have changed very little over the last two decades and are shown in Fig. 38.1.

The optimal antithrombotic regimen for patients with mechanical prostheses would minimize thromboembolic risk at an acceptable cost of bleeding. This decision is not straightforward because thromboembolic risk among patients with prosthetic mechanical heart valves is not uniform, varying based on numerous patient- and valve-related risk factors [6]. However, because most data on antithrombotic regimens in patients with mechanical valve prostheses are based on observational studies, estimates of thrombotic and bleeding risk are relatively imprecise. In the present article, we review the available evidence regarding the choice of anticoagulation strategy choices among patients with mechanical heart valves.

Pathophysiology

Risk Factors for Thrombosis

In addition to the substantial morbidity associated with cardiac surgery, the most feared complications after MHV replacement include major stroke, systemic embolization, and valve thrombosis. Risk is greatest in the immediate postoperative period and diminishes thereafter [7]. Physiologic changes in the coagulation cascade and platelet activation after implantation contribute to the heightened blood thrombogenicity following MHV surgery. Damaged perivalvular tissue and the prosthetic surface, for example, lead to activation of factor XII and initiation of the coagulation cascade [8]. This leads to subsequent platelet aggregation; platelet deposition may be visualized on the Dacron sewing ring as early as 24 h after surgery [9]. Shear forces generated by the mechanical prosthesis lead to ongoing cycles of platelet activation and destruction, which ultimately contribute to shortened platelet survival and augment thromboembolic potential. The impact of platelet kinetics on thromboembolism after MHV replacement was elegantly demonstrated in

Table 38.1 Risk factors for thromboembolism with mechanical heart valves

Valve-related	Patient-related
Valve design:	Atrial fibrillation
Caged-ball > monoleaflet > bileaflet	History of thromboembolism
Valve position:	Depressed ejection fraction
Nonaortic[a] > aortic	Hypercoagulable state
Time from surgery:	Advanced age
Early > late	Left atrial diameter >50 mm
	Dense left atrial spontaneous echocontrast
	Mitral stenosis

Reprinted, with permission from Baber et al. [12]

[a]Nonaortic includes mitral, tricuspid, pulmonic, and multiple valves

a historical study by Harker et al. [10]. In this study, the investigators compared platelet survival between 20 patients with various types of heart valve prostheses (18 mechanical, 2 bioprosthetic). The authors found a linear relationship between the total prosthetic material surface area and decrease in platelet survival such that platelet survival was 2.6 ± 0.2, 5.2 ± 0.1, and 6.5 ± 0.2 days in patients with double-valve, mitral, and aortic prostheses, respectively. Shortened platelet survival also correlated linearly with the incidence of embolic events. In addition, treatment with dipyridamole or aspirin plus dipyridamole led to near-normalization in platelet survival among MHV recipients. These findings suggest that platelets are consumed after implantation of a MHV and the magnitude of consumption is directly related to the total surface area of prosthetic material. These experimental observations are also consistent with clinical data demonstrating that thromboembolic complications are higher in patients with either double-valve (aortic and mitral) or mitral prostheses compared to aortic mechanical valves alone [6]. In a separate study, Dewanjee et al. quantified platelet deposition in 22 dogs after implantation of Bjork-Shiley mitral valve prostheses [11]. Platelet deposition on the prosthetic components was significantly reduced in prosthesis-implanted animals treated with dipyridamole and aspirin compared to prosthesis-implanted, untreated dogs [11]. In aggregate, these studies underscore the pathologic role of platelet aggregation in MHV-associated thrombosis and the potential role of platelet inhibitors in lowering this complication.

Additional correlates of thrombosis after MHV replacement include factors such as valve type, position, amount of time from surgery, and patient-related variables (Table 38.1) [6, 13]. Each type of valve differentially influences blood flow and turbulence, which partially explains variations in thrombogenicity for each valve design. Caged-ball valves, for example, generate areas of stagnant and circumferential blood flow and are associated with the greatest thromboembolic risk [14]. In contrast, monoleaflet (single leaflet or

tilting disk) valves have a major and minor orifice that provide central blood flow and thus reduce thrombotic risk compared with caged-ball designs [15]. Tilting disk valves have an area of stagnant blood flow adjacent to the minor orifice and a lower regurgitant jet volume compared with bileaflet valves, which may account for a slightly higher risk of thromboembolism than bileaflet prostheses [15]. Bileaflet valves generate central, nonturbulent blood flow and are associated with the lowest risk of thromboembolism of all valve designs and are currently the most commonly implanted mechanical heart valves in the world. Valve position is also an important determinant of thrombotic risk as mechanical mitral prostheses are associated with an approximately twofold increased risk of thromboembolism compared with aortic prostheses [6]. This may be partially attributable to a higher prevalence of underlying risk factors among patients who undergo mechanical mitral valve replacement (i.e., atrial fibrillation [AF]) compared with those who undergo aortic valve replacement. In addition to valve-related risk factors, patient-related variables contribute to thromboembolic risk among patients with mechanical heart valves. These risk factors include AF, prior thromboembolism, low ejection fraction, hypercoagulable state, and advanced age (see Table 38.1).

Diagnosis/Management

Initiation of Anticoagulation Following Surgery

The immediate postoperative period after MHV surgery is associated with the greatest risk for both hemorrhagic and thrombotic complications [13, 16]. In addition to patient-related factors, this risk is attributable to incomplete endothelialization of the sewing ring or other valve surfaces, increased variability of anticoagulation in the initial months after surgery, and prothrombotic changes in the coagulation cascade and platelet activation occurring at this time. Given the substantial risk for thromboembolic complications in the immediate postoperative period and the amount of time required for oral vitamin K antagonists to achieve optimal anticoagulant effect, bridging with an antithrombotic agent is necessary after MHV replacement. Potential advantages of low-molecular-weight vs. unfractionated heparin in this setting include self-administration, predictable anticoagulant effect, and a better safety profile [17]. Moreover, low-molecular-weight heparins (LMWH) have demonstrated both safety and efficacy in other clinical scenarios requiring anticoagulation such as acute coronary syndromes and venous thromboembolism prophylaxis [18]. Whether or not these benefits also extend to MHV recipients, however, is unknown as most studies are limited by single-center or non-randomized design. In the largest study to date, Montalescot

Fig. 38.2 Rate ratios (95 % CI) for embolism associated with different antithrombotics, valve position, and type (Data abstracted from Cannegieter et al. [6]) *Boxes* represent point estimates and lines 95 % confidence intervals (*CI*)

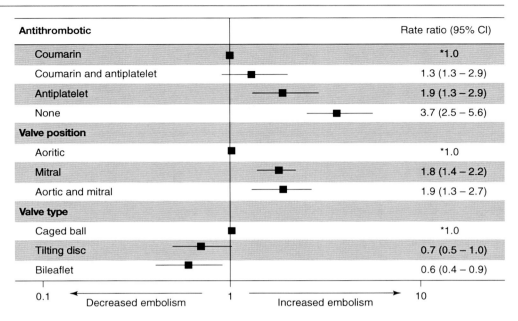

et al. compared the safety and efficacy of bridging with LMWH vs. unfractionated heparin in 208 patients after MHV replacement [19]. Most patients received single bileaflet valves in the aortic position. Although LMWH was associated with a more predictable and constant anticoagulant effect, the incidence of adverse events was very low with no differences between groups. In a separate single-center report, Fanikos et al. compared both clinical outcomes and economic costs between bridging with LMWH and unfractionated heparin in 63 patients after MHV replacement [20]. Similar to the findings of Montalescot et al., there were no significant differences in either thromboembolic or bleeding events between groups at 3 months of follow-up. Use of LMWH, however, was associated with a significantly shorter length of stay (6.6 ± 2.4 vs. 15.9 ± 10.7 days, $p < 0.001$) and lower total hospital costs ($\$29,141 \pm 11,415$ vs. $\$50,569 \pm 30,097$, $p < 0.001$). Pooling data from several observational studies, Kulik et al. [21] reported risk estimates for major embolism and hemorrhage in the first 30 days after mechanical valve replacement stratified by three commonly used antithrombotic regimens: oral anticoagulants alone (0.9 and 3.3 %), oral anticoagulants with intravenous unfractionated heparin (1.1 and 7.2 %), and oral anticoagulants with low-molecular-weight heparin ((LMWH) 0.6 and 4.8 %). Despite the limitations in the existing evidence base, current guidelines support the use of unfractionated heparin as a bridge to full anticoagulation with a vitamin K antagonist following surgery [22, 23]. Clearly, the optimal intensity of oral anticoagulation and the role of adjunctive heparin in the initial postoperative period after mechanical heart valve replacement are areas that require further investigation in adequately powered, prospective studies.

Chronic Oral Anticoagulation

Establishing reliable estimates of thromboembolic risk and the impact of antithrombotic therapy after MHV replacement is complicated by the marked clinical heterogeneity in the types of patients with advanced forms of valvular heart disease and the inclusion of different types of patients and/or valves within the same clinical study. In order to address these issues and provide more precise estimates of thromboembolic complications after implantation of a MHV, Cannegieter et al. pooled data from 46 studies involving over 13,000 patients [6]. Using meta-analytic techniques and multivariable Poisson regression, the investigators quantified the incidence of thromboembolic complications and the impact of various antithrombotic regimens on outcomes among patients undergoing MHV replacement in either the aortic, mitral, or both positions (Fig. 38.2) [6]. The incidence of major embolism among patients not receiving any antithrombotic therapy, antiplatelet therapy alone, and warfarin was 4.0, 2.2, and 1.0 per 100 patient-years, respectively. This risk also varied by valve type and position. A mechanical valve in the mitral position was associated with a twofold increased risk for major embolism vs. an aortic prosthesis. Moreover, a similar magnitude of incremental thrombotic risk was observed with caged-ball valves compared to either bileaflet or tilting disc valves. Based on these and other data, guidelines from multiple professional societies support the use of vitamin K antagonists for all patients with mechanical heart valve prostheses [22–24].

In a separate study, Cannegieter et al. also evaluated the impact of different international normalized ratio (INR) intensities on embolic and hemorrhagic complications in 1,608 patients following MHV replacement [25]. Most

Table 38.2 Contemporary guideline statements for a target INR for patients with mechanical heart valves

Valve position		Aortic			Mitral
Valve type		Bileaflet (e.g., St. Jude[a])	Monoleaflet (e.g., Medtronic Hall[b], Bjork-Shiley[c])	Caged-ball (e.g., Starr-Edwards[d])	
Management guidelines:					
ACC/AHA[e]	Target INR	2.0–3.0	2.0–3.0 Medtronic Hall; 2.5–3.5 other monoleaflet valves	2.5–3.5	2.5–3.5
	Aspirin	75–100 mg/day			
ACCP[f]	Target INR (range)	2.5 (2.0–3.0)	2.5 (2.0–3.0) Medtronic Hall; 3.0 (2.5–3.5) if additional patient risk factors[f]	3.0 (2.5–3.5)	3.0 (2.5–3.5)
	Aspirin	50–100 mg daily in patients at low risk of bleeding			
ESC[g]	Target INR	2.5–3.0	2.5–3.0 (Medtronic Hall); 3.0–3.5 (Bjork-Shiley and other monoleaflet valves)	3.5–4.0	3.0–4.0
	Aspirin	Consider in the presence of concomitant atherosclerotic disease and/or following embolic event in the setting of an adequate INR, in whom benefit outweighs risk of bleeding			

Modified from Baber et al. [12]

ACCP recommendations for older-generation prostheses based on 2008 document while recommendations for newer prostheses and aspirin from 2012 statement

ACC American College of Cardiology, *ACCP* American College of Chest Physicians, *AHA* American Heart Association, *ESC* European Society of Cardiology, *INR* international normalized ratio

[a]St. Jude Medical, Secaucus, NJ

[b]Medtronic, Minneapolis, MN

[c]Pfizer, New York, NY

[d]Edwards Laboratories, Irvine, CA

[e]Consider higher INR target with the following risk factors: prior thromboembolism or valve thrombosis, atrial fibrillation, left ventricular ejection fraction less than 35 %, or hypercoagulable state

[f]Consider higher INR target with the following risk factors: atrial fibrillation, anteroapical ST-elevation myocardial infarction, left atrial enlargement, hypercoagulability, or low ejection fraction

[g]Higher target INR is advised in patients with one or more of the following patient risk factors: previous thromboembolism, atrial fibrillation, left atrial diameter 0.50 mm, left atrial dense spontaneous contrast, mitral stenosis of any degree, left ventricular ejection fraction <35 %, or hypercoagulable state

patients (60 %) received an aortic prosthesis alone, and the most common type was a Bjork-Shiley tilting disc valve (65 %). In the overall population, the optimal INR range (in which bleeding and thromboembolic events were lowest) was between 2.5 and 4.9. Moreover, the association between INR intensity and clinical outcomes was modified by valve type. The optimal INR ranges for patients with caged-ball, tilting disk, and bileaflet valves were 4.0–4.9, 3.0–4.9, and 2.0–3.9, respectively (Table 38.2).

It is important to note that thromboembolic risk and anticoagulation requirements may have been overestimated in this study because most patients received older-generation tilting disk valves. Data from other randomized and single-center studies suggested that a lower INR target of 2.5 (range, 2.0–3.0) was efficacious in reducing thromboembolic events while reducing bleeding rates compared with higher INR targets among patients who mainly received mechanical bileaflet or Medtronic Hall tilting disk valves (Medtronic, Minneapolis, MN) in the aortic position [26–28]. In the study by Cannegieter et al., however, less than 20 % of patients received such bileaflet valves. In addition, the prevalence of AF was not reported in this study and may have also led to higher INR requirements. At present, current guidelines endorse a target INR of 2.5 for patients with mechanical bileaflet aortic or Medtronic Hall tilting disc valves

and no additional thromboembolic risk factors. Because mechanical caged-ball and mitral valves are more thrombogenic, however, a higher target INR is generally recommended [22–24, 29].

Adjunctive Antiplatelet Therapy

Antiplatelet therapy alone does not provide adequate protection against thromboembolic events or valve thrombosis among patients with mechanical heart valves, but may have a role as an adjunct to oral vitamin K antagonists in reducing thrombotic risk. In an observational study of 527 patients who underwent implantation of 590 St. Jude prostheses (232 aortic, 232 mitral, and 63 aortic and mitral), Czer et al. found that antiplatelet therapy alone was associated with a twofold increased risk for embolic events (3.2 %/patient-year) compared to warfarin therapy (1.5 %/patient-year) over an 8-year follow-up [30]. Antiplatelet therapy did yield some benefit, however, as thromboembolic risk was substantially higher in patients not receiving any drug therapy (18.9 %/patient-year). In addition, while valve thrombosis was rare (0.4 %/patient-year), this highly morbid complication exclusively occurred in patients not treated with effective warfarin therapy. Similarly, Ribeiro et al. also demonstrated that antiplatelet therapy alone was insufficient to prevent valve thrombosis in patients with St. Jude aortic prostheses [30]. Among 107 patients treated with antiplatelet therapy alone (aspirin and dipyridamole) after St. Jude mechanical aortic valve replacement, the investigators found that valve thrombosis occurred in five recipients over a mean follow-up of 22 months. As one person died after this complication, the case fatality rate for aortic valve thrombosis in this series was 20 %. Accordingly, all guidelines (American College of Cardiology/American Heart Association (ACC/AHA), European Society of Cardiology (ESC), and American College of Chest Physicians (ACCP)) are consistent in recommending vitamin K antagonists over antiplatelet agents alone as antithrombotic therapy in patients with MHV.

While there is general consensus on the importance of oral anticoagulation following MHV replacement, data on the potential benefits of adjunctive antiplatelet therapy on lowering embolic events is less consistent. In 1993 Turpie et al. reported the results of a landmark study comparing the safety and efficacy of adding aspirin (100 mg daily) vs. placebo in patients with prosthetic heart valves treated with chronic warfarin [31]. All patients either had a MHV or biological prostheses with high-risk features for thromboembolism, and approximately one-third of patients also had significant coronary artery disease (CAD). After an average of 2.5 years, aspirin use was associated with a large and significant reduction in major systemic embolism or vascular death (relative risk reduction [95 % CI]: 77 % [44–91 %], $p < 0.001$). The magnitude of benefit varied by the extent of underlying CAD as the absolute risk reductions in this endpoint in patients with abnormal and normal coronary arteries were 18.9 and 4.6 %, respectively. Bleeding was also significantly increased in the aspirin compared to placebo group (35.0 % vs. 22.0 %, $p = 0.02$). Similarly, in a meta-analysis combining data from 11 studies and 2,428 patients, Little et al. found that the addition of antiplatelet agents to oral anticoagulants reduced thromboembolic events and mortality in patients with mechanical heart valve prostheses compared with oral anticoagulants alone but at an increased cost of bleeding [32]. Although low-dose aspirin (100 mg/day) was associated with a reduction in mortality with no increase in bleeding, higher doses (≥ 500 mg/day) were associated with a significantly increased risk of bleeding without any mortality benefit. These findings are consistent with other data demonstrating that the clinical benefit of aspirin observed at lower doses (<150 mg/day) is attenuated by increased gastric toxicity and bleeding at higher doses. [33, 34] Both the ACC/AHA and ACCP guidelines provide level IB recommendations for the addition of low-dose aspirin to oral anticoagulants for patients with mechanical heart valves [22, 24]. In contrast, European guidelines emphasize that benefits with antiplatelet agents observed in studies of patients with both prosthetic heart valves and vascular disease cannot be extrapolated to those with prosthetic heart valves alone. As a result, aspirin is only recommended for those patients with mechanical heart valves who have additional vascular risk factors or following a thromboembolic event [23].

Anticoagulation Self-Monitoring

The therapeutic window for anticoagulation with vitamin K antagonists is narrow; INR levels below 2.0 increase the risk of thrombotic events, whereas levels over 4.5 are associated with an increased risk of hemorrhage [25]. Anticoagulation variability may be quantified by the time in therapeutic range (TITR) and has emerged as a strong correlate of both thromboembolic and bleeding complications after MHV replacement [35]. In a study involving over 1,400 patients who underwent single valve replacement with Medtronic Hall prostheses, Butchart et al. found that TITR was a strong and independent predictor of survival [35]. Survival at 15 years after aortic valve replacement in patients with low, intermediate, and high levels of anticoagulation variability was 59, 55, and 28 %, respectively. The analogous survival rates after mitral valve replacement were 56, 42, and 24 %, respectively. Moreover, anticoagulation variability emerged as an independent predictor of reduced survival after multivariable adjustment (Hazard Ratio (HR) 1.8, $p = 0.001$). The TITR also varies as a function of the monitoring environment, ranging from 55 to 60 % if anticoagulation is managed by general practitioners, 60–65 % in anticoagulation clinics, 70–75 % in clinical trials, and approaching 80 % in highly motivated individuals using a self-monitoring point-of-care test [36]. Advantages of INR self-monitoring over conventional laboratory-based methods include improved patient compliance, convenience, and greater frequency of monitoring. In the Early Self-Controlled Anticoagulation Trial I, Kortke et al. [37] found that the TITR was much higher in the self-management than the conventional group (79 % vs. 65 %). This translated into a reduction in thromboembolic events and a 23 % increase in survival in the self-management group [37, 38]. In addition to these clinical benefits, INR self-management is also associated with improved quality of life [39]. Similar findings have been reported in other groups of patients with mechanical heart valves or other indications for chronic oral anticoagulation [40]. Despite the clear benefits of INR self-management, barriers to widespread implementation of such programs include high costs along with patient training and education.

Interruption of Anticoagulation

Many patients with mechanical heart valves will be required to temporarily discontinue oral anticoagulation because of the need for surgical or other invasive procedures. Randomized studies evaluating different antithrombotic options in this setting are limited, and current recommendations are largely based on observational data and expert opinion [22, 23, 29]. Management decisions must be individualized to incorporate risks of surgical bleeding and valve-related thromboembolism. Several studies suggest that patients may be able to continue oral anticoagulants without interruption before procedures in which bleeding may be minimal or easily controlled, such as diagnostic endoscopy, cataract surgery, arthrocentesis, and dental extractions [41, 42]. However, antithrombotic therapy must be altered for surgical procedures in which bleeding may be associated with severe consequences. Despite limitations in existing data, American and European guidelines are relatively consistent on statements regarding anticoagulation interruption in patients with MHV. Recommendations for patients at low risk for thromboembolism (bileaflet aortic valves without other risk factors) are to discontinue warfarin 48–72 h before the procedure and to resume oral anticoagulation 24 h after surgery [22, 23]. In contrast, for patients at high risk for thromboembolism, current guidelines endorse using periprocedural intravenous unfractionated heparin as bridging therapy. High-risk patients include those with mechanical mitral prostheses or aortic prostheses with additional risk factors. Heparin should be administered from the time the INR becomes subtherapeutic until 4–6 h before the surgery and restarted as early as possible after surgery. A few studies also suggest that LMWH may be used as an alternative anticoagulant in this setting [43–45]. In one retrospective analysis, Spyropoulos et al. compared clinical outcomes and total health-care costs between bridging with LMWH and unfractionated heparin in patients on long-term oral anticoagulation [45]. Approximately 40 % of patients had a MHV, and the most common surgeries were either orthopedic or cardiothoracic. While there were no differences in the incidence of adverse clinical events at 30 days (34.6 % vs. 40.0 %, $p=0.67$), bridging with LMWH was associated with significantly lower total health-care costs ($18,511 vs. $31,625, $p<0.01$). These cost savings were primarily attributed to outpatient vs. inpatient bridging between groups. Despite these encouraging results, current ACC/AHA and ESC guidelines tend to emphasize the inherent limitations in existing data regarding the safety and efficacy of LMWH among patients with MHV and generally favor unfractionated heparin (Class I or IIa) over LMWH (Class IIb) as a bridging anticoagulant [22].

Pregnancy

Pregnancy is associated with alterations in hemostasis and coagulability that increase the risk of thromboembolic events among women with mechanical prosthetic heart valves [46, 47]. Estimates of maternal mortality in such patients vary between 1 and 4 %, with most deaths attributable to thrombotic complications [48, 49]. The possibility of fetal toxicity and changes in dose requirements of antithrombotic agents during pregnancy further complicate management decisions in this high-risk population. Warfarin crosses the placenta and is associated with teratogenicity and fetal bleeding [50, 51]. Embryopathy resulting from in utero exposure to warfarin appears to be greatest during the first trimester, particularly between weeks 6 and 12 of gestation. Heparin does not cross the placenta and is considered a safer alternative to warfarin in terms of fetal side effects, but may be less efficacious in reducing maternal thromboembolic risk compared with warfarin [48]. In addition, prolonged exposure to heparin is associated with thrombocytopenia and osteoporosis [52, 53].

In the absence of controlled clinical trials, current recommendations are based on limited, observational data. In a systematic review of 24 studies and over 900 pregnant women with mechanical prosthetic heart valves, Chan et al. [48] evaluated maternal and fetal outcomes according to the type of antithrombotic regimen used during pregnancy: oral anticoagulants alone, oral anticoagulants substituted with heparin during the first trimester, heparin throughout pregnancy, and antiplatelet agents alone. Rates of maternal thromboembolic complications in women who received heparin alone, oral anticoagulants with heparin substitution during the first trimester, and warfarin alone were 33.3, 9.2, and 3.9 %, respectively. The corresponding rates of congenital fetal anomalies were 0, 3.4, and 6.4 %, respectively. These data suggest that heparin alone provides inadequate protection against thromboembolism among pregnant women with mechanical prosthetic heart valves compared with warfarin-containing regimens. Compared to regimens using warfarin alone, substitution with heparin during the first trimester is associated with a reduction in embryopathy from 6.4 to 3.4 % but increased maternal thromboembolic risk from 3.9 to 9.2 %. LMWHs offer several advantages over other antithrombotics used during pregnancy because of a lack of fetal toxicity and a lower incidence of osteopenia and thrombocytopenia compared with unfractionated heparin [17, 54]. Although LMWH appears to be a safe and efficacious alternative antithrombotic agent in nonpregnant patients, its role in thromboprophylaxis among pregnant women with mechanical prosthetic heart valves remains controversial as several authors have reported fatal valve thrombosis in pregnant women receiving LMWH alone [55, 56].

Despite the inherent limitations and inconsistencies in the available data regarding the optimal antithrombotic regimen in pregnant women with MHV, professional societies share several similarities in respective guideline statements. All guidelines, for example, emphasize discontinuing warfarin and substituting with heparin prior to delivery due to the risks of both fetal and maternal hemorrhage with warfarin use at this time [22, 57, 58]. Moreover, aggressive dose adjustment with frequent therapeutic monitoring of heparin

Table 38.3 Summary of antithrombotic agents, monitoring parameters, and associated risk during pregnancy

Anticoagulant	Monitoring	Fetal risk	Maternal risk	Favored use in pregnancy[a]
Warfarin	INR: 2.5–3.5	Embryopathy	Spontaneous abortion	Second and third trimester
UFH	aPTT ≥ twice the control	Minimal	Valve thrombosis/embolism, osteoporosis, HIT	First trimester and delivery
LMWH	Anti-Xa levels: 0.7 and 1.2 U/mL	Minimal	Valve thrombosis/embolism	First trimester and delivery

INR international normalized ratio, *UFH* unfractionated heparin, *LMWH* low-molecular-weight heparin, *aPTT* activated partial thromboplastin time

[a]Favored use refers to balancing maternal thromboembolic and fetal risk with different regimens at different times during pregnancy and is based on guideline documents from ACC/AHA, ACCP, and ESC

(LMWH and unfractionated) is also consistently emphasized in different guideline statements. Alternatively, American and European societies primarily differ in emphasizing heparin substitution for warfarin during the first trimester, when risk for Coumadin embryopathy appears to be highest. Citing several studies suggesting this risk may be minimal at warfarin doses less than 5 mg daily [59, 60], recent European guidelines advocate continuing warfarin (Class IIa) over substitution with heparin (Class IIb) at doses under this threshold in the first trimester [58]. A Class IIa recommendation is made for heparin substitution at warfarin doses exceeding 5 mg daily. In contrast, ACC/AHA guidelines do not stratify based on warfarin dose requirements, providing a Class IIa recommendation for heparin substitution during weeks 6–12 [22]. In addition, ACCP guidelines only recommend warfarin throughout pregnancy in those patients at highest risk for thromboembolism (i.e., older-generation or mitral prostheses) [57]. Another difference exists in the role of adjunctive aspirin in pregnant women with MHV. While the ACC/AHA guidelines provide a Class IIa recommendation for aspirin use in the second and third trimester, the ACCP only recommends this therapy in the highest-risk patients. There are no specific recommendations on aspirin use in the most recent European guidelines due to lack of data. Table 38.3 provides a general summary of the different anticoagulant options during pregnancy based on major guideline documents.

Bleeding and Holding Anticoagulation

The combination of thromboembolic and bleeding complications accounts for 75 % of all adverse events associated with MHV [16]. Although excessive anticoagulation increases bleeding risk, rapid decreases in INR may also lead to thromboembolism if the INR falls below the therapeutic range. As a result, in patients with elevated INR (5–10) without any bleeding, both ACC/AHA and ESC guidelines recommend withholding warfarin with or without low-dose oral vitamin K [23, 61]. The INR should be reassessed within 24 h and therapy adjusted as needed. In the presence of active bleeding or extremely elevated INR (>10.0), fresh frozen plasma

may be administered. In general, parenteral vitamin K should be avoided as this increases the risk of overcorrection to a hypercoagulable state.

Atrial Fibrillation

Atrial fibrillation (AF) is a common cardiac arrhythmia that is associated with an increased risk of ischemic stroke and mortality [62]. Because risk factors for AF and many forms of valvular heart disease are similar, it is not surprising that AF is frequently observed among patients who require cardiac valve replacement. Multiple randomized controlled trials have evaluated various antithrombotic regimens among patients with AF and have demonstrated that adjusted-dose warfarin to an INR between 2.0 and 3.0 offers the greatest protection against ischemic events [63]. Extrapolating these results to patients with both AF and mechanical heart valves is problematic, as most AF trials excluded participants with "valvular" AF (AF in the presence of mitral stenosis or a prosthetic heart valve). Similarly, many studies evaluating antithrombotic regimens among patients with mechanical heart valve prostheses excluded those with AF, whereas others did not report results in subgroups with AF [26, 64]. No controlled clinical trial to date has assessed antithrombotic strategy in patients with both AF and mechanical heart valve prostheses. Despite the lack of conclusive evidence, current guidelines support increasing the intensity of oral anticoagulation for patients with mechanical heart valves in the presence of AF [22, 23].

Novel Anticoagulants

At present, vitamin K antagonists are the only approved oral anticoagulants for thromboprophylaxis in patients with MHV. The limitations of warfarin—its narrow therapeutic window, unpredictable pharmacologic response, and requirement for frequent monitoring—have prompted a search for new oral anticoagulants for various indications [65]. Several novel oral agents targeting the initiation or propagation of the coagulation cascade have been evaluated in clinical trials.

These include inhibitors of factor Xa and factor IIa (thrombin). Dabigatran, an oral direct thrombin inhibitor, was recently shown to be as effective as adjusted-dose warfarin in preventing stroke and systemic embolism among patients with AF [66]. Compared to warfarin, pharmacologic advantages of dabigatran include lack of food or drug interactions, a shorter half-life, and no monitoring of anticoagulant effect with routine blood tests. In addition to AF, dabigatran has shown similar efficacy to either warfarin or LMWH in the primary and secondary prevention of deep venous thrombosis following orthopedic surgery [67, 68]. Emerging experimental data also suggest a potential role for this novel oral anticoagulant in patients with MHV. In a swine animal model, McKellar et al. measured thrombus size and platelet deposition 30 days after implantation of bileaflet mechanical valve conduits [69]. Thrombus size was smallest in animals randomly allocated with dabigatran (19 ± 31) compared to either enoxaparin (121 ± 128) or no anticoagulation (638 ± 895), respectively. Similarly, platelet deposition was lower in the dabigatran vs. enoxaparin group (2.7×10^8 vs. 1.8×10^9, $p = 0.03$). Other investigators have reported similar results from in vitro experiments using the direct thrombin inhibitors argatroban and bivalirudin [70]. Factor Xa inhibitors, including rivaroxaban and apixaban, have also shown promising results in the treatment and prophylaxis of venous thromboembolic disease and are currently being evaluated in AF [71]. Whether or not these encouraging findings might also extend to humans with mechanical valve prostheses is the subject of ongoing investigation. It is important to emphasize that none of these novel anticoagulants have been evaluated among patients with mechanical heart valves and cannot be recommended as alternatives to vitamin K antagonists at this time.

Key Points

- MHV are inherently thrombogenic and the risk for thromboembolic complications varies as a function of both patient risk factors and valve parameters such as structural design, position, and time from surgery. Thrombotic risk is greatest in the immediate postoperative period and diminishes thereafter.
- All patients with MHV require lifelong anticoagulation with vitamin K antagonists.
- Adjunctive antiplatelet therapy with low-dose aspirin is also reasonable for patients with MHV, particularly in those with concomitant vascular risk factors.
- Interruption of anticoagulation is not necessary for minor procedures where risk of bleeding is minimal or can be easily controlled. In other surgical procedures with greater bleeding potential, bridging with unfractionated heparin is preferred over LMWH.
- Variability in anticoagulation is a major correlate of adverse events in patients with MHV and may be greatly improved with devices that facilitate patient self-monitoring.
- Pregnant patients with MHV require very close and aggressive monitoring of all antithrombotics that may be used: unfractionated heparin, LMWH, and oral vitamin K antagonists. Warfarin should be discontinued prior to delivery and substituted with heparin.

Summary of Key Guidelines

Key guideline statements from several professional societies (ACC/AHA, ACCP, and ESC) addressing anticoagulation therapy with mechanical heart valves are summarized in Table 38.2. In general, all organizations advocate higher intensity of anticoagulation with mitral vs. aortic mechanical prostheses and with monoleaflet vs. bileaflet valves in the aortic position. While adjunctive antiplatelet therapy is recommended in all patients with MHV in the ACC/AHA guidelines, aspirin is only recommended in patients with concomitant risk factors or at low risk of bleeding in the ESC and ACCP guidelines, respectively [22–24].

Current guidelines recommend frequent monitoring of anticoagulation therapy during pregnancy for women with mechanical prosthetic heart valves irrespective of the antithrombotic regimen chosen [22, 23]. Warfarin should be dose-adjusted to attain a target INR of 3.0 (range, 2.5–3.5), whereas the dose of unfractionated heparin should prolong the 6-h postinjection activated partial thromboplastin time to at least twice the control. Recommendations on LMWH suggest twice-daily administration to achieve an anti-Xa level of 0.7–1.2 U/mL 4–6 h after injection [22]. Heparin should also be substituted for warfarin 1–3 weeks before labor and delivery to minimize maternal bleeding and prevent fetal hemorrhage that might occur if the mother is taking warfarin during that time.

Bridging therapy with heparin may be required in patients with MHV requiring surgery or other invasive procedures. Certain low-risk procedures in which bleeding risk is minimal do not require interruption of anticoagulation (diagnostic endoscopy, cataract surgery, dental extraction). If needed due to bleeding risk at time of surgery, guidelines support interrupting anticoagulation and generally recommend bridging with unfractionated heparin over LMWH [22, 23].

References

1. Carapetis JR, Currie BJ, Mathews JD. Cumulative incidence of rheumatic fever in an endemic region: a guide to the susceptibility of the population? Epidemiol Infect. 2000;124:239–44.
2. Schoen F. Pathology of heart valve substitution with mechanical and tissue prostheses. In: Silver MD, Gotlieb AI, Schoen FJ, editors. Cardiovascular pathology. Philadelphia: Churchill Livingstone; 2001. p. 629–77.
3. Gott VL, Alejo DE, Cameron DE. Mechanical heart valves: 50 years of evolution. Ann Thorac Surg. 2003;76:S2230–9.
4. Vongpatanasin W, Hillis LD, Lange RA. Prosthetic heart valves. N Engl J Med. 1996;335:407–16.
5. Bokros JC. Carbon in prosthetic heart valves. Ann Thorac Surg. 1989;48:S49–50.
6. Cannegieter SC, Rosendaal FR, Briet E. Thromboembolic and bleeding complications in patients with mechanical heart valve prostheses. Circulation. 1994;89:635–41.
7. Heras M, Chesebro JH, Fuster V, et al. High risk of thromboemboli early after bioprosthetic cardiac valve replacement. J Am Coll Cardiol. 1995;25:1111–9.
8. Chesebro JH, Adams PC, Fuster V. Antithrombotic therapy in patients with valvular heart disease and prosthetic heart valves. J Am Coll Cardiol. 1986;8:41B–56.
9. Dewanjee MK, Trastek VF, Tago M, Kaye MP. Radioisotopic techniques for noninvasive detection of platelet deposition in bovine-tissue mitral-valve prostheses and in vitro quantification of visceral microembolism in dogs. Invest Radiol. 1984;19:535–42.
10. Harker LA, Slichter SJ. Studies of platelet and fibrinogen kinetics in patients with prosthetic heart valves. N Engl J Med. 1970;283:1302–5.
11. Dewanjee MK, Fuster V, Rao SA, Forshaw PL, Kaye MP. Noninvasive radioisotopic technique for detection of platelet deposition in mitral valve prostheses and quantitation of visceral microembolism in dogs. Mayo Clin Proc. 1983;58:307–14.
12. Baber U, van der Zee S, Fuster V. Anticoagulation for mechanical heart valves in patients with and without atrial fibrillation. Curr Cardiol Rep. 2010;12:133–9.
13. Butchart EG, Lewis PA, Kulatilake EN, Breckenridge IM. Anticoagulation variability between centres: implications for comparative prosthetic valve assessment. Eur J Cardiothorac Surg. 1988;2:72–81.
14. Yoganathan AP, He Z, Casey JS. Fluid mechanics of heart valves. Annu Rev Biomed Eng. 2004;6:331–62.
15. Butany J, Ahluwalia MS, Munroe C, et al. Mechanical heart valve prostheses: identification and evaluation. Cardiovasc Pathol. 2003;12:1–22.
16. Edmunds Jr LH. Thrombotic and bleeding complications of prosthetic heart valves. Ann Thorac Surg. 1987;44:430–45.
17. Weitz JI. Low-molecular-weight heparins. N Engl J Med. 1997;337:688–98.
18. Cohen M, Demers C, Gurfinkel EP, et al. A comparison of low-molecular-weight heparin with unfractionated heparin for unstable coronary artery disease. Efficacy and safety of subcutaneous enoxaparin in Non-Q-Wave Coronary Events Study Group. N Engl J Med. 1997;337:447–52.
19. Montalescot G, Polle V, Collet JP, et al. Low molecular weight heparin after mechanical heart valve replacement. Circulation. 2000;101:1083–6.
20. Fanikos J, Stapinski C, Koo S, Kucher N, Tsilimingras K, Goldhaber SZ. Medication errors associated with anticoagulant therapy in the hospital. Am J Cardiol. 2004;94:532–5.
21. Kulik A, Rubens FD, Wells PS, et al. Early postoperative anticoagulation after mechanical valve replacement: a systematic review. Ann Thorac Surg. 2006;81:770–81.
22. Bonow RO, Carabello BA, Chatterjee K, et al. 2008 focused update incorporated into the ACC/AHA 2006 guidelines for the management of patients with valvular heart disease: a report of the American College of Cardiology/American Heart Association Task Force on Practice Guidelines (writing committee to revise the 1998 guidelines for the management of patients with valvular heart disease): endorsed by the Society of Cardiovascular Anesthesiologists, Society for Cardiovascular Angiography and Interventions, and Society of Thoracic Surgeons. Circulation. 2008;118:e523–661.
23. Vahanian A, Baumgartner H, Bax J, et al. Guidelines on the management of valvular heart disease: The Task Force on the Management of Valvular Heart Disease of the European Society of Cardiology. Eur Heart J. 2007;28:230–68.
24. Whitlock RP, Sun JC, Fremes SE, Rubens FD, Teoh KH. Antithrombotic and thrombolytic therapy for valvular disease: antithrombotic therapy and prevention of thrombosis, 9th ed: American College of Chest Physicians evidence-based clinical practice guidelines. Chest. 2012;141:e576S–600.
25. Cannegieter SC, Rosendaal FR, Wintzen AR, van der Meer FJ, Vandenbroucke JP, Briet E. Optimal oral anticoagulant therapy in patients with mechanical heart valves. N Engl J Med. 1995;333:11–7.
26. Acar J, Iung B, Boissel JP, et al. AREVA: multicenter randomized comparison of low-dose versus standard-dose anticoagulation in patients with mechanical prosthetic heart valves. Circulation. 1996;94:2107–12.
27. Butchart EG, Lewis PA, Bethel JA, Breckenridge IM. Adjusting anticoagulation to prosthesis thrombogenicity and patient risk factors. Recommendations for the Medtronic Hall valve. Circulation. 1991;84:III61–9.
28. Hering D, Piper C, Bergemann R, et al. Thromboembolic and bleeding complications following St Jude Medical valve replacement: results of the German Experience With Low-Intensity Anticoagulation Study. Chest. 2005;127:53–9.
29. Salem DN, O'Gara PT, Madias C, Pauker SG. Valvular and structural heart disease: American College of Chest Physicians evidence-based clinical practice guidelines (8th edition). Chest. 2008;133:593S–629.
30. Czer LS, Matloff JM, Chaux A, De Robertis M, Stewart ME, Gray RJ. The St. Jude valve: analysis of thromboembolism, warfarin-related hemorrhage, and survival. Am Heart J. 1987;114:389–97.
31. Turpie AG, Gent M, Laupacis A, et al. A comparison of aspirin with placebo in patients treated with warfarin after heart-valve replacement. N Engl J Med. 1993;329:524–9.
32. Little SH, Massel DR. Antiplatelet and anticoagulation for patients with prosthetic heart valves. Cochrane Database Syst Rev 2003:CD003464.
33. Antithrombotic Trialists' Collaboration. Collaborative meta-analysis of randomised trials of antiplatelet therapy for prevention of death, myocardial infarction, and stroke in high risk patients. BMJ. 2002;324:71–86.
34. Patrono C. Aspirin and human platelets: from clinical trials to acetylation of cyclooxygenase and back. Trends Pharmacol Sci. 1989;10:453–8.
35. Butchart EG, Payne N, Li HH, Buchan K, Mandana K, Grunkemeier GL. Better anticoagulation control improves survival after valve replacement. J Thorac Cardiovasc Surg. 2002;123:715–23.
36. Ansell J, Hirsh J, Poller L, Bussey H, Jacobson A, Hylek E. The pharmacology and management of the vitamin K antagonists: the seventh ACCP conference on antithrombotic and thrombolytic therapy. Chest. 2004;126:204S–33.
37. Kortke H, Minami K, Breymann T, et al. INR self-management after mechanical heart valve replacement: ESCAT (early self-controlled anticoagulation trial). Z Kardiol. 2001;90 Suppl 6:118–24.
38. Koertke H, Zittermann A, Wagner O, Koerfer R. Self-management of oral anticoagulation therapy improves long-term survival in

patients with mechanical heart valve replacement. Ann Thorac Surg. 2007;83:24–9.

39. Sawicki PT. A structured teaching and self-management program for patients receiving oral anticoagulation: a randomized controlled trial. Working Group for the Study of Patient Self-Management of Oral Anticoagulation. JAMA. 1999;281:145–50.

40. Heneghan C, Alonso-Coello P, Garcia-Alamino JM, Perera R, Meats E, Glasziou P. Self-monitoring of oral anticoagulation: a systematic review and meta-analysis. Lancet. 2006;367:404–11.

41. Dunn AS, Turpie AG. Perioperative management of patients receiving oral anticoagulants: a systematic review. Arch Intern Med. 2003;163:901–8.

42. Wahl MJ. Dental surgery in anticoagulated patients. Arch Intern Med. 1998;158:1610–6.

43. Ferreira I, Dos L, Tornos P, Nicolau I, Permanyer-Miralda G, Soler-Soler J. Experience with enoxaparin in patients with mechanical heart valves who must withhold acenocumarol. Heart. 2003;89:527–30.

44. Kovacs MJ, Kearon C, Rodger M, et al. Single-arm study of bridging therapy with low-molecular-weight heparin for patients at risk of arterial embolism who require temporary interruption of warfarin. Circulation. 2004;110:1658–63.

45. Spyropoulos AC, Frost FJ, Hurley JS, Roberts M. Costs and clinical outcomes associated with low-molecular-weight heparin vs unfractionated heparin for perioperative bridging in patients receiving long-term oral anticoagulant therapy. Chest. 2004;125:1642–50.

46. Brenner B. Haemostatic changes in pregnancy. Thromb Res. 2004; 114:409–14.

47. Comp PC, Thurnau GR, Welsh J, Esmon CT. Functional and immunologic protein S levels are decreased during pregnancy. Blood. 1986;68:881–5.

48. Chan WS, Anand S, Ginsberg JS. Anticoagulation of pregnant women with mechanical heart valves: a systematic review of the literature. Arch Intern Med. 2000;160:191–6.

49. Elkayam U, Bitar F. Valvular heart disease and pregnancy: part II: prosthetic valves. J Am Coll Cardiol. 2005;46:403–10.

50. Ginsberg JS, Hirsh J, Turner DC, Levine MN, Burrows R. Risks to the fetus of anticoagulant therapy during pregnancy. Thromb Haemost. 1989;61:197–203.

51. Hall JG, Pauli RM, Wilson KM. Maternal and fetal sequelae of anticoagulation during pregnancy. Am J Med. 1980;68:122–40.

52. Douketis JD, Ginsberg JS, Burrows RF, Duku EK, Webber CE, Brill-Edwards P. The effects of long-term heparin therapy during pregnancy on bone density. A prospective matched cohort study. Thromb Haemost. 1996;75:254–7.

53. Warkentin TE, Levine MN, Hirsh J, et al. Heparin-induced thrombocytopenia in patients treated with low-molecular-weight heparin or unfractionated heparin. N Engl J Med. 1995;332:1330–5.

54. Harenberg J, Schneider D, Heilmann L, Wolf H. Lack of anti-factor Xa activity in umbilical cord vein samples after subcutaneous administration of heparin or low molecular mass heparin in pregnant women. Haemostasis. 1993;23:314–20.

55. Berndt N, Khan I, Gallo R. A complication in anticoagulation using low-molecular weight heparin in a patient with a mechanical valve prosthesis. A case report. J Heart Valve Dis. 2000;9:844–6.

56. Lev-Ran O, Kramer A, Gurevitch J, Shapira I, Mohr R. Low-molecular-weight heparin for prosthetic heart valves: treatment failure. Ann Thorac Surg. 2000;69:264–5; discussion 5–6.

57. Bates SM, Greer IA, Pabinger I, Sofaer S, Hirsh J. Venous thromboembolism, thrombophilia, antithrombotic therapy, and pregnancy: American College of Chest Physicians evidence-based clinical practice guidelines (8th edition). Chest. 2008;133:844S–86.

58. Regitz-Zagrosek V, Blomstrom Lundqvist C, Borghi C, et al. ESC guidelines on the management of cardiovascular diseases during pregnancy: the Task Force on the Management of Cardiovascular Diseases during pregnancy of the European Society of Cardiology (ESC). Eur Heart J. 2011;32:3147–97.

59. Cotrufo M, De Feo M, De Santo LS, et al. Risk of warfarin during pregnancy with mechanical valve prostheses. Obstet Gynecol. 2002;99:35–40.

60. Sillesen M, Hjortdal V, Vejlstrup N, Sorensen K. Pregnancy with prosthetic heart valves – 30 years' nationwide experience in Denmark. Eur J Cardiothorac Surg. 2011;40:448–54.

61. Bonow RO, Carabello BA, Kanu C, et al. ACC/AHA 2006 guidelines for the management of patients with valvular heart disease: a report of the American College of Cardiology/American Heart Association Task Force on Practice Guidelines (writing committee to revise the 1998 guidelines for the management of patients with valvular heart disease): developed in collaboration with the Society of Cardiovascular Anesthesiologists: endorsed by the Society for Cardiovascular Angiography and Interventions and the Society of Thoracic Surgeons. Circulation. 2006;114:e84–231.

62. Wolf PA, Abbott RD, Kannel WB. Atrial fibrillation as an independent risk factor for stroke: the Framingham Study. Stroke. 1991;22: 983–8.

63. Hart RG, Pearce LA, Aguilar MI. Meta-analysis: antithrombotic therapy to prevent stroke in patients who have nonvalvular atrial fibrillation. Ann Intern Med. 2007;146:857–67.

64. Fanikos J, Tsilimingras K, Kucher N, Rosen AB, Hieblinger MD, Goldhaber SZ. Comparison of efficacy, safety, and cost of low-molecular-weight heparin with continuous-infusion unfractionated heparin for initiation of anticoagulation after mechanical prosthetic valve implantation. Am J Cardiol. 2004;93:247–50.

65. Turpie AG. New oral anticoagulants in atrial fibrillation. Eur Heart J. 2008;29:155–65.

66. Connolly SJ, Ezekowitz MD, Yusuf S, et al. Dabigatran versus warfarin in patients with atrial fibrillation. N Engl J Med. 2009; 361:1139–51.

67. Eriksson BI, Dahl OE, Rosencher N, et al. Dabigatran etexilate versus enoxaparin for prevention of venous thromboembolism after total hip replacement: a randomised, double-blind, non-inferiority trial. Lancet. 2007;370:949–56.

68. Schulman S, Kearon C, Kakkar AK, et al. Dabigatran versus warfarin in the treatment of acute venous thromboembolism. N Engl J Med. 2009;361:2342–52.

69. McKellar SH, Abel S, Camp CL, Suri RM, Ereth MH, Schaff HV. Effectiveness of dabigatran etexilate for thromboprophylaxis of mechanical heart valves. J Thorac Cardiovasc Surg. 2011;141:1410–6.

70. Maegdefessel L, Linde T, Michel T, et al. Argatroban and bivalirudin compared to unfractionated heparin in preventing thrombus formation on mechanical heart valves. Results of an in-vitro study. Thromb Haemost. 2009;101:1163–9.

71. Lassen MR, Davidson BL, Gallus A, Pineo G, Ansell J, Deitchman D. The efficacy and safety of apixaban, an oral, direct factor Xa inhibitor, as thromboprophylaxis in patients following total knee replacement. J Thromb Haemost. 2007;5:2368–75.

Part VI

Cardiac Disease as a Source of Neurologic Sequelae

Evaluation of Patients with Suspected Cardiac Sources of Emboli

39

Adam A. Harris and David L. Brown

Abstract

The presentation of a patient with an acute arterial embolic event is not only dramatic for the acuity and severity of symptoms; it is also the harbinger of potentially life-threatening disease. Recognition of the many clinical manifestations that can result as emboli travel through the arterial system is the first step in the evaluation for cardiac sources of emboli. While nearly every organ in the body is a potential embolic target, the incidence of clinically apparent embolic events is approximately three times higher in the cerebral circulation than the peripheral circulation. The most common source of cardiac emboli is a left atrial thrombus due to atrial fibrillation, whereas the second most common source is a left ventricular thrombus following an acute myocardial infarction. Other etiologies include endocarditis, cardiac tumors, and aortic atherosclerosis. While a transthoracic echocardiogram (TTE) is the initial imaging test for most patients, transesophageal echocardiography (TTE) has been shown to be superior to TTE at detecting cardiac sources of emboli and is also more cost effective. Once a cardiac source of emboli is identified, management depends on the underlying etiology and patient comorbidities.

Keywords

Emboli • Thrombus • Stroke

Introduction

The presentation of a patient with an acute arterial embolic event is not only dramatic for the acuity and severity of symptoms; it is also the harbinger of potentially life-threatening disease. Because of the cardiovascular nature of the embolic syndromes, cardiologists are frequently the primary consultants for affected patients.

A.A. Harris, MD (✉)
Department of Internal Medicine, NYU Langone Medical Center,
550 1st Ave., New York, NY 10016, USA
e-mail: adam.harris@nyumc.org

D.L. Brown, MD, FACC
Division of Cardiology, Department of Medicine,
Stony Brook University School of Medicine, HSC 16-080,
Stony Brook, NY 11794, USA
e-mail: david.brown@stonybrookmedicine.edu

Therefore, recognizing the many clinical manifestations that can result as emboli travel through the arterial system is the first step in the evaluation for cardiac sources of emboli. While nearly every organ in the body is a potential embolic target, the incidence of clinically apparent embolic events is approximately three times higher in the cerebral circulation than the peripheral circulation [1, 2]. This may be due to the fact that most cerebral arteries are functional end arteries, whereas the peripheral circulation tends to have a rich anastomotic blood supply that can stave off clinically significant ischemia while the thrombus resolves. Other potential end organs of arterial emboli include the spleen, kidney, gut, eye, and, although commonly overlooked, the heart itself. Finally, diseases of the right heart can result in pulmonary emboli. The most common source of cardiac emboli is a left atrial thrombus due to atrial fibrillation (AF) [3], whereas the second most common source is a left ventricular (LV) thrombus following an acute myocardial infarction (MI) [1].

K. Stergiopoulos, D.L. Brown (eds.), *Evidence-Based Cardiology Consult*,
DOI 10.1007/978-1-4471-4441-0_39, © Springer-Verlag London 2014

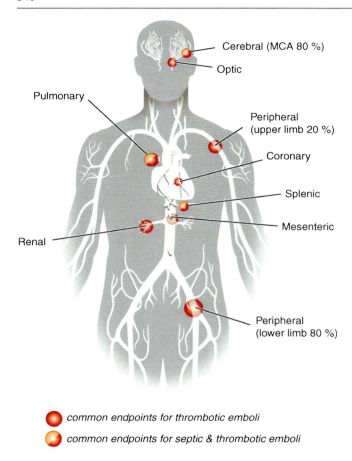

common endpoints for thrombotic emboli

common endpoints for septic & thrombotic emboli

Fig. 39.1 Common destinations for cardiac emboli

vertebral arteries. It is very rare for cardiac emboli to reach the anterior cerebral artery [8]. If the embolic thrombus is lysed quickly, only a transient ischemic attack (TIA) will occur. TIAs are defined as symptoms of stroke that last less than 24 h; however, most last less than 1 h. Patients with a history of TIA are at a very high risk for subsequent stroke, with an incidence of approximately 17 % by 90 days if untreated [9]. Immediate work-up and treatment of the underlying cause of embolism are imperative when TIA is suspected as the risk of subsequent stroke is highest in the days and weeks immediately after the TIA [10].

Peripheral Arterial Embolization

Cardiac emboli are by far the most common cause of peripheral artery embolization, with ischemic heart disease and AF accounting for approximately 80 % of cases. The lower extremities are involved in approximately 80 % of cases and the upper extremities in only 20 % [11]. As opposed to chronic limb ischemia in which collateral vessels develop over time to compensate for decreased antegrade flow, peripheral artery embolization results in an acute reduction of blood flow to the affected limb and is a medical emergency. Acute limb ischemia is a clinical diagnosis; symptoms include the 6 "Ps": pain, pulselessness, pallor, poikilothermia, paresthesias, and paralysis. Pain is generally the earliest and the most dominant symptom [12].

Other etiologies include endocarditis, cardiac tumors, and aortic atherosclerosis.

The cornerstone of the evaluation for cardiac sources of emboli is the echocardiogram. While a transthoracic echocardiogram (TTE) is the initial imaging test for most patients, transesophageal echocardiography (TEE) has been shown to be superior to TTE when evaluating for cardiac sources of emboli [4, 5] and is also more cost effective [6]. As a result, the evaluation for cardiac sources of emboli is the most common indication for using TEE [5]. Once a cardiac source of emboli is identified, management depends on the underlying etiology and patient comorbidities.

Clinical Syndromes of Cardiac Emboli
(Fig. 39.1)

Cerebral Vascular Accidents (CVA)

Embolisms of cardiac origin account for approximately 15–20 % of all ischemic strokes [7]. The overwhelming majority (80 %) of cardiogenic emboli lodge in the middle cerebral artery and its branches, while 10 % lodge in the posterior cerebral circulation and the remaining 10 % in the

Renal Emboli

The incidence of renal emboli in the general population is quite rare. In a study involving nearly 30,000 patients with AF followed for 13 years, the incidence of renal thromboemboli was only 2 % [3]. Symptoms of renal infarction are vague and overlap with more common conditions making the diagnosis difficult. Patients generally have abdominal or flank pain, nausea, and vomiting and may report hematuria. Laboratory findings can be helpful in raising suspicion for the diagnosis. Patients tend to have an elevated white blood cell count (WBC), elevated creatinine concentration, and markedly elevated serum lactate dehydrogenase (LDH). Finally, an elevation of urinary LDH is very suggestive of intrarenal pathology as LDH is generally too large to be filtered and its excretion is generally only increased in renal infarction and renal transplant rejection [13].

Splenic Emboli

Both splenic infarction and abscess should prompt evaluation for cardiac sources of emboli. Abscesses can present with persistent fever despite antibiotic therapy, left upper quadrant (LUQ) pain, and, sometimes, a left-sided plural effusion [14]. Splenic infarct presents similarly with LUQ pain, fever, LUQ tenderness, nausea and vomiting, elevated WBC count, and elevated LDH. The clinical presentation of splenic infarcts can be atypical, but the most consistent findings are LUQ pain and elevated LDH [15].

Optic Emboli

Central retinal artery occlusion is a relatively rare event, with an incidence of approximately 1.9 per 100,000 [16]. While the most common cause of retinal artery occlusion is carotid artery disease, cardiogenic sources may account for as many as 42 % of cases [17]. A cardiogenic source is more likely in younger patients and in patients with a history of cardiac disease such as AF or rheumatic heart disease [18]. Retinal artery emboli present clinically as acute onset, unilateral, painless, loss of vision. It is considered a form of stroke (if transient it is called amaurosis fugax) and should compel the clinician to investigate the source of the emboli to prevent other vascular events.

Mesenteric Emboli

Emboli to the mesenteric vasculature most commonly lodge in the superior mesenteric artery (SMA) because of its large caliber and the narrow angle of its departure from the aorta. Emboli to the SMA account for 5 % of peripheral emboli and approximately 50 % of cases of acute mesenteric ischemia [19]. Classic symptoms of mesenteric ischemia include nausea, vomiting, diarrhea, and acute periumbilical pain that appears "out of proportion" to the physical findings where tenderness is not prominent. The patient appears acutely ill and at least 50 % test positive for fecal occult blood with 15 % presenting with melena or hematochezia [20]. Acute mesenteric ischemia can be a catastrophic event, with mortality rates exceeding 60 % [21]. As such, when suspicion is high, physicians should have a low threshold for a definitive, invasive evaluation with angiography.

Pulmonary Emboli (PE)

While dislodged deep vein thrombi (DVT) are, by far, the most common cause of PE, cardiac sources of PE include right ventricular (RV) thrombi secondary to blood stasis, indwelling cardiac catheters, or pacemaker/defibrillator leads and right-sided endocarditis. In patients with right-sided endocarditis, which accounts for 5–10 % of cases of endocarditis [22], septic PE are common and can result in multiple pulmonary abscesses. The most common symptom

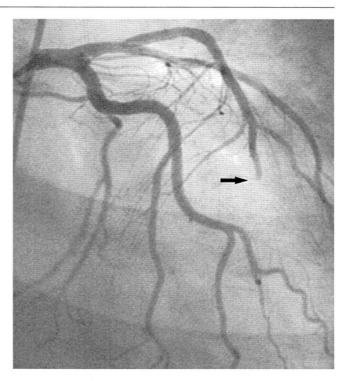

Fig. 39.2 Coronary angiogram showing normal coronary arteries with abrupt occlusion, as indicated by the *arrow*, (cut-off sign) of the distal left anterior descending coronary artery consistent with embolus (Reprinted with Permission Adachi and Kobayashi [88])

in such patients is fever. Other symptoms include dyspnea, pleuritic chest pain, cough, and hemoptysis [23]. Hypoxia and paradoxical emboli are also possible when right atrial pressures increase sufficiently to cause right-to-left shunting [24] in patients with an atrial septal defect or a patent foramen ovale.

Coronary Emboli

Approximately 4–7 % of patients with acute MI are found to have otherwise normal coronaries [25]. In such cases, emboli to the coronary arteries are an important consideration, especially in patients with underlying conditions that predispose to embolization such as AF. Coronary emboli are usually located in the left anterior descending (LAD) artery at the level of the distal epicardial and intramural branches (Fig. 39.2). This observation may be due to the aortic valve morphology which results in preferential blood flow into the left main coronary [26].

Etiology (Fig. 39.3)

There are three types of masses that can embolize from the heart: thrombotic, infectious, and neoplastic.

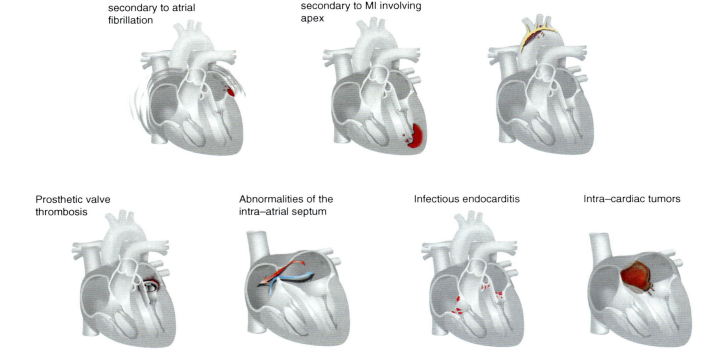

Fig. 39.3 Possible etiologies of cardiac emboli

Left Atrial (LA) Thrombi

A thrombus in the LA (Fig. 39.4) is the most common source of cardiogenic emboli. Most thrombi form in the LA appendage [27] secondary to blood stasis. Atrial fibrillation, rheumatic mitral stenosis, and LA enlargement are all conditions that predispose to stasis and subsequent thrombus formation. In the developed world, where rheumatic disease is less common, AF is the most common cause of LA thrombus formation [1, 3]. The association is so strong that in patients in sinus rhythm presenting with embolic strokes or TIA, only 1 % have LA thrombosis demonstrable by TEE as opposed to 14 % of those in AF [28]. Patients with dilated cardiomyopathy experience systemic emboli at a rate of approximately 4 % per year and more commonly are found to have thrombus in the LA rather than the LV suggesting that dilated cardiomyopathy is another important cause of LA thrombosis [29]. Mitral regurgitation does not appear to be associated with LA thrombus, possibly because the regurgitant flow prevents the stasis of blood in the LA [30].

Left Ventricular Thrombi

As in the case of LA thrombosis, LV thrombi also form under conditions of stasis. Ventricular aneurysms, diffuse ventricular hypokinesis (e.g., dilated cardiomyopathy), or segmental wall motion abnormalities (e.g., post-MI) are the main

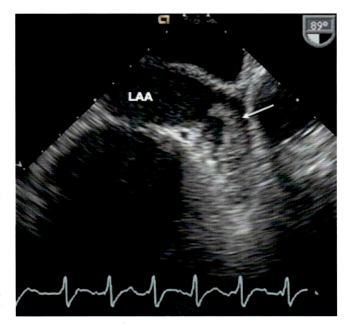

Fig. 39.4 Transesophageal echocardiogram showing left atrial thrombus (*arrow*) in the atrial appendage. This thrombus was visualized in two orthogonal views, using zoom mode and a high-frequency (7 MHz) transducer (Reprinted with Permission Otto [30])

causes of stasis in the LV. In the absence of an aneurysm or severe global or regional LV dysfunction, LV thrombi are unlikely to occur. Conversely, LV thrombi are most likely to

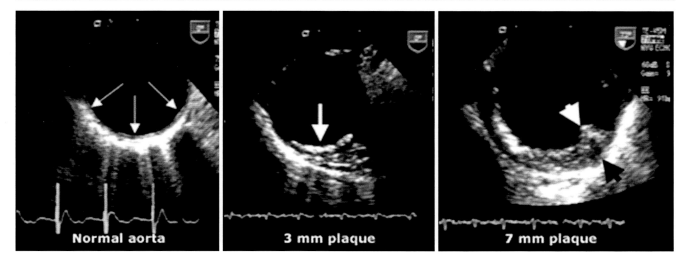

Fig. 39.5 Transesophageal echocardiograms of the thoracic aorta: *Left*: normal; *middle*: moderate (3 mm) plaque; and *right*: severe (7 mm) plaque (Reprinted with Permission Tunick [89])

occur in patients with large anterior wall infarction with apical wall motion abnormalities. LV thrombosis occurs in up to 46 % of these patients, while patients without apical involvement are at low risk for thrombosis. Thrombi tend to form between one and 11 days following an MI [31].

Aortic Atherosclerosis

Embolism related to aortic atherosclerosis can be secondary to either thromboembolism or atheroembolism (cholesterol embolism). Thromboembolism occurs when an aortic atherosclerotic plaque ruptures and the thrombus that forms at the site of rupture embolizes. These tend to be single large emboli with resulting clinical syndromes similar to those associated with cardiac emboli as noted above (TIA, stroke, limb ischemia, etc.). Atheroembolism, however, tends to result in multiple small artery occlusions leading to very variable clinical presentations. Vague symptoms such as fever, headache, and weight loss may be present, while more dramatic clinical presentations include "blue toe" syndrome, livedo reticularis, renal failure, and retinal ischemia [32]. Risk factors for embolization include characteristics of the plaque as observed on TEE (Fig. 39.5) and instrumentation during cardiac catheterization or surgery. Ulcerated, protruding, mobile plaques and plaques with thickness >4 mm are at the highest risk of embolism [33, 34].

Prosthetic Valve Thrombosis

The rates of prosthetic valve thrombosis range between 0.1 and 5.7 % per patient year depending on the valve characteristics [35]. Patients with bioprosthetic valves and those with mechanical valves with consistent therapeutic anticoagulation are at the lowest risk while patients with mechanical valves and inadequate anticoagulation and valves in the mitral position are at the highest risk. The risk of embolization in patients with mechanical valves is approximately 4 % per year without anticoagulation, 2 % per year on antiplatelet therapy, and 1 % per year on warfarin. Other risk factors for embolization such as AF and depressed LV function contribute to increased risks of embolization in patients who have undergone valve replacement [35]. However, it should be noted that the most common presenting symptom of prosthetic valve thrombosis is not an embolic event but rather congestive heart failure [36] due to an acute obstruction or restriction of valve opening.

Abnormalities of the Atrial Septum

Right-to-left shunting, which can occur in patients with a patent foramen ovale (PFO) or atrial septal defect (ASD), may lead to paradoxical emboli in which thrombi formed in the venous system cross the atrial defect to embolize systemically. A prerequisite for such an event is higher pressures in the right heart chambers than left. While several pathological conditions can increase right-sided pressures such as Eisenmenger syndrome or pulmonary hypertension from a variety of causes, right heart pressures can increase transiently under physiologic conditions, allowing the passage of paradoxical emboli from the venous to systemic circulations in otherwise normal patients. First, during the normal cardiac cycle, right atrial pressures transiently exceed left atrial during early systole. Second, under conditions where patients perform the Valsalva maneuver, there are two opportunities for right-to-left shunting. First, during straining, increased intrathoracic pressures disproportionately increase right heart pressure, and during release, the influx of venous blood again increases right-sided pressure above left-sided pressure

[37]. As such, patients who present with a history of straining immediately preceding an ischemic event should draw the clinician's attention to the possibility of paradoxical emboli.

It is estimated that approximately 25 % of the population has PFOs, and several studies have found an association between cryptogenic strokes (strokes with no clearly identifiable cause) and an increased prevalence of PFOs [38, 39]. Furthermore, patients with larger PFOs, patients in hypercoagulable states, patients with right-to-left shunting found on TEE, and patients with concurrent atrial septal aneurysms appear to have higher risks of embolism [40, 41]. However, population-based studies have not shown PFOs alone to be associated with statistically significant increases in the risk of stroke [42, 43]. This suggests that the role of PFO in cryptogenic strokes is likely only part of a multifactorial cascade that predisposes patients to paradoxical emboli.

Right Ventricular Thrombi

RV thrombi are quite rare but native RV thrombi can be seen in cases of severe RV dilatation or dysfunction and on indwelling catheters [30]. Another rare finding may be a floating RV thrombus. These likely represent thrombi in transit from the venous circulation and are associated with a high mortality. While native RV thrombi can be treated with anticoagulation, floating RV thrombi are an emergency and require emergent surgery or thrombolytic therapy [44].

Septic Emboli

Infectious intracardiac vegetations most commonly result from infective endocarditis (IE) on native valves. The infection likely begins with minor trauma secondary to the force of the valves opening and closing—which is supported by the relative frequency of the valves involved: mitral > aortic > tricuspid > pulmonic [45]—combined with transient bacteremia.

Although the brain and spleen are the most common sites of left-sided septic emboli, nearly any organ can be affected including the spinal cord, the paraspinal space, and the arteries themselves via the vasa vasorum which can lead to mycotic aneurysms [22]. Systemic embolization with subsequent abscess formation is a common cause of prolonged fever despite adequate antibiotic therapy. Right-sided IE commonly leads to septic pulmonary emboli with subsequent respiratory symptoms as noted above.

Nonbacterial Thrombotic Endocarditis (NBTE)

This entity, also known as marantic, Libman-Sacks, or verrucous endocarditis, refers to a large spectrum of valvular lesions that are usually associated with advanced malignancy

Table 39.1 Sensitivity and specificity of TTE and TEE in the evaluation of LA and LV thrombus formation

Test	Sensitivity (%)	Specificity (%)
LA thrombus		
TEE	99	100
TTE	53–63	95–99
CMR	100	94
LV thrombus		
TEE	40 ± 14	96 ± 3.6
TTE	92–95	86–88
CMR	88–93	85–99

Adapted from Otto [30]
TTE transthoracic echocardiogram, *TEE* transesophageal echocardiogram, *CMR* cardiac magnetic resonance imaging, *LA* left atrium, *LV* left ventricle

[46] and autoimmune conditions such as systemic lupus erythematosus. While rare, these vegetations have the potential for embolization.

Intracardiac Tumors

Primary cardiac tumors are very rare, with an incidence of only 0.06 % [47]. Only two types are associated with embolization: myxomas and papillary fibroelastomas. Myxomas are the most common type of cardiac tumor. They are benign tumors; most are located in the left atrium as a pedunculated growth off the atrial septum. The morphology of the tumor dictates the likelihood of embolization. Friable or villous myxomas, which account for 35 % of all myxomas, are more likely to embolize [48].

Papillary fibroelastomas are the second most common type of primary cardiac tumors. These are pedunculated tumors most commonly located on left-sided cardiac valves but can also be found on the endocardium itself. Again, it is a benign tumor that has the potential to cause serious morbidity and mortality from emboli. Tumor mobility is independently associated with increased risks of embolization [49]. The embolized material in myxomas or papillary fibroelastomas can be either pieces of the tumor itself or thrombi which form on the tumor and subsequently dislodge.

Evaluation

Echocardiography is the imaging modality of choice when evaluating for cardiac sources of emboli. As noted above, TEE has been found to be superior to TTE in the evaluation of the most common causes of cardiac emboli [4, 5] and has been shown to be more cost effective [6]. However, the superiority of TEE depends on the source of the emboli (Table 39.1). A TEE is performed by passing a modified gastroscope with an ultrasound transducer at its tip down the esophagus. The esophagus travels immediately posterior to the aortic arch and left atrium with minimal intervening tissue between the transducer and the heart, as opposed to TTE which has retrosternal airspace intervening. This close proximity allows for the use of high-frequency transducers which increase the spatial resolution of the resulting image. Therefore, TEE provides for improved detection of LA thrombi and tumors, PFOs, ASDs, valvular vegetations, atheromatous plaques within the aorta, and spontaneous left atrial echo contrast, which is a marker of blood stasis. On the other hand, TEE provides poor visualization of the LV apex, and as a result, when evaluating for LV thrombi (e.g., post-MI), TTE is still the imaging modality of choice.

It should be noted that TEE is an invasive procedure and therefore involves more risks than TTE. Minor complications occur in approximately 1/500 patients and include minor oropharyngeal trauma, transient bronchospasm, transient hypoxia (more likely in obese patients), nonsustained ventricular/atrial arrhythmias, and vomiting. More severe complications are rare but include esophageal perforation, gastrointestinal bleeding, pharyngeal hematoma, and methemoglobinemia [4, 50, 51]. Methemoglobinemia is a complication of the topical anesthetic benzocaine used for posterior pharyngeal anesthesia and is very rare, occurring in approximately 0.07 % of patients [52]. Endocarditis secondary to transient bacteremia during TEE is also rare; antibiotic prophylaxis is not recommended except in patients who are immunosuppressed and have prosthetic valves, cyanotic congenital heart disease, or a previous history of endocarditis [53].

As noted above, masses found in the heart may be of thrombotic, infectious, or neoplastic origin. However, since not all echo-dense objects found on echocardiogram are necessarily pathologic, one must be able to identify artifacts and normal variants to avoid misdiagnosis. Artifacts on echocardiogram in general lack clearly demarcated borders, do not have appropriate movement throughout the cardiac cycle, do not have clearly visualized attachment to the endocardial surface and cannot be seen in multiple views and different depths [54]. Also, normal anatomy may be misdiagnosed as intracardiac masses. These include normal trabeculae, aberrant chordae tendineae, the moderator band (especially in cases of right ventricular hypertrophy), or papillary muscles [30].

In situations in which TEE is inconclusive or cannot be performed, a cardiac magnetic resonance imaging (CMR) is a second-line option for the evaluation of cardiac sources of emboli. Studies have shown that for the detection of LV thrombi in post-MI patients, CMR has superior specificity with similar sensitivity [55] when compared to TTE, and is comparable to TEE for the evaluation of LA thrombi [56] (Table 39.1).

Left Atrial Imaging

TTE has two major limitations when evaluating the LA: first, in both the parasternal and apical views, the LA is in the far

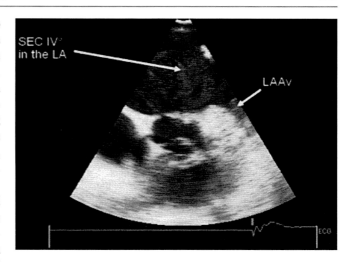

Fig. 39.6 Transesophageal echocardiography with dense spontaneous echo contrast (*SEC*). *LA* left atrium, *LAAv* left atrial appendage peak emptying velocity (Reprinted with Permission Bernhardt et al. [59])

field limiting the resolution of the image [30]; second, most atrial thrombi originate in the left atrial appendage [27], and TTE has poor visualization of the atrial appendage limiting its sensitivity for the diagnosis of LA thrombi [57].

As noted above, blood stasis is the major underlying cause of LA thrombosis, and it can be visualized on TEE with Doppler imaging or via the observation of spontaneous echo contrast (SEC) in the LA. On Doppler, flow velocity during LA contraction is normally above 0.4 m/s. Velocities lower than 0.4 m/s are associated with higher rates of thrombus formation [1].

SEC is best seen at high-frequency settings of TEE with low gain to be better able to distinguish SEC from noise artifact [1]. The echo density seen in SEC appears as white swirls (Fig. 39.6) and is thought to be the result of transient erythrocyte aggregation produced by interactions between erythrocytes and plasma proteins in low shear rate conditions [1, 58]. This hypothesis is supported by the finding that SEC is independently associated with hematocrit and fibrinogen levels in addition to stasis [58], suggesting that SEC also indicates a relatively hypercoagulable state. This finding helps to explain why SEC is so strongly associated with thrombus formation even when patients are on oral anticoagulation [59] and is an independent risk factor for thromboembolic events [60].

Imaging of the Atrial Septum

TEE also provides high-quality images of the atrial septum. TEE with bubble contrast, at rest, and with cough or Valsalva is the preferred method of evaluating right-to-left shunt (PFO or ASD) [5, 61] (Fig. 39.7). However, more recent studies have found TTE with Doppler and contrast to have similar sensitivity and specificity for the detection of PFO as TEE and can be used as an alternative approach [62, 63].

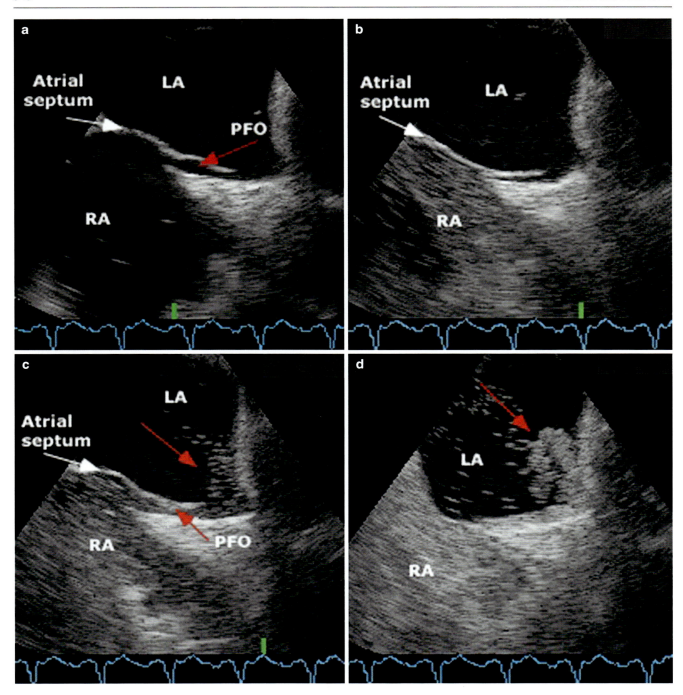

Fig. 39.7 Transesophageal echocardiography with contrast of a patent foramen ovale. The sequence of images shows the right and left atria during diastole (panel **a**); a flap of the atrial septum is seen covering the foramen ovale. There is opacification of the right atrium immediately after injection of agitated saline (panel **b**). Panel **c** shows the contrast passing through the right atrium (*RA*) to the left atrium (*LA*) through a patent foramen ovale (*PFO*) (*red arrow*). Panel **d** shows a large amount of contrast within the LA (*red arrow*) (Reproduced with Permission UpToDate, Waltham, MA 2012. Copyright © 2012 UpToDate, Inc.)

Valve Imaging

TEE has been found to be vastly superior to TTE in the evaluation of possible vegetations on native and prosthetic valves. Echocardiography, however, cannot distinguish between septic vegetations and NBTE [64].

Thoracic Aortic Imaging

TEE is the imaging modality of choice to evaluate the thoracic aorta for the potential source of embolism. TEE not only has been found to be highly sensitive and specific for detecting aortic atherosclerosis but is also able to define the morphologic characteristics of the plaque such as ulcerations, mobility, and thickness [65] which are predictors of the risk for embolization.

Left Ventricular Imaging

Given the high prevalence of LV thrombi after MIs that involve the apex, TTE should be preformed routinely on these patients to identify those at highest risk of embolization. Two characteristics have been found to be associated with greater risks for embolization: thrombus mobility and thrombus protrusion [66]. As noted above, LV imaging is best accomplished by TTE. However, the sensitivity of TTE may be decreased due to poor image quality in patients who are obese or have severe chronic pulmonary disease. Prominent LV trabeculae or papillary muscles can also cause suboptimal imaging. In such instances, intravenous contrast can be used to improve the sensitivity and specificity of the study [67]. It should be noted, however, that even in conditions in which a thrombus is not visualized, TTE can guide treatment by indicating patients at high risk of developing LV thrombi such as those with LV ejection fraction less than 40 %, apical wall motion abnormality, or aneurysm.

Management

Anticoagulation

The prevention or treatment of thromboembolism is accomplished through anticoagulation (vitamin K antagonists (VKA), direct thrombin inhibitors, and factor Xa inhibitors) or antiplatelet therapy. Anticoagulation is not benign and must be weighed against the risk of bleeding. Therefore, whether the practitioner chooses anticoagulation as opposed to antiplatelet therapy or a combined approach is dependent on the underlying etiology and the patient's risk factors for thrombus formation (Table 39.2):

Atrial Fibrillation

Being the most common cause of thromboembolism, AF has been extensively studied. Both acute and chronic AF have significant risk of thrombus formation [69], and thus, treatment is indicated in paroxysmal and persistent AF. The most popular and best-studied risk stratification calculator is the $CHADS_2$ score [70]. Its simplicity makes it quickly and easily applicable in the clinical setting. The score is calculated as follows: 1 point for congestive heart failure, 1 point for **h**ypertension, 1 point for **a**ge >75 years, 1 point for **d**iabetes, and 2 points for **s**troke or TIA; the sum of points is the total $CHADS_2$ score. As noted in Table 39.2, a $CHADS_2$ score of 0 can be managed with antiplatelet therapy or without any antithrombotic therapy; a score of 1 can be managed with aspirin or

Table 39.2 Recommendations for use of chronic antithrombotic therapy for various cardiac conditions

Disease comorbidities	Recommendation
Nonvalvular atrial fibrillation	
$CHADS_2$ score 0	Aspirin or no antithrombotic
$CHADS_2$ score 1	Aspirin or VKA
$CHADS_2$ score >1	VKA
Rheumatic mitral valve disease	
With atrial fibrillation, previous embolization, or atrial appendage thrombus or left atrial diameter >55 mm	VKA
Embolization or appendage clot despite INR 2–3	VKA plus aspirin
Aortic arch mobile atheroma	
Otherwise cryptogenic stroke or TIA	Aspirin or VKA
Patent foramen ovale	
Otherwise cryptogenic ischemic stroke or TIA	Aspirin
Indication for VKA (deep venous thrombosis or hypercoagulable state)	VKA
Mechanical heart value	
Aortic position, bileaflet, or Medtronic Hall tilting disk with normal left atrial size and sinus rhythm	VKA (INR 2.5, range 2–3)
Mitral position tilting disk or bileaflet valve	VKA (INR 3.0, range 2.5–3.50)
Mitral or aortic position, antero-apical myocardial infarct, or left atrial enlargement	VKA (INR 3.0, range 2.5–3.5)
Mitral or aortic position, with atrial fibrillation, or hypercoagulable state, or low ejection fraction, or atherosclerotic vascular disease	Aspirin plus VKA (INR 3.0, range 2.5–3.5)
Systemic embolization despite target INR	Add aspirin and/or increase INR: prior target was 2.5 increase to 3.0, range 2.5–3.5; prior target was 3.0 increase to 3.5, range 3–4
Bioprosthetic valve	
No other indication for VKA therapy	Aspirin
Infective endocarditis	Avoid antithrombotic agents
Nonbacterial thrombotic endocarditis	
With systemic embolization	Full dose unfractionated heparin or subcutaneous LMWH

Adapted from Smith et al. [68]
Dose of aspirin is 50–325 mg/day; target INR for VKA is 2.5 unless otherwise specified
INR international normalized ratio, *LMWH* low-molecular-weight heparin, *TIA* transient ischemic attack, *VKA* vitamin K antagonist

with VKA; a score of 2 or greater should be managed with VKA With a goal INR of 2–3. To help further stratify patients with a score of 0 or 1, the $CHADS_2$-VASc score was devised. Unlike the $CHADS_2$ score, it takes into account age 65–74, female sex, and vascular disease. If patients have any of these additional risk factors with a CHADS$_2$ score of 0, it is reasonable to maintain them on aspirin therapy while those with a score of 1 should be managed with VKA [71]. Finally, several recent trials [72, 73] have demonstrated that direct thrombin and Xa inhibitors are equally effective at preventing thromboembolism as VKA with similar bleeding risks. In all patients, when considering therapeutic options, the risk of stroke prevention must be balanced against the risk of bleeding.

Mechanical Valves

As noted above, mechanical valves are associated with a significant risk of thrombosis, and that risk is increased with mechanical valves in the mitral position and other comorbid conditions such as AF or low ejection fraction. These patients require lifelong anticoagulation and possibly antiplatelet therapy with INR goal depending on comorbid conditions (see Table 39.2). Of note, unlike patients with AF, the use of direct thrombin inhibitors and factor Xa inhibitors has not approved for use in patients with mechanical valves, and therefore, these drugs should not be used in patients with mechanical mitral valves.

Left Ventricular Thrombi

As noted above, as many as 46 % of patients with an anterior MI involving the LV apex eventually develop LV thrombi. In the absence of anticoagulation, approximately 10 % will have clinically evident CVAs [74]. Several studies [75–77] have shown that heparin followed by warfarin therapy in patients with LV thrombi decreases the incidence of CVA to 1–3 %. While the optimal duration of treatment has not been investigated, several studies have shown a reduced risk of embolization after 3 months [78]; thus, anticoagulation is recommended for at least 3 months. According to the 2012 American College of Chest Physicians guidelines on Antithrombotic Therapy and Prevention of Thrombosis, patients at high risk for thrombus formation and embolization should begin anticoagulation with VKA and aspirin early and continue for 3 months. After that point, VKA can be discontinued but aspirin should be continued. Patients considered high risk include those with documented LV thrombus on TTE, those with an LVEF less than 40 %, and those with an antero-apical wall motion abnormality or aneurysm [79].

Aortic Atherosclerosis

All patients with established atherosclerotic disease should be treated for secondary prevention of cardiovascular disease. This includes aspirin, statins, controlling hypertension, smoking cessation, and lifestyle modifications [80]. However, the use of anticoagulation has not been firmly established; the 2008 American College of Chest Physician guidelines on valvular and structural heart disease give a weak recommendation (grade 2C) for VKA therapy in patients with ischemic stroke associated with mobile aortic arch thrombi [81].

Cardiac Tumors

Surgical excision is the treatment of choice in the case of cardiac tumors. Cardiac myxomas are generally removed under cardiopulmonary bypass. In familial cases, myxomas have a high rate of recurrence (up to 22 %), but in sporadic cases the procedure is generally curative with a recurrence rate of only 1–2 % [82].

PFO/ASD Treatment

In patients who present with cryptogenic strokes or TIA and a PFO, two treatment options are available: antithrombotic therapy or percutaneous closure. In the PICSS (PFO in Cryptogenic Stroke Study) trial, there were no significant differences in the 2-year event rates among those treated with VKA as opposed to aspirin [83]. Given the risks of bleeding involved with anticoagulation, The 2012 American College of Chest Physicians guidelines recommend antiplatelet (aspirin and/or clopidogrel) therapy in these patients [84].

Whether percutaneous closure of a PFO is superior to medical therapy at preventing recurrent stroke is a topic of much debate. Recently the CLOSURE I (Evaluation of the STARFlex Septal Closure System in Patients with a Stroke and/or Transient Ischemic Attack due to Presumed Paradoxical Embolism through a Patent Foramen Ovale) trial found no benefit of percutaneous PFO closure over medical therapy (warfarin, aspirin, or both) [85]. However, there has been much controversy over the validity of the results [86], and thus, no clear recommendations can be made at this point. However, given that the results of this randomized trial showed no benefit of closure, patients should be treated medically or recommended to participate in ongoing PFO closure trials that are attempting to address some of the limitations of CLOSURE I. Percutaneous closure can be considered in patients who have events on antithrombotic therapy. On the other hand, in ASD, where left-to-right shunting may result in right heart failure, percutaneous or surgical closure is recommended for all adults who have right ventricular enlargement or other signs of overload regardless of symptoms of embolization [87].

Key Points
- The 3 types of masses that can embolize from the heart are thrombotic, infectious, and neoplastic.
- A left atrial thrombus is the most common source of cardiogenic emboli.

- The incidence of clinically apparent embolic events is approximately three times higher in the cerebral circulation as opposed to the peripheral circulation.
- Embolisms of cardiac origin account for approximately 15–20 % of all ischemic strokes.
- Cardiac emboli are the most common cause of peripheral artery embolization, with ischemic heart disease and AF accounting for approximately 80 % of cases.
- The symptoms of acute limb ischemia include the 6 "Ps": pain, pulselessness, pallor, poikilothermia, paresthesias, and paralysis.
- Other potential end organs of arterial emboli include the spleen, kidney, gut, eye, and, although commonly overlooked, the heart itself.
- Stasis of blood is the main risk factor for thrombosis; this commonly occurs in the LA secondary to AF and in the LV secondary to apical wall motion abnormalities post-MI.
- When evaluating cardiac sources of emboli, TTE is the test of choice to visualize the LV while TEE is the test of choice to visualize the LA, aortic arch and cardiac valves.
- Treatment of patients with cardiogenic emboli depends on the source and composition of the embolus and the bleeding risks of the individual patient.

References

1. Mark A, Diane KM, Marveen C, Mimi BC. Diagnostic medical sonography: echocardiography. 2nd ed. Philadelphia: Lippincott; 1999. p. 101–3.
2. Stratton JR. Common causes of cardiac emboli-left ventricular thrombi and atrial fibrillation [specialty conference]. West J Med. 1989;151:172–9.
3. Frost L, Engholm G, Johnsen S, Husted S. Incident thromboembolism in the aorta and the renal, mesenteric, pelvic, and extremity arteries after discharge from the hospital with a diagnosis of AF. Arch Intern Med. 2001;161(2):272–6.
4. Khandheria BK, Seward JB, Tajik AJ. Transesophageal echocardiography. Mayo Clin Proc. 1994;69(9):856.
5. Daniel WG, Mügge A. Transesophageal echocardiography. N Engl J Med. 1995;332(19):1268.
6. McNamara RL, Lima JA, Whelton PK, Powe NR. Echocardiographic identification of cardiovascular sources of emboli to guide clinical management of stroke: a cost-effectiveness analysis. Ann Intern Med. 1997;127(9):775.
7. Cerebral Embolism Task Force, Cardiogenic brain embolism. The second report of the Cerebral Embolism Task Force. Arch Neurol. 1989;46(7):727–743.
8. Kistler JP, et al. Cerebrovascular Diseases. In: Braunwald E, et al., editors. Harrison's principles of internal medicine. New York: McGraw-Hill; 1994. p. 2250.
9. Giles MF, Rothwell PM. Risk of stroke early after transient ischaemic attack: a systematic review and meta-analysis. Lancet Neurol. 2007;6(12):1063.
10. Van Wijk I, Kappelle LJ, Algra A, et al. Long-term survival and vascular event risk after transient ischaemic attack or minor ischaemic stroke: a cohort study. LiLAC study group. Lancet. 2005; 365(9477):2098.
11. Abbott W, Maloney R, McCabe C, et al. Arterial embolism: a 44 year perspective. Am J Surg. 1982;143:460.
12. Lin PH, Kougias P, Bechara C, Cagiannos C, Huynh TT, Chen CJ. Arterial disease. In: Brunicardi FC, Andersen DK, Billiar TR, Dunn DL, Hunter JG, Matthews JB, Pollock RE, editors. Schwartz's principles of surgery. 9th ed. New York: McGraw-Hill; 2010.
13. Korzets Z, Plotkin E, Bernheim J, Zissin R. The clinical spectrum of acute renal infarction. Isr Med Assoc J. 2002;4(10):781.
14. Johnson JD, Raff MJ, Barnwell PA, Chun CH. Splenic abscess complicating infectious endocarditis. Arch Intern Med. 1983; 143(5):906.
15. Lawrence YR, Pokroy R, Berlowitz D, Aharoni D, Hain D, Breuer GS. Splenic infarction: an update on William Osler's observations. Isr Med Assoc J. 2010;12(6):362.
16. Leavitt JA, Larson TA, Hodge DO, Gullerud RE. The incidence of central retinal artery occlusion in Olmsted County, Minnesota. Am J Ophthalmol. 2011;152(5):820.
17. Hayreh SS, Podhajsky PA, Zimmerman MB. Retinal artery occlusion: associated systemic and ophthalmic abnormalities. Ophthalmology. 2009;116(10):1928.
18. Recchia FM, Brown GC. Systemic disorders associated with retinal vascular occlusion. Curr Opin Ophthalmol. 2000;11(6):462.
19. Cappell MS. Intestinal (mesenteric) vasculopathy I. Acute superior mesenteric arteriopathy and venopathy. Gastroenterol Clin North Am. 1998;27(4):783–825.
20. Sreenarasimhaiah J. Diagnosis and management of intestinal ischaemic disorders. BMJ. 2003;326(7403):1372–6.
21. McKinsey JF, Gewertz BL. Acute mesenteric ischemia. Surg Clin North Am. 1997;77(2):307.
22. Habib G, Hoen B, et al. Guidelines on the prevention, diagnosis, and treatment of infective endocarditis (new version 2009): the Task Force on the Prevention, Diagnosis, and Treatment of Infective Endocarditis of the European Society of Cardiology (ESC). Endorsed by the European Society of Clinical Microbiology and Infectious Diseases (ESCMID) and the International Society of Chemotherapy (ISC) for infection and cancer. Eur Heart J. 2009;30(19):2369–413. Epub 2009 Aug 27.
23. Cook RJ, Ashton RW, Aughenbaugh GL, Ryu JH. Septic pulmonary embolism*: presenting features and clinical course of 14 patients. Chest. 2005;128(1):162–6.
24. Rob M, Brad M. Injection drug use and right sided endocarditis. Heart. 2003;89(5):577–81.
25. Waller BF. Atherosclerotic and nonatherosclerotic coronary artery factors in acute myocardial infarction. Philadelphia: Dabis; 1989. p. 29–104.
26. Kardasz I, De Caterina R. Myocardial infarction with normal coronary arteries: a conundrum with multiple aetiologies and variable prognosis: an update. J Int Med. 2007;261:4.
27. Orhan O, Eugene C. Novel approaches to stroke prevention in atrial fibrillation: introduction. Stroke. 2007;38:624–30.
28. Omran H, Rang B, Lüderitz B, et al. Incidence of left atrial thrombi in patients in sinus rhythm and with a recent neurologic deficit. Am Heart J. 2000;140(4):658–62.
29. Vigna C, Russo A, Loperfido F, et al. Frequency of left atrial thrombi by transesophageal echocardiography in idiopathic and in ischemic dilated cardiomyopathy. Am J Cardiol. 1992;70(18):1500.
30. Otto CM. Cardiac masses and potential cardiac "source of embolus". In: Textbook of clinical echocardiography. Philadelphia: Elsevier; 2009.

31. Richard AW, Frank ML, Joseph E, Morrison H, et al. Incidence of left-ventricular thrombosis after acute transmural myocardial infarction – serial evaluation by two-dimensional echocardiography. N Engl J Med. 1981;305:297–302.
32. Fine MJ, Kapoor W, Falanga V. Cholesterol crystal embolization: a review of 221 cases in the English literature. Angiology. 1987;38(10):769.
33. The French Study of Aortic Plaques in Stroke Group. Atherosclerotic disease of the aortic arch as a risk factor for recurrent ischemic stroke. N Engl J Med. 1996;334(19):1216.
34. Tunick PA, Perez JL, Kronzon I. Protruding atheromas in the thoracic aorta and systemic embolization. Ann Intern Med. 1991;115(6):423.
35. Vongpatanasin W, Hillis LD, Lange RA. Prosthetic heart valves. N Engl J Med. 1996;335(6):407.
36. Dürrleman N, Pellerin M, Bouchard D, Hébert Y, Cartier R, Perrault LP, Basmadjian A, Carrier MJ. Prosthetic valve thrombosis: twenty-year experience at the Montreal Heart Institute. Thorac Cardiovasc Surg. 2004;127(5):1388.
37. Langholz D, Louie EK, Konstadt SN, Rao TL, Scanlon PJ. Transesophageal echocardiographic demonstration of distinct mechanisms for right to left shunting across a patent foramen ovale in the absence of pulmonary hypertension. J Am Coll Cardiol. 1991;18(4):1112.
38. Cabanes L, Mas JL, Cohen A, Amarenco P, Cabanes PA, Oubary P, Chedru F, Guérin F, Bousser MG. Atrial septal aneurysm and patent foramen ovale as risk factors for cryptogenic stroke in patients less than 55 years of age. A study using transesophageal echocardiography. J Stroke. 1993;24(12):1865.
39. Di Tullio M, Sacco RL, Gopal A, Mohr JP, Homma S. Patent foramen ovale as a risk factor for cryptogenic stroke. Ann Int Med. 1992;117(6):461.
40. Schuchlenz HW, Weihs W, Horner S, Quehenberger F. The association between the diameter of a patent foramen ovale and the risk of embolic cerebrovascular events. Am J Med. 2000;109(6):456.
41. Wu LA, Malouf JF, Dearani JA, Hagler DJ, Reeder GS, Petty GW, Khandheria BK. Patent foramen ovale in cryptogenic stroke: current understanding and management options. Arch Intern Med. 2004;164(9):950.
42. Di Tullio MR, Sacco RL, Sciacca RR, Jin Z, Homma S. Patent foramen ovale and the risk of ischemic stroke in a multiethnic population. J Am CollCardiol. 2007;49(7):797.
43. Meissner I, Khandheria BK, Heit JA, Petty GW, Sheps SG, Schwartz GL, Whisnant JP, Wiebers DO, Covalt JL, Petterson TM, Christianson TJ, Agmon Y. Patent foramen ovale: innocent or guilty? Evidence from a prospective population-based study. J Am Coll Cardiol. 2006;47(2):440.
44. Chartier L, Béra J, Delomez M, Asseman P, Beregi JP, Bauchart JJ, Warembourg H, Théry C. Free-floating thrombi in the right heart: diagnosis, management, and prognostic indexes in 38 consecutive patients. Circulation. 1999;99(21):2779.
45. Shively BK, Crawford MH. Infective endocarditis. In: Crawford MH, editor. CURRENT diagnosis & treatment: cardiology. 3rd ed. New York: McGraw-Hill; 2009.
46. Deppisch LM, Fayemi AO. Non-bacterial thrombotic endocarditis: clinicopathologic correlations. Am Heart J. 1976;92(6):723.
47. Lam KY, Dickens P, Chan AC. Tumors of the heart. A 20-year experience with a review of 12,485 consecutive autopsies. Arch Pathol Lab Med. 1993;117(10):1027.
48. Pinede L, Duhaut P, Loire R. Clinical presentation of left atrial cardiac myxoma. A series of 112 consecutive cases. Medicine (Baltimore). 2001;80(3):159.
49. Gowda RM, Khan IA, Nair CK, Mehta NJ, Vasavada BC, Sacchi TJ. Cardiac papillary fibroelastoma: a comprehensive analysis of 725 cases. Am Heart J. 2003;146(3):404.
50. Mathur SK, Singh P. Transoesophageal echocardiography related complications. Indian J Anaesth. 2009;53(5):567–74.
51. Daniel WG, Erbel R, Kasper W, Visser CA, Engberding R, Sutherland GR, Grube E, Hanrath P, Maisch B, Dennig K. Safety of transesophageal echocardiography. A multicenter survey of 10,419 examinations. Circulation. 1991;83(3):817.
52. Kane GC, Hoehn SM, Behrenbeck TR, Mulvagh SL. Benzocaine-induced methemoglobinemia based on the Mayo Clinic experience from 28,478 transesophageal echocardiograms: incidence, outcomes, and predisposing factors. Arch Intern Med. 2007;167(18):1977.
53. Wilson W, et al. Prevention of infective endocarditis: guidelines from the American Heart Association: a guideline from the American Heart Association Rheumatic Fever, Endocarditis, and Kawasaki Disease Committee, Council on Cardiovascular Disease in the Young, and the Council on Clinical Cardiology, Council on Cardiovascular Surgery and Anesthesia, and the Quality of Care and Outcomes Research Interdisciplinary Working Group. Circulation. 2007;116(15):1736–54.
54. DeMaria AN, Blanchard DG. Echocardiography. In: Fuster V, Walsh RA, Harrington RA, editors. Hurst's the heart. 13th ed. New York: McGraw-Hill; 2011.
55. Srichai MB, Junor C, Rodriguez LL, Stillman AE, Grimm RA, Lieber ML, Weaver JA, Smedira NG, White RD. Clinical, imaging, and pathological characteristics of left ventricular thrombus: a comparison of contrast-enhanced magnetic resonance imaging, transthoracic echocardiography, and transesophageal echocardiography with surgical or pathological validation. Am Heart J. 2006;152(1):75.
56. Ohyama H, et al. comparison of magnetic resonance imaging and transesophageal echocardiography in detection of thrombus in the left atrial appendage. Stroke. 2003;34:2436–9.
57. Wolfgang A, Michael S, et al. Transesophageal two-dimensional echocardiography for the detection of left atrial appendage thrombus. J Am Coll Cardiol. 1986;7:1.
58. Ian BW, Colin CN, et al. Hematologic correlates of left atrial spontaneous echo contrast and thromboembolism in nonvalvular atrial fibrillation. J Am Coll Cardiol. 1993;21:451–7.
59. Bernhardt P, Schmidt H, Hammerstingl C, Lüderitz B, Omran H. Patients with atrial fibrillation and dense SEC at high risk a prospective and serial follow-up over 12 months with transesophageal echocardiography and cerebral magnetic resonance imaging. J Am Coll Cardiol. 2005;45(11):1807.
60. Daniel WG, Nellessen U, Schroder E, et al. Left atrial spontaneous contrast in mitral valve disease: an indicator for increased thromboembolic risk. J Am Coll Cardiol. 1988;11:1204–11.
61. Konstantinides S, Kasper W, Geibel A, Hofmann T, Köster W, Just H. Detection of left-to-right shunt in atrial septal defect by negative contrast echocardiography: a comparison of transthoracic and transesophageal approach. Am Heart J. 1993;126(4):909.
62. Trevelyan J, Steeds RP. Comparison of transthoracic echocardiography with harmonic imaging with transoesophageal echocardiography for the diagnosis of patent foramen ovale. Postgrad Med J. 2006;82(971):613–4.
63. Kerr AJ, Buck T, Chia K, Chow CM, Fox E, Levine RA, Picard MH. Transmitral Doppler: a new transthoracic contrast method for patent foramen ovale detection and quantification. J Am Coll Cardiol. 2000;36(6):1959.
64. Evangelista A, Gonzalez-Alujas MT. Echocardiography in infective endocarditis. Heart. 2004;90(6):614–7.
65. Vaduganathan P, Ewton A, Nagueh SF, Weilbaecher DG, Safi HJ, Zoghbi WA. Pathologic correlates of aortic plaques, thrombi and mobile "aortic debris" imaged in vivo with transesophageal echocardiography. J Am Coll Cardiol. 1997;30(2):357.

66. Keren A, Goldberg S, Gottlieb S, Klein J, Schuger C, Medina A, Tzivoni D, Stern S. Natural history of left ventricular thrombi: their appearance and resolution in the post-hospitalization period of acute myocardial infarction. J Am Coll Cardiol. 1990; 15(4):790.

67. Weinsaft JW, Kim RJ, Ross M, Krauser D, Manoushagian S, LaBounty TM, Cham MD, Min JK, Healy K, Wang Y, Parker M, Roman MJ, Devereux RB. Contrast-enhanced anatomic imaging as compared to contrast-enhanced tissue characterization for detection of left ventricular thrombus. JACC Cardiovasc Imaging. 2009; 2(8):969–79.

68. Smith WS, English JD, Johnston SC. Cerebrovascular diseases. In: Longo DL, Fauci AS, Kasper DL, Hauser SL, Jameson JL, Loscalzo J, editors. Harrison's principles of internal medicine. 18th ed. New York: McGraw-Hill; 2012.

69. Stoddard MF, Dawkins PR, Prince CR, Ammash NM. Left atrial appendage thrombus is not uncommon in patients with acute atrial fibrillation and a recent embolic event: a transesophageal echocardiographic study. J Am Coll Cardiol. 1995; 25(2):452.

70. Gage BF, Waterman AD, Shannon W, Boechler M, Rich MW, Radford MJ. Validation of clinical classification schemes for predicting stroke: results from the National Registry of Atrial Fibrillation. JAMA. 2001;285(22):2864.

71. Friberg L, Rosenqvist M, Lip GY. Evaluation of risk stratification schemes for ischaemic stroke and bleeding in 182,678 patients with atrial fibrillation: the Swedish Atrial Fibrillation cohort study. Eur Heart J. 2012;33(12):1500.

72. Connolly SJ, et al. Dabigatran versus warfarin in patients with atrial fibrillation (RE-LY). N Engl J Med. 2009;361:1139–51.

73. Manesh PR, et al. Rivaroxaban versus warfarin in nonvalvular atrial fibrillation (ROCKET-AF). N Engl J Med. 2011;365:883–91.

74. Fuster V, Halperin JL. Left ventricular thrombi and cerebral embolism. N Engl J Med. 1989;320:392–4.

75. Held AC, Gore JM, Paraskos J, Pape LA, Ball SP, Corrao JM, Alpert JS. Impact of thrombolytic therapy on left ventricular mural thrombi in acute myocardial infarction. Am J Cardiol. 1988; 62:310–1.

76. Natarajan D, Hotchandani RK, Nigam PD. Reduced incidence of left ventricular thrombi with intravenous streptokinase in acute anterior myocardial infarction: prospective evaluation by cross-sectional echocardiography. Int J Cardiol. 1988;20:201–7.

77. Eigler N, Maurer G, Shah PK. Effect of early systemic thrombolytic therapy on left ventricular mural thrombus formation in acute anterior myocardial infarction. Am J Cardiol. 1984; 54:261–3.

78. Furie KL, Kasner SE, et al. Guidelines for the prevention of stroke in patients with stroke or transient ischemic attack: a guideline for healthcare professionals from the American Heart Association/ American Stroke Association. Stroke. 2011;42(1):227.

79. Vandvik PO, Lincoff AM, et al. Primary and secondary prevention of cardiovascular disease: antithrombotic therapy and prevention of thrombosis, 9th ed: American College of Chest Physicians evidence-based clinical practice guidelines. Chest. 2012;141(2 Suppl):e637S.

80. Smith Jr SC, Benjamin EJ, et al. AHA/ACCF secondary prevention and risk reduction therapy for patients with coronary and other atherosclerotic vascular disease: 2011 update: a guideline from the American Heart Association and American College of Cardiology Foundation. Circulation. 2011;124(22):2458–73. Epub 2011 Nov 3.

81. Salem DN, O'Gara PT, Madias C, Pauker SG, American College of Chest Physicians. Valvular and structural heart disease: American College of Chest Physicians evidence-based clinical practice guidelines (8th edition). Chest. 2008;133(6 Suppl):593S.

82. Awtry EH, Colucci WS. Tumors and trauma of the heart. In: Longo DL, Fauci AS, Kasper DL, Hauser SL, Jameson JL, Loscalzo J, editors. Harrison's principles of internal medicine. 18th ed. New York: McGraw-Hill; 2012.

83. Homma S, Sacco RL, Di Tullio MR, Sciacca RR, Mohr JP, PFO in Cryptogenic Stroke Study (PICSS) Investigators. Effect of medical treatment in stroke patients with patent foramen ovale: patent foramen ovale in cryptogenic stroke study. Circulation. 2002; 105(22):2625–31.

84. Lansberg MG, O'Donnell MJ, Khatri P, Lang ES, Nguyen-Huynh MN, Schwartz NE, Sonnenberg FA, Schulman S, Vandvik PO, Spencer FA, Alonso-Coello P, Guyatt GH, Akl EA. Antithrombotic and thrombolytic therapy for ischemic stroke: antithrombotic therapy and prevention of thrombosis, 9th ed: American College of Chest Physicians evidence-based clinical practice guidelines. American College of Chest Physicians. Chest. 2012; 141(2 Suppl):e601S.

85. Furlan AJ, Reisman M, Massaro J, Mauri L, Adams H, Albers GW, Felberg R, Herrmann H, Kar S, Landzberg M, Raizner A, Wechsler L, CLOSURE I Investigators. Closure or medical therapy for cryptogenic stroke with patent foramen ovale. N Engl J Med. 2012; 366(11):991.

86. Johnston SC. Patent foramen ovale closure – closing the door except for trials. N Engl J Med. 2012;366(11):1048.

87. Warnes CA, Williams RG, Bashore TM, Child JS, Connolly HM, Dearani JA, del Nido P, Fasules JW, Graham Jr TP, Hijazi ZM, Hunt SA, King ME, Landzberg MJ, Miner PD, Radford MJ, Walsh EP, Webb GD. ACC/AHA 2008 guidelines for the management of adults with congenital heart disease: a report of the American College of Cardiology/American Heart Association Task Force on Practice Guidelines. Circulation. 2008;118(23):e714.

88. Adachi I, Kobayashi J, et al. Coronary embolism and subsequent myocardial abscess complicating ventricular aneurysm and tachycardia. Ann Thorac Surg. 2005;80:2366–8.

89. Tunick PA, Kronzon I. Vascular medicine: a companion to Braunwald's heart disease. Philadelphia: Elsevier; 2006. p. 677–687.

Sei Iwai

Abstract

Syncope is a transient loss of consciousness with loss of postural tone due to transient cerebral hypoperfusion with spontaneous recovery, usually after a short period of time. It is important to appreciate that not all transient loss of consciousness (TLOC) is due to syncope. The differential diagnosis for TLOC can be divided into cardiac and noncardiac causes. Cardiac causes which result in syncope can be broadly grouped into those due to autonomic nervous system dysfunction, cardiac arrhythmias, and obstruction to blood flow. Noncardiac causes of TLOC can be categorized into neurologic, metabolic, and psychogenic etiologies.

Syncope is a common reason for requesting a cardiology consultation. In general, there are two main reasons for evaluating patients who present with possible syncope. The first is to identify the underlying etiology of syncope, in order to initiate specific therapy aimed at the cause. The second reason is to better risk-stratify the patient, especially with respect to sudden death. Patients with structural heart disease are at higher risk for death following an episode of cardiac syncope.

This chapter reviews the differential diagnosis, pathophysiology, and steps to arrive at a diagnosis for the various etiologies of syncope and provides an evidence-based approach to management of these patients.

Keywords

Bradycardia • Electrophysiologic testing • Implantable cardioverter-defibrillator • Orthostatic hypotension • Pacemaker • Postural tachycardia syndrome • Sinus node dysfunction • Sudden cardiac death • Syncope • Tachycardia • Vasodepressor syncope • Ventricular tachycardia

Introduction

> Is syncope the same thing as sudden death except that you wake up?
>
> – Brian Olshansky, M.D. [1].

S. Iwai, MD, FACC, FHRS
Cardiac Electrophysiology,
Division of Cardiology, Westchester Medical Center,
New York Medical College,
100 Woods Road, Macy Pavilion,
111 Valhalla, NY 10595, USA
e-mail: iwais@wcmc.com

Syncope can be defined as transient loss of consciousness with loss of postural tone due to transient cerebral hypoperfusion with spontaneous recovery, usually after a short period of time. The term, syncope, is derived from the Greek term, *syncoptein*, which means "to cut short." It is important to appreciate that not all transient loss of consciousness (TLOC)

Table 40.1 Etiologies of loss of consciousness

Cardiac etiologies
   Autonomic nervous system dysfunction
      Reflex syncope
         Neurocardiogenic syncope
         Carotid sinus hypersensitivity
         Situational syncope (e.g., post-micturition)
      Postural tachycardia syndrome
      Orthostatic hypotension
   Arrhythmias
      Bradyarrhythmias
         Sinus node dysfunction
         2nd- or 3rd-degree AV block
      Tachyarrhythmias
         Supraventricular tachycardia
         Atrial fibrillation or flutter with rapid ventricular rates
         Ventricular tachyarrhythmias
   Obstruction to outflow
      Valvular disease
      Hypertrophic cardiomyopathy
      Myxoma
      Aortic dissection
      Pulmonary embolus
      Pulmonary hypertension
      Pericardial tamponade
      Congenital coronary anomalies
Noncardiac etiologies
   Neurologic
      Seizures
      Vertebral-basilar insufficiency
      Migraines
      Concussion
   Metabolic
      Hypoxemia
      Hypoglycemia
      Intoxication
      Medication-induced
   Psychogenic
      Hyperventilation
      Panic disorder

is due to syncope. The differential diagnosis for TLOC is quite lengthy and can be divided into cardiac and noncardiac causes (Table 40.1). Cardiac causes which result in syncope can be broadly grouped into those due to autonomic nervous system dysfunction, cardiac arrhythmias, and obstruction to blood flow. Noncardiac causes of TLOC can be categorized into neurologic, metabolic, and psychogenic etiologies. This chapter will focus on the cardiac causes.

Syncope is a common reason for a cardiology consultation. The estimated incidence of self-reported syncope is 6.2 per 1,000 person-years in the Framingham data [2].

In the United States, syncope accounts for approximately 3–5 % of emergency department visits and 1–6 % of urgent hospital admissions [3–7]. The age at first-time incidence of syncope is bimodal, with a high rate of occurrence in patients between 10 and 30 years of age and a subsequent decline after this. There is another peak after 65 years of age [8].

In general, there are two main reasons for evaluating patients who present with possible syncope. The first is to identify the underlying etiology of syncope in order to initiate specific therapy aimed at the particular cause. The second reason is to better risk-stratify the patient, especially with respect to sudden cardiac death (i.e., to identify when syncope was a spontaneously aborted cardiac arrest episode) but also regarding other significant adverse events and the likelihood of recurrent syncope. Soteriades et al. demonstrated that the underlying etiology of syncope has important implications on the likelihood of survival; patients with a cardiac etiology of syncope have the worst prognosis (Fig. 40.1) [2]. Furthermore, patients with structural heart disease are at higher risk for malignant causes of cardiac syncope. This group of patients includes those with a history of congestive heart failure or left ventricular dysfunction, electrocardiographic abnormalities such as atrial fibrillation, conduction system disease, nonsustained ventricular tachycardia, prolonged corrected QT interval, evidence of acute cardiac ischemia or acute or prior myocardial infarction, and/or significant valvular disease (Table 40.2).

Pathophysiology

The pathophysiology of syncope depends on the underlying etiology. The underlying pathophysiology of syncope due to cardiac arrhythmias or due to causes leading to obstruction to outflow is reduction in cardiac output and global cerebral hypoperfusion. Because the connection between the cause and effect of syncope in these cases is intuitive, attention will be focused on the pathophysiology of syncope due to autonomic nervous system dysfunction.

The nervous system (NS) in humans has two basic components that are functionally connected: (1) the central nervous system (i.e., the brain and spinal cord) and (2) the peripheral nervous system (ganglia and peripheral nerves) [10]. The peripheral NS is divided into the somatic and autonomic divisions. The somatic NS is involved with sensory information and muscle/limb position, whereas the autonomic NS involves the motor system for the viscera, smooth muscles of the body (including those of the vasculature), and the exocrine glands. The autonomic NS is comprised of three parts: (1) the sympathetic NS, (2) parasympathetic NS, and (3) enteric NS [11]. The sympathetic NS regulates the body's reaction to stress, the parasympathetic NS restores equilibrium to the resting state and conserves the body's resources, and the enteric NS controls gut function. The autonomic NS plays an important role in short- and long-term responses to

Fig. 40.1 Probability of survival, according to etiology of syncope. $p < 0.001$ for comparison between patients with and without syncope (Reproduced with permission from Kuriachan et al. [9])

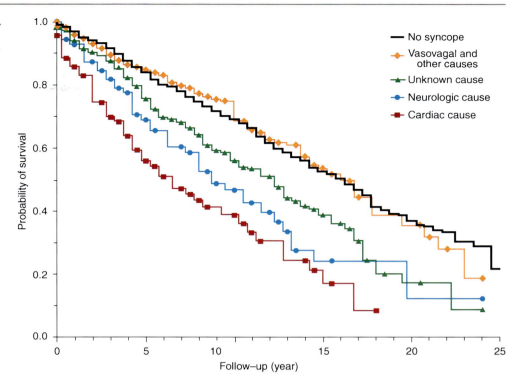

Table 40.2 Cardiac risk factors for malignant etiology of syncope

Congestive heart failure or left ventricular dysfunction

Abnormal 12-lead electrocardiogram

  Sinus bradycardia or pauses

  Bi- or trifascicular block

  2nd- or 3rd-degree atrioventricular block

  Atrial fibrillation

  Ventricular tachycardia (nonsustained or sustained)

  Prolonged corrected QT interval

  ST elevation or depression

  Ventricular preexcitation

  Evidence of Brugada pattern

  Evidence of arrhythmogenic right ventricular dysplasia/cardiomyopathy

  Early repolarization

Ischemic heart disease

  Myocardial infarction (acute or chronic)

  Myocardial ischemia

Significant valvular disease

Family history of premature unexplained or sudden death (before age of 50 years)

positional change. When one stands up from a supine position, approximately 300–800 cc of blood shifts abruptly downward to the legs and abdomen, due to gravity [12]. Almost 25 % of total blood volume can shift. This rapid decline in central blood volume results in a decline in venous return to the heart. As a result, stroke volume also declines. In addition to these volume shifts, upright posture also leads to a substantial increase in the transmural capillary pressure in the dependent areas of the body, which causes fluid filtration into the tissue spaces. This process equilibrates in approximately 30 min and can result in a decrease in plasma volume of up to 10 % [13]. To counteract the effects of these fluid shifts due to gravity, several cardiovascular counterregulatory systems must be activated to help maintain a steady level of arterial pressure and cerebral perfusion. Orthostatic stabilization is normally achieved in less than 1 min.

However, when these regulating systems do not compensate adequately, syncope can result, due to a cascade of events. In this situation, upright posture results in peripheral venous pooling with decreased venous return and a subsequent decline in arterial pressure and cardiac filling. This leads to an increase in ventricular contractility which activates pressure receptors in the carotid sinus and the aortic arch, as well as in the heart and lungs [14]. There is a "paradoxic" decline in sympathetic activity; vagal afferents in the atria and ventricles and mechanoreceptors combine to produce a tonic inhibitory effect on the nucleus tractus solitarii in the medulla [15]. Baroreceptors in the medulla activate cardiovagal neurons of the nucleus ambiguus and dorsal vagal nucleus and inhibit sympathoexcitatory neurons in the rostral ventrolateral medulla [16]. The final result is hypotension due to a combination of vasodilatation and bradycardia.

Continued upright posture results in activation of neurohumoral responses, the extent of which depends on the degree of volume depletion. Dehydration leads to more significant activation of the renin-angiotensin system and enhances vasopressin release. The inability of any of these factors to compensate could lead to syncope.

The best-appreciated form of syncope due to autonomic nervous system dysfunction is neurocardiogenic (i.e., vaso-vagal, vasodepressor, neurally mediated) syncope. This form of syncope tends to occur most frequently in younger patients and is often preceded by a prodrome of lightheadedness, nausea, and diaphoresis. Recovery of consciousness is usually rapid. A typical scenario is in the setting of orthostatic stress with venous pooling in the lower extremities. This results in increased ventricular contraction which results in activation of the mechanoreceptors. This surge of neural traffic to the brainstem provokes the aforementioned paradoxic withdrawal of sympathetic tone, leading to hypotension, bradycardia, and syncope [17]. Other triggers of neurocardiogenic syncope include emotional stress, pain, postprandial state, and coughing or micturition. Interestingly, Sutton and Petersen observed that responses seen during neurocardiogenic syncope and carotid sinus hypersensitivity are similar and may be part of the same disorder [18].

Chronic autonomic failure is another form of syncope due to autonomic nervous system dysfunction. One type of autonomic failure that has been the focus of attention in recent years is postural tachycardia syndrome (POTS). POTS includes a constellation of signs and symptoms of orthostatic intolerance, including fatigue, near syncope, lightheadedness, and exercise intolerance with tachycardia [19]. POTS is defined as presence of these symptoms with an increase in heart rate of 30 bpm (or heart rate above 120 bpm) occurring within 10 min of standing up in the absence of medications or debilitating conditions (e.g., prolonged bed rest). Other symptoms can include nausea, difficulty with concentration, tremulousness, and syncope. The symptoms are relieved by assuming a supine position. Most definitions of POTS also include a duration minimum of 3 months. The prevalence of POTS in the United States is estimated at 500,000 patients, and approximately one-quarter are disabled and unable to work [20]. Importantly, most patients with POTS do not have a significant decrease in blood pressure. Rather, they may exhibit no change, a small decrease, or even a small increase in blood pressure.

POTS can be categorized as either primary or secondary [21]. Primary POTS is not associated with other disease conditions, whereas secondary POTS is associated with other disease states. The most frequent form of primary POTS is the partial dysautonomic (PD) form, which has a 5:1 female-to-male ratio. These patients exhibit a mild form of peripheral neuropathy, with inability to maintain adequate vascular resistance during orthostatic stress and increased blood pooling in the dependent areas of the body. The extent of pooling increases over time, exceeding the compensatory effect of increase in heart rate. This form of POTS often follows a viral illness, pregnancy, sepsis, surgery, or trauma. Currently, it is thought that the PD form in many patients is due to an autoimmune process [22].

A less frequent form of primary POTS is the "hyperadrenergic" form [23]. These patients experience more gradual onset of symptoms, with symptoms including tremors, anxiety, and cold/clammy extremities while standing, as well as migraine headaches in the majority of patients. In addition, the hyperadrenergic form is often associated with orthostatic hypertension along with tachycardia and significantly elevated serum norepinephrine levels (>600 ng/mL) upon standing. These patients have a strong family history of the disorder. A single-point mutation that results in a poorly functioning reuptake transporter protein involved in recycling norepinephrine within the synaptic cleft has been reported in some patients [24].

Secondary POTS refers to conditions that produce a state of peripheral autonomic denervation or vascular unresponsiveness (with relative sparing of cardiac innervation). Secondary POTS is often seen in diabetes mellitus but also with amyloidosis, sarcoid, alcoholism, lupus, Sjögren syndrome, chemotherapy, and heavy-metal poisoning. In some cases, POTS can be part of a more severe autonomic nervous system disorder such as multiple system atrophy, pure autonomic failure, or a form of a paraneoplastic syndrome sometimes seen with certain adenocarcinomas. It is thought that these malignancies produce autoantibodies to acetylcholine receptors analogous to those seen in following viral syndromes [25].

Another entity, orthostatic hypotension, often accompanied by syncope, is due to an excessive fall in systemic pressure triggered by change in posture (i.e., sitting or standing up). Clinically significant hypotension is defined as a decrease in systolic blood pressure of at least 20 mmHg and/or a decrease in diastolic pressure of at least 10 mmHg within 3 min of standing. Orthostatic hypotension can be caused by impaired ability to increase vascular resistance, volume depletion/dehydration, venous pooling with decreased cardiac output, or impaired cardiac diastolic relaxation and can be precipitated by medications (diuretics, vasodilators, alcohol), by primary neurologic abnormality (Parkinson's disease, pure autonomic failure, or multiple system atrophy), or by acquired disease (diabetes mellitus).

Diagnosis

Initial Assessment

In the initial assessment of syncope, one should obtain a detailed history of the episode(s). This includes the general setting, precipitating factor(s), body position, activity level, duration of loss of consciousness, and associated symptoms. Frequency of episodes and severity (i.e., if there was associated trauma) are also important. If the episode was witnessed, the observers should be interviewed as well. Inquiry into recent illnesses or underlying medical conditions can also be helpful. A complete family history with respect to any known arrhythmias, syncope, or unexplained, sudden, or early deaths may also be relevant.

Syncope in the setting of exercise should be considered as having a potentially malignant etiology until proven otherwise. Potential causes of exertional syncope include infarct-related ventricular tachycardia, torsade de pointes (a specific form of polymorphic ventricular tachycardia in patients with long QT syndrome), ventricular arrhythmias due to catecholaminergic polymorphic ventricular tachycardia (CPVT), arrhythmias (especially atrial fibrillation [AF] with rapid conduction down an accessory pathway, also called "preexcited AF"), and significant valvular disease, including aortic and mitral stenosis. Other causes include congenital heart disease, anomalous coronary arteries, hypertrophic cardiomyopathy, arrhythmogenic right ventricular dysplasia/cardiomyopathy, and myocarditis.

Physical examination should include complete vital signs including orthostatic blood pressure measurements (and in certain cases, repeated measurements while standing for 2, 5, and 10 min), as well as an evaluation for evidence for structural heart disease. For example, a late-peaking systolic ejection murmur with absent A2 heart sound may be indicative of significant aortic stenosis, while a harsh systolic murmur that increases with Valsalva maneuver may indicate hypertrophic cardiomyopathy.

A complete blood count and metabolic profile should be obtained to evaluate for blood loss, dehydration, and electrolyte abnormalities. If the hyperadrenergic form of POTS is suspected, serum samples of norepinephrine, epinephrine, and dopamine levels should be obtained in the supine and upright positions. A 12-lead electrocardiogram (ECG) is also important to evaluate the underlying rhythm (and rate) and to look for evidence of conduction system disease, ventricular preexcitation, left ventricular hypertrophy, epsilon wave, repolarization abnormalities, or evidence of Brugada syndrome. An echocardiogram is also essential to evaluate for underlying structural heart disease. This should include evaluation of left ventricular function and wall thickness, presence of valvular disease, pulmonary hypertension, and pericardial effusion.

A (24- or 48-h) Holter monitor is only useful if patients have daily symptoms, which is quite unusual. Even external event monitors (small portable electrocardiographic recording devices), which can be carried for a month or longer, are rarely effective in capturing the underlying cardiac rhythm during a syncopal episode.

Tilt Table Testing

Frequently, a definite cause of syncope is not elucidated by the initial history and testing. Tilt table testing has traditionally been used to assess patients with suspected neurocardiogenic syncope. Various protocols have been proposed, including variation in tilt duration and facilitation with pharmacologic agents such as adenosine, isoproterenol, and nitroglycerin [26]. However, due to a lack of a "gold standard" for diagnosing neurocardiogenic syncope, interpretation of tilt table testing results has been limited by the inability to identify "false positives" and "false negatives." Utilizing observed diagnostic yield in a given population as a function of assumed population prevalence, Stein et al. [27] calculated "imputed sensitivity" of passive (i.e., drug-free) tilt testing of varying durations and concluded that it had limited sensitivity for diagnosing neurally mediated syncope. In fact, for populations with a pretest likelihood of 25–50 %, tilt testing results are inaccurate in up to two-fifths of patients.

For diagnosing POTS or orthostatic hypotension, however, tilt table testing remains a valuable tool to evaluate heart rate and blood pressure response to orthostatic stress.

Implantable Loop Recorder

In an effort to more effectively and efficiently provide a diagnosis in patients with unexplained syncope, Krahn et al. [28] randomized 60 patients to either "conventional" testing (which included external loop recorder, tilt testing, and electrophysiologic testing) to prolonged monitoring with an implantable loop recorder (ILR). Patients enrolled had recurrent unexplained syncope or a single episode that was associated with injury and, thus, warranted cardiovascular investigation. Prior to enrollment, they received 24 h of baseline outpatient or inpatient telemetry and transthoracic echocardiography. Patients were excluded if their left ventricular ejection fraction was less than 35 %. In the 30 patients randomized to ILR monitoring, a diagnosis was obtained in 14, including 10 with symptomatic bradycardia, 1 with supraventricular tachycardia, and 3 with vasovagal syncope. In contrast, in the "conventional" monitoring group, only 6 of 30 patients were diagnosed during follow-up (20 % for conventional arm vs. 52 % for ILR arm). One patient had symptomatic third-degree AV block (while wearing external loop recorder), 2 patients had a positive tilt test, and during electrophysiologic testing, 2 patients had significant AV node dysfunction while 1 had inducible ventricular tachycardia. Furthermore, 6 of the patients who were undiagnosed in the ILR arm at 1 year crossed over to the conventional arm, but only 1 was subsequently diagnosed (with sustained AV nodal reentry tachycardia with hypotension at electrophysiologic testing). Twenty-one crossed over from the conventional arm to the ILR arm; a diagnosis was made in 8 patients (4 with symptomatic bradycardia, 2 with tachycardia, and 2 with sinus rhythm with phasic motion artifact suggestive of seizure activity). The authors concluded that a prolonged monitoring strategy (with ILR) is more likely to provide a diagnosis than conventional testing in this patient population.

Further evidence of the utility of the ILR, as well as the lack of utility for tilt table testing, comes from the ISSUE (International Study on Syncope of Uncertain Etiology) investigators. In 1 substudy, the investigators implanted ILRs and followed patients with no structural heart disease and normal electrocardiogram with recurrent (≥3 episodes in prior 2 years). The results were similar in the "isolated" syncope group (who had negative tilt table tests) and the "tilt-positive" group, with 46 and 62 % of patients, respectively, having prolonged asystolic pauses, mainly due to sinus arrest (lasting a median of 31 s), preceded by progressive bradycardia or tachycardia-bradycardia (i.e., findings consistent with a vasodepressor etiology) [29].

It is important to appreciate that the findings on data collected from ILRs depend on the underlying patient substrate. This was demonstrated by another study by the ISSUE investigators, in which the mechanism of syncope was investigated in patients with a negative electrophysiology test and underlying bundle branch block pattern on electrocardiogram [30]. During a follow-up period of 3–15 months, syncope recurred in 22 of 52 patients (42 %), with the event being documented on ILR in 19 patients (after a median of 48 days). The most common etiology in this population was prolonged asystole (mainly due to AV block); this occurred in 17 patients. The remaining 2 patients had normal sinus rhythm or sinus tachycardia.

Electrophysiology (EP) Study

Electrophysiologic testing can be used to document sinus node, atrioventricular node, and His-Purkinje system dysfunction. However, despite its high specificity, the utility of EP testing is limited by its low sensitivity. Patients with bundle branch block are at higher risk of developing high-degree AV block. This risk is increased by a history of syncope or a prolonged His-ventricular (HV) interval during EP testing. The progression rate to AV block at 4 years was 12 and 24 % in patients with an HV interval of ≥70 and ≥100 ms, respectively [31]. EP testing can also be used to assess for inducibility of supraventricular tachycardia in patients with a prodrome of palpitations.

According to the 2006 American College of Cardiology (ACC)/American Heart Association (AHA)/European Society of Cardiology (ESC) guidelines [32]. EP testing is recommended in patients with syncope of unknown cause with impaired left ventricular function or structural heart disease (a Class I indication). Furthermore, EP testing can also be useful in patients with syncope when bradyarrhythmias or tachyarrhythmias are suspected and in whom noninvasive diagnostic studies are not conclusive (Class IIa indication).

The role of electrophysiology (EP) study in evaluating for ventricular arrhythmias as a potential cause of syncope has been evaluated by several studies. In patients with prior myocardial infarction and preserved left ventricular function, induction of sustained monomorphic ventricular tachycardia was found to be strongly predictive of the cause of syncope [33]. However, induction of ventricular fibrillation is considered a nonspecific finding [34]. Conversely, the absence of induction of ventricular arrhythmias may identify a group of patients at lower risk of arrhythmic syncope [35].

Patients with known coronary artery disease need to be investigated aggressively. In a study evaluating the long-term outcome of patients with coronary artery disease and unexplained syncope who were treated with an approach guided by electrophysiology study, Mittal et al. reported that EP study suggested a plausible diagnosis in 32 of 67 patients (48 %) with inducible monomorphic ventricular tachycardia being the most common abnormality [36]. Unfortunately, despite the presence of an implantable cardioverter-defibrillator (ICD) in this group, total mortality was high, with 1- and 2-year survival rates being only 77 and 45 %, respectively.

In patients with nonischemic dilated cardiomyopathy (NIDCM) presenting with syncope, the possibility of ventricular arrhythmias needs to be considered strongly. In a small study of 14 patients, Knight et al. [37] reported that 7 patients (50 %) in the group with syncope and NIDCM received appropriate implantable cardioverter-defibrillator (ICD) shocks (i.e., due to ventricular arrhythmias) during a mean follow-up period of only 24±13 months. In a control group of patients with NIDCM and prior cardiac arrest, 8 of 19 patients (42 %) had appropriate ICD shocks during a follow-up of 47±41 months. Among patients receiving appropriate ICD shocks, the mean time from ICD implant to first shock was 10±14 months in the group with syncope compared to 48±47 months in the control group (with prior cardiac arrest). Unfortunately, diagnosis of ventricular tachycardia is limited by the poor yield of EP testing in the NIDCM patient population [38]. Therefore, empiric ICD implantation is generally recommended in patients with NIDCM and syncope, rather than relying on electrophysiologic testing.

Management

The management of syncope is dictated by the level of suspicion for a malignant cause. Patients who have characteristics listed in Table 40.2 who present with syncope should be considered for hospital admission for further diagnostic evaluation and management. Other patients for whom hospitalization should be considered include those with severe anemia and electrolyte disturbances. Too often, however, patients without high-risk features are admitted via the emergency department for observation [39]. Some hospitals have created "syncope management units" (SMUs) in an attempt to better evaluate which patients require hospital admission. In the SEEDS (Syncope Evaluation in the Emergency Department Study) trial [40], a presumptive diagnosis was made in 67 % of patients assigned to an SMU compared with only 10 % of "standard care" patients.

Vasodepressor Syncope

A summary of various therapeutic modalities evaluated in randomized clinical trials to treat vasodepressor syncope is listed in Table 40.3, as modified from Kuriachan et al. [9]. Physical counterpressure maneuvers should be taught to all patients with vasodepressor syncope who have a prodrome and are often tired prior to medical therapy. Squatting, leg-crossing, arm-tensing, or handgrip maneuvers have proven useful in mitigating vasovagal episodes, reducing the total burden and recurrence rate of syncopal events. In the Physical Counterpressure Manoeuvres Trial (PC-Trial), counterpressure maneuvers increased recurrence-free survival (39 % relative risk reduction); syncope burden during follow-up was reduced from 51 to 32 % [41]. Brignole et al. also found that isometric arm contraction is capable of aborting impending vasovagal syncope [48]. During tilt table testing, handgrip maneuvers result in an increase in systolic blood pressure during symptoms of impending syncope compared to placebo (increase from 92 ± 10 mmHg to 105 ± 38 mmHg vs. decrease from 91 ± 11 mmHg to 73 ± 21 mmHg, respectively; $p = 0.008$). After training, handgrip maneuver was successful in 94/95 episodes (99 %).

"Tilt training" has also been proposed as a non-pharmacologic technique to reduce the recurrence of vasovagal syncope. Tilt training is thought to improve the neurovascular response to orthostatic stress and involves progressively longer periods of standing, with one's back leaning slightly against a wall. DiGirolamo et al. [49] followed 47 consecutive adolescents with recurrent syncope and positive tilt table test, according to their consent ("training" group; 24 patients) or refusal ("controls"; 23 patients) to enter a tilt training program. Interestingly, response to head-up tilt was reevaluated after 1 month, and 95.8 % of the training group became tilt-negative compared with 26.1 % of the control group ($p < 0.0001$). Furthermore, over a period of 18.2 ± 5.3 months, spontaneous syncope occurred in 56.5 % of the control group but in none of the training group ($p < 0.0001$).

Liberalization of salt and fluid intake is also encouraged in patients with suspected vasovagal syncope. Of course, this should be avoided in patients with hypertension, renal disease, congestive heart failure, or left ventricular dysfunction.

Regarding pharmacologic therapy, initial enthusiasm regarding the use of beta-adrenergic blockers diminished following the results of the first Prevention of Syncope Trial (POST) [42]. This was a randomized, placebo-controlled, double-blind study assessing the utility of metoprolol in vasovagal syncope. Metoprolol provided no benefit compared to placebo.

Table 40.3 Summary results of selected major randomized clinical trials of treatment for vasovagal syncope

Treatment	Reference number	Author	Patients	Clinical outcome	Effect	P value
Physical counterpressure maneuvers	[41]	VanDijk	223	Syncope recurrence	51 % control	0.005
					32 % PCM	
Metoprolol	[42]	Sheldon	208	Syncope recurrence	36 % controls	0.99
					36 % metoprolol	
Fluoxetine or propranolol	[43]	Theodorakis	96	Syncope or presyncope recurrence	41 % controls	<0.05
					51 % propranolol	
					22 % fluoxetine	
Midodrine	[44]	Qingyou	26	Syncope recurrence	80 % controls	0.023
					22 % midodrine	
Fludrocortisone	[45]	Salim	33	Syncope or presyncope recurrence	36 % controls	<0.04
					55 % fludrocortisone	
Pacemakers	[46]	Connolly	100	Syncope recurrence	40 % controls	0.14
					31 % pacing	
Pacemakers	[47]	Raviele	29	Syncope recurrence	38 % controls	Not stated
					50 % pacemakers	

Modified from Kuriachan et al. [9] with permission

Given that serotonin is important in the regulation of heart rate and blood pressure, it is reasonable to assume that it plays an important role in vasovagal syncope. However, a recent double-blind, placebo-controlled study found that fluoxetine, propranolol, and placebo had equal effects (although patients on fluoxetine had an improved quality of life and decreased syncope and presyncope) [43].

Midodrine, a peripherally active alpha-agonist, has been used to mitigate the reduction in peripheral sympathetic outflow that is responsible for venous pooling and vasodepression. After initial promising studies with midodrine on vasodepressor syncope, Qingyou et al. randomized 26 children with at least 3 episodes of syncope per year, in open-label fashion, to midodrine vs. conservative diet and posture training [44]. Clinical recurrence of syncope over 10 months of follow-up was 20 % vs. 80 % (midodrine vs. control groups, respectively). Importantly, midodrine should not be used in hypertensive patients.

Finally, fludrocortisone (a corticosteroid with mainly mineralocorticoid activity) has been used to try to treat vasodepressor syncope by increasing blood volume by sodium and water retention. Again, despite promising preliminary data, Salim and DiSessa found that children on fludrocortisone had more symptoms compared with those taking placebo [45]. The results of POST II, which is also investigating fludrocortisone in neurally mediated syncope have not been published yet [50].

Initial data regarding the utility of pacemakers for vasovagal syncope pointed to significant benefits in reduction of subsequent episodes. These pacemakers typically utilized a "rate-drop" feature, in which the pacemaker would sense a rapid drop in heart rate and pace at a rate of 100–110 bpm for a period of time (approximately 2 min) in an effort to counteract the bradycardic aspect of the episode. However, these studies were not blinded (i.e., patients knew whether or not they had a pacemaker implanted), and the benefit was likely, at least in part, due to a placebo effect. The second Vasovagal Pacemaker Study (VPS II) was a double-blind, placebo-controlled, multicenter, prospective study which randomized 100 patients with vasovagal syncope and positive tilt table test to dual-chamber pacing or sensing only, i.e., all patients had a pacemaker implanted [46]. There was no significant benefit to pacing after a 6-month follow-up period. Another double-blinded study, the Vasovagal Syncope and Pacing (SYNPACE) trial [47] also showed no significant benefit with dual-chamber pacing, although this trial was terminated early due to the results of VPS II. More recently, however, Brignole et al. found that dual-chamber pacing is effective in reducing the recurrence of syncope in patients over 40 years of age with severe asystolic neurally mediated syncope, with a 32 % absolute (and 57 % relative) reduction in syncope

recurrence [51]. Given these findings, while pacemaker implantation should not be used routinely in vasovagal syncope, a selected subgroup of patients with documented asystole during syncope might benefit from dual-chamber pacing.

Postural Tachycardia Syndrome (POTS)

Treatment for POTS, like most disorders, needs to be individualized for each patient. Removal of any medications that may be exacerbating the condition and identifying and treating any underlying medical condition which may be causing POTS (described earlier) are extremely important. Physical aerobic exercise and reconditioning should be encouraged for all POTS patients, along with gentle resistance training of the abdomen and legs (to strengthen the skeletal muscle pump). Fluid (approximately 2 l/day) and salt (3–5 g/day) can also be helpful, except in the hyperadrenergic form [21]. Waist-high elastic compression stockings providing 30 mmHg of ankle counter pressure are also useful in some cases. Regarding medical therapy, although no medication is approved by the US Food and Drug Administration for treatment of POTS, several have been tried "off-label," including fludrocortisone (0.1–0.2 mg daily), desmopressin (DDAVP; 0.1–0.2 mg qHS), midodrine (5–10 mg 3 times daily), methylphenidate (5–10 mg 3 times daily), and serotonin reuptake inhibitors. More recently, pyridostigmine (30–90 mg up to 3 times daily) has been found to be useful [52]. Other therapies that have been investigated include erythropoietin and octreotide (50–200 mg subcutaneously, 3 times daily). In the hyperadrenergic form, clonidine, labetalol, carvedilol, methyldopa, and phenobarbital have been tried.

It is important to remember that most patients with POTS following a viral syndrome recover over 2–5 years. In general, although some patients do not recover, younger patients appear to have a better prognosis. Unfortunately, those with the hyperadrenergic form often require long-term therapy.

Orthostatic Hypotension

Treatment of orthostatic syncope or hypotension should emphasize awareness of factors that can aggravate postural hypotension, maintenance of adequate hydration, compression stockings, and, possibly, "tilt training" as described previously. Adjustment of a patient's medical regimen may be necessary to eliminate diuretics and/or vasodilators, if possible, or addition of vasoconstrictors such as midodrine. In certain cases, medications such as erythropoietin, desmopressin, clonidine, and octreotide may be useful.

Patients with Structural Heart Disease

Treatment of syncope associated with structural heart disease may involve surgical correction, e.g., if it is due to severe aortic stenosis or to an atrial myxoma. If there is an acute etiology, such as myocardial infarction, myocardial ischemia, pericardial effusion with tamponade physiology, or pulmonary embolism, the underlying process needs to be addressed and treated. Patients with hypertrophic cardiomyopathy can have syncope due to vasovagal reasons but also from outflow tract obstruction or ventricular arrhythmias.

Determining whether a cardiac arrhythmia is the underlying etiology of syncope in these patients can be difficult. However, there are scenarios in which either pacemaker or ICD implantation is warranted, if suspicion is high and risk factors are present (see section "Summary of Key Guidelines"). For example, pacemaker implantation is recommended for patients with sinus node dysfunction and syncope of unexplained origin when clinically significant abnormalities of sinus node function are discovered or provoked during EP study; this is a Class IIa indication, and syncope of undetermined origin with clinically relevant, hemodynamically significant sustained VT or ventricular fibrillation induced at electrophysiological study is a Class I indication for ICD implantation [53].

Cardiac Arrhythmias in the Absence of Overt Structural Heart Disease

When supraventricular tachycardia or monomorphic ventricular tachycardia in the absence of structural heart disease is discovered either clinically or during EP testing and suspected to be the etiology of syncope, management often includes curative catheter ablation, although medical therapy can also be considered.

In some patients, ventricular arrhythmias due to a channelopathy or other familial cardiomyopathy can be the underlying etiology of syncope. The diagnosis and management of these patients is beyond the scope of this chapter. However, these include the long QT syndrome, Brugada syndrome, and polymorphic catecholaminergic ventricular tachycardia, which can present with sustained and nonsustained ventricular tachyarrhythmias. In addition, patients with arrhythmogenic right ventricular dysplasia/cardiomyopathy may only have subtle structural changes which are not readily apparent on routine diagnostic testing (typically detected with cardiac magnetic resonance imaging), especially early on in the disease process, and can present with syncope due to ventricular tachycardia.

Key Points

- Syncope is defined as transient loss of consciousness with loss of postural tone due to transient cerebral hypoperfusion with spontaneous recovery usually after a short period of time.
- Syncope is a common reason for requesting a cardiology consultation and accounts for 1–6 % of urgent hospital admissions.
- There are two main reasons for evaluating patients who present with possible syncope:
  - To identify the underlying etiology of syncope in order to initiate specific therapy aimed at the particular cause
  - To better risk-stratify the patient, especially with respect to sudden death
- The presence of structural heart disease is a key differentiating factor in the evaluation process, prognosis, and treatment of patients presenting with syncope.

Summary of Key Guidelines

Recommendations for permanent pacing in patients *with syncope*:

Class I Indication:

Sinus node dysfunction with:

Documented symptomatic bradycardia, including frequent sinus pauses that produce symptoms

Acquired atrioventricular (AV) block:

Third-degree and second-degree AV block at any anatomic level associated with bradycardia with symptoms (e.g., syncope)

Hypersensitive carotid sinus syndrome with:

Recurrent syncope caused by spontaneously occurring carotid sinus stimulation and carotid sinus pressure that induces ventricular asystole of more than 3 s

Class IIa Indication:

Sinus node dysfunction with:

Heart rate less than 40 bpm when a clear association between significant symptoms (e.g., syncope) consistent with bradycardia and the actual presence of bradycardia has not been documented

Syncope of unexplained origin when clinically significant abnormalities of sinus node function are discovered or provoked in electrophysiological studies

Chronic bifascicular block with:

Syncope not demonstrated to be due to AV block when other likely causes have been excluded, specifically ventricular tachycardia

Hypersensitive carotid sinus syndrome with:

Syncope without clear, provocative events and with a hypersensitive cardioinhibitory response of 3 s or longer

Class IIb Indication:

Hypersensitive carotid sinus syndrome with:

Significantly symptomatic neurocardiogenic syncope associated with bradycardia documented spontaneously or at the time of tilt table testing

Recommendations for permanent pacing in patients *with syncope*:

Following cardiac transplantation with:

Syncope even when bradyarrhythmia has not been documented

Class III Indication:

Sinus node dysfunction with:

Symptomatic bradycardia due to nonessential drug therapy

Hypersensitive Carotid sinus syndrome with:

Situational vasovagal syncope in which avoidance behavior is effective and preferred

Modified from Connolly et al. [46]

Recommendations for ICD implantation in patients *with syncope*:

Class I Indication:

Structural heart disease and spontaneous sustained ventricular tachycardia (VT)

Syncope of undetermined origin with clinically relevant, hemodynamically significant sustained VT or ventricular fibrillation induced at electrophysiological study

Class IIa Indication:

Unexplained syncope, significant left ventricular dysfunction, and nonischemic dilated cardiomyopathy

Hypertrophic cardiomyopathy and unexplained syncope

Long QT syndrome with syncope while receiving beta-blockers

Brugada patients with syncope

Catecholaminergic polymorphic VT patients with syncope while receiving beta-blockers

Class IIb Indication:

Advanced structural heart disease in whom thorough invasive and noninvasive investigations have failed to define a cause

Class III Indication:

Syncope of undetermined cause in a patient without inducible ventricular tachyarrhythmias and without structural heart disease

Modified from Connolly et al. [46]

References

1. Olshansky B. Is syncope the same thing as sudden death except that you wake up? J Cardiovasc Electrophysiol. 1997;8:1098–101.
2. Soteriades ES, Evans JC, Larson MG, et al. Incidence and prognosis of syncope. N Engl J Med. 2002;347:878–85.
3. Kapoor WN. Evaluation and outcome of patients with syncope. Medicine (Baltimore). 1990;69:160–75.
4. Day SC, Cook EF, Funkenstein H, et al. Evaluation and outcome of emergency room patients with transient loss of consciousness. Am J Med. 1982;73:15–23.
5. Kapoor WN, Karpf M, Wieand S, et al. A prospective evaluation and follow-up of patients with syncope. N Engl J Med. 1983;309:197–204.
6. Manolis AS, Linzer M, Salem D, et al. Syncope: current diagnostic evaluation and management. Ann Intern Med. 1990;112:850–63.
7. Manolis AS. The clinical spectrum and diagnosis of syncope. Herz. 1993;18:143–54.
8. Moya A, Sutton R, Ammirati F, et al. Guidelines for the diagnosis and management of syncope: the task force for the diagnosis and management of syncope of the European Society of Cardiology (ESC). Eur Heart J. 2009;30:2631–71.
9. Kuriachan V, Sheldon R, Platonov M. Evidence-based treatment for vasovagal syncope. Heart Rhythm. 2008;5:1609–14.
10. Kandel ER. The nervous system. In: Kandel ER, Schwartz JH, Jessell TM, editors. Essentials of neural science and behavior. Norwalk: Appleton and Lange; 1995. p. 71–88.
11. Benarroch E. The central autonomic network: functional organization, dysfunction and perspective. Mayo Clin Proc. 1993;68:988–1001.
12. Thompson WO, Thompson PK, Dailey ME. The effect of upright posture on the composition and volume of the blood in man. J Clin Invest. 1988;5:573–609.
13. Streeten D. Physiology of the microcirculation. In: Streeten D, editor. Orthostatic disorders of the circulation. New York: Plenum Medical; 1987. p. 1–12.
14. Jacobsen TN. Relative contributions of cardiopulmonary and sino-aortic baroreflexes in causing sympathetic activation in human skeletal muscle circulation during orthostatic stress. Circ Res. 1993;73:367–78.
15. Andresen MC, Kunze DL. Nucleus tractus solitarius: gateway to neural circulatory control. Annu Rev Physiol. 1994;56:93–116.
16. Dampney RA. Functional organization of central pathways regulating the cardiovascular system. Physiol Rev. 1994;74:323–64.
17. Kosinski D, Grubb BP, Temesy-Armos P. Pathophysiological aspects of neurocardiogenic syncope. Pacing Clin Electrophysiol. 1995;18:716–21.
18. Sutton R, Petersen M. The clinical spectrum of neurocardiogenic syncope. J Cardiovasc Electrophysiol. 1995;6:569–76.
19. Grubb BP, Karas B. Clinical disorders of the autonomic nervous system associated with orthostatic intolerance. Pacing Clin Electrophysiol. 1999;22:798–810.
20. Goldstein D, Robertson D, Esler M, et al. Dysautonomias: clinical disorders of the autonomic nervous system. Ann Intern Med. 2002;137:753–63.
21. Grubb BP. Postural tachycardia syndrome. Circulation. 2008;117:2814–7.
22. Vernino S, Low PA, Fealy RD, et al. Autoantibodies to ganglionic acetylcholine receptors in auto-immune autonomic neuropathies. N Engl J Med. 2000;343:847–55.
23. Vincent S, Robertson D. Hyperadrenergic postural tachycardia syndrome. In: Robertson D, editor. Primer on the autonomic nervous system. San Diego: Elsevier Academic Press; 2004. p. 344–5.
24. Shannon JR, Flattem NL, Jordan J, et al. Orthostatic intolerance and tachycardia associated with norepinephrine-transporter deficiency. N Engl J Med. 2000;342:541–9.
25. Klein CM, Vernino S, Lennon VA, et al. The spectrum of autoimmune autonomic neuropathies. Ann Neurol. 2003;53:752–8.
26. Benditt DG, Remole S, Bailin S, et al. Tilt table testing for evaluation of neurally-mediated (cardioneurogenic) syncope: rationale and proposed protocols. Pacing Clin Electrophysiol. 1991;14:1528–37.
27. Stein KM, Slotwiner DJ, Mittal S, et al. Formal analysis of the optimal duration of tilt testing for the diagnosis of neurally mediated syncope. Am Heart J. 2001;141:282–8.
28. Krahn AD, Klein GJ, Yee R, Skanes AC. Randomized assessment of syncope trial: conventional diagnostic testing versus a prolonged monitoring strategy. Circulation. 2001;104:46–51.
29. Moya A, Brignole M, Menozzi C, et al. Mechanism of syncope in patients with isolated syncope and in patients with tilt-positive syncope. Circulation. 2001;104:1261–7.
30. Brignole M, Menozzi C, Moya A, et al. Mechanism of syncope in patients with bundle branch block and negative electrophysiological test. Circulation. 2001;104:2045–50.
31. Scheinman MM, Peters RW, Suavé MJ, et al. Value of the H-Q interval in patients with bundle branch block and the role of prophylactic permanent pacing. Am J Cardiol. 1982;50:1316–22.
32. Zipes DP, Camm AJ, Borggrefe M, et al. ACC/AHA/ESC 2006 guidelines for management of patients with ventricular arrhythmias and the prevention of sudden cardiac death—executive summary. J Am Coll Cardiol. 2006;48:1064–108.
33. Olshansky B, Hahn EA, Hartz VL, et al. Clinical significance of syncope in the electrophysiologic study versus electrocardiographic

monitoring (ESVEM) trial. The ESVEM Investigators. Am Heart J. 1999;137:878–86.

34. Mittal S, Hao SC, Iwai S, et al. Significance of inducible ventricular fibrillation in patients with coronary artery disease and unexplained syncope. J Am Coll Cardiol. 2001;38:371–6.

35. Link MS, Kim KM, Homoud MK, et al. Long-term outcome of patients with syncope associated with coronary artery disease and a nondiagnostic electrophysiological evaluation. Am J Cardiol. 1999;83:1334–7.

36. Mittal S, Iwai S, Stein KM, et al. Long-term outcome of patients with unexplained syncope treated with an electrophysiologic-guided approach in the implantable cardioverter-defibrillator era. J Am Coll Cardiol. 1999;34:1082–9.

37. Knight BP, Goyal R, Pelosi F, Flemming M, et al. Outcome of patients with nonischemic dilated cardiomyopathy and unexplained syncope treated with an implantable defibrillator. J Am Coll Cardiol. 1999;33:1964–70.

38. Poll DS, Marchlinski FE, Buxton AE, et al. Usefulness of programmed stimulation in idiopathic dilated cardiomyopathy. Am J Cardiol. 1986;58:992–7.

39. Bartoletti A, Fabiani P, Adriani P, et al. Hospital admission of patients referred to the emergency department for syncope: a single-hospital prospective study based on the application of the European Society of Cardiology guidelines on syncope. Eur Heart J. 2006;27:83–8.

40. Shen SK, Decker WW, Smars PA, et al. Syncope evaluation in the emergency department study (SEEDS): a multidisciplinary approach to syncope management. Circulation. 2004;110:3636–45.

41. VanDijk N, Quartieri F, Blanc JJ, et al. Effectiveness of physical counterpressure maneuvers in preventing vasovagal syncope: the physical counterpressure manoeuvres trial (PC-trial). J Am Coll Cardiol. 2006;48:1652–7.

42. Sheldon R, Connolly S, Rose S, et al., and the POST Investigators. Prevention of syncope trial (POST): a randomized, placebo-controlled study of metoprolol in the prevention of vasovagal syncope. Circulation. 2006;113:1164–70.

43. Theodorakis GN, Leftheriotis D, Livanis EG, et al. Fluoxetine vs. propranolol in the treatment of vasovagal syncope: a prospective randomized, placebo-controlled study. Europace. 2006;8:193–8.

44. Qingyou Z, Junbao D, Chaoshu T. The efficacy of midodrine hydrochloride in the treatment of children with vasovagal syncope. J Pediatr. 2006;149:777–80.

45. Salim MA, DiSessa TG. Effectiveness of fludrocortisone and salt in preventing syncope recurrence in children: a double-blind, placebo-controlled randomized trial. J Am Coll Cardiol. 2005;45:484–8.

46. Connolly SJ, Sheldon R, Thorpe KE, et al., on behalf of the VPS II Investigators. The Second Vasovagal Pacemaker Study (VPSII): a double-blind randomized controlled trial of pacemaker therapy for the prevention of syncope in patients with recurrent severe vasovagal syncope. JAMA. 2003;290:1579–80.

47. Raviele A, Giada F, Menozzi C, et al., for the Vasovagal Syncope and Pacing Trial Investigators. A randomized double-blind, placebo-controlled study of permanent cardiac pacing for the treatment of recurrent tilt-induced vasovagal syncope. The vasovagal syncope and pacing trial (SYNPACE). Eur Heart J. 2004;25:1741–8.

48. Brignole M, Croci F, Menozzi C, et al. Isometric arm counter-pressure maneuvers to abort impending vasovagal syncope. J Am Coll Cardiol. 2002;40:2053–9.

49. DiGirolamo E, DiIorio C, Leonzio L, et al. Usefulness of a tilt training program for the prevention of refractory neurocardiogenic syncope in adolescents: a controlled study. Circulation. 1999;100: 1798–801.

50. Raj SR, Rose S, Ritchie D, et al., for the POST II Investigators. The second prevention of syncope trial (POST II)- a randomized clinical trial of fludrocortisone for the prevention of neurally mediated syncope: rationale and study design. Am Heart J. 2006;151(6):1186. e11–7.

51. Brignole M, Menozzi C, Moya A, et al., on behalf of the ISSUE-3 Investigators. Pacemaker therapy in patients with neurally mediated syncope and documented asystole: Third International Study on Syncope of Uncertain Etiology (ISSUE-3). A randomized trial. Circulation. 2012;125:2566–71.

52. Raj SR, Black BK, Biaggioni I, Robertson D. Acetylcholinesterase inhibition improves tachycardia in postural tachycardia syndrome. Circulation. 2005;111:2734–40.

53. Epstein AE, DiMarco JP, Ellenbogen KA, et al. ACC/AHA/HRS 2008 guidelines for device-based therapy of cardiac rhythm abnormalities: executive summary: a report of the American College of Cardiology/American Heart Association Task Force on Practice Guidelines (writing committee to revise the ACC/AHA/NASPE 2002 guideline update for implantation of cardiac pacemakers and antiarrhythmia devices) developed in collaboration with the American Association for Thoracic Surgery and Society of Thoracic Surgeons. J Am Coll Cardiol. 2008;51:2085–105.

Index

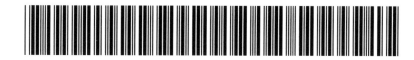